CURRENT THERAPY in REPTILE Medicine & Surgery

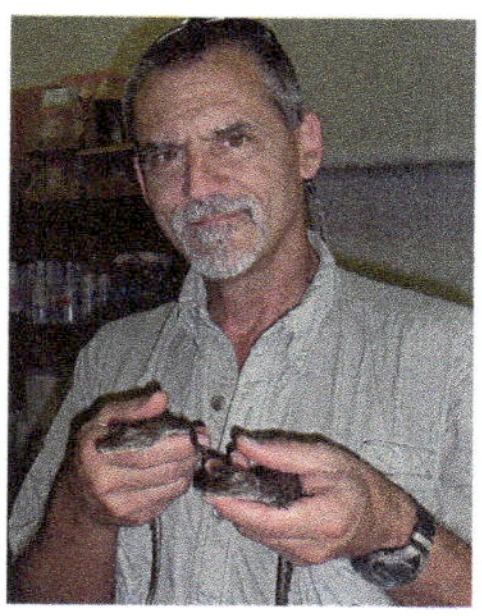

Photo credit: Jeanne Selander

Douglas R. Mader, MS, DVM, DABVP (Canine/Feline), DABVP (Reptile/Amphibian), DipECZM (Herpetology)

Fellow, Royal Society of Medicine

Marathon Veterinary Hospital
Sea Turtle Hospital
Marathon, Florida, USA

Courtesy Assistant Professor
Aquatic Animal Health
University of Florida, College of Veterinary Medicine
Gainesville, Florida, USA

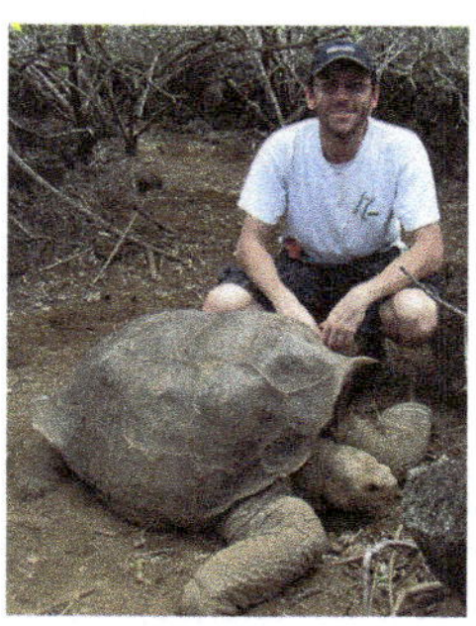

Photo credit: Dr. Joe Flanagan, Houston Zoo

Stephen J. Divers, BVetMed, DZooMed, DipECZM (Herpetology), DipECZM (Zoo Health Management), DACZM, FRCVS

Professor of Zoological Medicine
Department of Small Animal Medicine and Surgery
College of Veterinary Medicine
University of Georgia
Athens, Georgia, USA

ELSEVIER
SAUNDERS

ELSEVIER
SAUNDERS

3251 Riverport Lane
St. Louis, Missouri 63043

CURRENT THERAPY IN REPTILE MEDICINE AND SURGERY ISBN: 978-1-4557-0893-2

Notices

Knowledge and best practice in this field are constantly changing. As new research and experience broaden our understanding, changes in research methods, professional practices, or medical treatment may become necessary.

Practitioners and researchers must always rely on their own experience and knowledge in evaluating and using any information, methods, compounds, or experiments described herein. In using such information or methods they should be mindful of their own safety and the safety of others, including parties for whom they have a professional responsibility.

With respect to any drug or pharmaceutical products identified, readers are advised to check the most current information provided (i) on procedures featured or (ii) by the manufacturer of each product to be administered, to verify the recommended dose or formula, the method and duration of administration, and contraindications. It is the responsibility of practitioners, relying on their own experience and knowledge of their patients, to make diagnoses, to determine dosages and the best treatment for each individual patient, and to take all appropriate safety precautions.

To the fullest extent of the law, neither the Publisher nor the authors, contributors, or editors, assume any liability for any injury and/or damage to persons or property as a matter of products liability, negligence or otherwise, or from any use or operation of any methods, products, instructions, or ideas contained in the material herein.

Library of Congress Cataloging-in-Publication Data

Current therapy in reptile medicine and surgery / [edited by] Douglas R. Mader, Stephen J. Divers.
p. ; cm.
Includes bibliographical references and index.
ISBN 978-1-4557-0893-2 (hardcover : alk. paper)
I. Mader, Douglas R., editor of compilation. II. Divers, Stephen J., editor of compilation.
[DNLM: 1. Animal Diseases. 2. Reptiles. 3. Amphibians. 4. Analgesia--veterinary. 5. Anesthesia--veterinary. 6. Surgical Procedures, Operative--veterinary. SF 997.5.R4]
SF997.5.R4
639.3'78--dc23 2013030672

Vice President and Publisher: Linda Duncan
Content Strategy Director: Penny Rudolph
Content Manager: Shelly Stringer
Publishing Services Manager: Catherine Jackson
Senior Project Manager: Mary Pohlman
Design Direction: Ashley Miner

Printed in the United States of America

Last digit is the print number: 9 8 7 6 5 4 3

In Memoriam

During the writing of this edition, the herp and zoo world said "goodbye" to two most incredible individuals.

Dr. Greg Flemming, who penned three chapters in this edition, passed away while on a trip to Africa. Greg leaves a void that can never be filled, but his legacy will live on in all of our hearts.

Dr. Kevin Wright, author of two chapters, died just days after the 2013 Association of Reptilian and Amphibian Veterinarians annual meeting in Indianapolis, Indiana. Fortunately, Kevin got to spend time with many of his friends at the meeting, leaving many with fond memories.

Both of these veterinarians were icons in their field, leading the world in cutting-edge medicine, surgery, teaching, and leadership. Although there certainly will be future editions of *Reptile Medicine and Surgery,* without the contributions of Greg Flemming and Kevin Wright, they will never be the same.

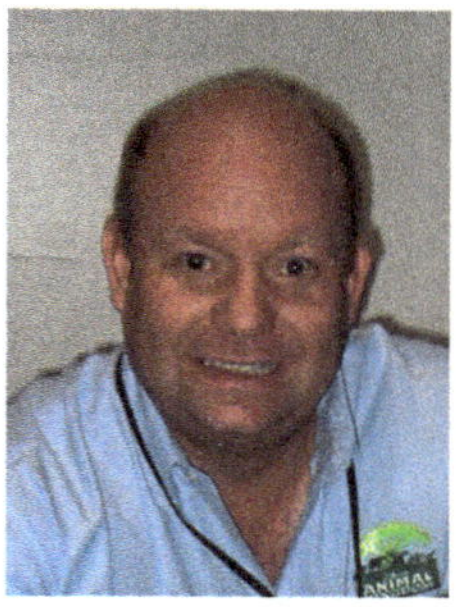

Greg Flemming
March 13, 1966 – March 9, 2013
(Photo courtesy Disney Animal Kingdom)

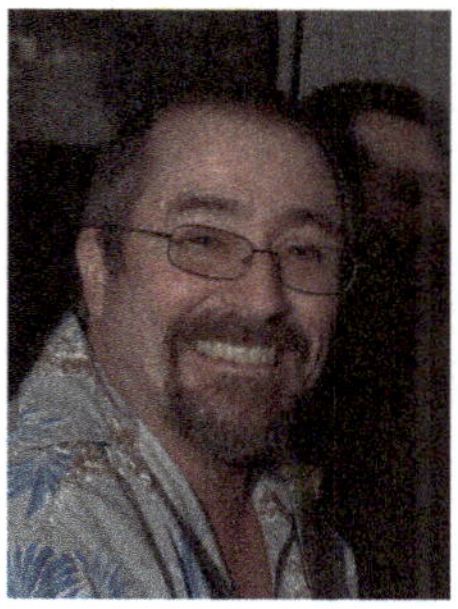

Kevin Wright
September 27, 1962 – September 26, 2013
(Photo courtesy Steve Barten, DVM)

Contributors

Kimberly M. Andrews, PhD, MS
Research Coordinator
Jekyll Island Authority Georgia Sea Turtle Center
Savannah River Ecology Laboratory
The University of Georgia
Savannah River Site
Jekyll Island, Georgia
Techniques for Working with Wild Reptiles

Stephen L. Barten, DVM
Vernon Hills Animal Hospital
Mundelein, Illinois;
Program Coordinator
North American Veterinary Community
Gainesville, Florida
Current Herpetologic Husbandry and Products

Terry W. Campbell, MS, DVM, PhD
Associate Professor
Clinical Sciences
Colorado State University
Fort Collins, Colorado
Clinical Pathology

James W. Carpenter, MS, DVM, DACZM
Zoological Medicine Service
Department of Clinical Sciences
College of Veterinary Medicine
Kansas State University
Manhattan, Kansas
Reptile Formulary and Laboratory Normals
Abridged Formulary for Amphibians

Ryan S. DeVoe, DVM, MSPVM, DACZM, DABVP (R/A)
North Carolina Zoological Park
Ashboro, North Carolina
Abridged Formulary for Amphibians

Stephen J. Divers, BVetMed, DZooMed, DipECZM (Herpetology), DipECZM (Zoo Health Management), DACZM, FRCVS
Professor of Zoological Medicine
Department of Small Animal Medicine and Surgery
College of Veterinary Medicine
University of Georgia
Athens, Georgia
Diagnostic Endoscopy
Endoscope-Assisted and Endoscopic Surgery
Video Telescopic Operating Microscope: A Recent Development in Reptile Microsurgery
Reptile Viruses

†Gregory J. Fleming, DVM, DACZM
Veterinarian
Department of Animal Health
Disney's Animals, Science, and the Environment
Lake Buena Vista, Florida
Current Herpetologic Husbandry and Products
Conditioning and Behavioral Training in Reptiles
New Techniques in Chelonian Shell Repair

Paul M. Gibbons, DVM, MS, DABVP (R/A)
Managing Director
Behler Chelonian Center
Turtle Conservancy
Ojai, California
Therapeutics
Reptile Formulary and Laboratory Normals

Chris Griffin, DVM, DABVP (Avian)
Owner/Medical Director
Griffin Avian and Exotic Veterinary Hospital
Kannapolis, North Carolina
Common Pathology and Diseases Seen in Pet Store Reptiles

Claudia Hochleithner, DVM
Tierklinik Strebersdorf
Vienna, Austria
Ultrasonography

Mason Holland, VMD, DACVR
Port City Veterinary Referral Hospital
Portsmouth, New Hampshire
Ultrasonography

Charles J. Innis, VMD, DABVP (R/A)
Director of Animal Health
Animal Health Department
New England Aquarium
Boston, Massachusetts
Conservation Issues

---

†Deceased.

Eric Klaphake, DVM, DABVP (Avian), DACZM, DABVP (R/A)
Associate Veterinarian
Cheyenne Mountain Zoo
Colorado Springs, Colorado;
Clinical Associate Professor of Veterinary Medicine
Western University of Health Sciences
Pomona, California
Specialization in Reptile Medicine
Reptile Formulary and Laboratory Normals

Kenneth L. Krysko, PhD, MS, BS
Collection Manager
Division of Herpetology
Florida Museum of Natural History
Department of Wildlife Ecology and Conservation
School of Natural Resources and Environment
University of Florida
Gainesville, Florida
Invasive and Introduced Reptiles and Amphibians

Douglas R. Mader, MS, DVM, DABVP (C/F, R/A) DipECZM (Herpetology)
Fellow, Royal Society of Medicine
Sea Turtle Hospital
Marathon Veterinary Hospital
Marathon, Florida;
Courtesy Assistant Professor
Aquatic Animal Health
University of Florida, College of Veterinary Medicine
Gainesville, Florida
Forensics in Reptile Investigation

Christoph Mans, med. vet
Clinical Instructor in Zoological Medicine
Special Species Health Service
Department of Medical Sciences
School of Veterinary Medicine
University of Wisconsin-Madison
Madison, Wisconsin
Anesthesia

Maud L. Marin, DMV, MSc, DACZM
Associate Veterinarian
Houston Zoo Inc.
Houston, Texas
Vacuum-Assisted Wound Closure in Chelonians

Rachel E. Marschang, PD, Dr.med.vet., DECZM (Herpetology), FTÄ Mikrobiologie, ZB Reptilien
Laboklin GmbH & C. KG
Stenbenstr 4, 97688
Bad Kissingen, Germany
Kleintierpraxis Dr. Grassmann
Leonberg-Höfingen, Germany
Clinical Virology
Reptile Viruses

Joseph R. Mendelson III, PhD
Director of Herpetological Research
Zoo Atlanta
Adjunct Professor
School of Biology
Georgia Institute of Technology
Atlanta, Georgia;
Research Officer
Amphibian Ark
Apple Valley, Minnesota
A New Era of Amphibian Taxonomy

Melinda D. Merck, DVM
Veterinary Forensics Consulting, LLC
Atlanta, Georgia
Forensics in Reptile Investigation

Nancy S. Mettee, DVM
Director of Sea Turtle Medicine
Wider Caribbean Sea Turtle Conservation Network
Staff Veterinarian
Pet Emergency of Martin County
Stuart, Florida
Vacuum-Assisted Wound Closure in Chelonians

Debra Lee Miller, BS, MS, DVM, PhD
Professor and Wildlife Pathologist
University of Tennessee
Knoxville, Tennessee
Ranavirus

Mark A. Mitchell, DVM, PhD, MS
College of Veterinary Medicine
Department of Veterinary Clinical Medicine
University of Illinois at Urbana-Champaign
Urbana, Illinois
Developing Your Reptile Medicine IQ: Learning How to Get the Most from and Contribute to the Herpetological Literature

Terry M. Norton, DVM, DACZM
Director and Veterinarian
Georgia Sea Turtle Center
Jekyll Island Authority
Jekyll Island, Georgia;
Wildlife Veterinarian
St. Catherines Island Foundation
Midway, Georgia
Vacuum-Assisted Wound Closure in Chelonians
Techniques for Working with Wild Reptiles

Dorcas P. O'Rourke
Professor and Chair
Department of Comparative Medicine
The Brody School of Medicine
East Carolina University
Greenville, North Carolina
Reptiles and Amphibians in Laboratory Animal Medicine

Lonny B. Pace, DVM, DACVECC
Owner
Emergency Veterinary Service
Riverside, California;
Staff
Emergency/Critical Care
Pet Emergency and Specialty Hospital
Thousand Oaks, California;
Staff
Emergency/Critical Care
Inland Valley Emergency Pet Clinic
Upland, California
Glossary

Jean A. Paré, DMV, DVSc, DACZM
Associate Veterinarian
Zoological Health Program Wildlife Conservation Society
Bronx, New York
Update on Fungal Infections in Reptiles

Chad Peeling
Operations Manager
Peeling Productions at Clyde Peeling's Reptiland
Allenwood, Pennsylvania
Exhibiting Amphibians

Allan P. Pessier, DVM, DACVP
Senior Scientist
Wildlife Disease Laboratories
Institute for Conservation Research
San Diego Zoo Global
San Diego, California
Infectious Diseases of Amphibians: It Isn't Just Redleg Anymore
Chytridiomycosis
Short Tongue Syndrome and Hypovitaminosis A

Jennifer B. Pramuk, BA, MA, PhD
Affiliate Curator
Burke Museum of Natural History and Culture
University of Washington
Curator
Animal Management
Woodland Park Zoo
Seattle, Washington
A New Era of Amphibian Taxonomy

Drury R. Reavill, DVM, DABVP (Avian), DACVP
Owner
Zoo/Exotic Pathology Service
West Sacramento, California
Common Pathology and Diseases Seen in Pet Store Reptiles

Robert N. Reed, PhD
Chief
Invasive Species Branch
U.S. Geological Survey
Fort Collins, Colorado
Invasive and Introduced Reptiles and Amphibians

Juergen Schumacher, Dr.med.vet., DACZM, DECZM (Herpetology)
Professor and Director
Avian and Zoological Medicine
Small Animal Clinical Sciences
College of Veterinary Medicine
The University of Tennessee
Knoxville, Tennessee
Anesthesia

Michelle L. Skurski
Zoological Manager of Behavioral Husbandry
Animals, Science and Environment Line of Business
Disney's Animal Kingdom
Bay Lake, Florida
Conditioning and Behavioral Training in Reptiles

Kurt K. Sladky, MS, DVM, DACZM
Clinical Associate Professor
Department of Surgical Sciences
School of Veterinary Medicine
University of Wisconsin
Madison, Wisconsin
Analgesia

Lora L. Smith, PhD
Associate Scientist
Herpetology
Joseph W. Jones Ecological Research Center
Newton, Georgia
Techniques for Working with Wild Reptiles

James F.X. Wellehan Jr., DVM, PhD, DACZM, DACVM (Virology, Bacteriology/Mycology)
Clinician
Zoological Medicine Service
Service Chief, Clinical Microbiology
Co-Director
Wildlife and Aquatic Veterinary Disease Laboratory
University of Florida
Gainesville, Florida
Clinical Aspects of Evolution in Reptile Medicine
Molecular Infectious Disease Diagnostics

†Kevin Wright, DVM DABVP (R/A)
Founder
Wright Bird and Exotic Pet Hospital
Mesa, Arizona
Amphibian Therapy
Abridged Formulary for Amphibians

Jeanette Wyneken, PhD
Associate Professor of Biological Sciences
Florida Atlantic University
Boca Raton, Florida
Computed Tomography and Magnetic Resonance Imaging

†Deceased.

Foreword

"The most abject reptile and torpid of beings distinguishes the hand that feeds it, and is touched with the feelings of gratitude."

The Reverend Gilbert White,
"The Natural History of Selborne" (1788)

Like the authors of this book, I have been fascinated by reptiles and amphibians—and, indeed, all wild animals—since my childhood. As a youngster, growing up in England, I caught lizards and snakes and retained them for periods of time in captivity before returning them to the wild. At university my long-suffering classmate had to share not only a bedroom with me and an African python but also a bath with my caiman. I have always kept notes about the animals I owned—and I have retained those detailed jottings and observations to this day.

In the 1950s and 1960s few veterinarians knew much about reptiles or their care. Those of us in Europe who kept reptiles and amphibians relied very much on the writings and lectures of that pioneer of lower vertebrate pathology, Dr. Edward Elkan, a medical man. I went to veterinary school expecting to be learning with, and from, people of like mind: alas, only a handful of students—and even fewer staff members—shared my passion for what are, after all, the most prevalent of all vertebrate animals, the nonmammalian species.

Over the past 40 years, the situation has changed beyond recognition. Initially, in the early 1970s, only a handful of veterinarians was actively involved in treating reptiles and amphibians, amongst them Oliphant Jackson and myself in Great Britain, Peer Zwart in The Netherlands, and (among others) Fred Frye and Elliott Jacobson in the United States. Subsequently other herpetologist-veterinarians joined the ranks, and over the decades reptile medicine has evolved to become a well-recognised and highly professional discipline. Doug Mader and Steve Divers are pioneers of this modern approach, and it is fitting that they should coauthor and edit this special edition of *Current Therapy in Reptile Medicine and Surgery*. In addition to their professional reputations, the two bring a transatlantic orientation to the publication. Doug Mader is an American who, despite the vicissitudes of living in a hurricane-prone location, loves living and working in Florida, with its ready access to wildlife and wild places. Steve Divers was brought up and received his initial veterinary training in England (his British friends quickly detect a London twang, even when he tries to disguise himself as an American!), and he retains strong links and affinity with Europe. This combination serves as a timely reminder that concern for the health, welfare, and conservation of reptiles needs to be promoted on an international scale if the remaining populations of these much maligned creatures are to survive and to thrive. Herpetological medicine demands the input of people from all over the world, not solely from relatively privileged, richer, "Western" countries. As one who continues to provide training in East Africa and elsewhere, I know that this book will be of value not only to those of us in North America and Europe but also to colleagues in far-flung parts of the globe, where so many fascinating and beautiful members of the classes Reptilia and Amphibia are to be found.

Reptile Medicine and Surgery has firmly established itself as a leading, authoritative text. I strongly recommend this *Current Therapy* edition and, on behalf of those who will read it, thank Doug Mader and Steve Divers as well as their contributors for a job that has been thoroughly and skilfully accomplished.

JOHN E. COOPER, DTVM, FRCPath, FSB, CBiol, FRCVS
RCVS Specialist in Veterinary Pathology
Diplomate, European College of Veterinary Pathologists
European Veterinary Specialist, Zoological Medicine
Honorary Research Fellow, Durrell Institute of
Conservation and Ecology (DICE)
The University of Kent, United Kingdom
Visiting Professor, Faculty of Veterinary Medicine
University of Nairobi, Kenya

Preface

This current edition of *Reptile Medicine and Surgery* was conceived during the 2011 North American Veterinary Conference in the speaker ready room at the Marriott World Center. Doug Mader approached Steve Divers and asked "What do you think about co-editing a new edition of *Reptile Medicine and Surgery* with me?" Steve, without really thinking it through, responded, "Great, count me in!"

It's amazing how a brief moment of excitement starts something that consumes a lot of your time for the foreseeable future. Later that week, we talked it over and sat down with Penny Rudolph of Elsevier to discuss the idea. It quickly became apparent that the vast majority of the content within the second edition was still as relevant today as it was when it was first published in 2006. Therefore, this new book could not be a replacement but rather a companion to that second edition, hence the *Current Therapy* concept. *Current Therapy in Reptile Medicine and Surgery* should, most definitely, sit right alongside the second edition on your bookshelf—if you don't have a second edition then your herpetologic library will remain incomplete.

We have tried to keep those essential elements that were instrumental in the success of the second edition. Specifically, we invited world-renowned specialists from both sides of the Atlantic to provide updates in those areas of herpetologic medicine and surgery that have seen the greatest growth and development over the past 7 years. Consequently, the author list is an inevitable Who's Who in reptile medicine and includes a variety of specialists from academia, private practice, and various zoo and research institutions. Indeed, many of these authors were involved in the original journal publications that first brought many of these new developments and concepts to light.

However, we trust that you will also notice that there have been some significant changes in the style of this current therapy. Most notably, color reproduction has become cheaper and has altered the landscape of medical publishing. We were, therefore, keen to see the inclusion of as many images as the publishers would possibly allow, and the diagnostic imaging and endoscopy chapters have probably been the greatest beneficiaries. In addition, significant advances and updates have been included for husbandry equipment, clinical virology, mycotic diseases, therapeutics, anesthesia and analgesia, and diagnostic endoscopy. There are also several new reptile topics that have been included for the first time, including veterinary specialization, common pathology and diseases seen in pet stores, clinical aspects of evolution, molecular infectious disease diagnostics, conditioning and behavioral training, endosurgery, vacuum-assisted wound closure, new techniques in chelonian shell repair, video telescope operating microscopy, laboratory animal medicine, working with wild reptiles, forensic investigation, and issues of species invasion and conservation. This current text also sees a significant expansion in amphibian material with additional chapters dedicated to amphibian diversity, exhibition, infectious and noninfectious diseases, and therapy. Despite these many advances, there is always scope for increasing and improving the scientific basis for our specialty. *The Journal of Herpetological Medicine and Surgery* is always looking for original research and clinical case publications, and an appendix on statistics and scientific writing has been specifically included to encourage all of us to submit material for peer review and publication.

Although it says Mader and Divers on the cover, there is absolutely no doubt that the quality and hence success of this book lies in the quality of its authors, and in that regard we feel proud of the contributions made by our colleagues and friends. We hope that you will consider this update a welcome addition to your library and that the pages quickly become tatty from frequent use by busy practitioners everywhere.

Douglas R. Mader
Stephen J. Divers

Acknowledgments

After nearly three decades in veterinary medicine I still look forward to going to work every day. Aside from the fact that I truly love what I do, I think that my main motivation is the idea that I can make a positive impact on the human–animal bond. Almost everybody reading this essay likely feels the importance of this bond, oddly enough, even with reptiles and amphibians. I suspect, no, I know, that there are many, many people who can't appreciate the impact that a herp can have on our lives.

Whether it is a pet snake or a wild crocodile, to those of us that love poikilotherms, there is something magical whenever we have an interaction. I have stewarded critters for my entire life—from dogs to cats to horses to birds to amphibians to herps. I have loved them all. I have also had my heart broken over many; dogs and cats shouldn't have such relatively short lives.

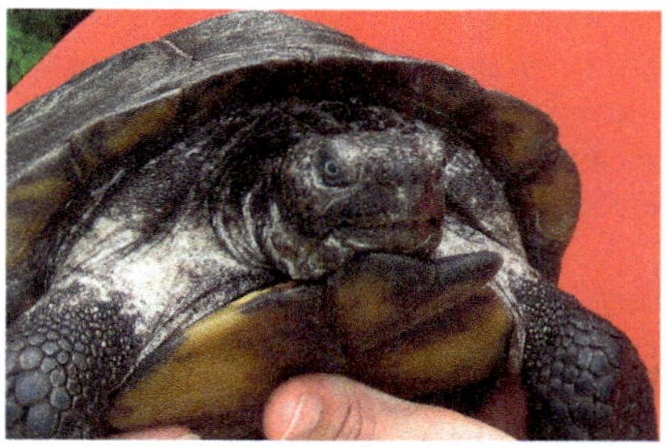

It is no surprise that the longest length of time that I have ever owned a pet was when I had a California Desert Tortoise. I acquired Dewe from an indigent client when I was a resident at the University of California, Davis, School of Veterinary Medicine and shared my life with him for 27 years. He was an adult when I got him, so I suspect he was more than 50 years old when he succumbed to hepatic adenocarcinoma.

Some may make the argument that I am reasonably good at what I do, and I certainly try really hard; however, even with my resume, I was not able to save Dewe when he fell ill. I drew on all of my experience, my knowledge, my high-end equipment, contacted my esteemed colleagues for consults and much, much more. It was all to no avail. I had to say goodbye.

I want to thank Dewe for 27 years of companionship. Dewe, you are the reason that I do what I do: writing the books and teaching others. I do what I do so others can share their lives with their Dewes.

Although Dewe provided me the motivation to tackle another edition of *Current Therapy in Reptile Medicine and Surgery*, it could not have happened without the assistance of several very special two-legged friends. First off, I have to give major props to my partner in editing, Dr. Stephen Divers. I could not have produced another edition without his friendship, collaboration, and input. Steve has a vast amount of knowledge and experience and his talent shines throughout this book.

Several individuals have helped review chapters, loaned me images, and much more. I am sure I will forget some, and I apologize in advance, but my sincere appreciation goes out to Dr. Karen Overall, Dr. Fred Frye, Dr. Len Marcus, Dr. Jim Wellehan, Dr. Stephen Barten, Dr. Richard Funk, Dr. Tim Tristan, Dr. Melinda Merck, Dr. Jackie Bruce, Dr. Molly Willett, Dr. Kristin Hall, Dr. Cathy Connelly, Dr. Jeanette Wyneken, Dr. Javier Nevares, Dr. Mark Mitchell, and Dr. Kevin Wright.

Many thanks to all the contributing authors. The level of intellect represented here is mind-boggling. Dr. Divers and I have managed to convince these busy individuals to share their skills with us and the rest of the herp world. Once you read this edition, you will realize what I am talking about.

Special thanks to Richie, Bette, Tom, and the crew at the Marathon Sea Turtle Hospital and Ryan at the Gumbo Limbo Nature Center for their support and endless supply of sea turtle cases over the past 19 years.

Bev, Pam, and the staff of Theater of the Sea have included me on their health care team and trusted me with their amazing collection over the years. The images on the cover of this book come from one of their charges—you take the best care of your collection! Thanks for letting me do what I do. You make it easy and fun to be a veterinarian.

I want to make a shout out to the Key West Aquarium, Dynasty Marine, Key West Butterfly conservancy, Key Deer Refuge, Everglades Alligator Farm, the Everglades Outpost, and the Monroe County Sheriff's Animal Farm for also trusting me with your valuable collections or charges.

The crew at Elsevier has been amazing to work with. Corralling Steve and myself is no easy task, and they have, for the most part, kept us in line. Shelly Stringer, Penny Rudolph, and Mary Pohlman, and the rest of the editorial staff, are all unmatched. Thank you all.

Finally, love and appreciation go to my family: Simon, Tracy, Stella, Atigun, Aragon, Puck, Pixel, and, most importantly, my partner in business and life, Gerry. You are the best.

Doug Mader

When I first sat down to write this I thought it would be short and sweet. However, as I started to recount the individuals that have played key roles in enabling me to succeed in zoological medicine, I quickly realized that the list was long, and the process humbling. There is no doubt that I am standing on the shoulders of many, and I pray for forgiveness if I forget anyone from these acknowledgments. Memory lapse is something that my wife tells me is becoming more frequent, or at least I think it was my wife that said it?!

My parents, Christine and Alan, are the most wonderful, loving parents a son could ask for, and my family was completed by a brother, Richard, and sister, Amanda. They all tolerated and even encouraged my childhood indulgences in pond dipping and keeping a host of exotic pets, including boa constrictors, leopard geckos, and green iguanas. My parents' interests in animals included their health and welfare and were obvious and infectious to me while growing up. My mother had an enviable collection of *Testudo* and *Geochelone* (which she ultimately translocated to a chelonian retirement community in the south of France), while I once caught my dad talking to one of my Boa Constrictors. I knew I always wanted to be in medicine, but there was a time when I was not sure whether it would be human or veterinary. To my surprise, my parents were delighted when I chose animals over humans! I don't tell them often enough how much they mean to me and how everything I have become is due to their support and encouragement. Thank you mum and dad.

I left home for the Royal Veterinary College in London, where Oliphant Jackson and John Cooper galvanized my interest in zoological medicine, specifically reptiles, and several of my classmates including Sharon Redrobe, Ian Foster, and Louise Rayment became staunch allies in the "exotic" group. As a student, I was fortunate to be trained by several notable clinical veterinarians, and of them, Dermod Malley, an enthusiastic and exuberant Irishman, was most influential. His kindness, enthusiasm, humor, and dedication to high-quality medicine were infectious.

I was afforded further support by my first employer, Philip Lhermette, who not only encouraged my exotic interests but also facilitated this new graduate's first endeavors into endoscopy. Indeed, I think we both catalyzed each other because Philip went on to develop one of the most successful companion endoscopy practices in the United Kingdom. I was also lucky to receive further training and mentorship from Fred Frye, Peer Zwart, John Cooper, and David Williams, all of whom I consider friends as well as colleagues.

It was soon after I graduated in 1994 that I came to my first Association of Reptilian and Amphibian Veterinarians (ARAV) meeting and met a young guy who has subsequently proven to be the most important professional acquaintance and friend I could ever hope to have. Dr. Scott Stahl immediately took this young Brit under his wing, we immediately became close friends, and have remained close ever since. Scott has taught me a lot about practical referral practice, as well as how to be a better person. I tried to teach him the rules of cricket but was unsuccessful. He is a valued research colleague, wet-lab co-instructor, and was the best man at my wedding. The ARAV conference times I have spent with him and my other ARAV friends, including Charles "Chuckles" Innis, Mark "Elvis" Mitchel, Kevin "Lick me" Wright, and many others, are memories that I continue to cherish.

I moved to the United States in 2001 and remain grateful for the opportunities afforded to me as a faculty member of the University of Georgia's College of Veterinary Medicine. Drs. Heather Barron, Nicole Northrup, Simon Platt, and Joerg Mayer, to name but a few, have made the University of Georgia a pleasurable and productive place to work. I am also grateful to all the past zoological medicine interns and the current residents, Drs. Rodney Schnellbacher, Laila Proenca, and Lara Cusack for keeping me honest and focused.

I am extremely grateful for the expertise, professionalism, and dedication to timelines that the authors displayed. An entire Elsevier editorial team was behind this book, but special thanks to Penny Rudolph, Mary Pohlman, and especially Shelly Stringer. My final professional acknowledgment goes to Douglas Mader. I first read an article of his when I was at vet school (yes, I am considerably younger), and from that point on he was a role model exemplifying the type of innovative and progressive clinician that I aspired to be. Thank you Doug for having faith in me. It was a real pleasure working with you, and I would gladly do it again.

No man is an island, and in 2010 I married the most caring and loving woman I have ever known. Leticia is my rock who stops me from spiraling out of control. She has enlightened me that there is more to life than work, and thanks to her I now enjoy evenings and weekends away from labs, computers, and endoscopes. Her thoughtful insights and advice have been of immense benefit to me, both personally and professionally. I have no doubt that her being a veterinary behaviorist may also have played a critical role (I don't know why, but when I hear that clicker I just come running?). In 2011, Leticia gave birth to our son, John-Eduardo, a real character from day one. In fact, now that I come to think of it, the 2011 North American Veterinary Conference was a critical meeting for me because it saw the inception of this book and the conception of my son. I am especially thankful that he slept 12 hours through the night from his second month; otherwise this book would have taken considerably longer to complete. Leticia and John, thank you for making my life complete and making everything worthwhile—Eu te amo!

Steve Divers

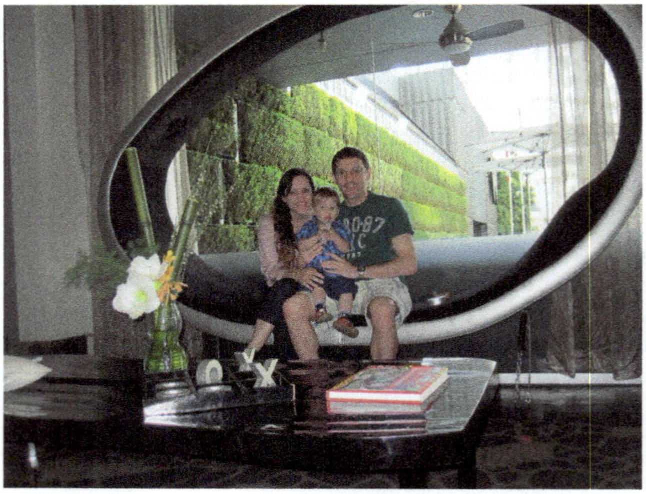

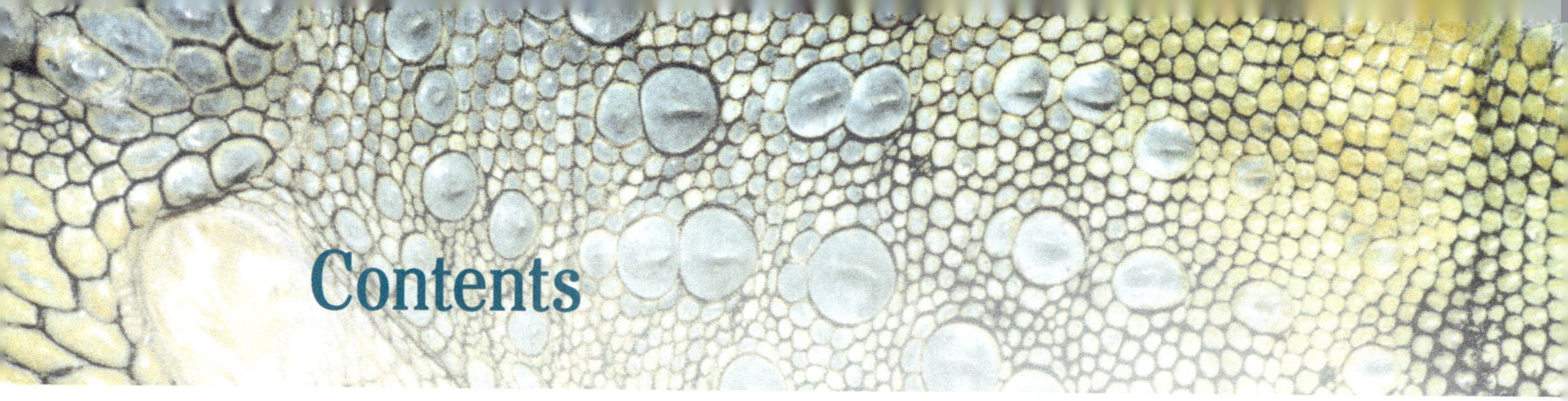

Contents

†Deceased

SECTION IV: ADVANCES IN BIOLOGY, CONSERVATION, LAW, AND RESEARCH

APPENDICES

Specialization in Reptile Medicine

Eric Klaphake

SPECIALIZATION

Receiving a veterinary degree in and of itself is an incredible achievement. However, there is always a push within any profession to "take things to another level," that is, to develop a higher level of expertise. At an initial level, this usually is addressed by reading journals, belonging to veterinary organizations, and attending conferences for continuing education. Over time, there can be a great drive to develop a niche within the profession, whether for the veterinary practice or an individual employed there. Part of this drive is for personal growth; in other cases, it may be more financially driven to develop a "product" for the practice that allows the practice to offer a service not otherwise available within the community. Legally and ethically, there are guidelines as to how one may advertize such a product. While beyond the scope of this chapter, the American Veterinary Medical Association's Web site (www.avma.org) provides such guidelines for the United States, and communicating directly with one's state veterinary board can also provide guidance as to how to advertize such skills. Ultimately, however, in both the United States and Europe, the term *specialist* is considered the gold standard for indicating the highest level of expertise.

A veterinarian graduate is legally able to treat any animal species, except human beings. However, most new graduates have developed a comfort level with a small subset of species, usually dogs and cats or horses or food animals. A relatively new area of veterinary focus involves exotic animals as pets, wildlife, or part of a larger public or private collection. In many ways, the irony of working with such a diverse collection of animals truly challenges an individual to be able to become a specialist; in some cases the phrase "jack-of-all-trades, master of none" is more applicable. These veterinarians know a little about a lot of species. Because this chapter resides within a herpetologic book, the discussion will be directed toward two different opportunities for specialization in reptiles and amphibians: becoming a Diplomate of the American Board of Veterinary Practitioners (Reptile/Amphibian) (ABVP R/A) or the American College of Zoological Medicine (ACZM) or becoming a Diplomate of the European College of Zoological Medicine (Herpetology) (ECZM).

COSTS OF SPECIALIZING

The efforts of getting accepted to and graduating from veterinary school can make one adverse to considering further sacrifice. Some people immediately transition from veterinary school to an internship and perhaps a residency. This can be one pathway for becoming a specialist and is often the fastest one, although by no means is it the only option available. So why become a specialist? In some fields, it can lead to a higher level of financial reward—either as a short-term bonus or reflected long-term in the form of greater overall production revenue, which hopefully translates into a higher base salary or greater compensation in a commission-style contract. One should be aware that at this time, within the field of zoological medicine, there is not always a direct correlation between specialization and salary increases. In academia, specialization is a requirement for promotion and tenure and salary increases are often guaranteed. In referral centers, and even some primary care practices, salary increases can be achieved by being able to charge higher fees and offering a greater range of specialized services.

A specialist is also more likely to be sought locally, nationally, or even internationally for guidance by general practitioners or other specialists. This may also translate into modest financial opportunities from speaking at veterinary conferences or writing articles or book chapters. Specialists may become recognized in their community as the "go to" person for the media, local schools, and nonprofit organizations seeking that expertise. Although this may be viewed either as a perk or a burden, it is part of the mantle of being a specialist. Specializing also opens new doors of opportunity professionally. Most academic positions require some level of specialization, as do many secondary or tertiary private practices. Zoos have been slower to recognize the need for and benefit of specialists, but that has begun to change rapidly within the past few years.

Nonetheless, specializing does not come without costs, some of which are tangible and others intangible. The first route of pursuing specialization is through an approved residency. The ACZM and ABVP Web sites can direct an interested individual to the location of these approved residencies. At the time of this writing, no approved ECZM residencies were available in herpetologic medicine. Approval can change rapidly based on changes of those in charge of such programs or an inability to meet the requirements of approved residencies. Likewise, new programs can be created just as quickly. Most of these residencies are quite competitive, so often an interested individual must begin the process by serving an internship or sometimes even two! This is an important cost consideration.

First, examine the loss of financial earning power. Most internships (1-year duration) pay approximately US $25,000 per year with some benefits, as of 2013. Some internships pay more, but one should evaluate the cost of living in the area, and usually the higher salary reflects such. Most residencies offer US $25,000 to $30,000 per year plus benefits and last 2 (ABVP) to 3 years (ACZM and ECZM). Compare this to the average starting salary for a private practitioner, approximately US $65,000 per year. Doing the math, one sacrifices from US $50,000 to $120,000 or more, depending on the length of training. With US veterinary student debt at ever-increasing levels, this should give individuals pause when considering this route to specialization. With some specialties such as surgery, one may quickly begin to recoup these financial losses, but this may not be so with ABVP (R/A) or ACZM. In Europe, the costs of veterinary education are generally much lower; therefore the financial burden of delayed salary may be less.

Second, internships and residencies often necessitate continued movement across the country—veterinary school to internship, to second internship, to residency location. Some residencies even require living at different locations each year. The costs of moving and locating new housing may be compounded by significant others or spouses finding new employment at each location, creating the necessity of a long distance relationship or even leading to the fracturing of relationships. Ancillary to this financial cost can be the emotional cost on relationships with significant others and children. As with veterinary school, hours are often long, with emergency shifts, "free time" spent writing papers, and the need to come in on "off days" to see unique cases.

With approved residencies, a resident should be in a stronger position to qualify to successfully sit on specialty boards. In some cases, mentorship can be a benefit, but one is advised not to have high expectations. Some programs may espouse these virtues, but the reality may be that there is little supervision and residents are left to figure things out for themselves, serving as cheap labor. One wishes this were not so, but I would be remiss if I did not acknowledge that many residents have completed their programs quite bitter about this aspect. However, if a resident goes into a residency recognizing that this opportunity will expedite the process, improve one's resume, and allow access to diagnostics, therapeutics, and unusual cases to which other practitioners will not be exposed, then it is unlikely the resident will become disillusioned or disappointed. Anything gained over and above that from a residency is simply a bonus. The reader should not feel that all approved residencies misrepresent what they offer, but it behooves an individual to diligently access the strengths and weaknesses of any program and not to be overly influenced by a program's reputation. Prospective applicants are strongly encouraged to talk to current or previous residents, and one should consider it a red flag if any program resists that open dialogue.

In theory, most approved residencies should allow for time to study for the specialty examination, prepare case reports or first author publications, and systematically review over the time of the entire residencies all of the didactic information to which one needs to be exposed. For example, the ACZM mandates a minimum of 5 hours of scholarly time away from clinical duties per week (approximately 30 days per year). In some cases, the opportunity to perform research may manifest itself, and, of course, completing a residency does enhance one's chance of employment in the academic sphere.

For either specialty, new employment opportunities may present themselves outside general practice, such as working in a zoo, for a nongovernmental organization often in field settings, as a federal or state wildlife veterinarian, as a teaching- or research-only academician, or as a referral specialist.

In the near future, all organizations should be completely paperless, so duplication of submissions will become unnecessary.

A *board* is of equal standing to a *college* with regard to specialization, according to the American Board of Veterinary Specialties (ABVS). The role of the ABVS or the EBVS is simply to maintain the standards established by each specialty, and they make no effort or claim that one board or college is equal to another regarding difficulty.

For all of the following organizations, check regularly with their Web sites to access the most current information regarding timelines, credentialing and re-credentialing requirements, and examination structure and content.

Procrastinating is common among many residency candidates, both those pursuing the practitioner routes and those in residencies. Mentors often have the job of motivating residents to receive their credentials and pass their examinations, but mentors and their programs also benefit in membership size by having more of their residents take and eventually pass boards. It is important for every individual to ascertain whether passing one of these examinations is a personal or career goal or whether they are only doing it for someone else. If potential applicants have no real interest in taking the examination, then they should forego it so that someone who is dedicated can take that valuable place.

One may never feel ready for such an examination, but a good course of action is to work on and complete the credentialing process and then focus on studying. Once one has committed to the field by becoming credentialed, the incentive to study and pass the examination becomes an intense motivator compared with studying for an examination sometime in the future. For credentialing, some may prefer to work through one case report or submit one publication at a time, whereas others may find it more efficient to work on several simultaneously. Having an online study group or a group to review case reports can be extremely helpful. ABVP does provide these, and further information is available on their Web site. Likewise, the ACZM offers dedicated short courses to aid candidates in examination preparation. Remember, both examinations only require a score of 65% to 70%, which is the usual pass/fail line. This type of score may feel like failure to many veterinarians, but this is the level at which most veterinarians score.

SPECIALTY BOARDS

The American Board of Veterinary Practitioners

The ABVP Web site is www.abvp.com (not .org). Their mission statement is "To advance the quality of veterinary medicine through certification of veterinarians who demonstrate excellence in species-oriented clinical practice." This specialty is focused more on the private practitioner, although other opportunities do abound. ABVP Diplomates have demonstrated excellence in the care of the total patient. Certification provides professional and public recognition of advanced knowledge, skills, and competency in a species category. Diplomate status is granted with approval of the ABVS. The organization began in 1978, and the first examination was given in 1981. In 2010, the first Reptile/Amphibian specialty examination was administered, and five individuals successfully passed the inaugural test. As of January 2013, approximately 900 Diplomates were in good standing across all species specialties, 13 of which were specialists in reptile and amphibian medicine.

Two paths qualify an individual to submit credentials. One must either have practiced a minimum of 5 years in any combination of practice that allowed the minimal amount of professional exposure and caseload of reptiles and amphibians as required, or have completed an ABVP R/A approved residency program. The applicant should contact the current ABVP R/A regent for current requirements at the time of application. As of 2013, the credentialing process timeline is a short, simple first-time application form, and the fee is due by September 1 of each year; this allows the candidate to take the examination no sooner than November of the following year if all requirements are met. The more complex credentials packet, which is described later, is due January 15 of the earliest year a candidate hopes to sit for the examination. The final evaluation of the credentials packet is completed and notification of acceptance or rejection (complete or partial) of that packet is provided to the candidate by June 1 of the earliest year a candidate hopes to sit. Studying then commences, and accepted candidates determine by September 1 if they will register for that year's examination or wait an additional year. Basic information regarding the contents of the 2012 Application and Credentials Packets can be found in Boxes 1 and 2.

One of the most challenging components of the credentials packet is the case report. As noted in Box 2, an applicant may submit one case report and a publication or two case reports. Selection of a case to report requires careful consideration. To demonstrate excellence in reptile and amphibian medicine and surgery, it behooves the candidate to show some breadth of expertise. Each case report's species should be different in that there is only one of each of the following: lizard, snake, chelonian, crocodilian, anuran, caudate, or caecilian. It is also preferable to have one case demonstrating medical expertise and the other demonstrating surgical expertise. The topic of each case should generally avoid obscure, new, or uncommon diseases; instead, show expertise at thoroughly working up a standard case. Case reports must have been personally seen and worked up by the applicant within the past 5 years. Each case report must have adequate literature review and demonstrate a logical thought process and well-defended decisions and diagnostic interpretations. Applicants should demonstrate their thought processes and what they know in the case report: significant presenting signs, diagnostic characteristics, problem lists, pathophysiology, differential diagnoses, treatments, and management options. Other directions that could have been taken in hindsight for the aforementioned components should also be discussed for a complete case report.

BOX 1 AMERICAN BOARD OF VETERINARY PRACTITIONERS APPLICATION FORM

- Due September 1
- Requirements
  - Contact information
  - Listing of current position(s)
  - Graduation year and school
  - Listing of state license(s)
  - Designation of specialty category to which you are applying
  - Fee
- Two copies of the application form should be submitted along with the fee

Important: Once the first-time application and fee are received, applicants have 3 years to complete the credentialing process. If not successfully completed in the allotted 3 years, the process starts over from the beginning with submission of a new application and fee.

BOX 2 AMERICAN BOARD OF VETERINARY PRACTITIONERS CREDENTIALS PACKET

♦ Due January 15	
♦ Veterinary diploma photocopy	Two copies
♦ Curriculum vitae	Two copies
♦ Synopsis of veterinary practice	Two copies
♦ Self-reported job experience	Two copies
♦ Continuing education documentation	Two copies
♦ Applicant evaluation forms (3)	One copy each
♦ Case reports (2)	Five copies each
OR	
♦ Case report (1) and publication (1)	Five copies each

More specific guidelines and example case reports are available on the Web site. Formatting is significantly different from most professional journals. The most common reason for failing to credential is inadequate case reports! *Both* case reports or *both* the case report and the publication must pass to qualify for the board certifying examinations.

It is highly advisable that applicants begin writing their case reports *before* submitting the application and application fee.

Study groups are available from ABVP and can help with the process of compiling a case report; taking advantage of this expertise and assistance is recommended. An outside review of the case report is also encouraged, but make sure that the individual is aware of the needed components of an ABVP case report. Grammar and syntax are important. Remember, this work represents the applicant's ability to become a Diplomate.

For the refereed (peer-reviewed) publication, the applicant must be the first author. The topic of publication must make a meaningful contribution to the literature of the species specialty and must be different than that of the case report. The publication must have be published no more than 5 years before the

January 15 deadline in a refereed English-language scientific journal. Conference proceedings, online publications, clinical vignettes, short/brief communications, serial features (e.g., ECG of the Month, Drug Topic of the Month, What's Your Diagnosis), and narrative review articles will *not* be accepted. If uncertain, one is advised to communicate directly with the executive director of ABVP, well before any deadlines, to determine clarification on this issue. Acceptance for publication in a refereed scientific journal does not guarantee that the manuscript will be admissible in lieu of an ABVP-style case report.

Once an individual is credentialed to take the examination, preparation for the examination becomes critical. The ABVP examination has two components. One is an all-day two-part (morning and afternoon) general multiple choice reptile/amphibian examination in which each question has one correct answer and two distracters. The second component is a practical examination with slide images to be identified or to be used to answer the associated question. Generally, this second component may be the night before the all-day examination or the morning after. This is clarified by the ABVP once one has been accepted for the examination. The ABVP examination takes place in the fall, and examinees are informed of their own score and of the pass score within 45 days of the examination.

The American College of Zoological Medicine

The ACZM Web site is www.aczm.org. Work began in 1977 to create ACZM. Established in 1983 by eight charter members, ACZM is an international specialty organization for certification of veterinarians with special expertise in zoologic medicine. Of note, zoologic medicine includes all exotic species, so a Diplomate is not restricted to being just a herp specialist. Six individuals sat for the first examination in 1984. ACZM became a stand-alone College in 1988. As of 2012, there were more than 130 Diplomates in the College. ACZM is responsible for establishing training requirements, evaluating and accrediting training programs, and examining and certifying veterinarians in the veterinary specialty of zoologic medicine. ACZM Diplomates foster high-quality medical care for non-domestic animals and are actively involved in the discovery of new knowledge in the discipline and the dissemination of this knowledge to the veterinary profession and public.

Eligibility for examination can occur either by practicing in 100% exotic or zoologic animal practices for at least 6 years, 50% for 12 years, or some combination thereof. Participation in an ACZM-approved residency program (3 years) can reduce the number of practice years needed to qualify to sit for the examination to a minimum of 4 years after graduation. Many residents find it difficult and daunting to take the examination that soon and may choose to wait an additional year or two.

Unlike ABVP, there is no case report component for qualifying; instead, the applicant for credentialing must have five, senior-authored (first author) peer-reviewed publications, and at least one must be original research, either prospective or retrospective. Papers must be fully accepted before the application deadline—a letter from the editor indicating this may be sufficient proof. Papers must make a meaningful contribution to the literature. Book chapters, review papers, and proceedings papers *are not* acceptable. See Box 3 for more general information regarding the credentialing application; however, always refer to the Web site for changes in the process, form, and requirements.

BOX 3 AMERICAN COLLEGE OF ZOOLOGICAL MEDICINE APPLICATION FORM

Requirements

- Confirmation of professional ethics
- Detailed curriculum vitae and copies of license and veterinary diploma
- Three letters of reference
- Indication of Day 2 subspecialty
- Application check
- Indication of whether examination will be taken this year or next year
- Copies of each of the five accepted or published, first-author peer-reviewed publications (at least one needs to be original research)
- Four copies of all of the above must be sent before March 31

BOX 4 AMERICAN COLLEGE OF ZOOLOGICAL MEDICINE DAY 1 EXAMINATION

Aquatic Animal Medicine

- Fish (47.5%), marine mammals (47.5%), invertebrates (5%): both captive (aquaria) and wild

Mammalian Medicine

- All captive terrestrial mammals

Wildlife Medicine

- Free-ranging wildlife, including mammals, birds, and herps

Avian Medicine

- Zoo and companion birds with an emphasis on captive animals

Herpetofauna Medicine

- Reptiles and amphibians, with an emphasis on reptiles; emphasis on captive animals

The ACZM examination also occurs over 2 days; however, it differs significantly from the ABVP examination. The examination takes 2 full days, and the total point allocation is 675 points. On Day 1, all candidates take five sections of the test: Avian, Herpetofauna, Mammal, Wildlife, and Aquatic. Box 4 shows the breakdown of the four components of the Day 1 sections. Continuation to Day 2 is contingent on passing all five Day 1 sections with a score of 65% or higher for each section. There are 75 multiple choice questions for each of the five Day 1 components, and each question has one right answer and four distractors. Thus, 49 of 75 questions must be answered correctly in each section. On both the ACZM and the ABVP examinations, questions may be disqualified for various reasons during the grading process; thus the actual number of correct answers needed to pass a section can have some variation, but 49 is a starting point.

There are still some encouraging rewards if three or four of the sections are passed. On returning the next year, examinees

BOX 5 AMERICAN COLLEGE OF ZOOLOGICAL MEDICINE DAY 2 EXAMINATION OPTIONS

Aquatic Animal Medicine

- Fish, marine, and aquatic mammals, aquatic invertebrates, aquatic birds, and aquatic reptiles, either free-ranging or captive (including zoologic and aquaculture institutions)

General Zoo

- Captive mammals, birds, reptiles, amphibians, and fish, with an emphasis on species kept in standard zoologic institutions.

Wildlife

- Free-ranging wildlife, including mammals, birds, and other

Zoological Companion Animal Medicine

- Major emphasis on companion birds, reptiles and amphibians, and mammals

only need to pass the remaining one or two sections to continue on to Day 2. However, failure to pass those final one or two components will cause the examinees to have to repeat all five sections of the Day 1 examination the next year if they so desire to continue with the attempts.

The Day 2 examination for ACZM is based on one of four options of a subspecialty—General Zoo, Zoological Companion Animal, Aquatics, or Wildlife. See Box 5 for more details of each. Obviously, reptiles and amphibians are a component of each of these four options; however, many examinees choose one of the first two options. Each option has four sections: a practical examination, an essay examination, a slide examination, and an advanced multiple choice examination (75 questions). One must pass with 65% or greater, but for Day 2, the score is cumulative. If examinees do not pass Day 2 on the first try, they return the following year for one last try. Failure on the second try for Day 2 requires the examinee to start completely over with passing Day 1, all sections, again.

The European College of Zoological Medicine

The ECZM is a European Veterinary Specialist College formed under the auspices of the European Board of Specialisation (www.eczm.eu). The ECZM evolved from the European College of Avian Medicine and Surgery (ECAMS), itself a veterinary specialist organization founded in 1993. ECAMS was an initiative of the European Committee of the Association of Avian Veterinarians, in response to a growing demand for better avian medical and surgical services for birds through specialization and a need to harmonize certification in this area. ECAMS became recognized as a fully functional College in 2005. In 2007, an initiative was commenced to broaden the membership and areas of specialty of ECAMS. The aims were to strengthen the College by increasing membership, provide the opportunity for those working at a specialist level within allied zoologic fields to gain recognition, and facilitate greater recognition of the clinical area by the profession within veterinary academia, by governments, and by the public. The result was that ECAMS changed to ECZM, and herpetologic medicine was added in April 2009. De facto recognition for this specialty is still being accepted until April 2014. Founding diplomates of these specialties are also in the process of creating residencies to facilitate training in these specialties.

The ECZM Web site provides detailed information about the ECZM, including the constitution, bylaws, and information brochures on all specialties, including herpetologic medicine. The latter contains information about requirements for admission to the College, a profile of the specialties, and application and examination procedures.

Currently, a specialist is only required to be active in the field for a minimum of 50% to 60% of the time. No herpetologic residencies currently exist, although efforts are under way to change this. In addition, although the herpetologic examination has not been finalized, the current ECZM examination structure comprises a 1-day examination for a total of 370 points.

ANNOTATED SUGGESTED READING LISTS

For ABVP, ECZM, and ACZM, these lists are provided to guide veterinarians studying for the examination. They are *not* a comprehensive listing of all available material but rather a guide to facilitate finding information in areas in which the candidate does not have extensive experience. Questions are taken from the extant literature and are not confined only to information from the work on the list. Not all chapters in listed textbooks are necessarily of significance for the examination. Questions based on journal articles emphasize literature from the past 5 years, although older references may also be included. It is recommended that candidates prioritize study material within the references suggested.

EXAMINATION PREPARATION

No perfect method exists for studying for these examinations: different systems work for different people. Some basic recommendations include the following: spend time reading (one of the main reasons for taking this examination is to give you the opportunity to, at least once, do a thorough review of the literature), start early (8 to 12 months before the examination), have a study plan, and have an examination-taking plan. Beyond these steps, what follows are some of the strategies that may help some individuals better direct their energies.

For ACZM credentialing, in most cases candidates likely have a good idea of whether they meet the requirements. However, with credentials submitted by March 31, that only leaves about 5 months until the examination. Thus some individuals indicate that they will take the examination the following year, giving themselves an 18-month time frame to study. For ABVP, notification of acceptance of credentials usually occurs in early summer, giving about 5 months until the next examination; in September, the option to postpone an additional 12 months is available. As previously mentioned, no matter how much time one has to study, one will likely never feel prepared enough.

Some examinees go into an examination with little or no preparation, using this strategy to see what they know and to analyze the question style to help preparation for the next year. Many current Diplomates in both organizations frown on this strategy; however, it has worked for some individuals. This can be an expensive endeavor for many individuals because the examination fee, plane ticket, hotel expenses, and even the stress of waiting another year before trying again does add up.

Using this strategy, one would need a multiyear examination plan from the beginning.

Another strategy often employed, particularly for the ACZM examination, is to try to pass the Day 1 examination in a multiyear approach. Again, while this strategy is not encouraged, it can be successful, particularly for those on the practitioner track, because these individuals often cannot devote large amounts of time to studying the enormous amount of information; however, if they perhaps focus on birds, reptiles, and fish, then a component of Day 1 might be passed. Disadvantages to this method include the cost of multiple examination site visits as already mentioned, the stress of not being done after the first attempt, and the possibility that the sections with increased focus are actually failed. Nonetheless, given the huge breadth of ever-increasing knowledge required for passing the ACZM examination, this technique has worked well for a growing number of examinees. The technique does not work well for the ABVP examination because the only partial one can get is either passing only the practical or only the multiple choice, so partial passage is more incidental in most cases.

For those attempting to pass one of the examinations completely in one try, the first step is developing a technique to organize the information. Organizing by taxonomic groups/populations is one technique used, and another is to skim through core topics and recent research and organize by information source.

Working with a good mentor can be helpful; however, mentors not familiar with the current examination can sometimes be extremely detrimental because they may direct the examinee to study topics on the examination that are no longer relevant. Some mentors also put too much emphasis on the core topics, leaving the candidate blindsided by the examination question coverage. Speaking candidly with individuals previously mentored by that person can be extremely helpful in evaluating whether that particular mentor will be helpful.

Practice examination questions from within a study group or that are completely self-created can help one to start thinking like an question writer and thus can help in determining whether a particular paper may have value from an examination standpoint. Reading papers and references from the standpoint of taking an examination versus evaluating those same sources for clinical information usually require an individual to look at those sources very differently. For either examination, assume that the results of a paper are valid, even if one personally disagrees. An exception to this is when another paper contradicts the other's findings; this controversy often leads to avoidance of that aspect of the topic for an examination question, although essay questions may touch on those controversies in the ACZM examination. Likewise, if findings are ambiguous or questionable, the results are not likely to be the focus of a question from that source.

For the ACZM Day 2 essay and practical portions, try to focus on the major topics in each area. For example, a question on amphibian surgery would be less likely than one on chytridiomycosis. Comparing and contrasting similar diseases are often a good way to cover such topics. Real-life scenarios (e.g., "You note a die-off of Wyoming toads. How would you work it up? Then compare and contrast two major diseases that might be involved here.") are always helpful. Essay questions may be of ancillary benefit to ABVP examinees, but learning format is not often helpful. Day 2 of the ACZM examination is used by many candidates as a core portion of their combined Day 2 points because these questions focus more on showing what you know (usually a lot) versus what you do not know. However, points will be deducted for wrong information, so writing down everything possible hoping that some part of it is correct is not a good strategy.

Develop a pacing strategy for the examination. Remember, even if only guessing, one will be "correct" 33% of the time for the ABVP and 20% of the time for ACZM/ECZM examinations. Examinees then just need to combine what they already know and what they still need to learn in the area for the additional 37% to 45% to score in the 65% to 70% range. This perspective can help keep a candidate calm when feeling overwhelmed by the amount of information. For essays, examinees should quickly read through all of them, skipping those on which they have little or no information; the more well-known questions (and therefore the greater sources of points) should be completely answered first. Time should be allotted at the end of each section for writing down something for those questions that one does not have much to add. For practicals on both examinations and the slide portion of Day 2 ACZM, one often cannot return to certain stations or images, or, if the latter is allowed, only a brief reassessment may be performed. Be careful about changing answers—sometimes first impressions are the best. However, also be careful about "easy question–answer" combinations; these are often screened from the question pools, so quick associations of terms may not be the correct answer.

Having a study group for either examination does seem to improve the success of examinees. Some partner with a single other person, others with a larger group. Communication can be weekly, monthly, or even just once. Some try to form study groups with individuals of different backgrounds professionally so that each person brings something different to the group. Others prefer groups of like-minded people, who study and organize their summarized information similarly. Again, there is no single solution; it is different for everyone.

Images for the practical in both examinations and the slide portion of the Day 2 component of the ACZM examination should be reviewed in atlases, textbooks, journal articles, and on the Web. Most actual images on the examinations are rarely in the public domain, but similar ones have often been contributed to the examination.

Some people like to take time off 1 to 4 weeks before the examination for review of all topics. Many practitioners do not have the luxury of such an option, but it may be helpful if possible. It is also important to realize that at this late stage of examination preparation, such reviews may help more by keeping a person focused and busy rather than allowing more time to gather novel information. Nonetheless, such reviews at the end or periodically throughout the study process may be helpful. It is very important to set a schedule so that one does not spend too much time on a particular topic or area and to also recognize that some topics of unfamiliarity may require greater energy and focus. Study groups often help keep one on schedule.

Do not panic during the studying process or during the examination, and try to stay positive. Everyone hits highs and, more commonly, lows during the process. Study group members can be helpful again in this regard. Also do not forget that these examinations are not life or death: failure is not the end of the world (I passed the ACZM examination on the second try and am aware of some extremely well-respected zoo veterinarians and private practitioners that took the examination more than one time). Make sure to dedicate time for family, pets, and a life outside of the examination process—no extra letter after one's name is worth that sacrifice or loss!

RE-CREDENTIALING

Currently, ABVP Diplomates are required to either retake the examination or re-credential via a point process every 10 years. Notification occurs in Year 8 to allow adequate time for this lengthy process and for second/third attempts if early failure occurs so that Diplomate status is not lost. Until recently, few U.S. veterinary specialties required this other than the ABVP. However, the ABVS is mandating such a process in the near future for all specialties, including ACZM from 2016. Current Diplomates would be grandfathered in, although they would be encouraged to engage in the process. Re-credentialing, other than retaking the examination, requires a significant amount of documentation of appropriate specialty continuing education in the previous 5 years, publications, appropriate lectures, writing examination questions, and doing topic summaries, among other options. Re-credentialing should not be left until the last minute; some ABVP Diplomates have lost their Diplomate status because they lacked enough points. Interestingly, ABVP offers points if one has taken the ACZM examination and passed since the Diplomate last credentialed. The ECZM also has a compulsory re-credentialing system, which requires active Diplomates to re-credential every 5 years.

ACKNOWLEDGMENTS

I would like to specially thank the Executive Director of ABVP, Marisa Hackemann, for development of much of this information. Other members of the ABVP Core of Regents over the years also helped develop the Policies and Procedures, the Applicant Handbook, and the PowerPoint used to promote ABVP that were a prominent source for this chapter. I would also like to give special thanks to the ABVP Credentialing and Examination Committees. Likewise, ACZM, their officers, and members of their Examination and Credentialing Committees contributed to this chapter. I particularly appreciate the help of Sonia Hernandez, Chris Handley, Jennifer Langan, Stephane Lair, and Stephen Divers, and Dr. Nico Shoemaker who reviewed the material for the ECZM.

SECTION I

ADVANCES IN REPTILE MEDICINE

CHAPTER 1

Current Herpetologic Husbandry and Products

Stephen L. Barten and Gregory J. Fleming†

Husbandry techniques and equipment for captive reptiles and amphibians have advanced at a rapid pace over the last several decades to parallel the ever-growing popularity of these animals as pets. Multiple books, journals, magazine articles, and booklets discussing herpetologic husbandry and herpetoculture have been published, not to mention the overwhelming amount of information available on the internet. Additionally, a large number of specialty companies and distributors furnish a wide and ever-changing array of supplies and equipment specifically designed for captive reptiles and amphibians, known colloquially as *herps*.

One of the major problems facing herpetoculture is that no standard of care exists when it comes to herpetologic husbandry. Most husbandry advice is subjective and based on experience rather than scientific data. Information sources can include professional herpetologists, herpetoculturists, hobbyists, veterinarians, books and magazines, the internet, and pet store employees. Obviously advice from such different sources sometimes can be conflicting, which is frustrating for a pet owner. Critical thinking must be used when assessing husbandry recommendations. The advice of a professional herpetologist or a herpetoculturist with years of experience keeping and breeding hundreds of specimens may carry more weight than that of someone without formal education or a pet store employee who has never kept the species in question. The adjective *proper* used to describe some aspect of herp husbandry, as in *proper cages, proper temperature*, or *proper diet*, is purely subjective and should not always be taken at face value.

Currently there is no government regulatory agency that monitors products manufactured for reptiles for safety or efficacy. Thus any manufacturer can make almost any claim they like without providing evidence for that claim. Unfortunately many products for herps may have questionable value and may be inappropriate or even dangerous to the reptiles for which they are intended. Likewise, with literally hundreds of species of reptiles with differing natural histories available in the pet trade, products intended for one species could be potentially harmful for another species.

It is important to utilize all available information to best care for reptiles in captivity. A great deal of published scientific information is available concerning herpetologic natural history, life histories, natural diets, and reproductive data. However, this information is often in the professional herpetologic literature, as opposed to veterinary or lay herpetologic literature. These professional sources should be sought out.

Herpetologic husbandry still boils down to providing an adequate enclosure, appropriate social groupings, temperature gradients to allow thermoregulation, humidity, and ultraviolet light sources and offering a balanced diet. These are the things that herpetoculturists strive for, and when they fall short it often results in medical conditions that can be resolved with proper knowledge of husbandry and enclosure design.

Herpetoculture, like everything else, is an ever-growing and expanding field. New products, new diets, and new techniques are being developed every year. The herpetologic veterinarian and herp keeper must keep abreast of new developments. The purpose of this chapter is to discuss recent trends and developments in herpetoculture and is not intended to be a comprehensive discussion of herpetologic husbandry.

ENCLOSURE TYPE

Many keepers, especially novice ones, have metaphoric blinders on and are only aware of what products they see on the shelves of local pet stores. They must be advised that alternatives to the traditional glass aquarium or terrarium exist for housing herps. A variety of plastic and fiberglass cages and tubs designed specifically to house captive reptiles are available from numerous manufacturers. Often these enclosures come in much larger sizes for lower prices than glass aquariums. Larger size allows for more aesthetically appealing displays. Additional advantages of plastic or fiberglass enclosures can include larger space for the herp, better escape prevention, better visual security, stackability, ease of attaching light and heat sources, better heat and humidity retention, and better thermoregulation on a vertical as well as horizontal axis. Likewise, plastic and fiberglass cages tend to be lighter in weight, more durable, and easier to clean than glass aquariums.

Besides enclosures for snakes and lizards, plastic and fiberglass tubs suitable for keeping aquatic and semiaquatic turtles are available. A number of manufacturers produce plain, round or rectangular tubs in sizes from 0.5 gallons to 5000 gallons (1.9 to 18,927 L) (Figure 1-1). Waterland Tubs (www.waterlandtubs.com) is a line of plastic tubs designed specifically for keeping aquatic and semiaquatic turtles. These tubs have a water side and an access ramp to a land side to allow for basking and egg laying. They come in multiple sizes up to 200 gallons (757 L). Waterland tubs are lightweight, can be placed outside, and can be modified to add bulk heads and drains to make cleaning easier.

†Deceased.

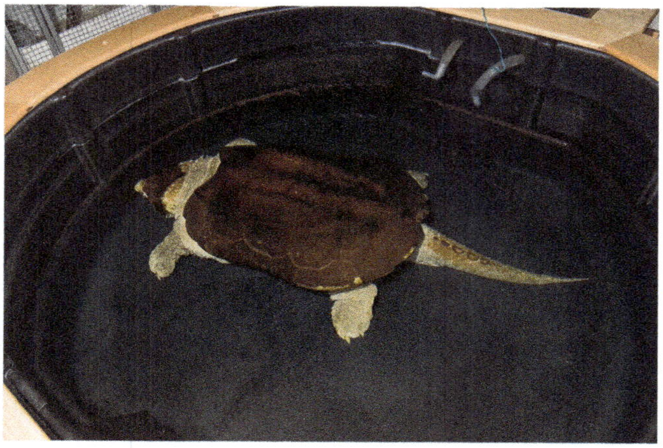

FIGURE 1-1 Large plastic and fiberglass tubs up to several thousand gallons are available to house aquatic turtles. This is a large Alligator Snapping Turtle *(Macrochelys temminckii)*. *(Photo courtesy Dr. Stephen L. Barten, Vernon Hills Animal Hospital, Mundelein, Ill.)*

WATER FILTRATION

Often temperature and lighting are considered when keeping captive reptiles; however, water filtration is commonly overlooked. Poor water quality may be one of the main reasons that aquatic reptiles and amphibians may not thrive in captivity and are considered "dirty" or hard to keep.

Any amphibian or aquatic or semiaquatic reptile species requiring something more than a water bowl for proper husbandry should have filtration included in their enclosure design. This can be as simple as an air pump and a sponge filter or as complicated as a wet-dry filter for larger systems. In any case, filtration has the goal of reducing biologic waste, including ammonia and its toxic by-products, through mechanical, biologic, and chemical filtration.

- Mechanical filtration—this includes pumps, canisters, and air lifts. Mechanical filtration is the physical action of moving water over media (e.g., protein skimmer foam or filter media). Mechanical filtration removes the large particulate matter in the water and also oxygenates the water.
- Biologic filtration—within a high surface area filter, on the gravel, and walls of the aquarium, live bacteria that are responsible for breaking down ammonia (produced by the reptile or amphibian) into nitrite and then nitrate, the least toxic form of nitrogenous waste. This process is called the nitrification cycle and takes about 21 days in most aquariums to become established in a new setup. Aquatic reptiles are not as sensitive to this cycle as fish and amphibians, which are exquisitely sensitive to ammonia and its by-products.
- Chemical filtration—activated carbon has great absorbency and is used to remove harmful chemicals and color compounds from water. Other examples are sodium hydroxymethylsulfinate and sodium thiosulfate, which remove ammonia and chlorine, respectively.

Most commercial filtration units combine all three filtration methods, which makes for a very powerful filtration system. Currently many fish filtration devices as well as specific reptile and turtle filtration options are commercially available. The reptile and turtle filtration units can work in shallow water, which is usually not the case with most fish filters. These filters are now easy to maintain and promote good health in aquatic reptilian and amphibian species.

Filtration alone is insufficient for maintaining adequate water quality in aquatic habitats. Frequent partial water changes and regular complete water changes also are necessary. Depending on the size of the aquarium and the number and size of inhabitants, one third of the water might be changed weekly, and all of the water should be changed once every month or two. Dechlorination by either aging or chemical means is important for amphibians and gilled inhabitants but less so for reptiles. New water added to the aquarium should be brought to the same temperature and pH as water already in the aquarium to prevent shock caused by sudden, dramatic differences.

Zoo Med Laboratories (3650 Sacramento Dr., San Luis Obispo, CA 93401, http://zoomed.com) has a complete line of terrariums, aquatic habitats, and filtrations for all species of reptiles. Exo Terra (Rolf C. Hagen [USA] Corp, Mansfield, MA 02048, http://www.exo-terra.com) has many filters and accessories for amphibian and aquatic reptile enclosures.

SPACE REQUIREMENTS

The once-popular practice, especially among snake and gecko keepers, of keeping dozens to hundreds of specimens in small, Spartan, laboratory-style cages with minimal space and few cage furnishings is falling out of favor. Minimalist cage design facilitates ease of maintenance for the keeper but provides little for the welfare or behavioral well-being of the animals. An important trend in herpetoculture is to downsize collections and provide spacious cages for the remaining specimens. Indeed, for observation and appreciation of a reptile's natural behavior, a more natural enclosure must be provided. An adult Cornsnake *(Pantherophis [Elaphe] guttatus)* or Kingsnake *(Lampropeltis getula)* might survive in a 20-gallon (76 L) aquarium but would thrive in a cage measuring 4 × 2 × 2 feet high (1.2 × 0.6 × 0.6 m high). Snakes and other reptiles in larger cages tend to be more active and have better muscle tone (Figure 1-2). Larger cages allow more cage furniture such as climbing branches, multiple hides, and larger water sources. They allow for wider thermal and humidity gradients and better thermoregulation. Larger cages allow for the use of ventilation fans and misters. Larger cages usually are more aesthetically appealing (Figure 1-3).

Some guidelines for cage size have been published.[1,2] One formula recommends that the length plus the width of a snake cage should at a minimum equal the length of the snake; thus a 4 × 2-foot (1.2 × 0.6 m) cage is the minimum size recommended for a 6-foot (1.8 m) long snake. Likewise large lizards should be housed in cages that are twice as long as the total length of the lizard; thus a 4-foot (1.2 m) wide cage is acceptable for a 2-foot (0.6 m) lizard (the minimum cage size should be 1.5 times as long as the length of the lizard).[3] The upper range of cage size is limited only by the spatial and financial restrictions of the owner. It is incorrect to assume that reptiles, being ectothermic, are sedentary and inactive. In fact, with adequate available space, most reptiles are highly active with complex behaviors.[4]

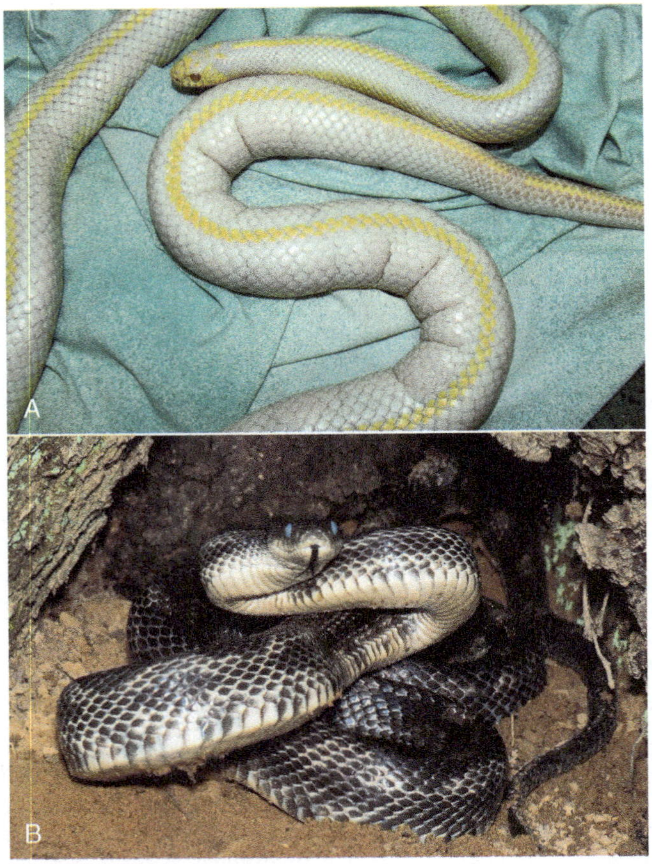

FIGURE 1-2 A, "Cage potato" Kingsnake *(Lampropeltis getula)* exhibiting poor muscle tone and obesity due to lack of exercise and overfeeding. **B,** A wild Midland Rat Snake *(Pantherophis* [*Elaphe*] *spiloides)* showing well-developed musculature as a result of a large home range and more frequent climbing and foraging than most captive snakes undertake. *(Photos courtesy Dr. Stephen L. Barten, Vernon Hills Animal Hospital, Mundelein, Ill.)*

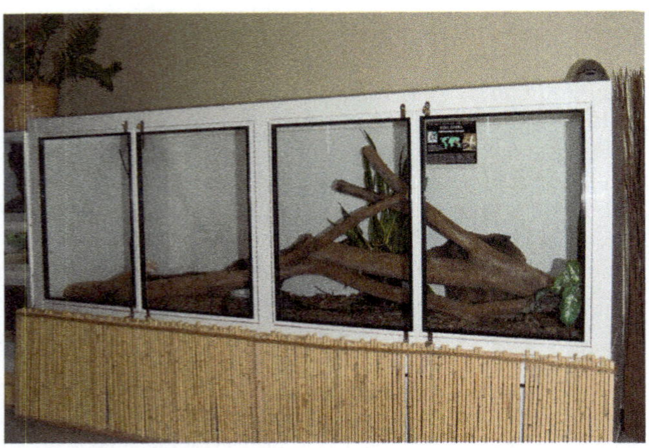

FIGURE 1-3 This plastic cage by Habitat Systems Ltd. (Des Moines, Iowa) located in a nature center measures 12 feet wide by 3 feet deep and 4 feet high (3.7 × 0.9 × 1.2 m) and houses a King Cobra *(Ophiophagus hannah)*, a large, very active species. Large reptile enclosures have many advantages and are preferred over small, minimalist setups. *(Photo courtesy Dr. Stephen L. Barten, Vernon Hills Animal Hospital, Mundelein, Ill.)*

A number of companies produce plastic or fiberglass enclosures in standard or custom designs for keeping reptiles and amphibians. Most of these companies have Web sites, and some offer free shipping. A variety of these products may be viewed at many of the large reptile shows held periodically around the country. A partial list of such companies in no particular order are included in Box 1-1.

SUBSTRATE

Zoos and nature centers often use natural substrates to line cages instead of newspaper, indoor/outdoor carpeting, bark chips, or gravel. Natural substrates are aesthetic, provide material for digging and other behaviors, hold moisture, and are absorbent. Materials that are small enough not to cause a blockage if ingested are recommended; in other words, avoid gravel and large bark and wood chips.

Natural substrates can be mixed and matched to meet the needs of various species. Commonly used materials that can be blended together in various combinations to meet the needs of the reptile or amphibian include beach sand, peat, top soil (with no insecticide or fertilizer), Eco Earth (compressed, expandable coconut fiber bedding; Zoo Med Laboratories Inc, San Luis Obispo, Calif, http://www.zoomed.com), and leaf mulch. For instance, a desert species might be kept on a mix with more sand and less soil, peat, and leaf mulch, while a forest species requiring more moisture might be kept on a mix with more leaf mulch, soil, and peat and less sand, if any. A topping of dead leaves adds aesthetic appeal, and the leaves decompose and add to the soil mix.

The substrate should be spot cleaned as necessary but raked weekly to aerate the mix. The entire mix should be replaced as necessary when soiled or fouled with waste or uneaten food.

Natural substrates have better aesthetic appeal and can be useful for maintaining environmental conditions, but they also can be implicated in veterinary issues. Wood chips or bark are not recommended because they often can be ingested or caught in the mouth of a lizard or snake. Gravel is ingested by aquatic turtles and can result in intestinal blockage. Sand substrates also can be ingested, causing intestinal blockage in tortoises, Bearded Dragons *(Pogona vitticeps)* and Leopard Geckos *(Eublepharis macularius)*. Most of these issues can be solved by providing balanced nutrition, an appropriate temperature gradient, and ultraviolet (UV) B light and by placing feed on large trays or bowls that keep the food material away from the substrate. In the case of large tortoises housed outside, small cement pads or flagstone pieces are recommended to keep food from contacting soil or sand. These feeding palates can be washed off or disinfected. In some cases, large tortoises housed in sandy areas can be fed psyllium that binds to the sand so that it is passed with the feces. In the author's (GJF) experience, a psyllium dose of 1 tsp/5 kg daily for 5 to 7 days repeated once a month has been beneficial.

NATURAL BACKGROUNDS

Various companies manufacture natural-looking backgrounds and cage furniture that make a cage more aesthetically appealing, provide more climbing and enrichment for the inhabitants, are sturdy, and yet are easy to clean and disinfect (Figure 1-4). The use of such backgrounds can make an ordinary enclosure a true showpiece and allow for visualization of

BOX 1-1 A PARTIAL LIST OF COMPANIES THAT PRODUCE PLASTIC OR FIBERGLASS ENCLOSURES IN STANDARD OR CUSTOM DESIGNS FOR KEEPING REPTILES AND AMPHIBIANS

Habitat Systems Limited, 4489 NW 2nd Ave, Suite 3B, Des Moines, IA 50313, http://www.habitatsystemsltd.com — reptile and amphibian enclosures

Animal Plastics, 6220 NW Beaver Dr., #1, Johnston, IA, 50131, http://www.animalplastics.com — reptile and amphibian enclosures

Vision Products Plus, Inc., 7453 Deering Ave, Canoga Park, CA, 91303, http://www.visionproducts.us — large range of single or stackable reptile enclosures and tortoise tubs

Neodesha Plastics, Inc. (NPI) Reptile and Snake Cages, P.O. Box 539, Neodesha, KS 66757, http://www.npicages.com — one-piece molded cages with slanted fronts for maximum viewing

Boaphile Plastics, P.O. Box 394, Cannon Falls, MN 55009, http://www.boaphileplastics.com — plastic reptile cages up to 8 feet (2.4 m) wide with single cage, multiunit stacks and rack systems

Glasscages.com, http://www.glasscages.com — custom glass and acrylic aquariums and terrariums, as well as backgrounds, stands, and supplies for all species of reptiles

Waterland Tubs, http://www.waterlandtubs.com — aquatic and semiaquatic turtle tubs with land and water sides and accessories

Pentair Ltd. (formerly Aquatic Eco-Systems, Inc.), 2395 Apopka Blvd., Apopka, FL 32703, http://www.aquaticeco.com/topics/1/Aquarium-Supplies — Plastic and fiberglass tubs and aquariums for aquatic species, along with an expansive catalog of supplies

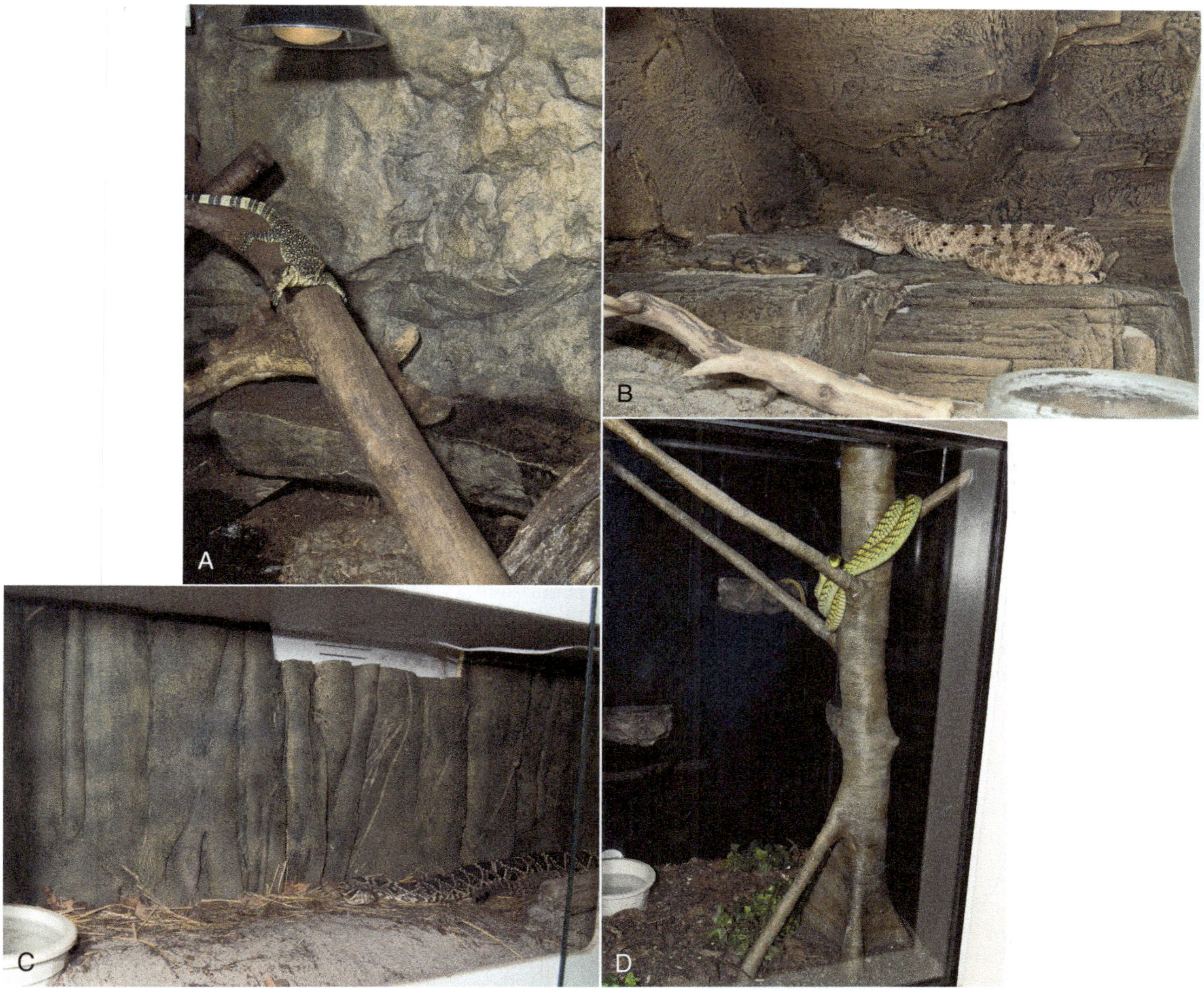

FIGURE 1-4 **A,** Natural-looking backgrounds enhance the aesthetic appeal of a herp display cage. The background in this Water Monitor's *(Varanus salvator)* large cage was custom made by Habitat Systems Ltd. (Des Moines, Iowa). **B,** This is a standard background from Aqua Terra (Baldwin Park, Calif) cut to fit the cage housing a Sidewinder Rattlesnake *(Crotalus cerastes).* **C,** A ventilation hole has been cut into this Aqua Terra natural background. The hole should be secured with mesh screen adhered to the back edge of the hole with silicone adhesive to prevent the snake from getting behind the background. The snake is an Eastern Diamondback Rattlesnake *(Crotalus adamanteus).* **D,** A fiberglass tree allows climbing by this Jameson's Mamba *(Dendroaspis jamesoni).* It looks natural yet can be securely anchored and easily cleaned and disinfected. *(Photos courtesy Dr. Stephen L. Barten, Vernon Hills Animal Hospital, Mundelein, Ill.)*

natural reptile behaviors (Figure 1-5). These backgrounds should be adequately secured, and care must be taken to block any access to the space behind the background. If a snake or lizard were to disappear into that space it may be necessary to tear down the entire enclosure to access the reptile. Any holes through the background for tubing or ventilation can be secured by affixing screen mesh over the hole using silicone adhesive applied to the rear of the background around the hole. Another potential hazard is improperly secured backgrounds or cage furniture made of heavy material that can fall and result in crushing injuries to enclosure inhabitants. A partial list of companies that provide these products in no particular order are included in Box 1-2.

AXIAL FANS TO IMPROVE VENTILATION

An important trend in herpetoculture is the use of ventilation fans for solid-sided cages. A focal heat source in a cage lacking ventilation eventually will heat the entire cage, minimizing thermal gradients and the ability of the cage inhabitant to thermoregulate. When ventilation is established, the focal basking site remains but the rest of the cage is cooler, allowing the reptile more thermoregulatory choices. In one case, three Eastern Indigo Snakes *(Drymarchon couperi)* kept in three identical cages were observed to bask under their heat lamps for only an hour each morning. Four-inch (10.2 cm) ventilation holes were cut in both ends of the 60 × 33 × 24 inch high (1.5 × 0.84 × 0.60 m high) enclosures, the holes were screened, and an axial fan was placed over the hole on the end with the heat lamp in each cage (Figure 1-6). It was directed to blow air out of the cage and pull air in from the far end. The fans were connected to the same timer as the heat lamps in the cages, so both fans and lamps were on the same 12-hour on/12-hour off cycle. The snakes were observed to increase their basking times to 4 to 5 hours daily after the addition of the axial fans (Carmichael R: Pers. com., Aug 26, 2011).

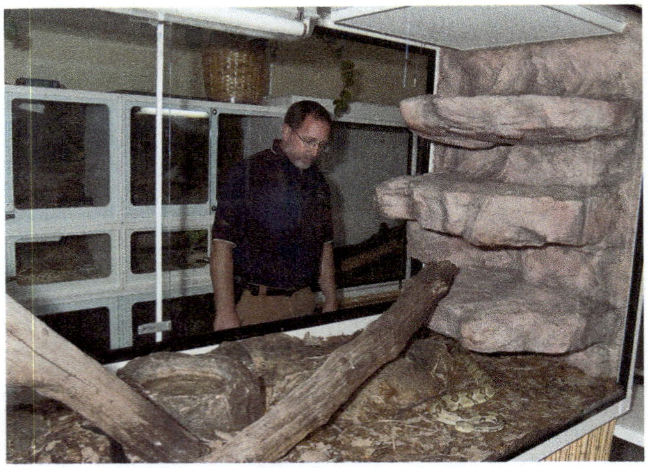

FIGURE 1-5 Natural-looking backgrounds allow captive reptiles to exhibit natural behaviors. The rock like shelves in this exhibit allow the Timber Rattlesnakes *(Crotalus horridus)* housed within to thermoregulate under the radiant heat panel attached to the cage ceiling by moving to higher and lower shelves. *(Photo courtesy Dr. Stephen L. Barten, Vernon Hills Animal Hospital, Mundelein, Ill.)*

Axial fans are small fans used to provide spot cooling for electronics like computers, telephones, cameras, and copy machines. They come in a variety of sizes based on voltage, mounting hole diameter, and airflow. Airflow is measured in cubic feet per minute (CFM), which is calculated by multiplying the air speed in feet per minute by the area in square feet. The strength of various fans can be compared by their CFM rating.

In general, to supply clean air requires four to eight air changes per hour. Kitchens can require 15 to 60 air changes per hour.[5] Presumably, heated reptile cages would require air exchanges at the upper end of this range to be effective. In the situation of a cage measuring 4 to 5 feet wide (1.2 to 1.5 m), an axial fan with a CFM of 55 will provide more than enough ventilation. A fan with a CFM of 105 is recommended for cages measuring 7 to 8 feet wide (2.1 to 2.4 m) (Wismann K: Pers. com., Aug 29, 2011). Fans with less power are recommended for species that require higher humidity, such as chameleons and tree frogs.

Axial fans are commercially available from a variety of manufacturers. One such company is Grainger (Lake Forest, Ill, http://www.grainger.com/production/info/axial-fans.htm). Customers must choose the appropriate style for their needs; choices include 115-volt AC, 230-volt AC and DC (battery)

BOX 1-2 A PARTIAL LIST OF COMPANIES THAT MANUFACTURE NATURAL-LOOKING BACKGROUNDS AND CAGE FURNITURE

Aqua Terra, Not Just Fish Inc., 14160 Live Oak Ave, Unit E, Baldwin Park, CA 91706, http://www.aquaterra-intl.com/index.html produces Naturalistic 3-D Backgrounds, a line of artificial backgrounds that mimic various rock or tree designs, with eight styles from which to choose. They are suitable for both aquariums and terrariums and come in modular sections that can be joined together to fit any size enclosure. They are easily cut to fit or allow for ventilation or filter hoses and can be adhered to the enclosure with silicone adhesive. An owner can install these backgrounds at home. The company also has modular rocks that can be used by themselves or joined with other rocks or with backgrounds for decoration or for use as hides.

Habitat Systems Limited, 4489 NW 2nd Ave, Suite 3B, Des Moines, IA 50313, http://www.habitatsystemsltd.com manufactures natural-looking fiberglass branches, trees, and logs, as well as hides and water bowls. They also produce unique fiberglass backgrounds for cages that mimic rock walls or other natural habitats.

Zoo Med Laboratories, 3650 Sacramento Drive, San Luis Obispo, CA 93401, http://zoomed.com has a complete line of terrariums, natural-looking backgrounds, aquatic habitats, and feeding and water bowls for all species of reptiles.

Glasscages.com, www.glasscages.com has a complete line of terrariums, artificial rocks, and backgrounds. The backgrounds can be used in aquatic and terrestrial setups and can be cut or drilled for custom applications.

fans in a variety of diameters. Cord sets are ordered separately, as are fan guards and filters.

Obviously, the enclosure ventilation holes must be screened to prevent the cage inhabitants from contacting the fan blades.

ULTRAVIOLET METERS

Over the last several decades, our understanding of the requirement for UV lighting to maintain healthy reptiles has grown. Most reptiles utilize UV wavelengths in the 290 nm to 320 nm range (UVB) for the synthesis of vitamin D_3, which is necessary for calcium metabolism. Calcium, vitamin D metabolism, and UVB have been discussed in detail elsewhere.[6-8] Likewise, much advice concerning the use of UVB lamps for captive reptiles to stimulate vitamin D_3 synthesis is available. While most if that advice is anecdotal, more and more scientific studies involving measurements of UVB irradiance and blood levels of vitamin D_3 in specific species are being completed every year.[9-14]

In general, four types of lamps are commonly used to provide UVB for captive herps. Fluorescent tubes provide diffuse light and little heat. Compact fluorescent bulbs produce a more concentrated area of UVB but also little heat. Fluorescent UVB lamps should be used in conjunction with another heat source for thermoregulation. Mercury vapor spot lights produce a focused beam of very bright light, strong UVB, and significant heat. Finally, mercury vapor flood lamps provide very bright light, strong UVB, and heat over a wider area than do spot lamps.[15]

The UVB output of a lamp in $\mu W/cm^2$ can be measured with a UVB meter. A number of companies produce UV meters for a variety of uses. UV meters are used to measure solar radiation, erythema dose, window and acrylic UV transmission, solar panel irradiance and power calculation, and UVB lamp intensity and aging. Specialized UVB lamps that might be monitored with a UVB meter include lamps for captive reptiles, aquariums, treatment of elevated bilirubin levels in premature infants, acne treatment, skin rejuvenation, tanning beds, as well as germicidal lamps.[16]A variety of UV meters are commercially available for different purposes and different types of lamps; some models are manufactured for more generalized use and some are for very specific applications. Consumers must research the specifications of a given UV meter to ensure that it meets their needs. The Solarmeter models 6.2 and 6.4 (Solartech, Inc, Harrison Township, Mich, http://www.solarmeter.com/) are manufactured specifically for use with reptile lamps and are popular among herpetoculturists. Model 6.2 measures UVB output in $\mu W/cm^2$, whereas Model 6.4 measures the specific UVB wavelengths that convert vitamin D_3 in human skin in IU D_3/min. The entire UVB spectrum does not produce vitamin D_3 equally, and peak production occurs at 298 nm; production of D_3 tapers off above and below this wavelength.[17,18] Because human skin is different than reptile skin (and reptile skin varies tremendously between reptile species), the amount of vitamin D_3 actually produced in a given reptile may differ from the meter reading. Because Solarmeter models 6.2 and 6.4 measure different variables, a given lamp with high output within the UVB range (290 to 320 nm) but lower output in the vitamin D_3 converting range (around 298 nm) could have a higher relative reading with a model 6.2 meter than a model 6.4 meter. However, because specific UVB requirements for various reptile species are unknown, these differences are more theoretical than practical.

UVB meters have a number of uses pertinent to reptile husbandry. The UVB output of the lamp being used should be measured to verify that it meets the targeted requirements of the species being kept. UVB measurements can be taken at varying distances and angles for a given lamp to produce a graph of the effective range of that lamp and help determine the best placement of basking perches.[19] The UVB output of a lamp degrades over time and drops below therapeutic levels before the lamp burns out. It is recommended that UVB lamps be replaced when their output drops below 70% of the initial readings for that lamp.[20] Finally, a UVB meter can be used to determine how much UVB is reaching a captive reptile through various cage materials, such as glass, plastic, acrylic, or screen,

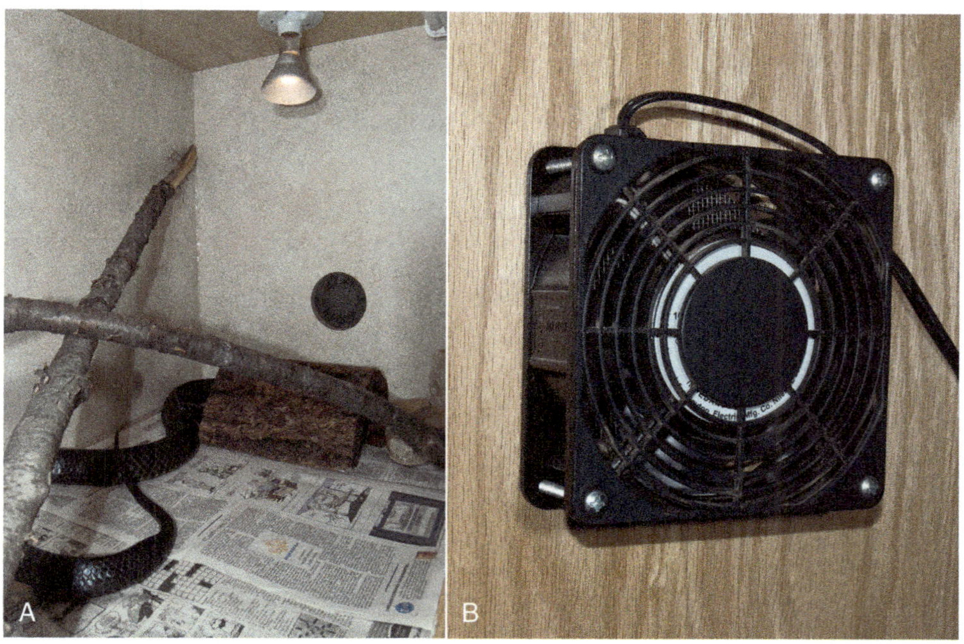

FIGURE 1-6 A, Indigo Snake *(Drymarchon couperi)* in a cage with ventilation holes on both ends and an axial fan to increase air flow over the basking site. **B,** The axial fan attached to the outside of one ventilation hole on the Indigo Snake cage. Note the screen mesh between the fan and the ventilation hole that keeps the snake out of the fan. *(Photo courtesy Dr. Stephen L. Barten, Vernon Hills Animal Hospital, Mundelein, Ill.)*

all of which absorb or reflect some UVB. These readings can be used to make appropriate adjustments in lamp strength and distance and can determine the need for reflectors.

Instructions for using a UV meter with captive reptiles are available from the manufacturer and online sites targeting reptile husbandry.[21] It is recommended that users wear UV eye protection and avoid looking directly into the lamp when taking measurements. Lamps should be allowed to warm up for a minimum of 5 minutes before readings are taken. Other lamps in the cage should be turned off as they may affect the readings. Readings should be taken at the same distance every time to allow accurate comparisons. A standard distance of 12 inches (30 cm) is commonly used, although using the recommended basking distance for mercury vapor lamps will give a more accurate reflection of the UV available to the reptile when the output of those lamps is measured. The recommended basking distance for mercury vapor lamps varies by the product but often is 24 inches (60 cm) or more. The meter is aimed directly at the lamp and moved slowly back and forth with tiny adjustments to find the highest reading, which is the number to record. Two or three readings are recommended to ensure that the alignment was as precise as possible. Different manufacturers or models of UVB meters can vary in their sensors, spectral sensitivity, or calibration and can thus produce different results from the same lamp.[17,22,23] Therefore, the readings from different models of UVB meter cannot be compared directly.

All reptiles need vitamin D. Some species may utilize oral sources of vitamin D_3, but most probably benefit from exposure to some amount of UVB. Species whose natural history involves basking in strong sunlight for hours every day almost certainly need more UVB than species that are normally nocturnal or crepuscular. Growing juveniles and gravid females may need more UVB than nonreproductive adults. Most reptiles avoid direct sunlight in the heat of midday, which can reach UVB levels of 350 to 450 $\mu W/cm^2$ in tropical settings.[24] However, even the shady areas to which these animals retreat have reflected UVB that can reach 30 to 50 $\mu W/cm^2$.[25] In general an attempt should be made to copy the UV exposure in nature for the species in question, and a UVB gradient should be provided to allow the animals themselves to determine their own UVB exposure. Panther Chameleons *(Furcifer pardalis)* regulate their exposure to UVB with great precision depending on dietary vitamin D_3 status; those with low D_3 intake bask in available UVB significantly more than those with high D_3 intake and through that behavior are able to maintain adequate D_3 levels.[26] Conversely, excessive amounts of UVB have been shown to cause disease. High levels of full spectrum light resulted in dermatitis and keratoconjunctivitis in a Blue-tongued Skink (*Tiliqua* sp.) and a Ball Python *(Python regius)*, which resolved once the new lights were removed from the enclosures.[27]

Examples of basking species with high UVB requirements include Bearded Dragons, Uromastyx (*Uromastyx* sp.), Chuckwallas *(Sauromalus obesus)*, and many tortoises.[24] Bearded Dragons given a UVB gradient were observed to spend most of their time basking in the range of 30 to 150 $\mu W/cm^2$ but occasionally would bask at 200 to 300 $\mu W/cm^2$.[24] It is recommended that Green Iguanas *(Iguana iguana)* be provided with 75 to 150 $\mu W/cm^2$ UVB in their basking areas for a minimum of 6 hours a day[25], longer if a UVB gradient and the ability to move out of the lamp beam is available. Mercury vapor lamps are needed to achieve such high UVB output.

Chameleons appear to have more sensitive skin and require lower levels of UVB; higher levels resulted in reduced egg hatchability in Panther Chameleons. It was recommended that species be provided with a gradient of 15 to 33 $\mu W/cm^2$ for 12 hours a day.[17] Another keeper recommended UVB gradients up to 30 $\mu W/cm^2$ for chameleons in general.[24]

Nocturnal and crepuscular species such as Leopard Geckos anecdotally thrive in captive environments with no UVB sources if supplemented with oral sources of vitamin D_3 but also will bask when given the opportunity. Low levels of UVB for brief periods of time might be useful in geckos with low dietary levels of vitamin D_3.[24]

Most snakes are kept successfully with only dietary sources of vitamin D_3 and no UVB, but some herpetoculturists recommend low levels of UVB for Diamond Pythons *(Morelia spilota spilota)* and various North American colubrid snakes including Indigo Snakes, Watersnakes (*Nerodia* sp.), and Greensnakes (*Opheodrys* spp.).[24,28,29] These recommendations are based on subjective keeper observations, and it is often stated that full spectrum light including UVB is not required but is recommended for these species. A recent study has shown that captive Cornsnakes exposed to UVB exhibited significant increases in plasma 25-hydroxyvitamin D_3 over Cornsnakes that did not have UVB exposure.[13]

MISTING SYSTEMS

Reptile and amphibian species with high humidity requirements present unique challenges to their keepers. Good ventilation is important with high humidity levels to prevent buildup of harmful bacteria and fungi. However, this necessitates the frequent replacement of moisture lost to evaporation, especially when supplemental heat also is used. Daily misting with a handheld plant sprayer often is not enough to meet the needs of such species and often is too infrequently utilized by the owners. Misting and fogging systems designed specifically for use with captive herps are available from many manufacturers to maintain humidity in enclosures (Figure 1-7).

In general, fogging machines increase humidity with low volumes of water and are designed for smaller cages (10 to 30 gallon; 38 to 114 L), whereas misting systems can provide high volume "rainlike" environments and are generally preferred for larger enclosures. With the advent of misting and fogging systems, keeping habitats damp is a more realistic goal. Currently, there are a number of products on the market that are designed for use with both single and multiple cages, and new products are introduced every year. Foggers and misters can be controlled with timers to spray for a preset number of minutes at preset intervals or with a humidistat (like a thermostat for humidity) connected to a hygrometer probe to spray as needed to maintain a preset humidity level.

- Most larger units have direct plumbing (Figure 1-8) or large water reservoirs. Water used in the reservoirs should be deionized or obtained by reverse osmosis if the residential water supply is rich in calcium or other minerals that result in water line and spray tip blockage. Sprayer tips also may be removed and soaked in vinegar to remove hard water scale.

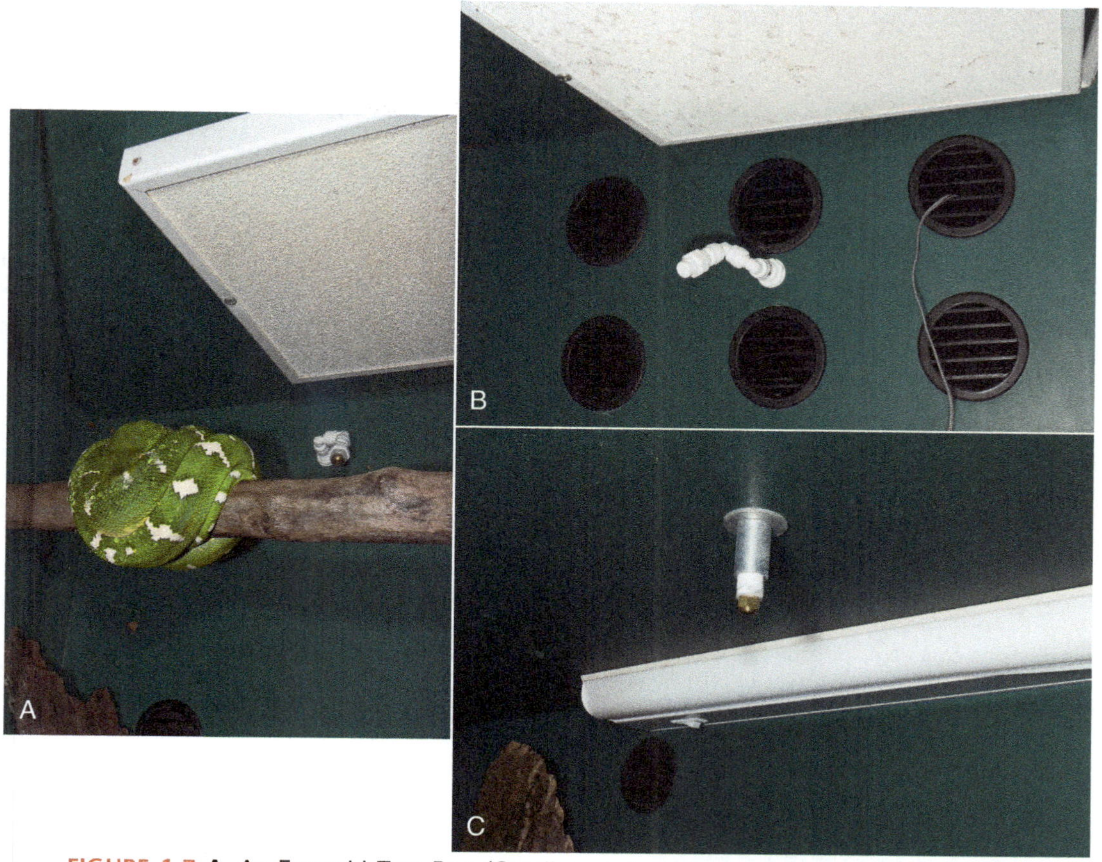

FIGURE 1-7 **A,** An Emerald Tree Boa *(Corallus caninus)* in an enclosure with a misting system. Note the white misting nozzle protruding from the back wall, the drops of water on the snake, and the radiant heat panel attached to the ceiling of the cage. **B,** This misting nozzle is in an enclosure for amphibians. Note the multiple ventilation holes to account for the high humidity levels, the radiant heat panel attached to the top of the cage, and the temperature probe wire that is attached to the thermostat that regulates the heat panel output. **C,** A different style of misting head. *(Photos courtesy Dr. Stephen L. Barten, Vernon Hills Animal Hospital, Mundelein, Ill.)*

- It also is important that the water reservoirs and lines be cleaned and disinfected on a routine schedule. There have been reports of disease in amphibian colonies and large herpetologic collections resulting from bacterial overgrowth in misting systems. Clean water in the reservoirs may foul over time and be a prime breeding zone for *Aeromonas* spp., *Pseudomonas* spp., and other pathogenic organisms. A 1:10 bleach solution or a 1% chlorhexidine solution can be used to flush the system, followed by thorough rinsing with clean water to prevent these disinfectants from coming into contact with live reptiles, amphibians, or plants.
- Large systems may also introduce large volumes of water into an enclosure, so adequate drainage must be provided. This may include a hole drilled into the enclosure with an attached drainage tube or an overflow bucket.

A partial list of companies providing misting products in no particular order are included in Box 1-3.

THERMOSTATS

Technological advances have resulted in ever more complex, precise, reliable, and safe environmental control units for herpetologic enclosures. Thermostats act as a regulator of power to heating devices such as lamps, heat tiles, and under-enclosure heat mats and come in three basic types.

Rheostat Thermostat

This most basic thermostat acts like a dimmer on a light source, regulating the power output to the heating devices. This thermostat allows you to dial the power to a specific heat source up or down. Units with dials or sliders have less precise control than digital units.

Thermostat

This device has a temperature setting and a temperature probe that monitors the environmental temperature. When the temperature rises above or falls below the set temperature, this type of thermostat turns the heating devices on or off at full power.

Proportional Thermostat

This most advanced type of thermostat works by continuously adjusting the amount of power delivered to the heater based on the set temperature and the reading from the attached temperature probe, as opposed to simply turning it on and off. This results in a more constant thermal environment and

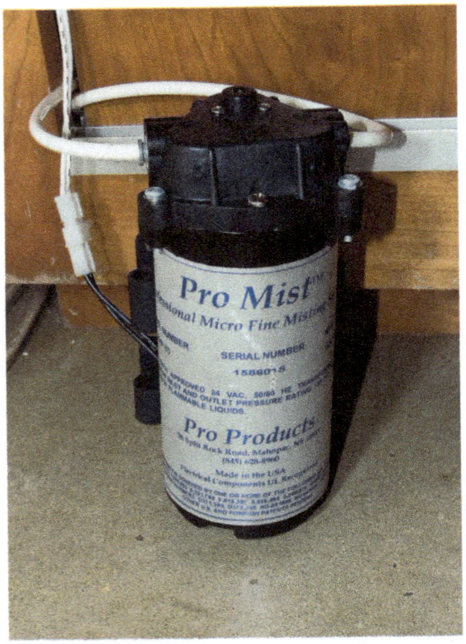

FIGURE 1-8 This mister is connected directly to a water line and mists several cages in the bank of enclosures. It normally is kept out of sight in the cabinet under the cages. *(Photo courtesy Dr. Stephen L. Barten, Vernon Hills Animal Hospital, Mundelein, Ill.)*

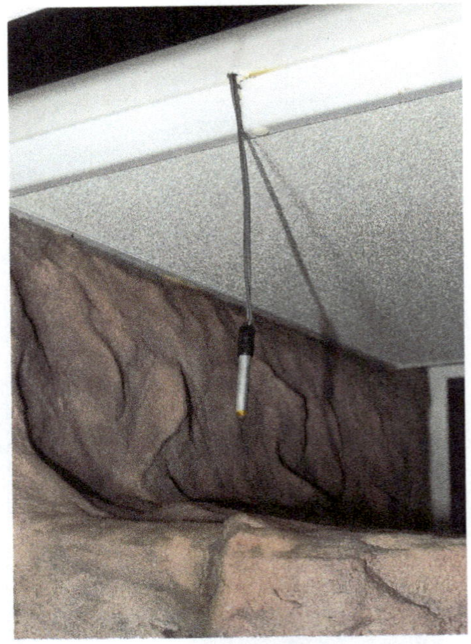

FIGURE 1-9 This temperature probe is connected to the thermostat that controls the output of the radiant heat panel in the background. *(Photo courtesy Dr. Stephen L. Barten, Vernon Hills Animal Hospital, Mundelein, Ill.)*

BOX 1-3 A PARTIAL LIST OF COMPANIES THAT MANUFACTURE MISTING SYSTEMS

Zoo Med, www.zoomed.com. This catalog lists a variety of misting options for the pet sector, including Habba Mist Automatic Misting Machine, Repti Fogger Terrarium Humidifier, The Big Dripper, Ultrasonic Humidifying Fogger, and the Misty Mountain Volcano.

Exo Terra, http://www.exo-terra.com. Products include the Monsoon RS 400 Rainfall System and an ultrasonic fog generator.

Mist King, Jungle Hobbies Ltd, www.mistking.com. A complete line of misting systems, nozzles, timers and controllers, pumps, valves, drains, tubing, and accessories is available.

Pro Products, www.pro-products.com. The Pro Mist microfine misting system includes four models to cover both small and large collections.

is reported to increase the life of heating devices, as the power is slowly modified versus constantly turning on and off. Many proportional thermostats have digital controlling units and have multiple settings that allow for specific control of day and night temperatures that can be user-set for any species.

Control displays for various thermostats can vary from simple dials to precise digital controls. It is important to consider where in the cage the temperature probe is placed. If the probe is placed near the focal hot spot or basking perch (Figure 1-9), the thermostat setting controls the hottest part of the cage. Conversely, if it is placed away from the heat source, the thermostat setting controls the background temperature and the hot spot may reach much higher temperatures.

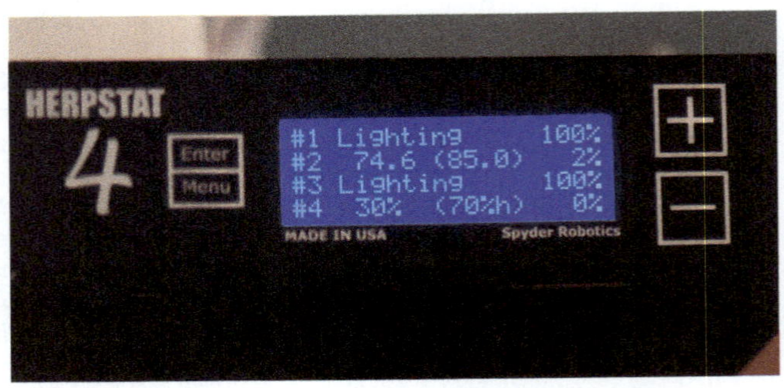

FIGURE 1-10 The control unit of the Spyder Robotics Herpstat 4 four-channel thermostat. *(Photo courtesy Dr. Stephen L. Barten, Vernon Hills Animal Hospital, Mundelein, Ill.)*

In some instances, thermostats have been combined with other functions. One such high-end unit is the Spyder Robotics Herpstat 4, (Spyder Robotics, LLC., Rochelle, Ill) a professional thermostat with four channels to control any combination of heating, cooling, lighting, and humidity of up to 400 watts per channel (Figure 1-10). This unit is a proportional thermostat but also can be set to nonproportional (on/off) mode. A number of special features exist including a safety relay that disconnects power to the outlets in the event of a system error to prevent overheating; an audible alarm in case of system error; temperature control between 40°F and 150°F (4°C and 65°C) within 0.1°; temperature and light ramping allowing user-set gradual warming and brightening of light over any set period of up to several hours to mimic sunrise and gradual cooling and dimming at night to simulate sunset; humidity settings controlling attached misters to run at set times or to match a preset humidity level with an optional humidity sensor; night temperature drop settings with built-in timers on all four channels; a cooling function controlling cooling equipment; and the ability to record high and low temperatures and time to allow tracking.

BOX 1-4 A PARTIAL LIST OF THERMOSTAT SUPPLIES

Spyder Robotics, http://spyderrobotics.com/products/herpstat_4.html. A multichannel, multidevice proportional thermostat is available.
Helix Controls, Inc, www.helixcontrols.com. Proportional thermostats, heating devices, and axial fans are available.
Zoo Med, www.zoomed.com. The catalog offers several models of both rheostat and on/off thermostats as well as the HygroTherm Humidity & Temperature Controller, an on/off thermostat with a humidity controller.

BOX 1-5 THERMAL/TEMPERATURE GAUGING PRODUCTS

TempGun, http://tempgun.com — infrared remote temperature sensor manufactured for use with captive reptiles
Zoo Med, www.zoomed.com — compact handheld reptile enclosure temperature gun
Rayteck, www.rayteck.com — complete range of industrial handheld thermal sensing units

The use of a thermostat is recommended for every enclosed herpetologic habitat. Most thermostats are rated for a safe maximum wattage for the heating devices they control; care must be taken not to overload the device. Larger units can control power to multiple enclosures. In any case, thermostat function should be checked on a routine basis with a thermometer or an infrared temperature sensor to compare set temperatures verses actual cage temperatures. Besides providing specific thermal habitats, thermostats also reduce the potential for overheating, and many have an internal power cutoff feature if they sense overheating or short circuit. A partial list of thermostat supplies is included in Box 1-4.

INFRARED REMOTE TEMPERATURE SENSORS

For years small thermometers have been placed at the upper corner of a reptile aquarium to indicate the temperature of the enclosure; however this is not an accurate portrayal of the thermal conditions in that enclosure. To better monitor temperatures across the thermal gradient of an enclosure and best meet the thermal needs of the inhabitants, other methods are now preferred. The use of noncontact infrared temperature sensors, with their compact size and inexpensive price, are now the gold standard for thermal environment monitoring in herpetoculture. The herp community refers to these devices as *temp guns*.

Infrared temperature guns measure the temperatures of objects, including substrates, basking perches, and animals themselves, through the emissivity (the relative ability of an object to emit energy from its surface by radiation) of an object or reptile. Water has low emissivity; thus measurements of water temperatures with infrared temp guns are not accurate. These devices can read a large range of temperatures; a typical range is −27°F to 428°F (−33°C to 220°C). Most units have a specific target area and the farther away from the target the device is held, the less precise the temperature reading. For example, a device with an infrared cone distance to spot ratio (D:S) of 6:1 means that at a distance of 6 inches (15 cm), the device is reading an area just 1 inch (2.54 cm) in diameter, and at a distance of 2 feet (61 cm), an area of just 4 inches (10 cm). Because infrared temp guns allow the specific temperature of any part of an enclosure to be measured, herpetoculturists can directly monitor and thus manipulate the environmental conditions of any enclosure (Box 1-5).

REFERENCES

1. Melissa Kaplan's Herp Care Collection Web site. Reptile housing: size, dimension and lifestyle. Available at: http://www.anapsid.org/enclsize.html. Accessed April 12, 2013.
2. *Draft code of practice for the private keeping of reptiles*. Sydney, NSW, Australia: Department of Environment, Climate Change and Water, NSW, 2009. Available at: http://www.environment.nsw.gov.au/resources/wildlifelicences/09675DraftReptiles.pdf. Accessed April 12, 2013.
3. de Vosjoli P. Designing environments for captive amphibians and reptiles. *Vet Clin North Am Exot Anim Pract* 1999;2:43–68.
4. Warwick C. Psychological and behavioural principles and problems. In: Warwick C, Frye FL, Murphy JB, eds. *Health and welfare of captive reptiles*. London: Chapman and Hall, 1995;205–238.
5. The Engineering Toolbox Web site. Air change rates for typical rooms and buildings. Available at: http://www.engineeringtoolbox.com/air-change-rate-room-d_867.html. Accessed September 11, 2011.
6. Gehrmann WH. Artificial lighting. In: Mader DR, ed. *Reptile medicine and surgery*, 2nd ed. St Louis, MO: Saunders Elsevier, 2006;1081–1084.
7. Mader DR. Metabolic bone diseases. In: Mader DR, ed. *Reptile medicine and surgery*, 2nd ed. St Louis, MO: Saunders Elsevier, 2006;841–851.
8. Holick MF. Vitamin D: importance in the prevention of cancers, type 1 diabetes, heart disease, and osteoporosis. *Am J Clin Nutr* 2004;79:362–371.
9. Ferguson GW, Brinker AM, Karsten KB, et al. Voluntary exposure of some western-hemisphere snake and lizard species to ultraviolet-B radiation in the field: how much ultraviolet-B should a lizard or snake receive in captivity? *Zoo Biol* 2010;29:317–334.
10. Ferguson GW, Gehrmann WH, Karsten KB, et al. Ultraviolet exposure and vitamin D synthesis in a sun-dwelling and a shade-dwelling species of *Anolis*: are there adaptations for lower ultraviolet B and dietary vitamin D_3 availability in the shade? *Physiol Biochem Zool* 2005;78:193–200.
11. Michael Burger R, Gehrmann WH, Ferguson GW. Evaluation of UVB reduction by materials commonly used in reptile husbandry. *Zoo Biol* 2007;26:417–423.
12. Acierno MJ, Mitchell MA, Roundtree MK, et al. Effects of ultraviolet radiation on 25-hydroxyvitamin D3 synthesis in red-eared slider turtles (*Trachemys scripta elegans*). *Am J Vet Res* 2006;67:2046–2049.
13. Acierno MJ, Mitchell MA, Zachariah TT, et al. Effects of ultraviolet radiation on plasma 25-hydroxyvitamin D3 concentrations in corn snakes (*Elaphe guttata*). *Am J Vet Res* 2008;69:294–297.
14. Ferguson GW, Gehrmann WH, Karsten KB, et al. Do panther chameleons bask to regulate endogenous vitamin D3 production? *Physiol Biochem Zool* 2003;76:52–59.
15. UV Guide Web site. The UV Guide Lighting Survey. Available at: http://www.uvguide.co.uk/lightingsurveyintro.htm. Accessed September 11, 2011.
16. Solartech, Inc Web site. Solartech Solarmeter Product Summary. Available at: http://www.solarmeter.com/products.php. Accessed October 17, 2011.
17. Ferguson GW, Gehrmann WH, Chen TC, et al. Effects of ultraviolet light exposure on reproductive success of the female panther chameleon (*Furcifer pardalis*) in captivity. *Zoo Biol* 2002;21:525–537.
18. Lindgren J, Gehrmann WH, Ferguson GW, et al. Measuring effective vitamin D3-producing ultraviolet B radiation using Solartech's Solarmeter 6.4 handheld, UVB radiometer. *Bull Chicago Herp Soc* 2008;43:57–62.

19. UV Guide UK. Make yourself a UVB spread chart. Available at: http://www.uvguide.co.uk/makingspreadcharts.htm. Accessed October 16, 2011.
20. Solartech, Inc. FAQ, When should lamps be replaced? Available at: http://www.solarmeter.com/faqs.html. Accessed October 17, 2011.
21. UV Guide Web site. Using the Solarmeter 6.2 UVB Meter. Available at: http://www.uvguide.co.uk/usinguvmeter.htm. Accessed September 11, 2011.
22. Gehrmann WH, Horner JD, Ferguson GW, et al. A comparison of responses by three broadband radiometers to different ultraviolet-B sources. *Zoo Biol* 2004;23:355–363.
23. Gehrmann WH, Jamieson D, Ferguson GW, et al. A comparison of vitamin-D synthesizing ability of different light sources to irradiances measured with a Solarmeter Model 6.2 UVB Meter. *Herp Rev* 2004;35:361–364.
24. UV Guide Web site. What UV light do reptiles need? Available at: http://www.uvguide.co.uk/whatreptilesneed.htm. Accessed September 11, 2011.
25. MacCargar R. Iguanas and artificial ultraviolet light: how and how much made simple—well, not exactly simple. *J Int Iguana Soc* 2003;10:82.
26. Karsten KB, Ferguson GW, Chen TC, et al. Panther chameleons, *Furcifer pardalis*, behaviorally regulate optimal exposure to UV depending on dietary vitamin D3 status. *Physiol Biochem Zool* 2009;82:218–225.
27. Gardiner DW, Baines FM, Pandher K. Photodermatitis and photokeratoconjunctivitis in a ball python (*Python regius*) and a blue-tongue skink (*Tiliqua* spp.). *Zoo Wildl Med* 2009;40:757–766.
28. AZA Snake TAG 2011. *Eastern Indigo Snake* (Drymarchon couperi) *Care Manual.* Silver Spring, Md: Association of Zoos and Aquariums, 2011. Available at: http://www.aza.org/uploadedFiles/Animal_Care_and_Management/Husbandry,_Health,_and_Welfare/Husbandry_and_Animal_Care/IndigoSnakeCareManual_2011.pdf. Accessed October 19, 2011.
29. Rossi JV. *Snakes of the United States & Canada. Natural history and care in captivity.* Malabar, Fla: Krieger Publishing Co, 2003.

CHAPTER 2

Common Pathology and Diseases Seen in Pet Store Reptiles

Drury R. Reavill and Chris Griffin

Evaluation of recently obtained reptiles from the growing population of captive-bred or wild-caught harvested animals available as pets can be daunting for most practitioners. The types of species presented for examination and the dizzying range of requirements for their needs—from husbandry to diet—can easily overwhelm the time constraints of a typical veterinary office call. In addition, the laboratory tests and parameters of health can vary tremendously across the numbers of reptile species kept as pets.

This chapter will present an overview of the types of reptiles currently in the pet trade, the recognized husbandry deficiencies, the diseases that do not commonly result in a need for pathologic evaluation, and those disease processes that can result in death. The data for the postmortem and, rarely, biopsy evaluations come from a review of reptiles (n = 349) sold through a pet store chain over the time period from 2003 to 2010 and submitted to one author's laboratory (DRR). The described husbandry and common conditions not associated with a need for pathologic sampling are collected from one exclusive exotic animal private practice (CG).

Understanding the types of conditions that could lead to disease and/or death can assist in determining which laboratory tests and/or husbandry/nutritional deficiencies to focus on within specific species.

SPECIES SUBMITTED FOR LABORATORY EVALUATION

Chelonians were the smallest group (14%) presented for necropsy and biopsy evaluation. The species included, in descending order of frequency, are as follows: Russian Tortoise (*Testudo horsfieldii*), Red-eared Slider (*Trachemys scripta elegans*), turtle (not specified), Malayan Box Turtle (*Cuora amboinensis*), box turtle (*Terrapin* spp.), African Sideneck Turtle (Pelomedusidae family), Marginated Tortoise (*Testudo marginata*), and Red-footed Tortoise (*Chelonoidis carbonaria*).

Lizards were the next largest group evaluated (31%). The species of lizards examined by necropsy and, infrequently, biopsy samples included the popular Leopard Gecko (*Eublepharis macularius*) (33%) and Bearded Dragon (*Pogona vitticeps*) (23%). The remaining species in descending numbers were Green Water Dragons (*Physignathus cocincinus*), common Green Iguana (*Iguana iguana*), gecko (not specified), anole (family Polychrotidae), Savannah Monitor (*Varanus exanthematicus*), lizards (not specified), Emerald Swift (*Sceloporus malachiticus*), Blue-tongued Skink (*Tiliqua* sp.), chameleon (not specified), and *Ameiva* (family Teiidae).

Snakes were the largest group evaluated (34%). The species of snake submitted for pathologic examination included, in descending order of frequency, are as follows: Ball Python (*Python regius*), "Red-tailed" Boa (*Boa constrictor constrictor*), Cornsnake (*Elaphe guttata*), snake (not specified), Ribbon Snake (*Thamnophis sauritus*), Milk Snake (*Lampropeltis triangulum*), Garter Snake (*Thamnophis* spp), and Green Tree Python (*Morelia viridis*).

Although many of the lizards and snakes were young animals (evidenced by size and the occasional yolk sac remnants observed on gross postmortem examination), the age of many of the chelonians was not determined (Figure 2-1).

The gender of each animal submitted was determined in most complete postmortems; however, there were rarely noted disease conditions linked to the reproductive tract. This is not unexpected given the age of the animals for sale in the pet trade.

These necropsy percentages may not exactly reflect the types of species seen in a busy private practice because submission depends on not only the perceived value of the animal but also the value of the postmortem findings.

HUSBANDRY-RELATED CONDITIONS

Deficiencies in husbandry are overwhelmingly the most common factor causing illnesses in captive reptiles. Overcrowding, exposure to sick animals (and their body fluids/excrements), poor nutrition, improper thermal gradients, and many other aspects of reptile care may constitute the basis of many of the illnesses that plague reptiles in the pet trade today (Figure 2-2). Many of the most popular reptiles are shipped to pet stores in containers that are either too small or have too many other of the same (or different) species and minimal, if any, thermal regulation. Many may be shipped from a breeder to a distribution center before being sent to a pet store, and many of these animals (usually younger animals) may not feel like eating for several days during this transition period. The basics of thermal support, humidity, feeding opportunities, hiding options, and a reasonable animal-to-space ratio may not always be provided, even within a pet store setting. All of these factors may trigger new conditions or flare-up of preexisting conditions. Examples may include adenoviral or coccidial infections in Bearded Dragons and cryptosporidial infections in Leopard Geckos.[1]

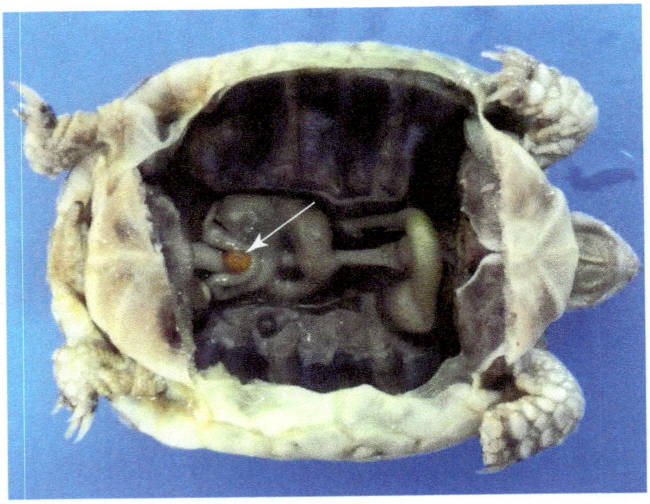

FIGURE 2-1 A yolk sac remnant *(arrow)* in a young Marginated Tortoise (*Testudo marginata*), formalin-fixed specimen.

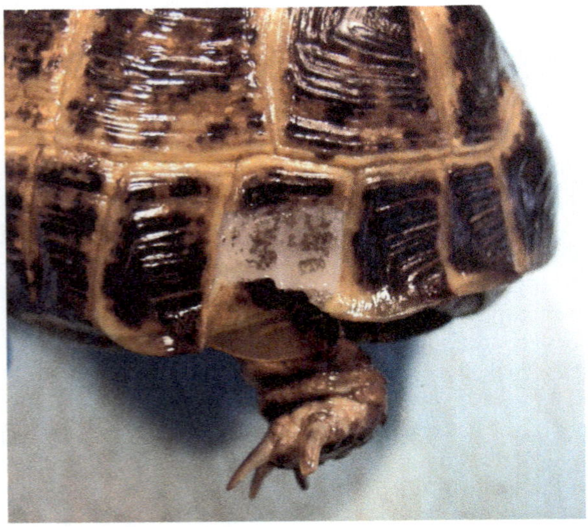

FIGURE 2-2 Shell damage during shipping of a Russian Tortoise *(Testudo horsfieldii)*.

The most important aspects of diagnosing sick reptiles in the pet store rely on the training of the employees/caretakers. Good observational skills and an understanding of basic health and behavior are paramount to early detection and evaluation of these reptiles in the veterinary hospital. Seeing a sick reptile 1 or 2 days into an illness often affords a much better prognosis than attending to a sick reptile 14 to 21 days into an illness.

When possible, diagnostics should be performed. These should include (but not be limited to) a thorough physical examination, fecal parasite examinations (e.g., direct, float, and/or special stains), laboratory analysis (complete blood count/chemistry profile) and histology/cytology, when indicated (Figure 2-3). Advanced diagnostics including cultures (bacterial and fungal), imaging (e.g., radiographs, ultrasound, magnetic resonance imaging [MRI], and computed tomography [CT]), and molecular testing (including polymerase chain reaction [PCR] testing) may also be indicated. Once a diagnosis is obtained, specific treatments, when available, should be recommended and pursued. While test results are pending, supportive care (including environmental support, fluids, nutritional [caloric and vitamin] support, and antibiotics, among others) should be instituted, as needed.

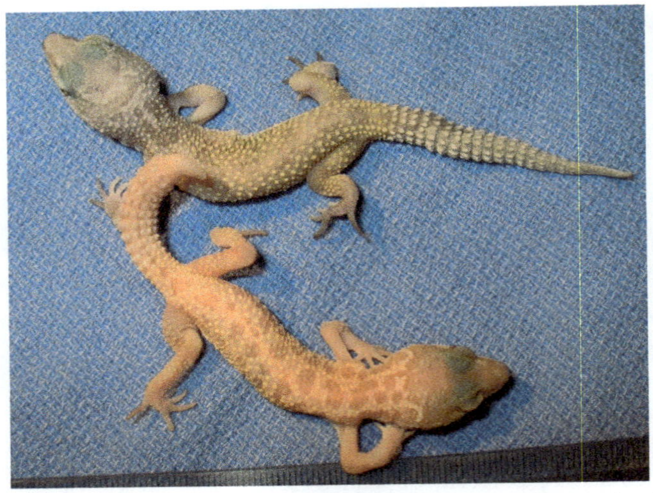

FIGURE 2-3 The physical examination will be determined by the type of animal and size. Evaluation of body condition, color, activity, swellings/masses, and integrity of the skin should be noted.

COMMON CLINICAL DISEASES

Many of the common presentations that are seen in practice are manageable, and many of these animals that are seen are not included in the necropsy numbers listed earlier in the chapter. The most common conditions that present are as follows:

In **tortoises**, poor nutritional status, failure to thrive, poor shell development, and anorexia are common conditions (Figure 2-4).

In **lizards**, parasites include coccidia, pin worms, and protozoans in Bearded Dragons, cryptosporidia are found in Leopard Geckos, and protozoans in most species. Gram-negative enteritis are common in many species. Nutritional secondary hyperparathyroidism (resulting in hypocalcemia and associated changes) is common in iguanas and has also been seen in Leopard Geckos (Figure 2-5). Ocular issues, including conjunctivitis from environmental factors (e.g., reptile bark) or retained sheds (possibly from humidity/hydration issues), are also common (Figure 2-6). Stomatitis is commonly seen in Water Dragons, Blue-tongued Skinks, Bearded Dragons, and Leopard Geckos. Adenovirus in Bearded Dragons may be more common than reported, and concurrent infections with adenovirus and parasites (e.g., coccidia and cryptosporidia) may lead to more severe signs and a greater chance of mortality.[2] *Failure to thrive,* a catch-all term used in captive animals to describe illnesses that are not specifically identified but compromise the animal, is seen in more "sensitive" species (e.g., most chameleon species, some geckos, uromastyx species, and in some areas, water dragons) (Figure 2-7).

In **snakes**, mites (*Ophionyssus* spp.), retained sheds, and dehydration are common in all species. Failure to feed

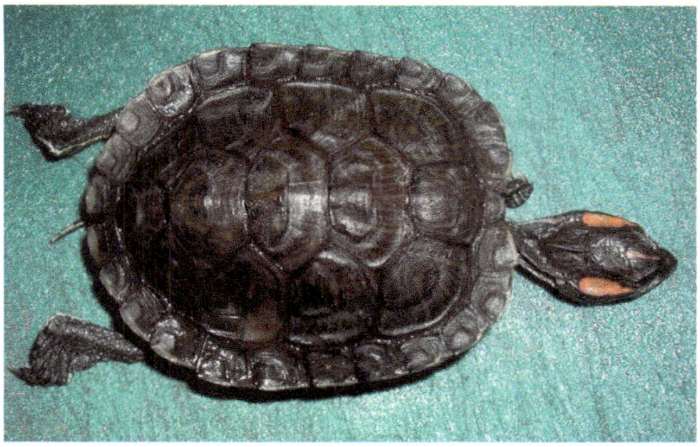

FIGURE 2-4 A Slider Turtle *(Trachemys scripta)* with significant loss of body condition and muscle wasting.

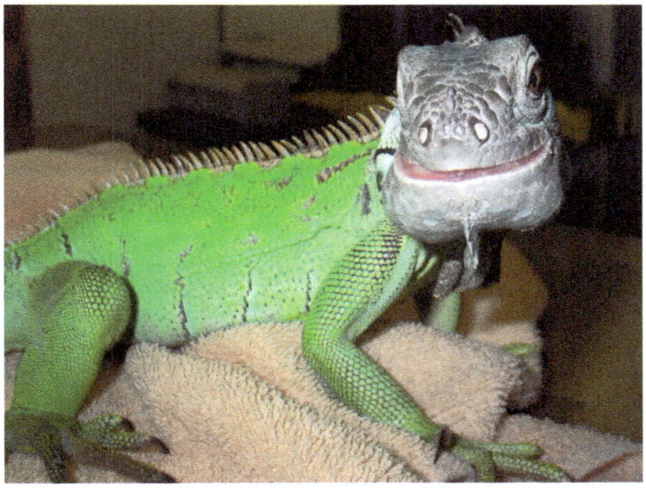

FIGURE 2-5 The bilateral swelling of the mandible in this common Green Iguana *(Iguana iguana)* is due to fibrous tissue attempting to stabilize the bones.

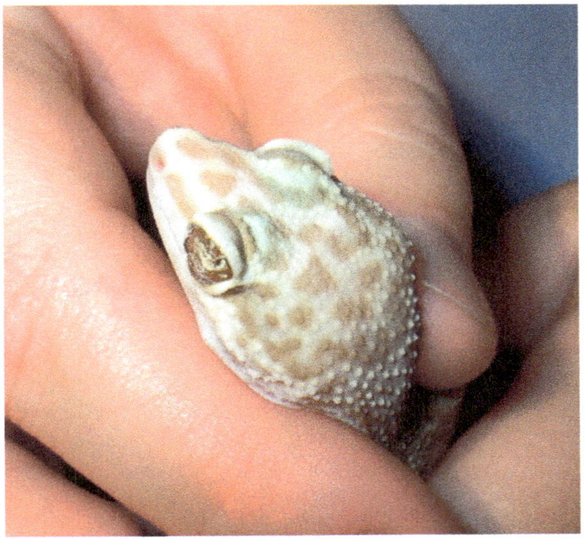

FIGURE 2-6 In Leopard Geckos *(Eublepharis macularius)*, the skin of the inner eyelid may be retained with an abnormal shed. Failure to shed this skin can result in an accumulation of keratin in the conjunctival sac, subsequent irritation, and infection.

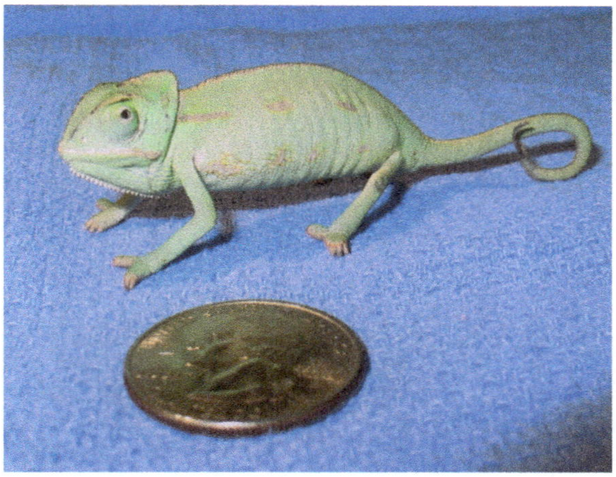

FIGURE 2-7 A poorly thriving chameleon with secondary diseases (necrosis of the tail tip).

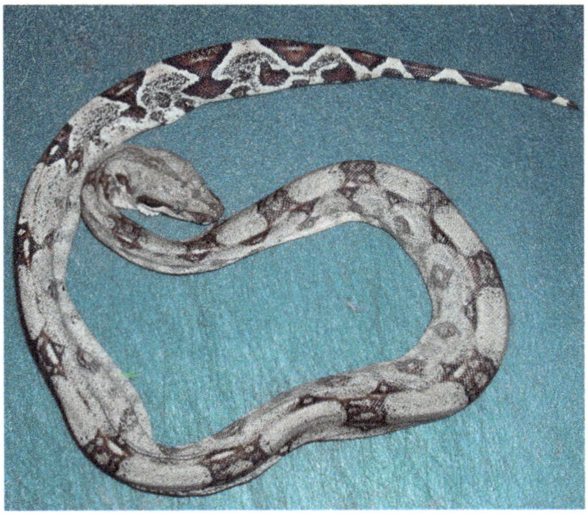

FIGURE 2-8 Significant loss of muscle mass and severe dehydration are evident in this Red-tailed Boa *(Boa constrictor constrictor)*.

(especially with shy species such as Ball Pythons) with resulting weight loss and/or failure to grow is common (Figure 2-8). Neurologic signs (weakness) associated with viral infections and other conditions, such as ectoparasites, may also be seen.

Diagnosis and treatment of the aforementioned conditions can be found in a variety of resources, including other sections of this book. The reader is referred to the appropriate chapters on specific diagnostic testing and therapeutics for these conditions.

Viral infections are probably more common than previously thought in all species of reptiles, and the work of some of our colleagues may shed light on this aspect of reptile disease in the near future.

Of all the presentations commonly seen, cryptosporidia (in any species) seems to be the most frustrating because the mortality rate is close to 100% in diagnosed patients, despite a variety of attempted treatments. Concurrent viral infections (e.g., adenovirus in Bearded Dragons) may increase the likelihood of mortality in these cases.

DISEASES IDENTIFIED POST MORTEM

Across reptile groups, the most commonly diseased organ system was the gastrointestinal tract. This suggests that close evaluation of the gastrointestinal system is a priority and also stresses that nutritional support is an essential part of the therapy. A table for each reptile group lists more specific morphologic and etiologic findings (Table 2-1).

CHELONIANS

Of the turtles and tortoises examined, the most common finding was chelonid herpesvirus infection of Russian Tortoises, which, in many cases, was from outbreaks involving multiple animals. Herpesvirus-associated rhinitis, stomatitis, glossitis, tracheitis, bronchopneumonia, and, uncommonly, necrotizing hepatitis have been reported in a number of tortoise species: Hermann's Tortoises *(Testudo hermanni)*, Afghan or Russian Tortoises, Spur-thighed Tortoises *(Testudo graeca)*, and Marginated Tortoises (Figure 2-9). This herpesviral infection is frequently complicated by secondary bacterial infections and generally results in severe debilitation of the tortoise. The transmission is most likely from infected carriers, although the pathogenesis of this viral infection has not been fully described. The early lesions in these Russian Tortoises were stomatitis and glossitis. This suggests that specifically testing for herpesvirus in tortoises with this presentation can help separate those animals with this typically fatal disease from those with other potentially treatable conditions.[3]

Nonspecific dermatitis (not involving the shell) was also a commonly recognized postmortem lesion, primarily in water turtles such as Red-eared Sliders (Figure 2-10). On the basis of the history, these lesions were suspected to be traumatic in origin and were slow to resolve with apparently adequate

TABLE 2-1

Summary of Disease Conditions Recognized by Pathologic Evaluation*

Lesions/Disease Agents	Chelonians (50/349)	Lizards (108/349)	Snakes (119/349)
Adenovirus[†] with associated lesions in the liver and/or intestines	—	26 (24%)	3 (2.5%)
Autolyzed sample[‡]	2 (4%)	3 (2.8%)	1 (0.8%)
Bacteremia	—	1 (1%)	4 (3.4%)
CANV[†] (fungal dermatitis)	—	22 (20.4%)	—
Debilitation, severe[§]	3 (6%)	12 (11.1%)	49 (41%)
Dermatitis, bacterial[†]	8 (16%)	9 (8.3%)	1 (0.8%)
Dermatitis, nonspecific[ǁ]	2 (4%)	7 (6.5%)	—
Dermatitis, other fungus (not CANV)	—	3 (2.8%)	1 (0.8%)
Encephalitis, nonspecific[ǁ]	—	2 (1.8%)	2 (1.7%)
Entamoeba	1 (2%)	1 (1%)	—
Enteritis and/or gastritis, cryptosporidia[†]	2 (4%)	48 (44.4%)	8 (6.7%)
Enteritis, coccidia	—	7 (6.5%)	—
Enteritis, nematodes	4 (8%)	8 (7.4%)	3 (2.5%)
Enteritis, nonspecific[ǁ]	5 (10%)	14 (13%)	52 (43.7%)
Enteritis, protozoal flagellates	—	2 (1.8%)	2 (1.7%)
Enteritis, trematodes	1 (2%)	2 (1.8%)	—
Hepatitis, nonspecific[ǁ]	1 (2%)	17 (15.7%)	8 (6.7%)
Herpesvirus[†] (including necrotizing hepatitis and stomatitis)	19 (38%)	—	—
IBD[†]	—	—	14 (12.8%)
Kidney, protozoal flagellates	—	5 (4.6%)	—
Mycobacteria[†]	1 (systemic) (2%)	—	—
Myocarditis, nonspecific[ǁ]	1 (2%)	2 (1.8%)	—
Pneumonia, fungal	—	1 (1%)	—
Pneumonia, nonspecific[ǁ]	5 (10%)	7 (6.5%)	9 (7.6%)
Renal urate tophi	—	1 (1%)	—
Sarcocyst within skeletal muscle	3 (6%)	—	—
Schistosomes	4 (8%)	—	—
Shell necrosis	2 (4%)	—	—
Skin mites	—	—	5 (4.2%)
Stomatitis, nonspecific[ǁ]	2 (4%)	—	—
Trematode, intestines	1 (2%)	—	—
Vacuolar hepatopathy	—	3 (2.8%)	—

CANV, Chrysosporium anamorph of *Nannizziopsis vriesii*; *IBD,* inclusion body disease.
*The numbers will not equal 100% because animals may have had more than one lesion.
[†]The etiology, in some cases, was confirmed by further diagnosis with polymerase chain reaction or cultures.
[‡]The submitted animal was too autolyzed to identify any lesions on histologic examination.
[§]Debilitation was determined by loss of coelomic cavity fat, muscle wasting, and hepatic atrophy.
[ǁ]No specific etiologic agent was identified.

therapy. Bacterial involvement in cases of dermatitis was based on the presence of bacteria identified in the inflammation and/or bacteria granulomas present within the dermis on histologic examination. Fungal dermatitis of chelonians was not identified in this collection of cases.

Sporadic findings of intestinal parasitism were noted. These included nematode, trematode, and cryptosporidial enteropathies.[4] A small number of tortoises and turtles also had a nonspecific enteritis in which a disease etiology was not identified.

Primary pneumonia was uncommon and was usually associated with a variety of systemic diseases.

A small number of the freshwater and box turtles (species not reported) had intravascular parasites consistent with spirorchid fluke eggs. Adult spirorchid flukes (blood flukes) inhabit the cardiovascular system (heart and blood vessels) of many freshwater and marine turtles. These are analogous to the schistosomes of birds and mammals. Eggs deposited by the adults are carried through the circulatory system and can block small blood vessels in many organs, producing microgranulomas. The eggs then migrate to the lumen of the intestines, which can lead to necrosis and bacteremia. In freshwater turtles, the intermediate host is a snail, of which at least one species has been identified, *Helisoma anceps*.[5] Because antemortem testing is unlikely to identify this infection in the individual animal, a postmortem diagnosis should warrant treatment for all exposed turtles in a collection.[6]

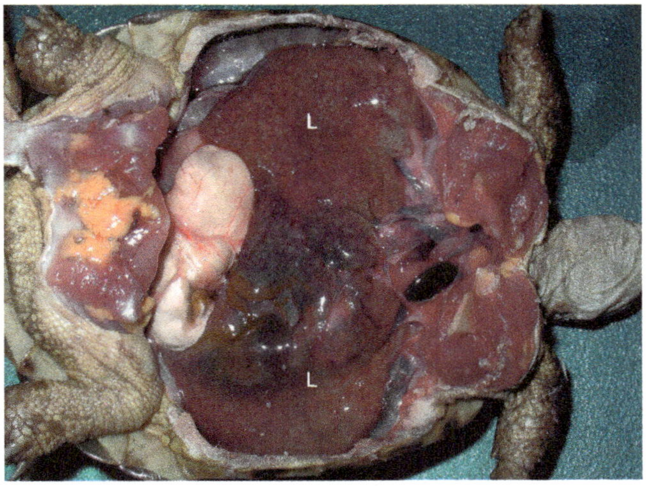

FIGURE 2-9 Russian Tortoise *(Testudo horsfieldii)* with multiple foci of hepatic necrosis due to herpesvirus. *L*, liver.

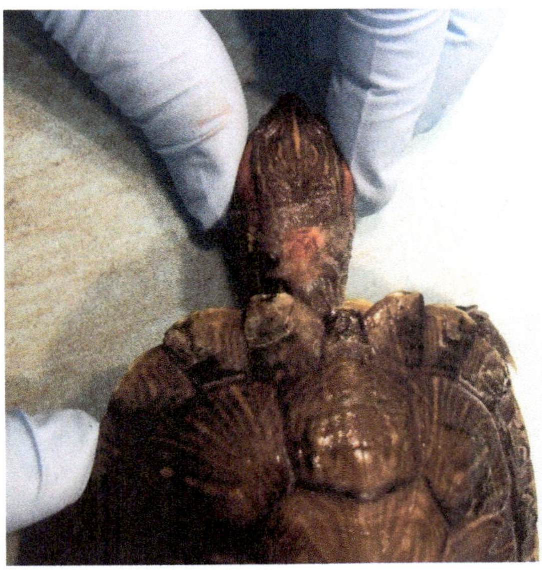

FIGURE 2-10 Erosive and ulcerative dermatitis on the dorsal neck, suspected to be caused by trauma from tank mates.

LIZARDS

Of the abnormalities reported in lizards, the most common finding was cryptosporidial enteritis and/or gastritis. This is most likely overrepresented because the most common lizards examined were Leopard Geckos; these lizards frequently were infected. Smaller numbers of Bearded Dragons and Water Dragons also had cryptosporidial enteropathies. Because these lizards were severely emaciated and dehydrated on postmortem evaluation, the cryptosporidial infections were deemed to be a significant contributor to disease and, ultimately, death (Figure 2-11).

Adenovirus infection involving the liver and gastrointestinal tract was common in Bearded Dragons that were examined. This viral infection has become established in lizard breeding colonies in the United States and can result in high mortality rates for stressed animals. The common clinical signs in young Bearded Dragons were progressive weakness and anorexia. Frequently, these emaciated lizards seen at postmortem examination had concurrent intestinal coccidial infections (Figure 2-12).

A fungal dermatitis consistent with *Chrysosporium* anamorph of *Nannizziopsis vriesii* (CANV) was the most common skin lesion in anoles, Ameiva, Bearded Dragons, common Green Iguanas, Water Dragons, and Curly-tailed Lizards. The lesions presented as multiple irregular patches of thickened skin supporting a hyperkeratotic exudate (Figure 2-13). The diagnosis was made by the fungal morphologic and histologic features of the lesions, although some cases were confirmed by culture and PCR. CANV has been described in Bearded Dragons and other lizards as a keratinophilic fungus that can result in a fatal granulomatous dermatitis (Figure 2-14).[7]

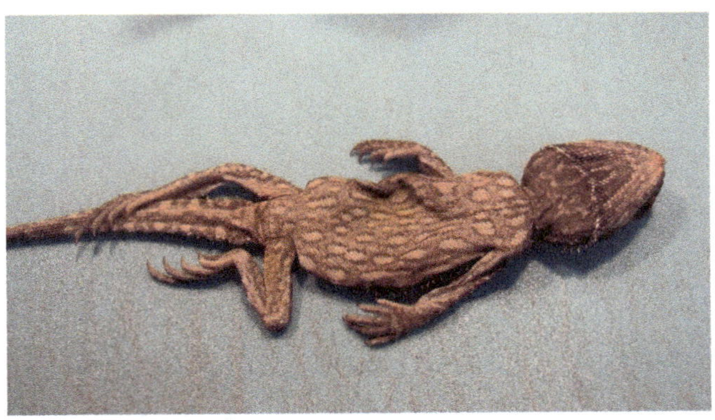

FIGURE 2-11 A Bearded Dragon *(Pogona vitticeps)* with enteric cryptosporidia. There is loss of body condition with muscle wasting and dehydration.

There were cases of bacterial dermatitis and some cases with no apparent etiologic agent. Both nonspecific hepatitis and enteritis were recognized as frequent lesions. The lack of etiologic agents could be due to attempts at antemortem therapies not reported in the clinical histories. Systemic debilitation, which contributed to decline and death, was characterized by hepatic atrophy and/or atrophy of the coelomic cavity fat pads.

SNAKES

Snakes were the largest group of reptiles submitted for histologic evaluation. Of these, generalized debilitation was a common presentation. Almost half of the animals had significant hepatic atrophy, as well as atrophy of the coelomic cavity fat pads. A nonspecific enteritis and/or enterocolitis was also a common finding that could be accounted for by poor husbandry such as inadequate heat and/or humidity.

Inclusion body disease of boids recently associated with the arenavirus was a frequent although not unexpected finding because the majority of snakes submitted were susceptible boids (Red-tailed Boa) (Figure 2-15).[8]

Skin mites and gastric cryptosporidia were not uncommon. Both these diseases are well-described in the literature.[9,10]

Knowing the common diseases in a population of animals and conducting a thorough examination with appropriate diagnostic testing can result in better health and care of the reptile pet and even a better reptile–human relationship for the reptile owner.

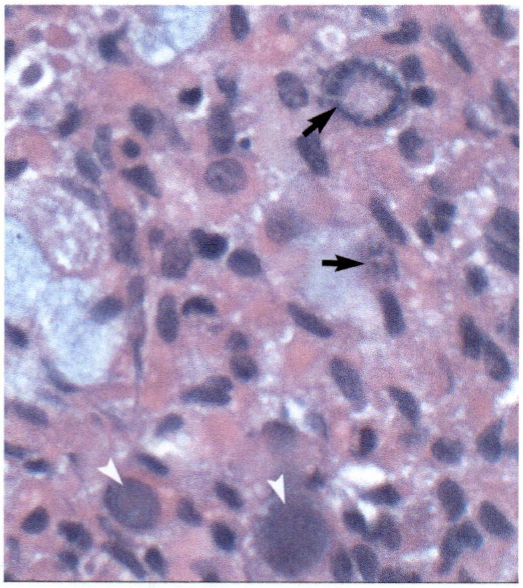

FIGURE 2-12 Histology of the intestinal mucosa of a Bearded Dragon *(Pogona vitticeps)* with coccidia *(black arrows)* and adenovirus *(white arrowheads)*. H&E stain; x40.

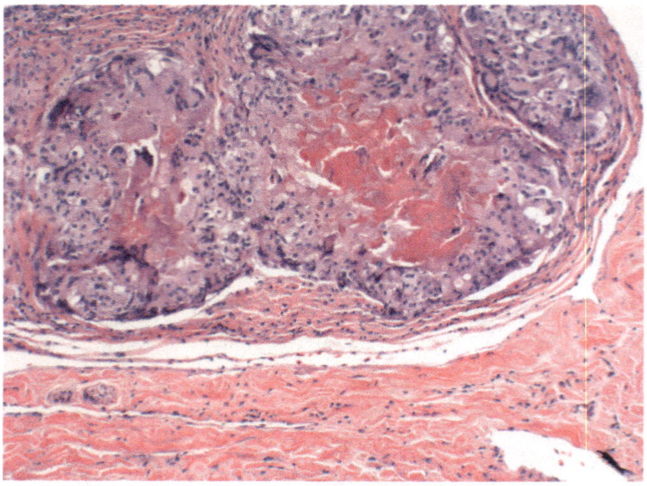

FIGURE 2-14 Fungal granulomas with a central core of bright eosinophilic debris surrounded by multinucleate giant cells and macrophages due to *Chrysosporium* anamorph of *Nannizziopsis vriesii* (CANV). H&E stain; x10.

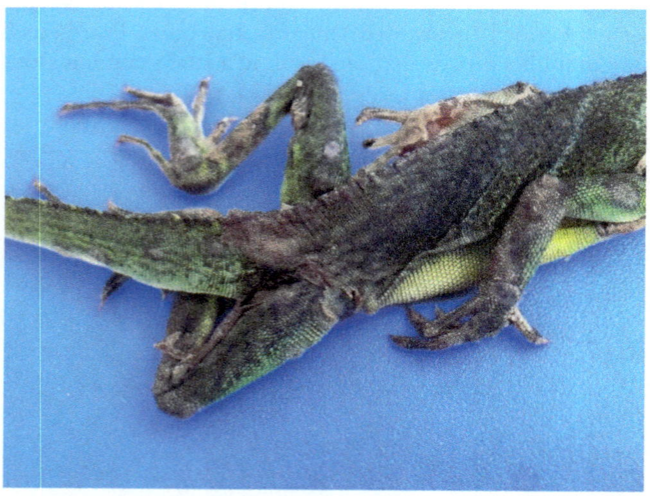

FIGURE 2-13 Green Water Dragon *(Physignathus cocincinus)* with multiple irregular foci of brown-gray hyperkeratotic plaques and dysecdysis due to *Chrysosporium* anamorph of *Nannizziopsis vriesii* (CANV).

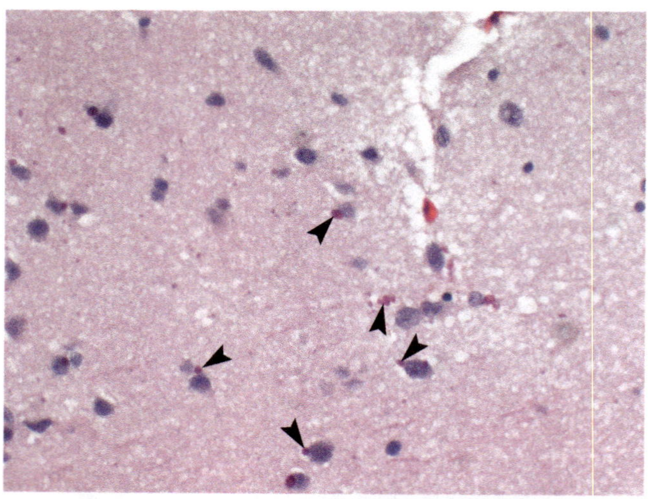

FIGURE 2-15 Round to oval intracytoplasmic viral inclusions *(arrowheads)* in the brain of a python (inclusion body disease). H&E stain; x40.

REFERENCES

1. Terrell SP, Uhl EW, Funk RS. Proliferative enteritis in leopard geckos (*Eublepharis macularius*) associated with *Cryptosporidium* sp. infection. *J Zoo Wildl Med* 2003;34:69–75.
2. Moormann S, Seehusen F, Reckling D, et al. Systemic adenovirus infection in Bearded Dragons (*Pogona vitticeps*): histological, ultrastructural and molecular findings. *J Comp Pathol* 2009;141:78–83.
3. McArthur S, Blahak S, Koelle P, et al. Chelonian herpesvirus. *J Herpetol Med Surg* 2002;12:14–31.
4. Griffin C, Reavill DR, Stacy BA, et al. Cryptosporidiosis caused by two distinct species in Russian tortoises and a pancake tortoise. *Vet Parasitol* 2010;170:14–19.
5. Holliman RB, Fisher JE. Life cycle and pathology of *Spirorchis scripta Stunkard*, 1923 (Digenea: Spirorchiidae) in *Chrysemys picta picta*. *J Parasitol* 1968;54:310–318.
6. Johnson CA, Griffith JW, Tenorio P, et al. Fatal trematodiasis in research turtles. *Lab Anim Sci* 1998;48:340–343.
7. Bowman MR, Paré JA, Sigler L, et al. Deep fungal dermatitis in three inland bearded dragons (*Pogona vitticeps*) caused by the *Chrysosporium* anamorph of *Nannizziopsis vriesii*. *Med Mycol* 2007;45:371–376.
8. Stenglein MD, Sanders C, Kistler AL, et al. Identification, characterization, and in vitro culture of highly divergent arenaviruses from boa constrictors and annulated tree boas: candidate etiological agents for snake inclusion body disease. *MBio* 2012;3:e00180–12.
9. Wozniak EJ, DeNardo DF. The biology, clinical significance and control of the common snake mite, *Ophionyssus natricis*, in captive reptiles. *J Herpetol Med Surg* 2000;10:4–10.
10. Richter B, Nedorost N, Maderner A, et al. Detection of *Cryptosporidium* species in feces or gastric contents from snakes and lizards as determined by polymerase chain reaction analysis and partial sequencing of the 18S ribosomal RNA gene. *J Vet Diagn Invest* 2011;23:430–435.

CHAPTER 3

Clinical Aspects of Evolution in Reptile Medicine

James F.X. Wellehan, Jr.

EVOLUTION

Evolution is an essential concept in biology. Indeed, when one considers definitions for life, perhaps the simplest and most elegant definition is that life consists of things that evolve. As medicine is a subfield of biology, evolution is central.

In comparative medicine, we often lack information on a given species, in areas including anatomy, physiology, microbiology, and pharmacology. When information is lacking on a given species, the best model to use is typically the closest relative from which data are available. This requires knowledge of species relationships. Because of ethical concerns, humans are not commonly used for experimentation; some common and appropriate laboratory models used are other primates or the closest relatives of the primates, rabbits and rodents. However, the understanding of animal classification that most current adults have been taught in grade school is fundamentally erroneous. Many commonly used terms, such as *reptile* or *lizard,* as they are generally interpreted, can lead to misunderstanding of relationships.

A definition is first necessary (Box 3-1). A *monophyletic group* is defined as a group that contains a common ancestor and all descendants. In comparative medicine, understanding what constitutes a monophyletic group is needed to understand relationships and to choose appropriate models. A group that is not monophyletic is called *paraphyletic.* Paraphyletic groups may not share a common ancestor or may exclude some descendants of the common ancestor. It is illogical to predict that paraphyletic groups would share characteristics that are not in nonmembers. Primates constitute a monophyletic group; when the primates except for humans are referred to, the term *nonhuman primates* is generally used. This qualification in the term helps the reader understand that a paraphyletic group is being referred to.

EVOLUTION OF TETRAPODS

When the evolution of the tetrapods (terrestrial vertebrates) is examined, both the fossil record and the even stronger evidence from nucleic acid sequence phylogeny analyses are in agreement on relationships.[1] The earliest divergence among the tetrapods is between the amphibians and the amniotes (Figure 3-1). The amniotes consist of the reptiles (including birds) and the mammals. The amnion was a major evolutionary advance, enabling the amniotes to have a completely terrestrial life cycle without the need to return to water for reproduction. This is also the first place in tetrapod evolution where common knowledge gives us fundamental errors. Herpetology is the study of nonavian reptiles and amphibians; it does not include mammals and birds. However, nonavian reptiles are far more fundamentally similar to birds and mammals than they are to amphibians, so it is not reasonable to expect nonavian reptile biology to resemble amphibian biology more closely than avian biology or mammalian biology. This is most medically apparent when looking at skin function, respiration, or reproduction.

AMNIOTES

The amniotes are then further divided into mammals and sauropsids (see Figure 3-1, shown in green). Within the sauropsids, the first group to diverge is the squamate (lizards and snakes)/sphenodontid (tuatara) clade. After this, the testudines (turtles) diverged, and the last two major sauropsid groups to diverge were the crocodilians and the dinosaurs, collectively known as the archosaurs. The recognition of dinosaurs as reptiles is widespread in our culture. However, what is not generally recognized is that dinosaurs are not extinct and that birds are the only surviving group of dinosaurs. This is supported both by the fossil record and by sequence data.[2] Part of this failure may be due to an erroneous picture of nonavian dinosaurs: they shared a number of traits with birds, including feathers,[3] and there is evidence they were warm blooded.[4] Nevertheless, although birds themselves constitute a monophyletic group, if birds are not considered to be part of the reptile group, then reptiles are not a monophyletic group. What we really mean by reptiles is sauropsids, and birds are a group of reptiles. The term *nonavian reptile* should be used if excluding birds from the reptiles, an awkward term indicating a logically awkward paraphyletic group.

CROCODILIANS AND BIRDS

Crocodilians and birds share a number of medically relevant similarities. In a mammal, a persistent right aortic arch is a developmental problem that obstructs the esophagus, and the left aortic arch is the main outflow for oxygenated blood from the heart. In archosaurs, the right aortic arch is the major outflow.[5] Unlike birds, crocodilians have retained their left aortic arch, but the function it serves is primarily to transport hypercapneic blood to the stomach, where it is used to create

BOX 3-1 DEFINITIONS

Agamids: The clade of lizards containing Bearded Dragons, Water Dragons, *Uromastyx* sp., and related species. Agamids are members of the larger clade Toxicofera.

Amniote: The clade of animals who undergo embryonic development in an amnion, consisting of the sauropsids and the mammals. The evolution of the amnion enabled reproduction in arid environments.

Amphisbaenids: The clade of squamates that are often called Worm Lizards. Many are legless.

Anguids: The clade of lizards containing Glass Lizards, Alligator Lizards, and related species. Anguids are members of the larger clade Toxicofera.

Archosaurs: The clade of reptiles whose surviving members are the crocodiles and birds.

Clade: A monophyletic group.

Definitive host: A host in which a pathogen has adapted to successfully propagate.

Dinosauria: The clade of reptiles containing the birds. Nonavian dinosaurs went extinct by the end of the Cretaceous period, 65 million years ago.

Helodermatids: The clade of lizards containing Gila Monsters and Beaded Lizards. Helodermatids are members of the larger clade Toxicofera.

Homeothermy: The trait of maintaining a constant body temperature, often above that of the environment.

Lacertids: The clade of lizards containing Jeweled Lacertas, Wall Lizards, and related species.

Monophyletic: Adjective describing a group that contains a common ancestor and all the descendents. A monophyletic group is also known as a clade.

Mutualistic: An ecologic relationship that benefits both organisms involved.

Paraphyletic: Adjective describing a group that is not monophyletic; the group's members do not share a common ancestor or exclude some descendants of a common ancestor.

Poikilothermy: The trait of depending on the environment for temperature regulation.

Sauropsid: The clade consisting of the reptiles, including squamates, tuataras, testudines, dinosaurs, and crocodilians. The term *reptiles* is often misunderstood not to include modern dinosaurs.

Sphenodontid: The reptile clade whose last surviving members are the tuatara in New Zealand.

Squamate: The clade of reptiles consisting of the lizards (including snakes).

Teiids: The clade of lizards containing tegus, ameivas, whiptails, caiman lizards, and related species.

Testudines: The clade of reptiles consisting of the turtles.

Tetrapod: The clade of animals containing all terrestrial vertebrates, including the reptiles, amphibians, and mammals. Along with lungfish and coelacanths, tetrapods are members of the larger clade Sarcopterygii (lobe-finned fish).

Toxicofera: The clade of lizards that possess venom apparatus, including snakes, iguanids, agamids, chameleons, monitors, helodermatids, and anguids.

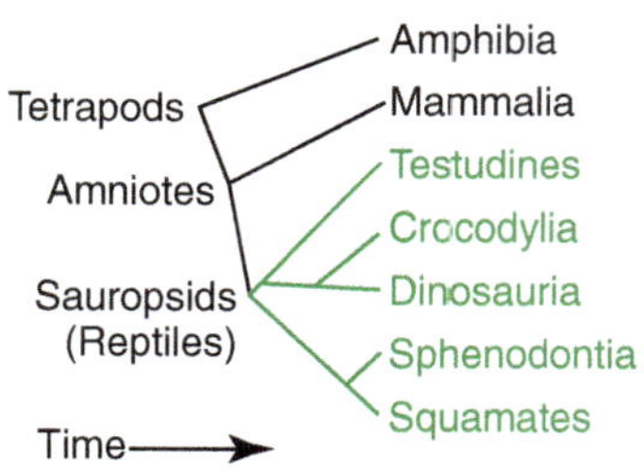

FIGURE 3-1 Phylogenetic tree of the tetrapods. Reptiles are in green.

an extraordinarily low gastric pH.[6] Indeed, crocodilians are one of the few groups of animals studied in which oral fluoroquinolones do not result in good blood levels, and it is possible that breakdown in the extremely acidic stomach may play a role in this.[7,8]

Both birds and crocodilians have four-chambered hearts. A four-chambered heart is not needed for separation of right and left blood flow, which is accomplished in nonarchosaur reptiles that lack a ventricular septum.[9] The major advantage of a ventricular septum is facilitation of pressure differentials between the left and right sides of the heart, as may be needed in an animal with a high metabolic rate. Ventricular septa evolved separately in archosaurs and mammals; both groups have warm-blooded members.

Crocodilians and birds also both have in common a respiratory system with unidirectional rather than tidal air flow, a much more efficient design than the mammalian lung.[10] An efficient respiratory system is also needed for a higher metabolic rate.

Ancestors of modern crocodilians from shortly after the divergence from dinosaurs were morphologically consistent with long-legged active terrestrial predators.[11] It is plausible that ancestral archosaurs were warm-blooded animals and that modern crocodilians lost homeothermy, which would be an evolutionarily disadvantageous trait for aquatic ambush predators.

When examined in detail, significant homologies between crocodilians and their closest extant relatives, the birds, become clear. However, the significant differences between birds and crocodilians are also obvious, and the clinician needs to be careful not to overextrapolate. The obvious differences between an alligator and a Fulvous Whistling Duck underscore the more cryptic but greater differences between an alligator and a tegu.

LIZARDS

Another prevalent error is the concept of lizards as a group distinct from snakes. In squamate evolution, the earliest divergence is the geckos, followed by the divergence of the skinks, night lizards, and plated lizards (Figure 3-2). The next groups to branch off were the teiids, lacertids, and amphisbaenids, and the remaining group, containing snakes, iguanids, agamids, chameleons, monitors, helodermatids, and anguids, is known collectively as the Toxicofera (see blue on Figure 3-2), named for the commonality of the presence of venom glands. There is

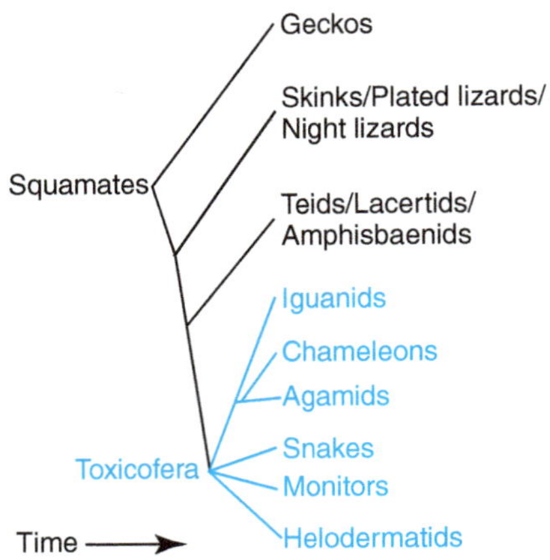

FIGURE 3-2 Phylogenetic tree of the squamates. Toxicofera are in blue.

a very nice image of the histologic features of Bearded Dragon venom glands in Fry et al.[12] Snakes diverge in the middle of the squamates, and if snakes are removed, then lizards are not a monophyletic group. Snakes are a group of lizards, and a Cornsnake is a better model for a Bearded Dragon than a Leopard Gecko.

CARING FOR CAPTIVE ANIMALS

It is critical, when caring for captive animals, to consider environments in which they have evolved. Eons of selective pressure have resulted in reptiles that have adapted to specific diets, habitats, and threats, and disease may result when captive conditions differ. Periodontal disease is common in lizards with acrodont dentition (agamids and chameleons) in captivity but not in the wild.[13] Infiltrative lipomas appear to be common in obese captive Cornsnakes.[14] Significant rostral trauma is common in water dragons and basilisks kept in glass enclosures without sufficient cover.

INFECTIOUS DISEASES

Evolution is also central to infectious disease. Multiple factors influence evolutionary rates, including selective pressures, generation times, and fidelity of copying genes. Microbes often have very short generation times. Ribonucleic acid (RNA) viruses, generally lacking proofreading, have high error rates when they make copies. As a result, evolution rates in microbes tend to be rapid, and RNA viruses are the most rapidly evolving organisms on the planet. This is useful for rapid adaptation to novel selective pressures, such as immune selection and antimicrobial use. To compensate, the most rapidly evolving genes in vertebrates are immune related.

MICROBES

Microbes are essential for all vertebrate life, for functions including digestion, nutrition, and defense. In veterinary school, we have all been taught Koch's postulates as criteria for establishing a microbe as a pathogen. Although Koch's postulates have their use, they frequently result in a false dichotomous understanding of microbes as either pathogenic or nonpathogenic. There is no such thing as a microbe that is always either a pathogen or a nonpathogen. There have been many asymptomatic human Ebola virus infections, and people have died of septicemia due to *Lactobacillus acidophilus*.[15,16] A microbe does not "want" to cause disease or not cause disease. All life on earth has been selected for billions of years to reproduce successfully, and this is all that matters from an evolutionary standpoint. If pathogenic traits provide an evolutionary advantage in a given situation, they will be selected for. If they provide a disadvantage, they will be selected against.

A number of important selective pressures affect microbes in a vertebrate host, including nutrient availability, temperature, competition with other microbes, the need to transfer to a new host, and the host immune system. A vertebrate host is a nutrient-rich environment. However, some nutrients may be sequestered; significant resources are spent by the host synthesizing transferrin, lactoferrin, and ferritin to make it unavailable. Many bacterial virulence pathways have evolved to access this sequestered iron.[17,18]

Homeothermic vertebrates also provide a highly temperature-controlled environment, whereas poikilothermic hosts require the ability to survive at different temperatures. Because of this, infectious disease manifestation may be highly temperature-dependent in poikilotherms.[19-21] This adds an extra dimension to disease ecology, especially with latent or persistent infections. Further investigation of the role of temperature in disease manifestation in poikilotherms is strongly indicated, especially with populations of many reptile species critically declining and likely to be affected by anthropogenic climate change.[22]

Competition is also a major selective pressure in a vertebrate; many organisms want to live in such a nutrient-rich environment. The majority of antimicrobials are derived from molecules secreted by other microbes to compete for ecologic niches. Animal guts are some of the most diverse and rich ecosystems to be found anywhere. Many organisms that have evolved in such a competitive environment have resistance to many antimicrobials; *Enterococcus* sp. is a classic example.

The limited lifespan of vertebrate hosts creates significant selective pressure toward the ability to move on to a new host. This often involves secretion of large amounts of microbes via respiratory discharge or diarrhea, but other routes occur, such as the simultaneous behavioral changes and salivary gland shedding of rabies or the use of insect vectors. Three fundamental strategies can be used to deal with limited host life spans. First, a microbe may survive well in the environment. Second, a microbe may adapt to a balance with the host environment. Finally, a microbe may move quickly to a new host.

Parasites often adapt to a balance with their hosts. Many parasites tend to have slower generation times compared with viruses or bacteria, which makes rapid reproduction and moving on to a new host less of a viable strategy. The costs of parasites to their definitive hosts are relatively minimal in many cases because it is advantageous to parasites to preserve their habitat. Bullfrog tadpoles carrying the pinworm *Gyrinicola batrachiensis* have better feed conversion and metamorphose earlier than uninfested controls, rendering the relationship mutualistic rather than parasitic.[23] However, for parasites with indirect life cycles, causing disease in an intermediate host may be advantageous. If a rodent carrying pentastomid larvae is debilitated, it is more likely to be eaten by a snake, completing the life cycle. This may also result in greater disease in accidental hosts.[24] Some parasites do survive well in the environment; this reduces the selective pressure not to harm the host. Parasites that survive well in the environment are much more likely to cause significant disease; perhaps the best known examples of this in reptiles are *Rhabdias* sp., which cause pulmonary disease in squamates that may be fatal.[25]

Most fungi also survive well in the environment, resulting in little selective pressure to keep their host alive. They compete significantly with bacteria for the same niches; this has resulted in the production of antibacterial compounds by fungi and antifungal agents by bacteria. The fungi are some of the closest relatives of animals; fungi, choanoflagellates, and metazoa (multicelled animals) form a clade known as the Opisthokonta.[26] An animal is much more closely related to a mushroom than it is to an oak tree. Antimicrobial drugs generally exploit differences in chemistry and metabolism between pathogen and host. Because fungi and vertebrate hosts diverged more recently, there are fewer differences to exploit, and antifungal drugs tend to have narrower therapeutic indices and use a smaller subset of mechanisms.

Bacteria constitute a large portion of the host ecosystem. There are far more bacterial cells in a normal vertebrate than there are vertebrate cells. Traditional approaches to examining bacterial diversity have depended on culture; this is a poor way of assaying diversity. Culture-independent methods, such as 16S polymerase chain reaction (PCR) and cloning, or high-throughput sequencing methods, have revealed that standard culture-based methods will detect between 1% and 10% of bacterial species present in most ecologic niches. As an understanding of further diversity has arisen, it becomes clearer that a vertebrate is a complex ecosystem.[27] This system may be very dynamic. The gut flora of Burmese Pythons changes significantly in response to feeding.[28] Postprandially, bacteria in the phylum Firmicutes ("classic" gram-positive bacteria, containing organisms such as *Clostridium, Lactobacillus,* and *Peptostreptococcus*) increase dramatically, while those in the phylum Bacteroidetes (primarily containing anaerobic gram-negative organisms such as *Bacteroides* and *Prevotella*) make up a greater percentage of the fewer species present after fasting. The gut flora did not significantly share species with prey mice, with the exception of the temporary postprandial establishment of *Lactobacillus* sp.

Ecologic disturbance may have significant negative impacts on many aspects of health. Damage to healthy gut flora by antibiotic use provides opportunity for invasive species; recent treatment with antibiotics markedly increases host susceptibility to *Salmonella*.[29] A 5-day course of ciprofloxacin will change human gut flora diversity and composition for several weeks, and the original composition may never reestablish.[30] In many ways, the use of broad-spectrum antibiotics for a bacterial infection in a vertebrate is analogous to starting a forest fire to get rid of coyotes. The ideal treatment for a bacterial pathogen would be as narrow-spectrum as possible, minimally disturbing the rest of the host ecosystem. Isoniazid, which targets only *Mycobacterium tuberculosis* and a few very closely related species and does not significantly affect many other *Mycobacterium* sp., is an excellent example. Unfortunately, current market forces have resulted in pharmaceutical companies developing antibiotics with as broad a spectrum as possible, and narrow spectrum antibiotics are often not put through further development and clinical trials.

Antibiotic use without consideration of microbial ecology and evolution rapidly leads to failure. Back in the 1980s, gentamicin was promoted for eradication of *Salmonella* from turtles.[31] Over the next few years, the *Salmonella* isolates from farmed turtles acquired a high rate of gentamicin resistance[32] and therefore posed a greater risk to human health than they had previously. Several studies have suggested that wild turtles may have a lower carriage rate for *Salmonella*.[33,34] The only realistic way to reduce the risk of *Salmonella* in farmed turtles over the long term is to alter the ecologic niche that it inhabits. Keeping farmed animals in high population densities increases contact rates, pathogen loads, and stress, lowering barriers to transmission. Increased ease of transmission reduces the selective pressure to keep the host alive and healthy. Reducing the risk of *Salmonella* in hatchling turtles probably means farming at lower densities and eliminating high-density turtle farming.[35]

VIRUSES

Viruses are strictly dependent on host cells for replication; this means that living in the environment as a strategy for dealing with limited host life spans is not a viable option. There are a number of important properties that affect viral evolution and ecology. Enveloped viruses are surrounded by a lipid envelope. This envelope is usually essential for invading a host cell. It is also easily damaged, which makes disinfection easier when dealing with an enveloped virus. Segmentation of viral genomes, allowing reassortment, may provide a hybrid advantage for crossing host species; this has been best studied in the Orthomyxoviridae.[36] Acquiring genes that are functional from a related virus is significantly more likely to be advantageous than random mutations; this is why animals and plants have sex. Throughout biology, hybridization is a factor allowing rapid nondetrimental change, allowing species to invade novel habitats.[37] New sites of infection or host species are novel virus habitats.

Nucleic acid type is another property with a major impact on viral evolution and ecology. Large deoxyribonucleic acid (DNA) viruses often adapt to a balance with their hosts. This usually involves latency or chronic infection, with a delicate balance with the host immune system. A larger number of genes is often used to maintain this balance. Because the viruses are larger and more complicated, they require more accurate replication to avoid accumulating lethal mutations. DNA viruses usually have much more accurate replication, with either host or viral proofreading mechanisms in place. Many DNA viruses evolve at rates not much more rapid than their hosts, which enables larger viral genomes with greater numbers of genes. Large DNA viruses, especially those with intranuclear replication, are the most host-specific viruses.[38] There is evidence that some of these viruses have codiverged evolutionarily along with their hosts; this evidence is strongest in the adenoviruses and herpesviruses. In Figure 3-3, a herpesvirus phylogenetic tree is shown. A potential root can be placed where the arrow is marked, representing an ancestral herpesvirus in an ancestral amniote. The earliest amniote divergence is between mammals and reptiles, as seen in Figure 3-1. All known members of the Betaherpesvirinae and Gammaherpesvirinae use mammal hosts, and the longer branch lengths in this area indicate that these viruses have diverged over a

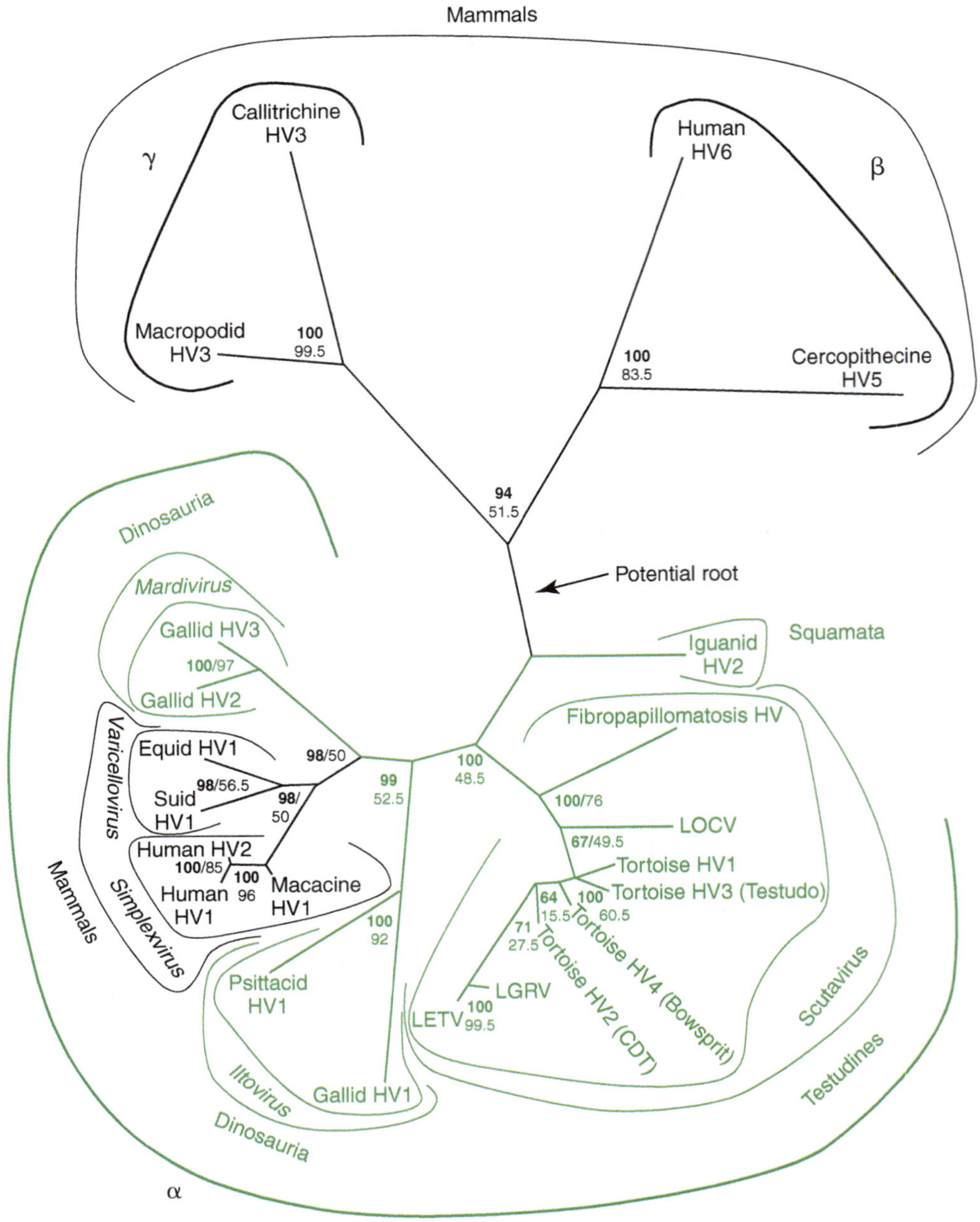

FIGURE 3-3 Phylogenetic tree of the Herpesviridae. Herpesviruses of reptile hosts are in green. Note similarity of branching pattern to that of the hosts.

longer period of time. Heading toward the Alphaherpesvirinae, the first agents to diverge infect squamates; the squamates are the earliest divergence within the reptiles. The next group to diverge is the scutavirus, infecting turtle/tortoise hosts; this is also consistent with host divergence patterns. There are no reliable crocodilian herpesvirus sequences available for comparison. *Mardivirus* and *Iltovirus* infect avian hosts. However, the mammalian alphaherpesviruses nest within the clade infecting avian hosts. The branch lengths within the mammalian alphaherpesviruses are relatively short, which indicates that these viruses have not diverged from each other to the same extent that mammalian herpesviruses in the other subfamilies have. One plausible explanation for this is that the mammalian alphaherpesviruses represent a host jump to mammals from the Dinosauria. Chickenpox, caused by the alphaherpesvirus human herpesvirus 3, may be a descendant of a dinosaurian virus and may be more aptly named than had been realized.

The complex coadaptation of some large DNA viruses provides selective advantage to causing minimal pathology in their hosts. A long-lived host may provide a suitable habitat for decades. However, this balance in a definitive host may not apply to other hosts. Hosts that are similar enough for a virus to infect but dissimilar enough for the intricate balance of latency/chronicity not to work may result in overwhelming and often fatal infection. The most significant pathology associated with herpesviruses is in aberrant hosts. A well-balanced host–virus relationship may actually be beneficial to the host. Columbid herpesvirus 1, endemic in Rock Doves, causes disease in squabs kept in stressful conditions, but the overall pathologic damage is relatively minimal. However, in raptors, which prey on Rock Doves, Columbid herpesvirus 1 causes an overwhelming infection that is rapidly fatal.[39] The advantage to the pigeon populations of killing off predators likely outweighs the disadvantage of minor disease in neonates.

RNA viruses reproduce less accurately. They generally lack proofreading and have the highest mutation rates of any organisms on the planet. These mutation rates mean that genetic complexity is not possible; the high error rates would render progeny requiring a large gene set nonviable. RNA viruses have small genomes and fewer genes. The advantage of such a high error rate is that RNA viruses are capable of rapidly outmaneuvering the host immune system. The strategy of RNA viruses is more likely to be rapid reproduction and moving to a new host. Because they have less complex relationships with their hosts, RNA viruses are much more capable of moving to new host species. This ability to move to new hosts reduces the selective pressure not to harm the host, and many RNA viruses are more pathogenic. A metaanalysis found that of the 20 virus families infecting the best-studied vertebrate host species, humans, four RNA virus families, Reoviridae, Bunyaviridae, Flaviviridae, and Togaviridae, accounted for more than half of emerging and reemerging viruses.[40] When one considers major viral human diseases that have recently emerged, high-profile diseases such as severe acute respiratory syndrome (SARS) (Coronaviridae), West Nile (Flaviviridae), influenza (Orthomyxoviridae), Ebola (Filoviridae), and Hendra (Paramyxoviridae) are all RNA viruses.

The retroviruses have RNA genomes and, when actively replicating, have very high mutation rates similar to other RNA viruses. However, retroviruses are unusual in that they reverse transcribe from RNA to DNA, and the DNA copy of their genome is then incorporated into the host genome. This has happened a lot over the course of evolution and makes retroviral discovery and diagnosis very challenging, not because they are hard to find but because they are widespread and present in such large numbers that it is difficult to sort out disease-associated virus from clinically irrelevant endogenous virus. Approximately 1% of the typical vertebrate genome encodes for vertebrate proteins, whereas 8% to 9% of the vertebrate genome is retroviral in origin. The diversity of retroviruses in reptiles is only beginning to be understood.[41] Because of the prevalence of retroviruses in their genomes, reverse transcriptase, the enzyme that converts viral RNA back to DNA, is commonly expressed in host cells. This has also resulted in less frequent incorporation of other viruses into host genomes, especially those that replicate in the nucleus. Bornaviruses, which have the uncommon trait for RNA viruses of nuclear replication, have been found to be incorporated into the genomes of many vertebrates, and bornaviral cDNA has been found in Gaboon Vipers.[42] Incorporation of inactive virus into host genomes complicates interpretation of nucleic acid–based diagnostics.

PATHOGENIC DISEASES

Several routine husbandry practices in the reptile trade create strong evolutionary selective pressures toward pathogenicity. First, overcrowding is common. It is unfortunately common and considered acceptable to house snakes in breeder racks, where enclosures that are smaller in dimension than the length of the snake are stored in vertical racks in close proximity. The stress of close confinement results in elevated corticosteroids and immunosuppression .[43] The design of these breeder racks makes good biosecurity practices impossible. High population densities lower transmission barriers, reducing pressure to keep hosts alive and selecting toward virulence.[44] It is also common in the reptile trade to select for color phases. This usually involves some degree of inbreeding to select for what are often recessive traits. A major driving force for the evolution of sex is acquisition of genetic diversity for immune function. Inbreeding results in selection for greater disease.[45] Finally, reptiles are still often wild-caught, and stressed wild-caught animals are brought to large distributors who have species from all over the world in the same facility with insufficient biosecurity. This is an ideal situation for pathogen host jumps, which is where the most dramatic disease is seen.[46] Mixing of species by the exotic animal trade has already proved disastrous, with the transferral of monkeypox from Gambian Pouched Rats to Prairie Dogs to humans.[47] An orthoreovirus was first isolated in 1996 from a Mediterranean Spur-thighed Tortoise *(Testudo graeca)* in Switzerland and later characterized by sequencing.[48] This virus has more recently been associated with a high mortality rate and syncytial cell enteropathy/hepatopathy in Leopard Geckos widely distributed in the United States.[49] This almost certainly represents a host jump at a breeding institution or distributor.

Reduction of the significant selective pressures toward highly pathogenic diseases involves major changes in the reptile industry. Genetic diversity in populations needs to be valued and monitored through appropriate use of studbooks and cooperative rather than competitive interactions with breeders. Breeding for mutations needs to be discouraged. Housing needs to be entirely revised so that larger enclosures for individual animals allow feeding and cleaning to be done without cross-contamination to other animals. Importation of wild animals for sale as pets needs to be strongly discouraged. Facilities need to focus on single species and have smaller numbers of animals at lower densities.

In conclusion, evolution is central to all areas of comparative medicine. It is critical for the reptile practitioner to take this into account, especially when dealing with herd health and infectious diseases.

REFERENCES

1. Hugall AF, Foster R, Lee MS. Calibration choice, rate smoothing, and the pattern of tetrapod diversification according to the long nuclear gene RAG-1. *Syst Biol* 2007;56:543–563.
2. Schweitzer MH, Zheng W, Organ CL, et al. Biomolecular characterization and protein sequences of the Campanian hadrosaur *B. canadensis*. *Science* 2009;324:626–631.
3. Xu X, Wang K, Zhang K, et al. A gigantic feathered dinosaur from the lower cretaceous of China. *Nature* 2012;484:92–95.
4. Eagle RA, Tütken T, Martin TS, et al. Dinosaur body temperatures determined from isotopic (^{13}C-^{18}O) ordering in fossil biominerals. *Science* 2011;333:443–445.
5. Eme J, Gwalthney J, Owerkowicz T, et al. Turning crocodilian hearts into bird hearts: growth rates are similar for alligators with and without right-to-left cardiac shunt. *J Exp Biol* 2010;213:2673–2680.
6. Farmer CG, Uriona TJ, Olsen DB, et al. The right-to-left shunt of crocodilians serves digestion. *Physiol Biochem Zool* 2008;81:125–137.
7. Helmick KE, Papich MG, Vliet KA, et al. Pharmacokinetics of enrofloxacin after single-dose oral and intravenous administration in the American alligator *(Alligator mississippiensis)*. *J Zoo Wildl Med* 2004;35:333–340.
8. Martelli P, Lai OR, Krishnasamy K, et al. Pharmacokinetic behavior of enrofloxacin in estuarine crocodile *(Crocodylus porosus)* after single intravenous, intramuscular, and oral doses. *J Zoo Wildl Med* 2009;40:696–704.

9. Jensen B, Nielsen JM, Axelsson M, et al. How the python heart separates pulmonary and systemic blood pressures and blood flows. *J Exp Biol* 2010;213:1611–1617.
10. Farmer CG, Sanders K. Unidirectional airflow in the lungs of alligators. *Science* 2010;327:338–340.
11. Riff D, Kellner AWA. Baurusuchid crocodyliforms as theropod mimics: clues from the skull and appendicular morphology of *Stratiotosuchus maxhechti* (Upper Cretaceous of Brazil). *Zool J Linnean Soc* 2011:163:S37–S56.
12. Fry BG, Vidal N, Norman JA, et al. Early evolution of the venom system in lizards and snakes. *Nature* 2006;439:584–588.
13. McCracken HE. Periodontal Disease in Lizards. In: Fowler ME, Miller RE, Donley S, eds. *Zoo and wild animal medicine: current therapy*. 4th ed. Philadelphia: WB Saunders Co, 1998;252–257.
14. Burkert, BA, Tully TN, Nevarez J, et al. Infiltrative lipoma in a corn snake, *Elaphe guttata guttata*. *J Herpetol Med Surg* 2002;12(3):33–35.
15. Leroy EM, Baize S, Volchkov VE, et al. Human asymptomatic Ebola infection and strong inflammatory response. *Lancet* 2000;355: 2210–2215.
16. Cannon JP, Lee TA, Bolanos JT, et al. Pathogenic relevance of *Lactobacillus*: a retrospective review of over 200 cases. *Eur J Clin Microbiol Infect Dis* 2005;24:31–40.
17. Haley KP, Skaar EP. A battle for iron: host sequestration and *Staphylococcus aureus* acquisition. *Microbes Infect* 2012;14:217–227.
18. Perry RD, Fetherston JD. Yersiniabactin iron uptake: mechanisms and role in *Yersinia pestis* pathogenesis. *Microbes Infect* 2011;13:808–817.
19. Klenk K, Snow J, Morgan K, et al. Alligators as West Nile virus amplifiers. *Emerg Infect Dis* 2004;10:2150–2155.
20. Rojas S, Richards K, Jancovich JK, et al. Influence of temperature on Ranavirus infection in larval salamanders *Ambystoma tigrinum*. *Dis Aquat Organ* 2005;63:95–100.
21. Goodwin AE, Merry GE. Mortality and carrier status of bluegills exposed to viral hemorrhagic septicemia virus genotype IVb at different temperatures. *J Aquat Anim Health* 2011;23:85–91.
22. Slenning BD. Global climate change and implications for disease emergence. *Vet Pathol* 2010;47:28–33.
23. Pryor GS, Bjorndal KA. Effects of the nematode *Gyrinicola batrachiensis* on development, gut morphology, and fermentation in bullfrog tadpoles (*Rana catesbeiana*): a novel mutualism. *J Exp Zool A Comp Exp Biol* 2005;303:704–712.
24. Brookins MD, Wellehan JF, Roberts JF, et al. Massive visceral pentastomiasis caused by *Porocephalus crotali* in a dog. *Vet Pathol* 2009;46: 460–463.
25. Langford GJ, Janovy J Jr. Comparative life cycles and life histories of North American *Rhabdias* spp. (Nematoda: Rhabdiasidae): lungworms from snakes and anurans. *J Parasitol* 2009;95:1145–1155.
26. Torruella G, Derelle R, Paps J, et al. Phylogenetic relationships within the Opisthokonta based on phylogenomic analyses of conserved single copy protein domains. *Mol Biol Evol* 2012;29:531–544.
27. Robinson CJ, Bohannan BJ, Young VB. From structure to function: the ecology of host-associated microbial communities. *Microbiol Mol Biol Rev* 2010;74:453–476.
28. Costello EK, Gordon JI, Secor SM, et al. Postprandial remodeling of the gut microbiota in Burmese pythons. *ISME J* 2010;4:1375–1385.
29. Croswell A, Amir E, Teggatz P, et al. Prolonged impact of antibiotics on intestinal microbial ecology and susceptibility to enteric *Salmonella* infection. *Infect Immun* 2009;77:2741–2753.
30. Dethlefsen L, Relman DA. Incomplete recovery and individualized responses of the human distal gut microbiota to repeated antibiotic perturbation. *Proc Natl Acad Sci U S A* 2011;108:4554–4561.
31. Siebeling RJ, Caruso D, Neuman S. Eradication of *Salmonella* and *Arizona* species from turtle hatchlings produced from eggs treated on commercial turtle farms. *Appl Environ Microbiol* 1984;47:658–662.
32. Diaz MA, Cooper RK, Cloeckaert A, et al. Plasmid-mediated high-level gentamicin resistance among enteric bacteria isolated from pet turtles in Louisiana. *Appl Environ Microbiol* 2006;72:306–312.
33. Richards JM, Brown JD, Kelly TR, et al. Absence of detectable *Salmonella* cloacal shedding in free-living reptiles on admission to the wildlife center of Virginia. *J Zoo Wildl Med* 2004;35:562–563.
34. Saelinger CA, Lewbart GA, Christian LS, et al. Prevalence of *Salmonella* spp in cloacal, fecal, and gastrointestinal mucosal samples from wild North American turtles. *J Am Vet Med Assoc* 2006;229:266–268.
35. Izadjoo MJ, Pantoja CO, Siebeling RJ. Acquisition of *Salmonella* flora by turtle hatchlings on commercial turtle farms. *Can J Microbiol* 1987;33:718–724.
36. Macken CA, Webby RJ, Bruno WJ. Genotype turnover by reassortment of replication complex genes from avian influenza A virus. *J Gen Virol* 2006;87:2803–2815.
37. Rieseberg LH, Kim SC, Randell RA, et al. Hybridization and the colonization of novel habitats by annual sunflowers. *Genetica* 2007;129:149–165.
38. Pulliam JR, Dushoff J. Ability to replicate in the cytoplasm predicts zoonotic transmission of livestock viruses. *J Infect Dis* 2009;199:565–568.
39. Pinkerton ME, Wellehan JF Jr, Johnson AJ, et al. Columbid herpesvirus-1 in two Cooper's hawks (*Accipiter cooperii*) with fatal inclusion body disease. *J Wildl Dis* 2008;44:622–628.
40. Woolhouse ME, Gowtage-Sequeria S. Host range and emerging and reemerging pathogens. *Emerg Infect Dis* 2005;11:1842–1847.
41. Jaratlerdsiri W, Rodríguez-Zárate CJ, Isberg SR, et al. Distribution of endogenous retroviruses in crocodilians. *J Virol* 2009;83:10305–10308.
42. Horie M, Honda T, Suzuki Y, et al. Endogenous non-retroviral RNA virus elements in mammalian genomes. *Nature* 2010;463:84–87.
43. Sykes KL, Klukowski M. Effects of acute temperature change, confinement and housing on plasma corticosterone in water snakes, *Nerodia sipedon* (Colubridae: Natricinae). *J Exp Zool A Ecol Genet Physiol* 2009;311:172–181.
44. Borovkov K, Day R, Rice T. High host density favors greater virulence: a model of parasite-host dynamics based on multi-type branching processes. *J Math Biol* 2012. doi: 10.1007/s00285-012-0526-9 [Epub ahead of print].
45. Morran LT, Schmidt OG, Gelarden IA, et al. Running with the Red Queen: host-parasite coevolution selects for biparental sex. *Science* 2011;333:216–218.
46. Pulliam JR. Viral host jumps: moving toward a predictive framework. *Ecohealth* 2008;5:80–91.
47. Bernard SM, Anderson SA. Qualitative assessment of risk for monkeypox associated with domestic trade in certain animal species, United States. *Emerg Infect Dis* 2006;12:1827–1833.
48. Wellehan JF Jr, Childress AL, Marschang RE, et al. Consensus nested PCR amplification and sequencing of diverse reptilian, avian, and mammalian orthoreoviruses. *Vet Microbiol* 2009;133:34–42.
49. Garner MM, Farina LL, Wellehan JFX, et al. Reovirus-associated syncytial cell enteropathy and hepatopathy in leopard geckos, *Eublepharus macularius*. In *Proceedings*. Conference of the Association of Reptilian and Amphibian Veterinarians, Milwaukee, Wisc, 2009;82.

CHAPTER 4

Molecular Infectious Disease Diagnostics

James F.X. Wellehan, Jr.

The development of molecular techniques has resulted in rapid advances in both our understanding of the diversity of infectious agents in reptiles and our ability to specifically and sensitively identify these agents in our patients. This has brought about a more nuanced understanding of the complex interactions between host, pathogen, coinfections, and environment in causing disease. Conversely, these techniques may not be understood by the practitioner and can lead to misinterpretation of results and bad clinical decisions. It is important for clinicians to understand the basics of molecular diagnostic testing, potential problems, common errors, and clinical implications of results.

SEROLOGY OR CULTURE COMPARED WITH MOLECULAR TECHNIQUES

When a clinician tests for infectious agents, it is first important to determine what information is being sought. Are you looking for a pathogen, such as a virus or bacterium, or are you looking for a reaction to a pathogen, such as an antibody response? The molecular testing emphasized in this chapter tests directly for the presence of a pathogen but does not give information about whether the host is actually suffering from disease. Immunologic testing gives evidence that an animal has had an immune response to a pathogen but does not give information about whether the pathogen is currently present. Tracking changes in immune response over time is typically needed to determine the current relevance of an immune response; this requires assaying the immune response at more than one time point.

For immunologic testing, it is also important to consider whether the patient has had time to develop an immune response to a pathogen. This may take several weeks in reptiles.[1] In acute infections, a specific immune response may not be present. There are large seasonal and temperature effects on the immune response of reptiles, as well as species differences.[2-4] Other factors, including reproductive status and exogenous corticosteroid administration, may also affect development of a measurable immune response.[5,6]

When a clinician tests for an immune response, it is also important to consider what aspect of the immune system is being measured. A humoral immune response primarily produces antibodies to fight pathogens extracellularly, whereas a cellular immune response primarily uses cytotoxic T cells to trigger self-destruction of host cells infected with pathogens. Cellular and humoral immune responses are often found together but not always. An animal may have a cellular immune response without a significant humoral immune response and vice versa. Most common assays measure humoral immunity. A cellular immune response is typically most protective for intracellular pathogens such as viruses. Many intracellular pathogens elicit a relatively poor humoral immune response; a study of Tortoise herpesvirus 3 (TeHV3) in Greek Tortoises *(Testudo graeca)* found that only three of four experimentally infected animals developed detectable humoral immune responses, and the responses in the three that did show a reaction were relatively transient.[7]

Another significant challenge with serologic assays is cross-reactivity with related antigens. In reptiles, the diversity of infectious agents that may be present is often not yet known. TeHV2 (endemic in California Desert Tortoises) is distinct from TeHV3 (endemic in Greek Tortoises) at a level greater than that seen between Human herpesvirus 1 (causing cold sores in humans but rapidly fatal in marmosets) and Macacine herpesvirus 1 (causing cold sores in Rhesus Macaques but rapidly fatal herpes B in humans). It is probable that the clinical significance of the different tortoise herpesviruses in different species is comparable.

Treating diverse herpesviruses as a single entity may lead to inappropriate management decisions. Before the diversity of tortoise herpesviruses was understood, a serosurvey of California Desert Tortoises using what was later shown to be TeHV3 as an antigen found that a number of California Desert Tortoises were seropositive; this was almost certainly cross-reactivity of antibodies to TeHV2 with TeHV3.[8] From a population management perspective, it is crucial to know which viruses are endemic in a host species and the pathogenic implications of these viruses in other potential contact species.

Similarly, hemagglutination inhibition assays for ophidian paramyxoviruses in the genus *Ferlavirus* show poor concordance between different assays using different isolates.[9] Recent work has expanded the known diversity of the genus *Ferlavirus*, and at least three distinct clades are known.[10] The seroreactivity of samples from different snakes to different paramyxovirus strains differs significantly (Wellehan J, et al: unpublished data), and this may account, at least in part, for the lack of concordance seen. Overall, few pathogen clades exist whose diversity in reptiles is well enough understood that a clinician could be confident of the specificity of a detected antibody. This limits the current utility of serologic diagnostics in reptile medicine.

Culture of a pathogen from a diseased animal is considered the gold standard for identification of infectious agents whenever possible. For some bacterial pathogens such as coliforms and pseudomonads, isolation and identification is fairly straightforward. However, successful culture conditions have yet to be determined for the vast majority of microbes. Typically, around 10% of bacterial species can be cultured in a given ecologic niche,[11] and success at culturing viruses or protozoa is even lower.

Even if an agent has been cultured, it is still necessary to identify it. Biochemical methods for bacterial identification have been the standard for the past century. These methods have been best developed for two phyla of bacteria: Proteobacteria, the "typical" gram-negative organisms, and Firmicutes, the "typical" gram-positive organisms. However, some of the most medically significant phyla in reptiles, such as Actinobacterium (containing *Mycobacterium, Devriesea, Dermatophilus,* and others) and Chlamydiae (containing *Chlamydophila* and others) are poorly identified by standard biochemical methods. Molecular methods involving nucleic acid sequencing are superior at identification.[12] The contrast is even more stark in molecular versus classic fungal identification, in which identification has been morphologic, which misses significant cryptic diversity. The most significant fungal pathogens of reptiles are *Chrysosporium* sp. These are commonly called anamorphs of *Nannizziopsis vriesii,* but there is no support for this when sequence data from these isolates are examined. Sequence-based identifications of *Chrysosporium* sp. in reptiles include identification of a *Chrysosporium* sp. related to but distinct from *Nannizziopsis vriesii* in Bearded Dragons *(Pogona vitticeps)*,[13] *Chrysosporium guarroi* in green iguanas *(Iguana iguana)*,[14] and *Chrysosporium ophiodiicola* in a Black Rat Snake *(Elaphe obsoleta)*.[15] To date, there are no reports in which available sequence data support identification as *Nannizziopsis vriesii*. Sequence-based identification methods should be used to identify any agent where there is reason to question identification by conventional means.

POLYMERASE CHAIN REACTION

Polymerase chain reaction (PCR) directly tests for the presence of nucleic acid from an infectious agent (pathogen). Like other pathogen isolation techniques, this requires that the clinician submit an appropriate sample that contains the actual pathogen. A negative test does not mean that the pathogen is not present elsewhere in the patient. Unlike pathogen isolation, with PCR, the suspected agent does not need to be viable.

The first step in sample processing is nucleic acid extraction. If a ribonucleic acid (RNA) template (typically an RNA virus) is to be amplified, the RNA will have to be transcribed into deoxyribonucleic acid (DNA), a process known as reverse transcription. DNA templates are used in PCR.

DNA is composed of two complementary strands oriented in opposite directions (Figure 4-1, *A*). Primers (short single-stranded segments of DNA) are designed to match the sequence of the two strands of pathogen DNA in a manner such that they face one another. The DNA is heated so that the two strands separate (Figure 4-1, *B*). The temperature is then decreased to an appropriate temperature for the primers to anneal (bind) with the DNA (Figure 4-1, *C*). If the primers

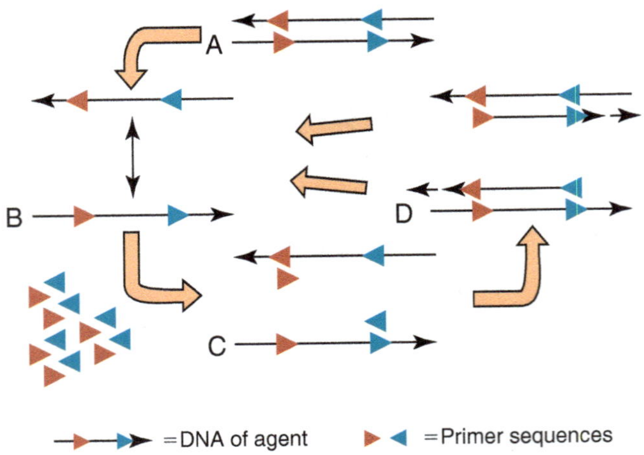

FIGURE 4-1 Polymerase chain reaction. **A,** Double stranded DNA of agent with known sequences *(in red and blue)* in opposite orientations on complementary strands. **B,** Nucleic acid is heated to separate the strands. **C,** DNA is cooled to an appropriate temperature for primers to bind to known sites. **D,** A high-temperature polymerase synthesizes a new complementary stand starting from the primer.

do not match with the DNA sequence, they will not anneal and no product will be formed.

The temperature is then increased to an appropriate temperature for thermostable DNA polymerase to extend the primer, making a matching strand for the DNA (Figure 4-1, *D*). The amount of DNA between the primers present is thus doubled. The cycle starts over again as the DNA is reheated to separate the strands. The cycle is repeated many times, and the amount of DNA increases geometrically.

The PCR product must then be validated, which means that it must be determined to be the appropriate product and not an accidental binding of the primers to an unexpected site on a different DNA template. Formerly, older validation methods were limited to measurement of the size of the product by gel electrophoresis or restriction fragment length polymorphism (RFLP). These methods are significantly less accurate than modern methods, such as sequencing or probe hybridization, and should no longer be considered acceptable.

The most definitive way to determine the identity of the PCR product is to sequence it. This was once expensive, but with the rapid improvements in sequencing technology that have taken place in the past decade, costs are now minimal.

Alternatively, a labeled piece of DNA containing part of the target sequence may be used to probe the PCR product. The probe must be designed to a sequence unique to the pathogen found within the PCR product. When done under the appropriate conditions, binding of the probe to the PCR product indicates that the PCR product is correct. Some protocols, such as quantitative PCR (qPCR), have the probe incorporated as the PCR is running, and this is discussed in the following section.

QUANTITATIVE POLYMERASE CHAIN REACTION

qPCR, also known as real-time PCR, is a PCR variant involving the use of a dye-labeled probe that binds to a sequence

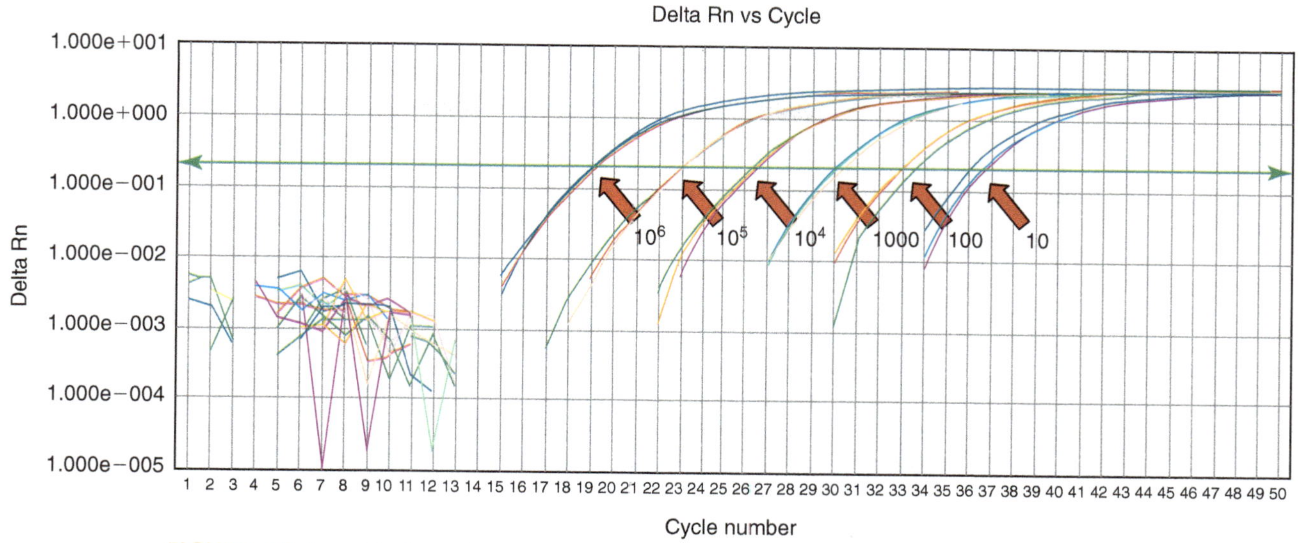

FIGURE 4-2 Quantitative polymerase chain reaction. The X axis shows number of cycles, and the Y axis shows fluorescence. Starting amounts of the different samples range from 10 to 1,000,000 copies. Larger starting amounts of template will result in fluorescence crossing the threshold at an earlier cycle number, enabling starting amount to be quantitated.

between the two primers. While there are qPCR techniques such as SYBR green that involve dye incorporation rather than use of a probe, these techniques are suboptimal because they do not provide the same degree of product validation. DNA polymerase, in addition to extending the primer to match the template DNA, also has exonuclease activity, which means that it will chew up any DNA in front of it that gets in the way as it is extending the primer. If the probe is bound to the template in front of the primer, the polymerase will chew through the probe, releasing the labeled dye. The dye released can be measured with a spectrophotometer. This has two distinct advantages. First, the validation of the PCR product is rapid and does not require further labor. For a product to be validated by sequencing, the PCR reaction must be confirmed as a single product by gel electrophoresis, appropriate bands must be cut out and purified from the gel, sequencing reactions must be run, electrophoresed, and edited, and then the sequence data must be analyzed, all of which is a significantly more complicated and labor intensive process. Validation in qPCR is done during the reaction, data output is simple, and no further steps are necessary. Second, the release of dye depends on the amount of template present, providing quantitative information. In Figure 4-2, a qPCR standard curve is shown. The horizontal axis is number of cycles, and the vertical axis is fluorescence. The arrows drawn on the figure indicate the number of template copies present in the initial reaction. When there are only 10 copies initially present, it takes approximately 37 cycles for the reaction to release enough dye to cross the threshold (green) line. When there are 1,000,000 copies initially present, the threshold is crossed after approximately 19 cycles, and intermediate numbers are spread evenly between. This provides a standard to which samples can be compared and also provides a control to ensure that reactions are working well and efficiently. Quantitative information can be clinically useful for determining whether loads are sufficient for consideration as a disease etiology and for following trends over time for assessment of a response to therapy. Well-designed qPCR is a highly useful tool for specific identification of a known agent.

CONSENSUS POLYMERASE CHAIN REACTION TECHNIQUES

Before primers can be designed, the nucleic acid sequence must be known. Some nucleic acid sequences are specific to a given species or even strain. Other nucleic acid sequences have stayed the same throughout evolution and are found across groups of related organisms. These are known as consensus sequences. Genes that are conserved throughout evolution are typically essential for function of the organism, such as ribosomal RNA (rRNA) or viral polymerases. Gene choice is critical and depends on the level of taxonomic resolution needed. Within adenoviruses, the polymerase is the most conserved gene, and primers have been designed that will amplify any adenovirus.[16] However, when Agamid adenovirus 1 was examined specifically in Bearded Dragons, all polymerase sequences obtained to date showed minimal variation, and it was necessary to obtain sequences from the hexon gene to differentiate strains.[17] Once consensus sequences have been identified, PCR primers can be designed in these conserved regions and used to amplify the more variable region between the consensus primers. In reptile medicine, many pathogens remain to be identified. If primers designed for conserved sequences are used in PCR, the PCR will amplify the DNA of all organisms containing the conserved sequence, which would provide the ability to identify novel pathogens in a known clade. Although consensus sequence PCR is useful for amplification of sequences from novel pathogens, the amplification of novel sequences does not lend itself to specific probe design, which eliminates qPCR as an option for this application. Consensus PCR should always be accompanied by sequencing of the PCR product.

ROLLING CIRCLE AMPLIFICATION

Rolling circle amplification (RCA) is a technique for amplification of small circular DNA genomes, as are found in several families of viruses, including papillomaviruses, polyomaviruses, anelloviruses, circoviruses, and tornoviruses. It does not require knowledge of any sequence from the agent. The technique involves a polymerase that moves around the circle as it synthesizes a complementary strand. When the beginning of the circle is reached, the polymerase continues around again, and the new strand is a long series of repeated copies of the circle. This strand is then cut with a restriction enzyme, which recognizes specific short four–base to six–base pair sequences. Because these sequences will be in the same place every time the circle is repeated, the restriction enzyme cuts the circle into a set of pieces of specific size. These pieces can then be cloned and used as a sequencing template. Because it does not require any known sequence, RCA has proven useful for obtaining sequence templates of divergent agents, such as tornoviruses in sea turtles.[18] However, this technique requires a significant amount of cloning and sequencing and is therefore highly labor intensive, raising costs.

HIGH THROUGHPUT SEQUENCING

The past decade has seen amazing advances in sequencing technology. Costs have been reduced by several orders of magnitude. New techniques, including pyrosequencing, Illumina sequencing, and SOLiD sequencing are capable of producing millions of sequences in a single run. This has enabled the development of metagenomics, in which nucleic acid representing an entire sample is sequenced rather than targeted amplification of a specific region. This enables an understanding of the diversity of complex and diverse environments such as the vertebrate gastrointestinal tract. The ability to obtain such datasets is a double-edged sword; while it provides the ability to obtain sequences from previously unknown and divergent pathogens, it requires the ability to recognize and sift these sequences from literally millions of nontarget sequences. This is a major bioinformatics challenge but has already resulted in significant advances in reptile infectious disease. Tornoviruses, divergent small circular viruses, were first identified using metagenomic techniques.[18] The previously known reptile paramyxoviruses were in the genus *Ferlavirus,* a clade in the subfamily Paramyxovirinae, containing other vertebrate paramyxoviruses such as *Morbillivirus* and *Respirovirus.* Metagenomic approaches enabled the identification of Sunshine virus from Australian pythons, a novel paramyxovirus that does not cluster within either known paramyxoviral subfamily and did not amplify with the use of consensus PCR methods based on all previously known paramyxoviruses.[19] Although costs for metagenomic methods are still considerable, they are decreasing rapidly, and what was once a $100,000 project a few years ago is a $1000 project now. It is only a matter of time before these techniques become clinically affordable.

SAMPLE COLLECTION PROCESS FOR NUCLEIC ACID–BASED DIAGNOSTICS

The first thing the practitioner needs to do is open a dialogue with the diagnostic laboratory. It is important first to understand what methodologies are offered, and ideally, peer-reviewed references describing testing methodologies should be provided to the clinician. Common problems and pitfalls should be discussed in advance, as well as limitations of diagnostic testing.

Histologic evaluation of a necropsy is often one indication that an agent requiring molecular testing is present. As such, while it is critical to collect a complete set of tissues in formalin for histologic evaluation, it is also important to save back another frozen set for further diagnostics as indicated by the histologic examination. Tissues should be routinely kept until histologic results have been received and there is no indication for further diagnostics, such as a collection-wide problem.

Sample choice is critical for nucleic acid–based diagnostics; the agent must be in the sample. This requires an understanding of the common distribution of the agent in the animal. Although plasma has historically been a common sample collected for infectious disease diagnostics because of the use of serodiagnostics, relatively few infectious agents are themselves commonly found in plasma, which makes it a suboptimal sample choice for testing for most reptile pathogens. A laboratory with significant clinical experience with a given reptile pathogen may be able to advise on sample choice.

PCR is a highly sensitive technique, and the potential for false-positive results from slight contamination anywhere in the process, from collection to laboratory, is high. As such, it is critically important that measures are taken to avoid contamination during sample collection and transport and that appropriate controls are run.

Transport is also crucial and needs to be discussed in advance with the laboratory. Agents such as RNA viruses, especially enveloped ones, tend to be significantly less environmentally stable. Media such as RNAlater (Life Technologies, Grand Island, NY) can be used to preserve viability of nucleic acids. Shipping on ice or even dry ice is often preferable. When same-day transport is not available, overnight shipping is indicated. The laboratory should be notified in advance so that potential problems can be identified and brought up with the shipping service on the same day if a delivery does not arrive.

It is an exciting time in reptile medicine. Molecular techniques are enabling us to begin to unravel the diversity of pathogens in reptiles and detect them in a clinically applicable fashion. An understanding of molecular diagnostic options and their clinical interpretation are essential in the armamentarium of the reptile practitioner.

REFERENCES

1. Lock BA, Green LG, Jacobson ER, et al. Use of an ELISA for detection of antibody responses in Argentine boa constrictors *(Boa constrictor occidentalis). Am J Vet Res* 2003;64:388–395.
2. el Masri M, Saad AH, Mansour MH, et al. Seasonal distribution and hormonal modulation of reptilian T cells. *Immunobiology* 1995;193:15–41.
3. Munoz FJ, De la Fuente M. The immune response of thymic cells from the turtle *Mauremys caspica. J Comp Physiol [B]* 2001;171:195–200.
4. Zapata AG, Varas A, Torroba M. Seasonal variations in the immune system of lower vertebrates. *Immunol Today* 1992;13:142–147.
5. Saad AH, el Deeb S. Immunological changes during pregnancy in the viviparous lizard, *Chalcides ocellatus. Vet Immunol Immunopathol* 1990;25:279–286.

6. Mondal S, Rai U. Dose and time-related in vitro effects of glucocorticoid on phagocytosis and nitrite release by splenic macrophages of wall lizard *Hemidactylus flaviviridis*. *Comp Biochem Physiol C Toxicol Pharmacol* 2002;132:461–470.
7. Origgi FC, Klein PA, Mathes K, et al. Enzyme-linked immunosorbent assay for detecting herpesvirus exposure in Mediterranean tortoises (spur-thighed tortoise [*Testudo graeca*] and Hermann's tortoise [*Testudo hermanni*]). *J Clin Microbiol* 2001;39:3156–3163.
8. Jacobson ER, Berry KH, Wellehan JFX, et al. Serological and molecular evidence for testudinid herpesvirus 2 infection in wild Agassiz's desert tortoises, *Gopherus agassizii*. *J Wildl Dis* 2012;48:747–757.
9. Allender MC, Mitchell MA, Dreslik MJ, et al. Measuring agreement and discord among hemagglutination inhibition assays against different ophidian paramyxovirus strains in the Eastern massasauga (*Sistrurus catenatus catenatus*). *J Zoo Wildl Med* 2008;39:358–361.
10. Abbas MD, Marschang RE, Schmidt V, et al. A unique novel reptilian paramyxovirus, four atadenovirus types and a reovirus identified in a concurrent infection of a corn snake (*Pantherophis guttatus*) collection in Germany. *Vet Microbiol* 2011;150:70–79.
11. Safaee S, Weiser GC, Cassirer EF, et al. Microbial diversity in bighorn sheep revealed by culture-independent methods. *J Wildl Dis* 2006;42:545–555.
12. Petti CA, Polage CR, Schreckenberger P. The role of 16S rRNA gene sequencing in identification of microorganisms misidentified by conventional methods. *J Clin Microbiol* 2005;43:6123–6125.
13. Abarca ML, Martorell J, Castellá G, et al. Dermatomycosis in a pet inland bearded dragon (*Pogona vitticeps*) caused by a *Chrysosporium* species related to *Nannizziopsis vriesii*. *Vet Dermatol* 2009;20:295–299.
14. Abarca ML, Castellá G, Martorell J, et al. *Chrysosporium guarroi* sp. nov. a new emerging pathogen of pet green iguanas (*Iguana iguana*). *Med Mycol* 2010;48:365–372.
15. Rajeev S, Sutton DA, Wickes BL, et al. Isolation and characterization of a new fungal species, *Chrysosporium ophiodiicola*, from a mycotic granuloma of a black rat snake (*Elaphe obsoleta obsoleta*). *J Clin Microbiol* 2009;47:1264–1268.
16. Wellehan JF, Johnson AJ, Harrach B, et al. Detection and analysis of six lizard adenoviruses by consensus primer PCR provides further evidence of a reptilian origin for the atadenoviruses. *J Virol* 2004;78:13366–13369.
17. Parkin DB, Archer LL, Childress AL, et al. Genotype differentiation of Agamid Adenovirus 1 in bearded dragons (*Pogona vitticeps*) in the USA by hexon gene sequence. *Infect Genet Evol* 2009;9:501–506.
18. Ng TF, Manire C, Borrowman K, et al. Discovery of a novel single-stranded DNA virus from a sea turtle fibropapilloma by using viral metagenomics. *J Virol* 2009;83:2500–2509.
19. Hyndman TH, Marschang RE, Wellehan JF Jr, et al. Isolation and molecular identification of sunshine virus, a novel paramyxovirus found in Australian snakes. *Infect Genet Evol* 2012;12:1436–1446.

CHAPTER 5

Clinical Virology

Rachel E. Marschang

A number of viruses have been shown to be important pathogens in reptiles. In other cases, the association between viral infection and disease is not clear, and the discovery of some viruses in reptiles has been incidental. Reptile virology is still a relatively young field and much remains to be discovered and understood. The clinical significance of viral infections appears to depend on many different factors including the virus family, the virus strain, the host species, factors affecting the host immune system, and additional infectious agents such as other viruses, bacteria, and parasites. Interpretation of diagnostic testing requires an understanding of the difference between infection and disease. Infection with a virus simply means that the virus has invaded and replicated in the body of the host. This may or may not lead to the development of disease. We are still in the process of understanding which viruses can be found in reptiles. It is even more difficult to interpret their clinical significance and to develop methods to detect them in infected reptiles, as well as deal with infected animals. This review will concentrate on the laboratory diagnosis of common viruses found in reptiles and possible interpretation of laboratory results. It is not meant as an overview of all viruses described in reptiles (an overview is provided in Appendix 2. See Jacobson[1] and Marschang[2] for comprehensive reviews of viruses detected in reptiles).

DIAGNOSIS OF VIRAL INFECTIONS IN REPTILES

Many different methods are available for the diagnosis of viral infections in reptiles. These include methods for the detection of viruses, viral proteins, or viral genomes and serologic methods for the detection of an immune response to viral infection. Which method should be used in a specific situation depends on many different factors. These include the host species, clinical observations, time since infection, virus species, reason for testing, and test availability, some of which, particularly time since infection and virus species, may not be known. The most common methods currently used for virus detection are polymerase chain reaction (PCR) and, in some countries, virus isolation in cell culture. Methods commonly used for the detection of an immune response against a specific virus include neutralization tests, enzyme-linked immunosorbent assays (ELISA), and (for paramyxovirus [PMV] infections) hemagglutination inhibition (HI) tests. None of the test systems available for reptile virology are fully standardized in that repeatability and reproducibility are not consistently studied. In addition, cross-reactivity and relationships between reptile viruses are not fully understood, and the specificity of some tests may therefore be lower than expected. To best use the test systems available and to interpret the results of these tests, clinicians should understand what each detects and the possibilities and limits of each. This chapter will present information on viruses commonly found in chelonians, squamate reptiles, and crocodilians, methods currently used to diagnose infection with these viruses, and interpretation of laboratory results.

VIRUSES OF CHELONIANS

A number of viruses have been described in chelonians. Among this group of animals, the viruses most commonly detected have been herpesviruses (HVs), which have been associated with various disease syndromes but have also been found in apparently healthy animals in some cases. HVs have been described most commonly in chelonians of the families Testudinidae (tortoises) and Cheloniidae (sea turtles). Other viruses that have been regularly detected in this group of animals are ranaviruses and picornaviruses. Individual reports have been published on the detection of adenoviruses (AdVs), PMVs, reoviruses, and papillomaviruses in chelonians. A list of viruses regularly detected in chelonians and methods for diagnostic testing can be found in Table 5-1.

HERPESVIRUSES

HVs are enveloped, double-stranded (ds) deoxyribonucleic (DNA) viruses. These viruses are relatively susceptible to disinfectants and are therefore easy to inactivate in the environment with the use of standard virucidal disinfectants. However, HV infections lead to lifelong latency. Latent virus remains inactive in infected cells—in the case of alphaherpesviruses, in neuronal cells. The virus can then begin to replicate again under some circumstances; thus an HV-infected animal that survives initial infection must be considered a lifelong carrier. HVs have been detected in many different species of turtles and tortoises as well as other groups of reptiles. In chelonians, HVs have been described in water turtles (Emydidae), tortoises, and sea turtles. In water turtles, the presence of HVs has been based on histologic detection of intranuclear inclusions and electron microscopy of infected tissues. Infections were associated with hepatic disease.[3-5]

TABLE 5-1

Diagnostic Methods Used for the Detection of Viruses of Chelonians

Virus Family	Virus Genus and Species	Host Species	Diagnostic Samples: Live Animals	Diagnostic Samples: Necropsied Animals	Virus Detection	Serology	References
Herpesviridae	"Chelonivirus": LETD virus	Green Sea Turtles *(Chelonia mydas)*	n.d.	Lung and trachea	PCR, virus isolation	ELISA	7, 20, 123
	LGRV	Loggerhead Sea Turtles *(Caretta caretta)*	n.d.	Material from lesions	PCR	n.d.	8
	LOCV	Loggerhead Sea Turtles	n.d.	Material from lesions	PCR	n.d.	8
	Fibropapillomatosis HV	Green Sea Turtles, Loggerhead Sea Turtles, Hawksbill Turtles *(Eretmochelys imbricate)*, Olive Ridley *(Lepidochelys olivacea)*	Fibropapillomas	Fibropapillomas	PCR	ELISA	1, 20
	TeHV1	Russian Tortoise *(Testudo horsfieldii)*	Oral swabs	Tongue (and other tissues)	PCR, virus isolation	NT, ELISA	13,21
	TeHV2	Desert Tortoise *(Gopherus agassizzii)*	n.d.	Tongue (and other tissues)	PCR	ELISA	12
	TeHV3	Many different species of Testudinidae	Oral swabs	Tongue (and other tissues)	PCR, virus isolation	NT, ELISA	13, 21
	TeHV4	Bowsprit Tortoise *(Chersina angulata)*	Oral swab	n.d.	PCR	n.d.	14
Iridoviridae	*Ranavirus*	Many different species of turtles and tortoises	Possibly oral and cloacal swabs, possibly peripheral leukocytes	Liver, gastrointestinal tract	PCR, virus isolation	ELISA	24, 26, 29, 31
Picornaviridae	Unclassified, called virus "X"	Many different species of Testudinae, most often Spur-thighed Tortoises *(Testudo graeca)*	Oral swabs	Intestine, tongue, trachea	Virus isolation	NT	34
Adenoviridae	*Siadenovirus*	Sulawesi Tortoise *(Indotestudo forsteni)*, Burmese Star Tortoise *(Geochelone platynota)*	Nasal flush, oral/nasal mucosal tissue, cho-anal swabs, cloacal swabs, plasma	Liver (and other tissues)	PCR	n.d.	38
	Unclassified	Box Turtle *(Terrapene ornata ornaae)*	n.d.	Liver	PCR	n.d.	41
Paramyxoviridae	*Ferlavirus*	Spur-thighed Tortoise *(Testudo graeca)*, Hermann's Tortoise *(Testudo hermanni)*, Leopard Tortoise *(Stigmochelys pardalis)*	n.d.	Several different tissues	RT-PCR, virus isolation	HI	49, 50, 52

ELISA, Enzyme-linked immunosorbent assay; HI, hemagglutination inhibition test; HV, herpesvirus; LETD, lung, eye, and trachea disease; LGRV, loggerhead genital-respiratory HV; LOCV, loggerhead orocutaneous HV; n.d., not described; NT, neutralization test; PCR, polymerase chain reaction; RT-PCR, reverse-transcriptase PCR; TeHV, testudinid herpesvirus.

In sea turtles, HV infections have been associated with skin lesions (gray patch disease), fibropapillomatosis, lung, eye, and trachea disease (LETD), loggerhead genital–respiratory HV (LGRV)-associated disease, and loggerhead orocutaneous HV (LOCV)-associated disease. Gray patch disease was the first HV-associated disease to be described in sea turtles and was found in aquaculture-reared young Green Sea Turtles *(Chelonia mydas)*.[6] Another HV-associated disease described in Green Sea Turtles was characterized by gasping, harsh respiratory sounds, buoyancy abnormalities, inability to dive properly, and the presence of caseated material on the eyes, around the glottis, and within the trachea. This disease was named LETD.[7] Two HV-associated disease syndromes have been described in wild-caught Loggerhead Sea Turtles *(Caretta caretta)*. Turtles infected with LGRV had ulcers in the trachea, around the cloaca, and on the base of the phallus. Turtles infected with LOCV had pneumonia and ulcers and cutaneous plaques covered with exudate in the oral cavity.[8] The most commonly described HV-associated disease in sea turtles is fibropapillomatosis (Figure 5-1). Fibropapillomatosis has been detected in Green, Loggerhead, Hawksbill *(Eretmochelys imbricata)*, and Olive Ridley *(Lepidochelys olivacea)* Sea Turtles around the world. Infected turtles develop fibropapillomas, and individual or multiple tumors can occur externally all over the body. Internal tumors are also possible. Although the fibropapillomatosis HV has never been isolated in cell culture, transmission of the disease is possible with the use of cell-free tumor extracts.[9]

In tortoises, HV infections have mostly been associated with diphtheroid-necrotizing stomatitis (Figure 5-2). This can be quite severe and often leads to the death of the affected animal. Rhinitis, conjunctivitis, cervical edema, anorexia, and lethargy are also frequently observed. Central nervous disorders such as paralysis and incoordination, as well as hepatitis, have also been described. Eosinophilic or amphophilic intranuclear inclusions are often detected in infected tissues, most commonly in epithelial cells of the tongue, oral mucosa, and upper respiratory tract as well as the gastrointestinal tract (Figure 5-3). Other tissues in which inclusions have been described include the urinary tract, the brain, the liver, and the spleen. In some cases, HV infections have also been detected in clinically healthy tortoises. Development of disease and prognosis appear to depend both on the host species and on the virus involved.[10] There are currently four different HVs that have been shown to infect tortoises. They have been named testudinid HV 1 to 4 (TeHV1 to 4).[2] TeHV1 was first detected in Russian Tortoises *(Testudo horsfieldii)* and Pancake Tortoises *(Malacochersus tornieri)* in Japan.[11] Similar viruses have also been found in tortoises in Europe. Although they have been detected in several different species, all cases so far have had direct contact with Russian Tortoises. TeHV1 is associated with stomatitis in infected animals but does not appear to cause high morbidity or mortality. TeHV2 was described in a California Desert Tortoise *(Gopherus agassizii)* in the United States. The animal exhibited anorexia, lethargy,

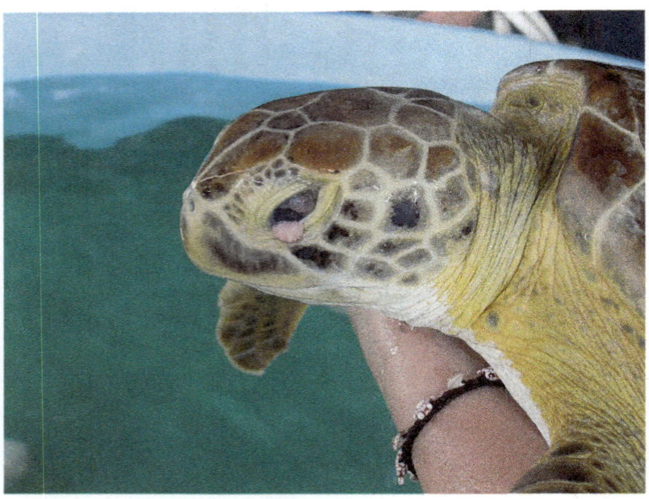

FIGURE 5-1 Green Turtle *(Chelonia mydas)* with fibropapillomas.

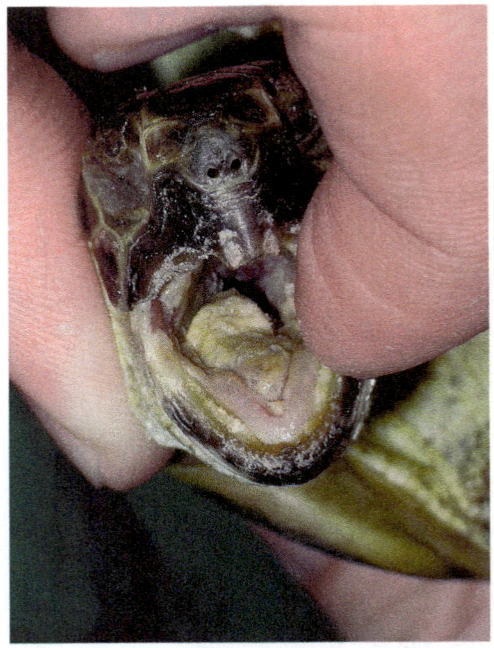

FIGURE 5-2 Russian Tortoise *(Testudo horsfieldii)* with herpesvirus infection. Severe stomatitis with diphtheroid plaques visible throughout the oral cavity. *(Photo courtesy of Dr. Volker Schmidt, Universität Leipzig, Leipzig, Germany.)*

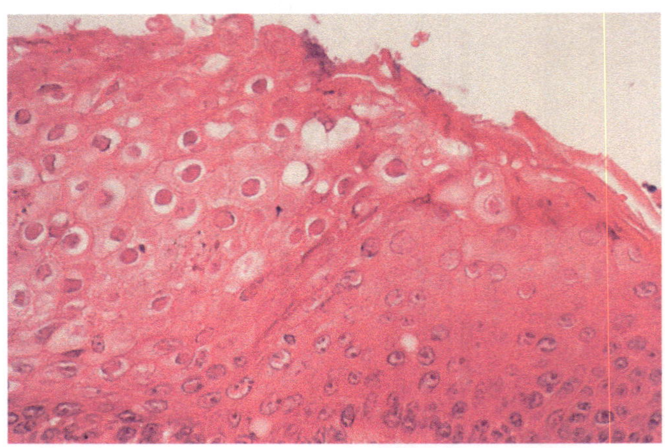

FIGURE 5-3 Herpesvirus infection in a tortoise *(Testudo hermanni)*. Photomicrograph of the epithelium of the tongue. Ballooning degeneration is evident in numerous epithelial cells. Large intranuclear inclusions are also visible in several cells. H&E stain, × 400. *(Photo courtesy Dr. Horst Posthaus, Universität Bern, Berne, Switzerland.)*

and yellow-white caseous plaques on the tongue and palate.[12] TeHV3 has been most frequently described in Mediterranean tortoises (Hermann's *[T. hermanni]*, Spur-thighed *[T. graeca]* and Marginated *[T. marginata]* Tortoises) and Russian Tortoises in Europe. It has also been detected in tortoises in the United States and in northern Africa. This virus is associated with severe disease and high morbidity and mortality, particularly in Hermann's and Russian Tortoises. Spur-thighed Tortoises develop disease less frequently and appear to be able to survive and carry the infection.[13] TeHV4 was detected in a clinically healthy Bowsprit Tortoise *(Chersina angulata)* in a zoo in the United States.[14]

DIAGNOSIS OF HERPES VIRUS INFECTIONS IN CHELONIANS

Virus Detection

Detection of viral DNA by PCR is the most commonly used method for detecting HVs in infected chelonians. A PCR using degenerate primers in a nested format targeting a highly conserved portion of the DNA polymerase gene has been used to detect HVs in many different chelonian species.[8,13,15] This method has been shown to be the most sensitive available for HV detection in tortoises. Other PCRs have been described targeting specific TeHVs.[16-18] All of these methods are, however, less sensitive than the nested PCR but more specific. This means that, although the nested PCR can detect all of the chelonian HVs tested so far, other methods are limited to one or two different virus species (e.g., only TeHV1 or only TeHV3), and other virus species will not be detected if these methods are used. Virus detection by PCR should be verified by additional methods (e.g., sequencing of the PCR product, especially when a PCR with degenerate primers is used). Virus isolation in cell culture has also been used to detect HVs in infected chelonians. LETD virus (LETV), TeHV1, and TeHV3 have all been isolated in cell culture (Figure 5-4, *B*). Isolation in cell culture is generally less sensitive than the nested PCR already described. It is time consuming and is offered by very few laboratories. It

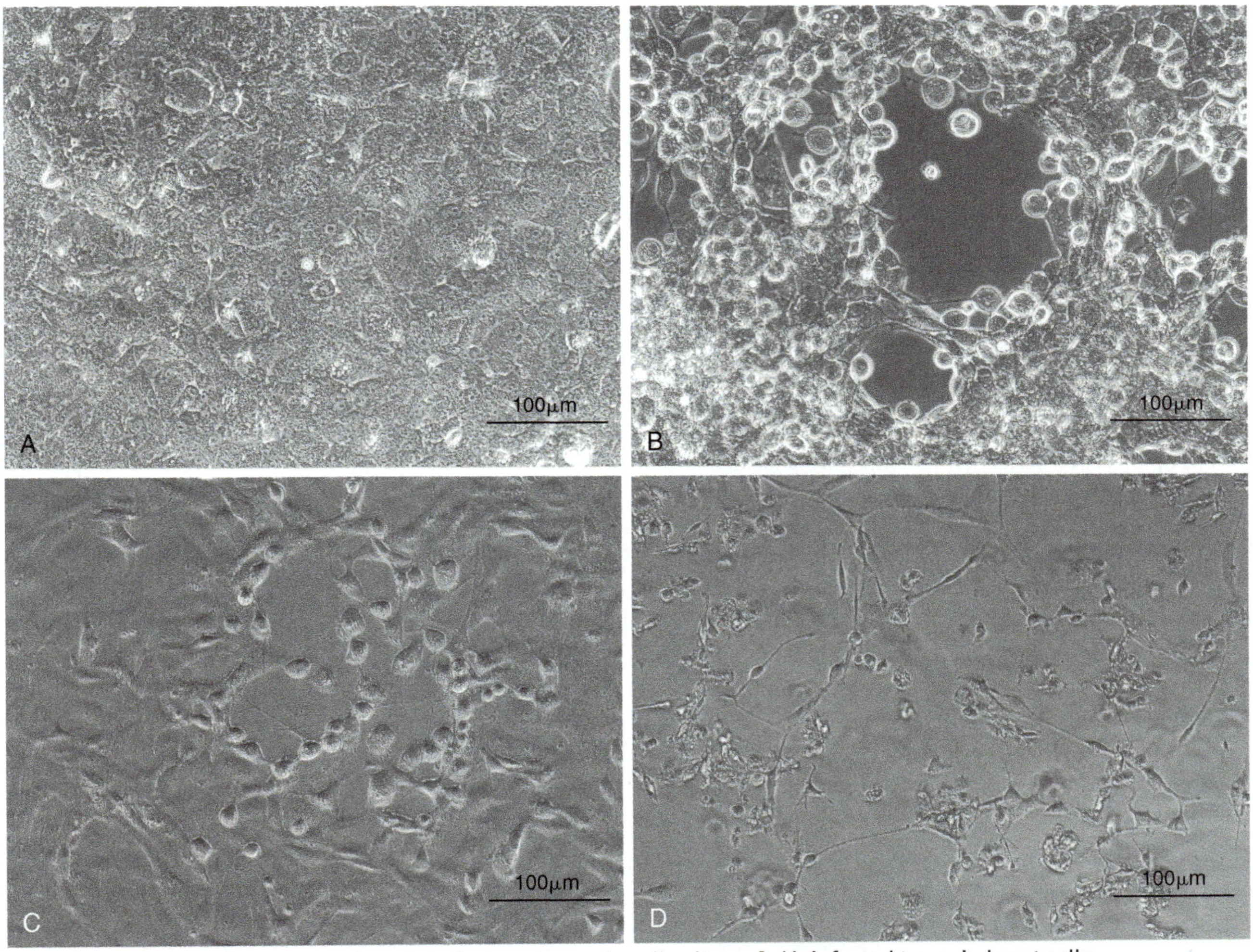

FIGURE 5-4 Isolation of chelonian viruses in cell culture. **A,** Uninfected terrapin heart cells (TH1), which are often used for the isolation of chelonid viruses. **B,** TH-1 infected with a testudinid herpesvirus 3 (TeHV3). This virus causes a cytopathic effect (CPE) with cell lysis and rounding of infected cells. **C,** TH1 infected with a ranavirus isolated from a Hermann's tortoise *(Testudo hermanni).* Ranaviruses from reptiles, amphibians and fish grow in a wide range of cell lines and cause CPEs with cell lysis and rounding of infected cells. **D,** TH1 infected with the picornavirus (virus "X"). This virus causes a CPE with cell lysis.

can be helpful for the detection of viruses other than HVs (e.g., picornaviruses; see further on), which may be important differential diagnoses for herpesviral disease or may be involved in disease processes. Samples for HV detection in chelonians should generally include tissues with lesions. For fibropapillomatosis, viral DNA can be detected in fibropapillomas removed from live or dead animals. In tortoises, HV DNA has been detected in oral swabs from live animals. Swabs should be taken from the base of the tongue and should include cellular material (Figure 5-5). In dead tortoises, the tongue is generally considered the best tissue for virus detection. Esophagus, stomach, intestine, trachea, liver, and brain can also be helpful in virus detection.

Serology

Detection of antibodies against HVs is particularly important because of the biologic properties of these viruses. Because HVs cause latent infections, any animal found to be serologically positive for HVs must be considered a lifelong carrier, even if the animal appears healthy. Serologic tests have been described for the detection of antibodies against fibropapillomatosis-associated HV and LETV in sea turtles and against TeHV1 and TeHV3 in tortoises.[19-21] An ELISA for the detection of antibodies against glycoprotein H of a chelonid fibropapillomatosis-associated HV has been described.[19] High seroprevalences were found in wild Green Sea Turtles in Florida and in Loggerhead Turtles using this method. Seropositivity did not correlate with clinical disease. However, testing for antibodies against this virus is not widely available.

An ELISA has also been described for the detection of antibodies against LETV. This ELISA was specific for LETV and did not detect antibodies against fibropapillomatosis-associated HV.[20] Virus neutralization tests and ELISAs have been described for the detection of antibodies against TeHV1 and against TeHV3. Virus neutralization tests are most commonly used in Europe, whereas ELISAs are used in the United States. Virus must be able to grow in cell culture for the development of a virus neutralization test. Virus neutralization testing with both TeHV1 and TeHV3 has shown that these viruses do not cross-react serologically; thus testing for antibodies against both is recommended in Europe. Detection of antibodies against these two viruses has been shown to depend on the tortoise species involved. Hermann's Tortoises, which are particularly susceptible to HV infection and disease, do not often develop neutralizing antibodies after infection. In contrast, antibodies are frequently detected in Spur-thighed Tortoises that have been infected. An ELISA has also been developed for the detection of antibodies against TeHV3 in tortoises.[21] This ELISA has also been adapted to detect antibodies against TeHV2 in California Desert Tortoises, on the basis of putative serologic cross-reactivity between TeHV2 and TeHV3.[12,22]

RANAVIRUSES

Ranaviruses belong to the family *Iridoviridae*, a group of large, dsDNA viruses infecting only ectothermic hosts including various invertebrates, fish, amphibians, and reptiles. Ranaviruses are enveloped but do not need their envelope to be infectious. In reptiles, ranaviruses have most commonly been detected in chelonians, although they have also been described in snakes and lizards. In chelonians, these viruses have been found in Russian Tortoises, Eastern Box Turtles *(Terrapene carolina carolina)*, Chinese Soft-shelled Turtles *(Pelodiscus sinensis)*, Hermann's tortoises, Red-eared Sliders *(Trachemys scripta elegans)*, Burmese Star Tortoises *(Geochelone platynota)*, Gopher Tortoises *(Gopherus polyphemus)*, Florida Box Turtles *(Terrapene carolina bauri)*, Egyptian Tortoises *(Testudo kleinmanni)*, a Leopard Tortoise *(Stigmochelys pardalis)*, Marginated Tortoises, and Spur-thighed Tortoises.[23-30] Ranavirus infection in chelonians has been associated with lethargy, anorexia, nasal discharge, conjunctivitis, severe subcutaneous cervical edema, ulcerative stomatitis, and "red-neck disease" (Figure 5-6). Histologically, infected animals have been found to have hepatitis, enteritis, and pneumonia. Infected cells, particularly epithelial cells of the gastrointestinal tract and hepatocytes, may have basophilic intracytoplasmic inclusions. In a transmission study with Box Turtles *(Terrapene ornata ornata)* and Red-eared Sliders, intramuscular injection of a ranavirus isolated from a Burmese Star Tortoise led to disease, including lethargy, anorexia, ocular discharge, conjunctivitis, and oral plaques, and death of the animals in some cases.[24]

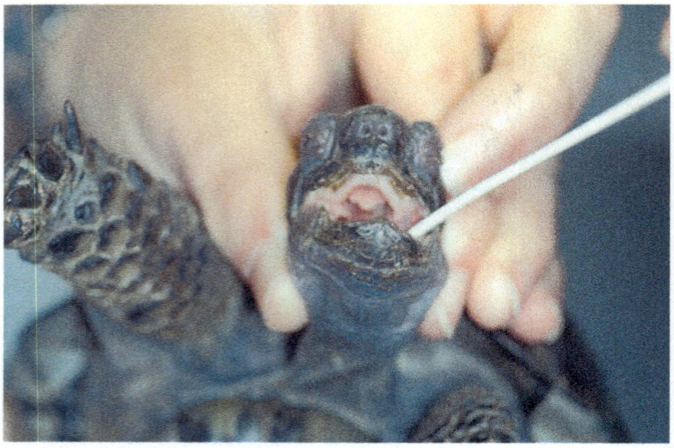

FIGURE 5-5 Spur-thighed Tortoise *(Testudo graeca)*. Oral swabs can be used to diagnose several different viral infections in live tortoises, particularly herpes, picorna, and ranavirus infections.

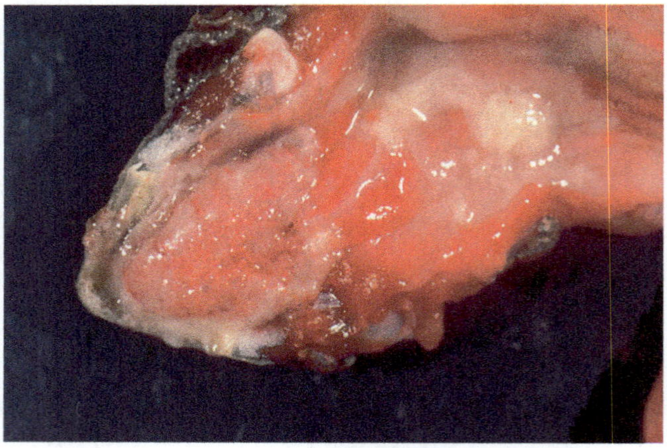

FIGURE 5-6 Hermann's Tortoise *(Testudo hermanni)* infected with a ranavirus. Severe stomatitis. *(Photo courtesy Dr. Horst Posthaus, Universität Bern, Berne, Switzerland.)*

Ranaviruses do not appear to be species specific and can be transmitted between animal species and possibly even between different classes of animals.

DIAGNOSIS OF RANAVIRUS INFECTIONS IN CHELONIANS

Ranaviruses grow well in cell culture and can be grown on a wide range of cell lines from reptiles, fish, mammals, and birds if the cells are kept at appropriate temperatures (below 32°C or 89.6°F) (see Figure 5-4, *C*). Virus isolation on cell culture is a sensitive method for the detection of ranaviruses. PCRs for the detection of viral DNA have also been used to diagnose ranavirus infections in chelonians. The gene most frequently targeted is the major capsid protein (MCP) gene.[23,26] This gene is highly conserved in ranaviruses and is therefore a good target for virus detection. PCR-positive reactions are generally specific, but confirmation of product identity by sequencing is recommended. Other PCRs, including real-time PCRs, have been described for the detection of ranaviruses in amphibians and fish but have not yet been used for ranavirus detection in chelonians. Samples for the detection of ranaviruses in dead chelonians should include liver and gastrointestinal tract. Spleen and kidney may also be virus positive.[24] In a transmission study viral DNA was detected in oral and cloacal swabs from intramuscularly infected Red-eared Sliders as early as 5 days postinoculation (p.i.) and until 26 days p.i. or until the animals died or were euthanized.[24] Both oral swabs and blood have been used to detect ranavirus in free-ranging Eastern Box Turtles in the United States, whereas oral and cloacal swabs have been used for the detection of viral DNA in naturally infected tortoises in Germany.[29,31]

Serology

Little work has been done studying the immune response of reptiles to ranaviral infection. An ELISA for the detection of anti ranavirus antibodies in Burmese Star Tortoises, Gopher Tortoises, and Eastern Box Turtles has been developed.[32] The assay is able to detect antibodies in all three species. Testing of 1000 Gopher Tortoises from the eastern United States showed a low prevalence of anti ranavirus antibodies of 1.5% overall, whereas prevalence in a group of 55 Eastern Box Turtles that had survived an outbreak of ranavirus infection 1 year previously was 1.8% (one positive). The authors postulated that the low prevalence rates detected may underestimate the true prevalence of infection, as ranavirus infections in chelonians are often associated with high mortality rates and the antibody response is unknown.[32] This ELISA has also been adapted for the detection of anti ranavirus antibodies in *Testudo* spp. in Europe.[29]

PICORNAVIRUSES

Picornalike viruses are frequently found in tortoises in Europe. The family *Picornaviridae* contains small single-stranded (ss), nonenveloped ribonucleic acid (RNA) viruses that can be relatively resistant to disinfection and can persist for extended periods of time in the environment. In tortoises, picornalike viruses have been detected by isolation in cell culture with the use of chelonian cell lines. Because of difficulties in characterizing these viruses, they have been called virus "X".[33] These viruses have most frequently been isolated from Spur-thighed Tortoises. They are also found in Marginated Tortoises, Hermann's Tortoises, Leopard Tortoises, and Egyptian Tortoises. Clinical signs associated with infection include softening of the carapace in young animals, diphtheroid-necrotizing stomatitis, rhinitis, conjunctivitis, and ascites (Figure 5-7). Viruses have also been isolated from clinically healthy animals[34] (Heuser: Pers. com.). There are no typical histologic lesions associated with infection. Many tortoises infected with virus "X" are also infected with other infectious agents, including HVs and *Mycoplasma* spp. (Marschang RE, unpublished observations). A large part of the genome of one virus "X" isolate has recently been almost fully sequenced, showing that this is a novel picornavirus.[35,36] The sequence information now available will allow the development of new diagnostic tools, including reverse transcriptase PCR (RT-PCR) as well as the comparison of virus "X" isolates from different tortoise species, different geographic locations, and different years.

DIAGNOSIS OF PICORNAVIRUSES IN TORTOISES

The detection of virus "X"-like viruses in tortoises currently relies on isolation in cell culture. Virus can be isolated on TH-1 (American Type Culture Collection [ATCC] No. CCL-50) at 28°C (82.4°F). The virus causes a lytic cytopathic effect in infected cells (see Figure 5-4, *D*). Virus identification after isolation is difficult and relies on the typical cytopathic effect (CPE) and resistance to chloroform. Visualization of virions in infected cell cultures by electron microscopy is difficult. Although no RT-PCR is currently available for the detection of these viruses in clinical samples, primers are available that can be used to help identify the viruses after isolation in cell culture. PCR products can then be sequenced and compared with available sequence data. The best samples for virus detection in live animals are oral swabs. Virus can also be shed via the cloaca and the conjunctiva, so swabs from these areas may also yield positive results. In dead animals, samples from the entire gastrointestinal tract (tongue to cloaca) can all be used for virus detection. Virus is frequently also found in other tissues (including liver, kidney, heart, brain, and lung). Serologic detection of antibodies against virus "X" can be carried out using virus neutralization methods. Antibodies against this virus are frequently found in tortoises in Europe, and low

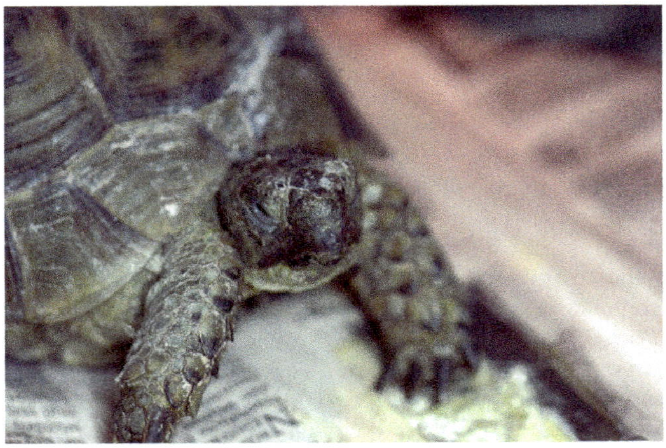

FIGURE 5-7 Spur-thighed Tortoise (*Testudo graeca*) with rhinitis. This animal was infected with a picornavirus ("virus X") as well as with a herpesvirus and mycoplasma.

titers have also been detected in wild-caught tortoises in Turkey.[37] It is unknown how closely related all virus "X" isolates are to one another, so cross-reactivity among these viruses and between these viruses and other picornaviruses is not yet understood.

OTHER VIRUSES DESCRIBED IN CHELONIANS

Adenoviruses

AdVs are nonenveloped, dsDNA viruses that have a relatively high resistance to inactivation and can be difficult to disinfect. In reptiles, they are most commonly detected in squamates, particularly agamids, but AdVs have recently also been described in several species of chelonians including Sulawesi Tortoises *(Indotestudo forsteni)*,[38] Impressed Tortoises *(Manouria impressa)*, a Burmese Star Tortoise,[39] a Leopard Tortoise[40], and a Box Turtle.[41] Infection in the Sulawesi Tortoises was associated with severe systemic disease and a mortality rate of 82%. Pathologic findings in infected tortoises were multifocal hepatic necrosis, amphophilic to basophilic intranuclear inclusions and diffuse hepatic lipidosis, myeloid necrosis in bone marrow, and severe necrotizing enterocolitis.[38] The Impressed Tortoises and the Burmese Star Tortoise were all exposed to infected Sulawesi Tortoises.[39] The Leopard Tortoise was also infected with a herpesvirus and had biliverdinuria, wasting, and episodes of hemorrhages.[40] The infected Box Turtle showed liver changes with cellular degeneration, pronounced vacuolization of the cytoplasm and pyknosis of nuclei, and inclusion bodies in some hepatocytes.[41] Diagnosis of AdVs is generally carried out with the use of PCR targeting a portion of the DNA polymerase gene.[42] This PCR uses degenerate primers and targets a highly conserved region of the genome and can therefore be used to detect a wide range of AdVs from different hosts. PCR products should therefore be sequenced to confirm the identity of the virus detected. In live animals, nasal flushes, oral/nasal mucosal tissue, choanal swabs, cloacal swabs, and plasma have all been successfully used to detect virus.[38] Liver tissue has been successfully used for virus detection in dead animals,[38,41] as have a number of other internal tissues.[38] The AdVs detected in chelonians so far do not appear to be closely related to the AdVs of squamates, and several appear to differ significantly from one another. No serologic test is currently available for the detection of antibodies against AdVs in chelonians.

Papillomaviruses

Papillomaviruses are nonenveloped dsDNA viruses with a circular genome. The papillomaviruses are highly host–species specific and tissue restricted. They generally cause benign tumors (warts, papillomas) in their natural hosts. Occasionally, they can also cause these lesions in related species. Papillomaviruses are highly resistant to inactivation and can persist in the environment for long periods of time. In chelonians, papillomaviruses have been described in Bolivian Side-neck Turtles *(Platemys platycephala)*[43], a Russian Tortoise,[44] a Loggerhead Turtle, and a Green Sea Turtle.[45] Skin lesions were reported in all but the Russian Tortoise, which had a history of stomatitis. In that case, papillomavirus-like particles were detected by electron microscopy in a lung wash but not in oral scrapings.[44] Diagnosis of papillomavirus infections has been mostly by detection of viral particles in infected tissues via electron microscopy. The complete sequences of the papillomaviruses of the Loggerhead and Green Sea Turtles have been determined, so future development of a diagnostic PCR is possible.[46] Tissues for analysis should include affected skin. Papillomaviruses do not generally grow well in cell culture, and no reptilian papillomavirus has been isolated. There is no serologic test available for the detection of antibodies against these viruses in chelonians.

Reoviruses

Reoviruses are nonenveloped RNA viruses with a dsRNA genome. There is only a single reported case of reovirus infection in a Spur-thighed Tortoise that was cachectic and had necrosis of the epithelium of the tongue. The virus was isolated from the tongue of that animal, as well as from several internal tissues.[34] A virus neutralization test has been used to detect antibodies against this virus in tortoises.[37]

Paramyxoviruses

PMVs are enveloped, ssRNA viruses. In reptiles, these viruses are most commonly detected in snakes, but they have also been described in lizards and tortoises. Most of the PMVs detected in reptiles so far have been classified in the new genus *Ferlavirus*.[47] In chelonians, PMV infections have been associated with dermatitis in a group of Spur-thighed Tortoises imported into Switzerland from Turkey.[48] In a Hermann's Tortoise and in a Leopard Tortoise, ferlavirus infection was associated with pneumonia. The Leopard Tortoise had been imported into Germany from Kenya several years previously and died with severe respiratory disease (Figure 5-8). A ferlavirus was detected in several internal tissues from that animal but not from the lung.[49] A Hermann's Tortoise is the only case in which a *Ferlavirus* from a tortoise has been isolated in cell culture so far.[50] Diagnosis of ferlavirus infection in tortoises can be carried out with the use of an RT-PCR targeting the L gene of ferlaviruses similar to the process for snakes.[51] This PCR often results in false-positive findings or products that are not the expected size and confirmation of positive results; therefore sequencing of PCR products is strongly

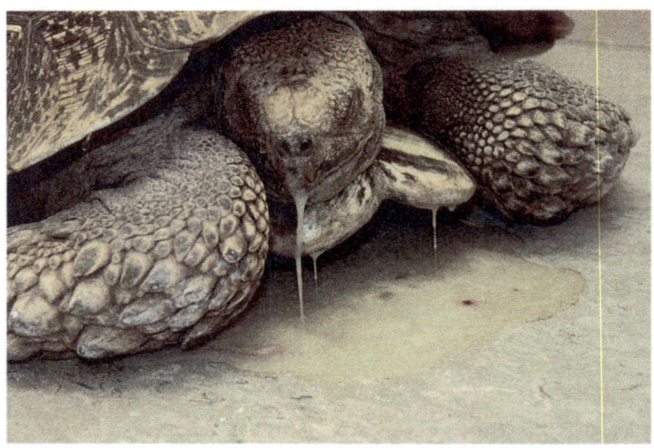

FIGURE 5-8 Leopard tortoise (*Stigmochelys pardalis*) with severe pneumonia. A ferlavirus was detected in this animal. *(From Papp T, Seybold J, Marschang RE. Paramyxovirus infection in a leopard tortoise* [Geochelone pardalis babcocki] *with respiratory disease.* J Herpetol Med Surg *2010;20:64-68. With permission.)*

recommended. Because ferlaviruses cause hemagglutination of chicken red blood cells, antibodies against these viruses in tortoises can be detected by HI assays, just as for snakes. Several different ferlaviruses have been detected in tortoises,[49,50] so the choice of antigen may affect test results. However, a study has indicated that there is significant serologic cross-reactivity between known ferlaviruses.[52]

VIRUSES OF SQUAMATES

A variety of viruses have been described in lizards and snakes. Lizards are not monophyletic, so relationships between some lizards (e.g., iguanids) and snakes are closer than between other lizard families. This is reflected in the relationships between the viruses infecting some of these animals. PMVs are well-known pathogens in viperid snakes but can also be found in other families of snakes as well as in lizards. Both AdVs and reoviruses are regularly detected in lizards and snakes. A list of viruses regularly detected in squamates and methods for diagnostic testing can be found in Table 5-2.

PARAMYXOVIRUSES

PMVs are enveloped viruses with a negative sense ssRNA genome. They are relatively unstable in the environment. Almost all PMVs detected in reptiles are classified in the genus *Ferlavirus*,[47] which contains PMVs detected in snakes, lizards, and chelonians. The ferlaviruses are named after the first PMV isolated from reptiles, Fer-de-Lance vipers in a Swiss serpentarium. During that outbreak in 1972, 87% of the snakes in one room died with dyspnea, opisthotonus, apathy followed by abnormal activity, mydriasis, and terminal convulsions.[53] Since then, ferlavirus outbreaks have been documented in numerous snake collections in North and South America and Europe. Common clinical signs described in infected snakes include abnormal posturing, regurgitation, anorexia, head tremors, abnormal respiratory sounds, and exudate in the oral cavity (Figure 5-9). In many cases, no clinical signs may be noticed, and infected animals may be found dead in their enclosures.[1,53,54] Severe disease has mostly been described in viperid snakes, but ferlaviruses have been found in snakes from the families Boidae, Elapidae, Colubridae, and Crotalidae.[1] Koch's postulates have been fulfilled for pulmonary lesions associated with ferlavirus infection in Aruba Island Rattlesnakes (*Crotalus durissus unicolor*). A ferlavirus isolated from several tissues of an Aruba Island Rattlesnake that died of the infection was inoculated intratracheally into four Aruba Island Rattlesnakes. Several snakes developed pulmonary symptoms including blood in the lungs, trachea, and oral cavity. The two animals that were not euthanized earlier died 19 and 22 days p.i.[55] Gross abnormalities are most consistently found in the lungs of infected snakes. Changes include congestion and hemorrhage. Histologic findings often show proliferative interstitial pulmonary disease with proliferation and vacuolation of epithelial cells lining the faveoli. In rare cases, intracytoplasmic inclusions can be seen in lining epithelial cells.[54,55] Although ferlaviruses are most commonly described in snakes, these viruses have also been detected in several species of lizard, including a Spotted False Monitor (*Callopistes maculatus*),[56] an Emerald Tree Monitor (*Varanus prasinus*),[57] a Flathead Knob-scaled Lizard (*Xenosaurus platyceps*),[58] and a group of Caiman Lizards (*Dracaena guianensis*).[59] Ferlavirus infections in lizards have been associated primarily with pneumonia, although virus infections in clinically healthy lizards have been documented. The viruses do not appear to be host specific, and transmission between different species of snakes and lizards as well as chelonians may be possible. There is no specific treatment available for ferlavirus infection in reptiles. The results of a single study attempting to vaccinate rattlesnakes against ferlavirus infection with the use of an inactivated cell culture isolate were equivocal, in that antibody responses were variable and transient.[60]

A PMV that differs distinctly from the ferlaviruses has recently been described in snakes in Australia. The virus has been preliminarily named Sunshine virus for the geographic location of the first isolation on the Sunshine coast of Australia. This virus was associated with neurorespiratory disease in Australian pythons.[61]

DIAGNOSIS OF PMV INFECTIONS IN SQUAMATES

Virus Detection

Ferlaviruses were first diagnosed in snakes with the use of isolation in cell culture followed by virus characterization.[62] Virus isolation has since been used in many cases to detect these viruses in clinical samples from snakes and lizards. Ferlaviruses can be isolated on Russell's Viper heart cells (VH2, ATCC, CCL-140) at 28°C (82.4°F) (Figure 5-10, *A*). They grow relatively slowly (7 to 14 days) and cause the formation of syncytia (Figure 5-10, *B*). A number of RT-PCRs have also been described for the detection of ferlaviruses in reptiles. The most sensitive test available to date is an RT-PCR targeting the large polymerase (L) gene.[50,51] This gene is relatively well conserved among PMVs, and the primers described for this RT-PCR have been able to detect all of the ferlavirus types detected to date. This RT-PCR can be used to detect ferlaviruses in tissues from dead animals or in samples from live animals. In live animals, oral and cloacal swabs, as well as transtracheal washes, can be used as diagnostic samples. Because oral and cloacal shedding can be inconsistent, it is recommended that a combined sample of both be submitted, possibly combined with fluid from a transtracheal wash for testing.[63] In dead animals, the highest viral load is found in the lung, and this tissue is recommended for testing.[64] The RT-PCR is not highly specific for ferlaviruses, and false-positive reactions have been shown to occur. For this reason, PCR products of the expected size (566 base pairs) should be sequenced.

Sunshine virus has been diagnosed in Australian pythons. It was originally isolated in VH2 from diseased and contact snakes. A PCR has also been described for the detection of this virus and has been used in Australia.[61]

Serology

Antibodies against ferlaviruses can be detected by HI tests. Ferlaviruses agglutinate chicken red blood cells, and antibodies against these viruses in plasma or serum will inhibit this reaction. HI testing has been used repeatedly to detect exposure to ferlaviruses in squamates, including wild-caught snakes and lizards.[54,57,58,65,66] Serologic cross-reactivity among ferlaviruses and between ferlaviruses and other PMVs is not fully understood, and some (but not all) ferlaviruses have been

TABLE 5-2

Diagnostic Methods Used for the Detection of Viruses of Squamates

Virus Family	Virus Genus and Species	Host Species	Diagnostic Samples: Live Animals	Diagnostic Samples: Necropsied Animals	Virus Detection	Serology	References
Paramyxoviridae	*Ferlavirus*	Many different snake and lizard species; most commonly viperid snakes	Oral and cloacal swabs, tracheal washes	Lung and other tissues	PCR, virus isolation	HI	50, 51, 54, 63
	Sunshine virus	Australian pythons (including a Black-headed Python *[Aspidites melanocephalus]* and a Jungle Carpet Python *[Morelia spilota cheynei]*)	n.d.	Brain, lung, liver, kidney	PCR, virus isolation	n.d.	61
Adenoviridae	*Atadenovirus*	Many different species	Cloacal swabs	Liver and intestine	PCR	NT (in snakes)	42, 82, 84
Reoviridae	*Orthoreovirus*	Many different species	Oral and cloacal swabs	Liver, intestine, lung (also other tissues)	PCR, virus isolation	NT	85, 93
Iridoviridae	*Ranavirus*	Green Pythons *(Morelia viridis)*, Leaf-tailed Gecko *(Uroplatus fimbriatus)*, Iberian Rock Lizard *(Lacerta monticola)*	Blood (optimal sample unknown)	Liver	PCR, virus isolation	n.d.	102, 103, 104
	Iridovirus (invertebrate iridoviruses, IIV)	Various lizard species including agamid, chameleonid, and iguanid lizards	Cloacal swab (CAVE – detected virus could originate from infected prey)	Intestine, skin, kidney, liver	PCR, virus isolation	n.d.	110
	Unclassified: Erythrocytic necrosis virus	Numerous species including Iberian Rock Lizard, and Ribbon Snakes *(Thamnophis sauritus sackenii)*	Erythrocytes	Erythrocytes	PCR, (generally diagnosed by histologic examination and EM)	n.d.	104, 113, 115
Herpesviridae	Unclassified	Various snake and lizard species	Gingival biopsy (area of lesion)	Material from lesions	PCR	n.d.	119, 120
Arenaviridae	Unclassified	Annulated Tree Boa *(Corallus annulatus)* and Boa Constrictors *(Boa constrictor)* with IBD	n.d.	Various tissues (brain, gastrointestinal tissue, heart, kidney, liver, lung, serum, blood cells)	PCR	n.d.	128

EM, Electron microscopy; HI, hemagglutination inhibition test; IBD, inclusion body disease; n.d., not described; NT, neutralization test; PCR, polymerase chain reaction.

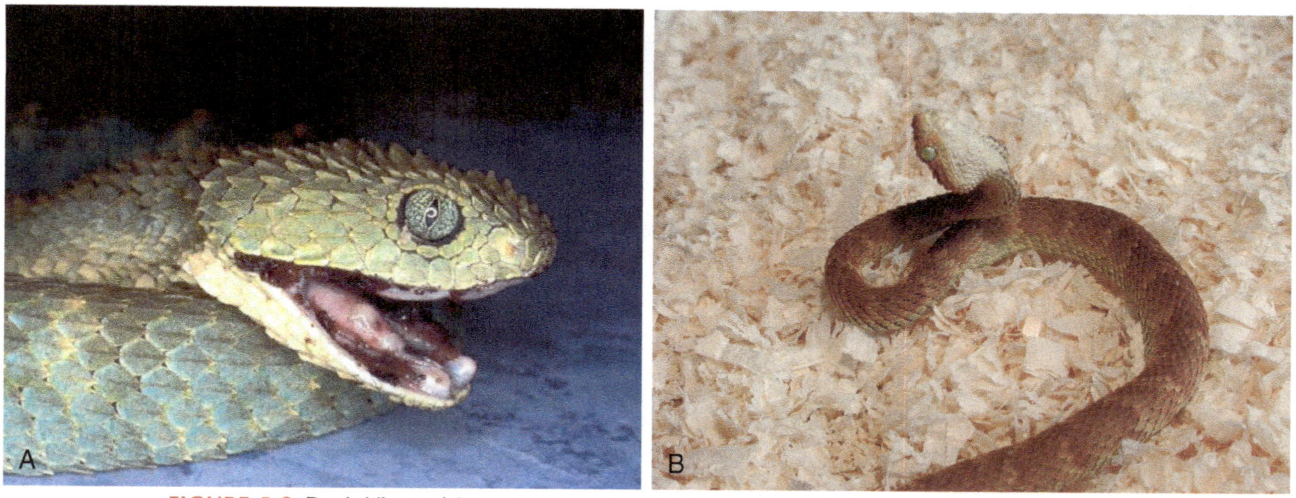

FIGURE 5-9 Bush Vipers (*Atheris squamigera*) infected with ferlaviruses. **A,** Dyspnea and bloody secretions in the oral cavity. **B,** Star gazing. *(Courtesy of Jutta Wiechert.)*

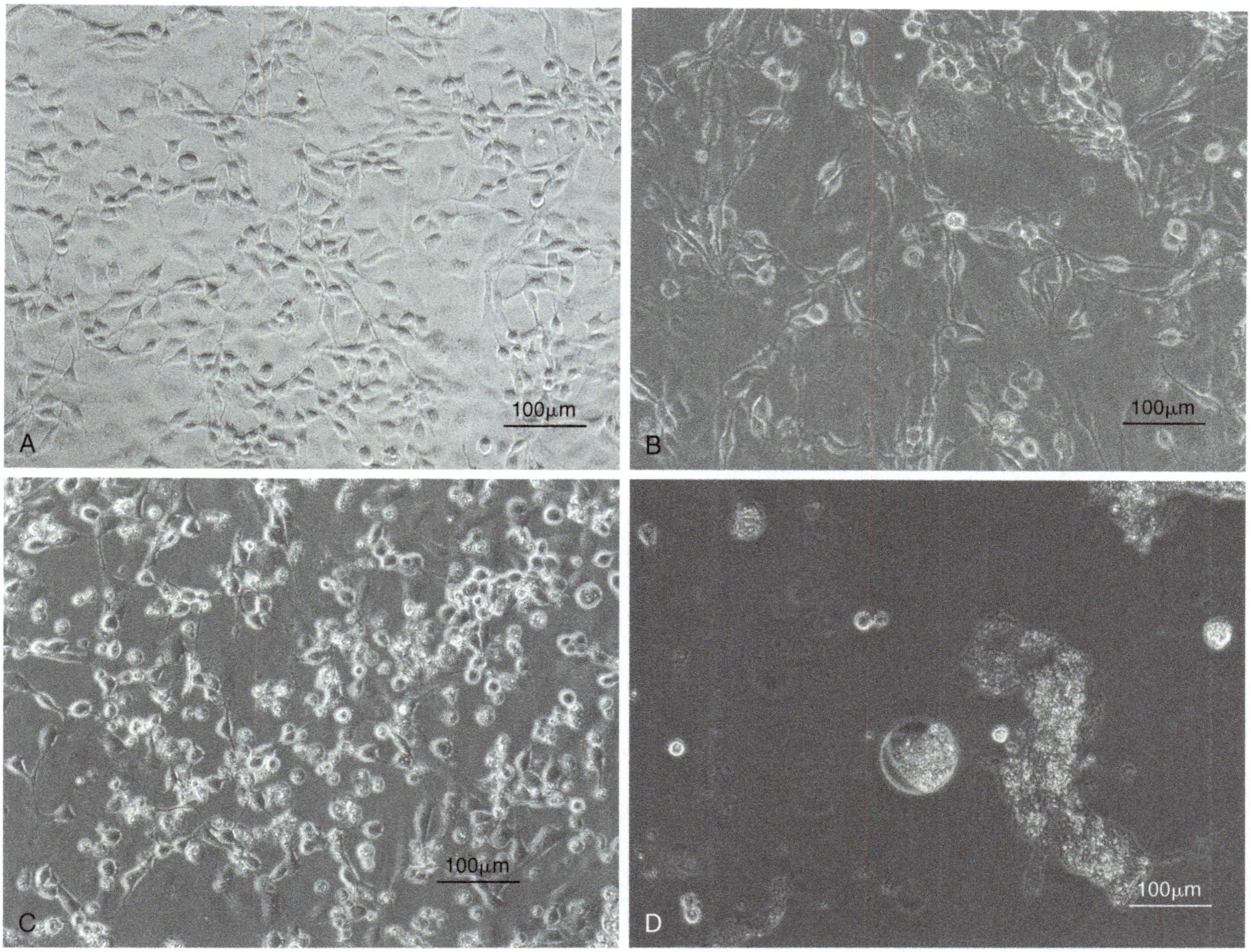

FIGURE 5-10 Isolation of snake viruses in cell culture. **A,** Uninfected viper heart cells (VH2), which are often used for the isolation of viruses from snakes. **B,** VH2 infected with a ferlavirus. This virus causes a cytopathic effect (CPE) with syncytia formation in infected cells. **C,** VH2 infected with an adenovirus isolated from a Boa Constrictor (*Boa constrictor*) (snake adenovirus 1). These viruses cause a CPE with cell lysis and rounding of cells. **D,** VH2 infected with a reovirus isolated from a Boa Constrictor. These viruses cause a CPE with the formation of giant syncytia.

shown to serologically cross-react with some avian PMVs. Cross-reactivity with avian PMV types 1, 3, and 7 have been demonstrated,[67,68] and avian PMV 1 and 7 have been used to screen snake sera for antibodies against PMVs.[65,68] Although serologic cross-reactivity exists between ferlaviruses, there is some indication that testing with different virus isolates will lead to different results. In a study comparing results of HI testing of plasma from Eastern Massasaugas (*Sistrurus catenatus catenatus*) from three different laboratories, different results were obtained from each; thus interpretation of results may be difficult.[69] Detection of anti PMV antibodies in squamates indicates that these animals have been exposed to ferlaviruses or serologically related viruses. Persistence of ferlavirus infection in reptiles has not been recorded, but there is clinical evidence that this may occur. It is not known how long virus replication and shedding may persist after the development of hemagglutination-inhibiting antibodies.

ADENOVIRUSES

AdVs are nonenveloped dsDNA viruses that can survive relatively long in the environment. Many AdVs appear to have coevolved with their hosts. All of the AdVs detected in squamates so far have belonged to the genus *Atadenovirus*, which is believed to have coevolved with reptiles.[70] This can be important in understanding the pathogenicity of the viruses because viruses that have coevolved with their hosts may not cause disease or may only cause disease in immune-suppressed animals or in conjunction with other infectious agents or other factors. In squamates, AdVs are most commonly found in agamids but have also been found in many other lizard and snake families. Clinical signs most commonly associated with AdV infection are gastrointestinal and neurologic, including anorexia, lethargy, wasting, head tilt, opisthotonus, and circling (Figure 5-11).[71-73] In individual cases, stomatitis,[74] dermatitis,[75] and pneumonia[76] have also been described. AdVs have also been detected in animals with no clinical signs of disease.[77-80] Koch's postulates have been fulfilled for an AdV-induced hepatic necrosis in a Boa Constrictor (*Boa constrictor*). In that case, hepatic necrosis was found in an adult boa constrictor that died after displaying regurgitation and a head tilt. An AdV was isolated from the liver and inoculated intracoelomically into a clinically healthy neonatal boa constrictor. The infected snake also developed hepatic necrosis and died, and an AdV was isolated from the liver.[71] Gross pathologic examination of animals that die with AdV infection can involve only the liver, which may be enlarged and have petechia or pale areas scattered throughout. Histologically, these animals generally have hepatic necrosis. The intestine is also frequently affected, and documented changes include dilatation of the duodenum and hyperemia of the mucosa. Basophilic intranuclear inclusions are often seen in hepatocytes and enterocytes,[72,81] (Figure 5-12) as well as in myocardial endothelial cells,[77] renal epithelial cells,[82] endocardium, epithelial cells of the lung,[80] and glial and endothelial cells in the brain.[73]

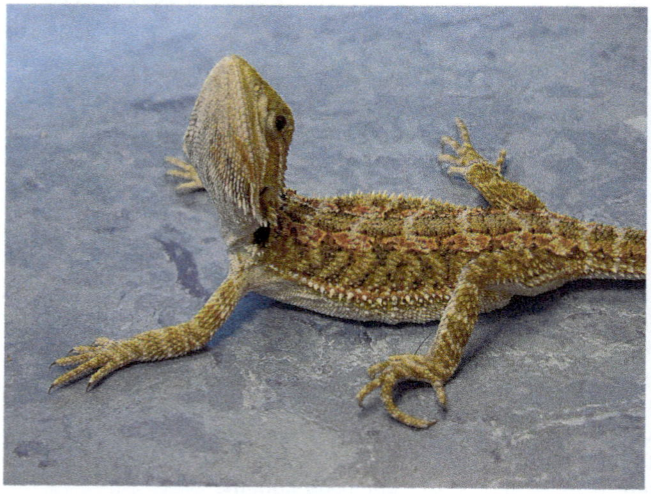

FIGURE 5-11 Bearded Dragon (*Pogona vitticeps*) infected with an adenovirus. This lizard showed neurologic signs including star gazing. *(Courtesy of Jutta Wiechert.)*

DIAGNOSIS OF ADENOVIRUSES IN SQUAMATES

Virus Detection

The most common, rapid, and sensitive method for the detection of AdVs in squamates is a PCR targeting the DNA polymerase gene.[42] This is a nested PCR technique using degenerate primers to target this highly conserved region of the viral genome. It has been used on a wide range of samples[83] and can detect not only AdVs of the genus *Atadenovirus*, which infect squamates, but also other AdVs. The PCR products can be directly sequenced, which is recommended because this PCR can also detect AdVs of prey animals.[84] Recommended samples for the detection of AdVs in lizards and snakes are cloacal swabs from live animals (Figure 5-13) and liver and intestine from dead animals. In some cases, AdVs can also be isolated from swabs or tissues in cell culture. To date, AdVs have almost exclusively been isolated from snakes[71,76,79,85,86] (see Figure 5-10, *C*), and two isolates have been obtained from helodermatid lizards.[83] These AdVs have been isolated on VH2 or iguana heart cells (IgH2, ATCC CCL-108). Isolation in cell

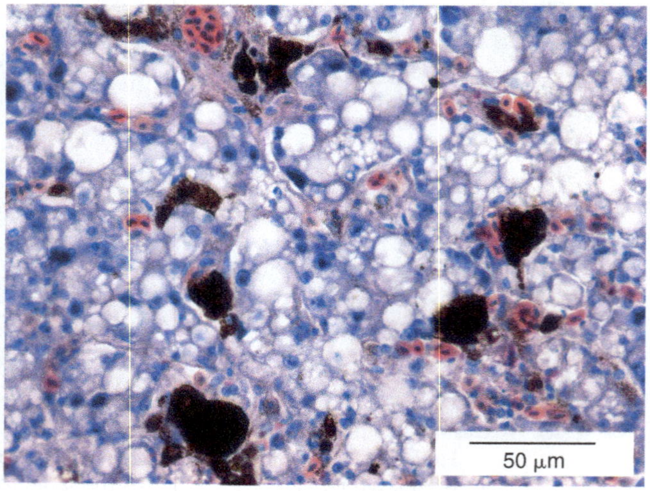

FIGURE 5-12 Bearded Dragon (*Pogona vitticeps*) infected with an adenovirus. Photomicrograph of the liver. Intranuclear inclusion bodies are visible in several cells. H&E stain. *(Photo courtesy Dr. Volker Schmidt, Universität Leipzig, Leipzig, Germany.)*

culture is generally slower and less sensitive than PCR. No AdVs have been isolated from nonhelodermatid lizards.

Serology

Little work has been done on the detection of antibodies against AdVs in reptiles. This is mostly due to the lack of virus isolates in cell culture, which makes the development of serologic tests difficult. Virus neutralization testing has been used for the detection of antibodies against a snake AdV (SAdV-1).[85,87] However, little is known about the serologic relationships among reptilian atadenoviruses. The main antigenic components of the AdVs are the fiber, hexon, and penton proteins that make up the icosahedral capsids of the virions.[70] The structures of these proteins vary between the different AdVs, and one study demonstrated genotypic differences in the hexon gene of agamid AdVs from captive Bearded Dragons *(Pogona vitticeps)* in the United States.[88] Serologic cross-reactivity between these different types is unknown. Because AdVs of different families of lizards appear to differ significantly on a genetic level, they may also differ serologically. Interestingly, there appears to be much less variation between snake AdVs, and the majority appear to be identical; thus the use of virus neutralization testing for the detection of antibodies against AdVs in snakes is possible.

REOVIRUSES

Reoviruses are nonenveloped viruses with a dsRNA genome that is segmented. They are quite stable in the environment. All reoviruses detected in reptiles so far have belonged to the genus *Orthoreovirus*. Reoviruses are frequently detected in both snakes and lizards. Clinically, reovirus infections have been associated with a wide range of clinical signs in squamates, ranging from sudden death to virus detection in apparently healthy animals. Specific clinical signs observed in infected animals have included papillomas in Green Lizards *(Lacerta viridis)*,[89] sudden death in Iguanas *(Iguana iguana)*,[90] pneumonia in a Spiny-tailed Lizard *(Uromastyx hardwickii)*,[91] enteropathy and hepatopathy in Leopard Geckos *(Eublepharis macularius)*,[92] enteritis in Chinese vipers *(Azemiops feae)*,[1] neurologic disease including incoordination, loss of proprioception, and convulsions in Prairie Rattlesnakes *(Crotalus viridis)*,[93] necrotizing hepatitis in Rough Green Snakes *(Opheodrys aestivus)*,[94] and fatal respiratory disease in Moellendorff's Ratsnakes *(Orthriophis moellendorffi)* and Beauty Ratsnakes *(Orthriophis taeniurus)*.[95] The reovirus isolated from that outbreak was inoculated intratracheally into a Black Ratsnake *(Pantherophis obsoletus obsoletus)*, which consequently died with pneumonia 26 days p.i. A reovirus was reisolated from the experimentally infected snake. In another transmission study, a reovirus that was isolated from a Boa Constrictor with inclusion body disease (IBD) was inoculated into two different groups of Boa Constrictors intratracheally, intracoelomically, and per os. No specific disease or pathology was observed in the infected animals, although virus was reisolated from the infected snakes up to 18 weeks p.i.[96] The clinical significance of reovirus infections is therefore not fully understood and may depend on the virus and the host, as well as other factors such as immune status, husbandry, and other infectious agents. Some genetic variation has been detected in reptilian reoviruses. These viruses do not appear to be species specific because related viruses have been found in various families of squamates and in a tortoise.[97,98]

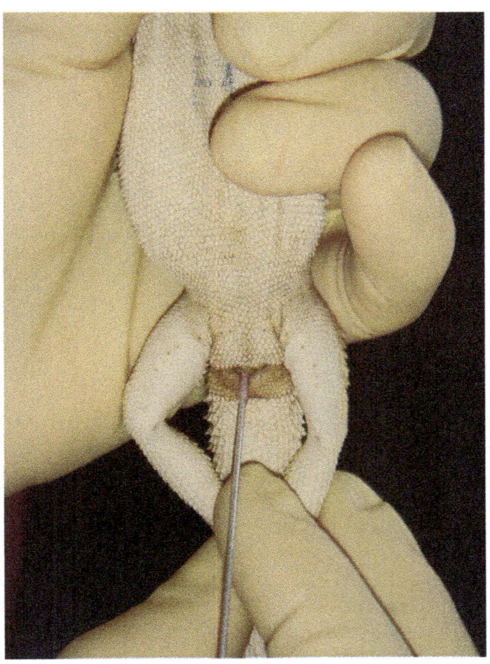

FIGURE 5-13 Bearded Dragon (*Pogona vitticeps*). Cloacal swabs are recommended for the diagnosis of adenovirus infections in live animals.

DIAGNOSIS OF REOVIRUSES IN SQUAMATES

Virus Detection

Reoviruses of squamates are relatively easily isolated in cell culture (VH2 and IgH2), in which they cause the formation of giant syncytia (see Figure 5-10, *D*). Virus has been isolated from oral and cloacal swabs from live snakes[86] and from liver, kidney, spleen, intestine, brain, and lung[86,90,92,93,95,99] of dead animals. An RT-PCR targeting the RNA-dependent RNA polymerase gene of *Orthoreovirus* and *Aquareovirus* has been described and used to characterize reoviruses isolated from various reptiles.[97,98] This RT-PCR has also been used to diagnose reovirus infections in tissues of infected snakes[94] but appears to be less sensitive than virus isolation in cell culture.[86]

Serology

Virus neutralization tests have been used to detect antibodies against reoviruses in snakes and lizards, and antibodies against reoviruses have been detected in wild-caught Green Iguanas, Utila Iguanas *(Ctenosaura bakeri)*, Spiny-tailed Iguanas *(C. similis)*, and Knob-scaled Lizards *(Xenosaurus grandis)*.[57,58] A study of the serologic cross-reactivity of six different reovirus isolates from lizards showed that at least three different serogroups exist; thus results of testing for antibodies using a virus neutralization test will depend on the virus used.[90]

IRIDOVIRUSES

The iridoviruses are large, dsDNA viruses that contain a lipid component. The family *Iridoviridae* is currently divided into five genera: *Iridovirus, Chloriridovirus, Ranavirus, Lymphocystivirus,* and *Megalocytivirus*.[100] Until recently, viruses of the genera *Iridovirus* and *Chloriridovirus* had only been described in invertebrates, whereas viruses of the genus *Ranavirus* have infected fish, amphibians, and reptiles. Viruses of the genera *Lymphocystivirus* and *Megalocytivirus* are found only in fish. The iridoviruses that have been described in squamates can be classified as ranaviruses, invertebrate iridoviruses, and erythrocytic viruses.

RANAVIRUSES

Members of the genus *Ranavirus* are common pathogens of amphibians, reptiles, and fish[101] and are one of the major causes of global amphibian die-offs.[102] In reptiles, ranaviruses have most commonly been detected in various chelonian species; however, squamates can also be infected, and ranaviruses have been found in Green Pythons *(Morelia viridis)* in Australia,[103] in a gecko *(Uroplatus fimbriatus)* in Germany,[104] and in an Iberian Rock Lizard *(Lacerta monticola)* in Portugal.[105] The Green Pythons showed ulceration of the nasal mucosa, hepatic necrosis, and severe necrotizing inflammation of the pharyngeal submucosa. In the gecko, infection was associated with granulomatous lesions in the tail and the liver. In the Iberian Rock Lizard, no overt disease was documented. That lizard had a high number of intracytoplasmic inclusion bodies in the erythrocytes, indicative of infection with an erythrocytic necrosis virus, which was also detected by PCR.

DIAGNOSIS OF RANAVIRUS INFECTION IN SQUAMATES

Ranaviruses infecting reptiles appear to be closely related to one another and to ranaviruses of amphibians. Methods for virus detection in squamates are identical to those described for virus detection in chelonians. Ranaviruses can be isolated in many different cell lines at 28°C (82.4°F) (see Figure 5-4, *C*). All published squamate ranaviruses have been detected with the use of virus isolation in cell culture. A number of PCRs are also available for the detection of ranaviruses in other animals. The highly conserved MCP gene is often targeted, and sequencing of a portion of this gene has been used to help identify and partially characterize all ranaviruses detected in snakes and lizards so far.[103-105] Samples for ranavirus detection in squamates should include liver tissue. A ranavirus has only been detected in a live lizard once, in the blood of the Portuguese Rock Lizard.[105] The optimal sample for the detection of ranaviruses in live squamates is unknown. No serologic test is available for the detection of antibodies against ranaviruses in squamates.

INVERTEBRATE IRIDOVIRUSES

Until recently, viruses of the genus *Iridovirus* had only been described in invertebrates, in which they can cause lethal infections in a wide range of host species.[106] At the end of the 1990s two research groups in Germany isolated and characterized iridoviruses from crickets (Orthoptera, Gryllidae) of the species *Gryllus campestris, Acheta domesticus,* and *Gryllus bimaculatus*.[107,108] In both cases, the insects derived from commercial breeders that produced crickets for the pet trade. Infected crickets showed hypertrophy and bluish iridescence of the affected fat body cells.[108,109]

Closely related or identical viruses have been detected in various lizard species in Europe. In 2001 a German group reported the isolation of invertebrate iridovirus (IIV)-like viruses from the lung, liver, kidney, and intestine of two Bearded Dragons, a chameleon *(Trioceros quadricornis)*, and from the skin of a Frill-necked Lizard *(Chlamydosaurus kingii)*. The Frill-necked Lizard showed poxlike skin lesions, and one of the Bearded Dragons had pneumonia. The other lizards had died with nonspecific clinical signs.[110] Since then, IIVs have been isolated or detected repeatedly in lizards from various sources, as well as from crickets (Marschang RE, unpublished observations, 2001-2013). It has been postulated that this virus has switched hosts from prey insects to the predator lizards, and a transmission study was able to demonstrate that an IIV isolated from a High-casqued Chameleon *(Trioceros hoehnelii)* was able to infect and cause disease in crickets *(Gryllus bimaculatus)*.[111] The clinical significance of IIV infection in lizards is not always clear because virus has been detected in clinically healthy animals, as well as in animals that were emaciated, had skin lesions (Figure 5-14), or died immediately. In some cases,

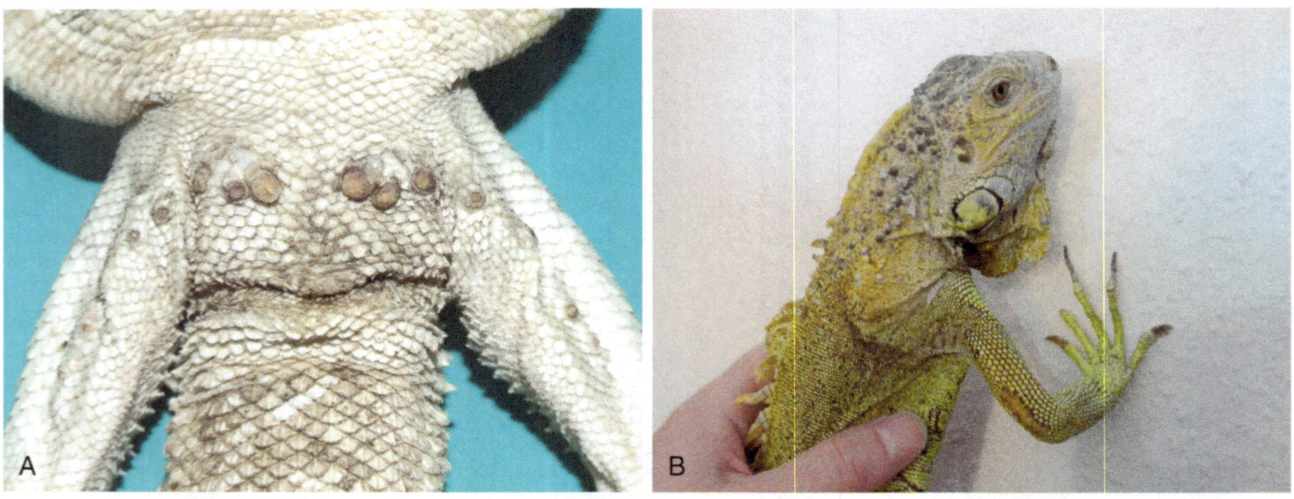

FIGURE 5-14 Invertebrate iridovirus (IIV) infections are often associated with skin lesions in infected lizards. **A,** Enlarged femoral pores in a Bearded Dragon (*Pogona vitticeps*) infected with an IIV. **B,** Skin lesion on upper right arm and loss of dorsal scales in a Green Iguana (*Iguana iguana*) infected with an IIV. *(**A,** Photo courtesy Dr. Karina Mathes, University of Veterinary Medicine Hannover, Germany.)*

other viruses have also been detected in infected lizards, especially AdVs, such that IIVs may be involved in multifactorial disease or they may be incidental.

DETECTION OF INVERTEBRATE IRIDOVIRUSES IN SQUAMATES

A number of methods have been developed for the detection of IIVs in lizards. These viruses grow well in a wide range of cell lines at 28°C (82.4°F), including cell lines from reptiles (e.g., TH1, VH2, and IgH2). Two different PCRs have been described for the detection of IIVs in samples from reptiles. Both target the highly conserved MCP gene. A nested PCR has been shown to be the most sensitive method described.[111] All of the methods used to detect IIV in samples from reptiles can also be used to detect these viruses in feed insects. In live lizards, IIVs are most commonly found in oral and cloacal swabs. However, because feed insects can be infected, detection of IIVs in these samples should be interpreted carefully: positive findings may represent contamination and not infection. In dead lizards, IIVs have most commonly been detected in intestines and skin. Again, interpretation of findings may be difficult. However, IIVs have also been detected in a number of internal tissues including kidney and liver. IIVs are often detected together with other infectious agents, particularly AdVs in agamids, and their clinical significance in infected lizards is not always clear.

ERYTHROCYTIC NECROSIS VIRUSES

Erythrocytic necrosis viruses cause intracytoplasmic inclusions in erythrocytes of fish, amphibians, and reptiles. These inclusions were originally believed to be parasites, but subsequently electron microscopy demonstrated crystalline arrays of virions.[112,113] Infected erythrocytes may show morphologic changes, and infected animals may be anemic. A transmission study has been carried out with blood from infected Iberian Rock Lizards and Iberian Emerald Lizards (*Lacerta schreiberi*) injected into uninfected lizards. The experimentally infected lizards developed intraerythrocytic inclusions. When lizards were kept at relatively low temperatures, the infection became systemic and resulted in death.[114] Erythrocytic necrosis viruses have been detected in wild-caught lizards and snakes worldwide.[105,115,116] No erythrocytic necrosis virus has been isolated in cell culture so far. Further characterization of these viruses has therefore been difficult. Partial sequences of the DNA polymerase gene are available from two erythrocytic necrosis viruses: one from a Ribbon Snake (*Thamnophis sauritus sackenii*) in Florida, United States, and one from an Iberian Rock Lizard in Portugal.[105,116] Both viruses have been shown to be related to viruses of the family *Iridoviridae* but may belong to a new genus. Infection with erythrocytic necrosis virus is currently diagnosed by the detection of intracytoplasmic inclusions in blood smears of infected animals, followed by electron microscopy and detection of virions with typical iridoviral morphology (Figure 5-15). Now that sequence information is available from two erythrocytic necrosis viruses, it may become possible to develop a diagnostic PCR for the detection of these viruses in reptiles.

HERPESVIRUSES

In snakes, reports of HV infection are rare and have been associated with decreased venom production in some venomous species, hepatic necrosis in juvenile Boa Constrictors, and gastrointestinal disease with mixed infections in several

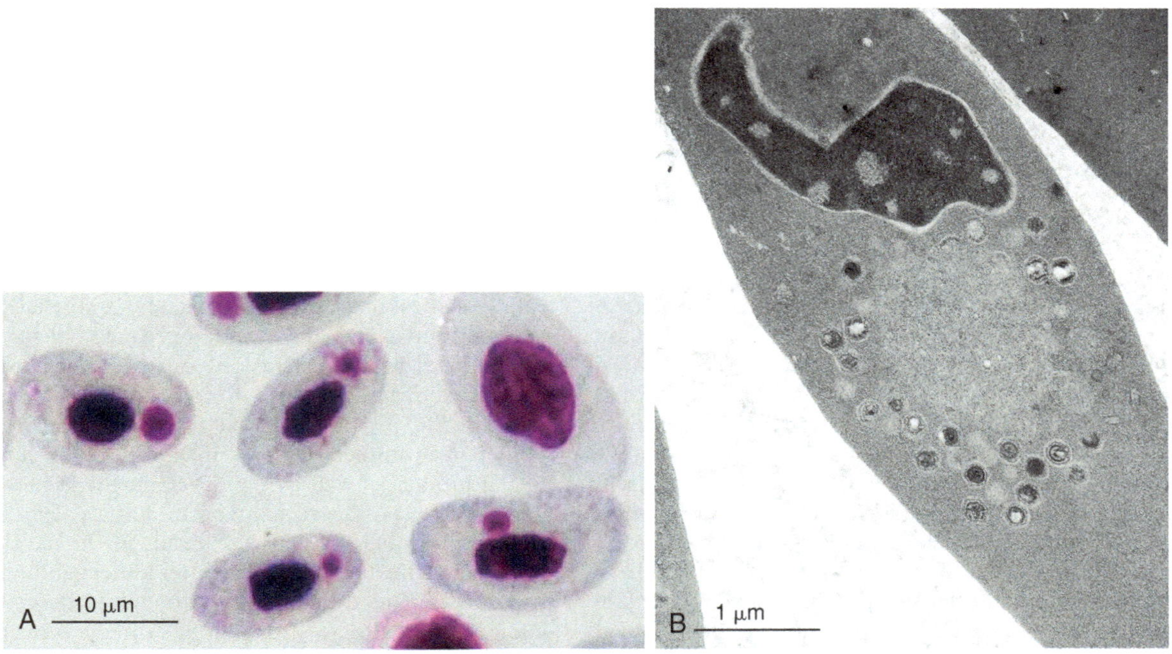

FIGURE 5-15 Iberian Rock Lizard *(Lacerta monticola)* erythrocytes with erythrocytic virus infection. **A,** Erythrocytic necrosis virus has caused intracytoplasmic inclusions in multiple erythrocytes. H&E stain. **B,** Transmission electron photomicrograph of the inclusion in an erythrocyte. The inclusions consist of viral precursors and viral particles in a crystalline array. *(**A** and **B**, Photo courtesy Antonio Pedro Alves de Matos, Curry Cabral Hospital, Lisbon, Portugal.)*

different snake species.[74,117,118] In lizards, HV infections have been associated with papillomas in Green Lizards.[89,119] Oral lesions have been described in Emerald Tree Monitor Lizards and Sudan and Black-lined Plated Lizards (*Gerrhosaurus major* and *Gerrhosaurus nigrolineatus*) infected with HVs,[120,121] and hepatic lesions have been described in Red-headed Agamas (*Agama agama*) and a San Esteban Chuckwalla (*Sauromalus varius*).[122,123] Diagnosis of HV infection in squamates has been carried out by electron microscopy, virus isolation in cell culture (in one case), and PCR. The PCR used was described for the detection of a wide range of HVs and is also used for the detection of HVs in chelonians.[124] No assay is currently available for the detection of antibodies against HVs in squamates.

INCLUSION BODY DISEASE

IBD is a disease of snakes of the families Boidae and Pythonidae that has been described worldwide in captive snakes. It is considered the most important worldwide disease of boid snakes.[125] The disease is characterized by the formation of intracytoplasmic inclusions in neurons and in epithelial cells of various organs. The etiology of IBD is unknown. It is believed to be a viral disease, but no etiologic agent has been definitively characterized yet. Retroviruses have been discussed as a possible cause of the disease.[126,127] Most recently, arenaviruses have been detected in IBD-positive snakes.[128] In that study, genetically variable arenaviruses were detected in 6 of 8 tested IBD-positive snakes and in none of 18 IBD-negative snakes. Viruses were detected by RT-PCR after sequencing of the genomes of two different viruses by metagenomics. They were also propagated in a cell line derived from the kidney of a Boa Constrictor.[128] The inclusions are made up of a unique protein (inclusion body disease protein, IBDP).[129] Some research into understanding the disease and the development of new diagnostic assays has focused on this protein, and monoclonal antibodies against IBDP have been produced.[125] IBD was originally most commonly detected in Burmese Pythons (*Python bivittatus*) but is now most commonly diagnosed in Boa Constrictors.[1] The host range also includes the Green Anaconda (*Eunectes murinus*), Yellow Anaconda (*Eunectes notaeus*), Rainbow Boa (*Epicrates cenchria*), Haitian Boa (*Epicrates striatus*), Madagascan Boa (*Acrantophis madagascariensis*), Annulated Tree Boa (*Corallus annulatus*), Indian Python (*P. molurus molurus*), Reticulated Python (*P. reticulatus*), and Ball Python (*P. regius*).[125,128] Clinical signs associated with IBD are variable and can range from subclinical carriers to severe neurologic disease and death. Common signs in infected Boa Constrictors include torticollis, disequilibrium, opisthotonus, inability to right itself, regurgitation, and flaccid paralysis (Figure 5-16). Other signs that may also be observed include stomatitis and pneumonia. Lymphoproliferative disorders and round cell tumors have also been described in infected snakes. Some snakes with IBD may die within weeks, but others may survive for extended periods of time. Diagnosis of IBD currently relies on the detection of typical eosinophilic to amphophilic intracytoplasmic inclusions in hematoxylin and eosin–stained tissue sections. In pythons, inclusions are most commonly found in neurons within the central nervous system. In Boa Constrictors, they can also be found in glial cells as well as in cells in the "esophageal tonsils," hepatocytes, pancreatic acinar cells, renal tubular epithelial cells, and epithelial cells lining the gastrointestinal and respiratory tracts (Figure 5-17).[125] In live boid snakes, inclusions can be detected in biopsies of the "esophageal tonsils," liver, and kidney. They can also be found in peripheral blood cells. The development of a monoclonal antibody against IBDP will allow further study of the protein as well as the development of more sensitive diagnostic tests. The recent detection of arenaviruses as possible etiologic agents may also result in the development of new diagnostic methods and a better understanding of disease transmission and development, although further study on the etiologic role of these viruses in this disease is needed.

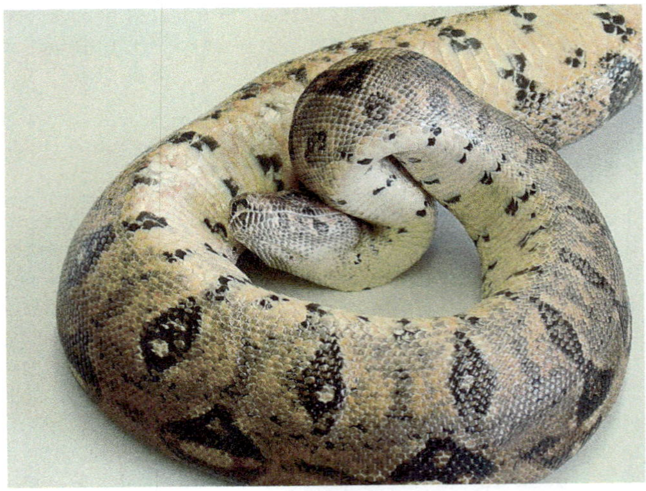

FIGURE 5-16 Boa Constrictor (*Boa constrictor*) with inclusion body disease (IBD). This snake was unable to right itself when placed in dorsal recumbency.

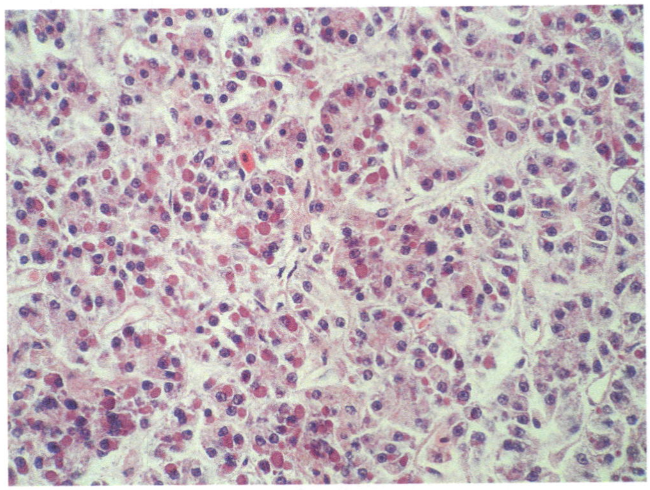

FIGURE 5-17 Boa Constrictor (*Boa constrictor*), inclusion body disease (IBD). Pancreas with multiple intracytoplasmic inclusion bodies. H&E stain, × 400. *(Photo courtesy Dr. Volker Schmidt, Universität Leipzig, Leipzig, Germany.)*

VIRUSES OF CROCODILIANS

Relatively little work has been done on viruses of crocodilians. There are, however, a number of viruses that have been shown to be important pathogens in this group of

TABLE 5-3

Diagnostic Methods Used for the Detection of Viruses of Crocodilians

Virus Family	Virus Genus and Species	Host Species	Diagnostic Samples: Live Animals	Diagnostic Samples: Necropsied Animals	Virus Detection	Serology	References
Poxviridae	Unclassified: Caiman pox virus	*Caiman crocodilus*	Skin lesions	Skin lesions	Histology and EM	n.d.	128, 130
	"Crocodylipoxvirus": Crocodilepox virus (CRV)	*Crocodylus* spp.	Skin lesions	Skin lesions	Histology and EM, PCR	n.d.	1, 134
Flaviviridae	*Flavivirus*: West Nile virus	*Alligator mississippiensis, Crocodylus niloticus*	Blood, serum, cloacal swabs	Liver, lung, blood	RT-PCR, virus isolation	NT, ELISA	139, 141, 144, 146

ELISA, enzyme-linked immunosorbent assay; n.d., not described; NT, neutralization test; PCR, polymerase chain reaction; RT-PCR, reverse-transcriptase PCR.

animals. The viruses most commonly reported in crocodilian species are poxviruses, which can cause outbreaks with skin lesions in captive caimans, crocodiles, and alligators. West Nile virus (WNV) has been shown to be pathogenic in crocodilians and can lead to high mortality rates in infected groups. This virus is also zoonotic, and it is possible for humans to become infected by close contact with infected crocodilians. A list of viruses regularly detected in crocodilians and methods for diagnostic testing can be found in Table 5-3.

POXVIRUSES

Poxviruses are large enveloped dsDNA viruses. Although they are enveloped and therefore should be relatively easy to disinfect, these viruses are often protected in the environment by sloughed skin cells. In this way they can persist for long periods of time, and it can therefore be challenging to fully decontaminate premises. Poxviruses are well-documented pathogens in crocodilians and have been associated with skin lesions in various species around the world. They were first reported associated with gray-white skin lesions over various parts of the body in captive Common Caimans (*Caiman crocodilus*) (Figure 5-18) in the United States[130] and have since been reported in this species in various other parts of the world.[131,132] Poxviruses have also been detected in Nile Crocodiles (*Crocodylus niloticus,*) as well as Saltwater Crocodiles (*Crocodylus porosus*) and Freshwater Crocodiles (*Crocodylus johnsoni*) in Australia.[133] Infected animals develop brownish wartlike skin lesions that can occur over the entire body (Figure 5-19). Infection is associated with high morbidity but low mortality.[134,135] Deeply penetrating skin lesions have also been described in infected crocodiles in Africa.[136] Poxvirus infection in crocodilians has generally been diagnosed on the basis of the detection of intracytoplasmic inclusions in hypertrophic epithelial cells followed by electron microscopic demonstration of viral particles within these inclusions or by electron microscopic detection of viral particles in unfixed scrapings from lesions.[1,136] After the determination of the entire genome sequence of a poxvirus from a Nile Crocodile (crocodilepox virus, CRV),[137] Huchzermeyer and colleagues[136]developed a PCR for the detection of this virus in scrapings from fresh lesions.

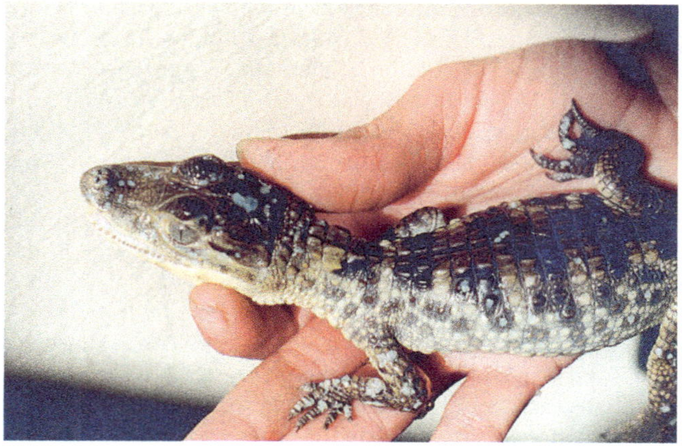

FIGURE 5-18 Caiman (*Caiman crocodilus*) with poxvirus infection. The skin lesions are covered with a white-gray crust. *(Photo courtesy Dr. Fritz W. Huchzermeyer, University of Pretoria, Onderstepoort, South Africa.)*

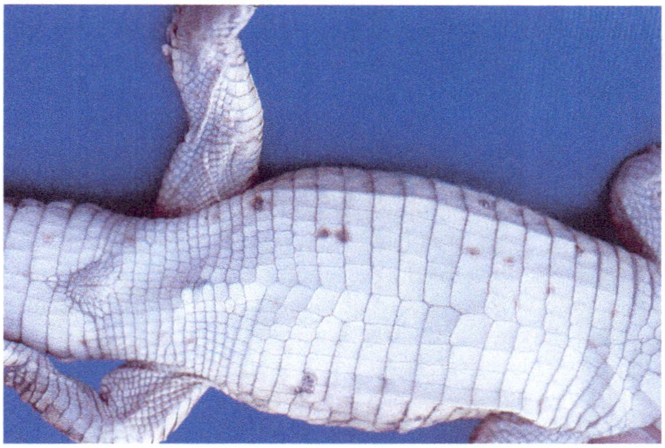

FIGURE 5-19 Nile crocodile (*Crocodylus niloticus*) infected with crocodile pox virus. Brownish lesions are seen on the abdominal skin. *(Photo courtesy Dr. Fritz W. Huchzermeyer, University of Pretoria, Onderstepoort, South Africa.)*

WEST NILE VIRUS

WNV is a mosquito-borne flavivirus (*Flaviviridae*) that can infect various species of mammals (including humans), birds, and reptiles. It primarily cycles between mosquitoes and birds, and other vertebrates are considered incidental hosts. WNV was first detected in Uganda in 1937. It is currently endemic in Africa, Europe, the Middle East, Asia, and North and Central America. It was first documented in North America in 1999, and epidemics caused by WNV have increased in southern Europe in recent years.[138,139] A number of arboviruses including WNV and other flaviviruses have been shown to be capable of infecting and causing viremia in different reptilian species. Most of these infections are not associated with disease. In crocodilians, however, WNV can lead not only to high titer viremias with potential for amplification and transmission to other animals but also to disease and death of the host. WNV infections in crocodilians, including American Alligators (*Alligator mississippiensis*) and Nile Crocodiles, have been reported in various states in the United States, Mexico, and Israel.[140-144] In some cases, these infections were associated with disease outbreaks on infected farms. Affected animals developed neurologic signs including anorexia, tremors, neck spasms, swimming on their sides, loss of leg control, spinning in the water, and opisthotonus. Oral lesions (stomatitis) were also noted. Death occurred 24 to 48 hours after the appearance of clinical signs. Juvenile alligators were most often affected.[140,141] WNV infection has also been associated with lymphohistiocytic proliferative cutaneous lesions in American Alligators. Lesions in infected animals were round to ovoid and restricted to the superficial dermis. The lesions were composed of large numbers of lymphocytes and macrophages. No virus was detectable in the lesions, but animals with lesions consistently tested positive for antibodies against WNV, and WNV RNA was detected in almost all skin and liver–brain samples tested.[145] Infection of crocodilians can occur by bite from infected mosquitoes, orally by consumption of contaminated meat (e.g., infected horses), and by contact with viremic tankmates.[141,146] The development and duration of viremia are dependent on ambient temperature.[146] Detection of WNV can be performed with the use of serum or whole blood in infected crocodilians. Viremic alligators have also been shown to shed virus via the cloaca, and cloacal swabs can be used to detect virus in some of these animals.[146] In dead animals, virus can be detected in a number of tissues including liver, lung, and blood. Liver has been shown to have the highest titers and yield the most positive results in American Alligators. Spinal cord and brain were found to be less often positive.[140,141] Virus detection has been carried out by isolation in cell culture (e.g., Vero cells) or by detection of viral RNA using RT-PCR. A number of RT-PCR protocols have been described for the detection of WNV RNA in various animals. WNV is currently grouped into five different lineages, and the choice of RT-PCR will affect which lineages can be detected. Lineage 1 is found in North America, southern Europe, Asia, and Africa, whereas lineage 2 is found in southern Africa and has recently also been found in Europe. Two real-time quantitative PCRs have been described for the combined detection of both lineages but have not been tested with crocodilian samples.[147] Antibodies against WNV can be detected in serum of infected crocodilians. In a transmission study with American Alligators, antibodies were detected within 25 days of virus detection in infected animals. Methods used for the detection of anti WNV antibodies have included a plaque reduction assay for the detection of neutralizing antibodies and an ELISA. The use of the plaque reduction assay is somewhat limited because it requires live virus and must therefore be carried out in a biosafety level 3 laboratory. An ELISA has been developed for the specific detection of antibodies against WNV in alligators.[148] In Europe, a competitive ELISA has been used for the detection of antibodies against WNV in many different mammalian and avian species (ID Screen West Nile Competition, ID VET, Montpellier, France) but has not been validated for use with reptilian samples. Antibodies against WNV can cross-react with antibodies against other related flaviviruses.

TREATMENT AND PROPHYLAXIS OF VIRAL DISEASE IN REPTILES

Treatment options for viral disease in reptiles remain severely limited, and little is known about the pharmacokinetics of antiviral substances available for mammalian species. Antivirals are therefore seldom used in reptile medicine. A possible exception is the use of acyclovir for the treatment of herpesviral disease in tortoises. However, dose, treatment schedule, and duration have not been sufficiently studied. Another approach that has been propagated for treatment of virus infection in reptiles is the use of immunomodulators, for example, Zylexis (Pfizer AG, Zurich, Switzerland), particularly in HV-infected tortoises. This approach is also experimental, and data on its effectiveness are lacking. Because many viral diseases of reptiles appear to be influenced by additional factors including husbandry and other infectious agents, optimization of conditions and treatment of other agents involved (e.g., bacteria and/or parasites) is warranted. Prophylactic measures should include an appropriate quarantine procedure, diagnostic testing, and barrier nursing of infected and contact animals. The length of quarantine is controversial and should depend on the reptile species involved. In species that brumate, a brumation period should be included in the quarantine period. Species should not be mixed during quarantine because any mixing of species can lead to transmission of infectious agents to more susceptible species. Appropriate disinfection protocols before and after quarantine are essential. Appropriate quarantine procedures may not protect a collection from the introduction of all infectious agents, especially agents that can persistently infect clinically healthy animals (e.g., HVs in some species of tortoises) or that are difficult to detect and have very long incubation periods (e.g., IBD in snakes). No vaccines are currently available for any of the viral diseases of reptiles.

REFERENCES

1. Jacobson ER. Viruses and viral diseases of reptiles. In: Jacobson ER, ed. *Infectious diseases and pathology of reptiles*. Boca Raton, Fla: CRC Press, Taylor and Francis Group, 2007;395-460.
2. Marschang RE. Viruses infecting reptiles. *Viruses* 2011;3:2087-2126.
3. Cox WR, Rapley WA, Barker IK. Herpesvirus-like infection in a painted turtle (*Chrysemys picta*). *J Wildl Dis* 1980;16:445-449.
4. Frye FL, Oshiro LS, Dutra FR, et al. Herpesvirus-like infection in two Pacific pond turtles. *J Am Vet Med A* 1977;171:882-884.
5. Jacobson ER, Gaskin GM, Wahlquist H. Herpesvirus-like infection in map turtles. *J Am Vet Med Assoc* 1982;181:1322-1324.
6. Rebel G, Rywlin A, Haines H. A herpesvirus agent associated with skin lesions of green sea turtles in aquaculture. *Am J Vet Res* 1975;36:1221-1224.
7. Jacobson ER, Gaskin JM, Roelke M, et al. Conjunctivitis, tracheitis, and pneumonia associated with herpesvirus infection in green sea turtles. *J Am Vet Med Assoc* 1986;189:1020-1023.

8. Stacy BA, Wellehan JFX, Foley AM, et al. Two herpesviruses associated with disease in wild Atlantic loggerhead sea turtles *(Caretta caretta)*. *Vet Microbiol* 2008;126:63-73.
9. Herbst LH, Jacobson ER, Moretti R, et al. Experimental transmission of green turtles fibropapillomatosis using cell-free tumor extracts. *Dis Aquat Organ* 1995;22:1-12.
10. McArthur S, Blahak S, Kölle P, et al. Roundtable: Chelonian herpesviruses. *J Herpetol Med Surg* 2002;12:14-31.
11. Une Y, Uemura K, Nakano Y, et al. Herpesvirus infection in tortoises *(Malacochersus tornieri* and *Testudo horsfieldii)*. *Vet Pathol* 1999;36:624-627.
12. Johnson AJ, Pessier AP, Wellehan JFX, et al. Identification of a novel herpesvirus from a California desert tortoise *(Gopherus agassizii)*. *Vet Microbiol* 2005;111:107-116.
13. Marschang RE, Gleiser CB, Papp T, et al. Comparison of eleven herpesvirus isolates from tortoises using partial sequences from three conserved genes. *Vet Microbiol* 2006;117:258-266.
14. Bicknese EJ, Childress AL, Wellehan JF Jr. A novel herpesvirus of the proposed genus *Chelonivirus* from an asymptomatic bowsprit tortoise *(Chersina angulata)*. *J Zoo Wildl Med* 2010;41:353-358.
15. Quackenbush SL, Work TM, Balazs GH, et al. Three closely related herpesviruses are associated with fibropapillomatosis in marine turtles. *Virology* 1998;246:392-399.
16. Murakami M, Matsuba C, Une Y, et al. Development of species-specific PCR techniques for the detection of tortoise herpesvirus. *J Vet Diagn Invest* 2001;13:513-516.
17. Teifke JP, Löhr CV, Marschang RE, et al. Detection of chelonid herpesvirus DNA by nonradioactive in situ hybridization in tissues from tortoises suffering from stomatitis-rhinitis complex in Europe and North America. *Vet Pathol* 2000;37:377-385.
18. Origgi F, Romero CH, Bloom DC, et al. 2004. Experimental transmission of a herpesvirus in Greek tortoises *(Testudo graeca)*. *Vet Pathol* 2004;41:50-61.
19. Herbst LH, Lemaire S, Ene AR, et al. Use of baculovirus-expressed glycoprotein H in an enzyme-linked immunosorbent assay developed to assess exposure to chelonid fibropapillomatosis-associated herpesvirus and its relationship to the prevalence of fibropapillomatosis in sea turtles. *Clin Vaccine Immunol* 2008;15:843-851.
20. Coberley SS, Herbst LH, Brown DR, et al. Detection of antibodies to a disease-associated herpesvirus of the green turtle, *Chelonia mydas*. *J Clin Microbiol* 2001;39:3572-3577.
21. Origgi FC, Klein PA, Mathes K, et al. Enzyme-linked immunosorbent assay for detecting herpesvirus exposure in Mediterranean tortoises (spur-thighed tortoise *[Testudo graeca]* and Hermann's tortoise *[Testudo hermanni]*). *J Clin Microbiol* 2001;39:3156-3163.
22. Jacobson ER, Berry K, Wellehan JFX Jr, et al. Serological and molecular evidence for tortoise herpesvirus 2 infection in wild desert tortoises, *Gopherus agassizii*. *J Wildl Dis* 2012;48:747-757.
23. Mao J, Hedrick RP, Chinchar VG. Molecular characterization, sequence analysis, and taxonomic position of newly isolated fish iridoviruses. *Virology* 1997;229:212-220.
24. Johnson AJ, Pessier AP, Jacobson ER. Experimental transmission and induction of ranaviral disease in western ornate box turtles *(Terrapene ornata ornata)* and red-eared sliders *(Trachemys scripta elegans)*. *Vet Pathol* 2007;44:285-297.
25. Chen Z, Zheng J, Jiang Y. A new iridovirus isolated from soft-shelled turtle. *Virus Res* 1999;63:147-151.
26. Marschang RE, Becher P, Posthaus H, et al. Isolation and characterization of an iridovirus from Hermann's tortoises *(Testudo hermanni)*. *Arch Virol* 1999;144:1909-1922.
27. Blahak S, Uhlenbrok C. Ranavirus infections in European terrestrial tortoises in Germany, in *Proceedings*. 1st International Conference on Reptile and Amphibian Medicine, Munich, Germany, 2010.
28. De Voe R, Geissler K, Elmore S, et al. Ranavirus-associated mortality in a group of eastern box turtles *(Terrapene carolina carolina)*. *J Zoo Wildl Med* 2004;35:534-543.
29. Uhlenbrok C. Nachweis von Ranavirusinfektionen bei Landschildkröten und Charakterisierung von VirusisolatenDetection of ranavirus infections in tortoises and characterisation of virus isolates. Vet. Med. Dissertation. Justus-Liebig-Universität, Giessen, Germany, 2010.
30. Benetka V, Grabensteiner E, Gumpenberger M, et al. First report of an iridovirus (Genus *Ranavirus*) infection in a leopard tortoise *(Geochelone pardalis pardalis)*. *Vet Med Austria/Wien Tierärztl Mschr* 2007;94:243-248.
31. Allender MC, Abd-Eldaim M, Schumacher J, et al. Ranavirus in free-ranging eastern box turtles *(Terrapene carolina carolina)* at rehabilitation centers in three southeastern US states. *J Wildl Dis* 2011;47:759-764.
32. Johnson AJ, Wendland L, Norton TM, et al. Development and use of an indirect enzyme-linked immunosorbent assay for detection of iridovirus exposure in gopher tortoises *(Gopherus polyphemus)* and eastern box turtles *(Terrapene carolina carolina)*. *Vet Microbiol* 2010;142:160-167.
33. Marschang RE, Ruemenapf TH. Virus "X": Characterizing a new viral pathogen in tortoises, in *Proceedings*. Association of Reptilian and Amphibian Veterinarians, Reno, Nev, 2002;101-102.
34. Marschang RE. Isolierung und Charakterisierung von Irido-, Herpes- und Reoviren aus Landschildkröten sowie Beschreibung eines nicht charakterisierten zytopathogenen Agens. Vet. Med. Dissertation, Giessen, Germany 2000.
35. Heuser W, Kaleta E, Giesow K, et al. Genome sequence of virus "X", a picornavirus isolated from a spur-thighed tortoise *(Testudo graeca)*, in *Proceedings*. EUROPIC 2010: XVI Meeting of the European Study Group on the Molecular Biology of Picornaviruses, St Andrews, UK 2010;Abstract H15;147.
36. Knowles, N. Tortoise picornavirus. Available at: http://www.picornaviridae.com/unassigned/tortoise_pv/tortoise_pv.htm. Accessed on April 9, 2013.
37. Marschang RE, Schneider, RM. Antibodies against viruses in wild-caught spur-thighed tortoises *(Testudo graeca)* in Turkey. *Vet Rec* 2007;161:102-103.
38. Rivera S, Wellehan JFX Jr, McManamon R, et al. Systemic adenovirus infection in Sulawesi tortoises *(Indotestudo forsteni)* caused by a novel siadenovirus. *J Vet Diagn Invest* 2009;21:415-426.
39. Innis CJ, Garner MM, Nordhausen RW, et al. Post-mortem detection of Sulawesi tortoise adenovirus-1 in two impressed tortoises *(Manouria impressa)* and a Burmese star tortoise *(Geochelone platynota)*, in *Proceedings*. Association of Reptilian and Amphibian Veterinarians, Milwaukee, Wisc, 2009;171-172.
40. Wilkinson R. Clinical pathology. In: McArthur S, Wilkinson R, Meyer J, eds. *Medicine and surgery of tortoises and turtles*. Chichester, UK: Blackwell Publishing, 2004;141-186.
41. Farkas SL, Gál J. Adenovirus and mycoplasma infection in an ornate box turtle *(Terrapene ornata ornata)* in Hungary. *Vet Microbiol* 2009;138:169-173.
42. Wellehan JFX, Johnson AJ, Harrach B, et al. Detection and analysis of six lizard adenoviruses by consensus primer PCR provides further evidence of a reptilian origin for the atadenoviruses. *J Virol* 2004;78:13366-13369.
43. Jacobson ER, Gaskin JM, Clubb S, et al. Papilloma-like virus infection in Bolivian side-neck turtles. *J Am Vet Med Assoc* 1982;181:1325-1328.
44. Drury SEN, Gough RE, McArthur S, et al. Detection of herpesvirus-like and papillomavirus-like particles associated with diseases of tortoises. *Vet Rec* 1998;143:639.
45. Manire CA, Stacy BA, Kinsel MJ, et al. Proliferative dermatitis in a loggerhead turtle, *Caretta caretta*, and a green turtle, *Chelonia mydas*, associated with novel papillomaviruses. *Vet Microbiol* 2008;130:227-237.
46. Herbst LH, Lenz J, Van Doorslaer K, et al. Genomic characterization of two novel reptilian papillomaviruses, *Chelonia mydas* papillomavirus1 and *Caretta caretta* papillomavirus 1. *Virology* 2009;383:131-135.

47. Kurath G. International Committee on Taxonomy of Viruses Web site. Available at: http://talk.ictvonline.org/files/proposals/taxonomy_proposals_vertebrate1/m/vert04/3859.aspx. Accessed June 28, 2011.
48. Zangger N, Müller M, Pagan O. Virale Dermatitis bei der Maurischen *(Testudo graeca)* und der Griechischen *(Testudo hermanni)* Landschildkröte in der Schweiz, in *Proceedings*. Fourth International Colloquium on Pathology and Medicine of Reptiles and Amphibians, Bad Nauheim, Germany 1991;25-29.
49. Papp T, Seybold J, Marschang RE. Paramyxovirus infection in a leopard tortoise *(Geochelone pardalis babcocki)* with respiratory disease. *J Herpetol Med Surg* 2010;20:64-68.
50. Marschang RE, Papp T, Frost JW. Comparison of paramyxovirus isolates from snakes, lizards and a tortoise. *Virus Res* 2009;144: 272-279.
51. Ahne W, Batts WN, Kurath G, et al. Comparative sequence analyses of sixteen reptilian paramyxoviruses. *Virus Res* 1999;63:65-74.
52. Marschang RE, Rösler R, Degan MA, et al. Detection of antibodies against paramyxoviruses in tortoises, in *Proceedings*. Association of Reptilian and Amphibian Veterinarians, Seattle, Wash, 2011.
53. Fölsch DW, Leloup P. Fatale endemische Infektion in einem Serpentarium. *Tierärztl Praxis* 1976;4:527-536.
54. Jacobson ER, Gaskin JM, Wells S, et al. Epizootic of ophidian paramyxovirus in a zoological collection: pathological, microbiological, and serological findings. *J Zoo Wildl Med* 1992;23:318-327.
55. Jacobson ER, Adams HP, Geisbert TW, et al. Pulmonary lesions in experimental ophidian paramyxovirus pneumonia of Aruba Island rattlesnakes, *Crotalus unicolor*. *Vet Pathol* 1997;34:450-459.
56. Ahne W, Neubert WJ. Isolation of paramyxovirus-like agents from teju *(Callopistes maculatus)* and python *(Python regius)*, in *Proceedings*. Second International Symposium on Viruses of Lower Vertebrates, Corvallis, Ore, 1991.
57. Gravendyck M, Ammermann P, Marschang RE, et al. Paramyxoviral and reoviral infections of iguanas on Honduran islands. *J Wildl Dis* 1998;34:33-38.
58. Marschang RE, Donahoe S, Manvell R, et al. Paramyxovirus and reovirus infections in wild-caught Mexican lizards (*Xenosaurus* and *Abronia* spp.). *J Zoo Wildl Med* 2002;33:317-321.
59. Jacobson ER, Origgi F, Pessier AP, et al. Paramyxovirus infection in caiman lizards *(Draecena guianensis)*. *J Vet Diagn Invest* 2001;13:143-151.
60. Jacobson ER, Gaskin JM, Flanagan JP, et al. Antibody responses of western diamondback rattlesnakes *(Crotalus atrox)* to inactivated ophidian paramyxovirus vaccines. *J Zoo Wildl Med* 1991;22: 184-190.
61. Hyndman TH, Marschang RE, Wellehan JFX, et al. Isolation and molecular identification of Sunshine virus, a novel paramyxovirus found in Australian snakes. *Infect Genet Evol* 2012;12:1436-46.
62. Clark HF, Lief FS, Lunger PD, et al. Fer de Lance virus (FDLV): a probable paramyxovirus isolated from a reptile. *J Gen Virol* 1979;44:405–418.
63. Pees M, Schmidt V, Marschang RE, et al. Examinations on the prevalence of viral infections in captive collections of boid snakes in Germany. *Vet Rec* 2009;166:422-425.
64. Blahak S. Untersuchungen zum Vorkommen von Paramyxoviren bei Schlangen und Charakterisierung ausgewählter Isolate. Dissertation. Justus-Liebig-Universität Giessen, Germany, 1994.
65. Lloyd C, Manvell R, Drury S, et al. Seroprevalence and significance of paramyxovirus titers in a zoological collection of lizards. *Vet Rec* 2005;156:578–580.
66. Allender MC, Mitchell MA, Phillips CA, et al. Hematology, plasma biochemistry, and antibodies to select viruses in wild-caught Eastern massasauga rattlesnakes *(Sistrurus catenatus catenatus)* from Illinois. *J Wildl Dis* 2006;42:107-114.
67. Blahak S. Isolation and characterization of paramyxoviruses from snakes and their relationship to avian paramyxoviruses. *J Vet Med B* 1995;42:216-224.
68. Manvell RJ, Geach M, Lewis JCM. Isolation of ophidian paramyxovirus type 7 from a reticulated python in the UK. *Vet Rec* 2000;147:696.
69. Allender MC, Mitchell MA, Dreslik MJ, et al. Measuring agreement and discord among hemagglutination inhibition assays against different ophidian paramyxovirus strains in the Eastern massasauga *(Sistrurus catenatus catenatus)*. *J Zoo Wildl Med* 2008;39:358-361.
70. Benkö M, Harrach B, Both GW, et al. Adenoviridae. In: Fauquet CM, Mayo MA, Maniloff J, et al, eds. *Virus taxonomy, eighth report of the international committee on taxonomy of viruses*. Amsterdam, Netherlands: Elsevier Academic Press, 2005;213-228.
71. Jacobson ER, Gaskin, JM, Gardiner CH. Adenovirus-like infection in a boa constrictor. *J Am Vet Med Assoc* 1985;187:1226-1227.
72. Kim D Y, Mitchell MA, Bauer RW, et al. An outbreak of adenoviral infection in inland bearded dragons *(Pogona vitticeps)* coinfected with dependovirus and coccidial protozoa (*Isospora* sp.). *J Vet Diagn Invest* 2002;14:332-334.
73. Raymond JT, Lamm M, Nordhausen R, et al. Degenerative encephalopathy in a coastal mountain kingsnake *(Lampropeltis zonata multifasciata)* due to adenoviral-like infection. *J Wildl Dis* 2003;39: 431-436.
74. Heldstab A, Bestetti G. Virus associated gastrointestinal disease in snakes. *J Zoo Anim Med* 1984;15:118-128.
75. Perkins LE, Campagnoli RP, Harmon BG, et al. Detection and confirmation of reptilian adenovirus infection by in situ hybridization. *J Vet Diagn Invest* 2001;13:365-368.
76. Juhász A, Ahne W. Physico-chemical properties and cytopathogenicity of an adenovirus-like agent isolated from corn snake *(Elaphe guttata)*. *Arch Virol* 1992;130:429-439.
77. Jacobson ER, Kollias GV. Adenovirus-like infection in a Savannah monitor. *J Zoo Anim Med* 1986;17:149-151.
78. Jacobson ER, Gardiner CH. Adeno-like virus in esophageal and tracheal mucosa of a Jackson's chameleon *(Chamaeleo jacksonii)*. *Vet Pathol* 1990;27:210-212.
79. Ogawa M, Ahne W, Essbauer S. Reptilian viruses: adenovirus-like agent isolated from royal python *(Python regius)*. *J Vet Med B Infect Dis Vet Public Health* 1992;39:732-736.
80. Schumacher J, Jacobson ER, Burns R, et al. Adenovirus-like infection in two rosy boas *(Lichanura trivirgata)*. *J Zoo Wildl Med* 1994;25:461-465.
81. Jacobson ER, Kopit W, Kennedy FA, et al. Coinfection of a bearded dragon, *Pogona vitticeps*, with adenovirus- and dependo-like viruses. *Vet Pathol* 1996;33:429-439.
82. Julian AF, Durham JK. Adenoviral hepatitis in a female bearded dragon *(Amphibolurus barbatus)*. *N Z Vet J* 1982;30:59-60.
83. Papp T, Fledelius B, Schmidt V, et al. PCR-sequence characterization of new adenoviruses found in reptiles and the first successful isolation of a lizard adenovirus. *Vet Microbiol* 2009;134:233-240.
84. Papp T, Robert N, Romanova I, et al. Nachweis von zwei verschiedenen Adenoviren bei einer Gruppe Königspythons, in *Proceedings*. 1. DVG Tagung über Vogel- und Reptilienkrankheiten, Leipzig, Germany, 2009.
85. Marschang RE, Michling R, Benkö M, et al. Evidence for widespread atadenovirus infection among snakes, in *Proceedings*. 6th International Congress of Veterinary Virology: Virus persistence and evolution (European Society for Veterinary Virology), Saint-Malo, France, 2003;152.
86. Abbas MD, Marschang RE, Schmidt V, et al. A unique novel reptilian paramyxovirus, four atadenovirus types and a reovirus identified in a concurrent infection of a corn snake *(Pantherophis guttatus)* collection in Germany. *Vet Microbiol* 2011;150:70-79.
87. Funk RS, Marschang RE, Romanova I, et al. Survey of native Arizona rattlesnakes for viral infections, in *Proceedings*. Biology of the Rattlesnakes, Tucson, Ariz, 2011.
88. Parkin DB, Archer LL, Childress AL, et al. Genotype differentiation of Agamid Adenovirus 1 in Bearded Dragons (Pogona vitticeps) in the USA by hexon gene sequence. *Infect Genet Evol* 2009;9:501-506.

89. Raynaud A, Adrian M. Cutaneous lesions with papillomatous structure associated with viruses in the green lizard *(Lacerta viridis Laur.)*. *C R Acad Sci Hebd Seances Acad Sci D* 1976;283: 845-847.
90. Blahak S, Ott I, Vieler E. Comparison of 6 different reoviruses of various reptiles. *Vet Rec* 1995;26:470-476.
91. Drury SE, Gough RE, Welchman D de B. Isolation and identification of a reovirus from a lizard, *Uromastyx hardwickii*, in the United Kingdom. *Vet Rec* 2002;151:637-638.
92. Garner MM, Farina LL, Wellehan JFX, et al. Reovirus-associated syncytial cell enteropathy and hepatopathy in leopard geckos *(Eublepharis macularius)*, in *Proceedings*. Association of Reptilian and Amphibian Veterinarians, Milwaukee, Wisc, 2009;82.
93. Vieler E, Baumgärtner W, Herbst W, et al. Characterization of a reovirus from a rattlesnake, *Crotalus viridis*, with neurological dysfunction. *Arch Virol* 1994;138:341-344.
94. Landolfi JA, Terio KA, Kinsel MJ, et al. Orthoreovirus infection and concurrent cryptosporidiosis in rough green snakes *(Opheodrys aestivus)*: pathology and identification of a novel orthoreovirus strain via polymerase chain reaction and sequencing. *J Vet Diagn Invest* 2010;22:37-43.
95. Lamirande EW, Nichols DK, Owens JW, et al. Isolation and experimental transmission of a reovirus pathogenic in ratsnakes (*Elaphe* sp.). *Virus Res* 1999;63:135-141.
96. Schragen S. Experimetelle Infektion von juvenilen *Boa constrictor* mit einem Orthoreovirusisolat. Vet. Med. Dissertation Justus-Liebig-Universität Giessen, Germany, 2006.
97. Wellehan JFX, Childress AL, Marschang RE, et al. Consensus nested PCR amplification and sequencing of diverse reptilian, avian, and mammalian Orthoreoviruses. *Vet Microbiol* 2009;133:34-42.
98. Marschang RE, Papp T. Isolation and partial characterization of three reoviruses from lizards. *J Herpetol Med Surg* 2009;19:13-15.
99. Ahne W, Thomsen I, Winton J. Isolation of a reovirus from the snake *Python regius*. *Arch Virol* 1987;94:135-139.
100. Chinchar VG, Essbauer S, He JG, et al. Iridoviridae. In: Fauquet CM, Mayo MA, Maniloff J, eds. *Virus taxonomy, eighth report of the international committee on taxonomy of viruses*. Amsterdam, Netherlands: Elsevier Academic Press, 2005;145-162.
101. Daszak P, Berger L, Cunningham AA, et al. Emerging infectious diseases and amphibian population declines. *Emerg Infect Dis* 1999;5:735-748.
102. Gray MJ, Miller DL, Hoverman JT. Ecology and pathology of amphibian ranaviruses. *Dis Aquat Org* 2009;87:243-266.
103. Hyatt AD, Williamson M, Coupar BEH, et al. First identification of a ranavirus from green pythons *(Chondropython viridis)*. *J Wildl Dis* 2002;38:239-252.
104. Marschang RE, Braun S, Becher P. Isolation of a ranavirus from a gecko *(Uroplatus fimbriatus)*. *J Zoo Wildl Med* 2005;36:295-300.
105. Alves de Matos AP, Caeiro MF, Papp T, et al. New viruses from *Lacerta monticola* (Serra da Estrela, Portugal): further evidence for a new group of nucleo-cytoplasmic large deoxyriboviruses (NCLDVs). *Microsc Micoranal* 2011;17:101-108.
106. Williams T. Forum: Natural Invertebrate Hosts of iridoviruses (Iridoviridae). *Neotrop Entomol* 2008;37:615-632.
107. Kleespies RG, Tidona CA, Darai G. Characterization of a new iridovirus isolated from crickets and investigations on the host range. *J Invertebr Pathol* 1999;73:84-90.
108. Just FT, Essbauer SS. Characterisation of an iridescent virus isolated from *Gryllus bimaculatus* (Orthoptera: Gryllidae). *J Invertebr Pathol* 2001;77:51-61.
109. Jakob NJ, Kleespies RG, Tidona CA, et al. Comparative analysis of the genome and host range characteristics of two insect iridoviruses: chilo iridescent virus and a cricket iridovirus isolate. *J Gen Virol* 2002;83:463-470.
110. Just F, Essbauer S, Ahne W, et al. Occurrence of an invertebrate iridescent-like virus (Iridoviridae) in reptiles. *J Vet Med B* 2001;48:685-694.
111. Weinmann N, Papp T, Alves de Matos AP, et al. Experimental infection of crickets *(Gryllus bimaculatus)* with an invertebrate iridovirus isolated from a high-casqued chameleon *(Chamaeleo hoehnelii)*. *J Vet Diagn Invest* 2007;19:674-679.
112. Stehbens WE, Johnston MRL. The viral nature of *Pirhemocyton tarentolae*. *J Ultra Mol Struct R* 1966;15:543-554.
113. Wolf K. Viral erythrocytic necrosis. In: Wolf K, ed. *Fish viruses and fish viral disease*. Ithaca, New York: Comstock Publishing Associates, 1988;389-398.
114. Alves de Matos AP, Paperna I, Crespo E. Experimental infection of lacertids with lizard erythrocytic viruses. *Intervirology* 2002;45: 150-159.
115. Telford Jr SR, Jacobson ER. Lizard erythrocytic virus in east African chameleons. *J Wildl Dis* 1993;29:57-63.
116. Wellehan JFX, Strik NI, Stacy BA, et al. Characterization of an erythrocytic virus in the family Iridoviridae from a peninsula ribbon snake *(Thamnophis sauritus sackenii)*. *Vet Microbiol* 2008;131: 115-122.
117. Simpson CF, Jacobson ER, Gaskin JM. Herpesvirus-like infection of the venom gland of Siamese cobras. *J Am Vet Med Assoc* 1979;175:941-943.
118. Hauser B, Mettler F, Rübel A. Herpesvirus-like infection in two young boas. *J Comp Pathol* 1983;93:515-519.
119. Literak I, Robesova B, Majlathova V, et al. Herpesvirus-associated papillomatosis in a green lizard. *J Wildl Dis* 2010;46:257-261.
120. Wellehan JFX, Johnson AJ, Latimer KS, et al. Varanid herpesvirus 1: a novel herpesvirus associated with proliferative stomatitis in green tree monitors *(Varanus prasinus)*. *Vet Microbiol* 2005;105:83-92.
121. Wellehan JFX, Nichols DK, Li L, et al. Three novel herpesviruses associated with stomatitis in Sudan plated lizards *(Gerrhosaurus major)* and a black-lined plated lizard *(Gerrhosaurus nigrolineatus)*. *J Zoo Wildl Med* 2004;35:50-54.
122. Watson GL. Herpesvirus in red-headed agamas *(Agama agama)*. *J Vet Diagn Invest* 1993;5:444-445.
123. Wellehan JFX, Jarchow JL, Reggiardo C, et al. A novel herpesvirus associated with hepatic necrosis in a San Esteban chuckwalla, *Sauromalus varius*. *J Herpetol Med Surg* 2003;13:15-19.
124. Van Devanter DR, Warrener P, Bennett L, et al. Detection and analysis of diverse herpesviral species by consensus primer PCR. *J Clin Microbiol* 1996;34:1666-1671.
125. Chang LW, Jacobson ER. Inclusion body disease, a worldwide infectious disease of boid snakes: a review. *J Exotic Pet Med* 2010;3:216-225.
126. Jacobson ER, Oros J, Tucker SJ, et al. Partial characterization of retroviruses from boid snakes with inclusion body disease. *Am J Vet Res* 2001;62:217-224.
127. Schumacher J, Jacobson ER, Homer BL, et al. Inclusion body disease in boid snakes. *J Zoo Wildl Med* 1994;25:511-524.
128. Stenglein MD, Sanders C, Kistler AL, et al. Identification, characterization, and in vitro culture of highly divergent arenaviruses from boa constrictors and annulated tree boas: candidate etiological agents for snake inclusion body disease. *MBio* 2012;3:e00180-12.
129. Wozniak E, McBride J, DeNardo D, et al. Isolation and characterization of an antigenically distinct 68-kd protein from nonviral intracytoplasmic inclusions in boa constrictors chronically infected with the inclusion body disease virus (IBDV: Retroviridae). *Vet Pathol* 2000;37:449-459.
130. Jacobson ER, Popp JA, Shields RP, et al. Poxlike skin lesions in captive caimans. *J Am Vet Med Assoc* 1979;175:937-940.
131. Penrith ML, Nesbit JW, Huchzermeyer FW. Pox virus infection in captive juvenile caimans *(Caiman crocodilus fuscus)* in South Africa. *J S Afr Vet Assoc* 1991;62:137-139.
132. Ramos MC, Coutinho SD, Matushima ER, et al. Poxvirus dermatitis outbreak in farmed Brazilian caimans *(Caimancrocodilus yacare)*. *Aust Vet J* 2002;80:371-372.
133. Buenviaje GN, Ladds PW, Martin Y. Pathology of skin diseases in crocodiles. *Aust Vet J* 1998;76:357-363.

134. Horner RF. Poxvirus in farmed Nile crocodiles. *Vet Rec* 1988;122:459-462.
135. Huchzermeyer FW, Huchzermeyer KDA, Putterill JF. Observations on a field outbreak of pox virus infection in young Nile crocodiles *(Crocodylus niloticus)*. *J S Afr Vet Assoc* 1991;62:27-29.
136. Huchzermeyer FW, Wallace DB, Putteril JF, et al. Identification and partial sequencing of a crocodile poxvirus associated with deeply penetrating skin lesions in farmed Nile crocodiles, *Crocodylus niloticus*. *Onderstepoort J Vet Res* 2009;76:311-316.
137. Afonso CL, Tulman ER, Delhon G, et al. Genome of crocodilepox virus. *J Virol* 2006;80:4978-4991.
138. Komar N. West Nile virus: epidemiology and ecology in North America. *Adv Virus Res* 2003;61:185-234.
139. Ulbert S. West Nile virus: the complex biology of an emerging pathogen. *Intervirology* 2011;54:171-184.
140. Jacobson ER, Ginn PE, Troutman JM, et al. West Nile virus infection in farmed American alligators *(Alligator mississippiensis)* in Florida. *J Wildl Dis* 2005;41:96-106.
141. Miller DL, Mauel MJ, Baldwin C, et al. West Nile virus in farmed alligators. *Emerg Infect Dis* 2003;9:794-799.
142. Nevarez JG, Mitchell MA, Kim DY, et al. West Nile virus in alligator ranches from Louisiana. *J Herpetol Med Surg* 2005;15:4-9.
143. Steinman A, Banet-Noach C, Tal S, et al. West Nile virus infection in crocodiles. *Emerg Infect Dis* 2003;9:887-889.
144. Farfán-Ale JA, Blitvich BJ, Marlenee NL, et al. Antibodies to West Nile virus in asymptomatic mammals, birds, and reptiles in the Yucatan Peninsula of Mexico. *Am J Trop Med Hyg* 2006;74: 908-914.
145. Nevarez JG, Mitchell MA, Morgan T, et al. Association of West Nile virus with lymphohistiocytic proliferative cutaneous lesions in American alligators *(Alligator mississippiensis)* detected by RT-PCR. *J Zoo Wildl Med* 2008;39:562-566.
146. Klenk K, Snow J, Morgan K, et al. Alligators as West Nile virus amplifiers. *Emerg Infect Dis* 2004;10:2150-2155.
147. Eiden M, Vina-Rodriguez A, Hoffmann B, et al. Two new real-time quantitative reverse transcription polymerase chain reaction assays with unique target sites for the specific and sensitive detection of lineages 1 and 2 West Nile virus strains. *J Vet Diagn Invest* 2010;22:748-753.
148. Jacobson ER, Johnson AJ, Hernandez JA, et al. Validation and use of an indirect enzyme-linked immunosorbent assay for detection of antibodies to West Nile virus in American alligators *(Alligator mississippiensis)* in Florida. *J Wildl Dis* 2005;41: 107-114.

CHAPTER 6

Update on Fungal Infections in Reptiles

Jean A. Paré

Fungi are ubiquitous on the skin of reptiles[1]; thus the mere isolation of a fungus from a lesion is clinically irrelevant if unsupported by compatible histopathologic findings. Morphologic characteristics of fungal elements in tissue sections are critical in assigning causality to isolates or dismissing them as contaminants. The literature is replete with cases of reptile mycoses in which various fungi were incriminated but for which causality was never established or even substantiated. Fungal identification was subjectively ventured based on hyphal or yeast morphologic features in histologic sections when material was unavailable for culture. Only when we possess a sound understanding of which fungi have in the past posed a threat to reptiles can we assign the "emerging" epithet to a fungal agent. For this to happen, we need to strictly consider cases in which identification and causality of an isolate were firmly or reasonably ascertained. When the existing literature pertaining to fungal disease in reptiles is objectively reviewed, only a few fungi have emerged as genuine repeat offenders. Common environmental organisms such as *Purpureocillium lilacinum* (formerly *Paecilomyces lilacinus*), *Fusarium solani* and other fusaria, *Metarhizium anisopliae, Beauveria bassiana,* various aspergilla, and yeast such as *Candida* or *Cryptococcus* can and will cause disease in reptiles under the right circumstances.[2,3] Pigmented fungi very rarely cause disease in squamates but, in contrast, are well-represented among agents of fungal disease in chelonians, especially tortoises and box turtles (*Terrapene* spp.). Infection with these opportunistic fungi is usually a result of overwhelming exposure, immune compromise, and stress from inadequate or substandard captive conditions, or any combination thereof. In wild chelonians and crocodilians, stressful climatic events such as cold spells or cold-stunning in sea turtles often precede systemic or pulmonary mycoses with otherwise fairly innocuous fungi. Similarly, in captive specimens, thermal extremes from mechanical breakdowns or other causes of environmental failure can subsequently lead to mycosis. Antifungal prophylaxis is routine in sea turtles recovering from cold spells, and it may be wise to do the same for other captive reptiles that have experienced accidental cooling events.

Of course, fungi other than those already listed can infect reptiles, and none among those is more of a threat than the fungus currently referred to as the "*Chrysosporium* anamorph of *Nannizziopsis vriesii*" (CANV), which we now know is an established cause of contagious, deep, and often fatal dermatomycosis in a variety of lizards and snakes and in crocodiles.[2,3] The CANV might not be a truly emerging reptile pathogen but rather one that has gone undiagnosed, misdiagnosed, or unrecognized for decades. Nevertheless, this fungus is the single most important fungal pathogen of reptiles, and research has demonstrated it may act as a primary pathogen.[4] More than 30 CANV isolates collected from various sources over the last 25 years have been catalogued, and all but one were retrieved from reptile lesions. Most of these were initially misidentified, often as *Trichophyton, Geotrichum, Malbranchea,* or as a distinct *Chrysosporium* species. Repeated attempts at mating isolates to yield a teleomorph have been unsuccessful, and although all reptile CANV isolates are morphologically indistinguishable from the true anamorphic stage of *Nannizziopsis vriesii,* they do differ slightly when examined at the molecular level (Hambleton S, Sigler L, and Paré JA: unpublished data). They are now known to represent an assembly of closely related fungi, many of which remain to be named (Hambleton S, Sigler L and Paré JA: unpublished data). *Chrysosporium ophiodiicola* and *Chrysosporium guarroi,* recently described agents of dermatomycosis in a Black Ratsnake *(Elaphe obsoleta)*[5] and a Green Iguana *(Iguana iguana)*,[6] respectively, are renamed fungi that would have previously fallen under the CANV group umbrella. CANV infection is contagious and typically occurs in captive reptiles as outbreaks of severe, progressive necrogranulomatous dermatitis that eventually disseminates. This fungus consistently expands its list of susceptible hosts. Recent additions include Broad-headed Snakes *(Hoplocephalus bungaroides)*,[7] Brown Anoles *(Anolis sagrei)*,[8] coastal Bearded Dragons *(Pogona barbata)*,[9] Leopard Geckos *(Eublepharius macularius)*,[10] and even Tuataras *(Sphenodon punctatus)*.[11] Of substantial concern is the recent identification of the CANV as a cause of severe disease in wild snakes, which carries significant conservation implications. The CANV, more precisely *C. ophiodiicola,* was strongly incriminated as the cause of disfiguring facial lesions in free-ranging Eastern Massasauga Rattlesnakes *(Sistrurus catenatus catenatus)*[12,13] in Illinois. Four snakes collected from the wild in southern Illinois over a period of 3 years as part of a health survey were compromised by deep, severe, very aggressive granulomatous infection resulting in effacement of normal facial and cranial anatomic structures.[12] The head of affected snakes becomes distorted from the infection, and the disease was dubbed *facial disfiguration syndrome* (FDS). The clinicopathologic picture was peculiarly yet strikingly consistent among affected snakes but was also identical to that of a Western Massasauga Rattlesnake (*Sistrurus catenatus*

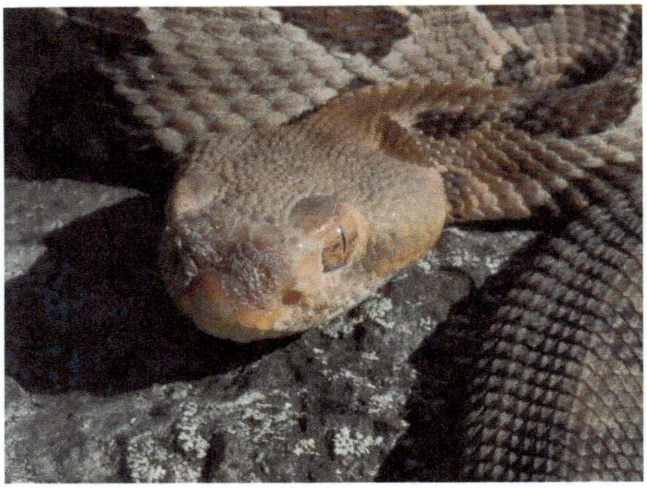

FIGURE 6-1 Wild juvenile Timber Rattlesnake *(Crotalus horridus)* with early *Chrysosporium ophiodiicola* infection, confirmed at the National Wildlife Health Center, Madison, Wisc. The rostrum is swollen, especially on the left side. Nasal, internasal, and loreal scutes are hyperkeratotic and necrotic, and the nares are effaced. *(Photo courtesy of J. Condon.)*

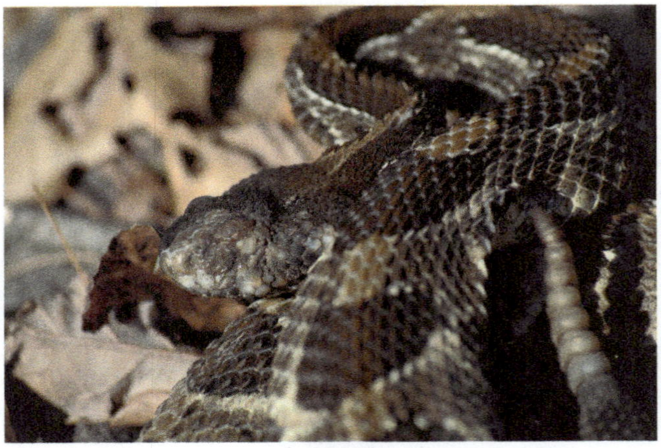

FIGURE 6-2 Wild adult Timber Rattlesnake *(Crotalus horridus)* with suspected *Chrysosporium ophiodiicola* infection. The whole side of the face is swollen and distorted. The eye is shrunken, and the spectacle is opaque. The supraocular and preocular scutes are necrotic and coalesced. The rostrum is rounded and swollen and covered with abnormal scales. *(Photo courtesy of J. Condon.)*

tergeminus) with extensive and invasive granulomatous fungal infection reported in 1979.[14] In the latter case, the description of the hyphae in tissue sections was not consistent with the presumptive diagnosis of *phycomycosis,* an obsolete term for *zygomycosis,* and this snake may well have been a misidentified case of *C. ophiodiicola* facial mycosis or FDS. Extensive dermatomycosis, very suggestive of FDS, has recently been observed in wild Timber Rattlesnakes *(Crotalus horridus)* in New England[13,15] (Figure 6-1). Necrogranulomatous lesions may not be limited to the face and may extend to the rest of the body. Snakes are typically found with lesions as they emerge from hibernacula in the spring, but some sick snakes are also seen basking outside dens in winter months (Condon J: Pers. com.,) (Figure 6-2). Infection progressively hinders feeding, and snakes become emaciated before they succumb. This disease might have substantially impacted northeastern Timber Rattlesnake populations. Investigations as to the causative agent are being conducted, but available data are also pointing to *C. ophiodiicola.* A wild Black Ratsnake and one of several Copperheads *(Agkistrodon contortrix)* with severe and ultimately fatal granulomatous skin disease in New Jersey were confirmed with *C. ophiodiicola* (Schantz K: unpublished data,) in the last 2 years. This spreading epidemic of fungal disease chiefly affects wild crotalid snakes but might have spilled over to sympatric Ring-necked Snakes *(Diadophis punctatus),* Black Racers *(Coluber constrictor),* Gartersnakes (*Thamnophis* sp.), and Watersnakes (*Nerodia* sp.) (Figure 6-3), all of which were seen with facial lesions consistent with CANV dermatitis. *C. ophiodiicola* is known from Europe and Australia and probably occurs worldwide (Sigler L and Paré JA: unpublished data), yet much remains to be known about this fungus and its impact on free-ranging animals. The ecologic niche of *C. ophiodiicola* and other CANV isolates remains unclear, but it has been implicated in the past as causing disease mostly in recently caught or newly imported terrestrial and aquatic reptiles. Treatment may be protracted, as lesions are often advanced by the time sick snakes are first observed. *C. ophiodiicola* does not grow or grows very poorly at 35°C, and this limited thermotolerance may partially account for some affected snakes with less severe lesions healing after emergence from the hibernaculum. Simple exposure to sunlight and warmer days would impede fungal growth and therefore disease progression, allowing animals to progressively improve with each shedding thereafter (Figure 6-4). In cases in which lesions are too extensive or deep, surgical debridement with topical care and long-term antifungal therapy are needed. Adjunct fluid therapy, as well as nutritional and thermal support, is usually initially indicated to stabilize the patient beforehand or concurrently with systemic medications and assist in recovery. Voriconazole, terbinafine, and itraconazole are all valid drug options, on the

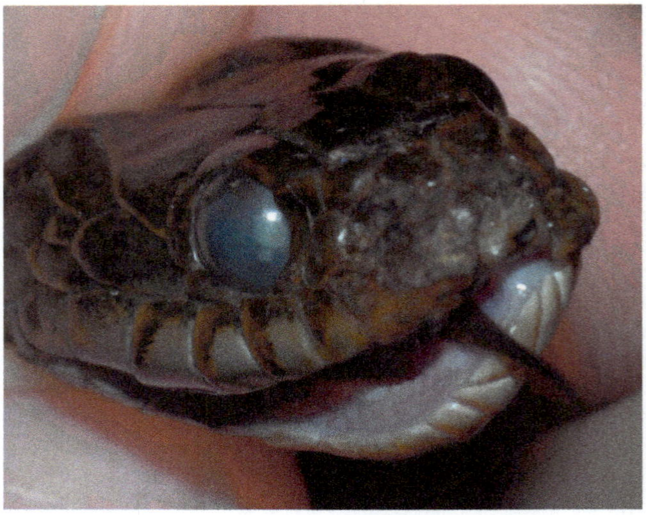

FIGURE 6-3 Wild adult Northern Watersnake *(Nerodia sipedon)* with *Chrysosporium ophiodiicola* infection, confirmed at the National Wildlife Health Center, Madison, Wisc. The rostral, nasal, internasal, and prefrontal scutes are necrotic and thickened. The nares are effaced. The snout is distorted and shortened. *(Photo courtesy of J. Condon.)*

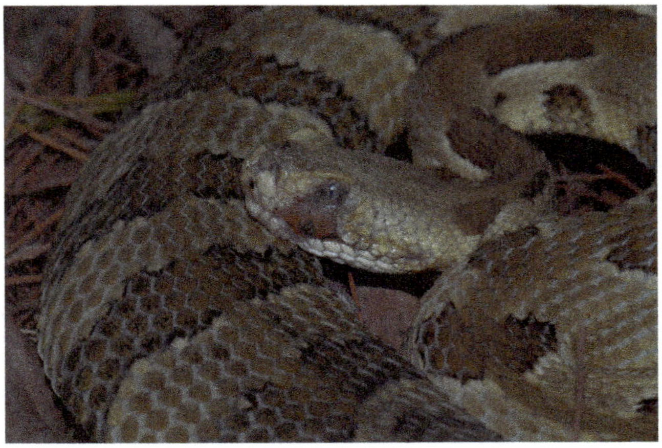

FIGURE 6-4 Wild adult Timber Rattlesnake *(Crotalus horridus)* with suspected *Chrysosporium ophiodiicola* infection. The subocular and upper labial scales have necrosed and sloughed, exposing the dermis. The rostrum is rounded and slightly distorted, possibly scarred from prior or deep infection. Lesions in this snake might be resolving. *(Photo courtesy of J. Condon.)*

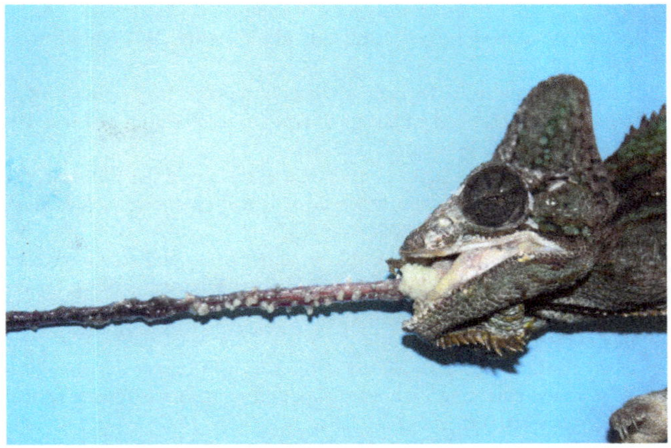

FIGURE 6-5 Cadaver of an adult Veiled Chameleon (*Chamaeleo calyptratus*) with *Chamaeleomyces granulomatis* infection. A myriad of smooth, spherical, cream-colored abscesses cover the entire length of the tongue. *(Photo courtesy Dr. Mads F. Bertelsen, Copenhagen Zoo, Copenhagen, Denmark.)*

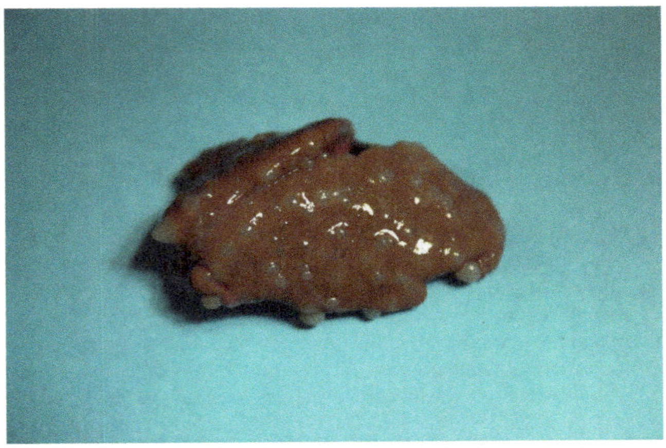

FIGURE 6-6 Liver of the same adult Veiled Chameleon *(Chamaeleo calyptratus)* in Figure 6-5 with *Chamaeleomyces granulomatis* infection. Note the miliary abscesses scattered across the hepatic parenchyma. *(Photo courtesy Dr. Mads F. Bertelsen, Copenhagen Zoo, Copenhagen, Denmark.)*

basis of prior CANV in vitro susceptibility studies.[16,17] Secondary bacterial infection may also need to be addressed.

C. guarroi causes a contagious, deep dermatitis in Green Iguanas that seems to be spreading in Europe and Asia through the pet trade. First reported in Spain,[6] it has also been documented in South Korea[18] and is likely more widespread in pet Green Iguanas than recognized. *Trichophyton mentagrophytes* var. *interdigitale*, the most common cause of human ringworm worldwide, was isolated from several farmed Green Iguanas in Iran[19] that were seen with crusting gray dermatitis, clinically very similar to that caused by *C. guarroi*. This report is unique in that it is the first unequivocally documented account of dermatophytosis in a reptile because all previous reports implicating any dermatophyte in reptile skin disease were questionable and likely misdiagnosed CANV infections. Green Iguanas with fungal dermatitis therefore might pose a zoonotic threat; thus fungal isolation appears mandatory to distinguish between disease caused by *C. guarroi* and *T. mentagrophytes* var. *interdigitale*. The corollary is that Green Iguanas may contract dermatophytosis from owners and handlers with tinea.

Another fungus, *Chamaeleomyces granulomatis,*[20] may qualify as an emergent agent of infectious disease in reptiles. This novel fungus has just recently been identified as the cause of disseminated infection in seven Veiled Chameleons *(Chamaeleo calyptratus)* in a Danish zoologic institution. Infection was characterized by conspicuous clusters of spherical, yellowish to cream, sometimes coalescing abscesses on the tongue, skin, and multiple viscera[20] (Figures 6-5 and 6-6). Eighteen Veiled Chameleons also were seen with this disease at a veterinary hospital over a period of 2 years.[21] The fatality rate was high because disease was often advanced at the time of presentation. A very similar disease was first reported more than 4 decades ago in 4 of 50 Jewelled Chameleons *(Furcifer lateralis)* imported to France from Madagascar.[22] The lizards were dying with identical lesions from *Paecilomyces viridis,* a fungus now synonymized with *C. granulomatis.*[20] This condition also resulted in multiple mortalities over years in a zoologic collection of Jackson's Chameleons *(Chamaeleo jacksonii)* in New Zealand (Potter: Pers. com.,).[23] The fungus often assumes a yeast phase in liver and other tissue, leading to some confusion when a mold is isolated. Some antibiotics may promote induction of the yeast phase of *C. granulomatis* in tissue.[24] Terbinafine may be the antifungal of choice, if the disease is caught early.[21] The source of the fungus and means of dissemination across animals within a collection remain unknown.

Undoubtedly, new fungal agents of infection in reptiles remain to be discovered. This will only happen if diligent care is taken by clinicians and pathologists to isolate and properly identify fungi that are truly causing lesions in reptiles, as confirmed histologically. Fungal isolates should be preserved in microfungus depositories so that they are available for eventual further examination.

REFERENCES

1. Paré JA, Sigler L, Rypien K, et al. Cutaneous mycobiota of captive squamate reptiles with notes on the scarcity of the *Chrysosporium* anamorph of *Nannizziopsis vriesii*. *J Herpetol Med Surg* 2003;13:10-15.

2. Paré JA, Sigler L. Fungal diseases of reptiles. In: Mader DR, ed. *Reptile medicine and surgery*, 2nd ed. Philadelphia: WB Saunders Co, 2002;217-226.
3. Paré JA, Jacobson EJ. Mycotic diseases of reptiles. In: Jacobson ER, ed. *Infectious diseases and pathology of reptiles: a color atlas and text.* Boca Raton, Fla: CRC Press, 2007;527-570.
4. Paré JA, Coyle KA, Sigler L, et al. Pathogenicity of the *Chrysosporium* anamorph of *Nannizziopsis vriesii* for veiled chameleons *(Chamaeleo calyptratus). Med Mycol* 2006;44:25-31.
5. Rajeev S, Sutton DA, Wickes BL, et al. Isolation and characterization of a new fungal species, *Chrysosporium ophiodiicola*, from a mycotic granuloma of a black rat snake *(Elaphe obsoleta obsoleta). J Clin Microbiol* 2009;47:1264-1268.
6. Abarca ML, Castellá G, Martorell J, et al. *Chrysosporium guarroi* sp. nov. a new emerging pathogen of pet green iguanas *(Iguana iguana). Med Mycol* 2010;48:365-372.
7. McLelland DJ, Johnson L, Reuter R. Fatal cutaneous mycosis in a broad-headed snake *(Hoplocephalus bungaroides)* caused by the *Chrysosporium* anamorph of *Nannizziopsis vriesii. Proc Wildl Dis Assoc Austral Tasmania Aust*, 2010: 55.
8. Burcham GN, Miller MA, Hickok TS. Pathology in practice. *J Am Vet Med Assoc* 2011;239:1305-1307.
9. Johnson RSP, Sangster CR, Sigler L, et al. Deep fungal dermatitis caused by the *Chrysosporium* anamorph of *Nannizziopsis vriesii* in captive coastal bearded dragons *(Pogona barbata). Aust Vet J* 2011;89:515-519.
10. Toplon DE, Terrell SP, Sigler L, et al. Dermatitis and cellulitis in leopard geckoes *(Eublepharis macularius)* caused by the *Chrysosporium* anamorph of *Nannizziopsis vriesii. Vet Pathol* 2012;Nov 16. [Epub ahead of print]
11. Masters NJ. Dermatomycosis caused by a *Chrysosporium* species in a captive tuatara *(Sphenodon punctatus)* in New Zealand, in *Proceedings.* International Conference on Diseases of Zoo and Wild Animals, Bussolengo, Italy, 2012;86.
12. Allender MC, Dreslik M, Wylie S, et al. *Chrysosporium* sp. infection in Eastern massasauga rattlesnakes. *Emerg Infect Dis* 2011;17:2383-2384.
13. Allender M, Dreslik MJ, Phillips CA, et al. Facial disfiguration syndrome in free-ranging snakes throughout the Eastern US: an emerging pathogen associated with *Chrysosporium. Proceedings.* American Association of Zoo Veterinarians, Oakland, Calif, 2012;93.
14. Williams LW, Jacobson EJ, Gelatt KN, et al. Phycomycosis in a western rattlesnake *(Sistrurus catenatus)* with infection of the telencephalon, orbit, and facial structures. *Vet Med Small Anim Clin* 1979;74:1181-1184.
15. McBride MP, Murray M, Wojick KB, et al. *Chrysosporium ophiodiicola* isolated from skin lesions in wild timber rattlesnakes *(Crotalus horridus)*, in *Proceedings.* Association of Reptile and Amphibian Veterinarians, Oakland, Calif, 2012;104-105.
16. Paré JA, Andes DR, and L Sigler. In vitro susceptibility of fungal isolates from reptiles to antifungal drugs, in *Proceedings.* American Association of Zoo Veterinarians, Omaha, Neb, 2005;124.
17. Hellebuyck T, Baert K, Pasmans F, et al. Cutaneous hyalohyphomycosis in a girdled lizard *(Cordylus giganteus)* caused by the *Chrysosporium* anamorph of *Nannizziopsis vriesii* and successful treatment with voriconazole. *Vet Dermatol* 2010;21:429-433.
18. Han JI, Lee SJ, Na KJ. Necrotizing dermatomycosis caused by *Chrysosporium* spp. in three captive green iguanas *(Iguana iguana)* in South Korea. *J Exotic Pet Med* 2010;19:240-244.
19. Khosravi AR, Shokri H, Rostami A, et al. Severe dermatophytosis due to *Trichophyton mentagrophytes* var. *interdigitale* in flocks of green iguanas *(Iguana iguana). J Small Anim Pract* 2012;53:286-291.
20. Sigler L, Gibas CFC, Kokotovic B, et al. Disseminated mycoses in veiled chameleons *(Chamaeleo calyptratus)* caused by *Chamaeleomyces granulomatis*, a new fungus related to *Paecilomyces viridis. J Clin Microbiol* 2010;48:3182-3192.
21. Schmidt V, Plenz B, Pfaff M, et al. Disseminated systemic mycosis in veiled chameleons *(Chamaeleo calyptratus)* caused by *Chamaeleomyces granulomatis. Vet Microbiol* 2012;16:145-152.
22. Ségretain G, Fromentin H, Destombes P, et al. *Paecilomyces viridis* nov. sp., dimorphic fungus agent of a generalized mycosis in *Chamaeleo lateralis* Gray. *Compt Rend Acad Sci (Paris)* 1964;259:258-261.
23. Gartrell BD, Alley MR, Geschke K. Disseminated mycosis in a Jackson's chameleon *(Chamaeleo jacksonii). N Z Vet J* 2004;52:51.
24. Samson RA. *Paecilomyces* and some allied hyphomycetes. *Stud Mycol* 1974;6:1-119.

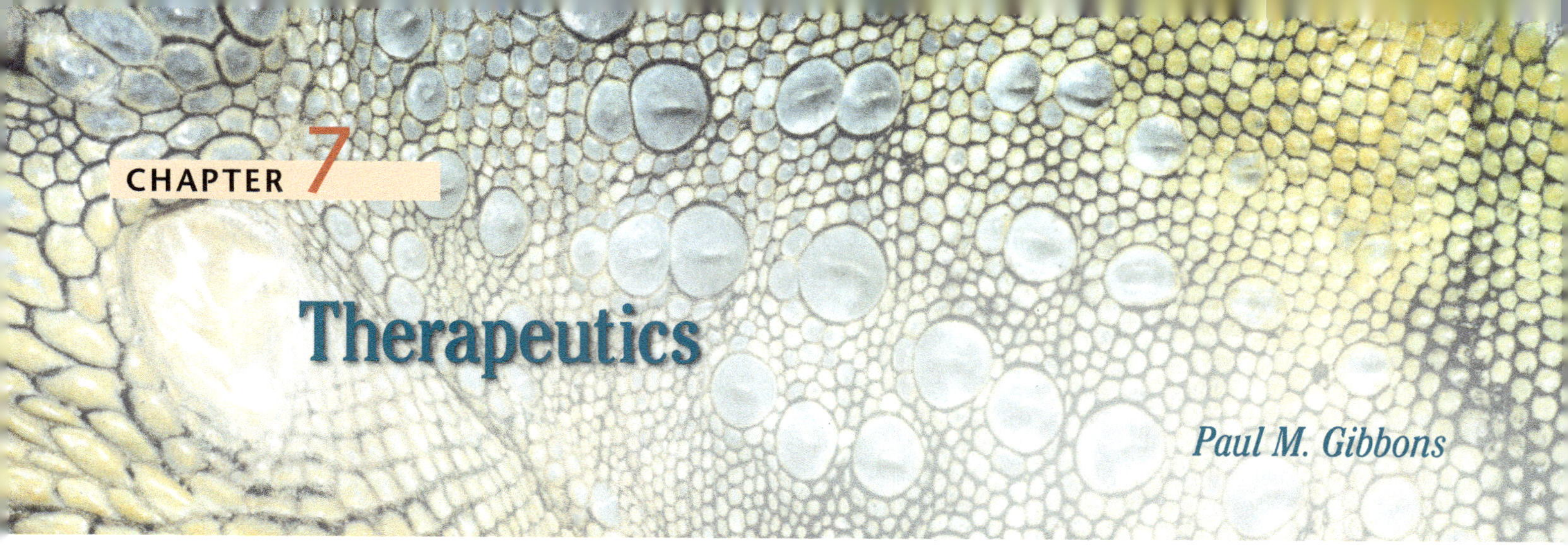

CHAPTER 7

Therapeutics

Paul M. Gibbons

DIAGNOSIS

The standard of today's reptile practice calls on clinicians to use an ever-increasing array of diagnostic tools to gather information and obtain a credible diagnosis. Few, if any, pathognomonic signs exist, and most clinical syndromes are not understood well enough to be able to define standard therapeutic protocols for a set of clinical signs without objective diagnostic information. For example, in the relatively distant past, clinicians treating reptiles would routinely administer parenteral calcium to Green Iguanas *(Iguana iguana)* with the chief presenting sign of muscle tremors; today we recognize that the risk of soft tissue mineralization and permanent damage to arteries, renal tubules, and other tissues almost always outweighs the potential short-term benefit. We know that administering calcium without knowledge of the patient's ionized calcium concentration is unwise. A problem-oriented diagnostic approach directed toward minimizing risk and maximizing therapeutic benefit is now the standard of reptile practice.

Similar to class Mammalia, class Reptilia includes a diverse group of species, each with a unique pharmacologic response to every chemotherapeutic agent. As a result, therapeutic safety and efficacy differ among species. Unlike mammals, conscious reptiles are ectothermic, so physiologic and biochemical processes are strongly influenced by body temperature.[1] Reasonable assumptions about each individual species' metabolism and immune response can therefore only be made under certain conditions. In most cases, the body temperature of a reptile patient must match that of the subjects in a given pharmacokinetic study for a treatment plan to be designed, although pharmacokinetics and pharmacodynamics do not necessarily differ at different temperatures.[2-5] Species-specific pharmacokinetics, pharmacodynamics, therapeutic efficacy, and environmental requirements must be known before administration of any drug can be considered. This is not only to predict absorption, distribution, metabolism, excretion, and the therapeutic window but also to meet the environmental needs of a reptile so that an appropriate immune response and healing can occur.[4,6-8] It remains true that, even though many pharmacokinetic studies have been published in reptiles, not all drugs have been studied in all of the species presented to reptile veterinarians. Published doses are available for many drugs, and these may have been selected empirically, may have been calculated with the use of allometric or other scaling technique, or may be from published pharmacokinetic research data collected from healthy animals under laboratory conditions. It is incumbent on the clinician to evaluate the probability that a published dose is likely to be effective in a particular species under the individual circumstances of a clinical case. Dosage, dosing interval, and administration route must be evaluated in light of the individual circumstances of each case. Consult up-to-date, peer-reviewed literature to identify species and their environmental needs, optimal body temperature, and the pharmacokinetics and pharmacodynamics of the drug in that species.[9] Consider how physical and physiologic changes caused by disease might affect absorption, distribution, metabolism, excretion, side effects, and required therapeutic levels of a drug.

Managed thermoregulation, hydration, and nutrition are paramount for safe, effective drug therapy. Thermal options and gradients must be provided for conscious, active reptiles to behaviorally thermoregulate, and body temperature should be monitored during therapy. In cases of weakness and decreased activity, the patient's thermoregulation should be actively managed as a part of the therapeutic plan. Dehydrated, anorexic reptiles may not absorb, distribute, metabolize, or eliminate chemotherapeutic agents in the same manner as the healthy animals tested under controlled conditions in pharmacologic research, so nursing care also must include management of fluids, electrolytes, and nutrition.[4,5,10]

Few therapeutic agents are approved for use in reptiles by the United States Food and Drug Administration (FDA), so almost all drug use is "extralabel." In the United States, the Animal Medicinal Drug Use Clarification Act of 1994 (AMDUCA) and the Minor Use and Minor Species Animal Health Act of 2004 (MUMS) serve as guides for extralabel drug use. Prescription drugs may be used to treat disease in reptiles under the supervision of a veterinarian if (1) they are approved by the FDA for any purpose in any species, (2) a valid veterinarian–client–patient relationship exists, and (3) the FDA has not specifically prohibited extralabel use of the drug. Certain medical record and prescription label requirements must be followed to meet the obligations of veterinary licensure.[11]

ADMINISTRATION AND DOSING

Dosage and route of administration are determined by the chemical, pharmacokinetic, and pharmacodynamic properties of each agent in each species. Much work has been done to understand the mechanism of action, therapeutic window, absorption, distribution, metabolism, and excretion variables of many drugs in many species of reptiles, although many questions remain unanswered and informed, empiric dosing is still used in many cases.[4,9] Veterinarians administer therapeutic agents to reptiles via oral, enteral via gavage, subcutaneous (SC), intramuscular (IM), intravenous (IV), intracoelomic, intratracheal, intrapulmonary, intraosseous, intraperitoneal, intrathecal, and intracardiac routes, as well as via nebulization. These administration routes have been described.[4]

Parenteral administration has proven to be more reliable than the enteral route for many drugs in reptiles.[4] Sufficient evidence exists to support administration of most parenteral drugs in the cranial half of the body when possible so that the first-pass effect for drugs that are eliminated via renal tubular excretion or hepatic metabolism is avoided. Venous blood from the caudal half of the body enters the caudal vena cava through either the renal portal system and peritubular capillaries or the hepatic portal system from the abdominal or mesenteric veins and through the hepatocellular parenchyma.[12,13] Administration in the caudal half of the body has proven to be acceptable for a few specific drugs and should be considered for those drugs in circumstances when the cranial half is not available for injections.[5,14,15] Dosing adjustments must be made to account for the effects of renal tubular or hepatic metabolism as determined in these reports. Intracoelomic administration of fluids or systemic drugs cannot be recommended, except in rare, specific cases in which other routes are unsatisfactory. Absorption across coelomic membranes is difficult to assess in clinical patients and is not guaranteed, particularly in cases of abnormal blood proteins, coelomitis, or ascites. Accidental needle puncture or laceration of an organ and accidental deposition of the agent into the intestines, reproductive tract, or urinary bladder rather than the coelomic space have been observed and probably occur undetected in many cases; adverse effects have been reported.[16] Some therapeutic challenges in reptiles can be overcome by novel approaches to drug administration, including osmotic pump, dermal patch, depot formulation, cardiac access port, and topical administration.

Osmotic Pump

Alzet osmotic pumps (Durect Corp., Cupertino, Calif.) (Figure 7-1) are implanted, miniature infusion pumps designed for continuous infusion of therapeutic agents to unrestrained animals. They are available with fixed delivery rates between 0.11 and 10 μL per hour and delivery durations between 1 day and 6 weeks. Marketed for laboratory animals, they range in size from 15 to 51 mm in length and 6 to 14 mm in diameter and have been used to deliver dozens of different therapeutic agents.[17] The "pumps" operate via an osmotic pressure difference between the tissue environment and a salt-containing osmotic sleeve. The high osmolality of the salt sleeve causes water to diffuse into the pump, across the outer semipermeable membrane and into the salt sleeve, which puts pressure on a flexible (impermeable) internal reservoir that contains the therapeutic agent. This pressure causes the agent to be expelled via a flow moderator at a controlled, predetermined, continuous rate that is independent of the chemical properties of the agent being dispensed. Different dosing rates can be achieved by varying the concentration of the agent used to fill the pump reservoir. Virtually any commonly used parenteral drug can be delivered by these pumps because they are loaded by the user just before the time of implantation.

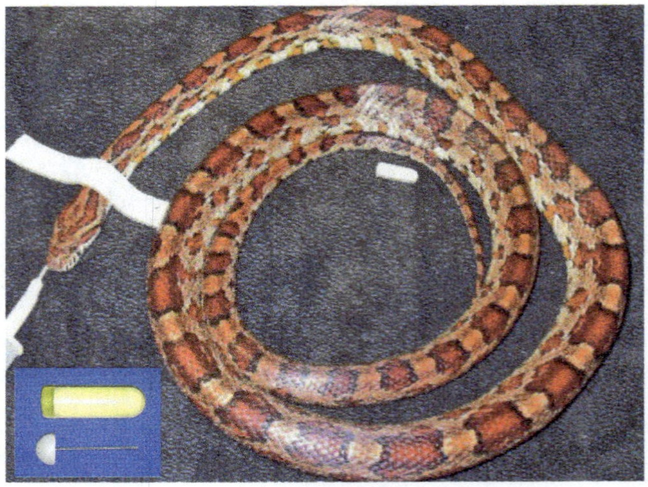

FIGURE 7-1 Alzet osmotic pumps (Durect Corp., Cupertino, Calif; model 1002 shown) can deliver medications continuously without the need for periodic injections. Although early clinical trials have not been successful, these do show promise for future drug delivery in reptiles that are difficult or dangerous to handle.

The use of osmotic pumps has been reported in Cornsnakes *(Elaphe guttata)*, Mojave Rattlesnakes *(Crotalus scutulatus)*, and Green Iguanas with amikacin, florfenicol, and gonadotropin-releasing hormone.[18-20] It is important to consider the tissue environment of the implant (availability of free water) and the pharmacokinetic and pharmacodynamic properties of the drug to be administered because some drugs, including amikacin, may be safer and more effective when administered in pulses rather than continuously.[21] In addition, substantial local necrosis and death occurred in five of six Mojave Rattlesnakes that were given florfenicol via subcutaneously implanted osmotic pumps.[20] In spite of disappointing results in recently published studies, further investigation using different implantation sites, other drugs, and other species should be considered. Implantable, bioresorbable devices also deserve consideration, particularly for use in treatment of dangerous and venomous animals in which multiple surgical procedures are impractical.[22]

Transdermal Patch

Fentanyl, scopolamine, nicotine, buprenorphine, naloxone, nitroglycerine, ketoprofen, and many other drugs can be delivered by transdermal patch to humans and domestic mammals. Recently, one study tested fentanyl that was suspended in an ethanol and cellulose gel and enclosed by a plastic barrier with a permeable adhesive membrane impregnated with a loading dose of fentanyl on Prehensile-tailed Skinks *(Corucia zebrata)*.[23] The study showed that all of the skinks in the study obtained measurable plasma concentrations of fentanyl within 24 hours of patch application, and fentanyl concentrations reached the human analgesic range by 36 hours. The most important finding of this study is that the scaled skin of Prehensile-tailed Skinks does not present an insurmountable barrier to systemic absorption of fentanyl delivered via transdermal patch. It is possible that other drugs could be delivered via transdermal patch, and further investigations are warranted in Prehensile-tailed Skinks and other species.

Depot Formulations

Numerous chemotherapeutic agents are available in long-acting formulations. Examples of long-acting formulations that have been used in reptiles include oxytetracycline, doxycycline, ivermectin, and leuprolide acetate.[24-27] Reports of pharmacokinetic studies of these formulations in reptiles provide support for the use of long-acting oxytetracycline for treatment of mycoplasmosis in American Alligators *(Alligator mississippiensis)* but not the other drugs.[24-27]

Vascular Access Ports

Vascular access ports are used to repeatedly collect blood samples or administer IV medications over time. They are particularly useful in pharmacokinetic studies and for cancer chemotherapy. Several authors have placed the rubber stopper from an evacuated blood collection vial into a round plastrostomy drilled ventral to the cardiac ventricle in tortoises. This has been used to collect multiple blood samples over time and can lead to myocardial fibrosis.[28,29] Vascular access ports were placed into the common carotid artery to study blood gasses in seven Green Iguanas and remained functional in most cases for several weeks.[30] A vascular access port (CompanionPort, Norfolk Medical Products Inc., Skokie, Ill) was placed into the ventral abdominal vein in a Green Iguana for lymphoma chemotherapy.[31] This port was replaced after 28 days because of dermal necrosis over the port, and the second port was used for 6 months without a complication.[31]

Topical Administration

Numerous topical medications are used in reptiles, primarily to treat wounds or skin disease. Ivermectin, ophthalmic drugs, disinfectants, creams, ointments, and lavage solutions are all applied via the topical route. These applications are generally intended to deliver local therapy, and systemic uptake is usually an undesired side effect. Recently, several topical preparations for systemic therapy have been evaluated. Topical administration is ideal for antiparasitic agents because most traditional antiparasitic drugs are delivered via orogastric intubation, which can be difficult in some lizards and many chelonians. Two antiparasitic products have been evaluated for systemic uptake of topical preparations. A commercially available topical treatment for intestinal parasites containing imidacloprid and moxidectin (Advantage multi/Advocate, Bayer, Shawnee Mission, Kans) is available for domestic companion animals. The product was applied to the skin of Frilled Dragons *(Chlamydosaurus kingii)* and Bearded Dragons *(Pogona vitticeps)*. After treatment, the feces no longer contained *Kalicephalus* spp. or oxyurid ova.[32] The safety of this imidacloprid/moxidectin topical formulation was not evaluated, and pharmacokinetic research is needed. A commercially available topical preparation containing emodepside and praziquantel (Profender, Bayer HealthCare, Shawnee Mission, Kans) was tested for absorption, elimination time, and efficacy in several lizards, snakes, and chelonians.[33,34] Both drugs were absorbed via the skin, except emodepside in a Red-eared Slider *(Trachemys scripta elegans)* that was returned to the water about 1 hour after application.[33,34] Treatment with emodepside/praziquantel at doses much greater than those used in mammals was followed by a marked decrease in the number of nematode ova in feces within 48 hours. Similarly, no adverse effects were observed and fecal nematode egg counts decreased after treatment in a relatively large (n = 417), uncontrolled clinical trial of emodepside/praziquantel in species from four different reptilian families.[35] The safety of this topical combination should be specifically studied because it holds great promise.

As opposed to these promising therapeutic innovations, several techniques that were proposed and have not gained broad clinical acceptance include percloacal deworming of tortoises, intrapulmonic therapy in chelonians, and intracoelomic administration of anesthetic agents.[36-38]

Antibiotics

Several antibiotics are currently used in reptile antibacterial therapy. Many pharmacokinetic studies have been published, so background information is available for assisting in selection of dose and dosing interval for several drugs in a number of species, although more research is necessary in the most common species presented to reptile veterinarians. A number of individual circumstances guide antibiotic selection in each case. Empiric antibiotic selection may be necessary in critical cases and should be based on the prevalence of specific pathogenic organisms for the disease syndrome, antimicrobial spectrum of activity, distribution of the antimicrobial to the diseased tissues, potential side effects, metabolic and excretory pathways, volume of the formulation necessary to deliver the necessary dose, dosing interval, and ease of administration. In many cases antibiotics can be withheld until culture and sensitivity results are available and antimicrobials are selected accordingly. Selection of antibiotics with a narrow spectrum of activity may help reduce the risk of therapy shifting the balance between enteropathic and commensal bacteria in the favor of the pathogens with the potential risk of infection. Multiple antimicrobials may be used to combat resistant strains of bacteria, and current guidelines for achieving synergy should be followed.[39]

Antibiotics often used in reptile medicine include amikacin, azithromycin, ceftazidime, ciprofloxacin, clarithromycin, danofloxacin, enrofloxacin, marbofloxacin, metronidazole, oxytetracycline, piperacillin, ticarcillin, trimethoprim/sulfamethoxazole, and tylosin. Most of these have been in use for decades and have been previously described.[4] Information presented here is limited to agents with recent advances.

Azithromycin is an azalide, a subclass of macrolide antibiotics that exert their bacteriostatic effect by inhibiting protein synthesis by binding to the 50S ribosome.[40,41] It concentrates in phagocytes and fibroblasts, which may increase its distribution to inflamed tissues. It is available as an oral suspension, oral tablets, and an IV injection and, as a dihydrate, is soluble in water. On administration it is widely distributed in human tissues but not cerebrospinal fluid. Its antimicrobial activity is pH-related and appears to be reduced with decreasing pH. It is eliminated unchanged via biliary and some urinary excretion in humans. Renal impairment has a minor effect on elimination. Drug–drug interactions are minor and not sufficient to warrant altered dosing. Its antimicrobial spectrum includes many gram-positive and gram-negative agents, including aerobes such as *Staphylococcus* spp., *Streptococcus* spp., *Haemophilus* spp., *Bordetella* spp., *Neisseria* spp., and *Moraxella* spp.; anaerobes including *Peptostreptococcus* spp. and *Prevotella bivia,* and other notable bacteria including *Legionella pneumophila, Chlamydophila* spp., *Mycoplasma* spp. Azithromycin demonstrates cross-resistance with erythromycin-resistant gram-positive strains; most strains of *Enterococcus faecalis* are resistant, and methicillin-resistant staphylococci are also resistant. Hepatotoxicity has been reported in humans, and azithromycin could cause reversible nonregenerative anemia in reptiles. It can contribute to dysbiosis and overgrowth of enteropathogens. Oral preparations should not be given concurrently with aluminum-containing or magnesium-containing antacids or phosphate binders.[40] In a single-dose pharmacokinetic study in Ball Pythons *(Python regius),* the authors found that the drug is distributed and excreted similar to humans, and the dose, 10 mg/kg per os (PO), is given at different frequencies based on the location of the infection: skin, every 3 days; respiratory tract, every 5 days; and liver/kidneys, every 7 days.[42]

Ceftazidime is a semisynthetic, broad-spectrum, bacteriocidal, beta-lactam antibiotic for parenteral administration.[43] It exerts its effect by disrupting the synthesis of the peptidoglycan layer in bacterial cell walls. It is highly stable to most clinically important beta-lactamases, either plasmid or chromosomal, so it is active against many organisms that are resistant to penicillins and other cephalosporins. Solutions for injection range from light yellow to amber depending on the diluent and volume used, and the pH ranges from 5 to 8. It is administered either IV or IM, is minimally metabolized, and is primarily excreted unchanged in urine. The dose should be reduced in patients with renal insufficiency, and in humans, elevated levels of ceftazidime can cause neurologic signs. Prolonged therapy with ceftazidime may lead to a fall in prothrombin activity, and vitamin K therapy may be needed.[43] It can contribute to dysbiosis and overgrowth of enteropathogens such as *Clostridium difficile.* It is active against numerous bacteria. Gram-negative aerobes include *Acinetobacter* spp., *Citrobacter* spp., *Enterobacter* spp., *Escherichia coli*, *Haemophilus* spp., *Klebsiella* spp., *Neisseria* spp., *Morganella* spp., *Proteus* spp., *Providencia* spp., *Pseudomonas* spp., *Salmonella* spp., *Shigella* spp., *Serratia* spp., and *Yersinia enterocolitica*. Gram-positive aerobes include *Staphylococcus* spp., and *Streptococcus* spp. Anaerobes include *Bacteroides* spp. (although many strains of *Bacteriodes fragilis* are resistant), *Clostridium* spp. (but not *C. difficile*), *Peptococcus* spp., and *Peptostreptococcus* spp. It is synergistic with aminoglycosides against *Pseudomonas aeruginosa* and the enterobacteriaceae. It is synergistic with carbenicillin against *P. aeruginosa*. It is not active against methicillin-resistant strains. A single-dose pharmacokinetic study was performed in five snake species kept at 30°C (86°F) in which the half-life of 20 mg/kg IM was 24 hours and a dosing interval of 72 hours was proposed at that temperature.[44] A single-dose pharmacokinetic study in Loggerhead Sea turtles *(Caretta caretta)* maintained at 22° to 26°C (75°F) found a serum half-life of 19 to 20 hours, and the authors proposed a dose of 22 mg/kg every 72 hours.[45] In a single-dose pharmacokinetic study of ceftazidime 22 mg/kg IM at the same time as fluconazole 21 mg/kg SC in cold-stunned Kemp's Ridley Sea turtles *(Lepidochelys kempii)* maintained at 21° to 24°C,[46] two of the turtles died during the study, and *E. faecalis* was cultured from the blood and lung of one of them. The maximum concentration (C_{max}) was similar to the study in Loggerhead Sea turtles (61.3 μg/mL versus 69.9 μg/mL, respectively), but the half-life in Kemp's Ridley Sea turtles was more than double that of Loggerheads (43.9 versus 19.1 hours, respectively).[45,46] Ceftazidime is widely prescribed to numerous species in reptile clinical medicine because of its broad-spectrum, low administration volume (when diluted to 100 mg/mL) and prolonged dosing interval of 48 to 72 hours. Further research with boids, lizards, tortoises, and freshwater turtles is needed to determine appropriate dosing in these species.

Clarithromycin is a semisynthetic, bacteriostatic, macrolide antibiotic that inhibits protein synthesis by binding to the 50S ribosome.[47] It is soluble in acetone, slightly soluble in methanol, ethanol, and acetonitrile, and practically insoluble in water. It is available in the United States as immediate-release tablets, extended-release tablets, and granules for oral suspension. It is rapidly absorbed from the gastrointestinal tract in humans, with approximately 50% bioavailability, and it is metabolized by the liver into 14-hydroxy clarithromycin, which is also microbiologically active. Clarithromycin and the 14-hydroxy metabolite distribute readily into human tissues and fluids; intracellular concentrations were greater than serum concentrations but cerebrospinal fluid was not tested.[47] Both clarithromycin and the 14-hydroxy metabolite are excreted primarily in urine. The antimicrobial spectrum includes a variety of gram-positive and gram-negative bacteria as well as *Mycobacterium avium* complex bacteria. Clarithromycin has been shown to be active against *Staphylococcus* spp., *Streptococcus* spp., *Haemophilus* spp., *Moraxella* spp., *Mycoplasma* spp., *Chlamydophila* spp., various mycobacteria, and *Helicobacter pylori* (particularly when in combination with amoxicillin and either omeprazole or lansoprazole). It may also be effective against aerobes including *Bordetella* spp. and *Pasteurella* spp., and anaerobes including *Clostridium perfringens, Peptococcus niger, Propionobacterium acnes,* and *Prevotella melaninogenica (Bacteroides melaninogenicus)*. Most methicillin and oxacillin-resistant isolates are resistant to clarithromycin. Side effects may include hepatotoxicity, and hepatic enzymes should be tested before and monitored during therapy. It should not be administered concomitantly with several drugs including colchicine, anticoagulants, statins (HMG-CoA reductase inhibitors), cisapride, terfenadine, pimozide, or astemizole. Clarithromycin may affect metabolism or serum concentrations of midazolam, alprazolam, digoxin, theophylline, itraconazole, carbamazepine, omeprazole, and ranitidine. It should not be used in gravid or pregnant animals. It can contribute to dysbiosis and overgrowth of enteropathogens such as *C. difficile.* Clarithromycin may be used to treat severe cases of mycoplasmosis in tortoises.[48,49] A recent long-term dosing study showed that clarithromycin therapy can be safe and effective (at resolving clinical signs but not eliminating the organism) in Desert Tortoises *(Gopherus agassizii)* when 15 mg/kg clarithromycin oral suspension (50 mg/mL Biaxin oral suspension, Abbott Labs, Abbott Park, Ill) is administered by gavage every 3.5 days (every 84 hours).[50] This dose results in median clarithromycin concentrations in plasma that rose from 3.32 μg/mL at 14 days to 4.79 μg/mL at 6 months, which is above the proposed target range of 2.0 μg/mL; no 14-hydroxy clarithromycin was detected.[50] The study also showed that per rectum administration did not achieve plasma concentrations in the target range when given every 12 hours for 48 hours followed by every 24 hours for 8 days.[50]

Danofloxacin mesylate is a synthetic fluoroquinolone for SC injection in cattle.[51] It exerts its bacteriocidal activity by inhibiting the bacterial DNA gyrase enzyme to block DNA replication. The FDA-approved label dose is 8 mg/kg once or 6 mg/kg repeated in 48 hours for bovine respiratory disease associated with *Mannheimia (Pasteurella) haemolytica* and *Pasteurella multocida*. It is rapidly absorbed, highly bioavailable, distributed widely in tissues, and has concentrations exceeding that in plasma. Danofloxacin has a half-life in cattle of 3 to 6 hours and has negligible accumulation. It can cause a transient local tissue reaction at the injection site. It is active against gram-negative and gram-positive bacteria.[51] Like other fluoroquinolones, danofloxacin causes articular chondropathy in adult animals at doses exceeding 18 mg/kg and should be used with caution in juveniles. A study assessing the effects of concomitant treatment with ivermectin and danofloxacin in sheep showed that the danofloxacin elimination half-life and systemic exposure (area under the curve [AUC]) increased.[52] A pharmacokinetic study in healthy and experimentally infected chickens with *P. multocida* showed that a dose of 5 mg/kg via gavage was sufficient to provide tissue levels above the minimum inhibitory concentration (MIC) of the organism; tissue levels were less in infected chickens but still above the MIC.[53] A single-dose pharmacokinetic study was performed in Loggerhead Sea turtles after IV, IM, and SC administration of 6 mg/kg.[54] Elimination half-life was 18.7 hours after SC administration and 14.7 hours after IM administration. Maximum plasma concentration and time to maximum concentration after SC and IM administration were similar for both routes (approximately 10 μg/mL and 1.5 hours, respectively). The authors speculate that danofloxacin 6 mg/kg IM or SC every 48 hours could be safe and effective against bacteria with an MIC ≤0.5 μg/mL in Loggerhead Sea turtles and called for a multidose pharmacokinetic study to test the hypothesis.[54] Danofloxacin has been administered at 6 mg/kg SC every 48 hours for 30 days to treat chronic mycoplasmosis in *Gopherus* species tortoises.[9]

Marbofloxacin is a synthetic, broad-spectrum, bacteriocidal fluoroquinolone antibiotic approved by the FDA for skin and soft tissue infections in dogs and cats and for urinary tract infections in dogs.[55] It is available as an oral tablet in the United States and Europe and as an injectable product in Europe. Its antimicrobial action is via inhibition of DNA gyrase, like other fluoroquinolones. It is soluble in water, but solubility decreases in alkaline conditions. Marbofloxacin is rapidly and almost completely absorbed from the gastrointestinal tract after oral administration to fasted dogs and cats. Bioavailability in dogs is 94%. Ten percent to 15% is metabolized by the liver in dogs. Approximately 40% of the oral dose is excreted unchanged in the urine of dogs, and 70% of the drug (85%) and its metabolites (15%) are excreted in the urine of cats. The remainder is eliminated in feces via biliary excretion. Marbofloxacin is bacteriocidal against a broad range of gram-negative and gram-positive organisms including *Staphylococcus* spp., *E. coli, Proteus mirabilis, Streptococcus* spp., *P. multocida, E. faecalis, Klebsiella pneumonia, Pseudomonas* spp., *Corynebacterium* spp., and *Bacillus* spp. Divalent cations diminish the absorption of fluoroquinolones, including calcium, magnesium, aluminum, and zinc, and drugs including sucralfate, so concomitant administration is contraindicated. Marbofloxacin, like other quinolones, is contraindicated in immature animals because it can cause articular chondropathy, and it should be avoided in animals with known central nervous system disorders. Pharmacokinetic studies have been performed in Ball Pythons, Loggerhead Sea turtles, and Red-eared Sliders, and its metabolites have been studied in Ball Pythons.[56-60] In the Ball Python, 10 mg/kg was administered IV or PO to animals maintained at 30°C, and testing continued for only 24 hours, so the half-life could not be calculated; however, the authors proposed a dosage of 10 mg/kg every 48 hours.[59] The pharmacokinetic studies in Loggerhead Sea turtles maintained at 26° to 28°C included dosing of 2 mg/kg IM, IV, and PO. While maximum concentrations and half-life differed somewhat among administration routes, the authors proposed administration of 2 mg/kg every 24 hours is sufficient for all three administration routes.[56,57] Marbofloxacin, 2 mg/kg, was administered IV and IM to Red-eared Sliders in the forelimbs and hindlimbs. Bioavailability was 77% for IM forelimb and 63% for IM hindlimb administration, but no significant difference was found for AUC, clearance, or half-life between locations. The authors determined that IV administration of 2 mg/kg every 24 hours is appropriate at this dose for organisms with an MIC ≤1μg/mL, and IM administration of 2 mg/kg every 24 hours is appropriate for organisms with an MIC ≤0.25μg/mL.[58] Higher doses should be investigated.

Metronidazole is an oral, synthetic, nitroimidazole antiprotozoal and antibacterial agent. It is bacteriocidal against obligate anaerobes (MIC ranging from 0.25 to 8 μg/mL) and is protozoacidal against numerous protozoa with an in vitro MIC of ≤1μg/mL.[61] The antimicrobial action targets DNA synthesis, in that metronidazole acts as an electron acceptor in the phosphoroclastic reaction and causes breaks in the adenine–thymine base pairing. Although resistance is uncommon, it can occur. Metronidazole is available as an IV infusion (metronidazole HCl) and as oral tablets (metronidazole base) in the United States. Metronidazole is a basic compound with a pKa value of 2.62; it is moderately soluble in water (approximately 10 mg/mL at 25°C) at pH 2.5 to 8.0; the pH of the IV infusion is 5.8.[61,62] Oral suspensions using pH-appropriate suspending agents can be procured from licensed compounding pharmacies and are generally the most appropriate formulation for accurate dosing in reptile patients. Metronidazole is well-absorbed after oral administration and is widely distributed to most body tissues and fluids.[62] The major route of elimination of metronidazole and its metabolites is via the urine (60% to 80% in humans), and fecal excretion accounts for 6% to 15% of the dose.[61,62] Metabolism to the 2-hydroxymethyl metabolite occurs, and decreased plasma clearance occurs in patients with decreased liver function but not in patients with renal insufficiency. Side effects are primarily gastrointestinal in humans, although neurotoxic, hepatic, and hematopoietic effects can occur. They include nausea, vomiting, and ataxia, reversible neutropenia, dysuria, yeast overgrowth, encephalopathy, seizures, and peripheral neuropathy. Metronidazole potentiates the effect of coumarin anticoagulants, and concomitant administration with drugs that induce microsomal liver enzymes (e.g., phenytoin or phenobarbital) may accelerate the elimination of metronidazole. Drugs that decrease microsomal liver enzymes (e.g., cimetidine) may prolong its half-life and decrease its plasma clearance.[61] It should be used with caution in patients with blood dyscrasia, and it may cause mild leukopenia. It is contraindicated in the first trimester of human pregnancy. Elevated liver enzyme activities in plasma have been reported in reptiles.[4] Serious toxic side effects in reptiles can occur at doses between 40 and 100 mg/kg.[4,63] Metronidazole is bacteriocidal against (1) gram-negative anaerobic bacilli including *Bacteroides* spp. (including *B. fragilis* group) and *Fusobacterium* spp., (2) gram-positive anaerobic bacilli including *Clostridium* spp. and *Eubacterium* spp., and (3) gram-positive anaerobic cocci including *P. niger* and *Peptostreptococcus* spp.[61] It is trichomonacidal and amoebacidal for protozoa with in vitro MIC ≤1μg/mL.[61] Pharmacokinetic studies in Red-eared Sliders, colubrid snakes *(Elaphe guttata* and *Elaphe obsoleta)*, and Green Iguanas have been published.[16,64-66] In Red-eared Sliders, a single intracoelomic dose of 20 mg/kg was administered; the maximum plasma concentration was 25 μg/mL at 5 hours after injection, and the elimination half-life was 27 hours.[16] The authors suggest an intracoelomic dosage of 20 mg/kg every 48 to 72 hours, depending on the MIC of the organism it is directed against, but caution that adverse effects did occur; thus the intracoelomic route may not be safe. In colubrid snakes, single doses of 20, 50, 100, and 150 mg/kg PO have been studied, and multiple 20-mg/kg doses have also been studied.[64,65] The maximum plasma concentration varies from 12.8 μg/mL after 20 mg/kg PO every 48 hours for 6 days to 2039 μg/mL after a single dose of 150 mg/kg PO. The half-life was 15 hours after the first 20-mg/kg dose, 23 hours after the sixth dose, and 26 hours after the 150-mg/kg dose.[64,65] No clinically significant adverse behavioral, hematologic, or biochemical effects were observed other than mildly elevated plasma lactate dehydrogenase activity after the last 20-mg/kg dose and mildly decreased glucose after the 50- and 150-mg/kg single doses.[64,65] Taken together, the results support a dosage of 20 mg/kg every 48 hours in *Elaphe* spp. snakes. Higher doses should be reserved for resistant infections so that the risk of adverse effects is avoided. A pharmacokinetic study of a single 20-mg/kg dose followed by 20 mg/kg every 24 hours for 10 days in Green Iguanas found a maximum plasma concentration (C_{max}) of 7.6 μg/mL after the single dose with a half-life of 12.7 hours and a C_{max} of 22.8 μg/mL after 10 days.[66] No adverse hematologic, biochemical, or behavioral effects were observed after the 10-day treatment trial. The authors concluded that 20 mg/kg every 48 hours would be sufficient for "most" infections and that the dosing frequency could be increased to every 24 hours for resistant strains with MICs ≥8 μg/mL.[66]

Antiviral Agents

Numerous viruses infect reptiles, and a causal relationship between disease and the viral pathogen has been established for a few; diagnostic tests are currently available for several of them.[67,68] Nursing care is the mainstay of antiviral therapy for individuals, and immune-stimulators and antiviral drugs may be useful in some cases.[69] Vaccine trials have shown promise for poxvirus in crocodilians but not herpesvirus in tortoises or paramyxovirus in snakes.[4,67,70] Reptiles testing positive for a virus should be isolated from uninfected reptiles to prevent further transmission. A few antiviral drugs have been evaluated for reptiles and may help improve an individual patient's clinical condition; however, in general, antiviral drugs are not expected to eliminate infection, and it is possible that a reptile could shed infective virus after treatment. Antiviral agents that have been evaluated in reptiles include acyclovir, ganciclovir, and valacyclovir.[71-73]

Acyclovir is a synthetic purine nucleoside analogue that interferes with nucleic acid synthesis and is active against herpesviruses.[74] The inhibitory activity is highly selective because of an affinity for thymidine kinase encoded by herpesviruses, which phosphorylates acyclovir into a nucleotide analogue that is further converted by a series of enzymes into acyclovir triphosphate. Acyclovir triphosphate stops replication of herpesviral DNA by competitive inhibition of viral DNA polymerase, incorporation into and termination of the growing DNA chain, and inactivation of viral DNA polymerase.[72,74] Acyclovir is available in tablets, capsules, oral suspension, and by injection. Its average bioavailability after oral administration is 10% to 20%, and food does not affect absorption. The elimination half-life and total body clearance of acyclovir are dependent on renal function in humans, and the dose should be reduced in patients with renal insufficiency.[74] Coadministration of probenecid with acyclovir increases the elimination half-life of acyclovir. Adverse effects are rare in humans. An in vitro study of acyclovir efficacy against a herpesvirus isolated from a Hermann's Tortoise *(Testudo hermanni)* indicated that 50 μg/mL reduced the virus content of cultures to below the limit of detection.[71] The pharmacokinetics of acyclovir in Marginated Tortoises *(Testudo marginata)* over a 24-hour period after 80 mg/kg PO every 24 hours for 7 days have been reported.[73] The maximum plasma concentration occurred 6.9 ± 4.2 hours after administration and was 1.40 ± 0.45 μg/mL; the tissue concentrations were not evaluated.[73] The elimination half-life was 8.9 ± 3.8 hours, and the authors proposed that a higher milligram dose be administered every 12 to 24 hours. A recently published study[72] on the pharmacokinetics of acyclovir in North American Box Turtles *(Terrapene carolina)* after a single oral dose of 40 mg/kg valacyclovir (the esterified form that is rapidly converted to acyclovir after oral administration) found the elimination half-life to be 14.6 hours, and the C_{max} of 1.94 μg/mL was reached 13.0 ± 7 hours after administration. Prolonged lethargy was noted in one turtle after receiving the dose of valacyclovir. The authors proposed that a dosage of valacyclovir of 40 mg/kg PO every 24 hours would be sufficient to achieve a steady-state level above 0.8 μg/mL in plasma. It is possible the proposed doses of valacyclovir in the Common Box Turtle and acyclovir in the Marginated Tortoise may be sufficient to treat herpesvirus in tortoises even though plasma levels are much lower than the necessary in vitro inhibitory concentration because acyclovir concentrates in herpesvirus-infected tissues; the MIC in humans is 0.45 μg/mL, 3 μg/mL in horses, and 18 μg/mL in cats. A topical preparation is also available (5% acyclovir, Zovirax, GlaxoSmithKline, Inc., Research Triangle Park, NC). A few clinicians suggest it may be useful in treatment of herpesvirus stomatitis in tortoises.[75,76] Further research measuring the tissue levels of acyclovir achieved in herpesvirus-infected tissue after oral administration and the efficacy of treatment are necessary. Valacyclovir may also have some effect on iridoviruses, and further research is warranted.[72]

Ganciclovir is a synthetic guanine derivative that is active against human cytomegalovirus and herpesvirus.[77] Its mechanism of action is similar to acyclovir. It has a solubility of 2.6 mg/mL in water at 25°C and pKa values of 2.2 and 9.4. As the monosodium salt, ganciclovir sodium, it has a solubility of approximately 6 mg/mL at 37°C. When reconstituted with water, the pH of the IV solution is 11. The in vitro MIC for cytomegalovirus ranges from 0.02 to 3.48 μg/mL. Ganciclovir inhibits mammalian cell proliferation at concentrations as low as 30 μg/mL. It is eliminated primarily via the kidneys, so the dosage should be reduced in patients with renal insufficiency. Viral resistance to ganciclovir has been found in humans that have never been treated with it before.[77] Pharmacokinetics have not been studied in reptiles, but an in vitro study showed that it was effective at 25 and 50 μg/mL against a herpesvirus cultured from a Hermann's Tortoise.

Antifungal Agents

Fungal infections are common enough in reptiles that antifungal therapy has become a routine part of clinical practice. Similar to antibiotics, antifungal agents are best selected in response to a specific etiologic diagnosis. Fungal culture should precede therapy, but antifungal sensitivity testing is not practical in most cases. Empiric selection of antifungal drugs may be necessary while awaiting culture results, which can take weeks. Selection should be based on the prevalence of a specific fungal organism for a disease syndrome, antifungal spectrum of activity, distribution of the antifungal drug to the diseased tissues, potential side effects, metabolic and excretory pathways, volume of the formulation required to deliver the necessary dose, dosing interval, and ease of administration. Multiple antifungal drugs may be used concomitantly to overcome the limitations of one drug alone or to expand the spectrum of activity. Topical agents are frequently combined with systemic agents for severe fungal dermatitis (e.g., *Chrysosporium* anamorph of *Nannizziopsis vriesii* [CANV]). A vaccine trial showed no difference between dermatologic lesions or septicemia between vaccinated and control Bearded Dragons experimentally infected with CANV.[78] This review is limited to those agents in which new information is available.

Amphotericin B is a polyene antifungal produced from a strain of *Streptomyces nodosus*. It acts to increase membrane permeability by binding to sterols in cell membranes of sensitive fungi. It also binds to the sterols in vertebrate cell membranes, which is believed to account for its toxicity in animals and humans. It is available as an injectable product and in lipid complex.[79] The lipid complex formulation has increased peak concentration, clearance time, volume of distribution, and terminal elimination half-life when compared with amphotericin B desoxycholate.[79] Several drugs interact with amphotericin B when used concomitantly. These include antineoplastic chemotherapeutics, corticosteroids, cyclosporin A, digitalis glycosides, flucytosine, imidazole antifungal agents (e.g., ketoconazole, clotrimazole, and fluconazole), other nephrotoxic agents, tubocurarine, and zidovudine.[79] Treatment can cause increases in levels of blood urea nitrogen, uric acid, aspartate aminotransferase, alanine aminotransferase, alkaline phosphatase, lactate dehydrogenase, and amylase. Treatment can cause decreased blood phosphorus and increases or decreases in blood glucose levels. It is likely to cause nephrotoxicosis in reptiles and is contraindicated in reptiles with renal insufficiency.[80] It is active against species of *Aspergillus, Blastomyces, Candida, Coccidioides, Cryptococcus,* and *Histoplasma* in mammals. Resistance can occur, particularly with prolonged therapy. The in vitro MIC against CANV cultured from captive lizards was 2 μg/mL.[81] There are clinical reports of its use in nebulization, intratracheal, and intrapulmonary therapy in reptiles.[63,82,83]

Itraconazole is a synthetic triazole antifungal agent. It exerts its antifungal action by inhibiting ^{14}C-demethylation of ergosterol, a cell wall component of fungi. It is available in capsules and oral solution. It is insoluble in water, slightly soluble in alcohols, and freely soluble in dichloromethane. It has a pKa of 3.70 and a log–log(n-octanol/water) partition coefficient of 5.66 at pH 8.1. The oral solution has a target pH of 2 and should be taken under fasting conditions for best absorption in humans, as opposed to the capsules, which should be taken with food because low pH is required for absorption.[84] It is metabolized by the cytochrome P450 isoenzyme system (CYP3A4), which results in several metabolites, primarily hydroxyitraconazole. It may undergo saturable metabolism with multiple doses, and the dosing interval may be longer than predicted by single-dose pharmacokinetic studies.[81,84] About 40% of the dose is excreted as inactive metabolites in urine, up to 18% is excreted unchanged in feces, and less than 0.03% is excreted unchanged in human urine. Itraconazole is widely distributed to tissues, especially lipophilic organs including skin. It is minimally distributed to aqueous humor of the eye, cerebrospinal fluid, urine, and saliva when inflammation is not present.[85] Because it is primarily metabolized by the liver, blood levels should be monitored in patients with hepatic insufficiency, and dosing intervals should be adjusted to maintain blood levels above the MIC of the target fungus. It is active against species of *Blastomyces, Aspergillus, Histoplasma, Coccidioides, Cryptococcus, Paracoccidioides, Sporothrix,* and *Trichophyton*. It can be active against some isolates of *Candida,* but many are resistant. It is not active against *Zygomycetes, Fusarium, Scedosporium,* and *Scopulariopsis*. It has been used to effectively treat CANV infections in reptiles. Itraconazole can cause rapid hepatotoxic effects including liver failure and death in humans, and its use is contraindicated in patients with hepatic insufficiency.[84] It can cause anorexia and weight loss in Bearded Dragons. In one treatment trial, five of seven Bearded Dragons died on days 5, 20, 22, 36, and 54 of treatment with itraconazole oral solution (Sporanox, Janssen-Cilag, Berchem, Belgium) 5 mg/kg every 24 hours PO, although histopathologic evidence of hepatotoxicity was absent.[81,86] Itraconazole accumulates over time in CANV-infected Bearded Dragons, reaching a steady-state plasma concentration of 4 to 8 μg/mL after approximately 10 days.[81] In vitro MIC_{90} of itraconazole for CANV cultured from infected Bearded Dragons was 0.25 μg/mL.[81] The fungus could no longer be cultured from lesions after 4 weeks of treatment. In a different treatment trial, seven Bearded Dragons were successfully treated for CANV with itraconazole (and clotrimazole), but six were euthanized.[87] A group of Green Anacondas (*Eunectes murinus murinus*) infected with CANV were treated with itraconazole (Sporanox Oral Solution, OrthoBiotech, Raritan, NJ) at one of two dosages, either 10 mg/kg every 48 hours for 14 days or 10 mg/kg every 24 hours for 7 days then every 48 hours for 7 days; plasma levels of itraconazole reached 4.3 to 9.0 μg/mL and persisted for at least 14 d after treatment.[88] A series of cases showed that itraconazole was effective without adverse effects at metabolically scaled doses (0.5 to 1.7 mg/kg PO every 53 to 75 hours for 148 to 184 days) in the treatment of *Aspergillus* spp. in two lizard species and two snake species (total of seven cases).[89] Therefore, because itraconazole appears to be well-absorbed after oral administration, has efficacy against fungal infections, and is of questionable safety, further pharmacokinetic studies, preferably in fungus-infected patients, are warranted.

Voriconazole is a triazole antifungal agent that exerts its antifungal effect by inhibiting fungal cytochrome P450-mediated 14 alpha-lanosterol demethylation, which is essential for ergosterol inhibition. It is more selective for fungal than mammalian cytochrome P450 enzyme systems.[90] It is available as a lyophilized powder for IV infusion, film-coated tablets for oral administration, and as a powder for oral suspension.[90] Pharmacokinetics in humans are similar after the oral and IV routes, and maximum plasma concentrations are achieved 1 to 2 hours after dosing.[90] It is widely distributed into tissues and is metabolized by cytochrome P450 enzymes to metabolites including N-oxide voriconazole, which has minimal antifungal activity and accounts for 72% of the circulating metabolites.[90] It is eliminated primarily via hepatic metabolism; less than 2% of the oral dose is excreted unchanged in the urine of humans, and more than 80% of the metabolites are recovered in the urine. Doses should be adjusted accord to plasma levels of the drug in patients with hepatic insufficiency. No adjustment is necessary in patients with renal insufficiency after oral administration, but IV administration should be avoided because the IV vehicle (sulfobutyl ether beta-cyclodextrin sodium) accumulates. The terminal elimination half-life is dose dependent because the pharmacokinetics of voriconazole are nonlinear. Serious drug interactions occur with concomitantly administered agents that are also metabolized via the cytochrome P450 enzyme system. Side effects in humans include visual disturbances, gastrointestinal disturbances, hepatic toxicity, fetal toxicity in pregnant women, and electrocardiac disturbances. It is effective against species of fungi including *Aspergillus, Candida, Fusarium* (except *Fusarium solani*), and *Scedosporium*. Drug resistance has not been studied thoroughly, but strains that are resistant to fluconazole or itraconazole may also show reduced sensitivity to voriconazole.[90] In vitro voriconazole sensitivity (MIC_{90}) of CANV that was isolated from captive lizards was 0.0625 μg/mL.[81]

When used for treatment of CANV in Bearded Dragons, only one of seven died compared with five of seven treated with itraconazole; in those that survived, the disease was cleared with treatment of voriconazole (Vfend, Pfizer, Ixelles, Belgium) 10 mg/kg PO every 24 hours for 4 to 9 weeks.[81] The steady-state plasma concentration of voriconazole was 3.4 to 5.7 μg/mL, but substantial interindividual variation was observed.[81] A Giant Girdled Lizard *(Cordylus giganteus)* was treated for CANV with voriconazole tablets (Vfend, Pfizer, Ltd, Sandwich, England) suspended in water, 10 mg/kg PO every 24 hours for 10 weeks.[91] This resulted in a steady-state plasma concentration of approximately 2.0 to 3.5 μg/mL after 3 days of treatment. In vitro MIC of the cultured CANV was 0.25 μg/mL for voriconazole. Weekly fungal culture of the skin wounds was negative during weeks 7 to 10 of treatment and for 3 weeks after treatment.[91] Pharmacokinetics of voriconazole were determined after a single SC injection (5 mg/kg) in Red-eared Sliders.[92] The maximum plasma concentration was greater than 1 μg/mL at 1 hour and 2 hours after injection. This route of administration is likely to require a much higher dose and short dosing interval to maintain a plasma concentration that is above the MIC of many organisms.[92]

Terbinafine hydrochloride is an allylamine antifungal agent. It can be fungicidal in vitro depending on the concentration and the fungal species.[93] Terbinafine exerts its antifungal action by inhibiting biosynthesis of ergosterol via inhibition of squalene epoxidase enzyme, which causes fungal death primarily due to increased membrane permeability from high concentrations of squalene but not ergosterol deficiency.[93] It is freely soluble in methanol and methylene, soluble in ethanol, and slightly soluble in water. Pharmacokinetics have not been studied in reptiles, but in mammals it is well-absorbed after oral administration; peak plasma concentrations generally occur within 2 hours after administration.[94] It is lipophilic and becomes concentrated rapidly in the stratum corneum of the skin; it has a terminal half-life of 200 to 400 hours in tissues such as adipose and skin, making it well-suited for treating fungal dermatoses.[94] It is metabolized in the liver via several CYP isoenzymes but not cytochrome P450; the metabolites have little antifungal activity.[93] It is primarily excreted in urine, and dosing should be adjusted in patients with renal insufficiency. Terbinafine is active against species of fungi including *Trichophyton, Candida, Epidermophyton,* and *Scopulariopsis*. In vitro sensitivity of CANV isolated from the skin of Bearded Dragons (MIC_{90}) to terbinafine was 2 μg/mL.[81] It has been administered to reptiles, but no pharmacokinetic data are available. Topically applied terbinafine (Lamisil, Novartis Farmaceutica, S.A., Barcelona, Spain) was administered concomitantly with topical chlorhexidine (Cristalmina solucion cutanea, Laboratorios Salvat A.A., Esplugues de Llobregat, Barcelona, Spain) and oral ketoconazole (Panfungol suspension, Doctor Esteve S.A., Barcelona, Spain) to treat CANV in a Bearded Dragon and two Green Iguanas.[95,96] The therapeutic combination brought about clinical resolution of CANV infection, but it is unclear what treatment effect could be attributed to terbinafine because of the confounding effects of the other therapeutic agents. Terbinafine was used to successfully treat *Exophiala oligosperma* phaeohyphomycosis of the carapace in an Aldabra Giant Tortoise *(Aldabrachelys [Geochelone] gigantea)*. Initially it was used topically in combination with oral itraconazole and then, because of lack of clinical response, switched to oral terbinafine (Lamisil, Norvartis Pharmaceuticals, East Hanover, NJ) 3.4 mg/kg PO every 24 hours for 15 months.[97] Plasma concentrations of terbinafine were not measured during treatment.

Antiparasitic Agents

A number of antiparasitic agents are currently being used to treat endoparasites and ectoparasites in reptiles. Effective treatment addresses the life cycle and ecology of the parasite. For example, it is essential to know what tissues it affects, whether it is directly transmitted, has intermediate hosts, has free-living life stages, and whether it participates in the transmission of other infectious agents. Treatment may or may not include antiparasitic drug therapy. Commonly used antiparasitic drugs include albendazole, fenbendazole, fipronil, ivermectin, metronidazole, oxfendazole, paromomycin, permethrin, ponazuril, praziquantel, pyrantel pamoate, toltrazuril, and trimethoprim/sulfas. Promising newer products include combinations of imidacloprid/moxidectin and emodepside/praziquantel that are administered topically (see previous sections in this chapter). This review is limited to a few notable agents about which there are recently published data. Topical treatment with imidacloprid/moxidectin (Advantage multi/Advocate, Bayer, Shawnee Mission, Kans) and emodepside/praziquantel (Profender, Bayer HealthCare, Shawnee Mission, Kans) show promise for the treatment of internal parasites in reptiles and have already been reviewed in this chapter.

Albendazole, fenbendazole, and oxfendazole are frequently used benzimidazole antiparasitic agents that exert their antiparasitic action by selectively binding and damaging tubulin, preventing tubulin polymerization and inhibiting microtubule formation.[98,99] At higher concentrations, benzimidazoles disrupt metabolic pathways within helminths and inhibit enzymes such as malate dehydrogenase and fumarate reductase. Fenbendazole is insoluble in water and only marginally absorbed after oral administration; peak blood levels of 0.07 to 0.11 μg/mL are seen in mammals, and up to 50% is excreted unchanged in the feces. The small amount of absorbed fenbendazole is metabolized by cytochrome P450 and other microsomal enzymes in the liver to metabolites including oxfendazole; some extrahepatic metabolism also occurs.[100] Benzimidazoles are effective against a range of nematodes, some trematodes, a few cestodes, and a few flagellated protozoans. Benzimidazole toxicity is generally rare in most species, but mortality has been reported, particularly after overdoses in birds and reptiles.[100-103] Relative toxicity of these anthelmintics in order of most toxic to least toxic appears to be albendazole >oxfendazole>fenbendazole.[104] Toxicosis leads to lesions that mimic radiation, which targets rapidly dividing cells including bone marrow and intestinal epithelium. They also cause hepatotoxicosis, teratogenic effects, and tumor promotion.[102] Benzimidazoles should be used with caution in gravid and pregnant animals and should be avoided in animals with septicemia. Fenbendazole and oxfendazole were compared with regard to their efficacy against intestinal oxyurid nematodes in Hermann's Tortoises after single oral doses of 100 mg/kg and 66 mg/kg, respectively.[105] Both treatments eliminated shedding of oxyurid ova in feces after 32 days, and a second treatment was not necessary.

Toltrazuril and its principle metabolite ponazuril are triazinetrione antiprotozoal compounds with activity against several genera of the Apicomplexa including *Eimeria, Isospora, Hepatozoon, Toxoplasma, Sarcocystis, Neospora,* and possibly others.[106-108] Ponazuril is available as an oral paste (Marquis, 15% w/w, Bayer Animal Health, Shawnee Mission, Kans) in the United States, and it can be compounded into an oral suspension by a licensed pharmacist. Toltrazuril is available outside of the United States as a solution for the drinking water of poultry (Baycox solution 2.5% and 10%, Bayer) and as an oral suspension (Baycox 2.5 and 5% suspension, Bayer). The pH of ponazuril oral paste is 5.7 to 6, and the pH of 2.5% toltrazuril solution is 8 to 10. Toltrazuril is rapidly metabolized in the liver to the sulfone derivative, ponazuril.[108] These drugs exert a coccidiocidal effect on intracellular coccidial stages by interfering with division of the nucleus, amino acid and fatty acid metabolism, and the electron transport system of mitochondria through ballooning of the endoplasmic reticulum and, in macrogametes, by damaging the wall-forming bodies.[106,107,109] There is no effect on oocysts. An additive effect can be achieved by concomitant administration of toltrazuril with an ionophore in the treatment of coccidiosis in poultry.[107] A concentration of 0.1 to 1.0 μg/mL ponazuril is sufficient to kill *Sarcocystis neurona,* which causes equine protozoal myeloencephalitis (EPM) when horses serve as aberrant hosts for the organism. The peak serum concentration was 5.6 μg/mL 18 days after oral administration in horses, and the peak concentration in cerebrospinal fluid was 0.21 μg/mL after 15 days.[106] The elimination half-life in horses is about 4.5 days. Acute toxicity of toltrazuril in rats, mice, and chickens required overdoses of 100 times the recommended therapeutic dose, with an LD_{50} range of 1600 to 5000 mg/kg; no observable effect occurred in mammals after a ponazuril dose of 90 mg/kg.[107,109] A 2-day treatment of toltrazuril in the drinking water (7 mg/kg) is sufficient to treat intestinal coccidiosis in poultry, and daily oral administration of ponazuril (5 mg/kg) for 28 days is recommended for treatment of EPM in horses.[106,107] A clinical trial in chameleons reported that toltrazuril was effective at eliminating shedding of coccidium, and no side effects were observed.[110] Similarly, a pilot study in Bearded Dragons reported that coccidian oocysts were found on fecal flotation before treatment with ponazuril 30 mg/kg PO every 48 hours for two treatments but not after.[111] An incidental finding in a group of 10 Bearded Dragons in an experimental cryptosporidiosis/paromomycin study was that treatment of a naturally occurring coccidiasis (presumed *Isospora amphiboluri*) with ponazuril (Marquis, Bayer, Inc., Montreal, Quebec, Canada) 30 mg/kg PO every 48 hours for three treatments and then again after 3 months 30 mg/kg every 48 hours for six treatments was not effective.[112] Histologic examination of the intestines immediately after the second treatment period showed mild to moderate intracellular *Isospora* in the enterocytes of all but one of the 10 dragons.[112] Toltrazuril (Baycox 5%, oral suspension, Bayer Vital GmbH, Germany), 15 mg/kg, every 48 hours for 30 days, and ponazuril (90 mg/mL compounded), 30 mg/kg PO every 24 hours for 4 days and repeated for 2 to 4 treatments at least 2 weeks apart, have been used to treat intranuclear coccidiosis of testudines in several species of tortoise, and both drugs appear to be associated with improved survival, cessation of shedding (negative results on polymerase chain reaction testing after treatment), and resolution of clinical signs in cases that are treated early in the course of the disease.[113] Controlled clinical trials and pharmacokinetic studies are needed for ponazuril and toltrazuril in reptiles.

Paromomycin is an oral aminoglycoside antiparasitic agent closely related to neomycin. Like all aminoglycosides, it exerts its cidal effect by binding to the 16S ribosomal RNA subunit to inhibit protein synthesis. Paromomycin is very soluble in water but, similar to other aminoglycosides, is poorly absorbed after oral administration, except in cases of severe intestinal ulceration. It is eliminated almost exclusively unchanged in the feces. It has antibacterial activity, which is a side effect when used to treat intestinal amoebiasis, cutaneous leishmaniasis, or cryptosporidiosis. Intestinal dysbiosis can occur when used for prolonged periods at high doses. Paromomycin has been used with limited success in reptiles to treat refractory intestinal amoebiasis and cryptosporidiosis.[112,114-118] Treatment with paromomycin 100 mg/kg PO every 24 hours for 7 days, then every 84 hours for 90 days in a group of Hermann's Tortoises with cryptosporidiosis initially controlled clinical signs and shedding, but the disease recrudesced after 9 months.[114] A colony of Leopard Geckos *(Eublepharis macularius)* with naturally occurring cryptosporidiosis were treated with 50 to 800 mg/kg paromomycin (Humatin, Parke-Davis, Morris Plains, NJ) PO every 24 hours; the treatment was associated with improvement in clinical signs and reduced oocyst shedding that returned when treatment was suspended.[118] In a different clinical trial, treatment of four Leopard Geckos with paromomycin (100 mg/kg every 24 hours for 7 days, and then every 84 hours for 72 days) brought about improvement of clinical signs and negative fecal examinations in three of the geckos but did not eliminate infection.[115] Two Gila Monsters *(Heloderma suspectum)* with naturally occurring cryptosporidium infection were treated with paromomycin at a dosage of 300 to 360 mg/kg PO every 48 hours for 14 days, which was repeated at 6 months; fecal samples were negative for cryptosporidia after 2 weeks of treatment and for at least 1 year.[117] A group of 10 hatchling (1-month-old) Bearded Dragons were experimentally infected with *Cryptosporidium* from a naturally infected adult, and five of them were treated with paromomycin (Humatin 250 mg capsules, Erfa, Montreal, Quebec, Canada) in saline (500 mg/5 mL) 100 mg/kg every 24 hours for 7 days, followed by every 84 hours for 72 days; the other five Bearded Dragons served as controls.[112] This treatment did not control shedding of the organism into the feces, so a second round of treatment with 360 mg/kg every 48 hours for 10 days was administered. This second treatment regimen did eliminate the cryptosporidia: infection was present in four of five control Bearded Dragons and in none of five treated Bearded Dragons on histologic examination of the gastrointestinal tract.[112]

Analgesic Agents, Anesthetics, and Chemical Restraint

See Chapter 18 for information about analgesic agents and Chapter 12 for anesthetics and methods of chemical restraint.

Antiinflammatory Agents

Meloxicam is a member of the enolic acid group of nonsteroidal antiinflammatory drugs (NSAID) that exhibits antiinflammatory, analgesic, and antipyretic activities.[119] It is available in tablets or a suspension for oral administration. Meloxicam is practically insoluble in water, has higher solubility in strong acids and bases, and pKa values of 1.1 and 4.2. Its mechanism of action is via inhibition of cyclooxygenase (COX) (prostaglandin synthetase), which results in reduced prostaglandins, thromboxanes, and prostacyclin; it is considered COX-2 preferential but is not COX-2 specific.[120] It is well-absorbed after oral administration, and the serum concentration first peaks in 4 to 5 hours in fasted humans then has a second peak resulting from enterohepatic cycling at 12 to 14 hours after administration.[119] It is highly bound to plasma proteins and is widely distributed to tissues, including synovial fluid. Meloxicam is extensively metabolized in the liver via cytochrome P450 and other enzymes, and the metabolites have no known pharmacologic activity.[119] Equal amounts are excreted in urine and feces, predominantly in the form of metabolites; the mean elimination half-life ranges from 15 to 20 hours in humans.[119] Similar to other NSAIDs, meloxicam has adverse effects in mammals that can include gastrointestinal ulcers, hypertension, acute renal failure, hepatic dysfunction, respiratory depression, coma, convulsions, cardiovascular collapse, and cardiac arrest, but short-term dosing studies in dogs have not demonstrated any untoward renal or hepatic toxicity.[119,120] It should not be administered concomitantly with other NSAIDs, angiotensin-converting enzyme inhibitors, anticoagulants, corticosteroids, furosemide, digoxin, fluconazole, or other nephrotoxic drugs.[119,120] Pharmacokinetic studies have been reported in reptiles. Meloxicam (Metacam, injectable solution, 5 mg/mL, Boehringer Ingelheim España, SA, Sant Cugat del Vallès, Barcelona, Spain) was administered to healthy Red-eared Sliders by IV (0.22 mg/kg), IM (0.5 mg/kg), and oral (0.5 mg/kg) routes.[121] The drug was rapidly eliminated after IV injection and was rapidly absorbed with good bioavailability after IM and oral administration. Individual variation was substantial after oral administration, so the authors concluded that the IM route is preferable.[121] Pharmacokinetics were determined in Green Iguanas after administration of 0.2 mg/kg meloxicam via IV and oral routes, toxicity was assessed after 1 or 5 mg/kg PO every 24 hours for 12 days.[122] Pharmacokinetic variables were similar between the two administration routes, except that the maximum plasma concentration was greater after IV administration (0.6 μg/mL) than after oral administration (0.2 μg/mL). No histologic evidence of toxicity was found after administration of the high doses. The authors concluded that 0.2 mg/kg IV or PO would result in plasma concentrations above 0.1 μg/mL for 24 hours.[122]

REFERENCES

1. Huey RB. Temperature, physiology, and the ecology of reptiles. In: Gans C, Pough FH, eds. *Biology of the reptilia 12, physiology C.* New York: Academic Press, 1982;25-91.
2. Johnson JH, Jensen JM, Brumbaugh GW, et al. Amikacin pharmacokinetics and the effects of ambient temperature on the dosage regimen in ball pythons (*Python regius*). *J Zoo Wildl Med* 1997;28(1):80-88.
3. Caligiuri R, Kollias GV, Jacobson E, et al. The effects of ambient temperature on amikacin pharmacokinetics in gopher tortoises. *J Vet Pharmacol Ther* 1990;13:287-291.
4. Mitchell MA. Therapeutics. In: Mader DR, ed. *Reptile medicine and surgery*. St. Louis: Saunders Elsevier, 2006;631-664.
5. Sykes JM, Greenacre CB. Techniques for drug delivery in reptiles and amphibians. *J Exotic Pet Med* 2006;15:210-217.
6. Evans EE, Cowles RB. Effect of temperature on antibody synthesis in the reptile, *Dipsosaurus dorsalis*. *Proc Soc Exp Biol Med* 1959;101:482-483.
7. Zimmerman LM, Vogel LA, Bowden RM. Understanding the vertebrate immune system: insights from the reptilian perspective. *J Exp Biol* 2010;213:661-671.
8. Martin LB. Stress and immunity in wild vertebrates: timing is everything. *Gen Comp Endocrinol* 2009;163:70-76.
9. Gibbons PM, Klaphake EA, Carpenter JW. Reptiles. In: Carpenter JW, ed. *Exotic animal formulary*. 4th ed. St. Louis: Elsevier, 2012;83-182.
10. Norton TM. Chelonian emergency and critical care. *Semin Avian Exotic Pet Med* 2005;14:106-130.
11. American Veterinary Medical Association Web site. Animal Medicinal Drug Use Clarification Act. Available at: https://www.avma.org/KB/Resources/Reference/Pages/AMDUCA.aspx. Accessed Oct 10, 2012.
12. Holz P. Renal anatomy and physiology. In: Mader DR, ed. *Reptile medicine and surgery*. 2nd ed. St. Louis: Sauders Elsevier, 2006;135.
13. Schaffner F. The liver. In: Gans C, Gaunt AS, eds. *Biology of the reptilia volume 19, morphology G visceral organs*. Ithaca, NY: Society for the Study of Amphibians and Reptiles, 1998;485-531.
14. Sladky KK, Mans C. Clinical anesthesia in reptiles. *J Exotic Pet Med* 2012;21:17-31.
15. Holz P, Barker IK, Burger JP, et al. The effect of the renal portal system on pharmacokinetic parameters in the red-eared slider (*Trachemys scripta elegans*). *J Zoo Wildl Med* 1997;28:386-393.
16. Innis C, Papich M, Young D. Pharmacokinetics of metronidazole in the red-eared slider turtle (*Trachemys scripta elegans*) after single intracoelomic injection. *J Vet Pharm Theraput* 2007;30:168-171.
17. Durect Corporation Web site. Alzet osmotic pumps. Available at: http://www.durect.com/wt/durect/page_name/alzet. Accessed Oct 10, 2012.
18. Phillips JA, Alexander N, Karesh WB, et al. Stimulating male sexual behavior with repetitive pulses of GnRH in female Green Iguanas, *Iguana iguana*. *J Exp Zool* 1985;234:481-484.
19. Sykes JM, Ramsay EC, Schumacher J, et al. Evaluation of an implanted osmotic pump for delivery of amikacin to corn snakes (*Elaphe guttata guttata*). *J Zoo Wildl Med* 2006;37:373-380.

20. Sykes JM, Folland D, Bemis D, et al. Osmotic pump delivery of florfenicol or amikacin in Mojave rattlesnakes *(Crotalus scutulatus)* with *Salmonella arixonae* osteomyelitis, in *Proceedings*. 15th Annu Conf Assoc Reptilian Amphibian Vet 2008;29-30.
21. Avent ML, Rogers BA, Cheng AC, et al. Current use of aminoglycosides: indications, pharmacokinetics and monitoring for toxicity. *Int Med J* 2011;41:441-449.
22. Tobias IS, Lee H, Engelmayr GC, et al. Zero-order controlled release of ciprofloxacin-HCl from a reservoir-based, bioresorbable and elastomeric device. *J Control Release* 2010;146:356-362.
23. Gamble KC. Plasma fentanyl concentrations achieved after transdermal fentanyl patch application in prehensile-tailed skinks, *Corucia zebrata*. *J Herpetol Med Surg* 2008;18:81-85.
24. Kirchgessner M, Mitchell M, Domenzain L, et al. Evaluating the effect of leuprolide acetate on testosterone levels in captive male green iguanas *(Iguana iguana)*. *J Herp Med Surg* 2009;19:128-131.
25. Sutherland-Smith M, Miller JA. Use of long-acting ivermectin suspension in snakes, in *Proceedings*. Ann Conf Am Assoc Zoo Vet 1994;98-101.
26. Johnson-Delaney CJ. *Chlamydophila psittaci* in a commercial colony of veiled chameleons, in *Proceedings*. 16th Annu Conf Assoc Reptilian Amphibian Vet 2009;149-152.
27. Helmick KE, Papich MG, Vliet KA, et al. Pharmacokinetic disposition of a long-acting oxytetracycline formulation after single-dose intravenous and intramuscular administrations in the American alligator *(Alligator mississippiensis)*. *J Zoo Wildl Med* 2004;35:341-346.
28. Rooney MB, Levine G, Gaynor J. Sevoflurane anesthesia in desert tortoises *(Gopherus agassizii)*. *J Zoo Wildl Med* 1999;30:64-69.
29. Wimsatt J, Johnson JD, Mangone BA. Use of a cardiac access port for repeated collection of blood samples from desert tortoises *(Gopherus agassizii)*. *Contemp Top Lab Anim Sci* 1998;37:81-83.
30. Hess JC, Grimm KA, Benson GJ, et al. The use of vascular access ports in nonanesthetized green iguanas *(Iguana iguana)* to collect baseline arterial blood gas parameters. *Vet Anesth Analg* 2005;32:18.
31. Folland DW, Johnston MS, Thamm DH, et al. Diagnosis and management of lymphoma in a green iguana *(Iguana iguana)*. *J Am Vet Med Assoc* 2011;239:985-991.
32. Groza A, Mederle N, Darabus G. Advocate-therapeutical solution in parasitical infestation in frillneck lizard *(Chlamydosaurus kingii)* and bearded dragon *(Pogona vitticeps)*. *Lucrari Stiintifice - Universitatea Stiinte Agricole Banatului Timisoara, Med Vet* 2009;42:105-108.
33. Mehlhorn H, Schmahl G, Frese M, et al. Effects of a combination of emodepside and praziquantel on parasites of reptiles and rodents. *Parasitol Res* 2005;97(Suppl 1):S65-S69.
34. Schilliger L, Betremieux O, Rochet J, et al. Absorption and efficacy of a spot-on combination containing emodepside plus praziquantel in reptiles. *Rev Med Vet (Toulouse)* 2009;160:557-561.
35. Brames H. Efficacy and tolerability of Profender in reptiles: spot-on treatment against nematodes. *Exotic DVM* 2008;10:29-34.
36. Innis C. In my experience: per-cloacal deworming of tortoises. *Bull Assoc Reptil Amphib Vet* 1995;5:4.
37. Divers SJ. The diagnosis and treatment of lower respiratory tract disease in tortoises with particular regard to intrapneumonic therapy, in *Proceedings*. 5th Annu Conf Assoc Reptilian Amphibian Vet 1998;95-98.
38. Milne V, Hoover J, Snider T, et al. Intracoelomic administration of propofol in hatchling green iguanas, *Iguana iguana*. *J Herpetol Med Surg* 2006;16:20-26.
39. Pena-Miller R, Lahnemann D, Schulenburg H, et al. The optimal deployment of synergistic antibiotics: a control-theoretic approach. *J R Soc Interface* 2012;9:2488-2502.
40. Pfizer Labs. Zithromax (azithromycin tablets and azithromycin for oral suspension) package insert. New York: Pfizer Labs, 2012.
41. APP Pharmaceuticals. Azithromycin for injection package insert. Schaumburg, Ill: APP Pharmaceuticals, LLC, 2008.
42. Hunter RP, Koch DE, Coke RL, et al. Azithromycin metabolite identification in plasma, bile, and tissues of the ball python *(Python regius)*. *J Vet Pharmacol Ther* 2003;26:117-121.
43. Sagent Pharmaceuticals. Ceftazidime for injection, USP package insert. Schaumburg, Ill: Sagent Pharmaceuticals, Inc., 2012.
44. Lawrence K, Muggleton PW, Needham JR. Preliminary study on the use of ceftazidime, a broad spectrum cephalosporin antibiotic, in snakes. *Res Vet Sci* 1984;36:16-20.
45. Stamper MA, Papich MG, Lewbart GA, et al. Pharmacokinetics of ceftazidime in loggerhead sea turtles *(Caretta caretta)* after single intravenous and intramuscular injections. *J Zoo Wildl Med* 1999;30:32-35.
46. Innis CJ, Ceresia ML, Merigo C, et al. Single-dose pharmacokinetics of ceftazidime and fluconazole during concurrent clinical use in cold-stunned Kemp's Ridley turtles *(Lepidochelys kempii)*. *J Vet Pharmacol Ther* 2012;35:82-89.
47. Abbott Laboratories. Biaxin (clarithromycin) package insert. North Chicago, Ill: Abbott Laboratories, 2012.
48. Johnson JD, Mangone BA, Jarchow JL. A review of mycoplasmosis infections in tortoises and options for treatment, in *Proceedings*. 5th Annu Conf Assoc Reptilian Amphibian Vet. 1998;89-92.
49. Wimsatt J, Johnson J, Mangone BA, et al. Clarithromycin pharmacokinetics in the desert tortoise *(Gopherus agassizii)*. *J Zoo Wildl Med* 1999;30:36-43.
50. Wimsatt J, Tothill A, Offermann CF, et al. Long-term and per rectum disposition of clarithromycin in the desert tortoise (Gopherus agassizii). J Am Assoc Lab Anim Sci 2008;47:41-45.
51. Pfizer. Advocin (danofloxacin mesylate) package insert. New York: Pfizer Animal Health, 2011.
52. Ballent M, Lifschitz A, Virkel G, et al. In vivo and ex vivo assessment of the interaction between ivermectin and danofloxacin in sheep. *Vet J* 2012;192:422-427.
53. Zeng Z, Deng G, Shen X, et al. Plasma and tissue pharmacokinetics of danofloxacin in healthy and in experimentally infected chickens with *Pasteurella multocida*. *J Vet Pharmacol Ther* 2011;34:101-104.
54. Marin P, Bayon A, Fernandez-Varon E, et al. Pharmacokinetics of danofloxacin after single dose intravenous, intramuscular and subcutaneous administration to loggerhead turtles. *Caretta caretta*. *Dis Aquat Organ* 2008;82:231-236.
55. Pfizer. Zeniquin (marbofloxicin). Exton, Pa: Pfizer Animal Health, 2004.
56. Lai OR, Marin P, Laricchiuta P, et al. Pharmacokinetics of marbofloxacin in loggerhead sea turtles *(Caretta caretta)* after single intravenous and intramuscular doses. *J Zoo Wildl Med* 2009;40: 501-507.
57. Marin P, Lai OR, Laricchiuta P, et al. Pharmacokinetics of marbofloxacin after a single oral dose to loggerhead sea turtles *(Caretta caretta)*. *Res Vet Sci* 2009;87:284-286.
58. Lai O, Laricchiuta P, Putignano C, et al. Pharmacokinetics, pharmacokinetic/pharmacodynamic integration and dosage regimen of marbofloxacin in red-eared slider *(Trachemys scripta elegans)*. *Proc Int Zoo Wildl Res Berlin* 2007;43:273-275.
59. Coke RL, Isaza R, Koch DE, et al. Preliminary single-dose pharmacokinetics of marbofloxacin in ball pythons *(Python regius)*. *J Zoo Wildl Med* 2006;37:6-10.
60. Hunter RP, Koch DE, Coke RL, et al. Identification and comparison of marbofloxacin metabolites from the plasma of ball pythons *(Python regius)* and blue and gold macaws *(Ara ararauna)*. *J Vet Pharmacol Ther* 2007;30:257-262.
61. Teva Pharmaceuticals. Metronidazole tablets USP. Sellersville, Pa: Teva Pharmaceuticals USA, 2012.
62. Rediguieri CF, Porta V, Nunes DSG, et al. Biowaiver monographs for immediate-release solid oral dosage forms: metronidazole. *J Pharm Sci* 2011;100:1618-1627.
63. Jacobson ER. Use of chemotherapeutics in reptile medicine. In: Jacobson ER, Kollias GV, eds. *Exotic animals*. New York: Churchill Livingstone, 1988;35-48.
64. Bodri M, Rambo T, Wagner R, et al. Pharmacokinetics of metronidazole administered as a single oral bolus to red rat snakes, *Elaphe guttata*. *J Herpetol Med Surg* 2006;16:15-19.

65. Kolmstetter CM, Cox S, Ramsay EC. Pharmacokinetics of metronidazole in the yellow rat snake, *Elaphe obsoleta quadrivitatta. J Herpetol Med Surg* 2001;11:4-8.
66. Kolmstetter CM, Frazier D, Cox S, et al. Pharmacokinetics of metronidazole in the green iguana, *Iguana iguana. Bull Assoc Reptilian Amphibian Vet* 1998;8:4-7.
67. Marschang RE. Viruses infecting reptiles. *Viruses-Basel* 2011;3:2087-2126.
68. Ariel E. Viruses in reptiles. *Vet Res* 2011;42:100-112.
69. Muschenich M, Blahak S. Ranaviral disease in Hermann's tortoises *(Testudo hermanni). Praktische Tierarzt* 2011;92:381-389.
70. Horner RF. Poxvirus in farmed Nile crocodiles. *Vet Rec* 1988;122:459-462.
71. Marschang RE, Gravendyck M, Kaleta FF. Herpesviruses in tortoises: investigations into virus isolation and the treatment of viral stomatitis in *Testudo hermanni* and *T. graeca. Zentralbl Veterinarmed B* 1997;44:385-394.
72. Allender MC, Mitchell MA, Yarborough J, et al. Pharmacokinetics of a single oral dose of acyclovir and valacyclovir in North American box turtles (*Terrapene* sp.). *J Vet Pharmacol Ther* 2013;36:205-208.
73. Gaio C, Rossi T, Villa R, et al. Pharmacokinetics of acyclovir after a single oral administration in marginated tortoises, *Testudo marginata. J Herpetol Med Surg* 2007;17:8-11.
74. GlaxoSmithKline. Zovirax (acyclovir) capsules product information. Research Triangle Park, NC: GlaxoSmithKline, 2008.
75. Cooper J, Gschmeissner S, Bone R. Herpes-like virus particles in necrotic stomatitis of tortoises. *Vet Rec* 1988;123:544.
76. Frye FL. *Reptile care: an atlas of diseases and treatments.* Neptune City, NJ: T.F.H. Publications, Inc, 1991.
77. Genetech USA. Cytovene-IV (ganciclovir sodium for injection) package insert. South San Francisco, Calif: Genentech USA, Inc., 2010.
78. Van Waeyenberghe L, Pasmans F, Hellebuyck T, et al. Infections with the *Chrysosporium* anamorph of *Nannizziopsis vriesii* in bearded dragons *(Pogona vitticeps)*: treatment and (experimental) vaccination. *Mycoses* 2012;55(IS s4):78-79.
79. Sigma-tau pharmaceuticals. Abelcet (amphotericin B lipid complex injection) package insert. Gaithersburg, Md: Sigma-tau Pharmaceuticals, Inc, 2012.
80. Fitzgerald KT, Vera R. Reported toxicities in reptiles. In: Mader DR, ed. *Reptile medicine and surgery.* 2nd ed. St. Louis: Saunders Elsevier, 2006;1068-1080.
81. Van Waeyenberghe L, Baert K, Pasmans F, et al. Voriconazole, a safe alternative for treating infections caused by the *Chrysosporium* anamorph of *Nannizziopsis vriesii* in bearded dragons *(Pogona vitticeps). Med Mycol* 2010;48:880-885.
82. Hernandez-Divers SJ. Pulmonary candidiasis caused by *Candida albicans* in a Greek tortoise *(Testudo graeca)* and treatment with intrapulmonary amphotericin B. *J Zoo Wildl Med* 2001;32:352-359.
83. Jenkins JR. A formulary for reptile and amphibian medicine, in *Proceedings.* Fourth Annu Avian/Exotic Anim Med Symp, University of California, Davis, 1991;24-27.
84. Janssen Pharmaceuticals. Sporanox (itraconazole) package insert. Beerse, Belgium: Janssen Pharmaceutica N. V., 2010.
85. Keller KA. Itraconazole. *J Exotic Pet Med* 2011;20:156-160.
86. Bowman MR, Pare JA, Sigler L, et al. Deep fungal dermatitis in three inland bearded dragons *(Pogona vitticeps)* caused by the *Chrysosporium* anamorph of *Nannizziopsis vriesii. Med Mycol* 2007;45:371-376.
87. Hedley J, Eatwell K, Hume L. Necrotising fungal dermatitis in a group of bearded dragons *(Pogona vitticeps). Vet Rec* 2010;166:464-465.
88. Bicknese E. Itraconazole treated CANV (*Chrysosporium* anamorph of *Nannizziopsis vriesii*) dermatitis in green anacondas *(Eunectes murinus murinus)*, in *Proceedings.* 16th Annu Conf Assoc Reptilian Amphibian Vet 2009;157-158.
89. Girling SJ, Fraser MA. Treatment of *Aspergillus* species infection in reptiles with itraconazole at metabolically scaled doses. *Vet Rec* 2009;165:52-54.
90. Pfizer. Vfend (voriconazole IV, tablets, oral suspension) package insert. New York: Roerig, Division of Pfizer, Inc, 2008.
91. Hellebuyck T, Baert K, Pasmans F, et al. Cutaneous hyalohyphomycosis in a girdled lizard *(Cordylus giganteus)* caused by the *Chrysosporium* anamorph of *Nannizziopsis vriesii* and successful treatment with voriconazole. *Vet Dermatol* 2010;21:429-433.
92. Innis C, Young D, Wetzlich S, et al. Plasma voriconazole concentrations in four red-eared slider turtles *(Trachemys scripta elegans)* after a single subcutaneous injection, in *Proceedings.* 15th Annu Conf Assoc Reptilian Amphibian Vet 2008;72.
93. Novartis Pharmaceuticals. Lamisil (terbinafine hydrochloride) tablets prescribing information. East Hanover, NJ: Novartis Pharmaceuticals Corporation, 2012.
94. Keller KA. Therapeutic review: terbinafine. *J Exotic Pet Med* 2012;21:181-185.
95. Abarca ML, Martorell J, Castella G, et al. Cutaneous hyalohyphomycosis caused by a *Chrysosporium* species related to *Nannizziopsis vriesii* in two green iguanas *(Iguana iguana). Med Mycol* 2008;46:349-354.
96. Abarca ML, Martorell J, Castella G, et al. Dermatomycosis in a pet inland bearded dragon *(Pogona vitticeps)* caused by a *Chrysosporium* species related to *Nannizziopsis vriesii. Med Mycol* 2009;20:295-299.
97. Stringer EM, Garner MM, Proudfoot JS, et al. Phaeohyphomycosis of the carapace in an Aldabra tortoise *(Geochelone gigantea). J Zoo Wildl Med* 2009;40:160-167.
98. Plumb DC. Fenbendazole. In: *Plumb's veterinary drug handbook.* 6th ed. Ames, Iowa: Blackwell Publishing Professional, 2008;376-379.
99. Pfizer. Valbazen (albendazole) oral suspension package insert. New York: Pfizer Animal Health, 2010.
100. Heggem B. Fenbendazole. *J Exotic Pet Med* 2008;17:307-310.
101. Neiffer DL, Lydick D, Burks K, et al. Hematologic and plasma biochemical changes associated with fenbendazole administration in Hermann's tortoises *(Testudo hermanni). J Zoo Wildl Med* 2005;36:661-672.
102. Alvarado TP, Garner MM, Gamble KC, et al. Fenbendazole overdose in four Fea's vipers *(Azemiops feae)*, in *Proceedings.* Annu Conf Am Assoc Zoo Vet 2001;28-29.
103. Howard LL, Papendick R, Stalis IH, et al. Benzimidazole toxicity in birds, in *Proceedings.* Annu Conf Am Assoc Zoo Vet 1999;36.
104. Capleton AC, Courage C, Rumsby P, et al. Prioritising veterinary medicines according to their potential indirect human exposure and toxicity profile. *Toxicol Lett* 2006;163:213-223.
105. Giannetto S, Brianti E, Poglayen G, et al. Efficacy of oxfendazole and fenbendazole against tortoise *(Testudo hermanni)* oxyurids. *Parasitol Res* 2007;100:1069-1073.
106. Marquis (15% w/w ponazuril) Antiprotozoal Oral Paste. Available at: http://bayer.naccvp.com/?m=product_view_basic&id=1040039&u=bayer&p=dvm. Accessed Oct 10, 2012.
107. Baycox Solution 2.5% for Coccidiosis Control in Poultry. Available at: http://www.baycox.es/index.php/fuseaction/download/lrn_file/Bayer_Baycox_Solution_25.pdf. Accessed Oct 10, 2012.
108. Plumb DC. Toltrazuril. In: *Plumb's veterinary drug handbook.* 6th ed. Ames, Iowa: Blackwell Publishing Professional, 2008;896-897.
109. Mitchell MA. Ponazuril. *J Exotic Pet Med* 2008;17:228-229.
110. Modry D, Sloboda M. Control of coccidiosis in chameleons using toltrazuril—results of an experimental trial, in *Proceedings.* 7th Int Symp Path Med Reptil Amphib (Berlin 2004) 2007;93-99.
111. Bogoslavsky B. The use of ponazuril to treat coccidiosis in eight inland bearded dragons *(Pogona vitticeps)*, in *Proceedings.* 14th Annu Conf Assoc Reptilian Amphibian Vet 2007;8-9.
112. Grosset C, Villeneuve A, Brieger A, et al. Cryptosporidiosis in juvenile bearded dragons *(Pogona vitticeps)*: effects of treatment with Paromomycin. *J Herpetol Med Surg* 2011;21:10-15.
113. Praschag P, Gibbons P, Boyer T, et al. An outbreak of intranuclear coccidiosis in *Pyxis* ssp. tortoises, in *Proceedings.* 8th Annu Symp Conserv Biol Tortoises Freshwater Turtles 2010;42-43.

114. Richter B, Rasim R, Vrhovec MG, et al. Cryptosporidiosis outbreak in captive chelonians *(Testudo hermanni)* with identification of two *Cryptosporidium* genotypes. *J Vet Diagn Invest* 2012;24:591-595.
115. Pantchev N, Ruschoff B, Kamhuber-Pohl A, et al. Cryptosporidiosis treatment in Leopard Geckos *(Eublepharis macularius)* with azithromycin (Zithromax (R)) and paromomycin sulfate (Humatin (R))— case reports and review of the literature. *Kleintierpraxis* 2008;53:95-104.
116. Raphael BL. Chelonians. In: Fowler ME, Miller RE, eds. *Zoo and wild animal medicine.* 5th ed. Philadelphia: Elsevier-Saunders, 2003;48-58.
117. Paré JA, Crawshaw GJ, Barta JR. Treatment of cryptosporidiosis in Gila monsters *(Heloderma suspectum)* with paromomycin, in *Proceedings.* 4th Annu Conf Assoc Reptilian Amphibian Vet 1997;23.
118. Coke RL, Tristan TE. *Cryptosporidium* infection in a colony of leopard geckos, *Eublepharis macularius*, in *Proceedings.* 5th Annu Conf Assoc Reptilian Amphibian Vet. 1998;157-163.
119. Boehringer Ingelheim Pharmaceuticals. Mobic (meloxicam) tablets prescribing information. Ridgefield, Conn: Boehringer Ingelheim Pharmaceuticals, Inc., 2012.
120. Plumb DC. Meloxicam. In: *Plumb's veterinary drug manual.* 7th ed. Ames, Iowa: Blackwell Publishing Professional, 2012;574-575.
121. Rojo-Solís C, Ros-Rodriguez JM, Valls M. Pharmacokinetics of meloxicam (Metacam) after intravenous, intramuscular, and oral administration in red-eared slider turtles *(Trachemys scripta elegans)*, in *Proceedings.* Joint Conf Am Assoc Zoo Vet Am Assoc Wildl Vet 2009;228.
122. Divers SJ, Papich M, McBride M, et al. Pharmacokinetics of meloxicam following intravenous and oral administration in green iguanas *(Iguana iguana). Am J Vet Res* 2010;71:1277-1283.

CHAPTER 8

Clinical Pathology

Terry W. Campbell

CLINICAL PATHOLOGY OF REPTILES

Blood is routinely collected from the reptilian patient for hematologic examination, and plasma biochemistry studies are performed for the purpose of health assessment and in the clinical diagnosis of disease. Blood samples collected from reptiles are often contaminated with lymphatic fluid. When this occurs, the sample is rendered useless for hematologic studies, except perhaps for evaluation of cell morphologic features. Lymphatic dilution of the blood sample also has an adverse effect on the biochemistry profile.

When evaluating the hematologic and biochemical responses of reptiles, one should consider the various normal physiologic and external factors that may enhance or inhibit these ectotherms' response to disease. These factors include age, gender, environment, season, and nutritional status.[1-4] Differences between captive individuals and free-ranging reptiles of the same species may be too great for use in comparison studies. It has been shown that captive-bred snakes tend to have significantly higher erythrocyte values, lower azurophil, heterophil, and punctate reticulocyte percentages, and higher lymphocyte numbers compared with wild-caught snakes.[5] Total leukocyte counts of captive male crocodiles were higher than those of females, whereas no differences between the sexes were observed in wild crocodiles of the same species.[6] The total leukocyte counts of foraging sea turtles were shown to be statistically lower than those for the nesting turtles that were likely fasting.[7] A marked seasonal variation was noted in all hematologic and blood biochemistry variables in turtles, except mean cell hemoglobin concentration, the relative monocyte and heterophil counts, and creatinine.[8] The influence of the normal physiologic and external factors was suspected to be responsible for the lack of significant differences in the packed cell volume, total protein concentration, and total leukocyte count between sick and healthy box turtles.[3] That significant hematologic changes in young crocodiles subjected to low temperature treatments occurred without any significant variation in corticosterone concentrations would suggest that the immunosuppressive effect of low temperature was independent of corticosterone concentrations and the hypothalamic–pituitary–adrenocortical axis.[9] All of these studies support the importance of knowing the various physiologic and external factors that might influence test results.

The cellular responses in reptilian blood, in particular, are less predictable than those of endothermic mammals and birds whose cellular microenvironments are more stable. The external factors mentioned earlier have a greater influence on the physiology and health of ectothermic vertebrates than they do on endotherms. Because species, age, gender, nutritional status, season, and physiologic status influence blood tests, interpretation of the hemogram and plasma biochemistry profiles becomes challenging. In addition, discrepancies among the results of various analytic methods should also be taken into consideration when one is comparing the results between studies.[7] Differences in test results may even occur between blood collection sites.[10] All of these factors make the creation of meaningful species-specific reference ranges difficult when compared with those of domestic mammals. An ideal reference interval for each analyte for a given species of reptile would take into consideration gender, age (size), body condition, parasite load, nutritional status, season, quality of habitat (captive versus wild), presence of environmental stressors, blood collection site, and analytic method. All of these things should be taken into consideration when interpreting hematologic and diagnostic chemistry data from a reptilian patient. The American Society for Veterinary Clinical Pathology has provided guidelines for the creation of reference intervals that includes the use of data obtained from a small number of individuals. These guidelines are available from http://www.asvcp.org/pubs/qas/index.cfm.

HEMATOLOGY

Evaluation of the hemogram and blood film is part of the laboratory evaluation of reptilian patients. Hematology is used to detect conditions such as anemia, inflammatory diseases, parasitemia, hematopoietic disorders, and hemostatic alterations. The hematologic evaluation of a reptilian patient may provide clues to its health status. Continued hematologic monitoring of the patient also provides important information regarding the patient's response to treatment or the progression of the disease. For example, lymphocytosis, heterophilia, and azurophilia in tortoises have been shown to occur concurrently with a resurgence of clinical signs in patients with upper respiratory disease, providing information regarding the status of the patients.[11]

The blood of reptiles contains nucleated erythrocytes, nucleated thrombocytes, heterophils, eosinophils, basophils, lymphocytes, and monocytes. The normal hematologic values of reptiles determined by different laboratories can vary significantly. This variation is likely caused by differences in blood sampling, handling, and analytic techniques. Other factors that are likely to contribute to the variation in the normal hematologic values of reptiles include variations in environmental conditions, physiologic status, age, gender, nutrition, and use of anesthetics. Published hematologic reference values for reptiles often fail to include information that may influence the hemogram, especially the environment of the population of reptiles used as normal controls. For these reasons, the published normal reference values of reptiles vary greatly compared with those of domestic mammals.

Routine evaluation of the reptilian hemogram includes determination of the packed cell volume (PCV), the total leukocyte counts, and a leukocyte differential and examination of the blood cell morphologic features on a stained blood film. The microhematocrit method is the quickest, most practical, and reproducible method for determination of the PCV and status of the reptilian erythron. The total leukocyte counts are determined with either manual methods or automated methods (erythrocytes only); the two commonly used methods for the determination of the total leukocyte count in reptilian blood are the semidirect method with phloxine B solution or the direct method with Natt and Herrick solution. The limitations for the semidirect method include increased errors in samples with low heterophil counts and the need for an accurate leukocyte differential. The limitations for the direct method include the use of manual diluting pipettes, the need to prepare the diluting solutions, and the difficulty in distinguishing between small lymphocytes and thrombocytes. Both methods require training and experience for consistent results.

Because of the limitations on obtaining total cell counts in reptilian blood, especially leukocyte counts, the evaluation of cell morphologic features is an important part of the assessment of the hemogram. Microscope slides containing reptilian blood films are commonly stained with Wright, Giemsa, or Wright/Giemsa for evaluation. Quick stains, such as Diff-Quik, can be used but have a tendency to damage some of the cell types (e.g., lymphocytes) and understain immature erythrocytes and lymphocytes.

A properly prepared blood film provides low numbers of smudge cells and an ample amount of monolayer areas for evaluating the cells. The coverslip-to-slide and the bevel-edge slide techniques can provide such quality.[12] Whenever possible, examination of blood films obtained from fresh non–anticoagulated blood is preferred. Ethylenediaminetetraacetic acid (EDTA), considered to be the anticoagulant of choice for hematologic studies, may cause the blood to lyse in some species of chelonians; therefore lithium heparin is typically used as an anticoagulant when blood is collected from those reptiles.[13,14] However, heparin often imparts a blue tinge to the overall staining of the blood film and causes clumping of leukocytes and thrombocytes, affecting cell counts.[15] If heparin is used as an anticoagulant for reptilian hematologic studies, the sample should be processed immediately so that its effects are minimized on the cells. If whole blood samples anticoagulated with lithium heparin or EDTA cannot be evaluated immediately, then the samples should be stored at 4°C and evaluated no longer than 24 hours after collection for best results.[16] Citrate used as an anticoagulant often results in significant cell lysis and should be avoided. The addition of albumin does not prevent cell lysis as others have suggested.[17]

REPTILIAN ERYTHROCYTES

Mature erythrocytes of reptiles are permanently nucleated, blunt-ended ellipsoids that are larger than erythrocytes of birds and mammals. The erythrocyte size for most reptiles ranges from a length by width of 14 × 8 μm to 23 × 14 μm and the length-to-width ratio of most reptile erythrocytes is 1.7 to 1.8.[17] Reptile erythrocytes that are round (length-to-width ratio, 1.5 or greater) rather than oval are rare and likely to occur in chelonians and some snakes.[17] The mean cellular volume (MCV) of most reptilian mature erythrocytes ranges between 200 and 1200 fL. The reptilian erythrocyte has a centrally positioned oval to round (especially chelonians) nucleus that is oriented along the cell's long axis. The nuclei often have irregular margins and contain dense purple chromatin. The cytoplasm appears orange-pink with Romanowsky stains such as Wright stain. Polychromatophilic erythrocytes have nuclear chromatin that is less dense and cytoplasm that is more basophilic than mature erythrocytes.

Reptiles have lower total erythrocyte counts (300,000 to 2,500,000 erythrocytes/μL) compared with mammals and birds.[18,19] An inverse relationship appears to exist between the total red blood cell count (TRBC) and the size of the erythrocytes.[18] Chelonians have the largest of the reptilian erythrocytes (MCV greater than 500 fL) and, as a result, the lower TRBC values (500,000 erythrocytes/μL or less). Lizards tend to have smaller erythrocytes (MCV less than 300 fL) than other reptiles; therefore they have higher total erythrocyte counts (1,000,000 to 1,500,000 erythrocytes/μL).[18,19] Snakes have lower TRBC values (700,000 to 1,600,000 erythrocytes/μL) than lizards but greater numbers than chelonians. The TRBC, hemoglobin concentration (Hb), and PCV values vary with a number of factors, such as environment (TRBC values are highest before hibernation and lowest immediately after hibernation), nutritional status; and gender (males tend to have higher TRBC values than females).[17-23]

The mean hemoglobin concentration (MCHC) is the red blood cell index denoting the proportion of an average erythrocyte that is composed of hemoglobin in grams per 100 red blood cells (gHb/100 RBC). The average MCHC for reptiles is 30% (range, 22% to 41%).[17,24,25] The hemoglobin concentration of reptilian blood generally ranges between 6 and 10 g/dL.[26] Most reptiles have multiple hemoglobin types, and considerable variation is seen in oxygen affinity between individual red blood cells.[27]

Immature erythrocytes are occasionally seen in the peripheral blood of reptiles, especially in young animals or those undergoing ecdysis. Immature erythrocytes are round to irregular cells with large round nuclei and basophilic cytoplasm (Figure 8-1). The nucleus lacks the dense chromatin clumping of the mature cell and has a characteristic checkerboard-like pattern. Immature erythrocytes frequently appear smaller than mature erythrocyte, probably because the final stage of erythrocyte maturation involves changing from a spherical cell, which appears small, to a flattened ellipsoid, which appears larger. In addition, the larger mature cell may contain more hemoglobin. Mitotic activity associated with erythrocytes is common in the peripheral blood of healthy reptiles.

Reticulocytes are detected by staining cells with a supravital stain, such as new methylene blue. They are a normal constituent of reptilian blood, representing 1.5% to 2.5% of

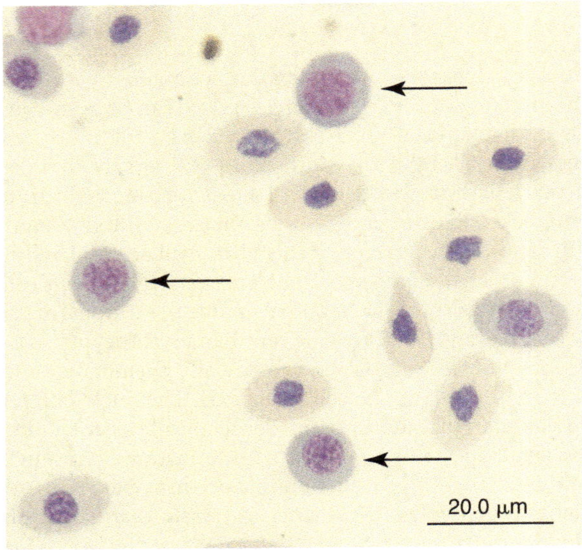

FIGURE 8-1 Immature (mid-polychromatic rubricytes) erythrocytes *(arrows)* in the blood film of Reeves' Turtle *(Mauremys reevesii)*; Wright-Giemsa stain × 1000.

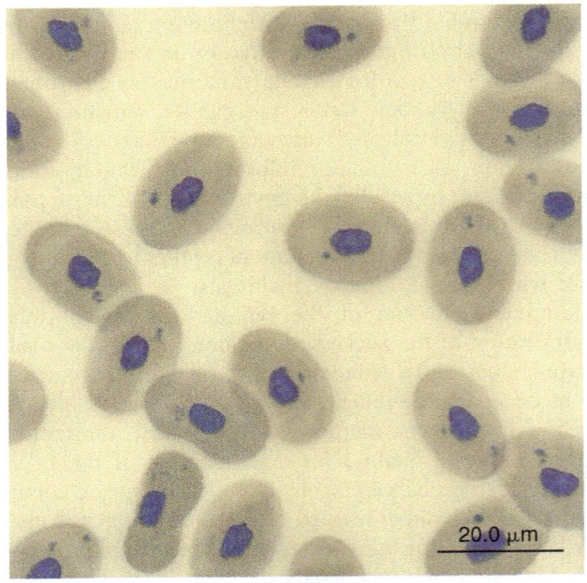

FIGURE 8-3 Erythrocytes containing irregular basophilic cytoplasmic inclusions considered to be artifact in the blood film of a Green Sea turtle *(Chelonia mydas)*; Wright-Giemsa stain × 1000.

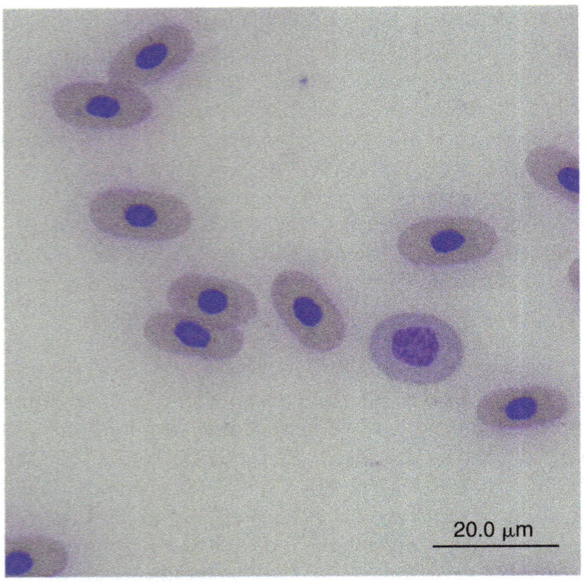

FIGURE 8-2 A polychromatic erythrocyte in the blood film of a Box Turtle *(Terrapene carolina triunguis)*; Wright-Giemsa stain × 1000.

the red blood cell population.[28,29] Reptilian reticulocytes that have a distinct ring of aggregated reticulum that encircles the red cell nucleus are likely the cells recently released from the erythropoietic tissues. Polychromatic erythrocytes account for less that 1% of the red blood cell population of most clinically healthy reptiles (Figure 8-2).

Round to irregular basophilic inclusions are frequently seen in the cytoplasm of erythrocytes in peripheral blood films from many species of reptiles (Figure 8-3). These inclusions most likely represent an artifact of slide preparation because blood films made repeatedly from the same blood sample often reveal varying degrees of these inclusions. Electron microscopy suggests these inclusions are degenerate organelles.[30] Other artifacts found in erythrocyte cytoplasm include vacuoles and refractile clear areas. These can be minimized with careful blood film preparation.

ERYTHROCYTE RESPONSES IN DISEASE

The normal PCV of most reptiles is approximately 30% (published ranges are 20% to 40%)[20,31,32] Therefore a PCV less than 20% is suggestive of anemia, and values greater than 40% suggest either hemoconcentration or erythrocytosis (polycythemia). Indicators of anemia include a decreased erythrocyte count, PCV, and hemoglobin concentration. The causes of anemia in reptiles are the same as those described for birds and mammals. The anemia can be classified as hemorrhagic (blood loss), hemolytic (increased red cell destruction), or depression anemia (decreased red cell production). Hemorrhagic anemias are usually caused by traumatic injuries or blood-sucking parasites; however, other causes, such as a coagulopathy or an ulcerative lesion, should be considered. Hemolytic anemia can result from septicemia, parasitemia, or toxemia. Depression anemias are usually associated with chronic inflammatory diseases, especially those associated with infectious agents. A low PCV without evidence of red blood cell regeneration supports the presence of a depression anemia—one likely associated with a chronic condition such as poor nutrition, chronic infectious or parasitic disease, immune deficiency related to a debilitated state, or a combination of any of these causes.[7] Other causes that should be considered for depression anemia in reptiles include chronic renal or hepatic disease, neoplasia, chemical contact, or possibly hypothyroidism.[33,34]

The degree of polychromasia or reticulocytosis in blood films of normal reptiles is generally low and represents less than 1% of the erythrocyte population. This may be associated with the long erythrocyte life span (600 to 800 days in some species) and therefore slow turnover rate of reptilian

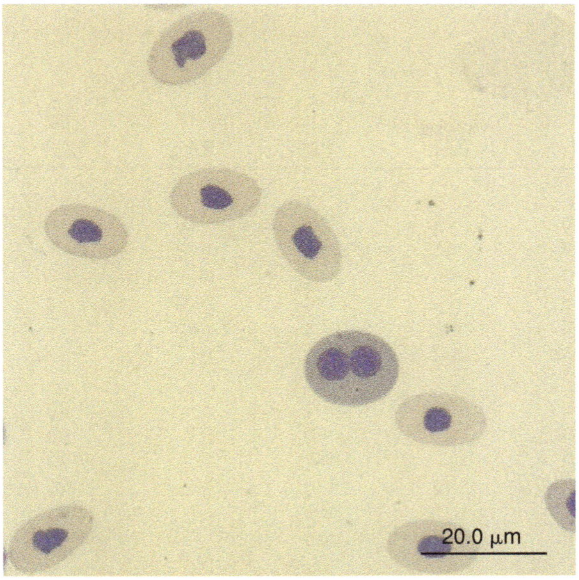

FIGURE 8-4 A binucleated erythrocyte likely representing accelerated erythropoiesis in the blood film of a Reeves' Turtle *(Mauremys reevesii);* Wright-Giemsa stain × 1000.

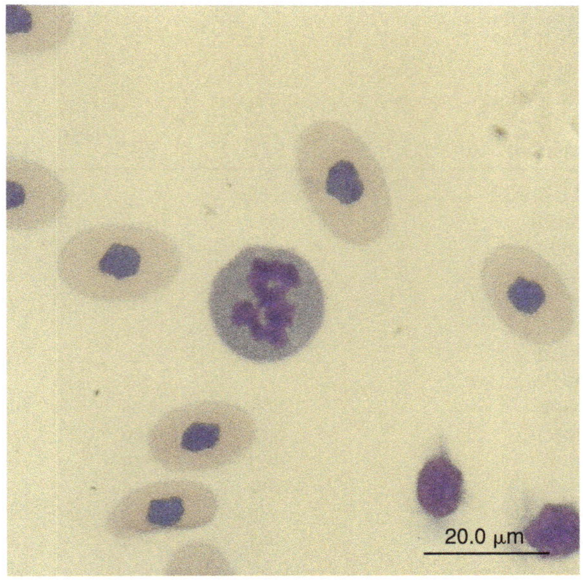

FIGURE 8-5 A mitotic figure likely associated with an erythrocyte and increased polychromasia likely representing accelerated erythropoiesis in the blood film of a Reeves' Turtle *(Mauremys reevesii);* Wright-Giemsa stain × 1000.

erythrocytes compared with those of birds and mammals.[18,20] The relatively low metabolic rate of reptiles may also be a factor. Young reptiles tend to have a greater degree of polychromasia than adults.

Slight anisocytosis and poikilocytosis are considered normal for most reptile erythrocytes. Moderate to marked anisocytosis and poikilocytosis are associated with erythrocytic regenerative responses and, less commonly, erythrocyte disorders. An increase in polychromasia and the number of immature erythrocytes is seen in reptiles responding to anemic conditions. The erythrocyte regenerative response in reptiles is expected to be slower than that of birds and mammals, which respond within 1 week to stimulus. The slow reptilian response (e.g., red cell numbers may return to normal in 4 months after repeated phlebotomy) may be related in part to the long transit time from the rubriblast stage to the mature erythrocyte stage and the long life span of the reptilian red blood cell.[35] Young reptiles or those undergoing ecdysis may also exhibit an increase in polychromasia and immature erythrocyte concentration. Erythrocytes exhibiting binucleation, abnormal nuclear shapes (anisokaryosis), or mitotic activity can be associated with marked regenerative responses (Figures 8-4 and 8-5). However, these nuclear findings may also occur in reptiles awakening from brumation or in association with severe inflammatory disease, malnutrition, and starvation.[36] Basophilic stippling usually suggests a regenerative response but is also seen in patients with iron deficiency and, possibly, lead toxicosis. Hypochromatic erythrocytes are associated with iron deficiency or chronic inflammatory disease (presumably in association with iron sequestration). Erythroplastids (anucleated erythrocytes) are an incidental finding (less than 0.5% of the erythrocytes) in reptilian blood.[37-39] A normocytic, hyperchromic anemia usually signals a regenerative anemia, whereas a normocytic, hypochromic anemia is often associated with infection or chronic inflammatory diseases.[40]

REPTILIAN LEUKOCYTES

The leukocytes found in the peripheral blood of reptiles are classified as granulocytes and agranulocytes (mononuclear leukocytes). The granulocytes of reptiles can be classified as heterophils, eosinophils, and basophils on the basis of their appearance in blood films stained with Romanowsky stains. The mononuclear leukocytes are classified as lymphocytes and monocytes.

Special stains (cytochemical staining techniques) are used to examine cellular constituents, such as enzymes, lipids, and carbohydrates. Peroxidase (PER; myeloperoxidase) is used as a marker for mammalian myeloid cells, such as neutrophils, eosinophils, and monocytes. Sudan Black B (SBB) stains lipids within neutrophils, eosinophils, and occasionally monocytes. Chloroacetate esterase (CAE) is a group of enzymes considered to be specific for mammalian neutrophils. Leukocyte alkaline phosphatase (LAP) is present in mammalian granulocytes and some subsets of lymphocytes. Periodic acid Schiff (PAS) staining is positive in a wide variety of mammalian blood cells and is used to differentiate granulocytic or megakaryocytic from lymphoid precursors.[41] Nonspecific esterases (NSE) and acid phosphatase (AP) staining of mammalian cells demonstrate unique staining characteristics. Toluidine blue (TB) is helpful in detection of mammalian basophils and mast cells. Some of these have been applied to reptilian blood cells in an effort to detect differences between normal cell types and similarities or differences between the hemic cells of different species (Table 8-1). The variation in cytochemical responses in these studies indicates that it is necessary to study species individually if meaningful clinical decisions are to be made.[42] Differences in cytochemical responses among the blood cells of various reptiles and even in studies that have used the same species might also be a reflection of differences in technique. Variations in the reactivity of a cell to the same cytochemical stain can occur with differences in pH, incubation temperatures, staining time, and reagents.[41,43] These factors add to the

TABLE 8-1

Summary of Selected Cytochemical Staining Reactions for Normal Leukocytes and Thrombocytes in Various Reptiles

Species/Cell	PER	SBB	CAE	AP	PAS	NSE	TB	LAP
GIANT LIZARD[42]								
Heterophil	pos	—	neg	neg	pos	pos	neg	—
Eosinophil	neg	—	pos	pos	neg	pos	neg	—
Basophil	neg	—	neg	neg	neg	±	pos	—
Lymphocyte	neg	—	neg	pos	neg	neg	neg	—
Mono/Azuro	neg	—	±	pos	neg	pos	neg	—
Thrombocyte	neg	—	neg	neg	neg	neg	neg	—
Iguana[23]								
Heterophil	pos	pos	neg	pos	pos	pos	—	neg
Eosinophil	neg	neg	neg	neg	neg	neg	—	neg
Basophil	neg	neg	neg	neg	±	neg	—	neg
Lymphocyte	neg	neg	neg	neg	neg	neg	—	neg
Mono/Azuro	neg	neg	neg	pos	±	pos	—	neg
Thrombocyte	neg	neg	neg	neg	pos	pos	—	neg
RAINBOW LIZARD[50]								
Heterophil	±	pos	—	pos	pos	pos	—	neg
Eosinophil	±	neg	—	pos	±	neg	—	neg
Basophil	neg	neg	—	neg	±	neg	—	neg
Lymphocyte	neg	neg	—	neg	neg	pos	—	neg
Mono/Azuro	±	±	—	pos	neg	neg	—	neg
Thrombocyte	pos	neg	—	neg	pos	pos	—	neg
King Cobra[5]								
Heterophil	—	pos	—	neg	neg	pos	—	—
Eosinophil	—	neg	—	neg	neg	neg	—	—
Basophil	—	pos	—	neg	pos	pos	—	—
Lymphocyte	—	neg	—	pos	pos	pos	—	—
Mono/Azuro	—	pos	—	neg	pos	pos	—	—
Thrombocyte	—	neg	—	neg	pos	neg	—	—
RATTLESNAKE[45]								
Heterophil	neg	neg	±	neg	±	±	neg	neg
Eosinophil	—	—	—	—	—	—	—	—
Basophil	neg	neg	neg	neg	pos	neg	neg	neg
Lymphocyte	neg	neg	neg	neg	neg	neg	neg	neg
Mono/Azuro	pos	pos	neg	neg	±	neg	neg	neg
Thrombocyte	neg	neg	neg	neg	±	±	neg	neg
GREEN TURTLE[46]								
Heterophil	neg	neg	neg	neg	pos	pos	—	—
Eosinophil	neg	neg	pos	neg	±	neg	—	—
Basophil	—	—	—	—	—	—	—	—
Lymphocyte	neg	neg	neg	neg	neg	neg	—	—
Mono/Azuro	neg	neg	neg	pos	pos	±	—	—
Thrombocyte	neg	neg	neg	neg	pos	pos	—	—
ASIAN POND TURTLE[8]								
Heterophil	±	—	—	—	neg	—	—	—
Eosinophil	pos	—	—	—	neg	—	—	—
Basophil	pos	—	—	—	neg	—	—	—
Lymphocyte	neg	—	—	—	neg	—	—	—
Mono/Azuro	neg	—	—	—	±	—	—	—
Thrombocyte	neg	—	—	—	pos	—	—	—
EUROPEAN POND TURTLE[44]								
Heterophil	neg	—	—	neg	±	±	neg	—
Eosinophil	neg	—	—	neg	neg	neg	neg	—
Basophil	neg	—	—	neg	neg	neg	pos	—
Lymphocyte	neg	—	—	neg	neg	neg	neg	—
Mono/Azuro	neg	—	—	±	neg	neg	neg	—
Thrombocyte	neg	—	—	neg	±	neg	neg	—

Continued

TABLE 8-1

Summary of Selected Cytochemical Staining Reactions for Normal Leukocytes and Thrombocytes in Various Reptiles—cont'd

Species/Cell	PER	SBB	CAE	AP	PAS	NSE	TB	LAP
MEDITERRANEAN POND TURTLE[44]								
Heterophil	neg	—	±	±	±	±	neg	±
Eosinophil	±	—	±	±	neg	pos	neg	±
Basophil	neg	—	±	±	neg	±	pos	±
Lymphocyte	neg	—	±	neg	neg	neg	neg	neg
Mono/Azuro	neg	—	±	±	±	pos	neg	±
Thrombocyte	neg	—	neg	neg	±	neg	neg	neg
TORTOISE[30]								
Heterophil	neg	neg	±	±	neg	±	neg	±
Eosinophil	pos	neg	±	neg	neg	neg	neg	neg
Basophil	neg	neg	neg	neg	neg	neg	pos	neg
Lymphocyte	neg	neg	neg	neg	neg	neg	neg	neg
Mono/Azuro	neg	neg	±	pos	neg	pos	neg	neg
Thrombocyte	—	—	—	—	—	—	—	—
ALLIGATOR[49]								
Heterophil	neg	—	neg	pos	pos	pos	—	—
Eosinophil	pos	—	neg	neg	pos	neg	—	—
Basophil	neg	—	neg	pos	pos	neg	—	—
Lymphocyte	neg	—	pos	pos	pos	pos	—	—
Mono/Azuro	neg	—	±	neg	pos	neg	—	—
Thrombocyte	neg	—	neg	neg	neg	neg	—	—

AP, Acid phosphatase; *CAE,* chloroacetate esterase; *LAP,* leukocyte alkaline phosphatase; *Mono/Azuro,* monocyte/azurophil; *neg,* no reaction; *NSE,* nonspecific esterase, *PAS,* periodic acid-Schiff; *PER,* peroxidase; *pos,* positive, easily detectable; *SBB,* Sudan black B; *TB,* toluidine blue; —, undetermined; ±, weak, focal, or occasional reactive.

difficulty when one compares the results of different studies, most of which have failed to use human controls to compare positivity and negativity.[44]

PER activity is present in the primary granules of mammalian neutrophils but absent in the heterophils of certain reptiles. The primary and secondary granules of mammalian neutrophils stain positive for SBB as do many reptilian heterophils, but this too varies among species. Mammalian neutrophils stain positive for CAE, a feature not common for reptilian heterophils. LAP activity, found in the secondary granules of neutrophils of many but not all species of mammals, is generally not a feature of reptilian heterophils. Neutrophils of some mammals stain positive for NSE, as do most reptilian heterophils that have been tested. AP and PAS activities are present in mammalian neutrophils but demonstrate variable staining among reptilian heterophils.

The PER activity of mammalian eosinophils occurs in different structures of the cell compared with the neutrophil, and not all mammalian eosinophils stain positive for this enzyme. Positive PER staining in reptilian eosinophils varies with the species. Mammalian eosinophils generally do not stain CAE positive; however, the eosinophils of some reptiles do. In general, reptilian eosinophils stain negative for SBB, LAP, and PAS (with the exception of alligators), and species variability exists in positive staining for AP and NSE.

Mammalian basophils generally stain negative for PER and SBB, as do reptilian basophils (with a few exceptions). Reptilian basophils usually stain negative for CAE, AP, NSE, and LAP, again with few exceptions. Many mammalian basophils, basophils of Desert Tortoises *(Gopherus agassizii)*, and basophils of alligators stain positive for TB.

Lymphocytes generally lack the positive reactivity of many of the cytochemical staining techniques used to identify mammalian granulocytes and monocytes. This is generally true for reptilian lymphocytes; however, exceptions exist, in that some species cells' react positively to AP, PAS, and NSE.

Monocytes of reptiles generally stain negative for TB and LAP and positive, although weakly at times, for SBB, CAE, and PER. They also demonstrate positive staining, depending on the species, for AP, PAS, and NSE.

Reptilian thrombocytes, like mammalian platelets, often stain positive for PAS. Positive staining for SBB, CAE, AP, TB, and LAP has not been reported in reptilian thrombocytes.

Reptilian heterophils are generally round cells with eosinophilic (bright or dull orange), generally fusiform cytoplasmic granules (Figures 8-6 through 8-9). The cytoplasm of normal heterophils is colorless. The mature heterophil nucleus is typically round to oval and eccentrically positioned in the cell, with densely clumped nuclear chromatin.[2,32,36,45-49] Some species of lizards have heterophils with lobed nuclei (Figure 8-10).[17,23] Heterophils range between 10 and 23 μm in size but vary between species and the individual blood sample.[17] Heterophil granules demonstrate heterogeneous electron microscopic morphologic features and cytochemical staining, indicating the presence of different granule types. The cytoplasmic granules of reptilian heterophils are usually PER negative, except for a few species of snakes and lizards.[18,30,48,50,51] The heterophil granules from the Green Iguana *(Iguana iguana)* stain strongly positive with benzidine peroxidase similar to mammalian neutrophils.[23] Reptilian heterophils do not stain for alkaline phosphatase.[30] These findings indicate that reptilian

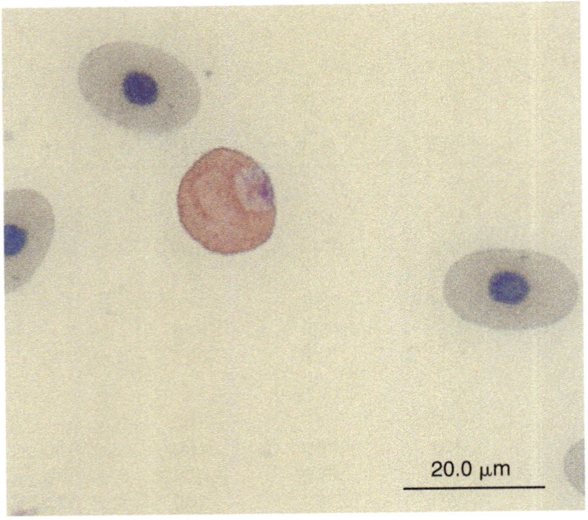

FIGURE 8-6 A heterophil in the blood film of a Wood Turtle *(Glyptemys insculpta)*; Wright-Giemsa stain × 1000.

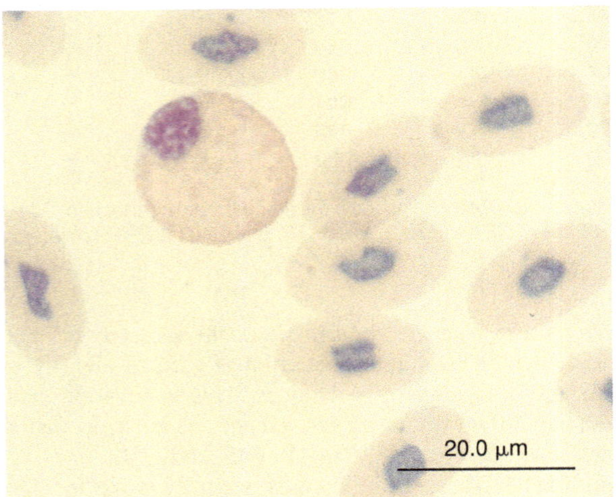

FIGURE 8-7 A heterophil in the blood film of a common Boa Constrictor *(Boa constrictor)*; Wright-Giemsa stain × 1000.

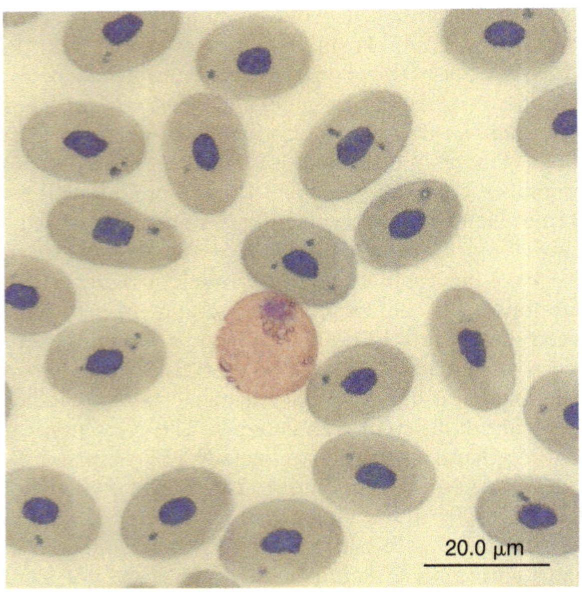

FIGURE 8-8 A heterophil in the blood film of a Green Sea turtle *(Chelonia mydas)*; Wright-Giemsa stain × 1000.

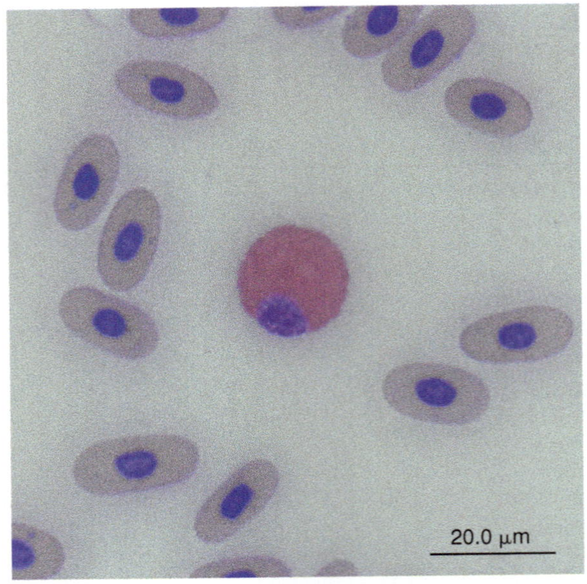

FIGURE 8-9 A heterophil in the blood film of a Box Turtle *(Terrapene carolina triunguis)*; Wright-Giemsa stain × 1000.

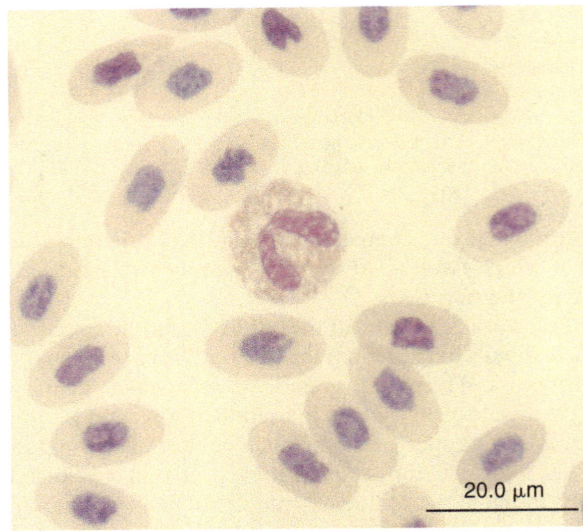

FIGURE 8-10 A heterophil in the blood film of a Green Iguana *(Iguana iguana)*; Wright-Giemsa stain × 1000.

heterophils are functionally equivalent to mammalian neutrophils but most likely behave like avian heterophils in that they rely more heavily on oxygen-independent mechanisms to destroy phagocytized microorganisms. The PER-positive heterophils of Green Iguanas suggest that these cells may possess bactericidal and oxidative properties similar to mammalian neutrophils.[23] The lack of cytochemical consistency in reptilian heterophils makes it difficult to develop guidelines in a related taxonomic group.[44]

Reptilian eosinophils are large round cells with spherical eosinophilic (typically brightly eosinophilic) cytoplasmic granules (Figures 8-11 and 8-12). The Romanowsky-stained granules of eosinophils found in the peripheral blood of some species of reptiles, such as the Green Iguana, stain blue (Figures 8-13 and 8-14). The cytoplasmic granules of eosinophils stain positive for PER in some species of reptiles, which allows easy differentiation between eosinophils

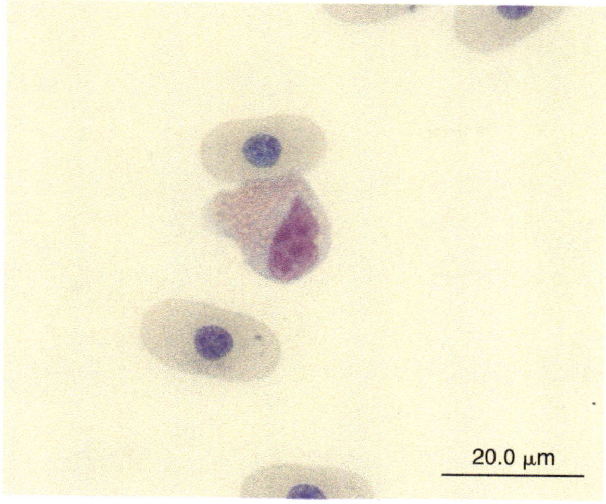

FIGURE 8-11 An eosinophil in the blood film of a Wood Turtle *(Glyptemys insculpta);* Wright-Giemsa stain × 1000.

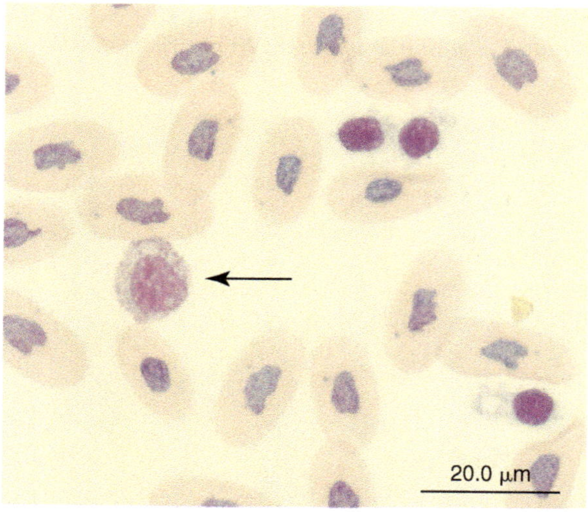

FIGURE 8-12 An eosinophil *(arrow)* and three thrombocytes in the blood film of a common Boa Constrictor *(Boa constrictor);* Wright-Giemsa stain × 1000.

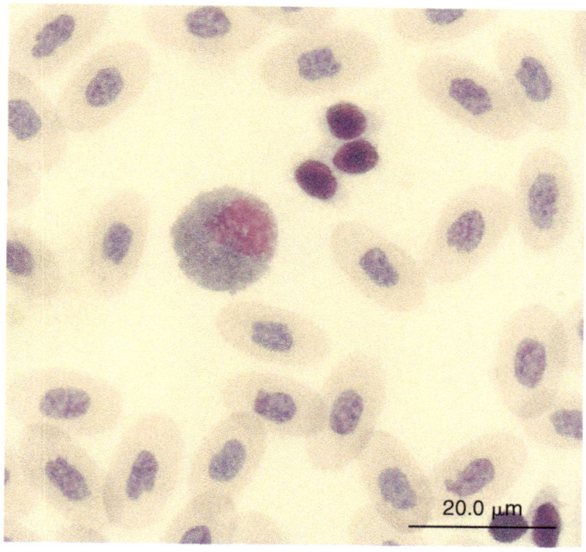

FIGURE 8-13 An eosinophil and three thrombocytes in the blood film of a Green Iguana *(Iguana iguana);* Wright-Giemsa stain × 1000.

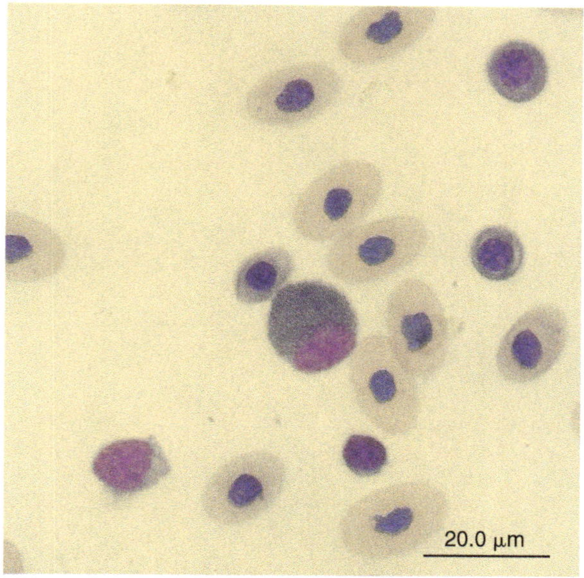

FIGURE 8-14 A cell resembling an iguana eosinophil in the blood film of a Reeves' Turtle *(Mauremys reevesii);* Wright-Giemsa stain × 1000.

and heterophils in those species with PER-negative heterophils.[30,52-54] The blue-staining granules of the Green Iguana eosinophils do not stain with PER or other common cytochemical stains.[23] As with heterophils, the size of eosinophils varies with species. For example, snakes tend to have larger eosinophils than do chelonians and lizards.[17] The nucleus of the reptilian eosinophil is typically centrally located in the cell and has a variable shape, ranging from slightly elongated to lobed. The variation in the cytochemical staining of reptilian eosinophils may be associated with the variability in cytochemical techniques.[44]

Reptilian basophils are usually small round cells containing basophilic metachromatic cytoplasmic granules, which often obscure the cell nucleus (Figures 8-15 through 8-18). When visible, the cell nucleus is slightly eccentric in position and not lobed. Basophils are easy to identify and stain strongly with TB stain.[41,44] Basophil granules are frequently affected by water-based stains, which cause them to partially dissolve. Alcohol fixation and the use of Romanowsky stains are preferred because they provide the best staining for reptilian basophils. Basophils vary in size according to the species of reptile but generally range between 7 and 20 µm.[17] Lizards tend to have small basophils, whereas turtles and crocodiles have large basophils.[17]

Reptilian lymphocytes resemble those of mammals and birds (Figures 8-19 through 8-21). They vary in size from small (5 to 10µm) to large (15µm).[17,18] Lymphocytes are round cells that exhibit irregularity when they mold around adjacent cells in the blood film or fold at their cytoplasmic margin (Figure 8-22). They have a round or slightly indented nucleus that is centrally or slightly eccentrically positioned in the cell. The nuclear chromatin of mature lymphocytes is heavily clumped. Lymphocytes typically have a large nucleus to cytoplasmic ratio

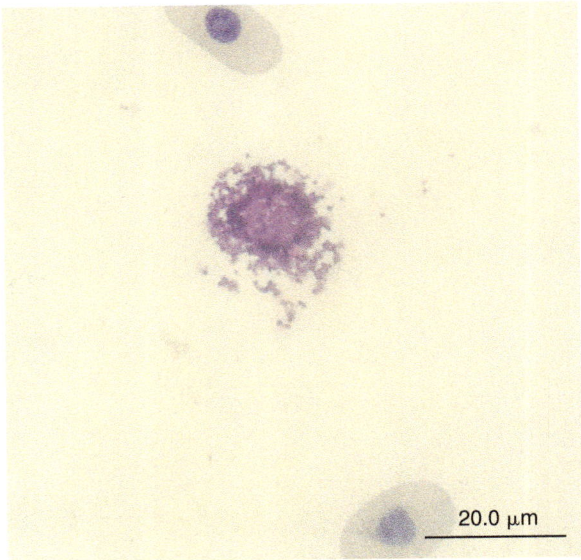

FIGURE 8-15 A ruptured basophil revealing its granules in the blood film of a Wood Turtle *(Glyptemys insculpta)*; Wright-Giemsa stain × 1000.

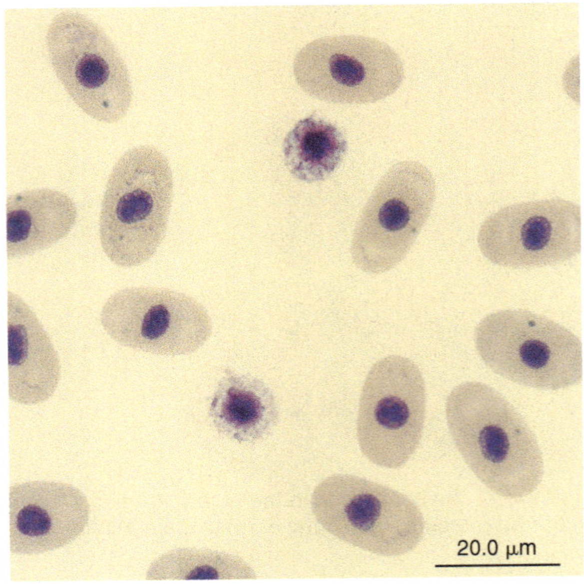

FIGURE 8-17 Two basophils in the blood film of a Painted Terrapin *(Callagur borneoensis)*; Wright-Giemsa stain × 1000.

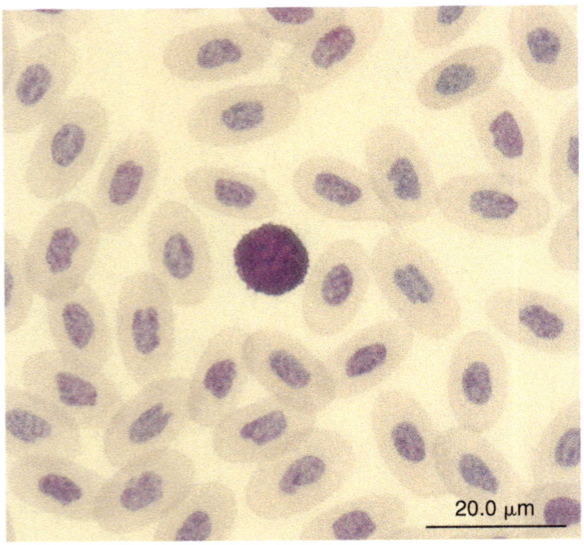

FIGURE 8-16 A basophil in the blood film of a Green Iguana *(Iguana iguana)*; Wright-Giemsa stain × 1000.

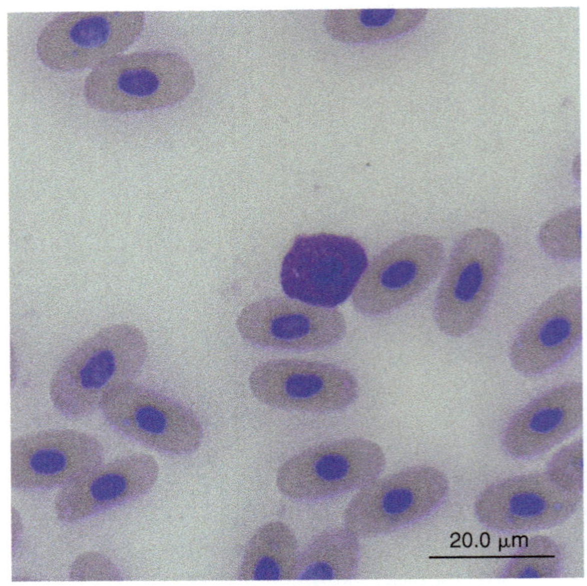

FIGURE 8-18 A basophil in the blood film of a Box Turtle *(Terrapene carolina triunguis)*; Wright-Giemsa stain × 1000.

(N:C). The typical small mature lymphocyte has scant slightly basophilic (pale blue) cytoplasm. Large lymphocytes have more cytoplasmic volume compared with small lymphocytes, and the nucleus is often pale staining. The cytoplasm of a normal lymphocyte appears homogeneous and lacks vacuoles and granules. Lymphocytes generally stain negative for nearly all of the cytochemical stains.

Lymphocytes in some species of reptiles may be difficult to differentiate from thrombocytes because cell size, appearance, and stain response are similar in both cells (Figure 8-23). The differentiation of these cells is made easier in species whose thrombocytes are characteristically elongated. In general, thrombocytes are slightly smaller than and often have a denser more compact nuclear chromatin pattern than lymphocytes. In addition, thrombocytes often have cytoplasmic vacuoles that are not usually present in inactivated lymphocytes.

Monocytes are generally the largest leukocyte in the peripheral blood of reptiles and resemble those found in the blood films of mammals and birds (Figures 8-24 through 8-28). They vary in shape from round to ameboid. The nucleus is variable in shape, ranging between round and oval to lobed. The nuclear chromatin of monocytes is less condensed and stains relatively pale compared with the nuclei of lymphocytes. The abundant cytoplasm of monocytes stains blue-gray, may appear slightly opaque, and may contain vacuoles or fine dust like eosinophilic or azurophilic granules. The monocytes of snakes often have a round to oval nucleus and contain abundant dust

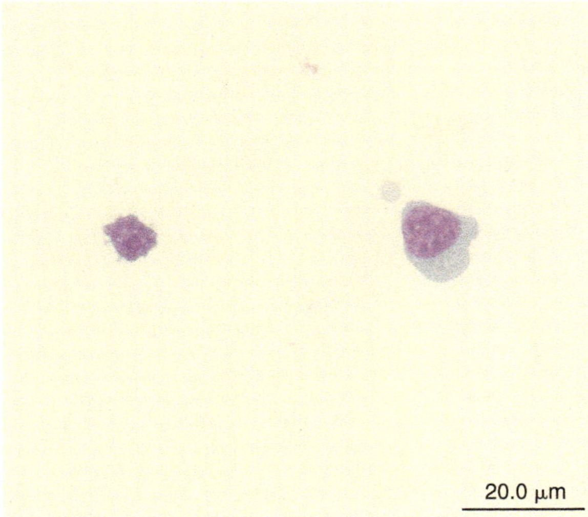

FIGURE 8-19 A large lymphocyte *(cell on the right)* and a small lymphocyte *(cell on the left)* in the blood film of a Wood Turtle *(Glyptemys insculpta);* Wright-Giemsa stain × 1000.

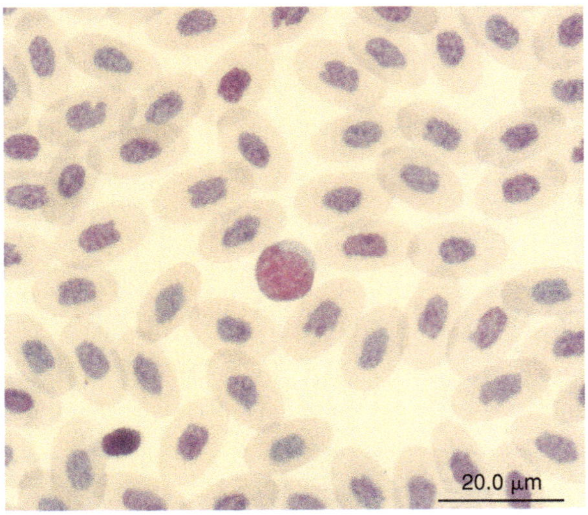

FIGURE 8-20 A lymphocyte in the blood film of a Green Iguana *(Iguana iguana);* Wright-Giemsa stain × 1000.

like azurophilic granules. Cytochemical staining of monocytes can vary among species, which may be related to variation in techniques. The monocytes of the Green Iguana stain positive with AP, alpha-naphthyl butyrate esterase, and PAS and negative with SBB and PER.[23] Snake monocytes with distinct azurophilic cytoplasmic granules (azurophils) stain positive for PER, SBB, and PAS.[23]

Morphologic differences have been detected in monocytes in the same blood sample of reptiles. This has led some to distinguish monocytes, identified as large cells with clear cytoplasm, from azurophils, identified as smaller cells with basophilic cytoplasm.[30,55] Similar morphologic variability has also been found in other cell types, such as thrombocytes, eosinophils, and heterophils.[44] Although monocytes that have an azurophilic appearance to the cytoplasm are often referred to as azurophils in the literature, the cytochemical and ultrastructural characteristics are often similar to monocytes and

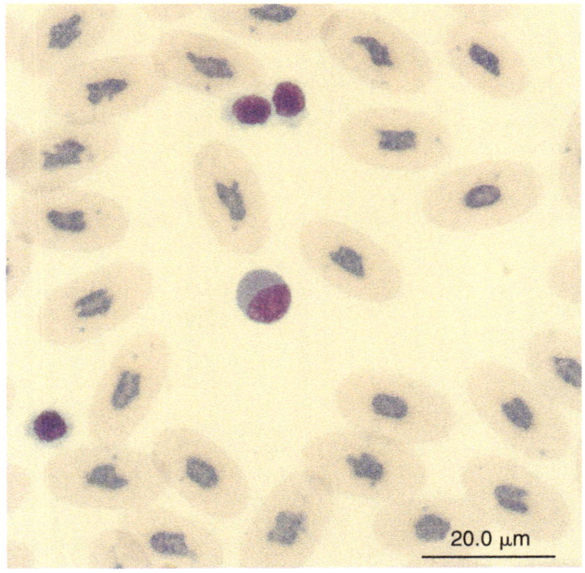

FIGURE 8-21 A large lymphocyte and thrombocytes (smaller cells) in the blood film of a common Boa Constrictor *(Boa constrictor);* Wright-Giemsa stain × 1000.

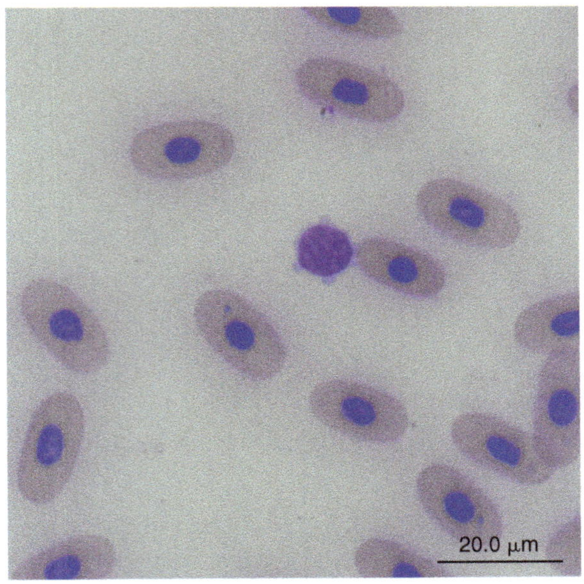

FIGURE 8-22 A small lymphocyte with scalloped cytoplasmic margins in the blood film of a Box Turtle *(Terrapene carolina triunguis);* Wright-Giemsa stain × 1000.

therefore should be reported as monocytes rather than as a separate cell type.[18,23,36,44,48] Therefore the term *azurophil* is not recommended when referring to reptilian monocytes. Instead, the term *azurophilic monocyte* can be used for monocytes with a basophilic cytoplasm and fine azurophilic granulation, if a distinction is desired.

LEUKOCYTE RESPONSES TO DISEASE

Because extrinsic factors, such as season, temperature, and specific stressors, such as capture, restraint, and confinement, can have a marked effect on the leukogram of reptiles,

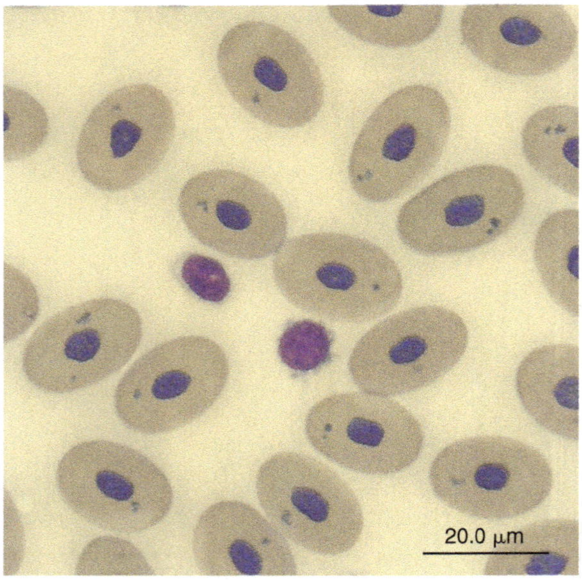

FIGURE 8-23 A lymphocyte and two thrombocytes in the blood film of a Green Sea turtle *(Chelonia mydas)*; Wright-Giemsa stain × 1000.

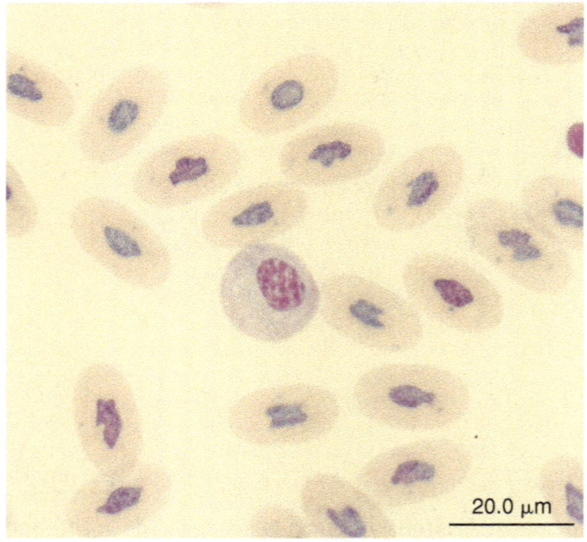

FIGURE 8-25 A monocyte in the blood film of a common Boa Constrictor *(Boa constrictor)*; Wright-Giemsa stain × 1000.

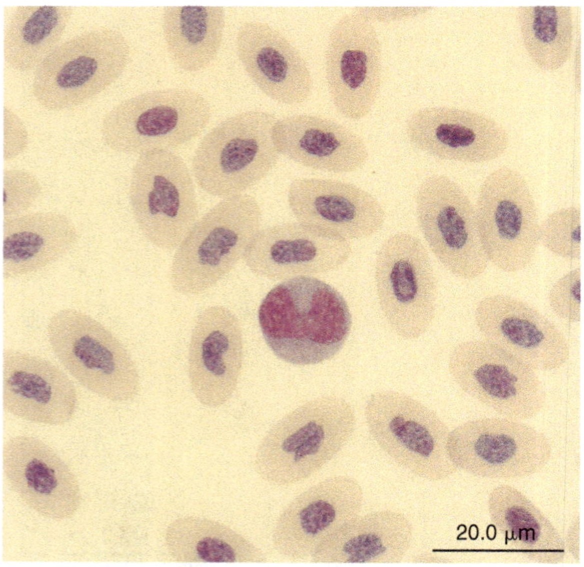

FIGURE 8-24 A monocyte in the blood film of a Green Iguana *(Iguana iguana)*; Wright-Giemsa stain × 1000.

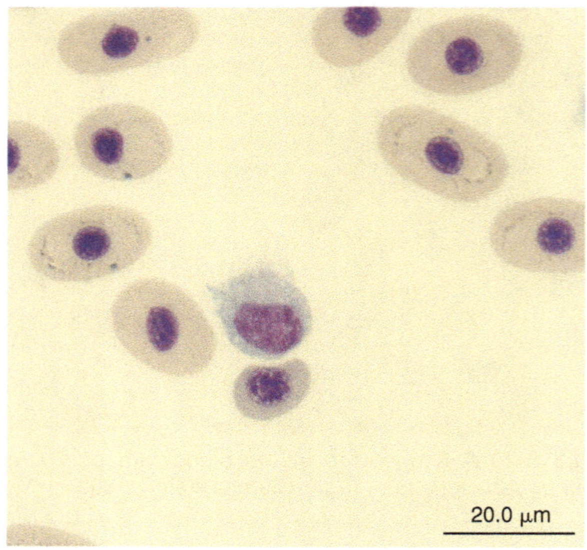

FIGURE 8-26 A monocyte in the blood film of a Painted Terrapin *(Callagur borneoensis)*; Wright-Giemsa stain × 1000.

it has been suggested that a total leukocyte count greater than 30,000 cells/μL would be required to indicate an inflammatory response associated with an infection.[4,9] However, regardless of the actual leukocyte count, the presence of toxic heterophils indicates a severe inflammatory response that is likely associated with sepsis.

The percentage of heterophils in the leukocyte differential of normal reptiles varies with species. Heterophils can represent up to 40% of the leukocytes in some healthy reptile species.[18,19,31,56-59] The concentration of heterophils in the peripheral blood is also influenced by seasonal factors. For example, heterophil concentration is highest during the summer and lowest during brumation.[19] Because the primary function of heterophils is phagocytosis, significant increases in the heterophil count of reptiles are usually associated with inflammatory disease, especially microbial and parasitic infections or tissue injury. Heterophil counts are expected to increase with tissue trauma associated with surgical procedures.[40] The lack of PER activity in most reptilian heterophils suggests little, if any, oxidative response to stimuli. Noninflammatory conditions that may result in heterophilia include stress (glucocorticosteroid excess), neoplasia, and heterophilic leukemia.

Heteropenia is indicative of either excessive peripheral utilization of heterophils or inadequate heterophil production. For example, heteropenia has been associated with drought and starvation in tortoises that may be physiologically compromised when entering hibernation.[60]

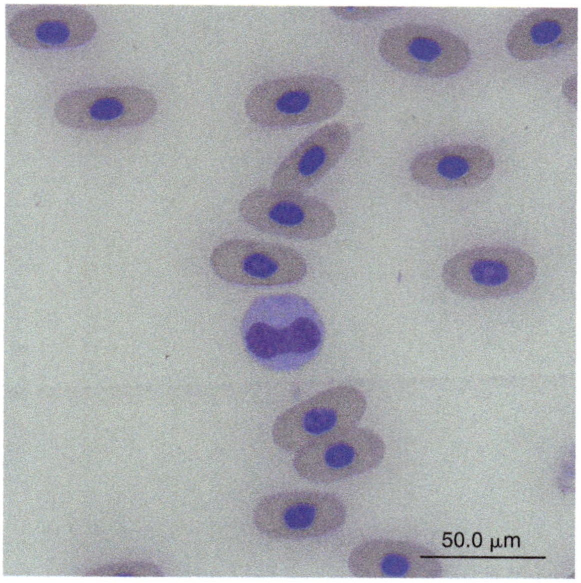

FIGURE 8-27 A monocyte *(center cell)* and small lymphocyte in the blood film of a Box Turtle *(Terrapene carolina triunguis);* Wright-Giemsa stain × 1000.

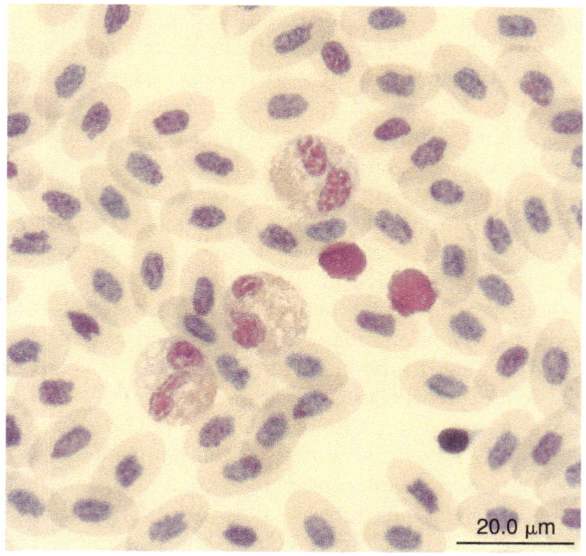

FIGURE 8-29 Toxic heterophils in the blood film of a Green Iguana *(Iguana iguana);* Wright-Giemsa stain × 1000.

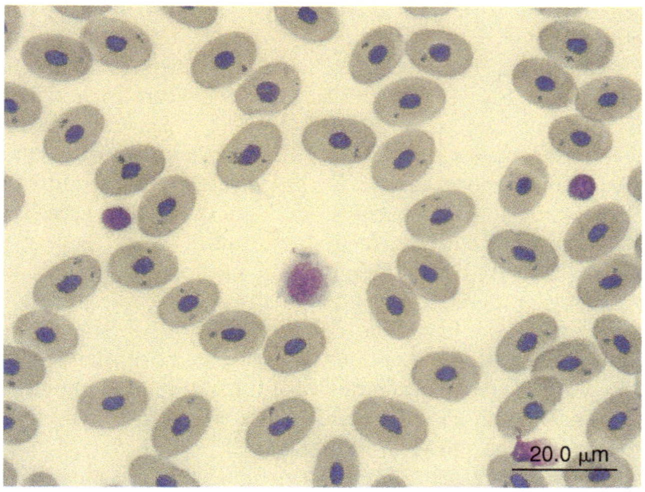

FIGURE 8-28 A monocyte *(center cell)*, a lymphocyte *(small cell on the right)*, and a thrombocyte *(small cell on the left)* in the blood film of a Green Sea turtle *(Chelonia mydas);* Wright-Giemsa stain × 1000.

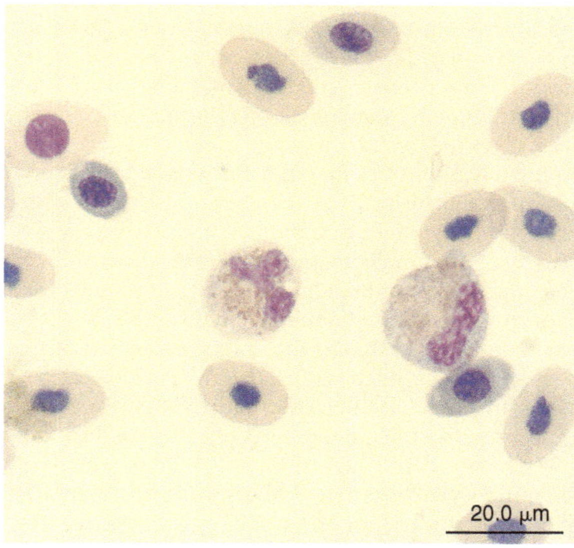

FIGURE 8-30 Toxic heterophils in the blood film of a Reeves' Turtle *(Mauremys reevesii);* Wright-Giemsa stain × 1000.

Heterophils may appear abnormal in reptiles with a variety of diseases. For example, heterophils may exhibit varying degrees of toxicity with inflammatory diseases, especially those involving infectious agents such as bacteria. Toxic heterophils exhibit an increase in cytoplasmic basophilia, abnormal granulation (i.e., dark blue to purple granules or granules with abnormal shapes and staining), and cytoplasmic vacuolation (Figures 8-29 and 8-30). Degranulated heterophils may be associated with artifacts of blood film preparation or may represent toxic changes. Nuclear lobation in species that normally do not have a lobated heterophil nucleus is also an abnormal finding suggestive of severe inflammation.

The number of circulating eosinophils in healthy reptiles is variable. In general, lizards tend to have low numbers of eosinophils compared with some species of turtles that can have up to 20%.[18,19,31,56-59] Like heterophils, the number of eosinophils present in the peripheral blood is influenced by environmental factors, such as seasonal changes. The number of eosinophils is generally lower during the summer and highest during brumation in some species.[19] Eosinophilia may be associated with parasitic infections and stimulation of the immune system.[59,61]

The percent of basophils in the differential leukocyte count of normal reptiles can range between 0 and 40%.[18,19,31,56-59] In general, variation in basophil concentration is less affected by seasonal changes, unlike acidophil concentrations, but this may vary with species.[17] Some species of reptiles have normally high numbers of circulating basophils. For example, some turtles typically have circulating basophil numbers that represent up to 40% of the leukocyte differential.[62,63] The reason for this is unknown. Reptilian basophils most likely function in a manner similar to those of mammals on the basis of cytochemical and ultrastructure studies. They appear to process surface immunoglobulins and release histamine on degranulation.[18,62,63] Immediately after surgical implantation of intracoelomic transmitters, snakes demonstrated higher basophil and lymphocyte counts, likely as part of the inflammatory response to the surgery.[40] Basophilia has also been associated with parasitic and viral infections.

Although variable, lymphocytes are generally considered to be the predominant leukocyte in the blood of reptiles. The lymphocyte concentration can represent more than 80% of the normal leukocyte differential in some species.[18] Lymphocyte numbers are influenced by a variety of environmental and physiologic factors. In general, juvenile reptiles tend to have higher lymphocyte counts compared with adults, and the lymphocyte concentrations decrease with age. As with heterophils and eosinophils, lymphocyte counts are also influenced by seasonal change: lymphocyte counts tend to be lowest during the winter and highest during the summer.[18,19,58] Temperate reptiles have a decrease or absence of lymphocytes during and after brumation.[64-67] Captive tropical reptiles may also show a decrease in circulating lymphocytes during the winter, despite lack of hibernation. Lymphocyte numbers may also be affected by gender in that differences may occur between males and females of some species. This does not hold true, however, for all reptiles; for example, no significant differences exist between sexes for free-ranging crocodiles.[6]

Reptilian lymphocytes function in a manner similar to those of mammals and birds. They have the same major classes of lymphocytes: B lymphocytes and T lymphocytes are involved in a variety of immunologic functions.[68] However, unlike birds and mammals, the immunologic responses of reptiles are influenced greatly by the environment.[69] For example, low temperatures may suppress or inhibit the immune response of reptiles.

Lymphopenia is often associated with malnutrition or is secondary to a number of diseases caused by stress and immunosuppression. A single hydrocortisone acetate dose (1mg/kg body weight) resulted in a 40% to 50% reduction of peripheral blood lymphocytes from lympholysis of lizards that lasted for approximately 4 weeks in one study.[70] Green Sea turtles with papillomas generally have total circulating white blood cell counts that are comparable to those of healthy individuals, but lower lymphocyte numbers indicate an alteration of the immune response.[71]

Lymphocytosis occurs during wound healing, inflammatory disease, parasitic infection (e.g., hemoparasites, anisakiasis, and spirorchidiasis), and viral infections. For example, the total leukocyte and lymphocyte counts were shown to be higher in *Hepatozoon*-positive snakes.[5] Compared with nesting and foraging sea turtles, stranded individuals tended to have higher lymphocyte counts.[7] Lymphocytosis also occurs during ecdysis.[32] The presence of reactive lymphocytes and, less commonly, plasma cells suggests stimulation of the immune system. These cells resemble those of mammals and birds. Reactive lymphocytes have more abundant, deeply basophilic cytoplasm compared with normal lymphocytes, and the nuclear chromatin may appear less condensed. Plasma cells have abundant intensely basophilic cytoplasm that contains a distinct Golgi zone and an eccentrically positioned nucleus.

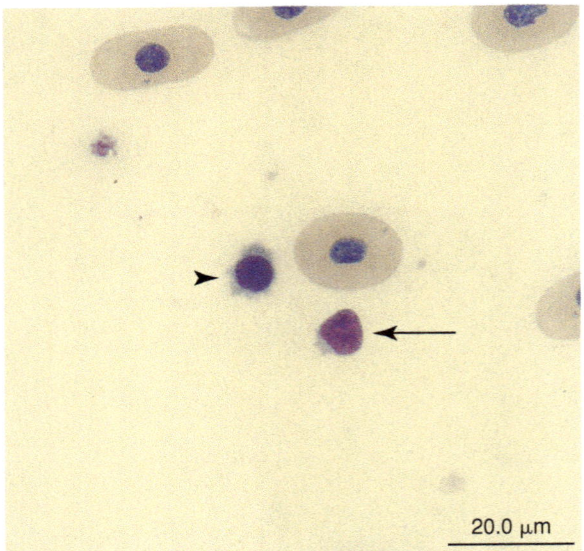

FIGURE 8-31 A thrombocyte *(arrowhead)* and a lymphocyte *(arrow)* in the blood film of a Wood Turtle *(Glyptemys insculpta);* Wright-Giemsa stain × 1000.

Leukocytosis with marked lymphocytosis can signal lymphoid leukemia.[34,72]

Monocytes generally occur in low numbers in the blood films of healthy reptiles and comprise between 0% and 10% of the leukocyte differential.[18,19,32,56-59,73] Snakes typically have monocytes with an azurophilic appearance to the cytoplasm (frequently referred to as *azurophils* in the literature).[36] The monocyte concentration changes little with seasonal variation.[19] Stranded sea turtles tend to have lower monocyte counts compared with foraging and nesting turtles.[7] Monocytosis is suggestive of inflammatory diseases, especially granulomatous inflammation. For example, it was shown that monocyte (azurophil) counts increased because of infection after surgical implantation of transmitters in the coelomic cavity of snakes rather than because of a simple reaction to the trauma of the surgical procedure alone.[40]

Although rare, some cases of leukemia have been reported in reptiles.[34,74-78] The myeloproliferative diseases of reptiles can be classified in the same manner as in mammals. Special cytochemical studies may be necessary to identify the abnormal cells.

THROMBOCYTES AND HEMOSTASIS

Thrombocytes of reptiles appear as elliptical to fusiform nucleated cells (Figures 8-31, 8-32, and 8-33). The centrally positioned nucleus has dense nuclear chromatin that stains purple, and the cytoplasm is typically colorless and may contain a few azurophilic granules. Activated thrombocytes are common and appear as clusters of cells with irregular cytoplasmic margins and vacuoles. Thrombocytes appear devoid of cytoplasm when aggregated. Reptilian thrombocytes often stain PAS-positive, which aids in distinguishing them from the PAS-negative lymphocytes; however, this does not hold true for all species.[23,42]

The actual thrombocyte concentration may be difficult to determine because thrombocytes tend to clump in vitro and when exposed to heparin. The thrombocyte concentration can be determined with the Natt and Herrick method for obtaining

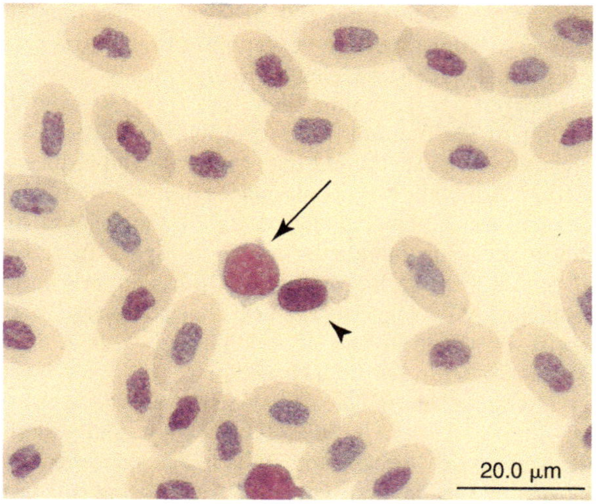

FIGURE 8-32 A thrombocyte *(arrowhead)* and a lymphocyte *(arrow)* in the blood film of a Green Iguana *(Iguana iguana)*; Wright-Giemsa stain × 1000.

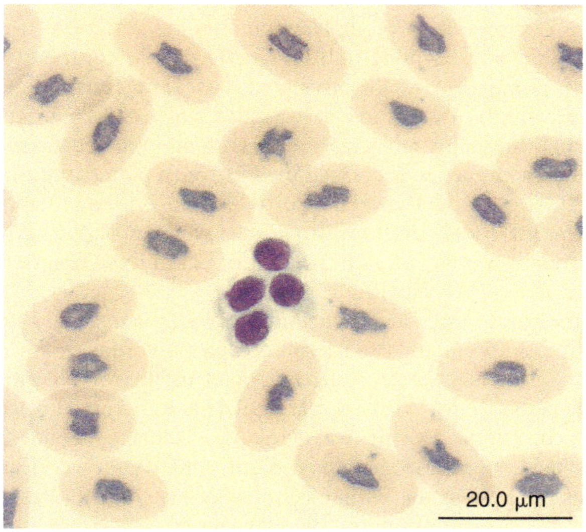

FIGURE 8-33 Thrombocytes clumped in the blood film of a common Boa Constrictor *(Boa constrictor)*; Wright-Giemsa stain × 1000.

erythrocyte and leukocyte counts. After the 1:200 dilution of the blood is prepared with Natt and Herrick solution and a Neubauer-ruled hemocytometer is charged, the number of thrombocytes in the entire central ruled area (central large square) are counted on both sides of the hemocytometer. The number of thrombocytes per microliter of blood is obtained by multiplying that number by 1000. A subjective thrombocyte concentration can be determined based on the number of thrombocytes that appear in a stained blood film and can be reported as reduced, normal, or increased. Thrombocytes typically occur in numbers that range between 25 and 350 thrombocytes per 100 leukocytes in the blood film of healthy reptiles.[18]

THROMBOCYTE RESPONSES TO DISEASE

Reptilian thrombocytes have a significant role in thrombus formation and function similarly to avian thrombocytes and mammalian platelets. The ultrastructure features of activated thrombocytes include pseudopodia with fine granular material and many fibrinlike filaments radiating between and around the cells.[18] Immature thrombocytes of reptiles resemble the immature thrombocytes of birds and, when present in blood film, represent a regenerative response. Thrombocytopenia of reptiles most likely occurs as a result of excessive peripheral utilization of thrombocytes or a decrease in thrombocyte production. Thrombocytes with polymorphic nuclei are considered abnormal and may be associated with severe inflammatory disease.[36]

CLINICAL CHEMISTRY PROFILES OF REPTILES

Lithium heparin is frequently used as an anticoagulant when blood is collected for biochemistry testing in reptiles. Collection of blood into lithium heparin allows for a greater sample volume per unit of blood compared with serum. This is especially significant in small sample volumes in which much of the sample is trapped in the clotted blood when serum is harvested. In addition, because clot formation in reptiles is unpredictable and often prolonged, significant changes may occur in some of the analytes, such as the electrolytes. The slow clotting is a result of the low intrinsic thromboplastin activity of reptilian blood and a strong natural circulating antithrombin factor, which is needed to compensate for the sluggish blood flow. Another advantage of the heparinized sample is that it can also be used for hematologic studies.

When faced with a small sample volume that precludes the use of a full diagnostic panel, the clinician must decide which tests are most beneficial in the evaluation of the reptilian patient. Blood biochemistry tests that appear the most useful in reptilian diagnostics include total protein, glucose, uric acid, aspartate aminotransferase (AST), calcium, and phosphorus. If a large sample size is available, then other tests that may prove useful include creatine, lactate dehydrogenase (LDH), creatine kinase (CK), albumin, sodium, potassium, chloride, total CO_2, and protein electrophoresis. Many modern blood chemistry analyzers require a small sample size (10 to 30 µL) to perform many of these tests. Commercial veterinary laboratories often offer chemistry profiles that require a minimal amount of serum or plasma (0.5 mL). Blood chemistry analyzers that use dry reagents and reflectance photometry for in-house testing may be used for reptile samples; however, studies have shown that less variance occurs among results from diagnostic laboratories, which is likely the result of the attention given to quality control. A great degree of heterogeneity in the performance of in-house analyzers, many failing to meet "world class standards" has been shown for a range of analytes.[79] The inadequacies in the performance of these analyzers usually go unnoticed by the clinician performing the analysis, who assumes the results provided on a specific patient can be believed, and likely impacts the clinical decision. In general, reference laboratories, especially those from veterinary teaching hospitals, are less likely to have unstable performances than in-clinic analyzers.[79] Because a significant variance in the blood biochemistry results occurs with the various analyzer methodologies, it is important to identify the specific methodology used when reporting and interpreting biochemical data because this magnitude of difference would influence interpretation of the test results and affect patient management.[80,81]

Ideally, plasma used for biochemical testing should be separated immediately (or within 5 to 6 hours) from the cellular component of the blood sample after blood collection. This may not be possible in field studies where a centrifuge is unavailable. In such situations, whole blood samples can be stored in a portable cooler up to 24 hours without appreciable change in select biochemical analytes.[6,82]

The plasma of most reptiles is colorless but may be colored in some species. For example, the carotenoid pigments in the diet of herbivores, such as the Green Iguana may color the plasma yellow to orange. The plasma of some snakes, such as pythons, may be greenish yellow due to dietary carotenoids and riboflavin. A few species of lizards may have green plasma because of normal high concentrations of biliverdin.[83]

Like the hematologic responses, the biochemical responses of reptiles are influenced by normal physiologic and external factors that may enhance or inhibit response to disease. These factors include species, age, gender, environment, season, and nutritional status and make interpretation of the blood biochemistry values of a reptilian patient a challenge.[1-4,84-86]

LABORATORY EVALUATION OF THE REPTILIAN KIDNEY

Blood biochemical testing for renal disease in reptiles is often based on diagnostic panels available for mammals. However, the detection of renal disease in reptiles is more difficult than it is in mammals because of the physiologic differences in their kidneys. The available commercial laboratory tests include blood urea nitrogen (BUN), uric acid, and creatinine.

The reptilian renal cortex contains only simple nephrons (called *cortical nephrons*) with a tubular system devoid of loops of Henle; therefore reptiles are unable to concentrate their urine.[87,88] The nitrogenous wastes excreted by the reptilian kidney include variable amounts of uric acid, urea, and ammonia, depending on the animal's natural environment. Freshwater turtles that spend much of their lives in water excrete equal amounts of ammonia and urea, whereas those with amphibious habits excrete more urea.[87] Sea turtles excrete uric acid, ammonia, and urea. Alligators excrete ammonia and uric acid. Terrestrial reptiles such as tortoises must conserve water, and ammonia, urea, and other soluble urinary nitrogenous wastes require large amounts of water for excretion. Therefore to conserve water, terrestrial reptiles produce more insoluble nitrogenous waste in the form of uric acid and urate salts, which are eliminated in a semisolid state.[88]

Although the reptilian kidney has moderate activities of LDH, AST, alanine aminotransferase (ALT), and CK, plasma activities of these enzymes do not increase with renal disease. Instead, detection of renal disease in reptiles depends on BUN, uric acid, and, when available, creatine concentrations.

BLOOD UREA NITROGEN

Unlike mammals, BUN and creatinine concentrations generally are poor indicators of renal disease in most reptiles. The normal BUN value of most reptiles is less than 10 mg/dL (3.57 mmol/L).[26,31,32,57,84-86,89-92] However, the plasma urea nitrogen concentrations may be more useful in the evaluation of renal disease among aquatic reptiles that primarily excrete urea. Because terrestrial reptiles primarily are uricotelic, the normal urea nitrogen concentration in these species is less than 15 mg/dL (<5.36 mmol/L), with the exception of terrestrial chelonians (especially desert species), which typically have plasma urea nitrogen concentrations that vary from 30 to 100 mg/dL (10.71 to 35.70 mmol/L).[84-87,90] This is considered to be a mechanism to elevate the plasma osmolarity and reduce water loss from the body.[57] The plasma osmolarity of freshwater turtles and crocodilians is approximately the same as that of common domestic mammals, but it is higher in terrestrial reptiles. An increase in plasma urea nitrogen concentration in reptiles may be suggestive of severe renal disease, prerenal azotemia, or a high dietary urea intake; however, it does not reliably increase under these conditions.

Free-ranging Desert Tortoises demonstrate a "water metabolism strategy" whereby BUN, uric acid, and osmolality values respond to the amount of available forage and water as determined by rainfall. Drought causes urine retention to conserve water and urea and can cause BUN values of up to 60 mg/dL (21.42 mmol/L) in healthy Desert Tortoises without clinical dehydration.[60] In a study,[93] free-ranging tortoises that exhibited increased plasma uric acid, sodium, and potassium concentrations with decreased osmolality and urea nitrogen were considered to be actively consuming water along with protein and electrolyte-rich forage. This is in contrast to the same population of tortoises that were not consuming significant amounts of food or water as suggested by increased plasma osmolality and urea nitrogen along with decreased uric acid concentration. Increased urea nitrogen concentration was considered to be a reflection of increased protein catabolism and perhaps dehydration. In another study, a high BUN concentration was a good indicator of decreased renal function but did not always predict mortality.[11]

Increased uric acid concentration was considered to be an indication of increased dietary protein intake. Tortoises that were feeding with restricted water intake revealed higher plasma osmolality with decreased BUN and increased uric acid concentrations. During wet seasons, plasma osmolality and uric acid, urea nitrogen, potassium, and sodium concentrations were lower than other seasons because of increased rates of water consumption and bladder emptying. Plasma concentrations of these analytes in captive tortoises having constant access to water are expected to resemble free-ranging tortoises in wet years.

CREATININE

Creatinine is a normal constituent of mammalian urine, but the amount formed in most reptiles is negligible (<1 mg/dL or 88.4 μmol/L).[2,32,57,90,94] Blood creatinine concentration is generally considered to be of poor diagnostic value in the detection of renal disease in reptiles. By contrast, the plasma creatine concentration may have diagnostic value in the detection of renal disease in some reptilian species, but the test is unavailable from most veterinary laboratories.

URIC ACID

Uric acid is the primary catabolic end product of protein, nonprotein nitrogen, and purines in terrestrial reptiles, and it represents 80% to 90% of the total nitrogen excreted by the kidneys.[20] Uric acid is formed by the breakdown of proteins by xanthine oxidase or by hydrolytic enzymes. In terrestrial reptiles, uric acid is further converted into urate (i.e., sodium and potassium urate), the salt form of uric acid. Urates are poorly water soluble and precipitate at low concentrations. Although uric acid is excreted by tubular secretion independent of the hydration status of the reptile, its elimination by the kidney is still influenced by dehydration. With normal hydration, the nephron actively excretes three times the amount of urates than it would in the dehydrated state.[88] The normal blood uric acid concentration in most reptiles is less than 10 mg/dL (594.8 μmol/L).Hyperuricemia is indicated by uric acid values of greater than 15 mg/dL (892.2 μmol/L) and is usually associated with renal disease. Renal diseases that are associated with hyperuricemia include severe nephritis, nephrocalcinosis, and nephrotoxicity. Hyperuricemia is neither a sensitive test nor a specific test for renal disease in reptiles. Hyperuricemia associated with renal disease most likely reflects the loss of two thirds (or more) of the functional renal mass. Hyperuricemia in reptiles can also be associated with gout or recent ingestion of a high-protein diet. Carnivorous reptiles tend to have higher blood uric acid concentrations than herbivorous reptiles, and their plasma uric acid concentrations generally peak the day after a meal, thereby resulting in a 1.5- to 2.0-fold increase in uric acid.[20]

Gout can result from an overproduction of uric acid (i.e., primary gout) or from an acquired disease that interferes with the normal production and excretion of uric acid (i.e., secondary gout). Conditions that result in secondary gout among reptiles include starvation, renal disease (especially tubular damage), severe and prolonged dehydration, and excessive dietary purines (i.e., herbivorous reptiles fed diets rich in animal proteins). In reptiles, nephritis has been implicated as the major cause of gout.[95] Hyperuricemia associated with renal disease and gout often results in greater than twofold increases in uric acid concentrations.

OTHER TESTS

The reptilian kidney has high ALT and alkaline phosphatase (ALP) activity.[96] Significant increases in the plasma activities of these enzymes, however, do not occur with renal disease because most of the enzymes released from damaged renal cells are released in urine, not in plasma.[96,97]

Reptiles rarely exhibit polyuria with renal disease. Therefore urinalysis is rarely performed to assess renal disease because of a lack of available urine to perform the tests.

The normal glomerular filtration rate based on iohexol clearance has been established for the Green Iguana and can be used to evaluate kidney function in that species.[98,99] Reported values are 14.78 to 18.34 mL/kg/h (mean and standard deviation, 16.56 ± 3.90 mL/kg/h).

CALCIUM AND PHOSPHORUS

Calcium

Both blood calcium metabolism and the amount of ionized calcium in reptilian plasma are mediated by parathormone (PTH), calcitonin, and activated vitamin D_3 (1, 25-dihydroxycholecalciferol).[100] Other hormones, such as estrogen, thyroxin, and glucagon, may also influence calcium metabolism in reptiles. The primary function of PTH is to maintain normal blood calcium levels by its action on bone, kidneys, and intestinal mucosa. Low blood levels of ionized calcium stimulate the release of PTH, which results in calcium mobilization from bone, increased calcium absorption from the intestines, and increased calcium reabsorption from the kidneys.

The exact role of calcitonin in reptiles is unknown, but it most likely has a physiologic role opposite that of PTH. Increases in the blood calcium level stimulate the release of calcitonin from the ultimobranchial gland, which inhibits calcium reabsorption from bone.

The active form of vitamin D_3 stimulates the absorption of calcium and phosphorus by the intestinal mucosa. Photochemical production of the active form of vitamin D_3 by exposure to ultraviolet radiation (wavelength, 290 to 320 nm) is believed to be essential for normal calcium metabolism in reptiles, especially basking species.

Gravid female reptiles generally have increased plasma or serum concentrations of total calcium, phosphorus, proteins, and globulins that are used as body stores that are mobilized during vitellogenesis, yolk production, and shell deposition. During egg development, female reptiles exhibit hypercalcemia in response to estrogen and reproductive activity.[26] The increase in total plasma calcium level is associated with an increase in protein-bound calcium during follicular development before ovulation, and the total plasma calcium level may increase by twofold to fourfold or more.

The normal plasma calcium concentration for most reptiles ranges between 8 and 11 mg/dL (2.0 to 2.7mmol/L), and it varies both with the species and the physiologic status of the reptile.[101] For example, some species of tortoises have low blood calcium concentrations (<8 mg/dL or 2.0 mmol/L).[2,9] Gender differences have been reported for plasma calcium concentration in free-ranging populations of reptiles where females exhibit significantly greater calcium concentrations than males. This difference is likely to be associated with reproductive activity (vitellogenesis) at the time of sample collection. Likewise, the calcium to phosphorus ratio (Ca: P) is affected by vitellogenesis. For example, foraging male and female Leatherback Sea turtles had an average Ca: P ratio of 0.60 compared with that of nesting females with a Ca:P ratio of 0.86.[102]

Regardless of age and gender, healthy reptiles have consistent plasma ionized calcium concentrations. For this reason, measurement of the ionized calcium concentration provides the best clinical picture of the physiologically active calcium in circulation in reptiles. For a reptile that has a normal total calcium concentration but that is suspected of having a calcium imbalance or for gravid females with hypercalcemia, evaluation of physiologically active calcium in the blood is vital for determining a therapeutic plan. The normal plasma ionized calcium concentration for healthy Green Iguanas has been determined to be 5.9 mg/dL ± 0.42 (1.47 ± 0.105 mmol/L).[103] With this knowledge, a precise evaluation of the calcium status provides assistance in the diagnosis of iguanas with renal disease and in those with seizure activity and allows for a better evaluation of the health status of the gravid female iguana.[103] The normal heparinized plasma ionized calcium concentration of captive tortoises (*Testudo* spp.) is 1.9 mmol/L (3.80 mEq/L) and is not affected by storage at 5°C for 48 hours.[104]

Hypocalcemia occurs in most reptiles when the plasma calcium concentration is less than 8 mg/dL (2.0 mmol/L).

Hypocalcemia can occur with dietary calcium and vitamin D_3 deficiencies, excessive dietary phosphorus, alkalosis, hypoalbuminemia, or hypoparathyroidism. Secondary nutritional hyperparathyroidism is a common disorder of herbivorous reptiles such as Green Iguanas.[105-109] Diets fed to captive herbivores are often deficient in calcium and contain excessive amounts of phosphorus. In addition, dietary deficiency in vitamin D_3 or lack of proper exposure to ultraviolet light predisposes reptiles to hypocalcemia. Juvenile reptiles (especially Green Iguanas) with secondary nutritional hyperparathyroidism commonly develop nutritional metabolic bone disease (NMBD) with fibrous osteodystrophy and pathologic fractures.[108] The clinical signs in adult reptiles with hypocalcemia include muscle tremors, paresis, and seizures. Carnivorous reptiles fed all-meat, calcium-deficient diets also develop hypocalcemia associated with nutritional imbalances in calcium and phosphorus. Secondary renal hyperparathyroidism may also result in hypocalcemia. Hypocalcemia associated with a low concentration of 25-hydroxycholecalciferol, a low level of ionized calcium, and metastatic calcification has been reported in a tortoise with primary hyperparathyroidism.[110]

Hypercalcemia in reptiles is indicated by a plasma calcium concentration of greater than 20 mg/dL (5.0 mmol/L). Marked hypercalcemia as indicated by a plasma calcium concentration greater than 40 mg/dL (10mmol/L) is generally associated with egg production in females but may also be caused by excessive supplementation with oral or parenteral vitamin D_3 or calcium.[105,111] Other differentials for hypercalcemia include primary hyperparathyroidism, pseudohyperparathyroidism, and osteolytic bone disease; however, these disorders are rarely reported in reptiles. A normal physiologic hypercalcemia is found in a few reptiles such as the Indigo Snake (*Drymarchon* spp.) in which the average plasma calcium value is 159 mg/dL (range, 30 to 337 mg/dL). The phosphorus concentration is also high in these snakes; the average is 35 mg/dL and the range is 8 to 69 mg/dL.[112]

Phosphorus

The normal plasma phosphorus concentration for most reptiles ranges between 1 and 5 mg/dL (0.3 and 1.6 mmol/L).[101] Gender differences have been reported for plasma phosphorus concentration in free-ranging populations of reptiles; females exhibit significantly higher concentrations than males. This difference is likely to be associated with reproductive (vitellogenesis) activity at the time of sample collection.

Hypophosphatemia may result from starvation or a nutritional deficiency of phosphorus. Hyperphosphatemia is indicated by a plasma phosphorus concentration of greater than 5 mg/dL (1.6 mmol/L). Disorders resulting in hyperphosphatemia include excessive dietary phosphorus, hypervitaminosis D_3, and renal disease. Rare causes of hyperphosphatemia include severe tissue trauma and osteolytic bone disease. In mammalian blood samples, an artifactual hyperphosphatemia can occur when serum or plasma is not promptly separated from the clot, thereby allowing phosphorus to be released from erythrocytes. A few studies have suggested this may be less likely with reptilian blood samples; however, hyperphosphatemia has been related to hemolysis in reptilian blood samples.[113] The ideal sample for biochemical testing is obtained by the immediate separation of the cells from plasma with no hemolysis.

LABORATORY EVALUATION OF THE REPTILIAN LIVER

Laboratory tests commonly found on mammalian biochemistry profiles that are used to evaluate the liver include enzymes, bilirubin, and cholesterol. These same tests are used in the assessment of the liver in reptiles, although few critical studies have examined the effectiveness of biochemical testing of reptilian blood to evaluate hepatic disease. LDH and AST activities are high in reptilian liver tissue, and increases in the plasma activities of these enzymes may suggest hepatocellular disease.[33,96,97] The plasma AST activity is not considered to be organ specific because activity for this enzyme can be found in many tissues. In general, normal plasma AST activity for reptiles is less than 250 IU/L. Increased plasma AST activity suggests hepatic or muscle injury. Generalized diseases such as septicemia or toxemia, however, may damage these tissues, thereby producing increased plasma AST activity. Increased AST activity in the plasma of healthy free-ranging tortoises may be related to muscle activity and injury due to increased male aggression during the breeding season. Hepatic lipidosis, degeneration, and hemosiderosis are commonly observed in tortoises and other reptiles secondary to anorexia, which may contribute to increased plasma AST, ALT, and ALP activities.[11]

The plasma LDH activity is also considered to have a wide tissue distribution in reptiles. Therefore increases in the plasma LDH activity (>1000 IU/L) may be associated with damage to the liver, skeletal muscle, or cardiac muscle. Hemolysis may also result in increased plasma LDH activity.

Like AST, plasma ALT is not considered to be organ specific in reptiles. The normal plasma ALT activity for reptiles is usually less than 20 IU/L. Although ALT activity occurs in the reptilian liver, increases in the plasma ALT activity may not be as reliable in the detection of hepatocellular disease compared with increases in the plasma AST or LDH activity. However, it has been suggested that elevated plasma ALT activity can be associated with a prolonged diet of unnatural foods, which causes liver disorders in captive tortoises.

ALP is also widely distributed in the reptilian body, and the plasma activity of this enzyme is not considered to be organ specific. Little information is available concerning the interpretation of increased plasma ALP activity in reptiles; however, increased activity may reflect increased osteoblastic activity rather than hepatobiliary disease. Increased plasma ALP has been associated with hyperparathyroidism and bone diseases, such as Paget's disease. Elevated plasma ALP activity and glucose concentration in the absence of liver pathology may be associated with high corticosteroid levels during periods of stress, such as occurs with the capture of healthy individuals.[114] Little to no gamma-glutamyltransferase activity is found in serum or tissues of reptiles; therefore plasma activities of this enzyme are not used for the detection of hepatobiliary disease in reptiles.[96]

Instead of bilirubin as with mammals, biliverdin, a green bile pigment, is generally considered to be the primary end product of hemoglobin catabolism in most reptiles. Green plasma results from the accumulation of biliverdin in reptilian blood, which is usually a pathologic finding that suggests hepatobiliary disease in these animals. A nonpathologic accumulation of biliverdin can occur in the blood of some reptilian species, such as arboreal scincid lizards (Scincidae) of the southwestern Pacific, which are rarely presented for clinical evaluation.[83] The physiologic advantage of this is not known. Biliverdin appears to be less toxic to tissues compared with bilirubin, and the normal biliverdin concentration in the plasma of some lizards (i.e., *Prasinohaema*) can be greater than 1000 μmol/L.[83,115]

Although an increased bile acid concentration is considered to be a specific test for hepatic insufficiency, a high (670 mg/mL) bile acid concentration associated with severe dehydration was reported in a tortoise.[11,113] In addition, postprandial bile acid (3α-hydroxy bile acid) concentrations increase significantly from preprandial concentrations (after a 48-hour fast) in the Green Iguana.[117]

Because the liver is the major site of cholesterol synthesis in animals, measurement of plasma cholesterol concentration can aid in the diagnosis of liver disease in reptiles. The normal cholesterol concentration of reptiles varies depending on the natural diet. In general, healthy herbivorous reptiles are expected to have lower normal cholesterol concentrations (77 to 270 mg/dL or 2 to 7 mmol/L) compared with that of omnivores and carnivores. Low-density lipoprotein (LDL) is the major carrier of cholesterol in the serum of tortoises (*Agrionemys horsfieldii*, *Testudo graeca*, and *Testudo hermanni*), and high-density lipoprotein (HDL) represents a minor carrier.[118] Female reptiles undergoing active vitellogenesis are expected to have higher cholesterol and triglyceride values along with higher total protein, albumin, and globulin values than males or reproductively inactive females.[7]

Although not fully studied, some forms of hepatic failure may lead to hypocholesterolemia because of decreased cholesterol synthesis. Bile is a major route of cholesterol excretion from the body; therefore, hypercholesterolemia may result from decreased cholesterol excretion as would occur with cholestasis. The plasma cholesterol concentration would not be expected to be a specific test for liver disease in reptiles because there are other nonhepatic disorders that can result in hypercholesterolemia. In addition, in many reptiles with liver failure, the plasma cholesterol concentrations have been normal.

LABORATORY DETECTION OF MUSCLE INJURY

CK is considered to be a muscle-specific enzyme and is used to test for muscle cell damage. It has been shown that although plasma CK activity may be muscle specific in iguanas, high values do not always indicate overt muscle disease.[4,119] Therefore, increases in the plasma CK activity can result from muscle cell injury or exertion. Increased plasma CK activity is frequently observed in reptiles that are struggling to resist restraint during blood collection or that are exhibiting seizure activity. Increased plasma CK activity resulting from muscle cell damage occurs with traumatic injury, intramuscular injections of irritating drugs or fluids, and systemic infections that affect skeletal or cardiac muscle. Brain tissue generally has high CK activity; however, whether brain lesions contribute significantly to plasma CK is not known.

Muscle injury also results in mild to moderate increases in plasma AST and LDH activities. These enzymes are not organ specific for muscle, however, and their activities could increase with hepatobiliary disease. When plasma CK activity is not increased during increased AST and LDH activity, hepatobiliary disease should be suspected. Damage to both liver and skeletal muscle can occur simultaneously, such as occurs with trauma and septicemia, which would result in elevated plasma AST, LDH, and CK activities.

LABORATORY EVALUATION OF PROTEINS

The plasma total protein concentration of healthy reptiles generally ranges between 3 and 7 g/dL (30 to 70 g/L).[101] Female reptiles demonstrate marked increases in their plasma total protein concentration during active folliculogenesis. This estrogen-induced hyperproteinemia is associated with increased levels of the proteins (primarily globulins) necessary for yolk production.[26] The plasma total protein concentration returns to normal after ovulation. Captive reptiles may exhibit greater plasma total protein concentrations when compared with the same free-living species because of prolonged high-protein diets.[109]

The biuret method is the most accurate for determining the plasma or serum total protein concentration. The refractometer method, however, is commonly used to rapidly estimate the plasma protein concentration in reptilian blood. Although the refractometric method tends to overestimate the total protein value, it is useful for clinical decision making.

Absolute concentrations of the various plasma proteins are obtained by determining the total protein concentration with the use of the biuret method in conjunction with electrophoretic separation of the proteins. Plasma protein electrophoresis has only recently been applied to the diagnosis of disease in reptiles. Electrophoretic data may be useful in diagnosing chronic and acute inflammation, chronic infection, nutritional, neoplastic, or metabolic disease, and early healing of trauma.[120-123] Elevations in serum globulin levels with subsequent decreases in the albumin/globulin (A/G) ratio are generally used as indicators of inflammation and infection in animals, including reptiles.[71,124,125] Because albumin concentrations obtained from chemical analyzers have not been validated for reptiles, protein electrophoresis provides a more accurate assessment of the serum or plasma albumin and globulin concentrations in reptilian blood. Individuals with a normal serum or plasma total protein concentration may have an alteration in the A/G ratio. For example, protein electrophoresis in sea turtles (with normal reference ranges) showed significantly higher protein fractions, except for gamma globulins, in healthy individuals compared with ill turtles.[126] In addition, the A/G ratio of Green Sea turtles with papillomas has been shown to decrease because of a decreased albumin concentration and increased gamma globulins.[71]

Increases in alpha-1 globulins have been reported to occur with acute inflammatory disease in snakes.[40] A decrease in beta globulins (proteins associated with iron and fat transport as well as involvement in blood clotting and inflammatory reactions) may indicate exhaustion of plasminogen, complement protein, or other components of this fraction resulting from prolonged inflammation and malnutrition associated with anorexia in snakes.[40] It is important to remember that hemolysis can caused an artificial increase in the gamma and beta fractions on the protein electrophoretogram, mimicking a chronic inflammatory condition.[127] Protein electrophoresis has also been recommended for serially evaluating the response to treatment.[128] For further development of its use as a diagnostic tool for reptiles, reference ranges that include age groups and environmental variables for many species need to be established.[121] For example, a positive correlation among total protein, alpha globulin, beta globulin, and gamma globulin concentrations and water temperature has been demonstrated in Loggerhead Sea turtles and between only total protein and alpha globulin concentrations and water temperature in Green Sea turtles.[126]

Hyperproteinemia is indicated by total protein values greater than 7 g/dL (70g/L) in most reptiles. Common causes of hyperproteinemia include dehydration or hyperglobulinemia associated with chronic inflammatory diseases. Hyperglobulinemia is a common feature of tortoises with chronic hepatic disease.[11] The alpha, beta, and gamma globulins may increase with infectious diseases; however, because normal values have not been established for many species of reptiles, the usefulness of this testing requires validation. A significant increase in total protein as measured by chemical analyzers can occur with hemolysis.[113]

Hypoproteinemia is indicated by a total protein value of less than 3 g/dL (30 g/L). A significantly low total protein concentration is commonly seen in reptiles with chronic malnutrition and gastrointestinal parasitism.[7] Other causes, however, such as malabsorption, maldigestion, protein-losing enteropathy, severe blood loss, and chronic hepatic or renal disease, should also be considered.

LABORATORY EVALUATION OF GLUCOSE METABOLISM

In general, the normal blood glucose concentration of most reptiles ranges between 60 and 100 mg/dL (3.33 to 5.55 mmol/L), but this is subject to marked physiologic variation.[101,129] The blood glucose concentration of healthy reptiles varies with species, nutritional status, and environmental conditions.[7] Glucose values are also affected by sample handling. For example, glucose concentration decreases significantly over time in heparinized blood samples; therefore immediate separation of blood cells from the plasma is important.[16] Reptiles have pancreatic beta and alpha cell types as a source of insulin and glucagon, respectively.[130] This suggests that their glucose metabolism is similar to that of mammals and other vertebrates. The actions of these hormones are affected by temperature as indicated by the variations in the normal oral glucose tolerance curves among species and with temperature. For example, an increase in temperature produces hypoglycemia in turtles but hyperglycemia in alligators.[129] In aquatic reptiles, hypoxia associated with diving results in a physiologic hyperglycemia because of anaerobic glycolysis. A significant gender difference in plasma glucose concentration has been observed in free-ranging tortoises in that males have higher concentrations than females.[93] The reason for this is not known.

Hypoglycemia in reptiles is commonly caused by starvation and malnutrition, severe hepatobiliary disease, and septicemia. Pancreatic disease, such as an islet cell tumor, should also be considered as a cause for a persistent hypoglycemia.[131] Clinical signs associated with hypoglycemia in reptiles include tremors, loss of righting reflex, torpor, and dilated, nonresponsive pupils.

In mammals, prolonged exposure of the serum or plasma to erythrocytes results in a glucose concentration that decreases at a rate of approximately 10% per hour. Limited studies have shown that this does not occur in reptiles. A significant decrease in plasma glucose concentration may not occur until erythrocytes have been in contact with the plasma for 96 hours.[82] This is likely a result of slower reptilian erythrocyte metabolism compared with that of mammals.

Hyperglycemia in reptiles often results from the iatrogenic delivery of excessive glucose. Hyperglycemia likely occurs with glucocorticosteroid excess.[132,133] Indications of this comes from studies in which a consistent rise in adrenal catecholamines, glucocorticoids, and glucose had been observed in a variety of free-ranging reptilian species subjected to periods of prolonged captivity.[4,134-138] Persistent, marked hyperglycemia and glucosuria are suggestive of diabetes mellitus, which is a rarely confirmed disorder of reptiles. Hyperglycemia has also been reported with pancreatitis in reptiles.[61,139]

LABORATORY EVALUATION OF ELECTROLYTES AND ACID–BASE

Water Balance

Species, diet, and environmental conditions such as temperature and humidity influence the water consumption of reptiles. Desert species require less water than temperate and tropical species. Some reptiles have developed methods for conserving water.[140] For example, tortoises and some lizards store water in the urinary bladder. Many reptiles can achieve water uptake through the cloaca by soaking.[87] Water also is conserved in reptiles by the elimination of nitrogenous waste in the form of uric acid and urate salts, which are excreted in a semisolid state.

Sodium and Chloride

Dietary sodium is absorbed in the intestines and transported to the kidneys, where it then is excreted or resorbed, depending on the reptile's need for sodium. Reptilian sodium and potassium metabolism involves an active renin–angiotensin system with direct action on osmoregulation.[141] Some reptiles have nasal salt glands that participate in the regulation of sodium, potassium, and chloride concentrations in the blood. Therefore disorders of the salt gland may affect the electrolyte balance.

The normal serum or plasma sodium concentration ranges between 120 and 170 mEq/L. The normal plasma sodium concentrations of tortoises and freshwater turtles range between 120 and 150 mEq/L (mmol/L).[101] Sea turtles tend to have higher normal sodium plasma concentrations, which range between 150 and 170 mEq/L (mmol/L). The normal plasma sodium concentrations of lizards range between 140 and 170 mEq/L (mmol/L), and those of snakes, such as boas and pythons, range between 130 and 160 mEq/L (mmol/L).[101]

Hyponatremia can result from excessive loss of sodium associated with disorders of the gastrointestinal tract (i.e., diarrhea), kidneys, or possibly, the salt gland. Iatrogenic hyponatremia can occur with overhydration when intravenous or intracoelomic fluids that are low in sodium are administered. Artifactual hyponatremia can occur with stored heparinized whole blood.[104]

Hypernatremia results from dehydration, either from excessive water loss or inadequate water intake, or from excessive dietary salt intake.

Chloride is the principle anion in the blood and, along with sodium, represents the primary osmotically active component of plasma in most reptiles. The normal serum or plasma chloride concentration of reptiles varies among species but generally ranges between 100 and 130 mEq/L (mmol/L).[142] Plasma chloride concentrations of turtles tend to range between 100 and 110 mEq/L (mmol/L), whereas those of most lizards and snakes range between 100 and 130 mEq/L (mmol/L).[101] The blood chloride concentration provides the least clinically useful information regarding the electrolytes.

Hypochloremia in reptiles is rare and, when present, is suggestive of the excessive loss of chloride ions or of overhydration with fluids that are low in chloride ions.

Hyperchloremia is associated with dehydration and, possibly, renal tubular disease or disorders of the salt glands.

Potassium

Normal serum or plasma potassium concentrations vary among reptilian species, but they generally range between 2 and 6 mEq/L (mmol/L). The normal plasma potassium concentration of most turtles, lizards, and snakes ranges between 2 and 6, 3 and 5, and 3 and 6 mEq/L (mmol/L), respectively.[101] The potassium concentration increased significantly over time in heparinized blood samples, indicating a need to quickly separate the cells from the plasma after blood collection.[16,104]

Plasma potassium concentration is highly dependent on dietary intake. For example, foraging turtles had higher potassium values than nesting and debilitated turtles because of decreased food intake and possible diarrhea in the latter group.[7]

Hypokalemia can result from inadequate dietary potassium intake or excessive gastrointestinal potassium loss. Hypokalemia can also be associated with severe alkalosis.

Hyperkalemia can be the result of decreased renal secretion of potassium. Hyperkalemia can also result from excessive dietary potassium intake or severe acidosis. The amount of potassium in erythrocytes also differs among reptiles; therefore the potential for artifactual hyperkalemia due to hemolysis varies with species.[113]

Electrolyte evaluation of reptiles provides useful clinical and prognostic information. In one study involving stranded sea turtles, the turtles that died had significantly greater plasma concentrations of sodium, chloride, potassium, calcium, phosphorus, and uric acid than did turtles that survived; during convalescence, the survivors had significantly lower glucose, sodium, and uric acid concentrations than the initial values.[143]

Acid–Base

The normal blood pH of turtles and most other reptiles ranges between 7.5 and 7.7 at 23°C to 25°C.[87,142] The normal blood pH of some snakes and lizards may fall below 7.4. The blood pH of reptiles is labile, however, and it changes with fluctuations in temperature. An increase in temperature or excitement may cause the blood pH to decrease.[144] The blood pH may increase to 7.7 to 7.8 during anesthesia. As in mammals, the oxygen dissociation curve for reptilian hemoglobin shifts to the left as the pH increases, thereby producing an increased affinity of hemoglobin for oxygen but a decreased release to tissues.

The buffering systems that regulate blood pH in mammals are most likely the same in reptiles; the bicarbonate–carbonic acid buffer system is the most important because of the rapid rate of CO_2 elimination via the lungs after conversion from H_2CO_3. Total plasma CO_2 or bicarbonate concentrations are rarely reported in reptiles; however, normal total CO_2 values for most reptiles are expected to range between 20 and 30 mmol/L.[101] High plasma CO_2 value are often a reflection of decreased respiratory ventilation in debilitated reptiles.[7]

A marked fasting physiologic metabolic alkalosis occurs in postprandial alligators because of an anion shift; bicarbonate replaces chloride in the blood as chloride is lost (as HCl) via gastric secretions.[129] Therefore a postprandial decrease of chloride and an increase of bicarbonate concentrations are seen in alligators and perhaps other reptiles.

Studies have shown that cold-stunned sea turtles are initially affected by metabolic and respiratory acidosis. When pH values returned to normal in these turtles, the ionized calcium concentrations were lower than convalescent concentrations; in addition, initial pH-corrected ionized magnesium concentrations were higher than convalescent concentrations.[143]

REFERENCES

1. Zaias J, Norton T, Fickel A, et al. Biochemical and hematologic values for 18 clinically healthy radiated tortoises *(Geochelone radiata)* on St Catherines Island, Georgia. *Vet Clin Pathol* 2006;35:321-325.
2. Campbell TW. Clinical pathology of reptiles. In: Mader DR, ed. *Reptile medicine and surgery.* 2nd ed. St. Louis: Saunders Elsevier, 2006;453-470.
3. Schrader GM, Allender MC, Odoi A. Diagnosis, treatment, and outcome of Eastern box turtles *(Terrapene carolina carolina)* presented to a wildlife clinic in Tennessee, USA, 1995–2007. *J Wildl Dis* 2010;46:1079-1085.
4. Scheelings TF, Jessop TS. Influence of capture method, habitat quality and individual traits on blood parameters of free-ranging lace monitors *(Varanus varius). Aust Vet J* 2011;89:360-365.
5. Salakij C, Salakij J, Apibal S, et al. Hematology, morphology, cytochemical staining, and ultrastructural characteristics of blood cells in king cobras *(Ophiophagus hannah). Vet Clin Pathol* 2002;31:116-126.
6. Padilla SE, Weber M, Jacobson ER. Hematologic and plasma biochemical reference intervals for Morelet's crocodiles *(Crocodylus moreletii)* in the northern wetlands of Campeche, Mexico. *J Wildl Dis* 2011;47:511-522.
7. Deem SL, Norton TM, Mitchell M, et al. Comparison of blood values in foraging, nesting, and stranded Loggerhead turtles *(Caretta caretta)* along the coast of Georgia, USA. *J Wildl Dis* 2009;45:41-56.
8. Chung CS, Cheng CH, Chin SC, et al. Morphologic and cytochemical characteristics of Asian yellow pond turtle *(Ocadia sinensis)* blood cells and their hematologic and plasma biochemical reference values. *J Zoo Wildl Med* 2009;40:76-85.
9. Turton JA, Ladds PW, Manolis SC, et al. Relationship of blood corticosterone, immunoglobulin, and haematological values in young crocodiles *(Crocodylus porosus)* to water temperature, clutch of origin and body weight. *Aust Vet J* 1997;l75:114-119.
10. López-Olvera JR, Montané J, Marco I, et al. Effect of venipuncture site on hematologic and serum biochemical parameters in Marginated tortoise *(Testudo marginata). J Wildl Dis* 2003;39:830-836.
11. Christopher MM, Berry KH, Henen BT, et al. Clinical disease and laboratory abnormalities in free-ranging Desert tortoises in California (1990–1995). *J Wildl Dis* 2003;39:35-56.
12. Perinan D, Hernandez-Diver SM, Hernandez-Diver SJ. Comparison of three different techniques to produce blood smears from green iguanas, *Iguana iguana. J Herpetol Med Surg* 2006;16:99-101.
13. Muro J, Cuenca R, Pastor J, et al. Effects of lithium heparin and tripotassium EDTA on hematologic values of Hermann's tortoises *(Testudo hermanni). J Zoo Wildl Med* 1998;29:40-44.
14. Martinez-Jimenez D, Hernandez-Divers SJ, Floyd TM, et al. Comparison of the effects of dipotassium ethylenediaminetetraacetic acid and lithium heparin on hematologic values in Yellow-blotched map turtles, *Graptemys flavimaculata. J Herpetol Med Surg* 2007;17:36-41.

15. Hanley CS, Hernandez-Divers SJ, Bush S, et al. Comparison of the effect of dipotassium ethylenediaminetetraacetic acid and lithium heparin on hematologic values in the green iguana *(Iguana iguana)*. *J Zoo Wildl Med* 2004;35:328-332.
16. Harr KE, Raskin RE, Heard DJ. Temporal effects of 3 commonly used anticoagulants on hematologic and biochemical variables in blood samples from macaws and Burmese pythons. *Vet Clin Pathol* 2005;34:383-388.
17. Saint Girons MC. Morphology of the circulating blood cell. In: Gans C, Parsons TC, eds. *Biology of the reptilia*. Vol 3. New York: Academic Press, 1970.
18. Sypik J, Borysenko M. Reptiles. In: Rowley AF, Ratcliffe NA, eds. *Vertebrate blood cells*. Cambridge, England: Cambridge University Press, 1988.
19. Duguy R. Numbers of blood cells and their variations. In: Gans C, Parsons TC, eds. *Biology of the reptilia*. Vol 3. New York: Academic Press, 1970.
20. Frye FL. Hematology as applied to clinical reptile medicine. In: Frye FL, ed. *Biomedical and surgical aspects of captive reptile husbandry*. 2nd ed. Vol 1. Malabar, Fla: Krieger Publishing Co, 1991.
21. Mussachia XJ, Sievers ML. Effects of induced cold torpor on blood of *Chrysemys picta*. *Am J Physiol* 1956;187:99-102.
22. Wojtaszek JS. Haematology of the grass snake *Natrix natrix natrix L*. *Comp Biochem Physiol A Comp Physiol* 1991;100:805-812.
23. Harr KE, Alleman AR, Dennis PM, et al. Morphologic and cytochemical characteristics of blood cells and hematologic and plasma biochemical reference ranges in Green Iguanas. *J Am Vet Med Assoc* 2001;218:915-921.
24. Ruiz G, Rosenmann M, Nunez H. Blood values in South American lizards from high and low altitudes. *Comp Biochem Physiol* 1993;106A:713-718.
25. Pough FH. Blood oxygen transport and delivery in reptiles. *Am Zool* 1980;20:173-185.
26. Dessauer HC. Blood chemistry of reptiles: physiological and evolutionary aspects. In: Gans C, Parsons TS, eds. *Biology of the reptilia*. Vol 3. New York: Academic Press, 1970.
27. Frische S, Bruno S, Fago A, et al. Oxygen binding by single red blood cells from the red-eared turtle *Trachemys scripta*. *J Appl Physiol* 2001;90:1679-1684.
28. Altland PD, Parker M. Effects of hypoxia upon the box turtle. *Am J Physiol* 1955;180:421-427.
29. Sheeler P, Barber AA. Reticulocytosis and iron incorporation in the rabbit and turtle: a comparative study. *Comp Biochem Physiol* 1965;16:63-76.
30. Alleman AR, Jacobson ER, Raskin RE. Morphologic and cytochemical characteristics of blood cells from the desert tortoise *(Gopherus agassizii)*. *Am J Vet Res* 1992;53:1645-1651.
31. Marks SK, Citino SB. Hematology and serum chemistry of the Radiated tortoise *(Testudo radiata)*. *J Zoo Wildl Med* 1990;21:342-344.
32. Wallach JD, Boever WJ. *Diseases of exotic animals, medical and surgical management*. Philadelphia: WB Saunders Co, 1983.
33. Keller JM, Kucklick JR, Stamper MA, et al. Associations between organochlorine contaminant concentrations and clinical health parameters in Loggerhead sea turtles from North Carolina, USA. *Environ Health Perspect* 2004;112:1074-1079.
34. Schilliger L, Selleri P, Frye FL. Lymphoblastic lymphoma and leukemic blood profile in a red-tail boa *(Boa constrictor constrictor)* with concurrent inclusion body disease. *J Vet Diagn Invest* 2011;23:159-162.
35. Altland PD, Thompson EC. Some factors affecting blood formation in turtles. *Proc Soc Exp Biol Med* 1958;99:456-459.
36. Hawkey CM, Dennett TB. Normal and abnormal red cells, granulocytes, lymphocytes, monocytes, and azurophils. In: Hawkey CM, Dennett TB, eds. *Color atlas of comparative veterinary hematology*. Ames, Iowa: Iowa State University Press, 1989.
37. Verma GK, Banerjee V. Intergeneric haematological studies in three selected reptiles: erythrocytes. *Indian J Anim Res* 1982;16:49-53.
38. Desser SS. Morphological, cytochemical, and biochemical observations on the blood of the tuatara, *Sphenodon punctatus*. *N Z J Zool* 1978;5:503-508.
39. Desser SS. Haematological observations on a hibernating tuatara, *Sphenodon punctatus*. *N Z J Zool* 1979;6:77-78.
40. Lentini AM, Crawshaw GJ, Licht LE, et al. Pathologic and hematologic responses to surgically implanted transmitters in Eastern Massasauga rattlesnakes *(Sistrurus catenatus catenatus)*. *J Wildl Dis* 2011;47:107-125.
41. Raskin RE, Valenciano A. Cytochemistry of normal leukocytes. In: Feldman BF, Zinkl JG, Jain NC, eds. *Schalm's veterinary hematology*. Philadelphia: Lippincot Williams and Wilkins, 2000;337-346.
42. Martínez-Silvestre A, Marco I, Rodriguez-Dominguez MA, et al. Morphology, cytochemical staining, and ultrastructural characteristics of the blood cells of the giant lizard of El Hierro *(Gallotia simonyi)*. *Res Vet Sci* 2005;78:127-134.
43. Andreasen CB, Latimer KS. Cytochemical staining characteristics of chicken heterophils and eosinophils. *Vet Clin Pathol* 1990;19:51-54.
44. Perpinán D, Sánchez C. Morphologic and cytochemical characteristics of blood cells from European pond turtle *(Emys orbicularis)* and the Mediterranean pond turtle *(Mauremys leprosa)*. *J Herpetol Med Surg* 2009;19:119-127.
45. Alleman AR, Jacobson ER, Raskin RE. Morphological, cytochemical staining, and ultrastructural characteristics of blood cells from eastern diamondback rattlesnakes *(Crotalus adamaneus)*. *Am J Vet Res* 1999;60:507-514.
46. Work TM, Raskin RE, Balazs GH, et al. Morphological and cytochemical characteristics of blood cells from Hawaiian green turtles. *Am J Vet Res* 1998;59:1252-1257.
47. Dotson TK, Ramsay EC, Bounous DI. A color atlas of the blood cells of the yellow rat snake. *Comp Contin Edu Pract Vet* 1995;17:1013-1016.
48. Montali RK. Comparative pathology of inflammation in higher vertebrates (reptiles, birds, and mammals). *J Comp Path* 1988;99:1-26.
49. Mateo MR, Roberts ED, Enright FM. Morphological, cytochemical, and functional studies of peripheral blood cells in young healthy American alligators *(Alligator mississippiensis)*. *Am J Vet Res* 1984;45:1046-1053.
50. Caxton-Martins AE, Nganwuchu AM. A cytochemical study of the blood of the rainbow lizard *(Agama agama)*. *J Anat* 1978;125: 477-480.
51. Taylor K, Kaplan HM. Light microscopy of the blood cells of *Pseudemys* turtles. *Herpetologica* 1961;17:186-192.
52. Garner MM, Homer BL, Jacobson ER, et al. Staining and morphologic features of bone marrow hematopoietic cells in desert tortoise *(Gopherus agassizii)*. *Am J Vet Res* 1996;57:1608-1615.
53. Cannon MS. The morphology and cytochemistry of the blood leukocytes of Kemp's ridley sea turtles *(Lepidochelys kempii)*. *Can J Zool* 1992;70:1336-1340.
54. Bounous DI, Dotson TK, Brooks RL, et al. Cytochemical staining and ultrastructural characteristics of peripheral blood leukocytes from the yellow rat snake *(Elaphe obsoleta quadrivittata)*. *Comp Haematol Int* 1996;6:86-91.
55. Anderson JL, Wack RF, Hatcher R. Hematology and clinical chemistry reference ranges for clinically normal captive New Guinea snapping turtles *(Elseya novaeguineae)* and the effects of temperature, sex, and sample type. *J Zoo Wildl Med* 1997;28:394-402.
56. Wood FE, Ebanks GK. Blood cytology and hematology of the green sea turtle, *Chelonia mydas*. *Herpetologica* 1984;40:331-336.
57. Jacobson ER, Gaskin JM, Brown MB, et al. Chronic upper respiratory tract disease of free-ranging desert tortoises, *Xerobates agassizii*. *J Wildl Dis* 1990;27:296-316.
58. Wright KM, Skeba S. Hematology and plasma chemistries of captive prehensile-tailed skinks *(Corucia zebrata)*. *J Zoo Wildl Med* 1992;23:429-432.
59. Mead KF, Borysenko M. Surface immunoglobulins on granular and agranular leukocytes in the thymus and spleen of the snapping turtle, *Chelydra serpentina*. *Dev Comp Immunol* 1984;8:109-120.

60. Christopher MM. Physical and biochemical abnormalities associated with prolonged entrapment in a desert tortoise. *J Wildl Dis* 1999;35:361-366.
61. Hidalgo-Vila J, Martínez-Silvestre A, Ribas A, et al. Pancreatitis associated with the helminth *Serpinema microcephalus* (Nematoda: Camallanidae) in exotic Red-Eared slider turtles (*Trachemys scripta elegans*). *J Wildl Dis* 2011;47:201-205.
62. Mead KF, Borysenko M, Findlay SR. Naturally abundant basophils in the snapping turtle, *Chelydra serpentina,* possess cytophilic surface antibodies with reaginic function. *J Immunol* 1983;130:384-390.
63. Sypek JP, Borysenko M, Findlay SR. Anti-immunoglobulin induced histamine release from naturally abundant basophils in the snapping turtle, *Chelydra serpentina. Dev Comp Immunol* 1984;8:358-366.
64. Wright RK, Cooper EL. Temperature effects on ectothermic immune responses. *Dev Comp Immunol* 1981;5(Suppl 1):117-122.
65. Hussein MF, Badir N, El Ridi R, et al. Effect of seasonal variation on the immune system of the lizard, *Scinus scinus. J Exp Zool* 1979;209:91-96.
66. Hussein MF, Badir N, El Ridi R, et al. Lymphoid tissue of the snake, *Spalerosophis diadema,* in the different seasons. *Dev Comp Immunol* 1979;3:77-88.
67. Hussein MF, Badir N, El Ridi R, et al. Differential effect of seasonal variation on lymphoid tissue of the lizard, *Chalcides ocellatus. Dev Comp Immunol* 1978;2:297-310.
68. Mansour MH, el Ridi R, Badir N. Surface markers of lymphocytes in the snake, *Spalerosophis diadema.* L. Investigation of lymphocyte surface markers. *Immunology* 1980;40:605-611.
69. Munoz FJ, Galvan A, Lerma M, et al. Seasonal changes in peripheral blood leukocyte functions of the turtle *Mauremys caspica* and their relationship with corticosterone, 17-beta-estradiol and testosterone serum levels. *J Vet Immuol Immunopathol* 2000;77:27-42.
70. Saad AH, el Ridi R, el Deeb S, et al. Effect of hydrocortisone on immune system of the lizard, *Chalcides ocellatus.* III. Effect on cellular and humoral immune responses. *J Dev Comp Immunol* 2000;10:235-245.
71. Cray C, Varella R, Bossart GD, et al. Altered in vitro immune responses in green turtles (*Chelonia mydas*) with fibropapillomatosis. *J Zoo Wildl Med.* 2001;32:436-440.
72. Orós J, Torrent A, de los Monteros AE, et al. Multicentric lymphoblastic lymphoma in a Loggerhead sea turtle (*Caretta caretta*). *Vet Pathol* 2001;38:464.
73. Otis VS. Hemocytological and serum chemistry parameters of the African puff adder, *Bitis arietans. Herpetologica* 1973;29:110-116.
74. Goldberg SR, Holshuh HJ. A case of leukemia in the desert spiny lizard (*Sceloporus magister*). *J Wildl Dis* 1991;27:521-525.
75. Langenberg JA, Teare JA, Carolan RJ, et al. Hematopoietic and lymphoreticular tumors in zoo animals. *Lab Invest* 1983;48:48A.
76. Frey FL, Carney J. Acute lymphocytic leukemia in a boa constrictor. *J Am Vet Med Assoc* 1973;163:653-654.
77. Frey FL, Carney J. Myeloproliferative disease in a turtle. *J Am Vet Med Assoc* 1972;161:595-599.
78. Schultze AE, Mason GL, Clyde VL. Lymphosarcoma with leukemic blood profile in a Savannah monitor lizard (*Varanus exanthematicus*). *J Zoo Wildl Med* 1999;30:158-164.
79. Rishniw M, Paul D, Maher T. The quality of veterinary in-clinic and reference laboratory biochemical testing. *Vet Clin Pathol* 2012;41:92-102.
80. Wolf KN, Harms CA, Beasley JF. Evaluation of five clinical chemistry analyzers for use in health assessment in sea turtles. *J Am Vet Med Assoc* 2008;233:470-475.
81. McCain SL, Flatland B, Schumacher JP, et al. Comparison of chemistry analytes between two portable, commercially available analyzers and a conventional laboratory analyzer in reptiles. *Vet Clin Pathol* 2010;39:474-479.
82. Eisenhawer E, Courtney CH, Raskin RE, et al. Relationship between separation time of plasma from heparinized whole blood on plasma biochemical analytes of loggerhead sea turtles (*Caretta caretta*). *J Wildl Dis* 2008;39:208-215.
83. Austin CC, Jessing KW. Green-blood pigmentation in lizards. *Comp Biochem Physiol* 1994;109A:619-626.
84. Lawrence K. Seasonal variation in blood biochemistry of long term captive Mediterranean tortoises (*Testudo graeca* and *T. hermanni*). *Res Vet Sci* 1987;42:379.
85. Samour JH, Hawkey CM, Pugley S, et al: Clinical and pathologic findings related to malnutrition and husbandry in captive giant tortoises (*Geochelone* spp.). *Vet Rec* 1986;118:299.
86. Rosskopf WJ. Normal hemogram and blood chemistry values for California desert tortoises. *Vet Med Sm Anim Clin* 1982;77:85.
87. Davies PMC. Anatomy and physiology. In: Cooper JE, Jackson OF, eds. *Diseases of the reptilia.* San Diego: Academic Press, 1981;9.
88. Dantzler WH. Comparative aspects of renal urate transport. *Kidney Int* 1996;49:1549-1551.
89. Chiodini RJ, Sunberg JP. Blood chemical values of the common boa constrictor. *Am J Vet Res* 1982;43:1701.
90. Taylor RW Jr, Jacobson ER. Hematology and serum chemistry of the gopher tortoise, *Gopherus polyphemus. Comp Biochem Physiol* 1982;72A:425.
91. Dawson WR. Physiological responses to temperature in the lizard *Eumeces obsoletus. Physiol Zool* 1960;33:87.
92. Mader DR, Hawath CC, Paul-Murphy J. The packed cell volume and serum chemistry of the gopher snake (*Pituophis melanoleucus catenifer*). *J Zoo Anim Med* 1985;16:139.
93. Dickenson VM, Jarchow JJ, Trueblood MH. Hematology and plasma biochemistry reference range values for free-ranging desert tortoises in Arizona. *J Wildl Dis* 2002;38:143-153.
94. Holz P, Holz RM. Evaluation of ketamine, ketamine/xylazine, and ketamine/medazolam anesthesia in red-eared sliders (*Trachemys scripta elegans*). *J Zoo Wildl Med* 1994;25:531-537.
95. Casimire-Etzioni AL, Wellehan JFX, Embury JE, et al. Synovial fluid from an African spur-thighed tortoise (*Geochelone sulcata*). *Vet Clin Pathol* 2004;33:43-46.
96. Ramsay EC, Dotson TK. Tissue and serum enzyme activities in the yellow rat snake (*Elaphe obsoleta quadrivittata*). *Am J Vet Res* 1995;56:423-428.
97. Boyd JW. Serum enzymes in the diagnosis of diseases in man and animals. *J Comp Pathol* 1988;98:381-404.
98. Hernandez-Divers SJ, Innis CJ. Renal disease in reptiles: diagnosis and clinical management. In: Mader DR, ed. *Reptile medicine and surgery.* 2nd ed. St. Louis: Saunders Elsevier, 2006;878-892.
99. Hernandez-Divers SJ, Stahl SJ, Stedman NL, et al. Renal evaluation in the healthy green iguana (*Iguana iguana*): assessment of plasma biochemistry, glomerular filtration rate, and endoscopic biopsy. *J Zoo Wildl Med* 2005;36:155-168.
100. Dubewar D. Effect of hypocalcemic and hypercalcemic substances on the parathyroid histology of the lizard, *Uromastyx hardwickii* (Gray). *Z Mikrosk Anat Forsch* 1979;93:315-320.
101. Stein G. Hematologic and blood chemistry values in reptiles. In: Mader DR, ed. *Reptile medicine and surgery.* Philadelphia: WB Saunders Co, 1996.
102. Harris HS, Benson SR, Gilardi KV, et al. Comparative health assessment of Western Pacific Leatherback turtles (*Dermochelys coriacea*) foraging off the coast of California, 2005–2007. *J Wildl Dis* 2011;47:321-337.
103. Dennis PM, Bennett RA, Harr KE, et al. Plasma concentration of ionized calcium in healthy iguanas. *J Am Vet Med Assoc* 2001;219: 326-328.
104. Eatwell K. Effects of storage and sample type on ionized calcium, sodium, and potassium in captive tortoises, *Testudo* spp. *J Herpetol Med Surg* 2007;17:84-91.
105. Frye FL, Centofanti BV. Successful treatment of iatrogenic (diet-related) hypervitaminosis D and hypercalcemia in an iguana (*Iguana iguana*), in *Proceedings.* 4th Int Colloq Pathol Therapeut Reptiles Amphibians, Bad Nauheim, Germany, 1991;244-250.
106. Mader DR. Metabolic bone diseases. In: Mader DR, ed. *Reptile medicine and surgery.* 2nd ed. St. Louis: Saunders Elsevier, 2006;841-851.

107. Marcus LC. *Veterinary biology and medicine of captive amphibians and reptiles*. Philadelphia: Lea & Febiger, 1981;1-5.
108. Boyer TH. Metabolic bone disease. In: Mader DR, ed. *Reptile medicine and surgery*. Philadelphia: WB Saunders Co, 1996.
109. Donoghue S, Langenberg J. Nutrition. In: Mader DR, ed. *Reptile medicine and surgery*. Philadelphia: WB Saunders Co, 1996.
110. Eatwell K. Hypocalcemia in a Tunisian tortoise. *J Herpetol Med Surg* 2008;18:117-122.
111. Bradford CM, Denver MC, Bronson E, et al. Hypercalcemia in prehensile-tailed skins *(Corucia zebrata)*. *J Herpetol Med Surg* 2009;19:57-59.
112. Drew ML. Hypercalcemia and hyperphosphatemia in indigo snakes *(Drymarchon corais)* and serum biochemical reference values. *J Zoo Wildl Med* 1994;25:48-52.
113. Benson KG, Paul-Murphy J, MacWilliams P. Effects of hemolysis on plasma electrolyte and chemistry values in the common green iguana *(Iguana iguana)*. *J Zoo Wildl Med* 1999;30:413-415.
114. Honeyfield DC, Ross JP, Carbonneau DA, et al. Pathology, physiologic parameters, tissue contaminants, and tissue thiamine in morbid and healthy central Florida adult American alligators *(Alligator mississippiensis)*. *J Wildl Dis* 2008;44:280-294.
115. Bissell DM. Heme catabolism and bilirubin formation. In: Ostrow JD, ed. *Bile pigments and jaundice: molecular, metabolic, and medical aspects*. New York: Marcel Dekker, 1986;133-156.
116. Divers S. Reptilian renal and reproductive disease diagnosis. In: Fudge A, ed. *Laboratory medicine—avian and exotic pets*. Philadelphia: WB Saunders, 2000;217-222.
117. McBride M, Hernandez-Divers SM, Koch T, et al. Preliminary evaluation of pre- and post-prandial 3α-hydroxy bile acids in the green iguana, *Iguana iguana*. *J Herpetol Med Surg* 2006;16:129-134.
118. Asadi F, Rostami A, Pourkabir M, et al. Serum lipid and lipoprotein profile of Asian tortoise *(Agrionemys horsfieldii)* in prehibernation state. *Comp Clin Pathol* 2007;16:193-195.
119. Wagner RA, Wetzel R. Tissue and plasma enzyme activities in juvenile green iguanas. *Am J Vet Res* 1999;60:201-203.
120. Tatum LM, Zaias J, Mealey BK, et al. Protein electrophoresis as a diagnostic and prognostic tool in raptor medicine. *J Zoo Wildl Med* 2000;31:497-502.
121. Zaias J, Cray C. Protein electrophoresis: a tool for the reptilian and amphibian practitioner. *J Herpetol Med Surg* 2002;12:30-32.
122. Gicking JC, Foley AM, Harr KE, et al. Plasma protein electrophoresis of the Atlantic loggerhead sea turtle, *Caretta caretta*. *J Herpetol Med Surg* 2004;14:13-18.
123. Machado CC, Silva LFN, Ramos PRR, et al. Seasonal influence on hematologic values and hemoglobin electrophoresis in Brazilian Boa, *Constrictor amarali*. *J Zoo Wildl Med* 2006;37:487-491.
124. Gumussoy KS, Uyanik F, Ataseve A, et al. Experimental *Aspergillus fumigatus* infection in quails and results of treatment with itraconazole. *J Vet Med Series B* 2004;51:34-38.
125. Harr K, Harvey J, Bonde R, et al. Comparison of methods used to diagnose generalized inflammatory disease in manatees *(Trichechus manatus latirostris)*. *J Zoo Wildl Med* 2006;37:151-159.
126. Osborne AG, Jacobson ER, Bresette MJ, et al. Reference intervals and relationships between health status, carapace length, body mass, and water temperature and concentrations of plasma total protein and protein electrophoretogram fractions in Atlantic loggerhead sea turtles and green turtles. *J Am Vet Med Assoc* 2010;237:561-567.
127. Roman Y, Bomsel-Demontoy M-C, Levrier J, et al. Effect of hemolysis on plasma protein levels and plasma electrophoresis in birds. *J Wildl Dis* 2009;45:73-80.
128. Hosseinzadeh Colagar A, Jafari N. Red blood cell morphology and plasma proteins electrophoresis of the European pond terrapin, *Emys orbicularis*. *Afr J Biotechnol* 2007;6:1578-1581.
129. Coulson RA, Hernandez T. *Biochemistry of the alligator*. Baton Rouge, La: Louisiana State University Press, 1964.
130. Kumar S, Khanna SS. Response of the blood glucose and the pancreatic islets of the lizard, *Uromastyx hardwickii* (Gray) to exogenous insulin. *Z Mikrosk Anat Forsch* 1977;91:131-143.
131. Naples LM, Langan JN, Mylniczenko ND, et al. Islet cell tumor in a Savannah monitor *(Varanus exanthematicus)*. *J Herpetol Med Surg* 2009;19:97-105.
132. Cuadrado M, Diaz-Paniagua C, Quevedo MA, et al. Hematology and clinical chemistry in dystocic and healthy post-reproductive female chameleons. *J Wildl Dis* 2002;38:395-401.
133. Swimmer JY. Biochemical responses to fibropapilloma and captivity in the green turtle. *J Wildl Dis* 2000;36:102-110.
134. Moore IT, Jessop TS. Stress, reproduction, and adrenocortical modulation in amphibians and reptiles. *Horm Behav* 2003;43:39-47.
135. Gregory LF, Schmid JR. Stress responses and sexing of wild Kemp's Ridley sea turtles *(Lepidochelys kempii)* in the northeastern Gulf of Mexico. *Gen Comp Endocrinol* 2001;124:66-74.
136. Jessop TS, Sumner JM, Limpus CJ, et al. Interplay between plasma hormone profiles, sex and body condition in immature hawksbill turtles *(Eretmochelys imbricata)* subjected to a capture stress protocol. *Comp Biochem Physiol A* 2004;137:197-204.
137. Jessop TS, Tucker AD, Limpus CJ, et al. Interactions between ecology, demography, capture stress, and profiles of corticosterone and glucose in a free-living population of Australian freshwater crocodiles. *Gen Comp Endocrinol* 2003;132:161-170.
138. Zachariah TT, Mitchell MA, Serra VF, et al. Acute corticosterone stress response to handling in four captive Gopher tortoises *(Gopherus polyphemus)*. *J Herpetol Med Surg* 2009;19:50-56.
139. Stahl JS. Diseases of the reptile pancreas. *Vet Clin North Am Exot Anim Pract* 2003;6:191-212.
140. Braysher ML. The excretion of hyperosmotic urine and other aspects of the electrolyte balance of the lizard *Amphibolurus maculosus*. *J Comp Biochem Physiol A* 1976;54:341-345.
141. Uva B, Vallarino M. Renin-angiotensin system and osmoregulation in the terrestrial chelonian *Testudo hermanni* Gmelin. *Comp Biochem Physiol A Comp Physiol* 1982;71:449-451.
142. Coulson RA, Henandez T. Reptiles as research models for comparative biochemistry and endocrinology. *J Am Vet Med Assoc* 1971;159:1672-1677.
143. Innis CJ, Ravich JB, Tlusty MF, et al. Hematologic and plasma biochemical findings in cold-stunned Kemp's ridley turtles: 176 cases (2001-2005). *J Am Vet Med Assoc* 2009;235:426-432.
144. Reeves RB. The interaction of body temperature and acid-base balance in ectothermic vertebrates. *Annu Rev Physiol* 1977;39:559-586.

CHAPTER 9

Computed Tomography and Magnetic Resonance Imaging

Jeanette Wyneken

The need for good anatomic information extends from the veterinary community to a diversity of basic research areas. Although detailed dissection of carcasses remains useful, suitable dissection material is not always available. While the dissection of fresh dead animals can provide a wealth of information, including identification of key landmarks, organ structure, and the overall arrangement of organ systems, the normal *in vivo* range of positions, shapes, and sizes of very dynamic organ systems and some vasculature cannot easily be seen in dead animals or even in "flat film" radiographs. Perhaps the most significant challenge that limits what can be learned from conventional radiography is the problem of superimposition of body parts. Within the past decade, the previously rare imaging methods of magnetic resonance imaging (MRI) and computed tomography (CT) have become much more accessible and somewhat more affordable. Recent advances in three-dimensional (3D) imaging and the availability of high-resolution diagnostic imaging tools[1-2] make visualizing reptilian anatomy and pathology not only possible but also accurate, even in the most unusual species. The 3D information that each can provide may improve diagnostics by allowing for evaluation of the extent of disease and accurate identification of adjacent organ systems.[3] Further, 3D imaging can guide treatment decisions and surgical solutions.[4] The following discussion provides descriptions of MRI and CT, suggested approaches to maximize the quality of the information obtained, and the basic background for understanding the images. Examples of each modality are provided to illustrate the characteristics of the more common imaging types while providing baseline reptile anatomy in several taxa. Some common problems associated with imaging are also discussed and illustrated.

As is common when new tools are embraced by a field, some early foundation studies using CT and MRI in reptile medicine differ greatly in resolution or scope of technique from what is currently available.[5-6] Others vary in anatomic accuracy.[7-9] Caution is merited with regard to some anatomic details of early CT and MRI studies, yet their methodologies often provide sound starting points. Hence, early studies made possible many of the improved techniques, high-resolution approaches, and modifications that are in contemporary use. Additionally, studies that verify image results with associated cadaveric anatomy[10] are particularly valuable when the structures are correctly identified.

BEFORE YOU START

Effective MRI or CT requires good communication with the technologist running the machines. Additionally, consultation with a radiologist or diagnostic imaging specialist should be considered essential when these modalities are used for disease diagnosis. First, find out if the technician is comfortable scanning a reptile. In most cases, it is a radiologic technologist, not the radiologist, who will run the machines. Not everyone is willing or able to work with reptile patients, particularly snakes. Thus, it is essential to ensure that the technologist is willing and able to focus on the study needed.

In terms of the study, there are a number of practical and necessary aspects to consider before starting. Discuss the following with the radiologic technologists who are trained in MRI and CT. They are likely to be your most effective resources because of their diverse experience with the equipment, as well as their training. Include the radiologist in the discussion if possible. Be sure to discuss the following:

- What is it that you need to see? Methods will differ for brain or spinal cord, air, bone, a mass (and if its consistency is important), blood flow, or fluid accumulation.
- What is the duration of the study? (Should you plan to sedate the animal or will it stay still long enough for the scan?)
- Does the animal have any metal in its body? (This may be a contraindication for MRI.)
- Will you need a contrast medium injected? (If so, be prepared to do so. The technologist is unlikely to know where the vessels are located.)
- Which plane(s) of view will be most informative? (Often, an axial series is best for high-resolution 3D reconstructions. However, a coronal (dorsoventral in a reptile) or sagittal series may also be essential to appreciate the extent of an injury or lesion.)
- What is the resolution of the images you need? (For example, small reptile patients or small structures require high-resolution scans; sequential images may be less than 1 mm apart. For larger patients, images in the series may be more than 5 mm from one another.)
- Do you need the whole animal scanned or just a part? (The time needed for the whole animal and the sizes of the data files are directly related to the volume scanned.)

- Will the scan expose the animal to excessive radiation? (For CT scans, size and resolution and machine type and age should be considered.)
- Do you need to do 3D reconstructions? If the data are to be used in a 3D reconstruction, the technologist will need to collect the data in ways that allow such reconstructions.

Addressing these questions before you start will enhance the quality of the results.

COMPUTED TOMOGRAPHY

CT, or computer-assisted radial tomography, provides 3D radiographs that use thousands of fast projections taken with a radiograph tube that spins around the subject.[1,11] The projections are organized as a series of two-dimensional (2D) images, similar to serial sections in a histologic study (or like slices of bread in a loaf). Computer software is used to reconstruct the 2D or 3D images of all or part of the animal. CT scans are particularly good for supplying details of structures that differ in density such as bones, eggs, scutes, or airways, and CT images eliminate superimposition of body parts. Recent advances in the machines and contrast media, as well as the software, make imaging of some soft tissues possible. Because the images are collected serially along the axis specified by the clinician, CT scans can provide flat section images that are dorsoventral, anteroposterior, or sagittal. The image data can also be assembled in 3D reconstructions[2] (Figure 9-1). CT image collection is fast (usually scan durations are measured in minutes or fractions of minutes). Resolution can be quite detailed. The necessary detail needs to be addressed so that the scan provides the resolution needed. CT data can be reviewed as serial sections (Figure 9-2) or reconstructed in a variety of ways to allow for the retention of 3D landmarks (see Figure 9-1). Virtual endoscopy is possible with the use of certain imaging modalities, with or without contrast solution (oral or intravenous) and the appropriate software.

Scan data are collected in series. The shorter the distance between scans, the greater the resolution (Figure 9-3). Sequential data series are assembled to form the 3D images. Consequently, any animal movement during the exposure period will produce a movement artifact in the images. When movement occurs during a scan, usually groups of sequential data are no longer in register with one another. For example, in Figure 9-4, *A*, the chameleon's tail shows a CT movement artifact; in Figure 9-4, *B* the turtle's anterior trunk shows a movement artifact due to breathing. If the area that moved is not part of the key study site, the scan may still be useful. However, for the most reliable scan quality, general anesthesia may be required.

Vasculature and organ systems (particularly hepatic, renal, and cardiopulmonary) may be visualized with injection of a radiopaque contrast medium. Many of the injection media currently available are of sufficiently low viscosity that they are suitable for small subjects. Viscosity of the contrast medium is important because of the small sizes of needles or cannulae used to deliver the solution. There are no systematic studies focused on identifying optimal dosages of CT contrast media in reptiles. A dose that is 25% to 35% of the human pediatric concentration of iopromide contrast medium (Ultravist Injection 370 mgI/mL at 1 to 2 mL/kg) can be used. The package

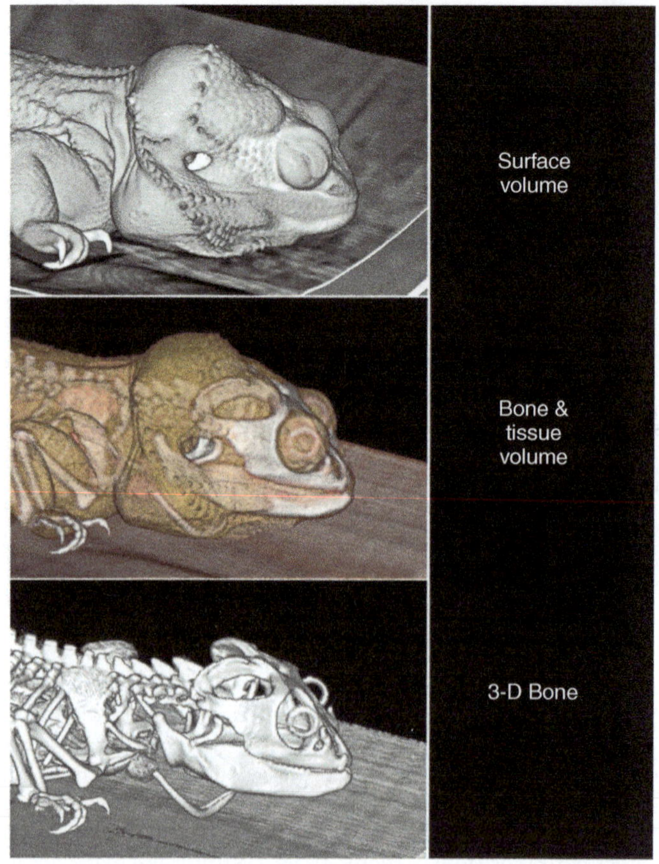

FIGURE 9-1 These lateral views of the head and torso of a Bearded Dragon *(Pogona vitticeps)* show the versatility of computed tomography (CT) data. They may be reconstructed in three dimensions to emphasize different structure densities and to allow understanding of external landmarks and the internal hard structures (the skeleton in this case). The same dataset from a single CT scan shows the results of three reprocessing modes. Different threshold settings allow the same dataset to be reconstructed as a surface image alone, showing the whole volume of the animal, a translucent tissue image of the whole volume with the skeleton also detected, and a three-dimensional image of the skeleton alone. Bony sutures are not seen in this image because their small size was below the level of sampling resolution. Cartilage cannot be seen when images are reprocessed for the bone but is included with other soft tissues reconstruction settings, which include some of the denser soft tissues. Bearded Dragon; snout-vent length, 22.5 cm.

information indicates that the maximum dose of Ultravist injection should not exceed 4 mL/kg.[12] This dose should provide adequate contrast for cardiac, renal, and vascular imaging in turtles and iguanas. Similarly, good results were obtained with an iodixanol contrast medium (Visipaque 270 [550 mg iodixanol/mL], GE Healthcare Inc., Princeton, NJ; in doses of 0.1 gI/kg body weight) in a Loggerhead Sea Turtle *(Caretta caretta)*. Other published studies that used other intravenous or enteric contrast material or higher doses had varied success.[6,10] A recent review[13] summarizes CT contrast media, their characteristics, and their effectiveness for various applications in small animals. Although focused mostly on mammals, it provides a good overview and perspective.

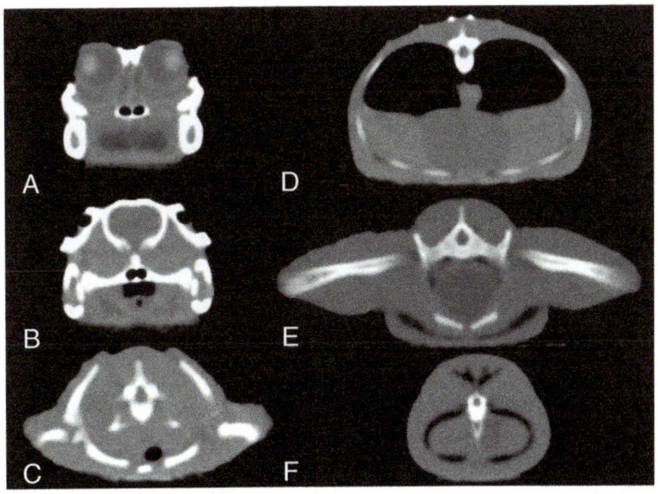

FIGURE 9-2 Two-dimensional axial computed tomographic images of several points along the body of an American Alligator *(Alligator mississippiensis)*. At the level of the eyes **(A)**, the jaws form the bony parts of the skull. Teeth can be seen extending from the lower jaw upward. The bony palate ventral to the choanae separates spaces that are the palatal vacuities. The vitreous and the tongue are darker. The lenses appear light. **B,** Posterior to the orbits, the palate is complete and the internal choanae can be seen joining the glottis. Dorsally is the oval braincase with posterior temporal bars extending ventrally and laterally. At the level of the shoulders **(C)**, the vertebrae are mostly surrounded by the scapulae and procoracoids. The single element ventral to the trachea is the interclavicle. **D,** Posterior to the forelimbs, the body wall is supported by dorsal ribs and ventral ribs. The sternum is not detected. The outline of the heart can be seen ventral to the paired lungs. Two osteoderms are visible dorsal to the trunk vertebra. **E,** The hindlimbs are supported by robust ilia articulating with sacral vertebrae. The anterior aspect of the paired pubic bones can be seen ventrally. **F,** The tail vertebra and ventral *y* shaped chevron bone are surrounded by muscle *(gray)* and tendon *(black)*. American Alligator; snout-vent length, 22 cm.

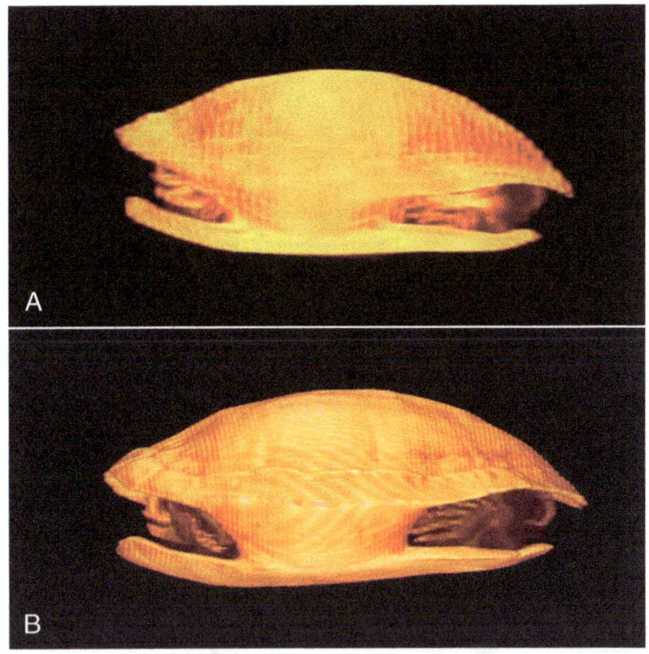

FIGURE 9-3 Image resolution of this Redear Slider *(Trachemys scripta)* CT improves with decreased spatial intervals. **A,** The sequential sections were three times farther apart than in *(B)*. **B,** Details of the skull, digits, and caudal vertebrae can be identified in this higher resolution scan. Redear Slider; straight carapace length, 24 cm.

A numbers of diverse reptilian studies using CT now have been published.[10,14-22] These studies represent both novel and traditional uses of the imaging tools. For example, the techniques used to diagnose disease in extant reptiles are now being applied to understand diseases of archosaurs that have long been extinct.[14-15] CT studies of modern reptiles and birds ("avian reptiles") are used commonly to understand the structure and function of fossilized avian and nonavian dinosaurs.[15] These various studies highlight the utility of CT in understanding both normal anatomy and pathology, and they put the historical occurrence of reptilian disease in perspective.[14,17-22]

MAGNETIC RESONANCE IMAGING

Advances in high-resolution MRI and the proliferation of MRI facilities have made machines accessible and their use as a standard diagnostic tool feasible. MRI scanning provides almost real-time images of live animals in a noninvasive or minimally invasive fashion. Usually the MRI is very good for visualization of soft tissues and fluids. Scan durations are somewhat slower than CT but do not rely on radiation or density differences in the tissues.

The most common diagnostic MRI machines are described by their format and magnet strength: open versus tunnel (closed), low-field versus high-field, respectively. The diameter, or distance, across the opening of a tunnel MRI machine is approximately 24 inches (60 cm), whereas the distance across an open MRI machine is often nearly 5 feet (1.5 m). High-field MRI machines, described by magnet strength in Tesla units (T), are usually 1.5T, although 3T machines are becoming more common clinically, and machines from 7T to 12T are in use in research facilities. The 3T and stronger machines can provide higher resolution, but the scans are more sensitive to movement, necessitating general anesthesia in most cases. Currently, open MRI machines are usually low-field (0.7T); the magnet strength and image resolution are usually not as great as those for tunnel MRI machines. However, recently, some new open MRI machines with openings of nearly 2.2 feet (67 cm) and 1.5T magnets provide options for larger patients.

All the MRI images included in this chapter were collected with a closed MRI. For large-bodied animals, the donut-shaped magnet and a receiver are housed together. For smaller animals or parts of the animal, smaller receivers, termed *coils,* may be used to provide clearer images by increasing the signal-to-noise ratio (Figure 9-5) and reducing artifacts. Head, knee, or wrist coils usually provide good quality images when the length of the animal or the region of interest is not great. Animals that move little when handled may need just minimal restraint. Others may be briefly sedated with a nonvolatile anesthetic. No metal can be on or in the animal because it may heat up during imaging and can cause discomfort or burns. Additionally, the signal from metals may leave large artifacts in the image, often obscuring the site of interest.

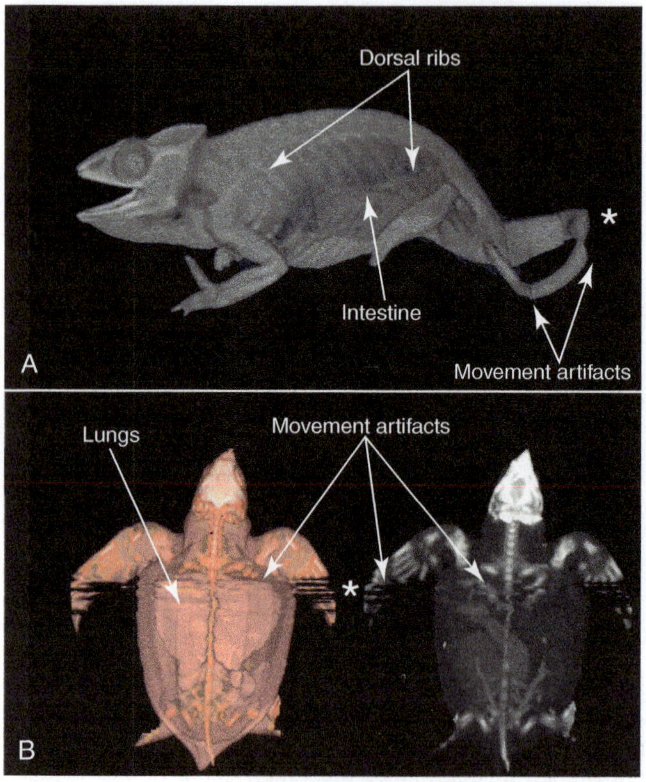

FIGURE 9-4 This set of three-dimensional (3D) computed tomographic (CT) images shows movement artifacts. Chameleons (Panther Chameleon *[Furcifer pardalis]*) have thin bones and large saclike lungs; both can be imaged with CT scans. These 3D reconstructions show both large areas of the body filled by the low-density field and the chameleon's numerous ribs that extend the entire length of the trunk. The dorsal ribs are jointed at their articulations with the spine, and with the ventral ribs (gastralia) from the belly. **A,** The data were reconstructed from 0.6-mm serial images and reprocessed so that both skeletal and airway data could be seen. Panther Chameleon; snout-vent length, 12.6 cm. **B,** Postprocessing of the turtle image data with false color highlights some skeletal and soft tissue structures such as lungs and parts of the intestine *(left)* that do not appear when the same dataset is reconstructed as a maximum intensity projection (MIP) 3D image *(right).* Movement artifacts (*) appear as discontinuous segments in the image associated with tail movement by the Chameleon **(A)** and breathing by a neonate Leatherback Sea Turtle *(Dermochelys coriacea)* **(B).** Straight carapace length, 6.2 cm.

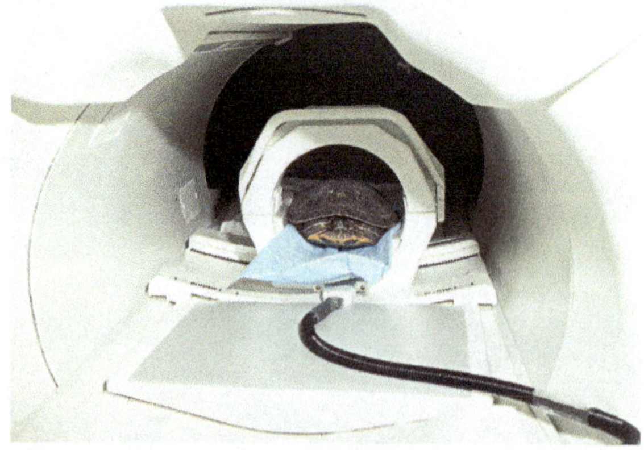

FIGURE 9-5 The closed magnetic resonance imaging machine has a donut-shaped magnet as its largest component. It produces, sends, and receives signals. For small-bodied animals like this turtle, a smaller receiver was mounted inside the gantry to provide better images.

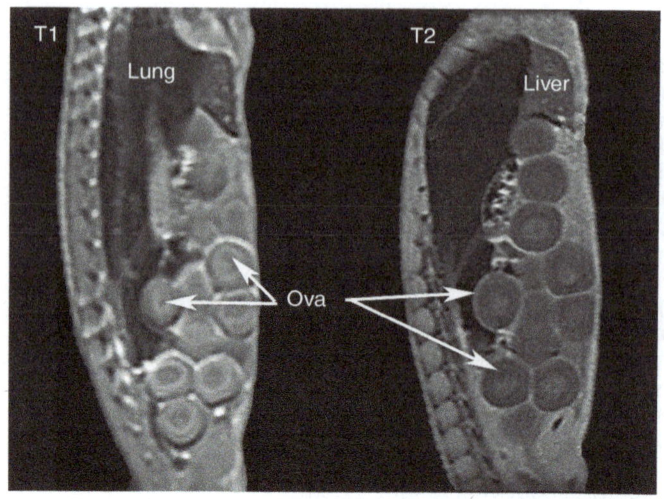

FIGURE 9-6 Two sagittal magnetic resonance images of a female Green Iguana *(Iguana iguana)* torso taken at roughly the same position. Cranial is toward the top of the image. In the T1 image *(left),* fat is bright, air is black, fluid (i.e., blood, edema, cerebrospinal fluid [CSF], or yolk) is dark, and cortical bone is dark. Parts of the spinal nerves can be seen as white dots running along the spine on the left side of the image. In T2 images, fluids are bright, fats are gray, and bone is dark. The posterior trunk vertebrae and vertebral muscles are easy to identify. This T2 scan *(right)* caught little blood flow (seen immediately to the left of the three more anterior ova). The more liquid centers of the yolked ova are clear in both images.

Because the MRI imaging is based on the responses of fluids, fats, or circulatory characteristics (e.g., flow rates),[1,6] this imaging modality is good for understanding the forms and positions of soft tissues, tracking changes, and identifying pathologic conditions. The pictures supply detailed landmarks and can provide an understanding of normal positions and sizes of soft tissues, such as the gastrointestinal tract, liver, and lung. MRI is also a good imaging choice for assessing neurologic conditions such as spinal cord injury, ischemic injury, or hydrocephalus. It is particularly effective for assessing the age of a lesion, tracking acute versus chronic conditions, extent of edematous change, assessing joint structure, damage, or disease, and tracing blood flow.

MRI is based on a set of techniques that uses the different biochemical and biophysical properties of the tissues in response to the magnetic pulses to produce images. An MRI machine focuses a magnetic field that rapidly spins around the subject.[1] Protons in tissues or liquids temporarily respond in tissue-specific ways to generate an image. Images are composed of a series of 2D images or "slices" that may be viewed alone or in 3D reconstructions.

The images can be collected in many different ways. For basic needs, two major categories of imaging modes can be used: T1-weighted and T2-weighted studies (Figure 9-6).

The terms refer to the images that result from tissue-specific biophysical properties of protons as they respond to magnetic fields. Often T1 scans are described as *anatomy scans* and T2 scans are *pathology scans*. Many special techniques for specific applications are based on variations of these two main types of imaging modalities and the tissue response characteristics that they emphasize. For those interested in the physical principles of MRI, several printed and online resources are available, and MRI machine characteristics are available at imaging facilities. For the purposes of this chapter, the essential difference is that, in T1 images, fat is bright, fluid (i.e., flowing blood, edema, cerebrospinal fluid [CSF]) are dark, and solid masses and cortical bone are dark. Bone marrow, because of the fat within, appears bright. T1 techniques are good for imaging brain and spinal cord because of the high levels of lipids in these regions. T2 techniques show fluids such as flowing blood and cysts as bright areas; pooling blood usually is dark gray, fats appear gray, and bone is dark. T2 imaging is good for visualizing circulation.[1] Several publications demonstrate the advantages of each of these two imaging modalities in diverse examples of reptiles.[23-27]

MRI scans are noisy as the magnetic pulses are delivered. It is not common to observe startle responses by lizards, turtles, or snakes to MRI noise; however, the potential exists, which may be another reason for considering sedation or anesthesia.

MRI may also be used to assess function. A fundamental concept of functional MRI (fMRI) is that it can detect areas with greater blood flow (presumably those areas are metabolically more active and demand more O_2) and higher concentration of deoxyhemoglobin. fMRI describes a set of imaging protocols used to assess organ function, reproductive condition, cardiopulmonary performance, blood flow patterns, metabolic activity, neural activity, or sites of fluid accumulation.[16-17,23-26] For example, identifying and assessing ischemic injury and chronic versus acute status of disease are common applications. In 2D and 3D pictures taken with fMRI, soft tissue functional anatomy or pathology with in vivo landmarks can be seen. This is particularly true in assessment of circulation or lack of circulation or with the results of angiogenesis. Gas and blood can be distinguished in some modalities. Pooling of blood or hematomas may be detected with or without intravenous contrast media. Gadolinium-positive contrast solution (dosed at 1 to 2 mL/kg) can give sufficient contrast to detail the circulation (Figure 9-7) in several species of turtles, pythons, and agamid lizards and causes no detectable adverse effects. This dose is similar to that which produces good results in dogs.[23]

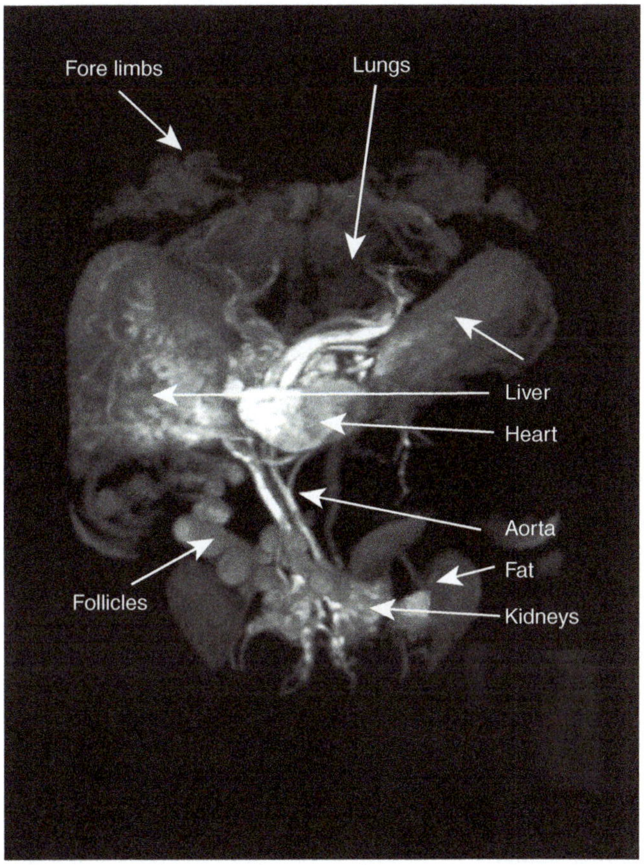

FIGURE 9-7 Soft tissue anatomy is outlined in this T2-weighted functional magnetic resonance imaging (fMRI) scan of a turtle; the vasculature is highlighted by gadolinium contrast medium. The heart plus the highly vascular liver, lungs, and kidneys are clearly outlined. Forelimbs are outlined less densely. The two systemic aortas join in the midbody as the single dorsal aorta. Follicles and fat pads are shown caudally. Redear Slider *(Trachemys scripta)*; straight-line carapace length unknown,

IMAGES, LANDMARKS, AND IMAGE PROCESSING

These two imaging methodologies can be used to complement one another and standard radiography in diagnostics, tracking the course of disease and guiding treatment decisions.[29,30] When coordination of views is important, photographing the position of the animal in the CT will help guide its position in MRI. (Note: some cameras will not work in presence of the MRI magnet so the CT image can be the guide for the MRI.) Taping markers on the animal can also be useful. For MRI, markers must be nonmetallic. The author has used elliptical Vitamin E capsules oriented with the long axis of the animal or at key intervals with good success. For CT, markers must be radiopaque; unopened syringe needles, or pieces of chalk taped to the body in the same locations work well.

Basic reptile skeletal structure, landmarks, and soft tissue anatomy are illustrated in a series of CT and MRI pictures (Figures 9-8 to 9-28). Image data were processed to maximize the landmark information with several different data processing modalities. The different processing options are presented, not only to enhance the reader's appreciation of reptilian anatomy but also to provide an introduction to the versatility of CT and MRI technologies.

MRI and CT studies often are supplied to the clinician as digital files on a CD or via online methods. The images usually are provided as digital imaging and communications in medicine (DICOM) files, which then can be viewed and manipulated to provide a variety of perspectives. Initial image formatting and organization is done with the CT or MRI scanner's software. Image manipulations then can be conducted with either the manufacturer's proprietary software or other image viewing and manipulation software. Most veterinary and medical machines are linked to a picture archiving and communication system (PACS) for medical records.

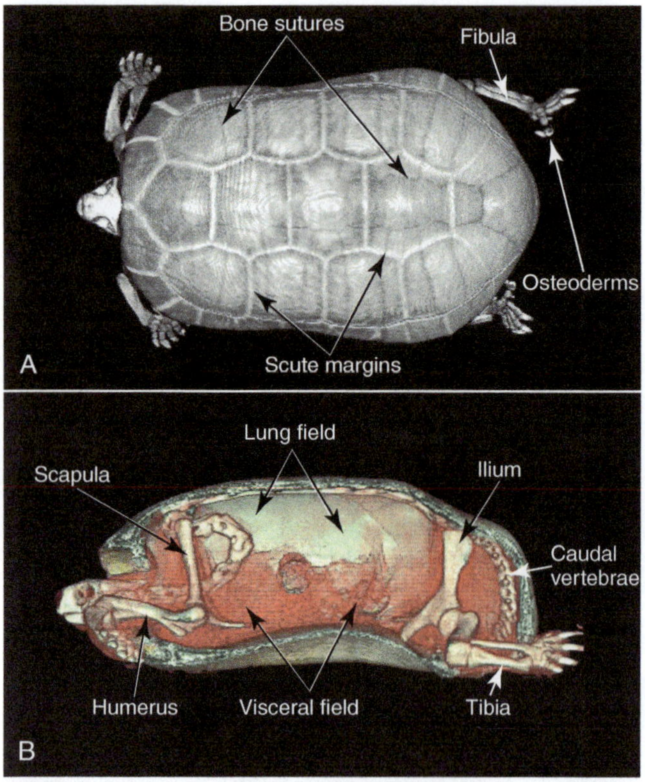

FIGURE 9-8 Computed tomography (CT) data can be reconstructed to show three-dimensional skeletal anatomy. **A,** This dorsal view of a tortoise shows both scute margins and bony sutures of the carapace. Osteoderms (ossified bones in the scales) also appear in this image along the hind feet. **B,** Postprocessing software allows for the reconstruction of the image series as a whole skeleton that can then be virtually cut using digital dissection to show internal anatomy. Adult Red-footed Tortoise *(Chelonoidis carbonaria)*; straight-line carapace length, unknown.

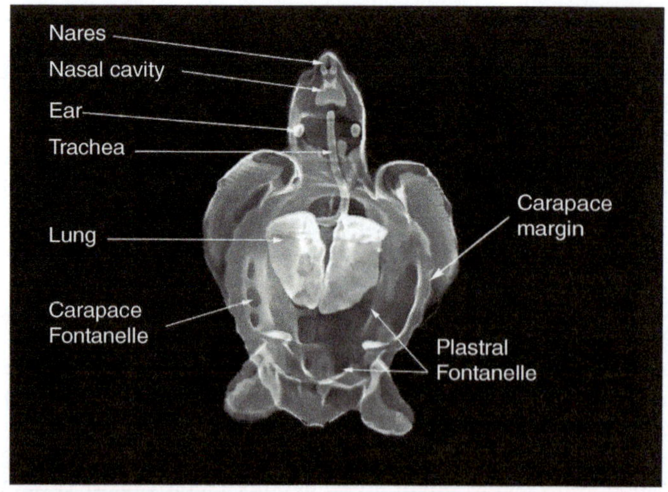

FIGURE 9-9 This computed tomography (CT) scan of a small juvenile sea turtle was reconstructed using image thresholds to make the bones and airways light and translucent, and provide the surface as an outline. The partial secondary palate of sea turtles allows the nares and nasal cavity to be seen clearly and separately from the trachea, which opens in the tongue. The lungs attach the carapace and along the vertebral column where their margin appears scalloped. Unossified fontanelles are in the margin carapace and make up the center of the plastron. The otic chamber *(labeled ear)* is air filled. Other areas of trapped air appear in the neck and inguinal pockets. Loggerhead Sea Turtle *(Caretta caretta);* straight-line carapace length, 6.3 cm.

The availability of good, user-friendly freeware medical image viewers for Windows or Macintosh computer systems include, but are not limited to, ezDICOM, (http://www.cabiatl.com/mricro/ezdicom/) or Agnosco DICOM viewer (www.e-dicom.com) for Windows. A robust open-source software, OsiriX, for Macintosh (http://www.osirix-viewer.com/) enables even novice users to explore and reconstruct their patient's data. These easy to use software resources allow the user to do basic viewing or work with the 2D and 3D images. More advanced versions of these software packages are available that provide more features, assurances, and precision. Each year more kinds of software or improved versions become available. All of the software options allow the user to adjust, at least, the contrast and black-to-white intensity (brightness) of the image.

Relatively few reptile image studies are conducted with correlated dissections.[7-10,27-28] In most cases such laborious anatomical verification is not essential because images can be processed to reveal deep structures in 3D. Although CT and MRI eliminate much superimposition, some structures are best seen after digital dissection of overlying structures. Digital dissection should be done after the data series is reassembled as a volume reconstruction. Working with the reconstruction as a black and white maximum intensity projection (MIP) image tends to be faster and less taxing on computer memory than working in a color volume or surface reconstruction. Working with brightness and contrast settings will allow the user to enhance the structures needed and deemphasize or eliminate those not needed. It is good practice to save the images periodically when doing a virtual dissection because it is easy to accidently remove information in one view that one needs in another view or to accidently cut out part of the image that is behind an area of interest.

Once the virtual dissection is complete, then various surface or volume-based renderings will provide the essential image information. Usually MIP images can be converted to surface or volume images. If images are provided as 3D reconstructions or .gif, .pdf, .jpg, or .png files, they usually cannot be processed further.

ACKNOWLEDGMENTS

The author thanks Fred Steinberg, MD, Medical Director, University MRI, Boca Raton, Florida, for providing access to his high-resolution CT and fMRI equipment and software. Gina Boykin, Andrew Kaufman, and Steve Rubel collected the images at University MRI. Dale Wilke at OMI of Jupiter, Florida taught the author much of what she knows about MRI techniques and procedures; he collected many of the turtle images presented here. The skills and assistance of these talented MRI and CT technologists and their willingness to work with reptiles are gratefully acknowledged. The author thanks the thoughtful reviewers, particularly Dr. Sam Silverman, for improving this chapter.

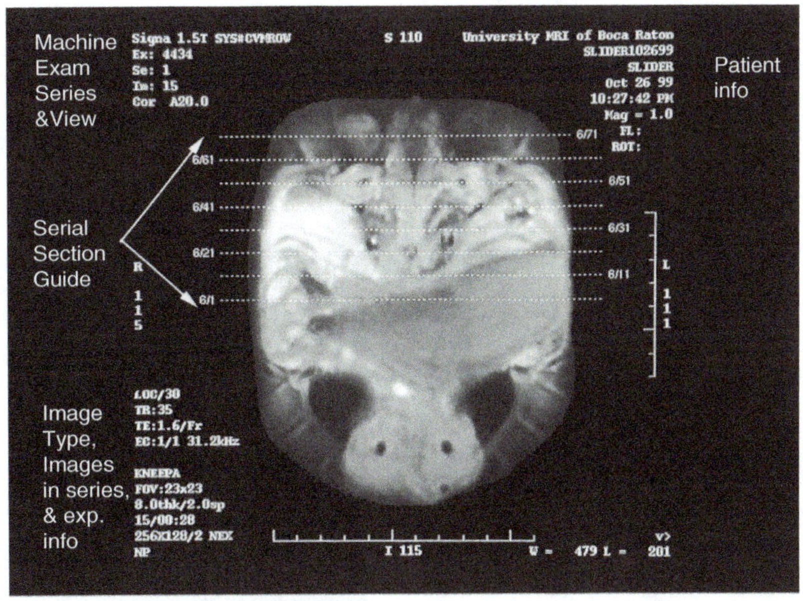

FIGURE 9-10 Both computed tomography (CT) and magnetic resonance imaging (MRI) are set up with a short exposure "scout image" on which a map of the imaging "slices" or sections (including their thickness) and extent is set. This image is often termed a *localizer* and is useful; it can be included with the films or files. The localizer provides the key to identifying where in the body the two-dimensional images were taken, in addition to patient information, the scan type, and number of sections in the examination. In this example, a frontal image of a Redear Slider from an MRI is used to map out an examination of transverse or axial images. The MRI scout image was used to set image collection for the cranial half of the turtle in a series of 80 slices or projections. This localizer maps them in groups of 10, starting at midbody and progressing toward the head. Because most commercially available MRI and CT machines have software specifically for human patients, one must carefully explain to the technician what planes of view are needed from the nonhuman patient. The images are often designated as if the animal were on its back so that its right may be on the left side of the image.

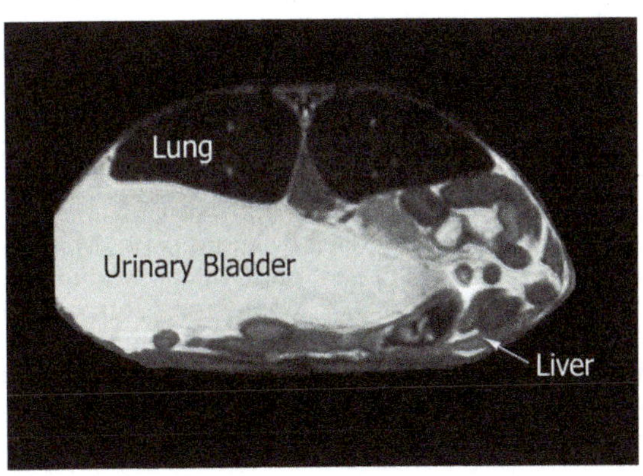

FIGURE 9-11 This T2-weighted magnetic resonance image is a transverse or axial section from the Slider midbody, designated by the line labeled *6/1* in the localizer image (see Figure 9-10). The turtle was oriented with the plastron down; left and right are not reversed in the image. At this level, the large fluid-filled urinary bladder extends anteriorly and occupies most of the left half of the image. Bone is barely visible as thin dark outline. Dorsally are the black spaces occupied by the lungs; within each lung, the paired pulmonary artery and vein can be seen as white dots. To the right are the gray intestines fat, intracoelomic fluid, and mesenteric blood are bright. The gray caudal tip of the liver is ventral. This image was magnified slightly in processing the data. Adult Redear Slider *(Trachemys scripta);* straight-line carapace length, unknown.

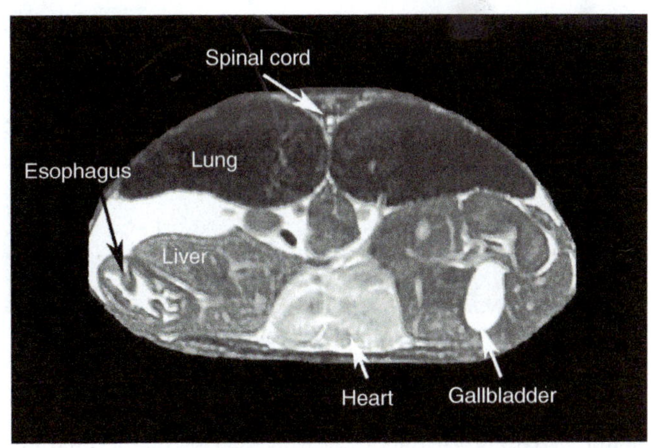

FIGURE 9-12 This magnetic resonance image section is 20 slices more cranial than section 1 (designated *6/21* in the localizer image, see Figure 9-10). At this level, the esophagus near the stomach can be seen to the left. The liver has two large lobes that fill much of the ventral half of the image and one small lobe dorsal to the heart. The heart is light gray and is found midventrally. The dark lungs are dorsal and abut the vertebrae. The spinal cord can be seen as a white dot between the medial and dorsal parts of the lungs. Blood, bile, pericardial fluid, and fat are bright.

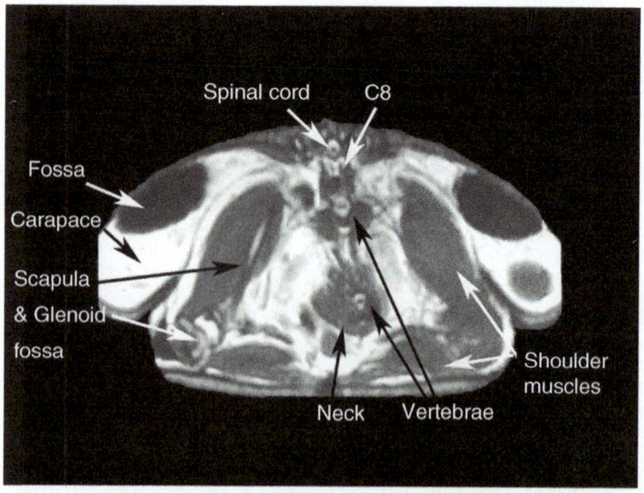

FIGURE 9-13 This magnetic resonance image section is 30 slices more cranial than section 21 (designated *6/51* in the localizer). At this level, the carapace appears to be "cut" transversely because of its curvature. The black spaces dorsolaterally are fossae where the forelimbs may retract. Medullary bone is bright. Muscle is dark gray. Both sets of shoulder muscles and the left scapula are in this plane. In the middle of the body is the retracted neck at the level where the vertebrae form an *s*-curve. As a result, parts of vertebrae C8, C7, or C6 and C3 are seen from dorsal to ventral. Fat and fluid are bright.

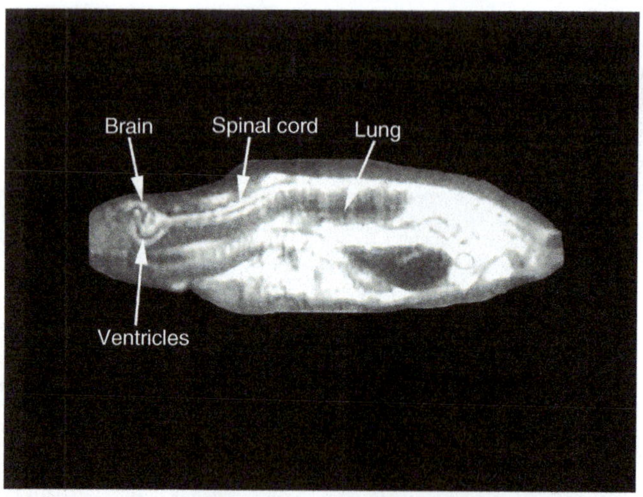

FIGURE 9-14 This T1-weighted magnetic resonance image of a posthatchling Leatherback Sea Turtle *(Dermochelys coriacea)* is a nearly midsagittal view. The brain and spinal cord are bright. The cerebrospinal fluid in the ventricles and the spinal canal appear dark gray. This species has a great deal of lipid in its shell and the residual yolk; hence, much of the body is bright. Gas appears black. Leatherback Sea Turtle; straight-line carapace length, 5.7 cm.

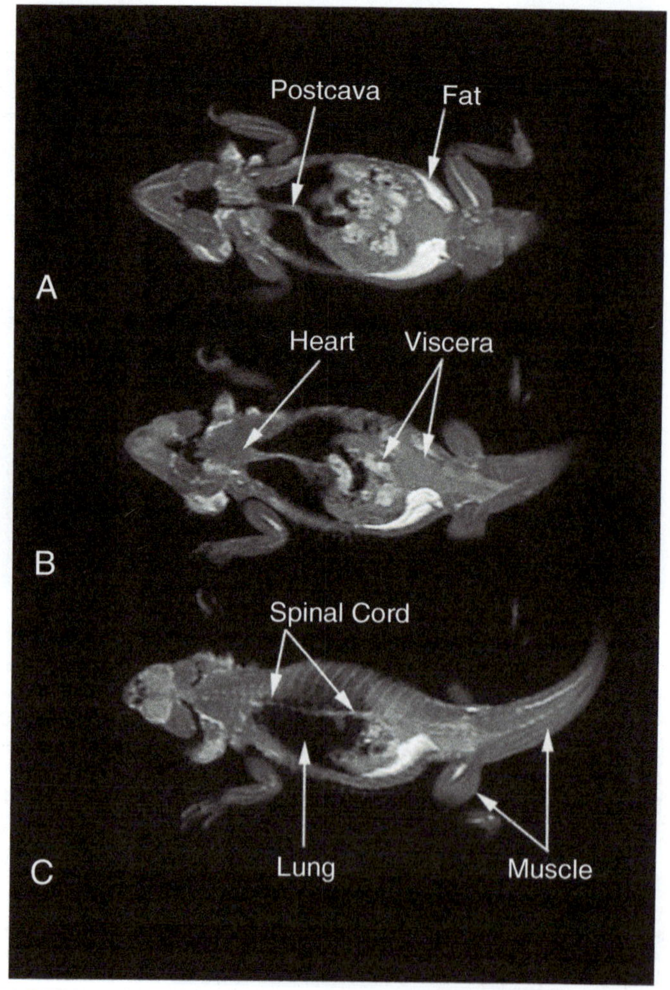

FIGURE 9-15 These three magnetic resonance images are of an adult male Bearded Dragon *(Pogona vitticeps)* viewed serially from ventral to dorsal in frontal sections. The exposures are T1-weighted, so fat is bright. Medullary bone also tends to be bright. Fluid and nonfatty tissues appear gray. Air in the lung fields appears black. The most ventral section **(A)** passes dorsal to the tongue and through the trachea, lungs, postcava, liver, viscera, and through the proximal tail. Long bones and muscles of the limbs can be seen. More dorsally **(B),** the lungs, pericardial sac, parts of the aortae, liver, viscera, and fat pads are clear. In the most dorsal view **(C),** the air-filled nasal passages, the eyes, left lung, parts of the spinal cord (light), abdominal fat pads, and tail muscles and tendons can be discriminated. Bearded Dragon; snout-vent length, 17.6 cm.

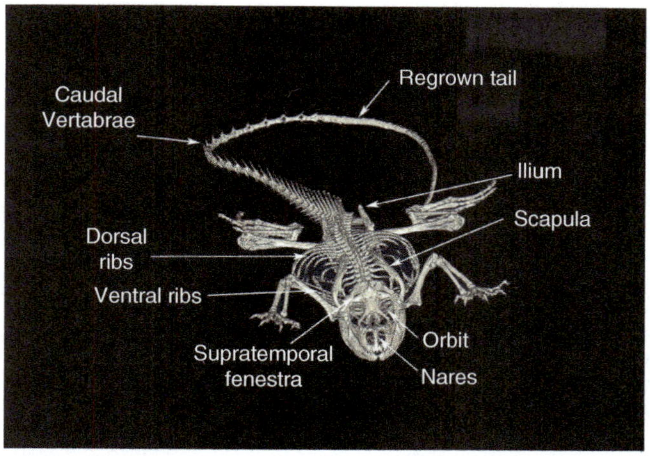

FIGURE 9-16 This three-dimensional reconstruction of an adult Green Iguana *(Iguana iguana)* skeleton shows normal anatomy, including the multiple fenestrae in the skull, arrangement of the vertebral spinous processes, and the dorsal girdle elements. A few common artifacts found in computed tomography images. First, rib elements appear to be missing laterally. The thinnest rib ends, and cartilaginous parts between the dorsal and ventral ribs are not detected in this kind of reconstruction. The thin nasal bones just behind the nares also appear to be missing. Their data fall outside of the threshold used by the software to make this kind of reconstruction. The striping that appears along the length of the skeleton is from reconstruction of sequential two-dimensional images. Green Iguana; snout-vent length, 41.8 cm.

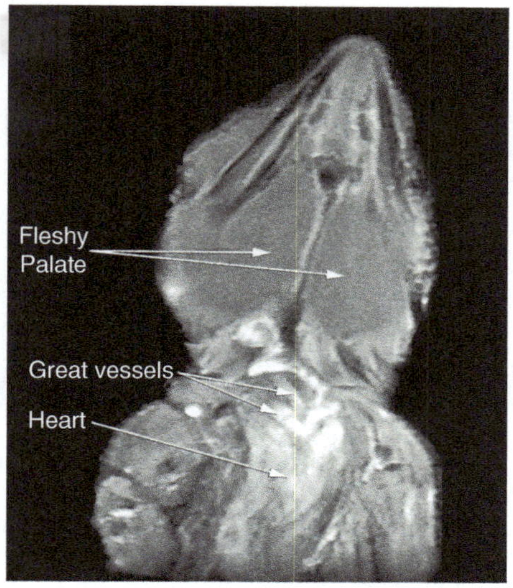

FIGURE 9-17 This two-dimensional frontal section functional magnetic resonance imaging scan was at the level of the primary palate of a Bearded Dragon *(Pogona vitticeps)*. Contrast medium shows that the great vessels are in the same plane. This is a T1-weighted image after gadolinium contrast medium was injected. Bearded Dragon; snout-vent length, 22.5 cm.

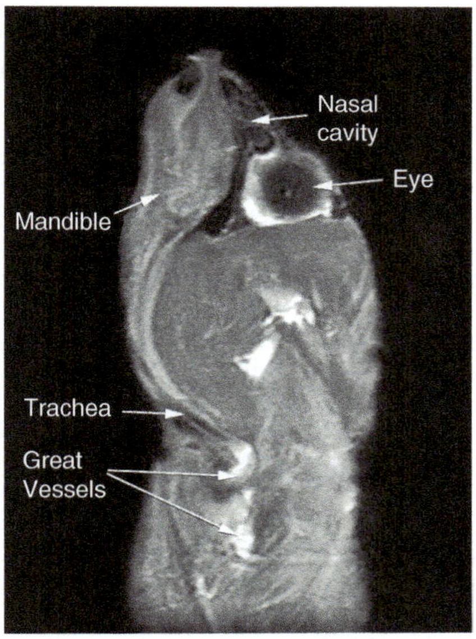

FIGURE 9-18 This two-dimensional parasagittal section functional magnetic resonance image shows muscle, the medial (buccal) edge of the lower jaw, and the nasal cavity. The synovial cavity of the jaw joint and part of the adjacent circulation (external jugular vein and ophthalmic veins) appear white. This is a T1-weighted image with gadolinium contrast medium in the vessels. Parts of the great vessels are caught in this plane of section, as is a small section of the trachea. Bearded Dragon *(Pogona vitticeps)*; snout-vent length, 22.5 cm.

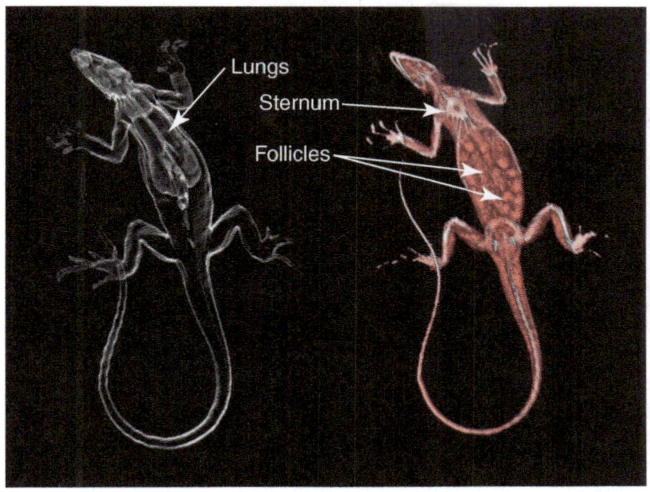

FIGURE 9-19 Green Iguana (*Iguana iguana*) computed tomography reconstructions showing lungs of an adult female with maturing follicles. The two reconstructed images are from the same scan data and view but was prepared with the use of a different combination of contrast and intensity. The artificial colors in the right image are from a soft tissue preset in the software that allowed the details of the follicles, some bones, and muscle to appear more clearly than in black and white MIP (maximum intensity projection) reconstruction. Green Iguana; snout-vent length, 41.8 cm.

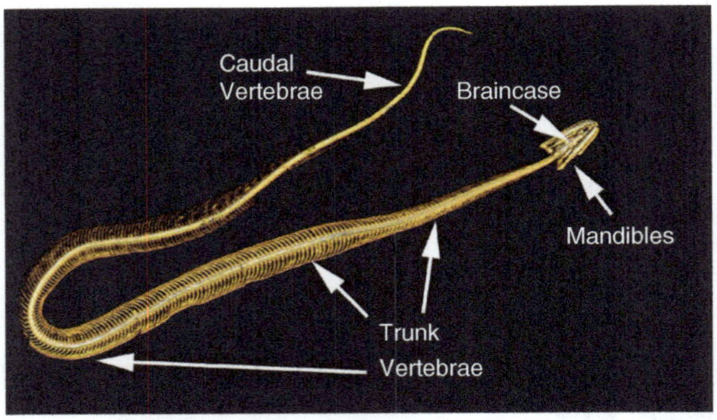

FIGURE 9-20 Ventral view of a Ball Python *(Python regius)* skeleton. The separate mandibles are easily seen, as are the hyoid components extending medially from the mandibles and passing almost parallel to the brain case. Snakes lack a secondary palate, so the roof of the mouth is also the floor of the braincase. Cervical vertebrae are limited to the anterior two and cannot be distinguished in this computed tomography reconstruction. Trunk vertebrae have ribs and extend most of the length of the snake. Snakes lack ventral ribs. Caudal vertebrae lack ribs. The slight shift in registration of the reconstructed sections in the midbody are associated with one breath taken by the snake during scanning. Adult Ball Python; snout-vent length, unknown.

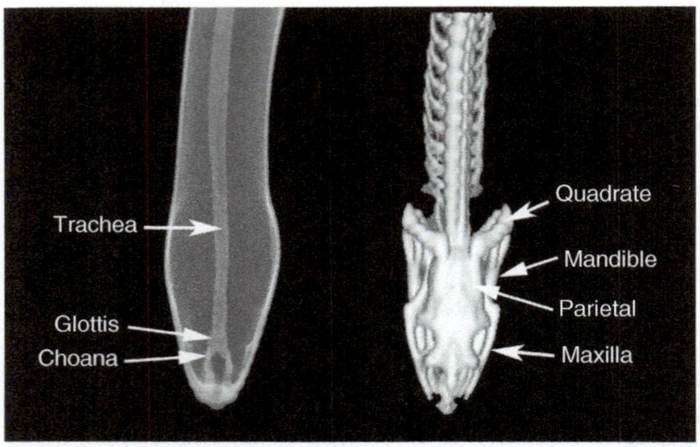

FIGURE 9-21 This close-up computed tomography scan of the head structure shows the relationship of the airways in a Cornsnake *(Elaphe guttata)* to its skull and neck. Although snakes lack a secondary palate, the airways through the choanae and to the glottis are clear. Snake skulls are highly kinetic. Joints between the parietals, quadrate, and mandibles contribute to the snake's large gape. Highly mobile maxillae assist in prey capture and manipulation for swallowing. No rigid joint is found between the two mandibles or the maxillae. Adult Cornsnake; snout-vent length, unknown.

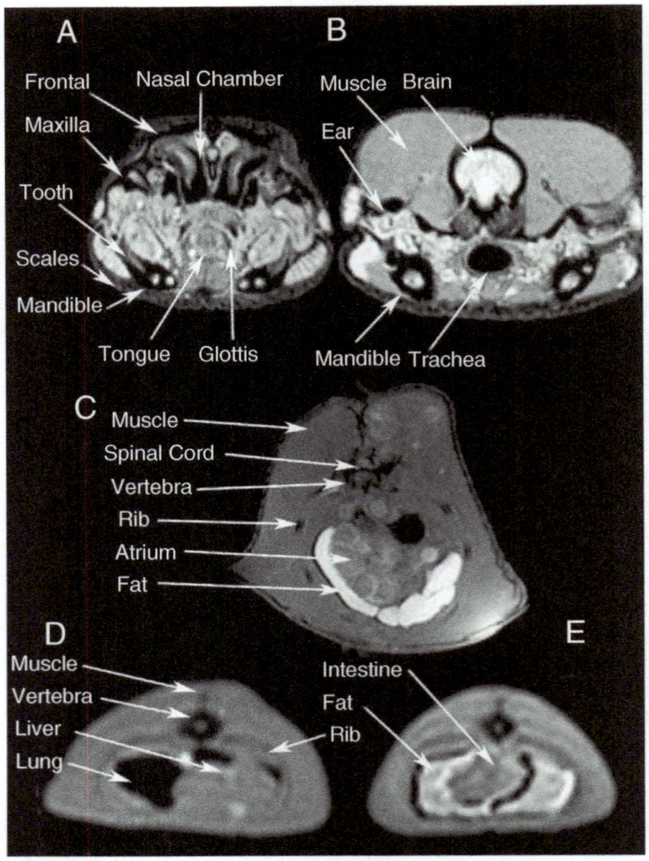

FIGURE 9-22 Burmese Python *(Python molurus)* axial composite magnetic resonance imaging (MRI) scan. MRI of whole snakes is difficult because of the tubular geometry of the animals. Often the snake must be examined in a series of sequential parts to obtain good image quality **(A** to **C)**. Snake images taken without the aid of a small imaging coil or those taken in an open MRI may be of limited value because they tend to have poor resolution due to high-noise, low-signal artifacts **(D** and **E)**. Few MRI tables have sufficient range to scan a whole snake or even part of a large snake, consequently the distance between the snake and receiver becomes maximized. This large distance leads to images with a great deal of noise and, hence, low image quality. Alternatively, one can scan snakes in small segments and use a small coil, but the entire animal (and sometimes the entire organ) cannot be examined in one scan. Here is a series that was taken using a coil receiver for images **A-C;** they are T1-weighted axial scans starting with the nasal passages and mouth structures **(A)**. **B,** More caudally along the head bone and air are dark, the brain is bright and muscles are various shades of gray. **C, D,** and **E,** Sections through the trunk show vertebrae and ribs as dark patches caught, in part, by the plane of view; the spinal cord is light. Fat and fluids also appear bright (**B, C,** and **E**). Adult male Burmese Python; total length, 2.9 m.

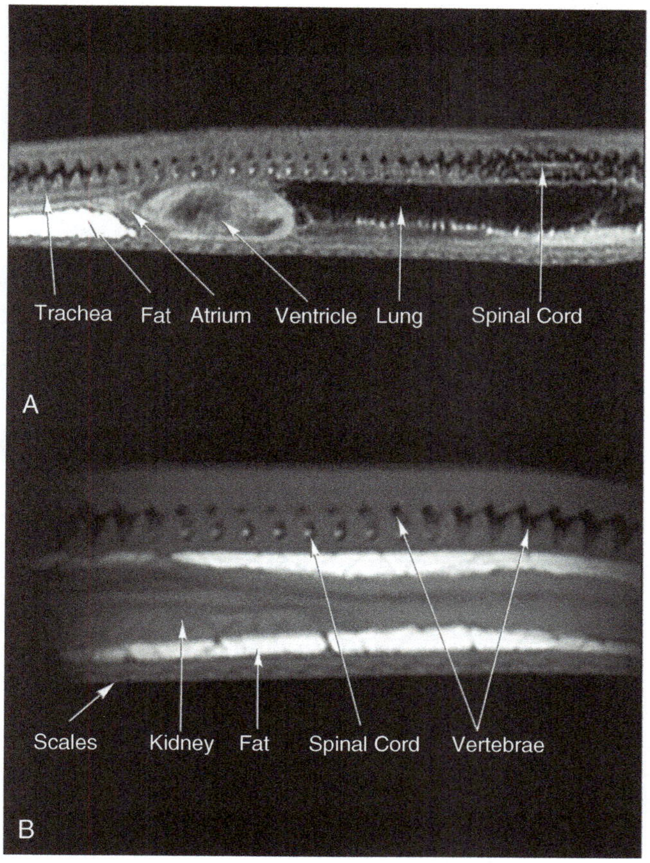

FIGURE 9-23 Burmese Python *(Python molurus)* magnetic resonance image; trunk composite. This composite of images taken in the sagittal or parasagittal planes shows major structures of the anterior **(A)** and posterior trunk **(B)**. The head is to the left in both images. These T1 images show the heart and lungs in less detail than the lobular kidney. Because the image was not synchronized with the heart beat, some movement artifacts occur in the anterior body. The thyroid and parathyroid glands occur in the region scanned in **(A)** but could not be distinguished from the fat with this imaging mode. Adult male Burmese Python; total length, 2.9 m.

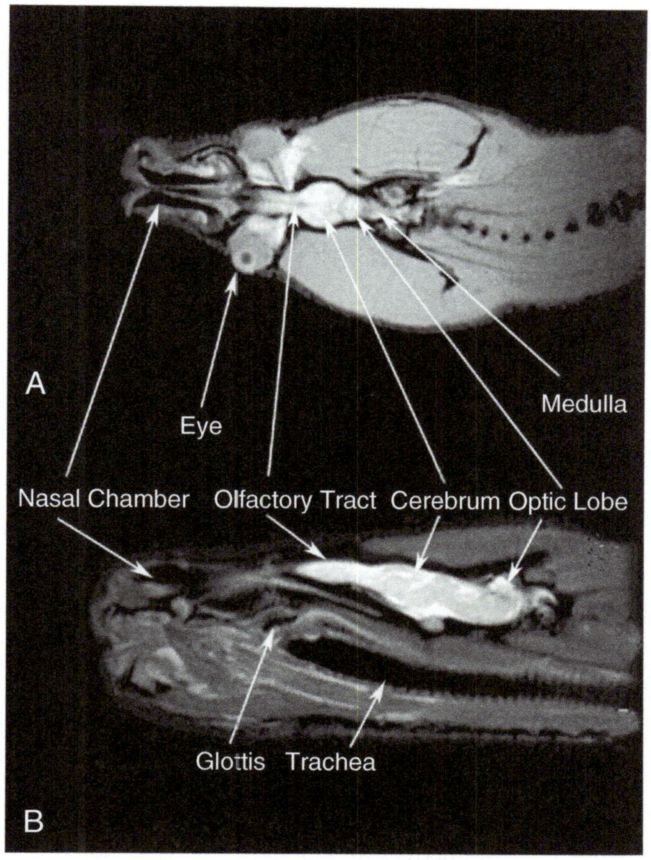

FIGURE 9-24 Burmese Python *(Python molurus)* head coronal and midsagittal magnetic resonance images. This pair of images shows the gross brain anatomy and some of the landmarks associated with the mouth. The two images show the muscle masses surrounding the braincase and brain **(A)** and the close proximity of the brain to the primary palate bones **(B)**. Adult male Burmese Python; total length, 2.9 m.

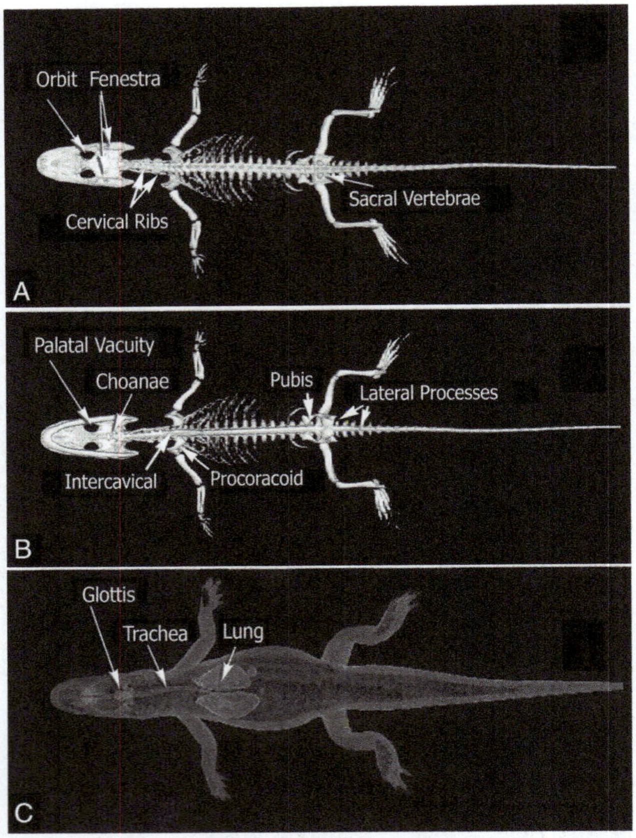

FIGURE 9-25 Computed tomography reconstructions of the skeleton and airways of a small juvenile American Alligator *(Alligator mississippiensis)*. **A,** In the dorsal view, alligator's diapsid skull form is demarked by paired superior and lateral fenestrae, which are located posterior to the large orbits. **B,** The ventral view shows the large secondary palate separating air and food passages. Paired palatal fenestrae (palatal vacuities) occur ventral to the orbits. The paired internal choanal openings appear unpaired along the midline because of the resolution of this scan. There are cervical ribs in the neck and normal dorsal ribs that articulate with the vertebrae. Both are seen in **A** and **B**. The sternum and thin ventral ribs were not detected in this scan for bone. The pectoral girdle of crocodilians is simple, with paired scapulae dorsally **(A)** and procoracoids ventrally; there is a primitive unpaired structure, the interclavicle located medially between the procoracoids, **(B)**. The pelvis is attached to the axial skeleton by robust sacral vertebrae **(A)**. The more proximal caudal vertebrae have prominent lateral processes; these processes are absent near the end of the tail (**A** and **B**). **C,** The glottis aligns with the choanae. The alligator's lungs occupy a relatively small volume in the body. Crocodilians have several types of ribs. American Alligator; snout-vent length, 22 cm.

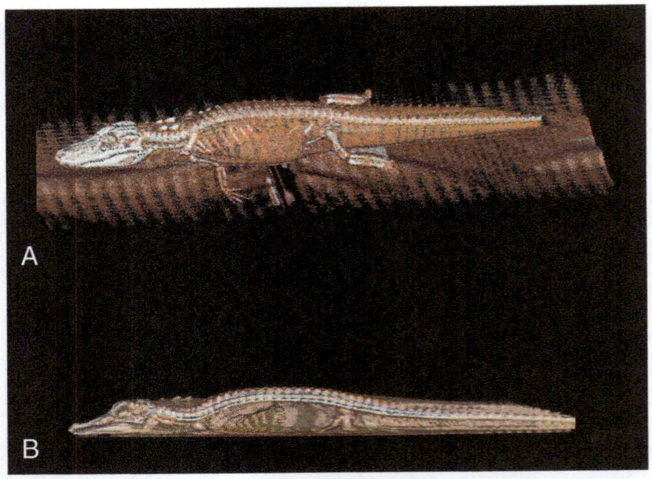

FIGURE 9-26 The computed tomography scan data are reconstructed in three dimensions. **A,** The bone and tissue together provide landmarks. **B,** The reconstruction was cut virtually with software then rotated into position to see the structures of interest. In this case, the midsagittal cut shows the skull's internal architecture, spine, lungs, and pelvis. In both views, the terminal tail vertebrae were beyond the scanned field. American Alligator *(Alligator mississippiensis)*; snout-vent length, 22 cm.

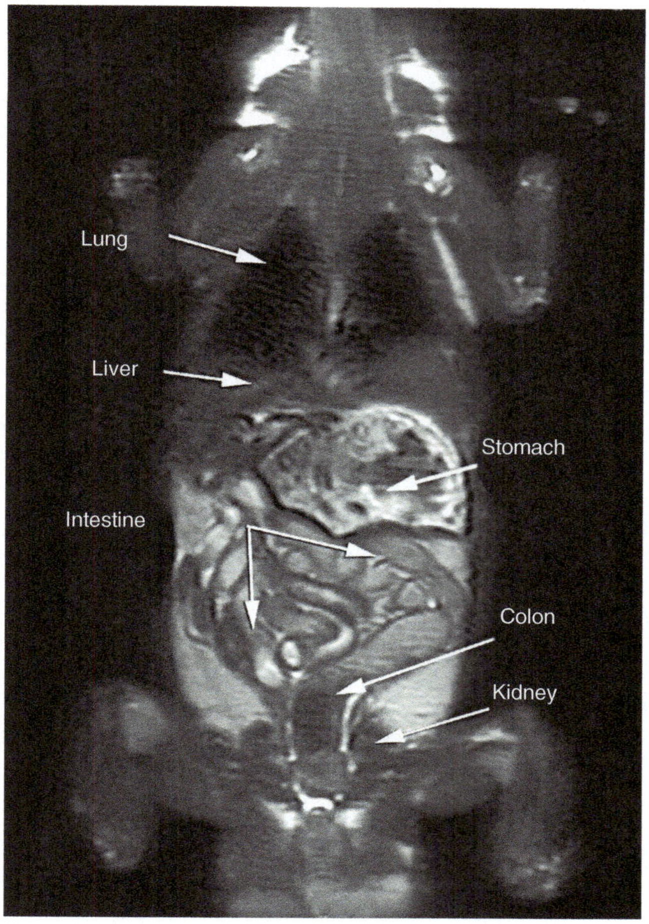

FIGURE 9-27 This T2-weighted magnetic resonance image of a juvenile American Alligator *(Alligator mississippiensis)* torso is a two-dimensional image. The plane of view is a thick frontal projection of the ventral one third of the animal. The gastrointestinal tract and its contents are clearly visible as light to medium gray. Fluids in the coelomic cavity and throat are bright. Fat is dark gray, and air is black. Portion of the kidneys are visible adjacent to the colon. American Alligator; snout-vent length, 29 cm.

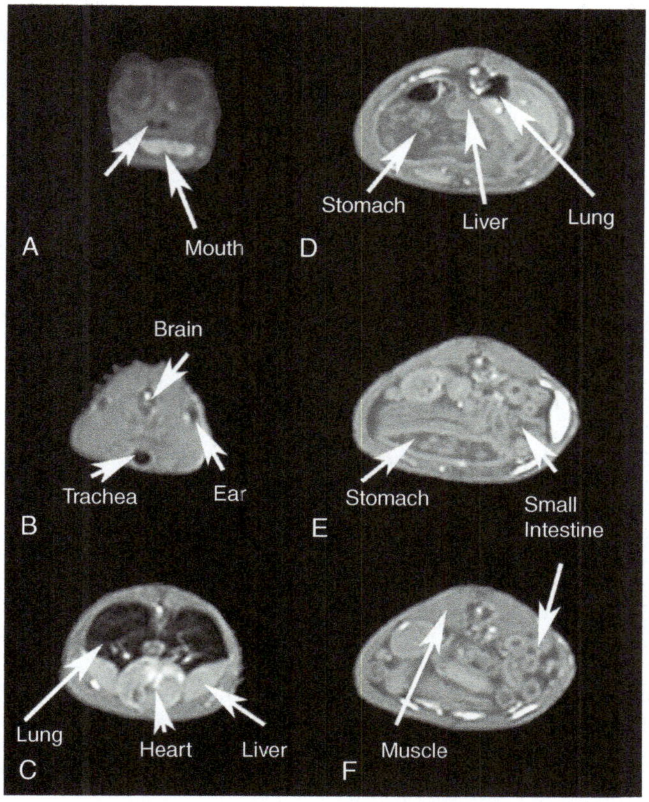

FIGURE 9-28 These axial magnetic resonance images (T2-weighted) are virtual sections of a small American Alligator *(Alligator mississippiensis)* and provide a survey of different parts of the animal from the head to the lower abdomen. The eyes appear as light gray ovals with dark gray centers (the vitreous); air in the nares, trachea, and ear cavities is black; and the brain is bright with gray surrounding bone (**A** and **B**). At the level of the heart, the great vessels and the pulmonary circulation appear bright; the lungs are black; muscles and liver appear gray; the spinal cord and cerebrospinal fluid (CSF) appear white **(C)**. At the midbody, the lung sections are small. The stomach and liver are large, and cross-sections of major vessels including the abdominal veins and aortae can be seen **(D)**. More posteriorly, the remainder of the gastrointestinal tract can be seen, as well as areas with bright coelomic fluid and blood in large vessels; gray back muscles occupy much of the dorsal body (**E** to **F**). Compare this composite with Figure 9-2 to see the differences in the two imaging modes. American Alligator; snout-vent length, 22 cm.

REFERENCES

1. Lee SH, Rao KCVG, Zimmerman RA. *Cranial and spinal MRI and CT*. 4th ed. Kingsport, Tenn, McGraw-Hill Professional, 1999.
2. Wu YT. From CT image to 3D model-creating physical models of patients through imaging. *Advanced Imaging-Fort Atkinson* 2001;16(8):20-23.
3. Mitchell MA. Managing the reptile patient in the veterinary hospital: establishing a standard of care model for nontraditional species. *J Exot Pet Med* 2010;19:56-72.
4. Stoskopf MK, Brown J, DeVoe R. Imaging in zoological medicine practice. *J Radiol* Nurs 2012;31:81-90.
5. Gumpenberger M, Henninger W. The use of computed tomography in avian and reptilian medicine. *Semin Avian Exot Pet Med* 2001;10:174-180.
6. Straub Jurina K. Magnetic resonance imaging in chelonians. *Semin Avian Exot Pet* Med 2001;10:181-186.
7. Valente AL, Cuenca R, Parga ML, et al. Cervical and coelomic radiologic features of the loggerhead sea turtle, *Caretta caretta*. *Can J Vet Res* 2006;70:285-290.
8. Valente AL, Cuenca R, Zamora MA, et al. Computed tomography of the vertebral column and coelomic structures in the normal loggerhead sea turtle *(Caretta caretta)*. *Vet J* 2007;174:362-370.
9. Valente AL, Marco I, Zamora MA, et al. Radiographic features of the limbs of juvenile and subadult loggerhead sea turtles *(Caretta caretta)*. *Can J Vet Res* 2007;71:305-313.
10. Banzato T, Selleri P, Veladiano IA, et al. Comparative evaluation of the cadaveric, radiographic and computed tomographic anatomy of the heads of green iguana *(Iguana iguana)*, common tegu *(Tupinambis merianae)* and bearded dragon *(Pogona vitticeps)*. *BMC Vet Res* 2012;8:53.
11. American Association of Physicists in Medicine (AAPM). *AAPM CT Lexicon Version 1.2*. College Park, Md: AAPM, 2012.
12. ULTRAVIST 2011. Bayer HealthCare Pharmaceuticals Web site. Available at: http://bayerimaging.com/index.php. Accessed April 14, 2012.
13. Pietsch H. CT contrast agents. In: Kiessling F, Pichler BJ, Hauff P, eds. *Small animal imaging*. Part 3. New York: Springer, 2011;141-149.
14. Reisz RR, Scott DM, Pynn BR, et al. Osteomyelitis in a Paleozoic reptile: ancient evidence for bacterial infection and its evolutionary significance. *Naturwissenschaften* 2011;98:551-555.
15. Witmer LM, Ridgely RC, Dufeau DL, et al. Using CT to peer into the past: 3D visualization of the brain and ear regions of birds, crocodiles, and nonavian dinosaurs. In Endo H, Frey R, eds. *Anatomical imaging: towards a new morphology*. New York: Springer, 2008;67-87.
16. Ziegler A, Kunth M, Mueller S, et al. Application of magnetic resonance imaging in zoology. *Zoomorphology* 2011;130:227-254.
17. Raiti P, Haramati N. Magnetic resonance imaging and computerized tomography of a gravid leopard tortoise *(Geochelone pardalis pardalis)* with metabolic bone disease. *J Zoo Wildl Med* 1997;28: 189-197.
18. Abou-Madi N, Scrivani PV, Kollias GV, et al. Diagnosis of skeletal injuries in chelonians using computed tomography. *J Zoo Wildl Med* 2004;35: 226-231.
19. Pees M, Kiefer I, Ludewig E, et al. Comparative use of modern imaging techniques for the diagnosis of pneumonia in three Indian pythons *(Python molurus)*. *Vet Comp Orthopaed* 2006;2006:275-282.
20. Mackey EB, Hernandez-Divers S, Holland M, et al. Clinical technique: application of computed tomography in zoological medicine. *J Exot Pet Med* 2008;17:198-209.
21. Pees M, Kiefer I, Thielebein J, et al. Computed tomography of the lung of healthy snakes of the species *Python regius, Boa constrictor, Python reticulatus, Morelia viridis, Epicrates cenchria*, and *Morelia spilota*. *Vet Radiol Ultrasound* 2009;50:487-491.
22. Roger Wilkinson R, Hernandez-Divers S, Lafortune M, et al. Diagnostic imaging techniques. In: McArthur S, Wilkinson R, Meyer J, eds. *Medicine and surgery of tortoises and turtles*. Oxford, England: Blackwell Publishing Ltd, 2008;187-238.
23. Jordin D, Green MS, Reed A, et al. Two- and three-dimensional MR coronary angiography with intraarterial injections of contrast agent in dogs: a feasibility study. *Radiology* 2003;226:272-277.
24. Gavin PR, Bagley RS. *Practical small animal MRI*. Ames, Iowa: Wiley-Blackwell, 2009.
25. Fleming GJ, Lester NV, Stevenson R, et al. High field strength (4.7t) magnetic resonance imaging of hydrocephalus in an African grey parrot *(Psittacus erithacus)*. *Vet Radiol Ultrasound* 2003;44:542-545.
26. De Decker S, Gielen IMVL, Duchateau L, et al. Agreement and repeatability of linear vertebral body and canal measurements using computed tomography (CT) and low field magnetic resonance imaging (MRI). *Vet Surg* 2010;39:28-34.
27. Arencibia A, Hidalgo MR, Vázquez JM, et al. Sectional anatomic and magnetic resonance imaging features of the head of juvenile loggerhead sea turtles *(Caretta caretta)*. *Am J Vet Res* 2012;73:1119-1127.
28. Jones MEH, Werneburg I, Curtis N, et al. The head and neck anatomy of sea turtles (Cryptodira: Chelonioidea) and skull shape in testudines. *PLoS ONE* 2012; 7(11): e47852. doi:10.1371/journal.pone.0047852
29. Steeil JC, Schumacher J, Hecht J, et al. Diagnosis and treatment of a pharyngeal squamous cell carcinoma in a Madagascar ground boa (*Boa madagascariensis*). *J Zoo Wildl Med* 2013;44(1):144-151.
30. Lim CK, Kirberger RM, Lane EP, et al. Computed tomography imaging of a leopard tortoise (*Geochelone pardalis pardalis*) with confirmed pulmonary fibrosis: a case report. *Acta Vet Scand* 2013;55:35:1-6.

RECOMMENDED READING

Kardong KV. *Vertebrates: comparative anatomy, function, evolution*. 6th ed. New York: McGraw-Hill Co, 2011.

Kiessling F, Pichler BJ, Hauff P, eds. *Small animal imaging*. Part 3. New York: Springer, 2011;141-149.

Romer AS. *The vertebrate body*. Philadelphia: WB Saunders Co, 1970.

Witherington D, Wyneken J. Chelonian anatomy. *Exotic DVM* 2003;4:35-41.

Witherington D, Wyneken J. Snake anatomy. *Exotic DVM* 2003;5:38-42.

Wyneken J. *Guide to the anatomy of sea turtles*. NMFS Tech Publication NOAA Tech, Memo NMFS-SEFSC-470, 2001.

Wyneken J. Respiratory anatomy: form and function in reptiles. *Exotic DVM* 2001;3:17-22.

Wyneken J. The external morphology, musculoskeletal system, and neuro-anatomy of sea turtles. In: Lutz P, Musick J, Wyneken J, eds. *The biology of sea turtles*. Vol. II. Boca Raton, Fla: CRC Press Inc, 2003.

Wyneken J. The skeleton—imaging in vivo. In: Wyneken J, Musick J, Lohmann K, eds. *The biology of sea turtles*. Vol. III, Boca Raton, Fla: CRC Press Inc, 2013.

CHAPTER 10

Ultrasonography

Claudia Hochleithner and
Mason Holland

Ultrasound has been used in small animal medicine routinely for more than 20 years. It is likely the most important imaging modality other than radiography. Early sonographers of reptile patients adapted this procedure to the special anatomic situations encountered within the wide range of this class.[1-4] With continuing advances in ultrasound machines and transducers, the often small size of reptilian or amphibian patients is less of an obstacle. It is possible to perform ultrasound even in small geckos or chameleons, with transducer frequencies of 10, 12, or even 18 MHz. However, several unique considerations still must be kept in mind during ultrasound evaluation of these species.

EQUIPMENT

Given the advances in ultrasound technology and equipment over the last several decades, good-quality scanners with high-frequency transducers are available for a reasonable price. A single typically recommended ultrasound equipment setup does not exist because of the wide range of anatomic situations that may be encountered in reptiles. One example of a standard machine is MyLab30Gold Vet (Haslauer-Medizintechnik/Esaote Europe). Depending on the body shape and size, linear, convex, and sector probes may be used (Figure 10-1). For snakes and lizards the linear transducers are generally recommended (Figure 10-2). For chelonians, a sector transducer or convex transducer with a small footprint is advantageous because it fits in the small sonographic windows cranial and caudal to the thoracic limbs and cranial of the pelvic limbs. The frequency of the transducer depends on the size of the animal to be examined. High-frequency transducers have the advantage of superior spatial resolution, yielding excellent detail of superficial structures but have a limited depth of penetration. Lower frequency transducers, although lacking in fine anatomic resolution, have the ability to penetrate deeper into tissue. In small lizards, therefore, high-frequency transducers (10 to 18 MHz) yield the best results. In larger lizards, such as iguanas, 7.5 to 10 MHz linear or convex transducers are recommended. For larger patients such as giant tortoises, frequencies from 2.5 to 5 MHz are recommended.[5-14]

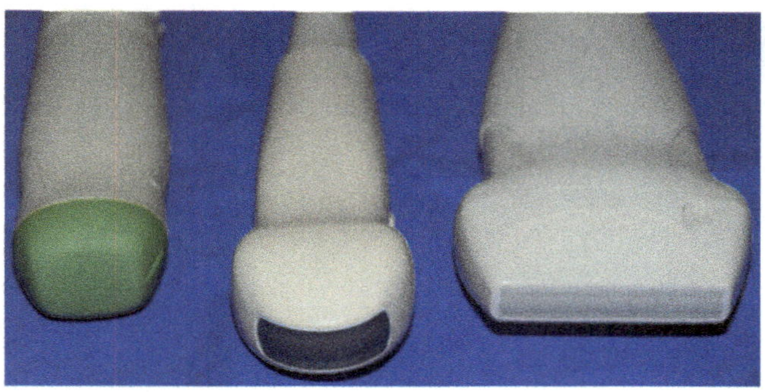

FIGURE 10-1 Ultrasound probes from left to right: phased array probe 5 to 7.5 MHz; microconvex probe 5 to 8 MHz; linear probe 10 to 18 MHz from Haslauer-Medizintechnik/Esaote Europe.

Special Considerations

Not only must the equipment and sonography suite be adapted to the special situations presented by reptile patients but the practitioner must also be aware of the wide variation in norms among the various species that may be encountered. There is a tendency to overinterpret normal structures in unfamiliar species, and whenever possible, known standards should be consulted, whether it be a different animal of the same or similar species or a published description of normal findings in that species.

It is difficult to accumulate expertise and perform a thorough evaluation when sonographic evaluations are limited

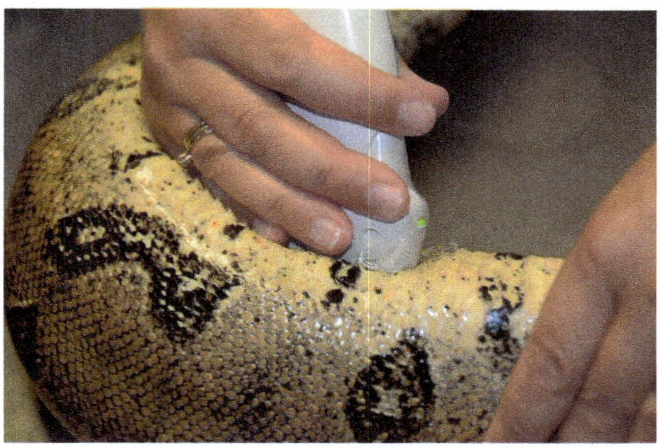

FIGURE 10-2 Performing ultrasound with a linear probe on a Boa Constrictor in a longitudinal plane; the green light indicates the cranial orientation of the indicator mark.

to short periods of available time between appointments. Ultrasonography, especially in unfamiliar species, is not a quick procedure. Therefore the office should be comfortable for the sonographer and the client, as well as for the persons handling the patient. A dim but not completely darkened room provides the best environment for viewing the monitor during the examination.

Proficiency in reptile ultrasonography is not easily acquired. Basic technical ultrasound skills needed to use the equipment and accurate interpretation of the findings are necessary. It is very advantageous to have experience in small animal ultrasonography in order to gain familiarity with the scanning technique and operation of the machine. Small animal patients are, in general, easier to evaluate and have a more uniform, familiar anatomy.[1-4] When the sonographer has accumulated this basic knowledge, the variable reptile anatomy and the unique sonographic appearances of reptile organs are more easily interpreted. Published literature describing the different reptilian species must be available, and special knowledge should be acquired during seminars, conferences, and laboratories. To improve image interpretation skills, one may also evaluate the organs of postmortem specimens in a water bath (Figure 10-3). This reduces artifacts caused by skin, scales, and other surrounding tissues and allows a more thorough evaluation of the viscera. Any abnormalities detected can be correlated with histopathologic findings (Figure 10-4,) to clarify the etiology of the disease process.

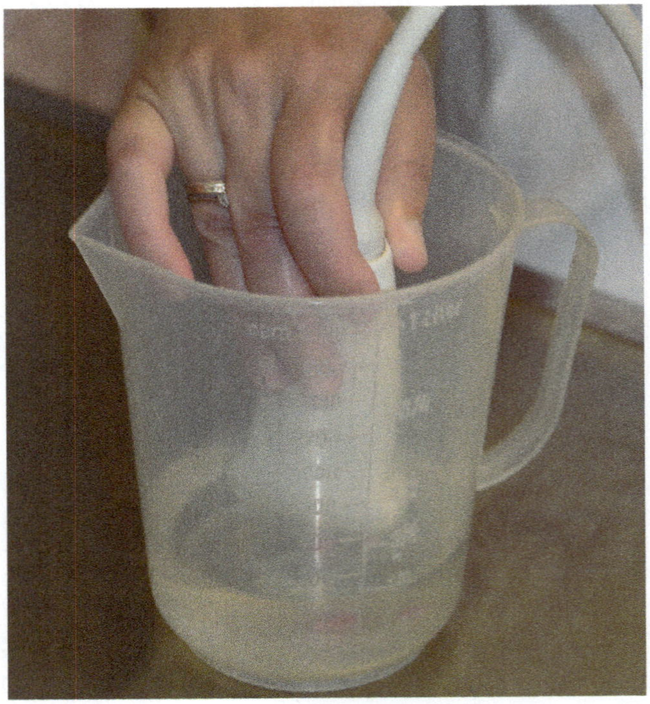

FIGURE 10-3 Water bath for investigating postmortem organs or tumors after surgery; results can be compared with histopathologic findings or can be used for self-training.

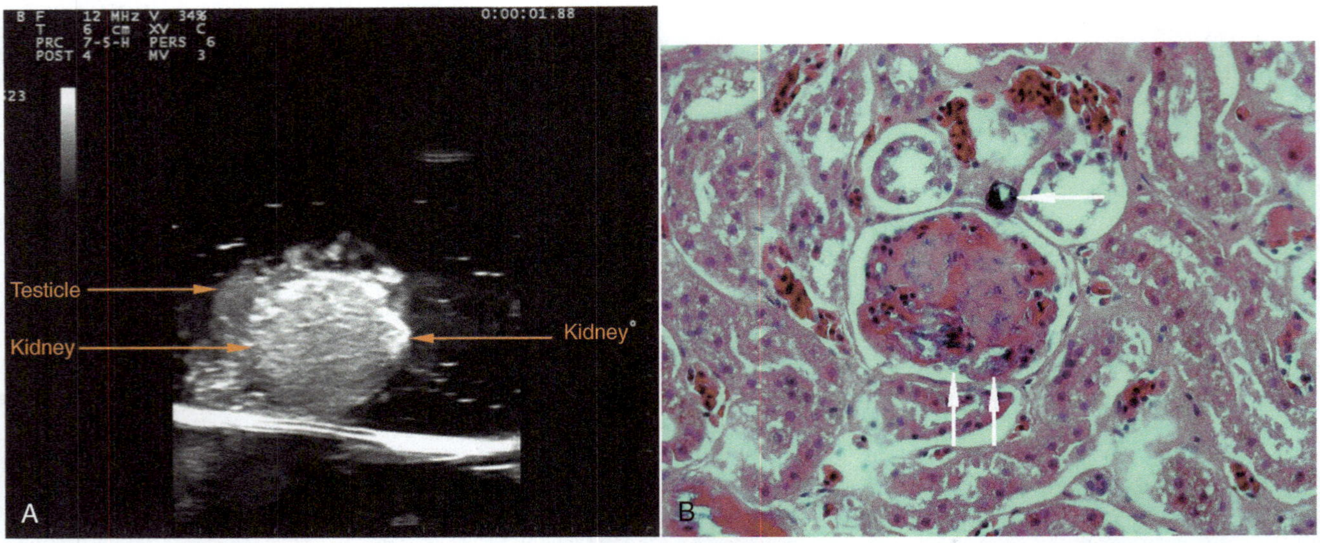

FIGURE 10-4 **A,** Post-mortem kidney and testicle ultrasound image in water bath; Greek Tortoise *(Testudo hermanni).* **B,** Histopathologic diagnosis of changes in kidney of the Greek Tortoise from **A.** Section of the kidney with calcium microlite *(a)* and dusty deposition of calcium within the glomerulus *(b).* Magnification, ×400. *(Dr. Anna Kuebber-Heiss, Research Institute of Wildlife Ecology, University of Veterinary Medicine Vienna.)*

PATIENT PREPARATION

Positioning of the patient must be adapted to what the patient will tolerate while allowing access to the anatomic regions of interest. Typically, dorsal recumbency is the most useful position, but an upright position may also be helpful, especially in weak lizards and in iguanas (Figure 10-5). Large snakes need more personnel to hold them comfortably for this procedure. In aggressive reptiles, sedation should be used to minimize the stress for the animal and the risk to the patient or the technicians.

It is important to develop a routine scanning technique that covers all typically visible organs so that an important sonographic finding is not missed. Whenever possible, each organ should be scanned in two planes: usually transverse and sagittal/longitudinal. Oblique scanning planes are also frequently used to evaluate organs and pathology of variable shape and anatomic location. The probe should always be held in the same fashion such that the sonographer is oriented to the spatial relationship between the tissues being scanned and their appearance on the screen.[5-9,13,14] Standard convention dictates that when the patient is in dorsal recumbency, the head is on the left side or facing away from a right-handed sonographer and the transducer is gripped so that the indicator of the probe shows either cranially or to the right side of the patient's body (Figures 10-6 through 10-9). When this technique is used, the left side of the image on the monitor is cranial in a longitudinal/sagittal view and represents the patient's right in a transverse view (Figure 10-10).

The body shape of the snake lends itself to examination from cranial to caudal in longitudinal and transverse scanning planes. In chelonians, there are only three accessible sonographic windows: cranial to the forelimb beside the neck (to investigate the heart and the liver), in the axillary region (for the heart and the liver), and in the inguinal, prefemoral window (to assess the intestine, urogenital tract, and the bladder) (Figure 10-11). In soft-shelled chelonians, it is possible to scan the coelomic viscera through the plastron. This is occasionally

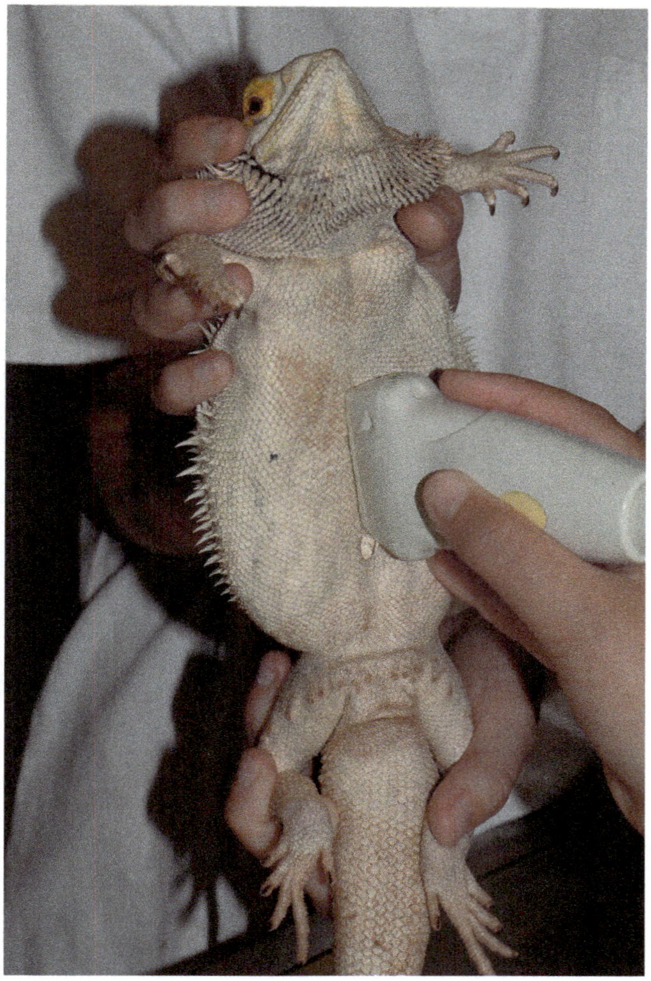

FIGURE 10-5 Upright positioning for weak patients. A Bearded Dragon *(Pogona vitticeps)* is held while ultrasound is performed.

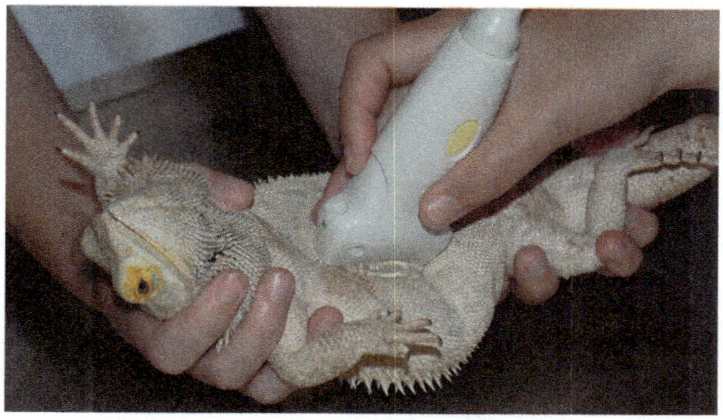

FIGURE 10-6 Positioning of the probe in a longitudinal view of a Bearded Dragon *(Pogona vitticeps)*.

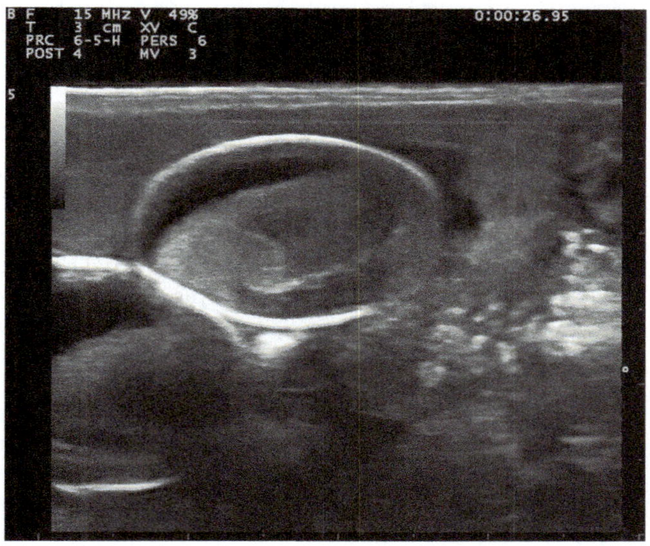

FIGURE 10-7 Sagittal plane image of an egg in the Bearded Dragon *(Pogona vitticeps)* from Figure 10-6. The hyperechogenic oval structure is the shell, the hypoechoic part is the albumin, and the rest of the content is the developing vitellogenic mass, shortly before being oviposited.

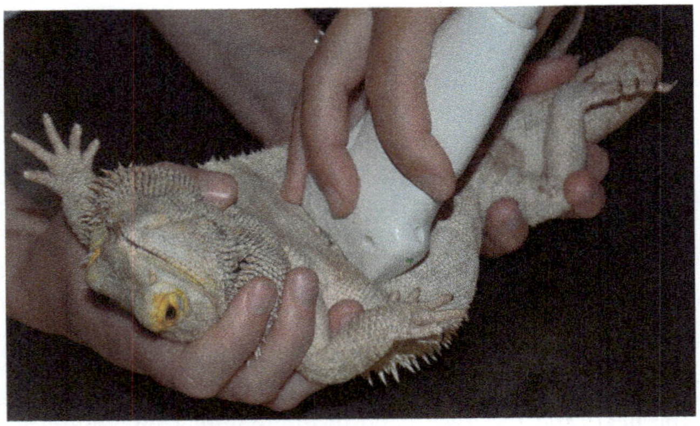

FIGURE 10-8 Positioning of the probe in a transverse imaging plane in a Bearded Dragon *(Pogona vitticeps)*.

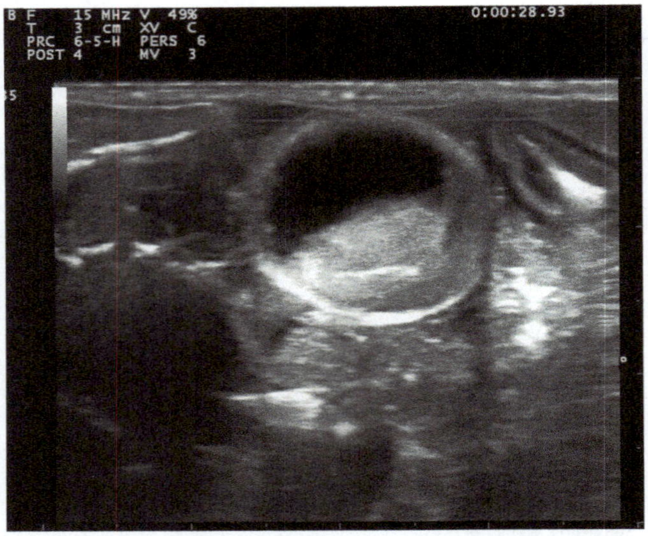

FIGURE 10-9 Transverse plane image of an egg in the Bearded Dragon *(Pogona vitticeps)* from Figure 10-8.

also possible in diseased chelonians if they have a poorly mineralized plastron (Figure 10-12).

Ample coupling gel must be applied to the skin surface. A gel bottle warmer should be used to prevent cooling of the patient. Better images can be obtained if the skin is moistened with warm water before the coupling gel is applied because contact is improved and trapped air bubbles that attenuate the sound beam are reduced. In chelonians and small patients, a stand-off pad to fill the space between the skin and the transducer surface may be helpful. An examination glove filled with warm water is a useful and substitutes for an inexpensive stand-off pad that can easily conform to the desired shape (Figure 10-13). Coating the standoff pad with coupling gel further enhances the image quality.

If the pressure of the probe on the patient's body is excessive, artifacts and inaccurate findings may result; excessive transducer pressure can result in compression and displacement of organs from their normal position, especially in snakes.

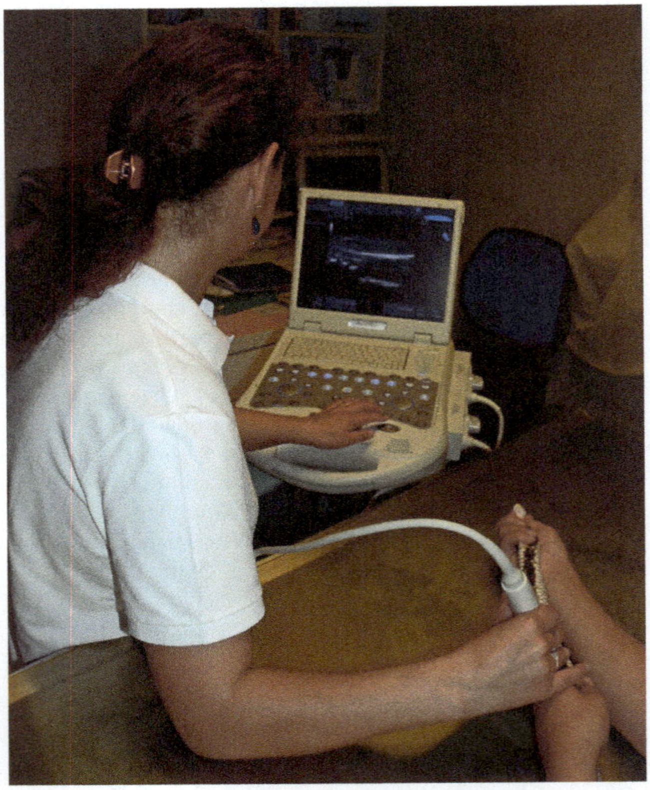

FIGURE 10-10 In dorsal recumbency, the head of the reptile is on the left side or facing away from a right-handed sonographer, so the indicator of the probe shows either cranially (in this picture) or to the right side of the patient's body.

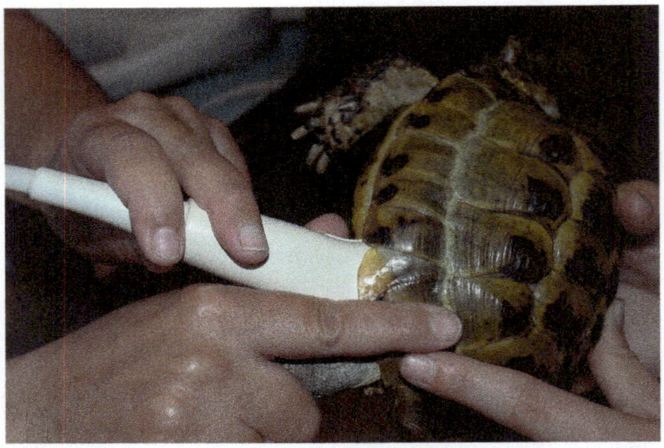

FIGURE 10-11 Prefemoral window to assess the intestine, urogenital tract, and the bladder in tortoises.

Although ultrasound is an excellent tool to investigate the organs of the coelomic cavity, some circumstances can complicate this procedure. Patients undergoing or soon to be undergoing ecdysis are poor candidates because air between the layers of the skin attenuates the majority of the sound beam, resulting in poor penetration of deeper tissues. Some species with ossified scales (e.g. *Tiliqua* spp. and *Heloderma* spp.) are also poor candidates because the ossified scales hinder penetration of the ultrasound beam.

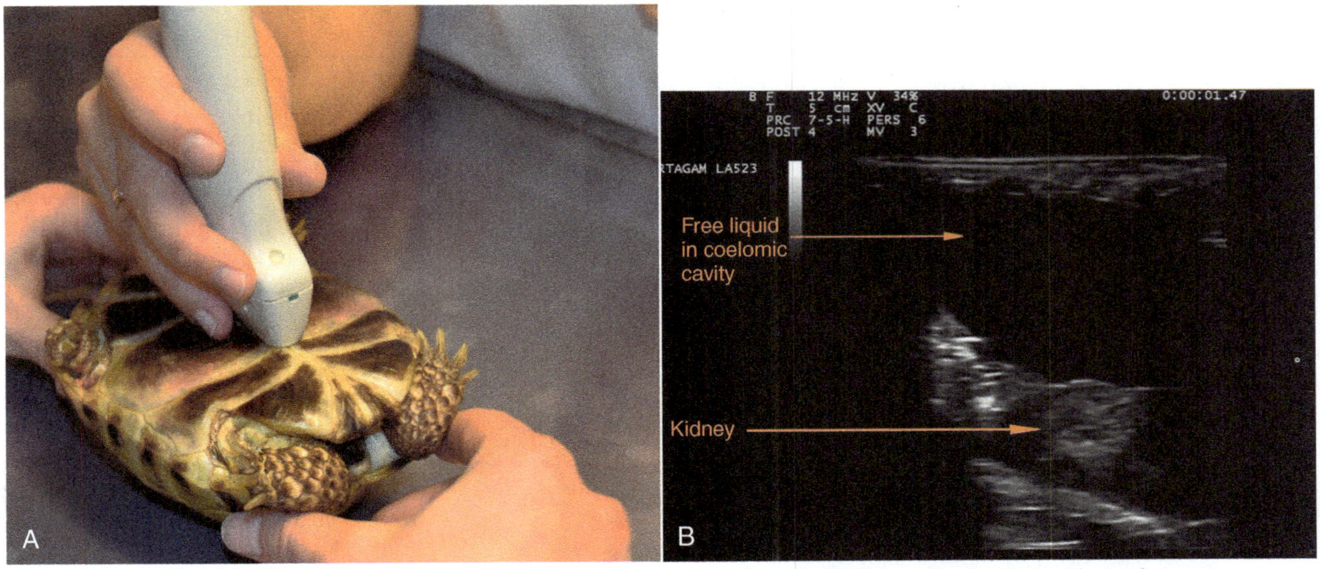

FIGURE 10-12 **A,** In diseased tortoises, it may be possible to scan the coelomic viscera through the plastron. **B,** Ultrasound image of the coelomic cavity of a diseased tortoise with renal failure due to secondary nutritional hyperparathyroidism combined with mismanagement of husbandry.

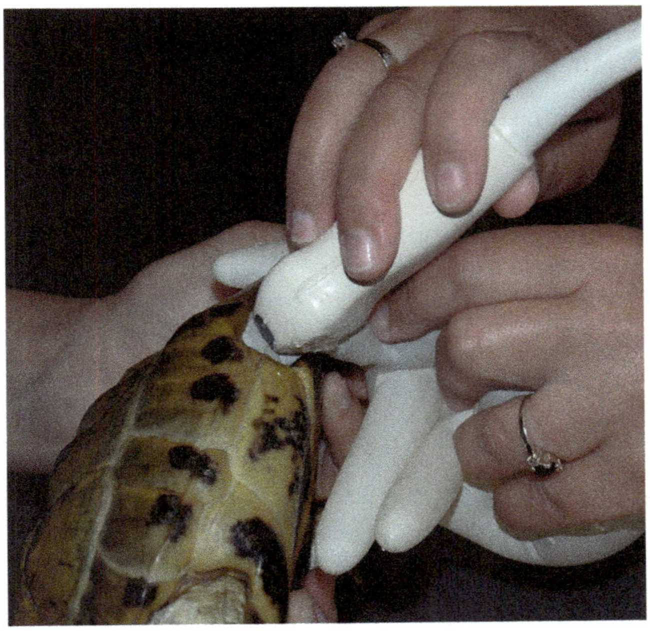

FIGURE 10-13 In tortoises, an examination glove filled with warm water can be used as a stand-off pad in the prefemoral window.

SCANNING PATTERN

The geometrically simple shape of the **snake** lends itself to the most straightforward method of sonographic examination. The heart is a useful starting point for establishing appropriate depth and settings on the machine. Blood in the vessels and chambers should be slightly hypoechoic to the cardiac muscle, and the valves should appear as hyperechoic lines. The body must to be scanned in saggital, transverse and dorsal (coronal) views caudally to the level of the cloaca (Figure 10-14).

In **lizards**, the liver and the gallbladder should be evaluated first. Adjustments should be made to the machine to at this time to tune image quality before proceeding to the rest of the exam. Next, the examination should move cranially to investigate the heart and then back again caudally with transverse and longitudinal views to investigate the fat bodies, gastrointestinal tract, gonads, bladder, and, finally, the kidneys.

Chelonians, except for soft-shelled species, are a little more challenging because they only have three useful acoustic windows to the coelomic cavity.[12]

The individual coelomic viscera are investigated by measuring the size, shape, and margination of each organ. Changes in echogenicity, either focal or diffuse, can be visualized and interpreted. The gastrointestinal tract is investigated as in small animals for motility, mural thickness, patency, and foreign content. With high-frequency transducers, intestinal wall layering can be appreciated (Figure 10-15).

The gonads are to be evaluated for size and shape in order to interpret the reproductive stage in both sexes. The kidneys are monitored for size and changes in echogenicity. The urinary bladder, when present, should be investigated for foreign material (e.g., calculi or ectopic eggs). Free coelomic fluid can be detected and assessed for echogenicity, amount, and cellular or solid content.

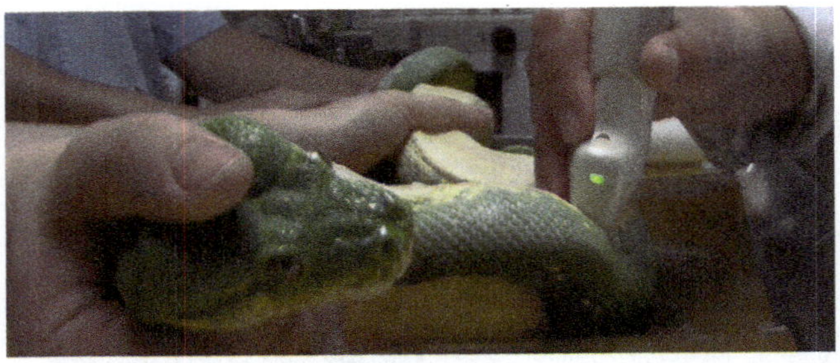

FIGURE 10-14 The simple shape of the snake lends itself to the most straightforward method of sonographic examination from cranial to caudal. All three planes should be scanned: sagittal, transverse, and dorsal.

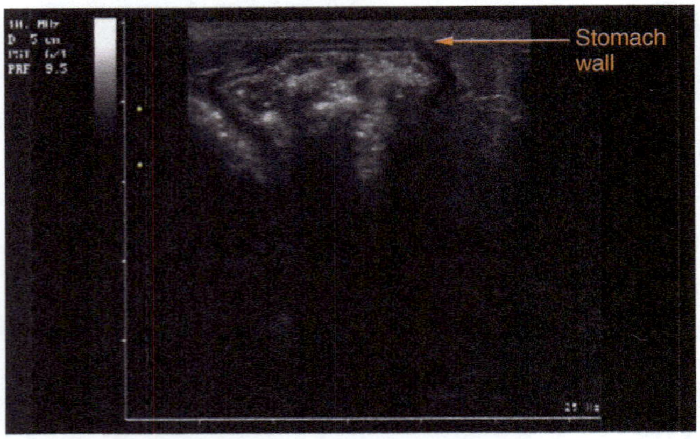

FIGURE 10-15 Ultrasound image of the different layers of the wall of the stomach of a Savannah Monitor *(Varanus exanthematicus)*. The first layer is the small hyperechoic line of the serosa, followed by the low echogenic muscularis layer; next is the higher echogenic submucosa, then the less echogenic mucosa, and the last layer is the highly echogenic mucosal surface, beneath which is seen the content of the stomach as an heterogeneous mass with some parts showing distal attenuation of the ultrasound beam (gas).

INDICATIONS

Ultrasound is often used as a tool for further imaging of a suspected abnormality, although, in many circumstances, ultrasonography has a clear advantage over radiology or endoscopy and may be chosen as the primary imaging modality.

Coelomic enlargements of unclear origin (e.g., tumors and ascites), along with reproductive monitoring, are the most common indications for ultrasonography. Any kind of enlargement on the animal's body can be scanned and interpreted to better characterize the nature of the swelling. Ultrasound-guided aspirates and biopsies may also be performed, but the need for these procedures should be evaluated in conjunction with possible risks such as organ perforation and hemorrhaging.[15,16] Reptile echocardiography is a relatively young field, but with improving equipment and continuing publications, the practical clinical utility of this will continue to increase.

THE HEART

Reptilian hearts, except those of the crocodilians, have three chambers: two atria and one (normally) thick-walled ventricle, which should not be mistaken for hypertrophic cardiomyopathy. The ventricle is divided by muscular septae in three subchambers: the cavum venosum, cavum pulmonale, and cavum arteriosum. The blood flows from the sinus venosum where the venae cavae join before emptying into the right atrium. From the right atrium, the deoxygenated blood flows to the cavum venosum and further on to the cavum pulmonale, which is the most ventral portion of the chamber. From there, blood passes via the pulmonary arteries to the lung. Oxygenated blood flows from the venae pulmonales to the left atrium and from there to the cavum arteriosum. During systole, the blood is circulated through the still partially contracted cavum venosum in the main circulation arteries.[17-20] All reptiles also have paired aortic arches, which are united to the aorta dorsalis. The atrioventricular valves are aligned such that they partially occlude the interventricular canal during atrial systole. During ventricular systole, they should prevent regurgitation of blood from the ventricle to the atria.

The most useful plane for investigating the reptilian heart is the sagittal plane (Figure 10-16, *A, B*). The second plane is the short-axis view, which is obtained by holding the transducer in a tranverse position, scanning the heart and the vessels from caudal to cranial (Figure 10-16, *C, D*). If the heart is cranially positioned, as it is in many lizards, it may be easier to view the heart from the left or right axillary region. For tortoises, the cervicobrachial window is applicable (Figure 10-17).

Changes in the size and the shape of the heart, contractility, and the pericardium can be assessed. A small amount of anechoic fluid in the pericardial space is normal (Figure 10-18).

Congenital and infectious diseases resulting in cardiac changes, such as endocarditis and myocarditis, have been described in the literature. Valvular disease, myocardial abnormalities, atrial thrombi, and neoplasia can be detected. The development of heart failure can be monitored with Doppler and M-mode measurements.[21-25] Uric acid crystal deposition within the myocardium or in the pericardial sac due to gout can be visualized (Figure 10-19).

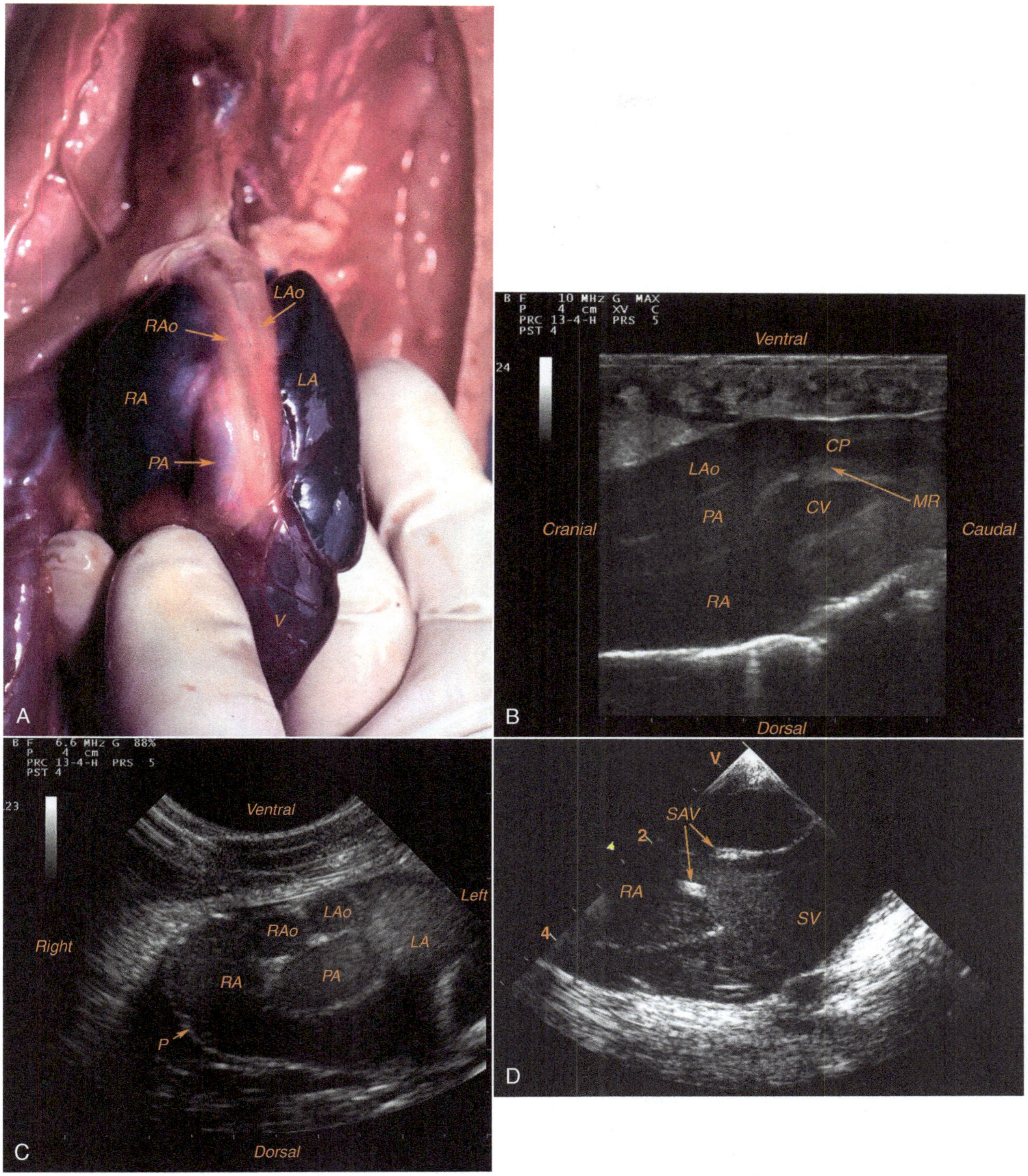

FIGURE 10-16 **A,** Ventral aspect of the heart in a Burmese python *(Python molurus bivittatus)* after resection of the pericardial sac. **B,** Echocardiographic examination in a Red-tailed Boa *(Boa constrictor imperator).* Long-axis view, right atrioventricular section. **C,** Echocardiographic examination in a Ball Python *(Python regius).* Short-axis view, transarterial section "Mickey Mouse Head" section (Photographs A-C courtesy L. Schilliger.) **D,** Echocardiographic examination in a Burmese Python *(Python molurus bivittatus).* Short-axis view, transatrial section (thickness because of suspected endocarditis). (Photograph courtesy V. Cherboul.) *CP,* Cavum pulmonale; *CV,* cavum venosum; *LA,* left atrium; *LAo,* left aortic arch (left aorta); *MR,* muscular ridge; *P,* pericardium; *PA,* pulmonary artery; *RA,* right atrium; *RAo,* right aortic arch (right aorta); *SAV,* sinoatrial valves; *SV,* sinus venosus; *V,* ventricle.

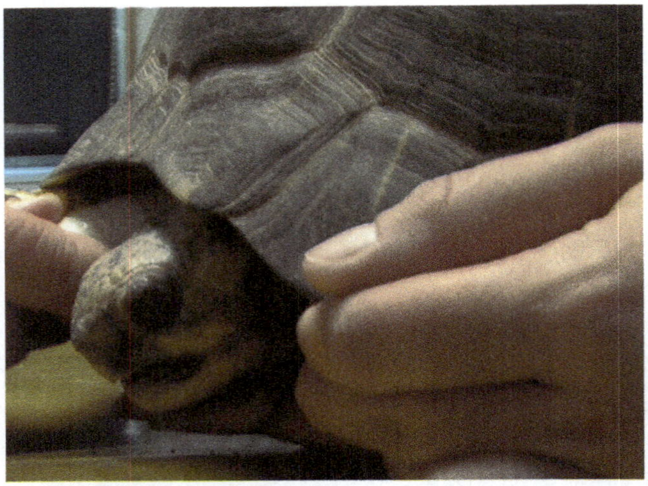

FIGURE 10-17 For investigation of the heart in tortoises, the transducer is placed into the cervicobrachial window on both sides.

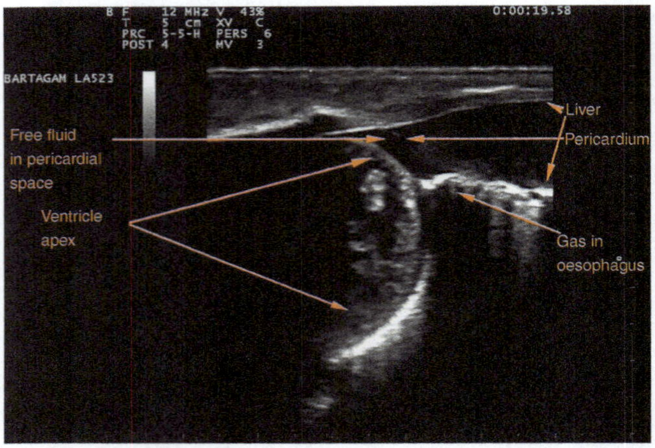

FIGURE 10-18 Free fluid in the pericardial space can be monitored during routine investigation. In this Green Iguana *(Iguana iguana)*, the amount is slightly increased because of early cardiac and renal failure.

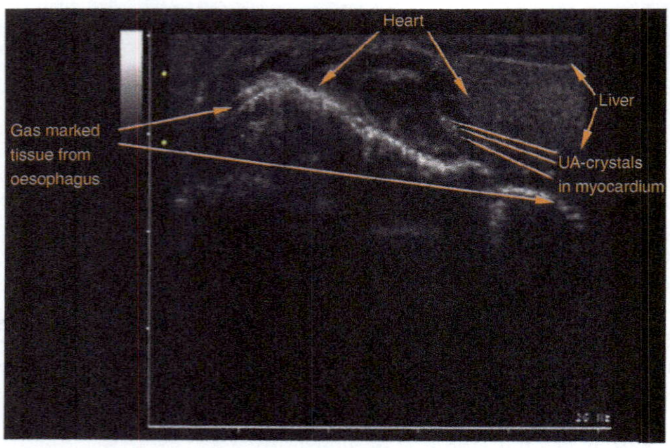

FIGURE 10-19 Mineralization, presumably uric acid crystal deposition in a Black-headed Monitor *(Varanus tristis)* due to renal disease can be seen in the myocardium as hyperechoic foci.

THE LIVER

The liver is characterized by a homogenous hypoechoic texture with anechoic vessels. In lizards and chelonians, the liver is bilobed. The anechoic gallbladder is attached to the right lobe[8,26] (Figure 10-20). With proper equipment, the portal vein, hepatic veins, and the caudal vena cava can be individually assessed (Figure 10-21).

In snakes, the liver extends caudally from the level of the lungs, where it occupies approximately the middle third of the length of the body. Two large vessels (the Vena hepatica portalis located dorsally, and the Vena hepatica ventrally) run from cranial to caudal through the length of the organ (Figure 10-22). The anechoic gallbladder is not associated with the hepatic parenchyma as it is in lizards and chelonians. Rather, the gall bladder is caudal to the liver and is visible as an anechoic round or slightly oval structure[8,9] (Figure 10-23). The liver can usually be easily differentiated from the fatbody (Figure 10-24).

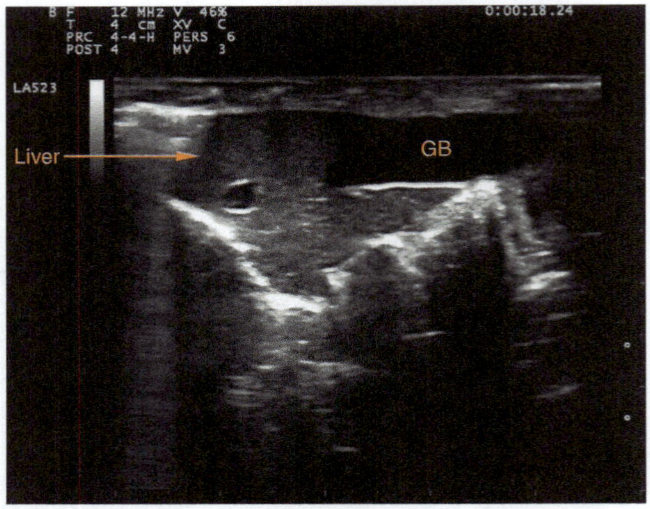

FIGURE 10-20 Ultrasound image of the homogenous hypoechogenic texture of the liver with the anechoic gallbladder attached to the right lobe in a Green Iguana *(Iguana iguana)*. *GB*, Gall bladder.

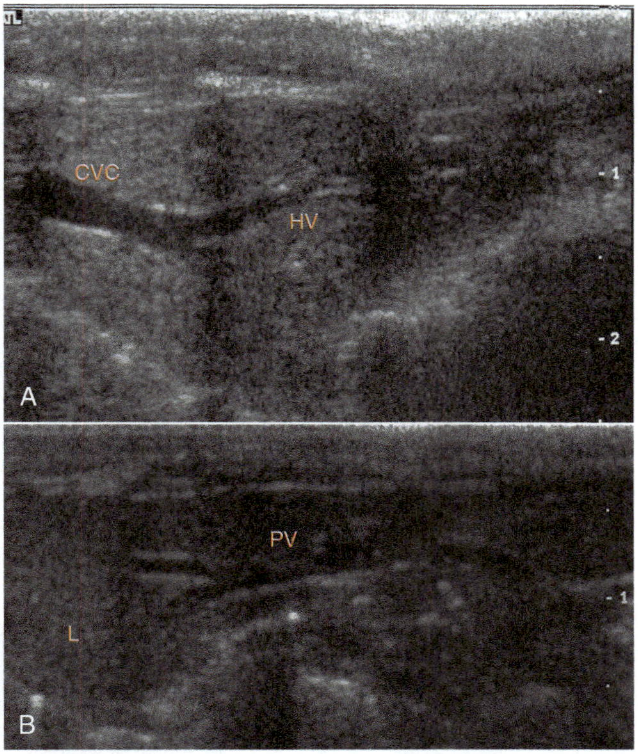

FIGURE 10-21 **A,** Oblique plane ultrasound image showing a hepatic vein *(HV)* entering the caudal vena cava *(CVC)* within the liver of a healthy Green Iguana *(Iguana iguana).* **B,** Sagittal plane ultrasound image showing the portal vein *(PV)* in a healthy Green Iguana originating in the caudal coelom and arborizing into the liver *(L)* on the left side of the image. *((Photo courtesy Dr. Mason Holland, Portsmouth, NH.)*

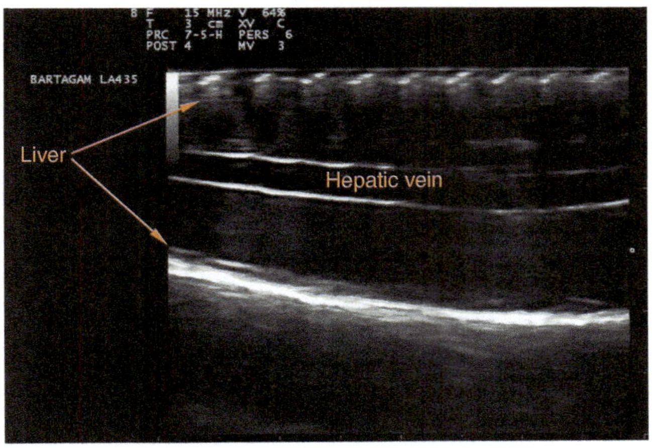

FIGURE 10-22 Sagittal plane image of the homogenous hypoechoic liver with the central hepatic vein in a Ball Python *(Python regius).* In this image, only the ventral Vena is seen as the probe is held slightly paramedian.

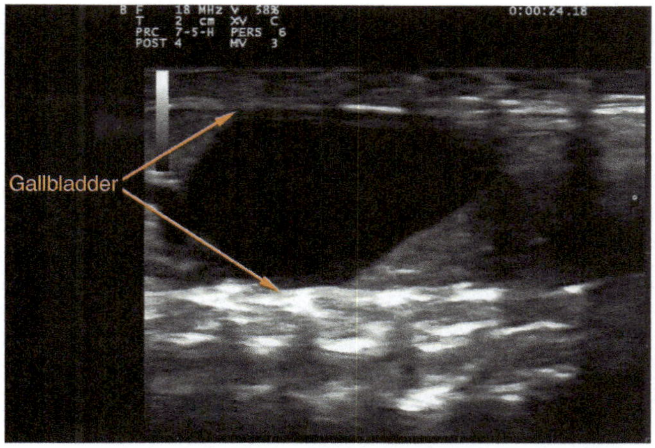

FIGURE 10-23 The gallbladder of snakes, here a Western Hognose *(Heterodon nasicus),* appears as a round to oval anechoic structure caudally separated from the liver.

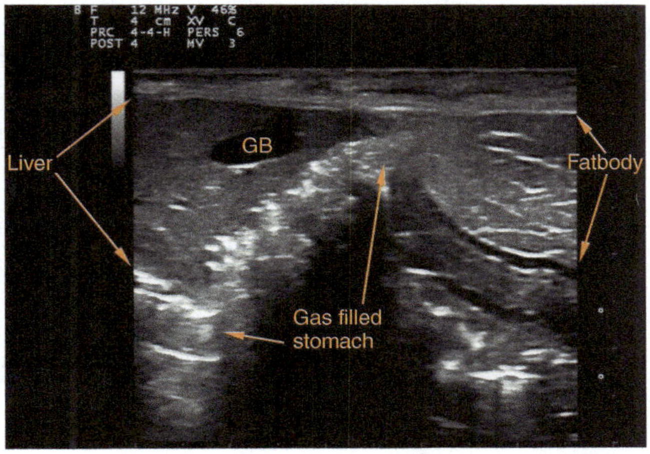

FIGURE 10-24 Ultrasound image of the echotexture of the liver in comparison with the higher echogenicity of the fatbody and the characteristic hyperechoic lines in between the fat in a Green Iguana *(Iguana iguana).* Between the liver and the fatbody is the gas-filled stomach, causing distal attenuation of the ultrasound beam. *GB,* Gall bladder.

Size and echotexture of the liver should be assessed; changes can be either focal, multifocal (Figure 10-25), or diffuse throughout the organ. These changes can be distinctly or indistinctly marginated, which can give a hint to the underlying process. Hyperechogenicity and enlargement of the liver are seen in connection with fatty liver degeneration (Figure 10-26). An heterogeneous pattern of the liver parenchyma with anechoic areas is common with focal necrosis or inflammation. Anechoic round or oval structures can be visualized in connection with cystic change (Figure 10-27). Hyperechoic particles in the gallbladder can be visualized as signs of thickening of the bile. Hyperechoic and heteroechoic lesions, usually focal and occasionally attached to the gallbladder, may represent abscessation[14] (Figure 10-28).

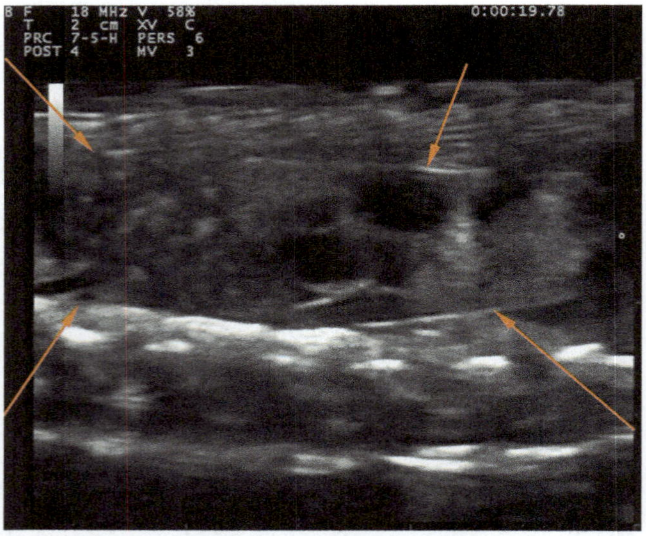

FIGURE 10-25 Ultrasound image of the liver (margins indicated with *arrows*) of a Western Hognose *(Heterodon nasicus)* showing a highly heterogenous pattern through the whole liver with round to oval anechoic structures—cystic changes. On histopathologic examination, it was diagnosed as liver carcinoma with cystic abnormalities.

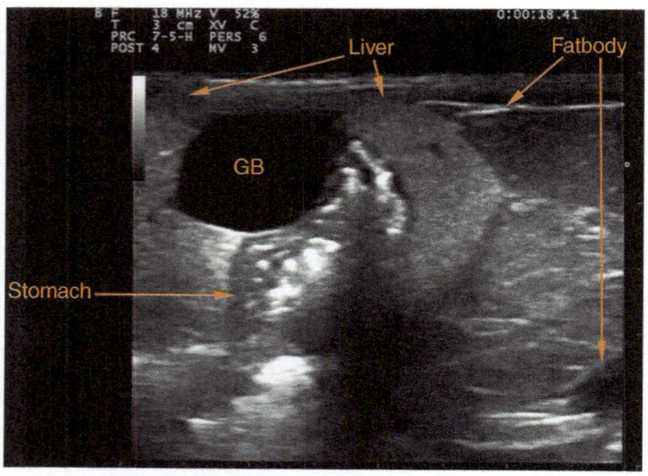

FIGURE 10-26 Sagittal plane image of fatty liver degeneration in a Bearded Dragon *(Pogona vitticeps)*. The liver shows greater echogenicity than the fatbody. In the middle of the figure, deep to the gallbladder, the stomach filled with ingesta and gas is visible. *GB*, Gall bladder.

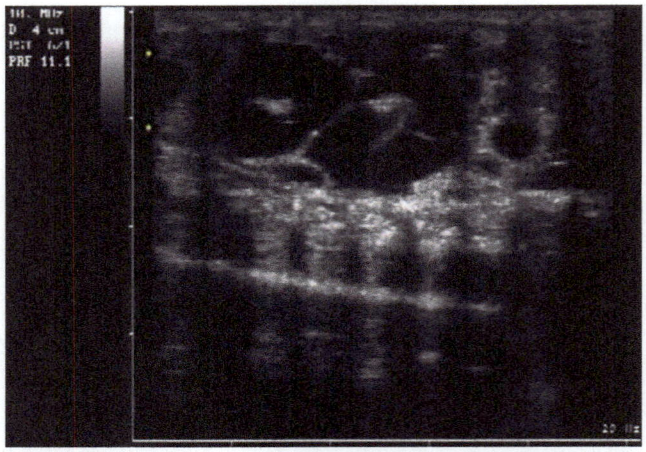

FIGURE 10-27 Ultrasound image of multiple anechoic structures in the liver of a Kingsnake (*Lampropeltis* sp.)—cysts, sagittal plane. On histopathologic examination, the changes in the liver were determined to represent cystic adenocarcinoma.

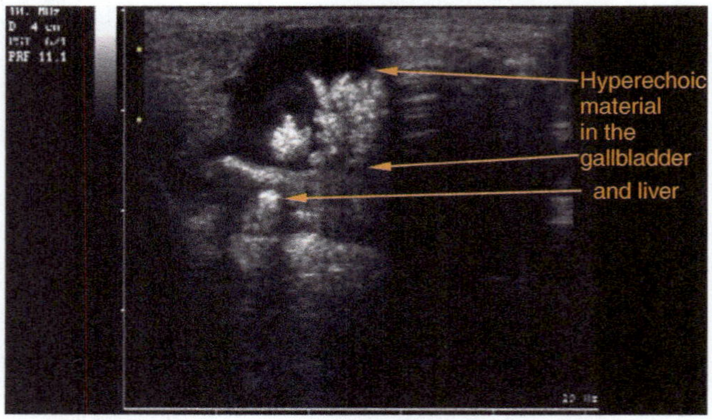

FIGURE 10-28 Ultrasound image of hyperechoic material in the lumen of the gallbladder and the surrounding liver tissue secondary to an abscess in a Bearded Dragon *(Pogona vitticeps)*.

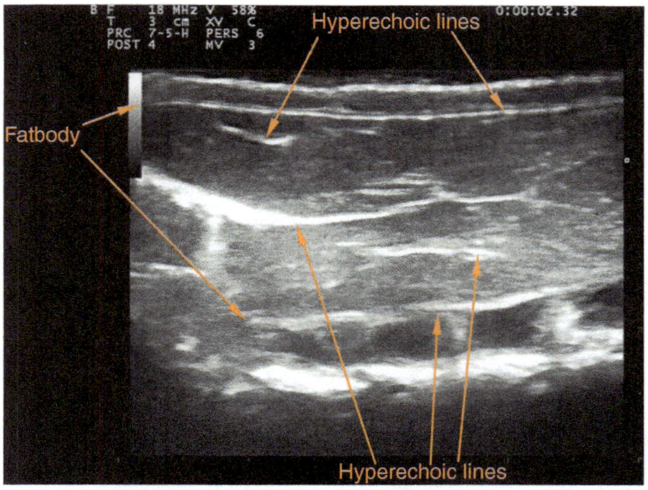

FIGURE 10-29 Ultrasound image of the fatbody in a Bearded Dragon *(Pogona vitticeps)* with normal hyperechoic lines in between the fat.

THE FATBODY

The fatbody varies in size and shape depending on the species and body condition of the patient. Normally, they are paired structures that lie laterally within the coelom, extending cranially from the region of the heart and liver to the caudal abdominal region. They show a greater echogenicity than the liver and curvilinear hyperechoic septae between fat lobules (Figure 10-29). Internal vasculature of the fat bodies will be less than that seen within the liver, which is useful to differentiate these two structures. The size of the fatbodies can give a good general assessment of the body condition of the animal (from emaciation through obesity). If a small amount of free fluid is present in the coelomic cavity (a common, normal finding), the fatbodies are easily distinguished. Abscesses or granulomas can be visualized as round, sometimes hyperechoic, sharply delineated structures with central hypoechoic/anechoic regions. Dystrophic mineralization or crystal formation in the fat pads are discernable by evidence of hyperechoic foci.

GASTROINTESTINAL TRACT

The gastrointestinal tract and the relationship between the size of the different portions varies greatly depending on whether the reptile is a herbivore, omnivore, or carnivore. In carnivorous reptiles, the stomach is large, and longitudinal folds can be visualized; the intestine is smaller and shorter compared with herbivorous animals. In herbivores, the stomach is smaller, has a thin wall, and the intestine is elongated with mucosal folds. Depending on the size of the animal and the frequency of the transducer, intestinal wall layering can be visualized, similar to mammals and birds (Figure 10-30). Changes in motility, foreign bodies, and large amounts of gas or impacted ingesta (such as sand impaction) can be visualized. Intestinal gas typically results in complete reflection of the ultrasound beam, preventing assessment of deeper tissues and evaluation of deeper structures. This is especially true in herbivorous species.

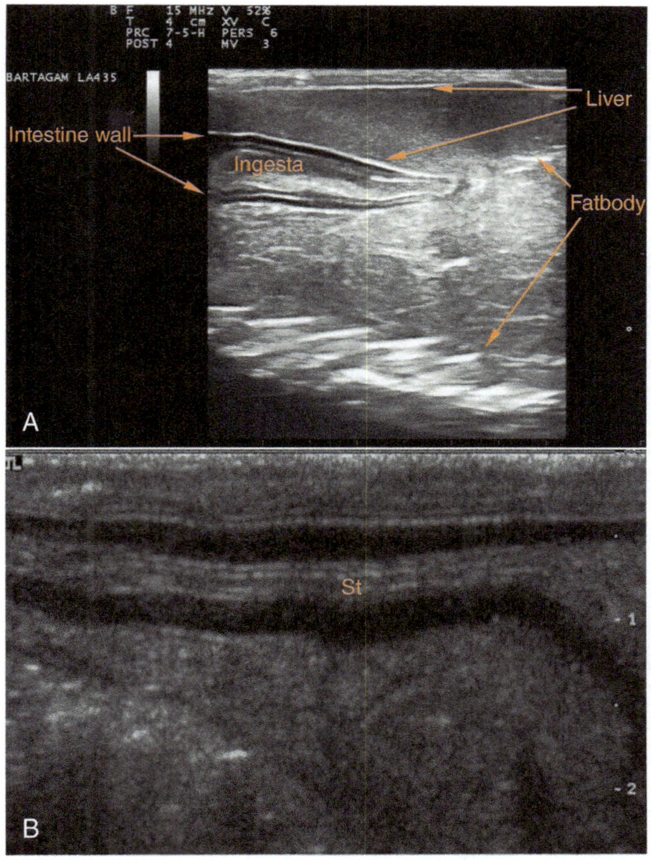

FIGURE 10-30 A, Sagittal plane image of a portion of the intestine in a Bearded Dragon *(Pogona vitticeps)* filled with ingesta. Intestinal layering is visible. The first small hyperechoic layer next to the liver is the small line of the serosa, followed by the low echogenic muscularis layer; next is the higher echogenic submucosa, the low echogenic mucosa, and the highly echogenic mucosal surface, beneath which is seen the content of the intestine (ingesta) as an heterogeneous mass. Below the ingesta is the intestine wall: small highly echogenic line of the mucosal surface, the low echogenic pattern of the mucosa, and the higher echogenic submucosa, followed by the low echogenic muscularis layer; next to the fatbody, as the last outside layer, is the small hyperechoic line of the serosa. **B,** Sagittal ultrasound image of the pyloric portion of a nondistended stomach (St) in a normal Green Iguana *(Iguana iguana)* showing prominent wall layering. A thick hypoechoic muscularis layer is present. Orad is to the right of the image.

Because ultrasound is often used as a further diagnostic tool after radiology, it should be performed before intestinal contrast studies. Barium has the same effect as gas or stones in the gastrointestinal tract, absorbing and reflecting the sound beam and limiting evaluation (Figure 10-31). Iodinated contrast media is, however, typically sonolucent.

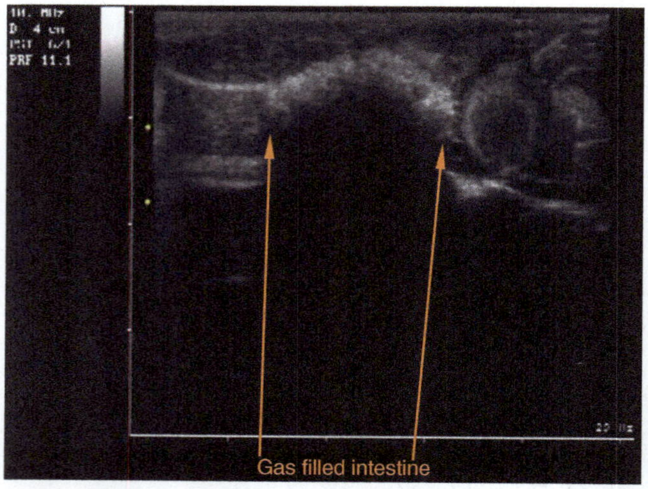

FIGURE 10-31 Ultrasound image of gas in the intestine with (distal) attenuation of the ultrasound beam in a Bearded Dragon *(Pogona vitticeps)*.

THE SPLEEN

The spleen is difficult to visualize because the organ is often located deep to the intestine, and evaluation is frequently limited by the presence of intestinal gas. Depending on the species, it is round to oval and of variable, generally small size; the texture is homogenous with medium echogenicity and fine granular echotexture similar to the testes[5-10,13,14,26] (Figure 10-32). In male Green Iguanas scanned during breeding season (early winter in the northern hemisphere), the spleen may be more easily seen because much of the adjacent intestine is displaced by hypertrophy of the adjacent testes[19] (Figure 10-33).

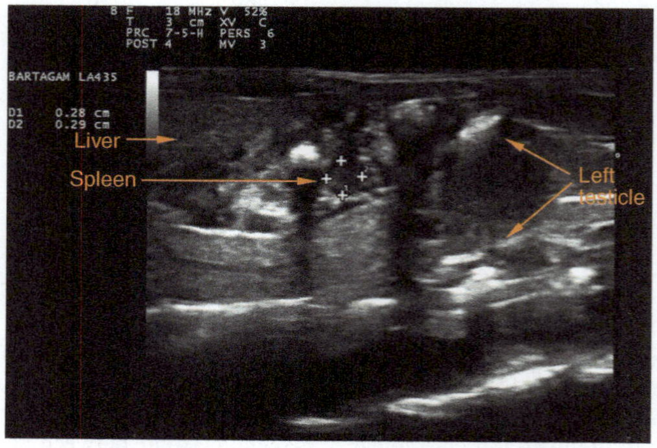

FIGURE 10-32 Ultrasound image of the spleen (+) in a Bearded Dragon *(Pogona vitticeps)* with adjacent intestine, liver, and left testis.

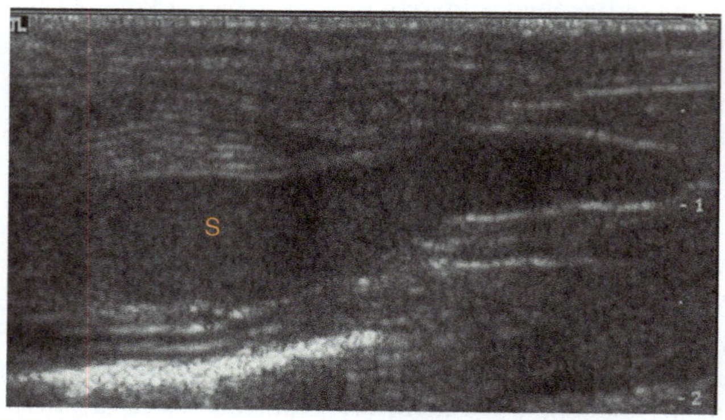

FIGURE 10-33 Sagittal image of the spleen *(S)* in a healthy male Green Iguana *(Iguana iguana)*. Physiologically enlarged testes have displaced overlying intestine but are not visible in this image because they were displaced from the plane by transducer pressure.

THE GONADS

Ultrasonography is the imaging modality of choice for evaluation of reproductive function, stage, and disease. Other applications include gender determination, evaluation of reproductive potential, and directing and assessing the efficacy of therapeutic interventions.[26-31]

Juvenile gonads are poorly visualized because they are obscured by intestine and are frequently small in size (Figure 10-34). The gonads lie in the last third of the body lateral to both sides of the abdominal aorta, and the right gonad is slightly cranial to the left. Depending on the age of the patient and stage of the reproductive cycle, the testes are ovoid and vary in size from barely visible to clearly obvious; they are especially pronounced in Bearded Dragon and Green Iguanas during breeding season (Figure 10-35). They show a fine, granular, homogeneous echo texture, are isoechoic to slightly hyperechoic to liver.

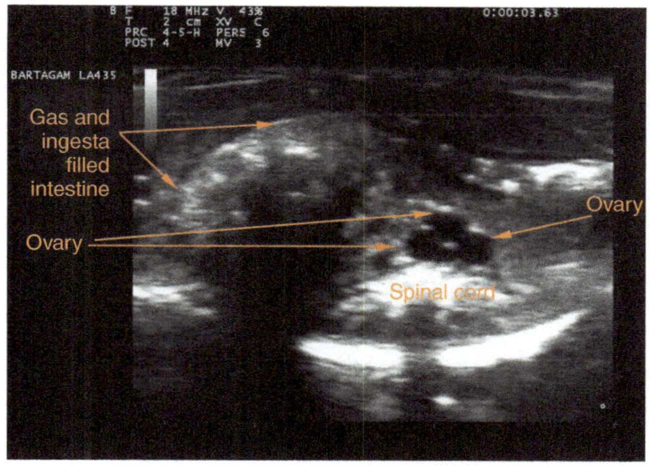

FIGURE 10-34 Ultrasound image in a transverse plane of the ovary as round anechoic structures ventral and lateral to the spinal cord in a 9-month-old Lawson's Dragon *(Pogona henrylawsoni).*

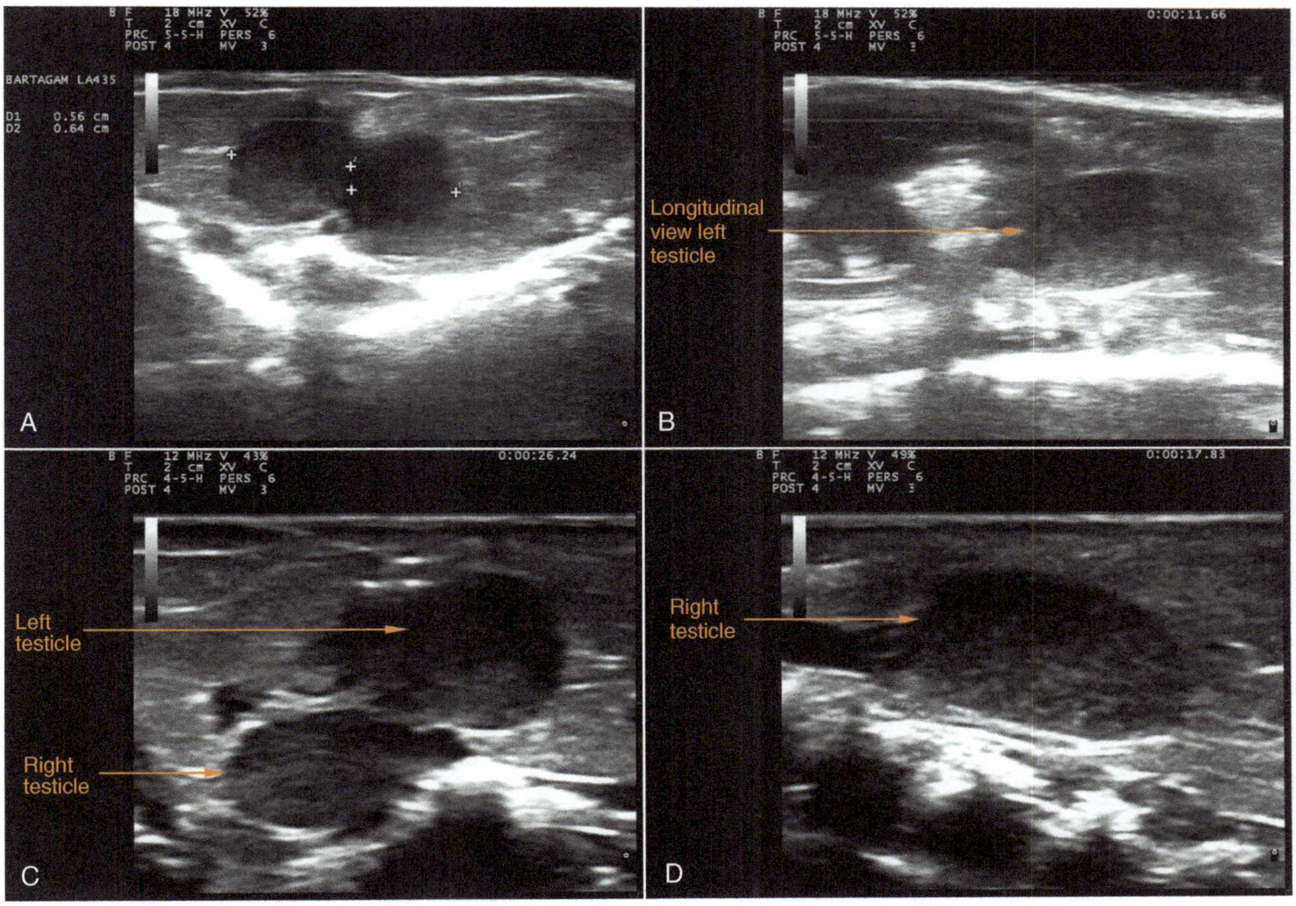

FIGURE 10-35 **A,** Transverse plane image of the testes in a 9-month-old Lawson's Dragon *(Pogona henrylawsoni).* The right testis lies slightly cranial to the left, showing finely granular and homogenous echotexture. **B,** Longitudinal ultrasound image of the left testis in the Lawson's Dragon *(P. henrylawsoni)* from **A. C,** Transverse plane ultrasound image of the testes in an adult reproductively active Bearded Dragon *(Pogona vitticeps).* **D,** Longitudinal view of the right testicle in the Bearded Dragon *(P. vitticeps)* of **C.**

The **ovaries** may be visualized, depending on their size. At the beginning of the reproductive cycle, the follicles are round and anechoic. In tortoises, they show higher echogenicity at this early stage. The size varies from one to a few millimeters (Figure 10-36). Before ovulation they grow to large round structures, and their echogenicity increases. In snakes, many anechoic, round structures can be visualized before ovulation, depending on the size of the snake (up to 2 cm in diameter in large pythons). In the late preovulatory state, nearly the entire coelomic cavity may be filled with rounded follicles (Figure 10-37). After ovulation, the ova elongate, and a slightly hyperechoic wall is produced. Depending on the species, the wall of the ova will range from noncalcified to calcified (Figure 10-38). The inside of the egg can be monitored, depending on the degree of calcification. At the beginning of pregnancy, the content can be distinguished as an anechoic layer of albumin and the hyperechoic yolk (Figure 10-39). Occasionally, a small embryo can be visualized. In ovoviviparous snakes, the development of the embryos can be monitored by the stage of development, activity, and heart beat (Figure 10-40).

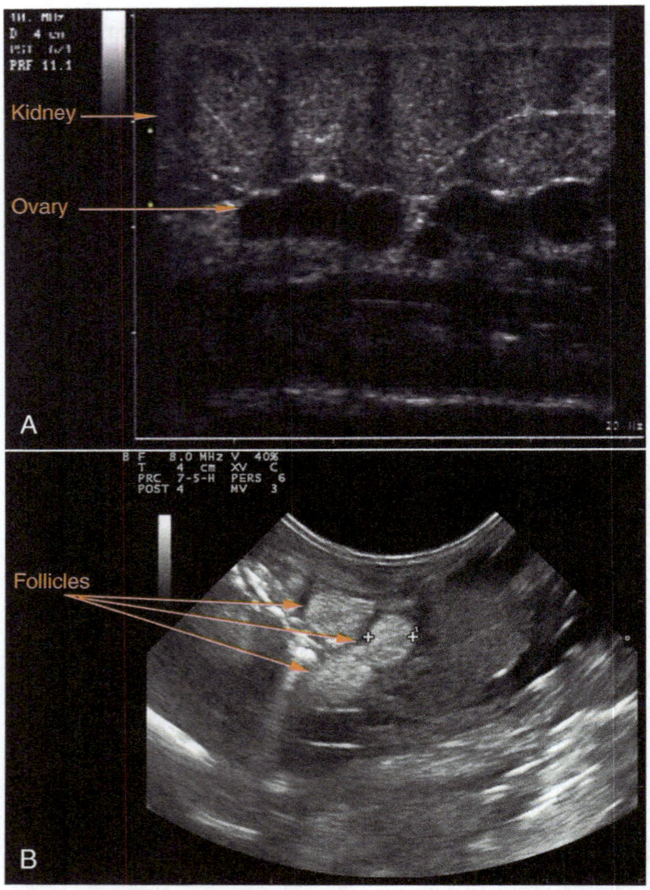

FIGURE 10-36 **A,** Longitudinal slightly paramedian ultrasound image of the ovary in a Green Tree Python *(Morelia viridis).* This is the beginning of the reproductive cycle, and different sizes of round, anechoic structures are aligned cranially to caudally. Laterally to the ovary, the right kidney is visualized. **B,** Ultrasound image of the follicles in a Red-eared Slider *(Trachemys scripta elegans).* In tortoises, unlike snakes and lizards, the follicles already show a higher echogenicity at this early stage.

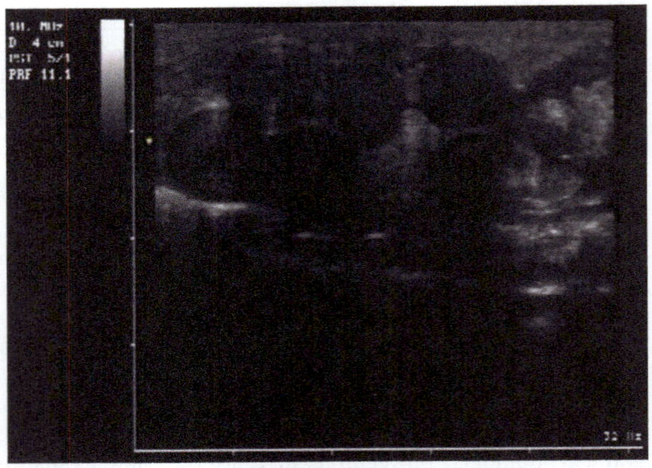

FIGURE 10-37 Ultrasound image of the ovary before ovulation in a Bearded Dragon *(Pogona vitticeps).* Round structures are starting to change from anechoic to more echogenic content. In this case, the Bearded Dragon developed preovulatory follicle stasis due to management problems in the environment.

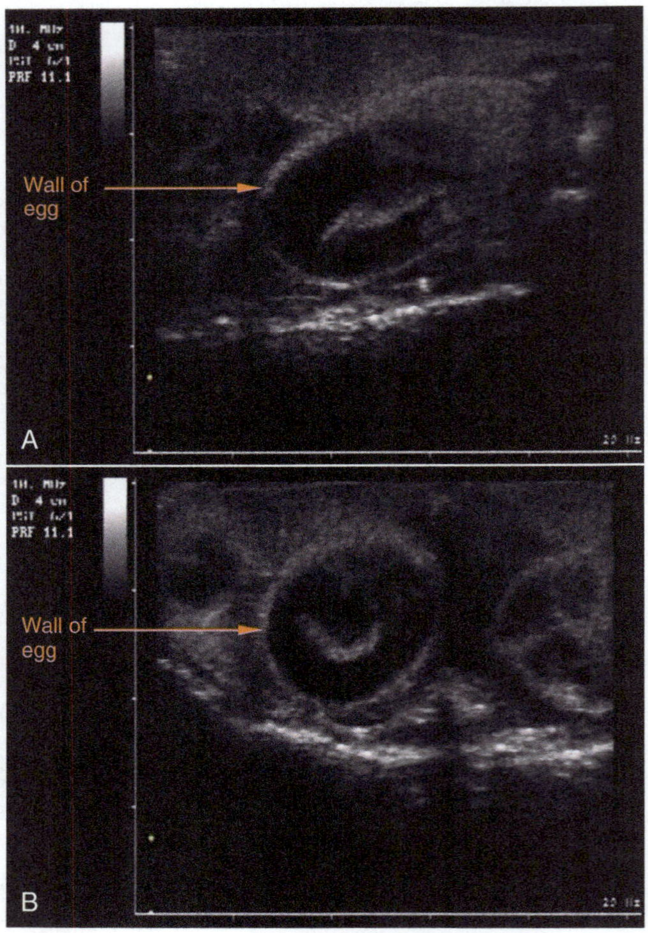

FIGURE 10-38 **A,** Ultrasound image (sagittal plane) of a more mature egg with higher wall echogenicity in a Bearded Dragon *(Pogona vitticeps).* **B,** Ultrasound image of the same egg in **A,** in a transverse plane.

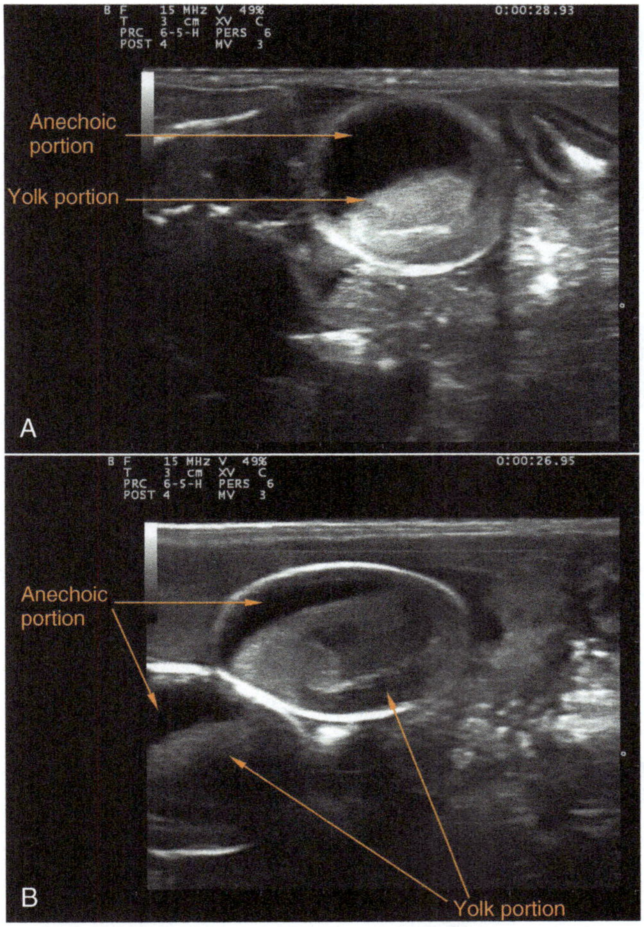

FIGURE 10-39 **A,** Ultrasound image of eggs in a Bearded Dragon *(Pogona vitticeps)* in a transverse plane with differentiation of the yolk portion (more echogenic) from the albumin, visualized as the anechoic part of the egg. **B,** Ultrasound image of one of the eggs from **A** in a Bearded Dragon in a sagittal plane with differentiation of yolk portion and anechoic part of the egg.

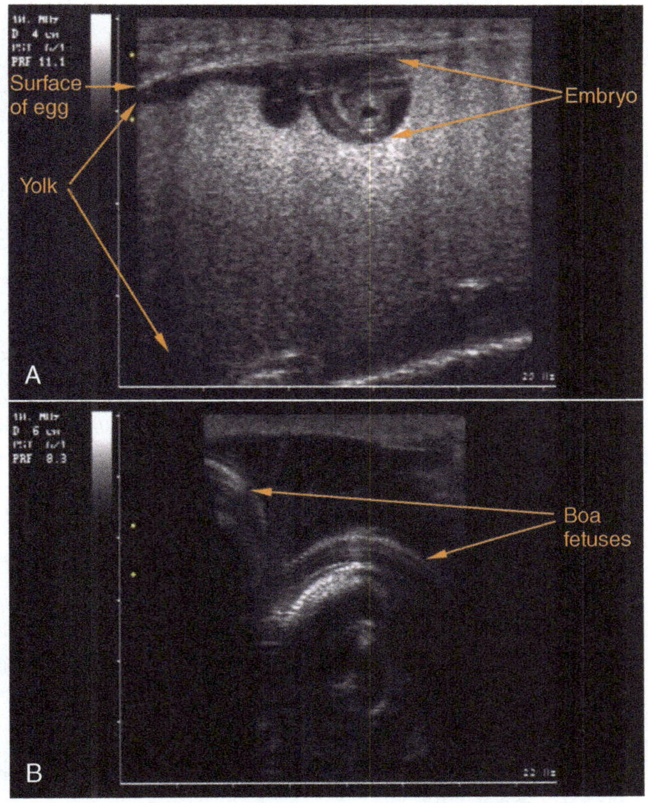

FIGURE 10-40 **A,** Ultrasound image of an egg filled with highly echogenic yolk and a small embryo developing in a Ball Python *(Python regius).* **B,** Ultrasound image just before birth in an ovoviviparous Boa Constrictor; it is also possible to see the movements of the fetuses and the beating hearts at this stage.

Pathologic changes can be monitored in all stages of the reproductive cycle. It is important to distinguish preovulatory from postovulatory status for detection of follicle stasis and egg binding. Normally, preovulatory follicles are uniform, round, and either anechoic or hypoechoic. As the follicles remain unovulated, more echogenic layers appear. In addition, the echogenicity changes to an heterogeneous pattern, the surface of the follicles is no longer smooth and well-demarcated, and anechoic fluid around the follicles can be visualized with echogenic free-floating particles in this fluid, indicating inflammation (Figure 10-41).

After ovulation, the ova change to a more elliptical, echogenic structure. The wall of the egg is normally smooth, and irregularity of the surface can suggest chronicity and prognosis in egg binding. An heterogeneous pattern of the content of the egg combined with free fluid in either the uterus or the coelomic cavity generally indicates a reduced reproductive prognosis. Pyometra after multiple problems with egg binding has been evaluated (Figure 10-42).

Ultrasound may also be useful in monitoring pathologic changes in the gonads. Gonadal origin of coelomic tumors is often difficult to confirm because of the variable appearance of the gonads, and this may be a diagnosis of exclusion, after successful identification of other normal-appearing coelomic structures (Figure 10-43).

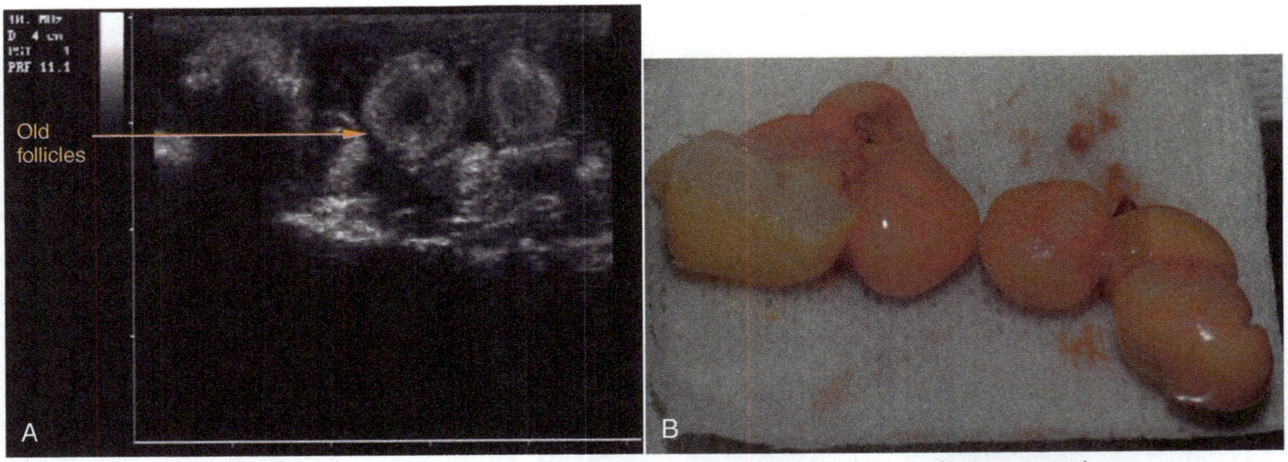

FIGURE 10-41 **A,** Ultrasound image of older preovulatory follicles before surgery in a Bearded Dragon *(Pogona vitticeps)*. The echogenicity increases and becomes slightly heterogeneous with aging of the follicles. **B,** Preovulatory follicle stasis in the Bearded Dragon from **A**. The content of the follicles firms with progression of stasis.

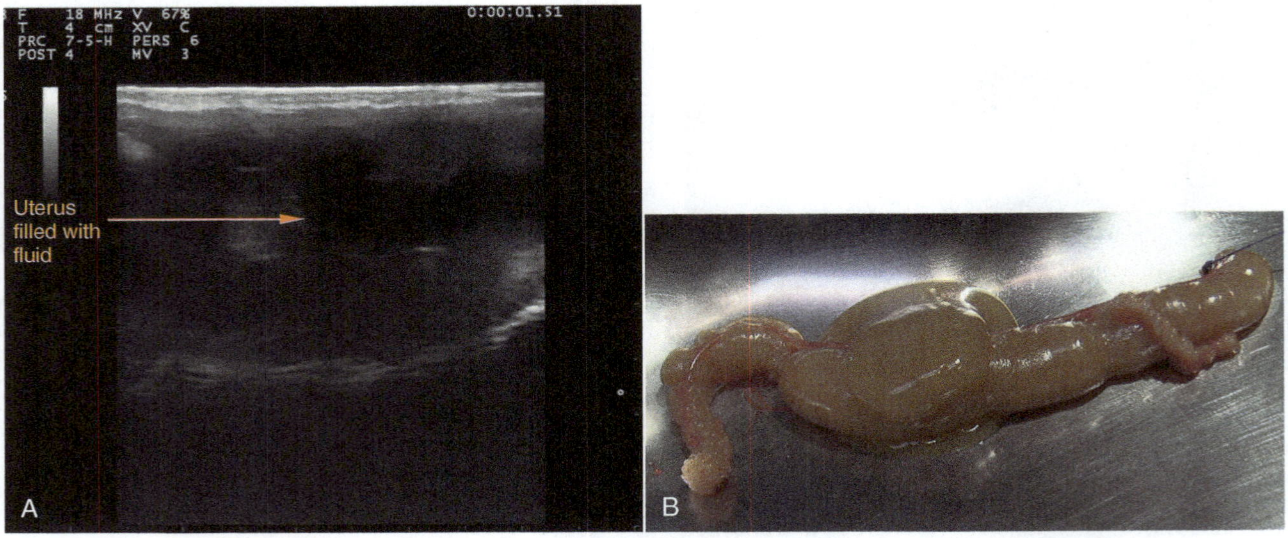

FIGURE 10-42 **A,** Ultrasound image of the abdomen of a Veiled Chameleon *(Chamaeleo calyptratus)*. The curved tubular structure with anechoic content visualized on the left side of the caudal coelom represents an accumulation of purulent material in the salpinx. **B,** Salpinx from the Veiled Chameleon in **A** filled with purulent exudate after surgery.

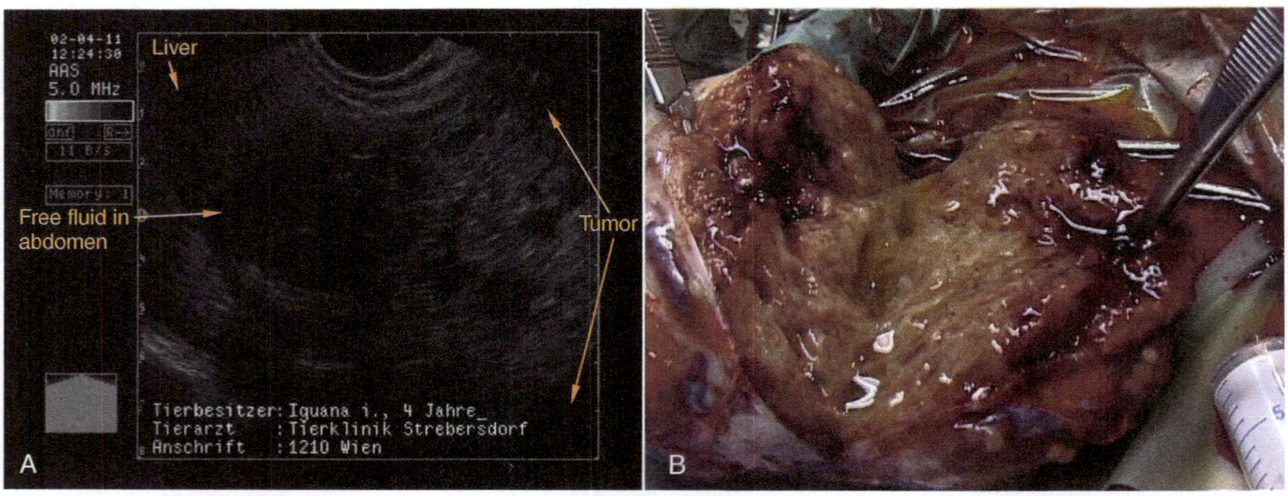

FIGURE 10-43 **A,** Ultrasound image of an heterogeneous mass with anechoic patches distributed multifocally throughout the mass. A large amount of anechoic free fluid was found in the coelomic cavity of this Green Iguana *(Iguana iguana)*. **B,** After aspiration of 750 mL free fluid and surgical removal of the tumor, the tissue was histologically investigated. The diagnosis was a cystic adenocarcinoma of the ovary of the Green Iguana from **A**.

URINARY BLADDER

The urinary bladder, when present, lies in the caudal portion of the coelomic cavity and has a thin, smooth, hyperechoic wall. The content is anechoic with hyperechoic particles or larger aggregates (uric acid particles) (Figure 10-44).[32] Urate aggregates show a typical snowflake-like pattern, especially when the patient is moved. Calculi can be distinguished by their more solid structure and the distal shadowing of the ultrasound beam. Pathologic changes can be seen in tortoises with egg retention or dystocia. Eggs may occasionally retropulse back into the bladder as they pass through the urodeum. They appear as large, round, multilayered structures within the urinary bladder. In these cases, the outer surface of the egg shows an irregular wall, with internal echogenic material. The urinary bladder wall may also be thickened because of mechanical irritation (Figure 10-45).

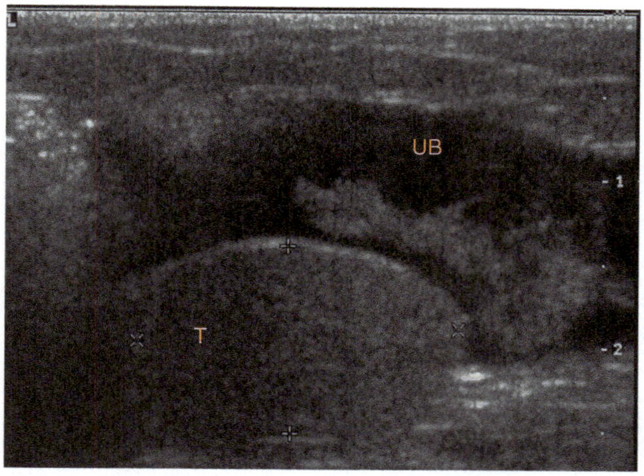

FIGURE 10-44 Sagittal plane ultrasound image in a healthy Green Iguana *(Iguana iguana)* showing an aggregate of echogenic urates suspended within the urinary bladder *(UB)*. A testis can also be seen *(T)*. The urinary bladder is thin walled and conforms to the surrounding organs.

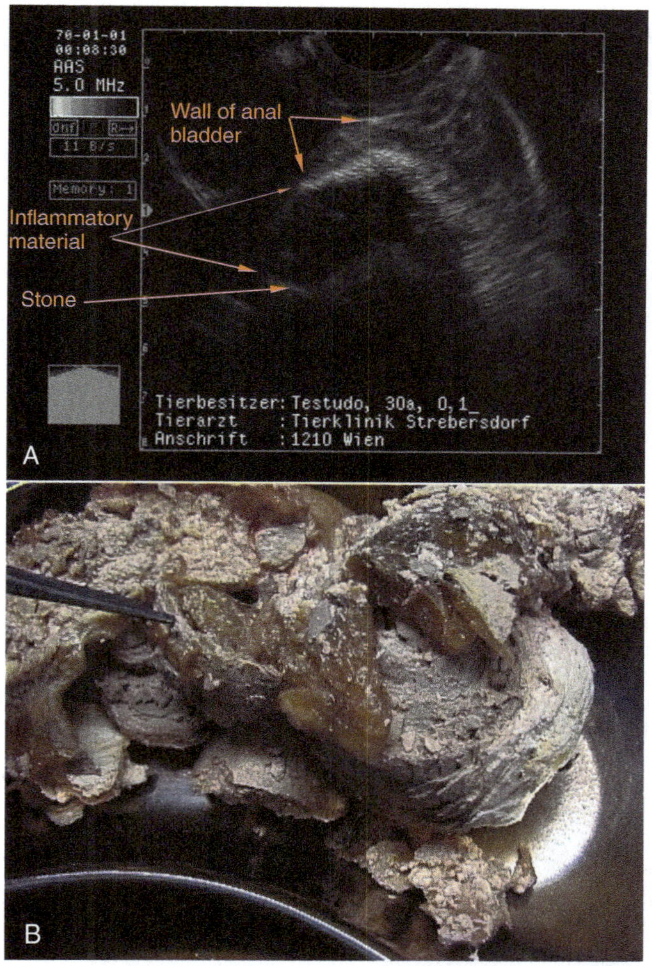

FIGURE 10-45 **A,** Ultrasound image of the anal bladder in a 30-year-old Greek Tortoise *(Testudo hermanni)*. The hyperechoic tissue of the anal bladder is thickened, and a calculus is visible as a line with distal extinction of the ultrasound beam. Between the two structures is a thick layer of inflammatory reaction and fibrin. **B,** The calculus with gel-like material on the surface. The cause of the calculus was determined to be the long-term presence of an egg in the lumen of the anal bladder.

THE KIDNEYS

The kidneys show a higher echogenicity than the liver and the fatbody, with a clear granular echotexture and a distinctly marginated surface. In snakes, they are elongated and lobes can be visualized; however, no hyperechoic septae can be visualized, unlike in the fatbody, which allows differentiation of these structures. In some lizards, like the common Green Iguana or the Bearded Dragon, the kidneys lie within the pelvis and are not easily seen (Figure 10-46). In other groups, such as the varanids, the kidneys are midcoelomic and are readily scanned.

In patients with intrapelvic kidneys, when renomegaly is present, the cranial poles of the kidneys can be visualized just cranial to brim of the pelvis[26,33] (Figure 10-47). In the iguana, an acoustic window just caudal to the pelvis may provide the best visualization of the kidneys.

Often large hyperechoic granules due to renal failure/gout can be detected and monitored in enlarged kidneys (Figure 10-48). Anechoic spherical structures, occasionally multifocal throughout the organ, indicate cystic changes (Figure 10-49). Mineralization, with the characteristic appearance of distal attenuation of the ultrasound beam, can be seen; tumors may also be detected (Figure 10-50).

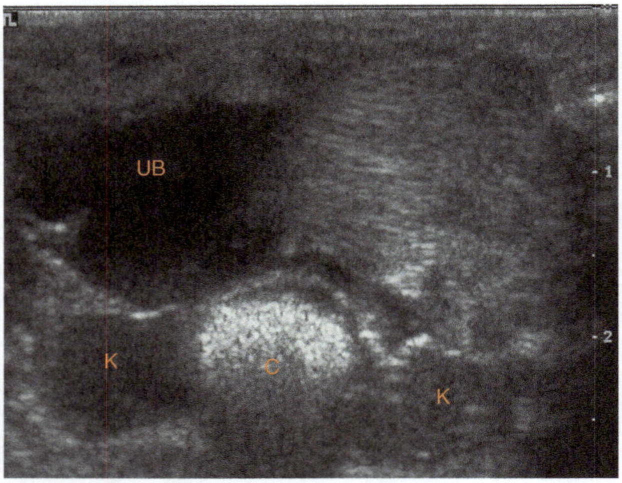

FIGURE 10-46 Transverse plane ultrasound image in a healthy Green Iguana *(Iguana iguana)*. The cranial poles of the kidneys *(K)*, which lie within the pelvic cavity in this and similar species, can occasionally be seen by angling the transducer caudally at the pelvic inlet, as in this image. *C,* Colon; *UB,* urinary bladder.

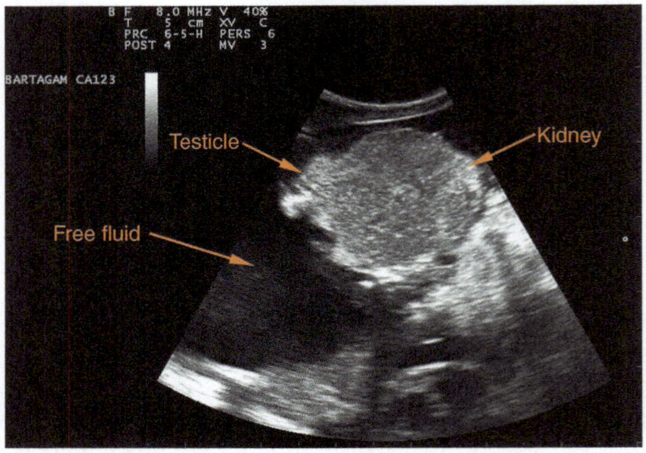

FIGURE 10-48 Ultrasound image of an enlarged kidney in a Greek Tortoise *(Testudo hermanni)* with large hyperechoic granules in the tissue, as a result of renal failure. A large amount of free fluid was found in the coelomic cavity (same tortoise as Figure 10-12).

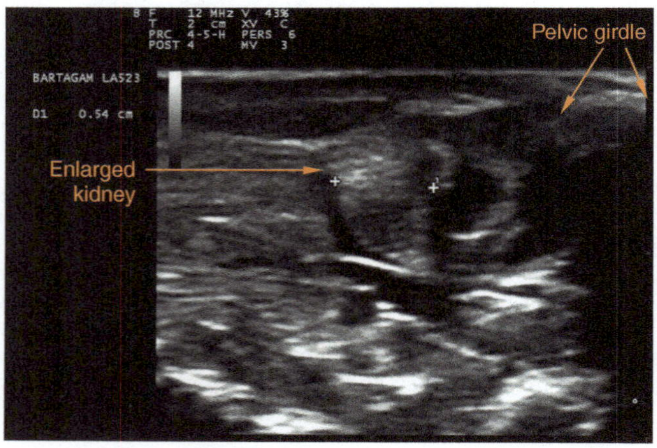

FIGURE 10-47 Ultrasound image of an enlarged kidney (+) in a Bearded Dragon *(Pogona vitticeps)* protruding cranially from the pelvic cavity.

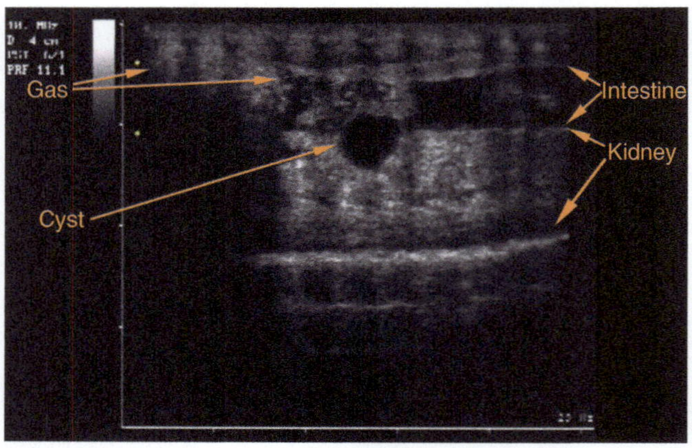

FIGURE 10-49 Ultrasound image of the kidney of a Kingsnake (*Lampropeltis* sp.) with anechoic spherical structures in the tissue. A cystic abnormality of the renal tubules is seen on the surface of the kidney (same animal as Figure 10-27). The intestine is filled cranially (on the left of the picture) with gas and caudally with fluid ingesta.

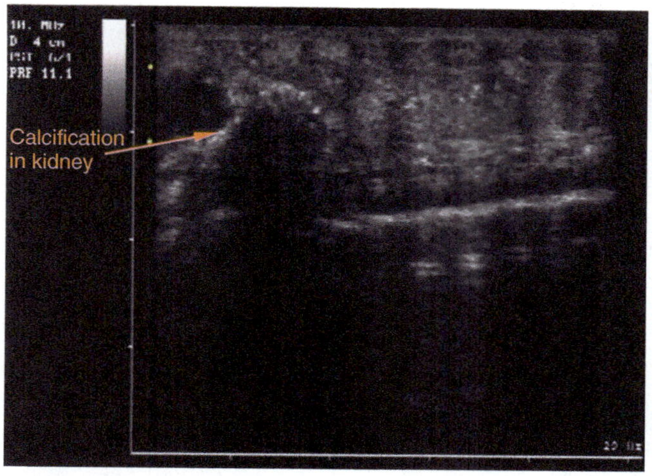

FIGURE 10-50 Ultrasound image of the kidney of the Kingsnake (*Lampropeltis* sp.) from Figure 10-27 and 10-49. The whole organ shows a slightly heterogeneous pattern. Focally there is a highly echogenic structure with distal attenuation of the ultrasound beam. On histopathologic examination, the changes in the kidneys were consistent with cystic adenocarcinoma with focal calcifications.

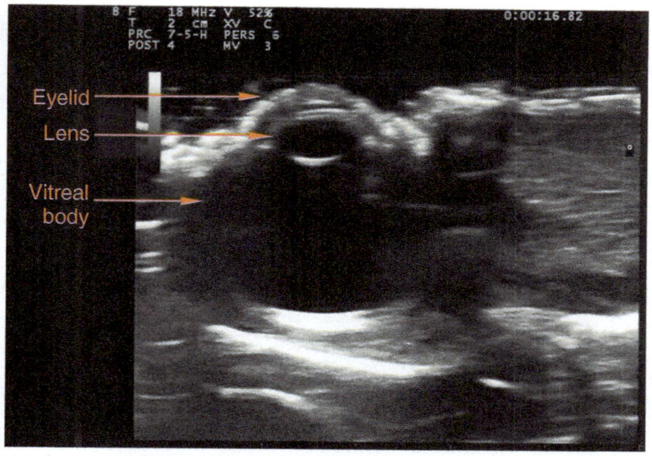

FIGURE 10-51 Ultrasound image with an 18 MHz transducer of a healthy eye in a Veiled Chameleon *(Chamaeleo calyptratus).* The most superficial echogenic structure is the eyelid; the lens appears as an oval, anechoic structure with thin hyperechoic margins; the vitreal body is anechoic; and there is a round border to the fundus.

THE EYE

Because of the small size of the normal reptilian eye, high-frequency transducers with a small footprint should be used to obtain a good image of the structures of the eye and the surrounding tissues. The coupling gel and the probe can be placed either directly on the cornea, the spectacle, or the eyelids (as in chameleons). Both eyes should always be investigated in sagittal, dorsal, and transverse planes for a thorough evaluation and bilateral comparison.

The image of the normal cornea and the attached spectacle in snakes is a small, parallel, hyperechoic two-lined structure. Posterior to the cornea, the anechoic anterior chamber is visible. The lens is an oval, anechoic structure with thin hyperechoic margins. The iris is slightly heterogenous of medium echogenicity, and, especially in small reptiles, not easily distinguished from the ciliary body. The vitreal body should be anechoic, and the fundus of the globe should be uniformly concave. The conus papillaris is visualized as a higher echogenic structure reaching from the posterior pole of the wall into the vitreal body. Its size ranges from a small structure to a large structure reaching almost to the posterior lens capsule wall (Figure 10-51).

Changes associated with dysecdysis in snakes, intraocular hemorrhage, abscesses, and tumors of the structures of the eye and the orbit can be visualized (Figure 10-52).

Probes with frequencies from 40 to 60 MHz will give even more detailed images. In ophthalmology, this technique is referred to as *ultrasound biomicroscopy.*[33]

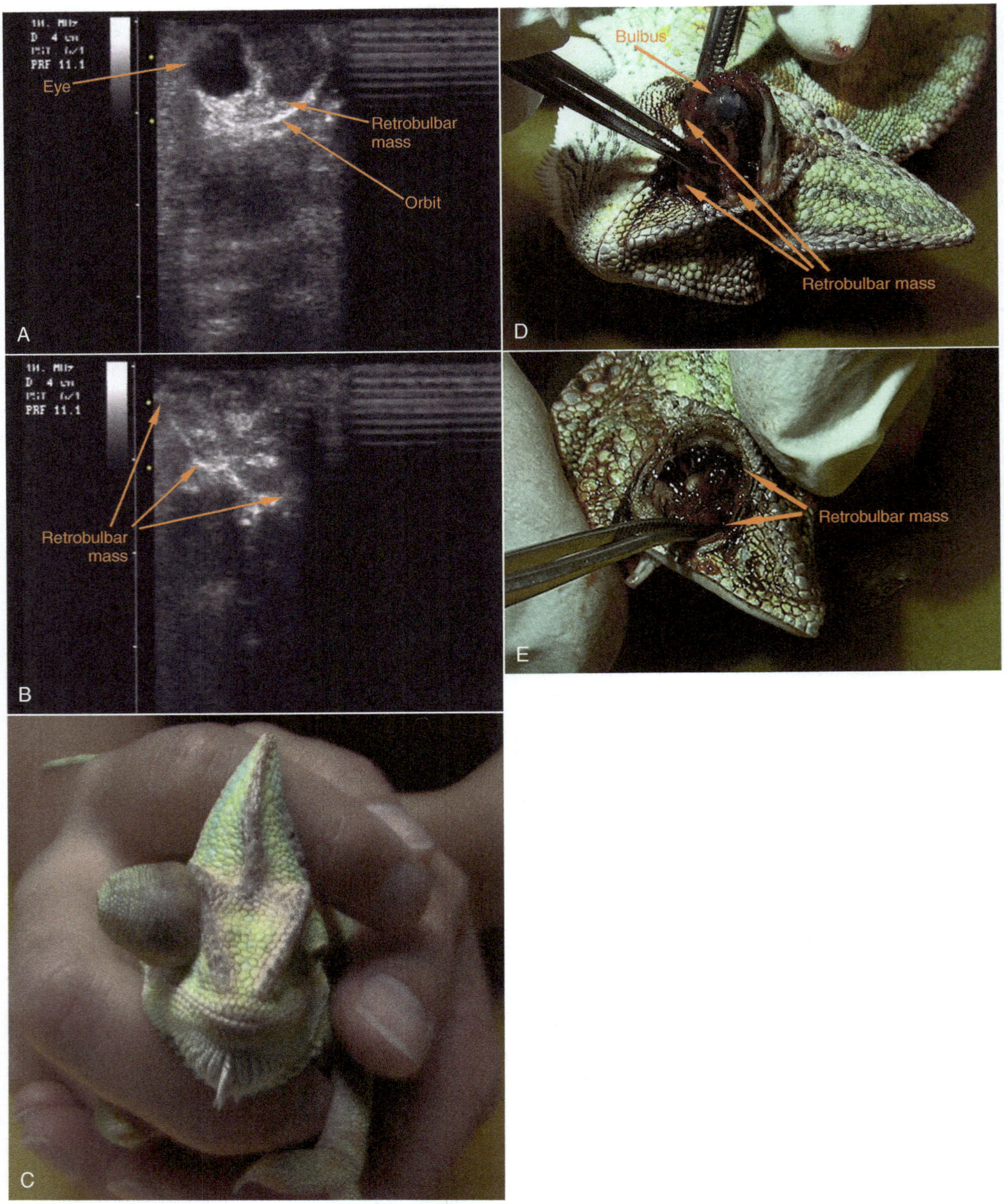

FIGURE 10-52 **A,** Ultrasound image with an 10 MHz transducer of an abnormal posterior wall of the globe in a different Veiled Chameleon *(Chamaeleo calyptratus).* There is a large heterogenous hyperechoic mass visible posterior to the globe. **B,** Ultrasound image of the heterogeneous hyperechoic retrobulbar mass from the Veiled Chameleon in **A**. On histopathologic examination, it was diagnosed as soft tissue sarcoma. **C,** Retrobulbar tumor in the Veiled Chameleon from **A** and **B**. **D,** Postmortem view from the head of the same Veiled Chameleon from **A-C** after opening the eyelid cranially and lifting up the bulbus. The retrobulbar mass had already spread underneath the eyelid. **E,** Postmortem view from the head of the same Veiled Chameleon from **A** through **D** after removal of the bulbus to get a view of the orbit, which is completely filled with the retrobulbar mass.

REFERENCES

1. Fritsch R, Gerwing M. *Sonografie bei Hund und Katze*. Stuttgart, Germany: Enke, 1993.
2. Nyland TG, Mattoon JS. *Small animal diagnostic ultrasound*. 2nd ed. Philadelphia: WB Saunders Co, 2002.
3. Poulsen Nautrup C, Tobias R. *Atlas und Lehrbuch der Ultraschalldiagnostik bei Hund und Katze*. 4. Auflage, Hannover, Germany: Schlütersche Verlagsgesellschaft, 2007.
4. Barr F, Gaschen L. *BSAVA Manual of canine and feline ultrasonography*, Quedgeley, Gloucester, England: British Small Animal Veterinary Association, 2011.
5. Göbel T, Schildger BJ, Spörle H. Propädeutik und diagnostische Verfahren bei Reptilien. *Prakt Tierarzt* 1990;3:14-25.
6. Schildger BJ, Caesares M, Kramer M, et al. Technique of ultrasonography in lizards, snakes and chelonians. *Semin Avian Exot Pet Med* 1994;3:147-155.
7. Tenhu H, Schildger BJ, Geyer B. Ultraschalluntersuchungen des Grünen Leguans *(Iguana iguana)*. *Verh ber Zootiere* 1995;37:319-232.
8. Schildger BJ, Tenhue H, Kramer M, et al. Ultraschalluntersuchungen bei Reptilien. *Berl Münch Tierärztl Wschr* 1996;109:136-141.
9. Hernandez-Divers SM, Hernandez-Divers SJ. Diagnostic imaging of reptiles. *In Pract* 2001;23:370-391.
10. Sainsbry AW, Gilig C. Ultrasonographic anatomy and scanning technique of the coelomic organs oft Bosc Monitors *(Varanus exanthematicus)*. *J Zoo Wildlife Med* 1991;22:421-433.
11. Caesares M, Rübel A, Honegger RE. Observations on the female reproductive cycle of captive giant tortoises (*Geochelone* spp.) using ultrasound scanning. *J Zoo Wildl Med* 1997; 28:267-273.
12. Pennick DG, Stewart JS, Paul-Murphy J, et al. Ultrasonography of the California desert tortoise *(Xerobates agassizi)*: anatomy and applications. *Vet Radiol* 1991;32:112-116.
13. Schumacher J, Toal RL. Advanced radiography and ultrasonography in reptiles. *Semin Avian Exot Pet Med* 2001;10:162-168.
14. Krautwald-Junghanns ME, Pees M, Reese S, et al. *Atlas der bildgebenden Diagnostik bei Heimtieren*. Hannover, Germany: Schlütersche Verlagsgesellschaft, 2009.
15. Isaza R, Ackerman N, Schumacher J. Ultrasound-guided percutaneous liver biopsy in snakes. *Vet Radiol Ultrasound* 1993;6:452-454.
16. Hernandez SJ, Stahl SJ, McBride M, et al. Evaluation of an endoscopic liver biopsy technique in green iguanas. *J Am Vet Med Assoc* 2007;230:1849-1853.
17. Snyder PS, Shaw NG, Heard DJ. Two-dimensional echocardiographic anatomy of the snake heart *(Python molurus bivittatus)*. *Vet Radiol* 1999;40:66-72.
18. Girling SJ, Hynes B. Cardiovascular and haemopoietic system. In: Girling SJ, Raiti P, eds. *BSAVA Manual of Reptiles*. 2nd ed. Quedgeley, Gloucester, England: British Small Animal Veterinary Association, 2004;243-260.
19. Schilliger L, Cherboul V, Tessier D. Standardizing two-dimensional echocardiographic examination in snakes. *ICE Proc* 2005:63-74.
20. Kik MJ, Mitchell MA. Reptile cardiology: a review of anatomy and physiology, diagnostic approaches, and clinical disease. *Semin Avian Exot Pet Med* 2005;14:52-60.
21. Jacobson ER, Homer B, Adam W. Endocarditis and congestive heart failure in a Burmese python *(Python molurus bivittatus)*. *J Zoo Wildl Med* 1991;22:245-248.
22. Clippinger TL. Aortic stenosis and atrio/ventricular dilatation in a green iguana *(Iguana iguana)*. *Am Assoc Zoo Vet* 1993:390-393.
23. Rishniw M, Carmel BP. Atrioventricular valve insufficiency and congestive heart failure in a carpet python. *Aust Vet J* 1999;77:580-583.
24. Redrobe SP, Scudamore CL. Ultrasonographic diagnosis of pericardial effusion and atrial dilation in a spur-thighed tortoise *(Testudo graeca)*. *Vet Rec* 2000;146:183-185.
25. Schilliger L, Tréhiou-Sechi E, Petit AMP, et al. Double valvular insufficiency in a Burmese python (*Python molurus bivittatus*, Linneaus, 1758) suffering from concomitant bacterial pneumonia. *J Zoo Wildl Med* 2010;41:742-744.
26. Holland MF, Hernandez-Divers S, Frank PM. Ultrasonographic appearance of the coelomic cavity in healthy green iguanas. *J Am Vet Med Assoc* 2008;233:590-596.
27. Rostal DC, Robeck TR, Owens DW, et al. Ultrasound imaging of ovaries and eggs in Kemp's Ridley sea turtles *(Lepidochelys kempii)*. *J Zoo Wildl Med* 1990;21:27-35.
28. Anderson NJ, Williams J, Sargartz JE, et al. Ovarian teratoma in a green iguana *(Iguana iguana)*. *J Zoo Wildl Med* 1996;27:90-95.
29. Love NE, Douglass JP, Lewbart G, et al. Radiographic and ultrasonographic evaluation of egg retention and peritonitis in two green iguanas *(Iguana iguana)*. *Vet Radiol Ultrasound* 1996;37:68-73.
30. Mehler SJ, Rosenstein DS, Patterson JS. Imaging diagnosis—follicular torsion in a green iguana *(Iguana iguana)* with involvement of the left adrenal gland. *Vet Radiol Ultrasound* 2002;43:343-345.
31. Pees M, Hänse M, Schlömer J, et al. Legenot bei Reptilien. *Tierärztl Prax* 2010;38:69-72.
32. Canny C. Gross anatomy and imaging of the avian and reptilian urinary system. *Semin Avian Exot Pet Med* 1998;7:72-80.
33. Hollingsworth SR, Holmberg BJ, Strunk A, et al. Comparison of ophthalmic measurements obtained via high-frequency ultrasound imaging in four species of snakes. *Am J Vet Res* 2007;68:1111-1114.

CHAPTER 11

Conditioning and Behavioral Training in Reptiles

Gregory J. Fleming[†] *and*
Michelle L. Skurski

Reptiles historically have carried the stigma of being unintelligent, uncharismatic, and easy to care for, with minimal husbandry needs. Nothing could be further from the truth. Animal caretakers now recognize a need for all animals to be able to perform biologically appropriate behaviors in captive environments, including reptiles. The environment provided should be determined by the animals' natural and individual histories. Training and enrichment are great ways to provide reptiles with the opportunity to display their natural behaviors and allow for people who keep reptiles to interact with these animals and observe their behavior close at hand.

Animal enrichment and training have become a normal routine in most zoological and aquarium facilities and can also be implemented in private homes. The concepts of training and enrichment are interrelated. In recent years, many professional animal-care facilities have seen improvements in the health and well-being of captive reptiles by providing an environment where reptiles can make choices. For example, natural behaviors such as foraging, climbing, digging, or swimming cannot take place if animals are housed in a plastic box. With a small amount of effort, private owners can successfully encourage these same behaviors and choices in their captive reptiles.

ENRICHMENT

Enrichment is more than just placing a new branch or a plant in a reptile's environment. Although there are many different definitions of enrichment, for the sake of consistency, we will follow the definition used by the Association of Zoos and Aquariums (AZA):

> *"Enrichment is a process for improving or enhancing animal environments and care within the context of their inhabitants' behavioral biology and natural history. It is a dynamic process in which changes to structures and husbandry practices are made with the goal of increasing behavioral choices available to animals and drawing out their species-appropriate behaviors and abilities, thus enhancing animal welfare."*
>
> **AZA/Behavior Scientific Advisory Group, 1999**

In practice, enrichment means encouraging species-appropriate behaviors and providing the animal with choices in every aspect of reptile husbandry, from food presentation to housing. The diversity of reptile habitats, microhabitats, and ecosystems, as well as the range and complexity of their behaviors, can actually increase the opportunities for enrichment to enhance the animals' lives.

Based on the aforementioned definition, there are three main goals for enrichment:

1. To promote species-appropriate behaviors
2. To provide behavioral opportunities
3. To provide animals with control over their environment

All three of these goals require a clear understanding of the animals' natural history. This information is critical to making the enrichment successful. Based on the natural history, each enrichment initiative should have a behavioral goal. One benefit of setting behavioral goals for enrichment is that it offers a way to measure our success. For example, a client may want to encourage an overweight arboreal snake to climb and utilize more of the enclosure. The question the client would ask is, "Did the addition of branches into the snake enclosure encourage the snake to climb and utilize the enclosure?" If the answer is yes, the behavioral goal was achieved. If the answer is no, then other options such as platforms, heat sources, or even different types of branches may be explored to encourage the snake to climb (Figure 11-1).

Another behavioral goal may be to encourage an animal to forage. For instance, natural scents can be provided by dragging a prey item through the enclosure to leave a scent trail that can stimulate the reptile to forage. Sometimes the scent just needs to be novel to engage the reptile. Keepers have successfully utilized a cinnamon scent trail scattered throughout an enclosure to encourage foraging in a Komodo Dragon.

Choice of housing, enclosure furnishings, and behavioral opportunity depend on whether the reptile is arboreal, terrestrial, aquatic, or semiaquatic. Something as simple as providing different levels in an enclosure can encourage exploration and foraging. Many species of monitor lizard are known to stand bipedal to forage in the wild. This behavior can be recreated through minor alterations of an enclosure and delivery of food to the animal (Figure 11-2). Although animals in the wild seem to exhibit this behavior without much effort, a monitor lizard in captivity may need to be encouraged to stand through small and successive approximation. Captive lizards are likely novices at standing and will need to develop the skills and physical ability to accomplish some behavioral goals.

The way in which food is presented can also provide behavioral opportunity. Multiple behaviors can be encouraged by

[†] Deceased.

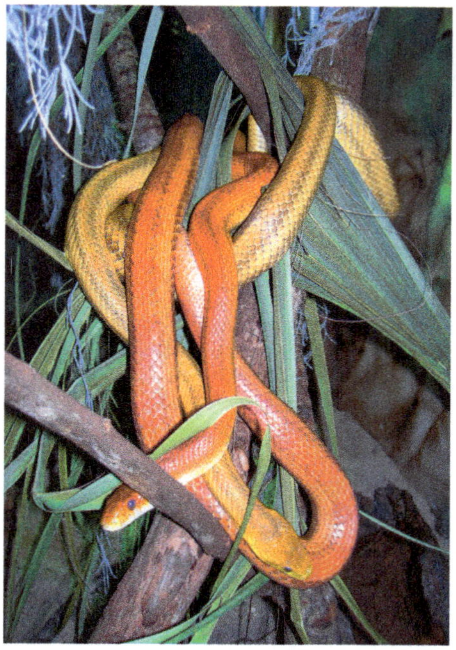

FIGURE 11-1 Cornsnakes *(Pantherophis guttatus)* utilizing natural climbing materials.

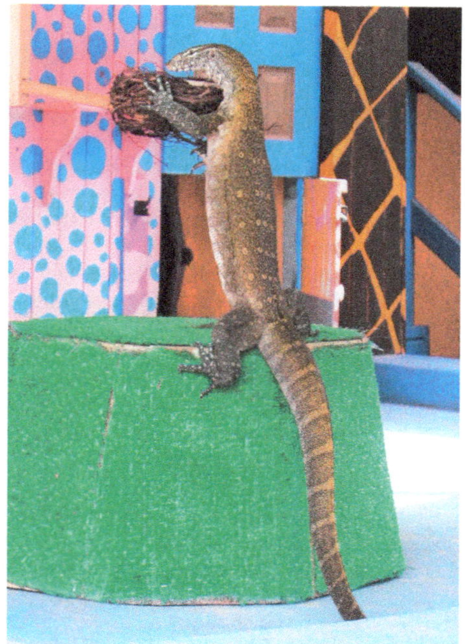

FIGURE 11-2 A Nile Monitor *(Varanus niloticus)* standing bipedal to acquire a food item.

varying the size of the food item, the placement or location of the food, and the time of day of the feeding. For example, tree pythons are nocturnal; as such, their activity level typically increases at night. During the more active periods, foraging and hunting behaviors will be displayed. Therefore feeding during these periods could encourage active behaviors that stimulate and exercise the snake.

Providing complexity and choices to an environment can be achieved through addition of or changes to rocks, branches, plants, light, and substrate within an enclosure. Providing choices for and control over thermoregulation opportunities is vital for the reptiles. Opportunities for thermoregulation can be provided with the use of lights, undercage heat pads, water of different or variable temperatures, and heat-emitting ceramic bulbs. Recently, improvements in technology allow changes in the temperature and humidity of captive enclosures by the minute. Environmental temperature and humidity may be altered on a daily basis, which allows for natural changes in the animal's environment that mimic a natural sunrise or an afternoon rainstorm.

Offering different levels in an enclosure provides reptiles an opportunity to utilize heat and light sources to varying degrees. Understanding the general environment for the reptile in the wild is not enough; a reptile caretaker must dig a bit deeper to meet the animal's needs. For instance, the animal could come from the desert but spend the majority of its day burrowed underground escaping from the sun and heat. In this case, the assumption that the animal would need a very warm, barren environment would take into account only a part of its natural history. Providing a way to escape the heat would also be vital to this animal's well-being. Appropriate lighting is essential not only for health but also for enriching a reptile's life.

Encouraging your clients to study the natural history of the species they care for will be the first step in the creation of a successful enrichment program for their reptiles. Enrichment done appropriately will improve the health and well-being of the animal, enhance their welfare, and assist in facilitating their care. To find some additional examples of enrichment ideas, see Disney's Animal Programs' enrichment Web site at www.animalenrichment.org.[1]

TRAINING

Since the early 1990s, there has been a dramatic increase in the use of operant conditioning techniques to train exotic animals for husbandry purposes. These animal training techniques can assist in facilitating day-to-day care, routine medical procedures, and management of reptiles. The act of training becomes enrichment for both the animal and the keepers as they interact. Any reptile brought into clinics, such as dendrobatid frogs, Bearded Dragons, Green Iguanas, monitor lizards, boas and pythons, and turtles and tortoises, can be trained to calmly and voluntarily enter a crate instead of being physically restrained for crating. Reptiles can also be trained to accept various veterinary procedures such as ultrasounds, nail clipping, blood draws, or even being medicated. Reptiles with chronic conditions requiring regular visits and or treatments can be trained to cooperate for many types of procedures. This kind of training allows for treatment with little to no stress to the animals and client.

To create a well-thought-out behavioral plan for a reptile, many facilities use the "SPIDER" framework[2] taught in several courses given by the AZA. The SPIDER framework includes setting goals, planning, implementing, documenting, evaluating, and readjusting (Table 11-1). More information on this process can be found at www.animaltraining.org.[3]

The first step (*S*) in the SPIDER process is setting goals. It is beneficial to start a training program by determining the overall behavioral goals (i.e., detailing the specific behaviors to be trained). During this goal-development process, it is important

TABLE 11-1

SPIDER Framework

Step	SPIDER Framework Details	Example
Setting Goals	Detail the specific behaviors to be trained.	Train the monitor lizard to enter a crate voluntarily and be calm and comfortable in the crate.
Planning	Create a series of steps for shaping the behavior. Plan who will be training the animal, when the animal will be trained, and any equipment or tool needed to achieve the training plan.	Wait for the lizard to move toward the crate; use crickets to reinforce. Continue to reinforce movements toward the crate until the lizard enters the crate. Reinforce calm behavior inside the crate by continuing to provide crickets. Close the door to the crate and continue to provide crickets for calm behavior.
Implementing	Train the behavior over many sessions, advancing only when the animal is ready. Ensure clear communication among participants regarding training steps and timelines.	The lizard's two owners will each train crating for two sessions per week. They will review each other's notes before each session. The crate will not be lifted with the lizard inside until the lizard has successfully entered the crate and remained inside calmly with the door closed for 10 minutes.
Documenting	Create a historical document that tracks the progress of the animal and shows trends in behavior.	Each of the owners will take notes on their training sessions, including a rating of the session and comments on the lizard's progress.
Evaluating	Review the documentation and training plan.	After 3 weeks, the lizard has not yet completely entered the crate.
Readjusting	Make any changes necessary to achieve the behavioral goals.	The owners decide to adjust the plan and begin placing a few crickets at the back of the crate to encourage the lizard to enter completely. Once this occurs, they will continue to provide crickets if the lizard remains calmly in the crate.

to include all parties involved with the management of the animals. Goals should be based on the joint needs of owners, veterinary staff, and the reptile. For example, if the monitor lizard can shift into a crate for transport to the veterinarian, the lizard is more easily crated and less distressed when in the crate. This outcome facilitates a better veterinary evaluation. The goals in this case would then be to train the monitor lizard to enter a crate voluntarily and be calm and comfortable in the crate.

The next step *(P)* is planning. This is where a training plan is created for the behavior. The training plan is a series of steps for shaping the behavior. The plan is meant to be a guide or a way for the trainer to think through the process before beginning to training an animal. If crate training is used as the example, the first step is to reinforce being comfortable with the crate itself. This process starts with providing positive reinforcement when the animal merely approaches the crate, which could occur randomly, and then slowly encouraging the animal to enter the crate. The reinforcer or reward for learning to tolerate and enter the crate could be small bits of a highly desirable food that are delivered as soon as the reptile approaches and/or moves closer to the entry of the crate.

The third step *(I)* is implementing. The behavior should be trained over a period of many sessions, and training should advance only when the animal is ready. If more than one trainer is involved, having clearly laid out plans, assignments, and timelines helps to facilitate a smooth process. Defining roles and creating clear avenues of communication among all participants is also important.

Before the training is implemented, a decision should be made regarding how the training sessions will be documented *(D)*. Videotaping sessions is an easy way to document and track progress of training. Taking notes, including session ratings and comments, is another useful way to document and track training outcomes. The goals of documenting are to create a historical document, track the progress of the animal, and look for trends in behavior.

The last two steps of the SPIDER process, evaluating *(E)* and readjusting *(R)*, require reviewing the documentation and training plan and making any changes necessary to achieve the behavioral goals. For more information on how to apply this process, visit Disney's Animal Programs Web site or www.animalenrichment.org1 or www.animaltraining.org.[2]

PRACTICAL EXAMPLES OF TRAINING AND ENRICHMENT

Nile Monitor

Be creative when developing your training and enrichment program. Creating unique and complex environments for reptiles in the home is not only enriching for the owners because they can see their animals perform natural behavior but also beneficial physically and mentally to the animals. Training a monitor to enter a crate on cue may be a safer alternative to physically restraining the reptile. It is certainly less stressful for both the caretaker and the lizard. A Nile Monitor *(Varanus niloticus)* has been trained to enter a crate voluntarily for transport (Figure 11-3). This trained behavior also allows the keepers to clean the enclosure safely.

Amphibians

Conditioning and behavioral shaping techniques can also be applied to amphibians. Dendrobatid frogs can be trained to associate feeding with the sound of a clicker. Once the clicker is sounded, the frogs will come out of hiding and look for food. A small plastic box with fruit flies can be added to the enclosure. Once the frog has moved into the box, the fruit flies

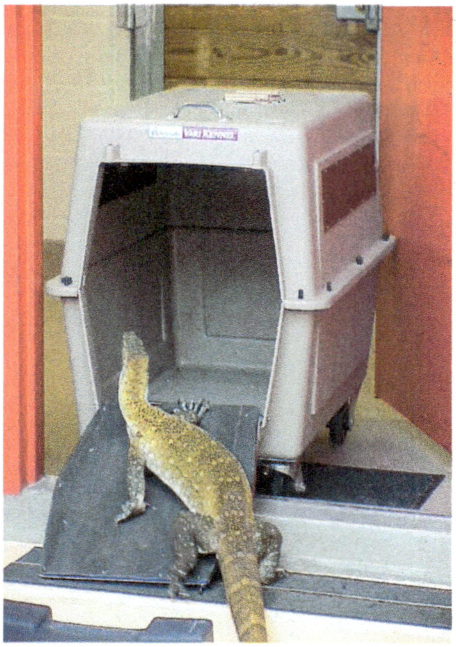

FIGURE 11-3 A Nile Monitor *(Varanus niloticus)* being cued to move into a transport crate.

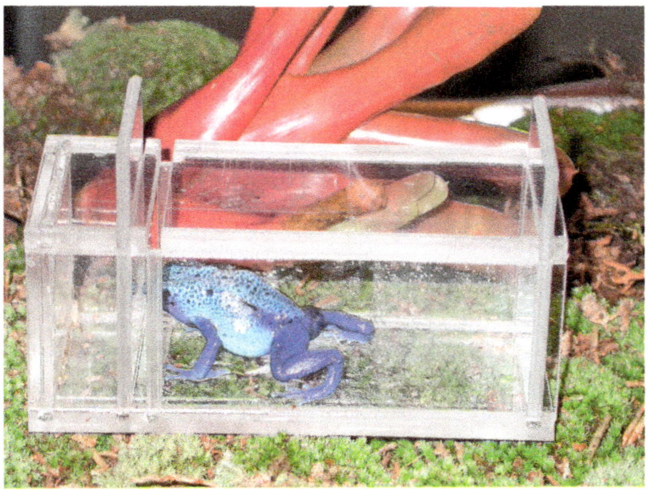

FIGURE 11-4 A Blue Poison Dart Frog *(Dendrobates azureus)* shifting into a transport crate. Note the fruit flies behind the shift door.

are released, reinforcing the frog's behavior (Figure 11-4). This allows for the owner to see each animal up close and remove the animal from the enclosure for transport, weighing, or veterinary examination.

Venomous Snakes

Training snakes to shift into a box is helpful, especially when dealing with venomous reptiles (Figure 11-5). Once the snake is safely in the holding box, a handling tube can be attached to the box and the snake can enter the tube. The husbandry staff then detaches the tube from the box with the snake gently restrained by the tube. This technique allows safe and humane examination or treatment (Figure 11-6). The snake does not come into direct contact with the handlers, making the entire procedure safer and less stressful for both the snake and the handlers.

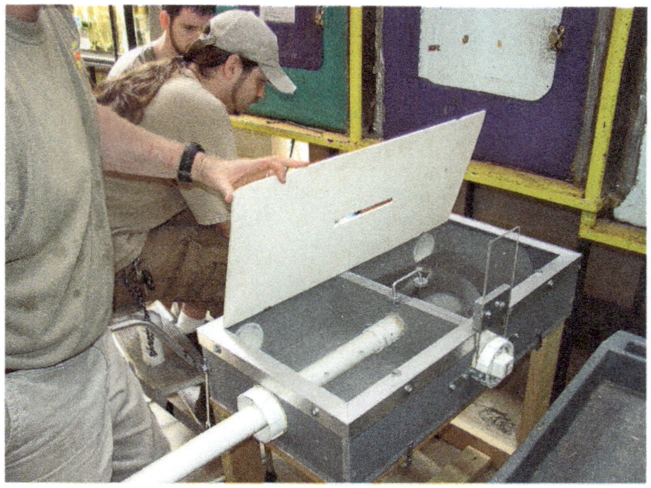

FIGURE 11-5 A Black Mamba *(Dendroaspis polylepis)* has shifted from his enclosure to the holding box. A handling tube is attached to the side of the box. Once this is attached, the door will open and the snake will move into the tube. *(Photo courtesy Dr. Brad Lock, Zoo Atlanta, Atlanta, Ga.)*

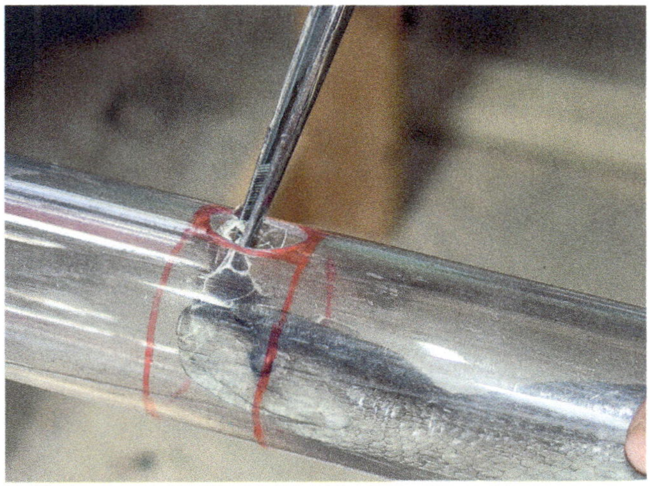

FIGURE 11-6 Once the snake is in the handling tube, the veterinarian can remove the retained eye cap without sedation. *(Photo courtesy Dr. Brad Lock, Zoo Atlanta, Atlanta, Ga.)*

REVIEW

The key to creating a successful training and enrichment program with a reptile is to develop the knowledge of the reptile's natural history. This is critical for understanding the needs and capabilities of the reptile and, ultimately, improves the reptile's welfare. Useful natural history information includes how the reptile thermoregulates, the preferred optimum body temperature range for the species, normal activity levels for the reptile, diel cycle (is the reptile diurnal or nocturnal?), natural diet and foraging style, and whether the reptile is arboreal, terrestrial, aquatic or semiaquatic. This information will help to prepare your clients to properly care for a reptile.

Consulting with a veterinarian can be helpful in deciding on proper enrichment objectives and appropriate behaviors to train for daily activity and medical procedures. In any case, training and enrichment can only benefit both the owner and the reptile by providing a closer relationship and a fuller enriching life for both participants.

ACKNOWLEDGMENT

Special thanks to Dr. Karen Overall for reviewing this chapter.

REFERENCES

1. Disney's Animal Programs: Enrichment Program Web site. Available at: http://www.animalenrichment.org. Accessed Apr 18, 2012.
2. Mellen J, MacPhee MS. Philosophy of environmental enrichment: past, present, and future. *Zoo Biol* 2001;20:211-226.
3. Disney's Animal Programs: Training Program Web site. Available at: http://www.animaltraining.org. Accessed Apr 18, 2012.

SECTION II

ADVANCES IN ANESTHESIA, SURGERY, AND ANALGESIA

CHAPTER 12

Anesthesia

Juergen Schumacher and
Christoph Mans

Safe and effective anesthesia of the reptilian patient is a requirement for procedures including physical examination of large or dangerous species, collection of diagnostic samples, application of various imaging modalities, and surgical procedures. The anesthetic management of the reptilian patient, including the design of the anesthetic protocol, represents unique challenges due to marked anatomic and physiologic differences between taxa. The response to commonly used anesthetic agents and dosages is often variable between taxa, and individual differences are also often seen. Commonly, anesthetic and analgesic protocols, including monitoring techniques to evaluate cardiopulmonary performance established in domestic animals, are applied to the reptilian patient; however, these techniques are often of limited value and should be interpreted with caution. Monitors such as pulse oximeters and blood gas analyzers are not calibrated for reptilian species, and their unique cardiopulmonary anatomy and physiology may produce erroneous values in an anesthetized reptile. More research needs to be conducted in the field of reptile anesthesia, including determining normal values for cardiovascular and respiratory function and response to anesthetic agents, so that values derived from monitoring devices can be accurately interpreted. In particular, conscious baseline cardiopulmonary values need to be established for common species. The design of a safe and effective anesthetic protocol requires a thorough understanding of anatomy and physiology, especially with regard to the cardiopulmonary system.

Comprehensive reviews of reptile anesthesia and analgesia, including cardiopulmonary anatomy and physiology and selection of effective drugs and dosages for various species, have been published previously.[1-8] An update on analgesic techniques is provided in Chapter 18, whereas this chapter reviews and highlights the current knowledge of reptile anesthesia, the effects of anesthetic agents on cardiopulmonary performance, and the application and limitation of monitoring techniques in reptile anesthesia.

PREANESTHETIC EVALUATION

A thorough and complete evaluation of the patient should be conducted so that an effective anesthetic and analgesic protocol can be designed. A complete history and critical review of husbandry practices including diet, temperature, and humidity should be obtained because they will provide valuable information on the health status of the patient. The medical record of the patient should be reviewed, followed by a complete visual and physical examination. Particular attention should be paid to evidence of systemic disease, as well as signs of cardiovascular or respiratory compromise, which would affect the patient's performance under anesthesia.

Diseases of the respiratory tract are commonly seen in reptiles and may affect both the upper and lower respiratory tract.[9] Most commonly, a viral or bacterial cause is identified, and the patient may require effective antimicrobial therapy before induction of general anesthesia. Determination of respiratory rate and effort will provide limited information on the presence of respiratory tract disease. Imaging modalities such as radiography or computed tomography and collection of diagnostic samples will assist in identifying the severity and etiology of respiratory tract disease.

Assessment of cardiovascular performance should be part of the physical examination. Unfortunately, few studies have determined normal values for cardiovascular performance (e.g., heart rate and arterial blood pressures) in reptiles. Although reference values for various cardiac variables need to be established in common reptile species, determination of heart rate and rhythm, radiographic evaluation of cardiac morphologic characteristics, and echocardiography will give valuable information on cardiac performance and abnormalities. Reviews of reptile cardiology, including anatomy, physiology, and diagnostic procedures, have been published previously.[10,11]

Diagnostic samples such as fecal screens and hematologic and plasma biochemistry panels should be evaluated to determine the health status of the reptile. Reference values for common reptile species have been published and may provide important information on organ function and the presence of infectious and noninfectious disease processes. Imaging modalities such as radiography, ultrasonography, computed tomography and magnetic resonance imaging are performed as indicated by medical history and physical examination findings.

SUPPORTIVE MEASURES

Many reptiles require supportive care before anesthesia because of underlying chronic disease processes and dehydration, which can often be identified during the preanesthetic evaluation. Effective fluid therapy is indicated for correcting fluid and electrolyte imbalances and returning the patient to a normovolemic state. Intravenous (IV) or intraosseous (IO)

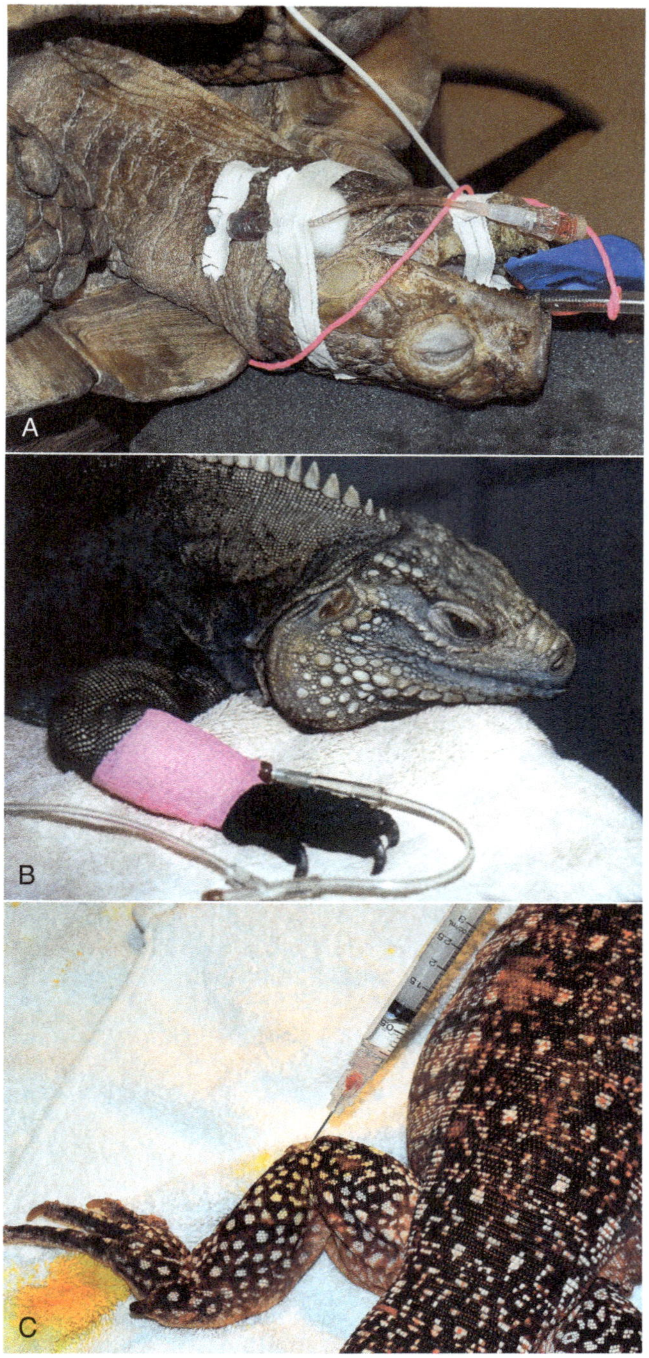

FIGURE 12-1 Intravascular access in reptiles. **A,** Intravenous catheter in the jugular vein of an African Spurred Tortoise *(Centrochelys sulcata).* **B,** Intravenous catheter in the cephalic vein of a Rock Iguana *(Cyclura spp.) (Photo courtesy Dr. Douglas R. Mader, Marathon Veterinary Hospital, Marathon, Fla.)* **C,** Intraosseous catheter placement in the left tibia of a Red Tegu *(Tupinambis rufescens).* Correct intraosseous catheter placement is confirmed by aspiration of hemorrhagic aspirate (needle hub), consistent with bone marrow.

fluid therapy is most effective and should be administered as a constant rate infusion if vascular or intraosseous access has been established (Figure 12-1). IV catheters can be placed percutaneously in the jugular veins of chelonians (Figure 12-1, *A*) and in ventral tail veins of lizards. After cut-down techniques, IV catheters can also be placed in the cephalic and ventral abdominal veins of lizards (Figure 12-1, *B*) or in the jugular veins of snakes. In lizards, the tibia is a common site for IO catheterization (Figure 12-1, *C*) when IV access is not possible.

In cases of suspected or confirmed bacterial and fungal infections, effective antimicrobial/antifungal therapy should be initiated before the anesthetic event but preferably after the collection of material for culture and sensitivity testing. Particular attention should be paid to signs of respiratory or cardiovascular compromise because these will affect the anesthetic plan, including selection of drugs, dosages, and monitoring equipment, and the requirement for supportive care measures during anesthesia, such as intermittent positive pressure ventilation (IPPV).

ANALGESIA

Until recently, relatively little work had been done to determine effective drugs and dosages in commonly kept reptile species. Reptiles are a diverse group of animals with often pronounced taxonomic differences in response to analgesic agents and dosages. Therefore application of drugs and dosages derived from one species to another should be done with caution. It is well-known that application of preemptive analgesia in mammals is more effective in the management of pain and should likewise be provided to reptiles undergoing potentially painful procedures.

A balanced analgesic regimen takes advantage of distinct analgesic pathways and may include the systemic administration of different classes of analgesics (e.g., nonsteroidal antiinflammatory drugs [NSAIDs] and opioids) and/or the provision of local anesthetics. At present, local anesthetic regimens are not commonly utilized in reptiles. Although little data are available on effective drugs, dosages, and techniques, local anesthesia in combination with systemic analgesic therapy offers the advantages of reduced dosages for systemic analgesic agents and will reduce maintenance requirements during general anesthesia. The same principles established in domestic animals should be followed and should include administration of lidocaine or preferably the longer acting bupivacaine at the surgery site. Advanced techniques such as spinal anesthesia have been investigated and are described further on. It should be part of the anesthetic protocol to provide preoperative, intraoperative, and postoperative analgesia. Opioid agents are most effective in controlling acute pain resulting from trauma and surgery, whereas NSAIDs are most commonly used for the management of chronic pain.[1,12-14]

Common opioid analgesic agents used in reptiles to manage acute pain include morphine (1 to 2 mg/kg) and hydromorphone (0.5 to 1 mg/kg).[1,13] At present, the most common NSAID used in reptiles is meloxicam at 0.2 mg/kg IV, intramuscularly (IM), or per os (PO) every 24 to 48 hours. For further information on effective pain management and protocols see Chapter 18.

SEDATION

Sedation is commonly used in human and domestic animal veterinary medicine to facilitate diagnostic sample collection, medical treatment, and positioning for diagnostic imaging (Figure 12-2, *A-C*). *Sedation* is defined as a state of drug-induced altered consciousness that allows the patient to better

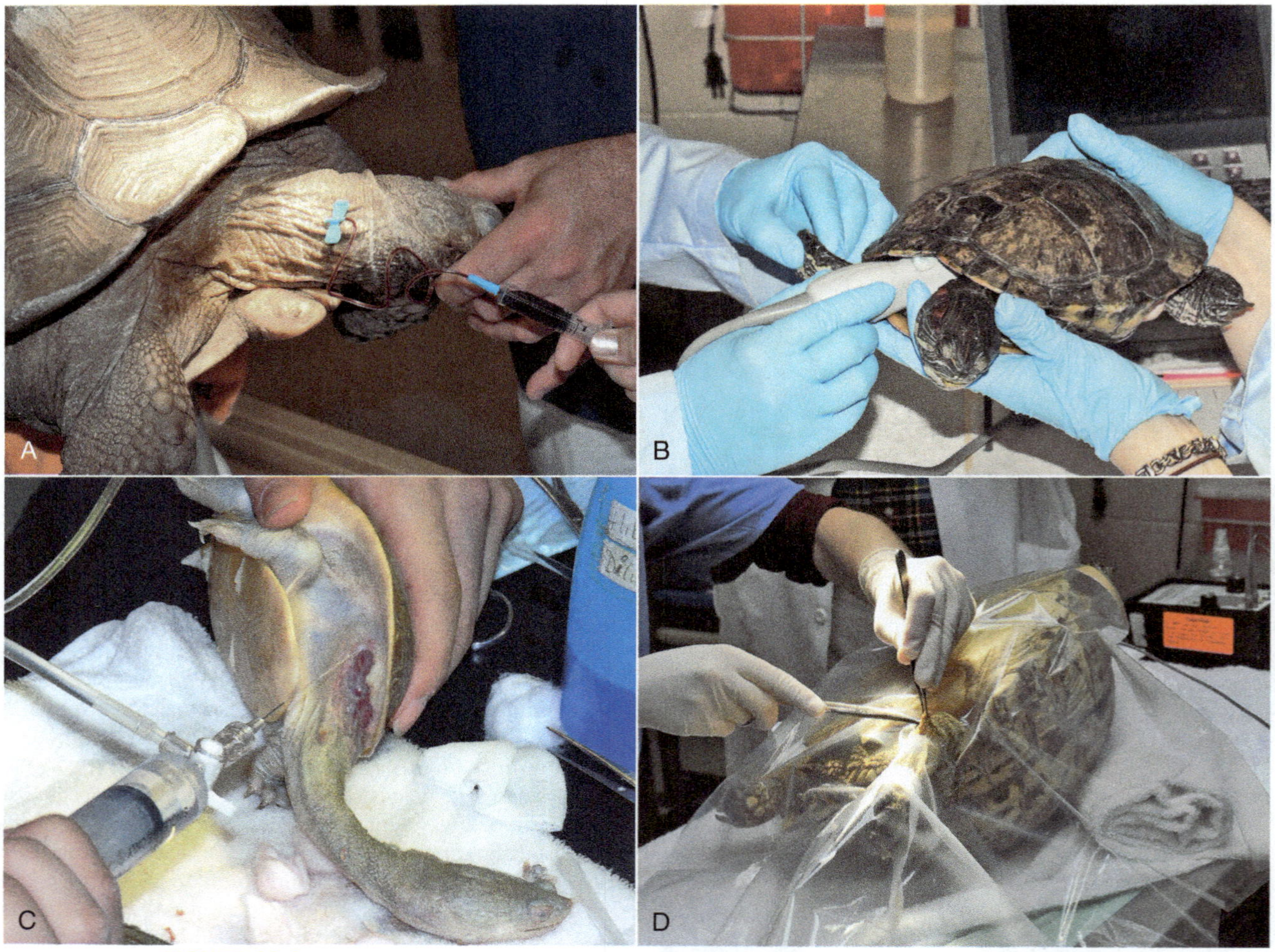

FIGURE 12-2 Procedural sedation in chelonians. In all animals, spontaneous respiration was maintained and a response to painful stimulation could be elicited. **A,** Blood collection from the right jugular vein of a sedated African Spurred Tortoise *(Centrochelys sulcata)*. **B,** Echocardiography in a sedated Red-eared Slider *(Trachemys scripta elegans)*. **C,** Wound debridement and lavage in a sedated Side-necked Turtle (*Chelodina* spp.). **D,** Surgical skin abscess removal under local lidocaine anesthesia in a sedated Leopard Tortoise *(Stigmochelys pardalis)*.

tolerate stressful or unpleasant procedures without depressing protective airway reflexes or having a significant cardiopulmonary depressant effect.[15] Currently, diagnostic procedures are often performed in conscious reptiles or under general anesthesia. For sedation of reptiles, a variety of injectable anesthetic drugs at lower subanesthetic doses can be used alone or, preferably, in combination.[16-19] Drugs used for sedation should be short-acting or reversible, so that prolonged or unpredictable recoveries are avoided. Sedative drugs should be chosen based on the desired level of sedation (mild to deep), the general condition of the patient, and the diagnostic and/or therapeutic procedure to be performed. Commonly used sedative protocols are summarized in Table 12-1. Under sedation, spontaneous respiration should be maintained and reptiles should respond to painful stimulation (e.g., toe pinch). The combination of procedural sedation, with either local or spinal anesthesia, offers the possibility of performing surgical or invasive procedures that would otherwise only be possible under general anesthesia (Figure 12-2, *D*). When sedation is combined with local or spinal anesthesia, the dose of general anesthetic drugs can be reduced, which will lead to reduced cardiovascular depression, more rapid recoveries, and potentially fewer anesthetic complications compared with general anesthesia.

REGIONAL ANESTHESIA AND ANALGESIA

Local Anesthesia

Local anesthesia is currently underutilized in reptile medicine but offers significant benefits, such as the ability to reduce the depth of general anesthesia or sedation for certain surgical procedures. In some cases, local anesthesia can be used solely in manually restrained or sedated animals for minor surgical procedures (see Figure 12-2, *D*).[20] Common indications for the use of local anesthetics as part of an anesthetic protocol in reptiles (see Table 12-2) include distal limb surgery, tracheal or lung washes, or infiltration of incision sites before coeliotomy. Lidocaine and bupivacaine are readily available in

TABLE 12-1

Sedation Protocols Commonly Used in Reptiles

	Dose (mg/kg)	Route	Species	Comments	Reference
CHELONIANS					
Midazolam	2	SC	Red-eared Slider Turtle	Mild sedation, inconsistent effects, completely reversible	17
Dexmedetomidine + midazolam	0.1 + 1	SC	Red-eared Slider Turtle, North American Box Turtles	Mild to moderate sedation, completely reversible; rapid recovery after reversal	*
Dexmedetomidine + midazolam + ketamine	0.1 + 1 + 2	SC	Red-eared Slider Turtle	Moderate sedation, partially reversible; rapid recovery after reversal, suitable for intrathecal injection and endotracheal intubation	24, 33
Medetomidine + ketamine	0.1 + 5	IM	Red-eared Slider Turtle	Deep sedation, suitable for intubation	36
Medetomidine + ketamine + morphine	0.15 + 2.5 + 1	SC	African Spurred Tortoise	Deep sedation to light anesthesia, partially reversible; rapid recovery after reversal	41
Medetomidine + midazolam + morphine	0.2 + 2 + 1	SC	African Spurred Tortoise	Deep sedation to light anesthesia, completely reversible; rapid recovery after reversal	41
Alfaxalone	10	IM	Red-eared Slider Turtle	Moderate sedation, suitable for intubation	49
Alfaxalone	10 and 20	IM	Horsfield's tortoises	Moderate to deep sedation, intubation not possible in about half of the tortoises	51
Propofol	2 to 5	IV		Moderate sedation; light anesthesia	5
LIZARDS					
Dexmedetomidine + midazolam	0.1 + 1	SC	Bearded Dragon, Green Iguana	Moderate sedation, completely reversible; rapid recovery after reversal	*
Dexmedetomidine + midazolam + ketamine	0.05 to 0.1 + 1 + 3	SC	Bearded Dragon, *Uromastyx*, Blue Iguana	Moderate to deep sedation, partially reversible; rapid recovery after reversal	*
Alfaxalone	10	IM	Green Iguana	Light to moderate sedation, maximum effect after approximately 5 min; duration of effect, approximately 10 min	50
Alfaxalone	9	IV	Australian lizards	Induction agent; maintain with gaseous anesthetic	52
Propofol	3 to 5	IV, IO		Deep sedation to light anesthesia	5
SNAKES					
Midazolam	1 to 2	SC, IM		Mild sedation, inconsistent effects	5
Tiletamine/zolazepam (Telazol)	2 to 5	SC, IM	Large snakes	Mild to moderate sedation, endotracheal intubation	6
Ketamine	5 to 10	SC, IM		Mild to moderate sedation, endotracheal intubation	6
Propofol	3 to 5	IV		Moderate sedation to light anesthesia	5, 20

*Mans C: Pers. com.

IM, Intramuscular; *IO,* intraosseous; *IV,* intravenous; *SC,* subcutaneous.

Atipamezole is used to antagonize medetomidine/dexmedetomidine in 1:1 volume, SC or IM. Flumazenil is used to antagonize midazolam: 0.01 to 0.1 mg/kg SC, IM, or IV. Nalaxone is used to antagonize morphine or hydromorphone: 0.04 to 0.2 mg/kg SC, IM, or IV.

most veterinary clinics, and both are effective local anesthetics in reptiles. The toxic dosages for local anesthetics have not been determined in reptiles. In mammals, toxic dosages for lidocaine have been reported to range from 5 to 20 mg/kg.[20] Although toxic dosages in reptiles are unknown, care should be taken not to exceed those dosages used in mammals, particularly in small reptile patients, so that systemic side effects can be avoided.

Spinal Anesthesia

In mammals and humans epidural anesthesia and spinal anesthesia (which is also known as intrathecal or subdural), are two estabilished forms of regional anesthesia of the spinal cord and nerves. In particular, epidural anesthesia is common practice. These techniques offer substantial advantages if used as part of a balanced anesthetic protocol: they reduce the amount of general anesthetics needed to perform certain surgical

TABLE 12-2

Anesthetic Protocols Commonly Used in Reptiles

	Dose (mg/kg)	Route	Species	Comments	Reference
CHELONIANS					
Medetomidine + midazolam + ketamine + morphine	0.15 + 2 + 2.5 + 1	SC	African Spurred Tortoise	Light anesthesia, reversible, rapid recovery, maintain with gaseous anesthetic, if necessary	41
Medetomidine + midazolam + ketamine + hydromorphone	0.15 + 0.5 + 10 + 0.5	SC	African Spurred Tortoise	Surgical anesthesia, maintain with gaseous anesthetic, if necessary	*
Medetomidine + ketamine	0.2 + 10	IM	Red-eared Slider Turtle	Surgical anesthesia, partially reversible	36
Medetomidine + ketamine	0.1 + 10	IV	Galapagos Tortoise	Surgical anesthesia, partially reversible	40
Medetomidine + ketamine + morphine	0.1 + 10 + 1.5	IM	Map Turtle	Surgical anesthesia; administration of nalaxone recommended if recovery is slow or to prevent renarcotization	37
Propofol	2 to 10	IV		Induction agent; use lower dose in large tortoises	5, 20
Propofol	10 to 20	IV	Red-eared Slider Turtle	Light anesthesia for approximately 60 min (10 mg/kg) or 90 min (20 mg/kg)	42
Alfaxalone	20	IM	Red-eared Slider Turtle	Induction agent; light anesthesia for 28 ± 13 min at 20°C	49
LIZARDS					
Alfaxalone	20 to 30	IM	Green Iguana	Induction agent, effect after about 5 min; duration of effect, 20 to 40 min	50
Alfaxalone	10	IV	Green Iguana	Induction agent; maintain with gaseous anesthetic	53
Propofol	5 to 10	IV, IO	Green Iguana	Induction agent, apnea common, requires intubation and IPPV	20, 79
SNAKES					
Propofol	3 to 10	IV, IC		Induction agent; maintain with gaseous anesthetic	5, 59
Alfaxalone	9	IV	Australian snakes	Light anesthesia, endotracheal intubation	52
Tiletamine/ zolazepam (Telazol)	2 to 6	IM		Induction agent; maintain with gaseous anesthetic	5
ALL REPTILES					
Isoflurane	2% to 5%			Induction, 5%; maintenance, 2% to 3%	5, 20
Sevoflurane	2.5% to 8%			Induction, 7% to 8%; maintenance, 2.5% to 4.5%	5, 20

*Mans C: Pers. com.

IC, Intracardiac; *IM,* intramuscular; *IO,* intraosseous; *IPPV,* intermittent positive pressure ventilation; *IV,* intravenous; *SC,* subcutaneous.

Atipamezole is used to antagonize medetomidine/dexmedetomidine in 1:1 volume, SC or IM. Flumazenil is used to antagonize midazolam: 0.01 to 0.1 mg/kg SC, IM, or IV. Nalaxone is used to antagonize morphine or hydromorphone: 0.04 to 0.2 mg/kg SC, IM, or IV.

procedures. Consequently, the dose-dependent cardiorespiratory depressant effects of general anesthetics are reduced, and in addition, improved and often longer term analgesia can be provided. Different classes of anesthetics and analgesics can be injected epidurally or intrathecally, which results in either desensitization of motor and sensory fibers (local anesthetics) or a sensory block only (i.e., opioid analgesics) without an effect on motor function. In humans and mammals, possible indications for epidural or spinal anesthesia include surgical procedures involving the tail, perineum, genitals, hindlimbs, and caudal abdomen.[21,22]

Regional anesthesia and analgesia of the spinal cord is currently in its infancy in reptiles and has only been reported in turtles and tortoises.[23-26] In chelonia, epidural anesthesia is not possible due to the lack of a sufficiently developed epidural space. However, a well-developed intrathecal (subdural) space, which directly surrounds the spinal cord and is filled with cerebrospinal fluid (CSF), is present (Figure12-3) and allows for intrathecal administration of various anesthetic and analgesic drugs. Because of the presence of the carapace and the fusion of the vertebral column to the carapace, access to the intrathecal space is limited in chelonia to the cervical and coccygeal vertebrae. Only intrathecal injections in the coccygeal area are of clinical interest.

In chelonia, the cloaca, genitalia, and hindlimbs are innervated by caudal branches of the sacral plexus and coccygeal nerves.[27,28] The sacral plexus arises from spinal nerves XVII through XXI, located at the last dorsal and sacral vertebrae[28,29] Within the sacral plexus, the nerves interconnect and subdivide several times before terminating in the inguinal, pelvic,

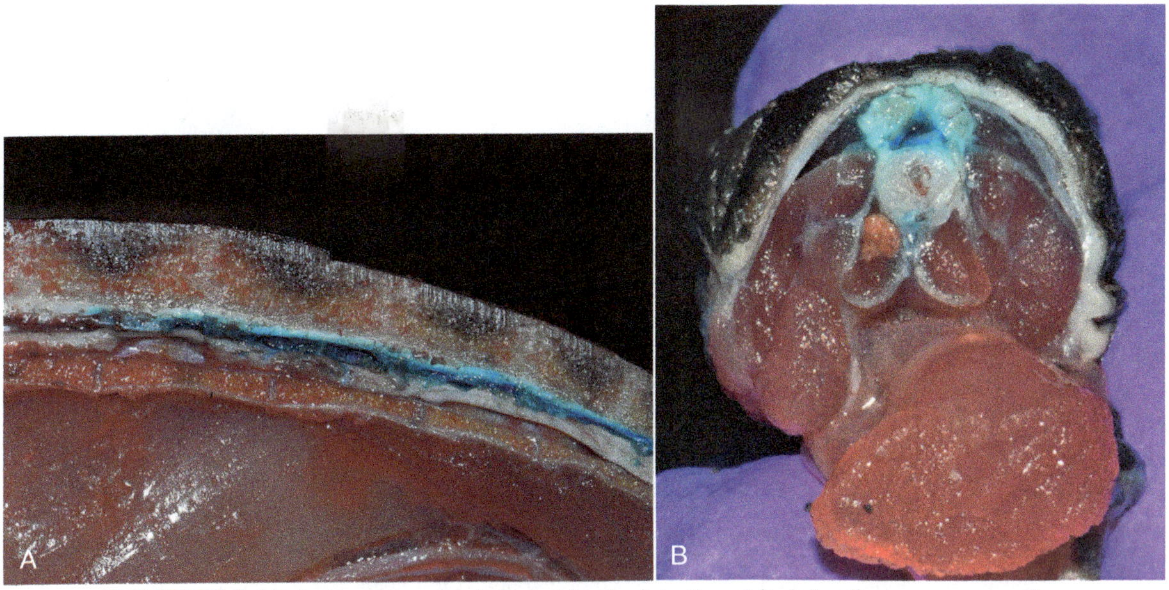

FIGURE 12-3 Methylene blue dye injected in the intrathecal (subdural) space surrounding the spinal cord in Red-eared Slider *(Trachemys scripta elegans)* carcasses. **A,** Cross-section of the proximal tail base. Note the close proximity of the skin overlying the neural arch dorsally. **B,** Sagittal view of the spinal canal at the level of the last dorsal and sacral vertebrae.

and hind leg muscles.[28,29] Therefore the temporary desensitization of these nerves by intrathecal injection of local anesthetics and analgesics can provide regional anesthesia and analgesia sufficient for a multitude of surgical procedures involving the cloaca, urinary bladder, genitals, and hindlimbs in turtles and tortoises. More cranial spreading of intrathecally administered anesthetics will lead to desensitization of spinal nerves located more cranially, which supply the prefemoral fossae and caudal coelomic organs, and potentially allow for surgical procedures via the prefemoral approach.

While anecdotal reports on the use of spinal anesthesia in chelonians exist, the clinical application has only been published in male Galapagos tortoises *(Chelonoidis [Geochelone] nigra)* with a body weight of 32 to 97 kg.[25] In these conscious tortoises 20G, 3-cm hypodermic needles were placed in the mid to distal dorsal coccygeal region after aseptic preparation (Figure 12-4, *A*). Needle placement was performed through an intervertebral space, which was identified by palpation. Correct intrathecal needle placement was confirmed by aspiration of CSF before intrathecal injection of 2% lidocaine at an average dosage of 0.8 mg/kg (0.04 mL/kg body weight or 1 mL of 2% lidocaine per 20 to 25 kg body weight). In all 15 animals, the level of regional anesthesia was graded as excellent and allowed for successful completion of phallectomy in all tortoises. At the reported dosage, no hindlimb paralysis was induced and no side effects were noticed. Repeated administration of local anesthetics into the intrathecal space after placement of an indwelling intrathecal catheter has also been reported in a Galapagos tortoise (body weight, 105 kg) for management of chronic cloacal prolapse.[26]

Research into the feasibility and efficacy of spinal anesthesia in Red-eared Sliders *(Trachemys scripta elegans)* has been performed.[23,24] Spinal anesthesia was successfully induced in turtles of both sexes, with body weights ranging from 0.5 to 1.0 kg. Injections were performed in sedated turtles, which allowed for proper restraint of the tail and correct intrathecal injection at the level of the mid to proximal coccygeal vertebrae. The turtles were positioned in horizontal ventral recumbencey and the tails were aseptically prepared before insertion of 28G needles, attached to 0.5-mL insulin syringes (Figure 12-5).[23,24] After penetration of the neural arch, the needle was advanced into the intrathecal space and careful aspiration was performed. If significant amounts of blood are aspirated, then the needle has been inadvertently placed in the prominent intravertebral venous plexus surrounding the intrathecal space. The needle position is readjusted until no aspiration of blood occurs, followed by injection of anesthetic and analgesic drugs over approximately 3 to 5 seconds. Successful intrathecal injection and induction of spinal anesthesia was confirmed by complete motor block (relaxation) of the tail, cloacal sphincter, and hindlimbs. A fast onset period was observed within 1 to 5 minutes. Following the initial injection of either preservative-free lidocaine (4 mg/kg, 2%) or bupivacaine (1 mg/kg, 0.5%) spinal anesthesia was successfully induced in about half of the turtles. In turtles in which no spinal anesthesia was induced after the initial injection, a second intrathecal injection of the same drug and dose was administered 15 minutes later. The repeated intrathecal injection increased the overall success rate to approximately 80% to 90 %.[23,24] In male and female Red-eared Sliders, the duration of motor block of the tail, cloacal sphincter, and hindlimbs was approximately 1 hour following lidocaine injection (4 mg/kg, 2%).[23,24] Intrathecal bupivacaine injection (1 mg/kg, 0.5%) in male Red-eared Sliders led to motor block of the tail, cloacal sphincter, and hindlimbs lasting approximately 2 hours.[24] A large variation in duration of spinal anesthesia was reported in male and female turtles. A possible explanation for this high degree of variation is the well-developed and prominent intravertebral venous plexus, which is located within the spinal canal directly overlying the intrathecal space predominately dorsally and laterally. Therefore a shorter duration of spinal anesthesia was attributed to a partial intrathecal dose delivery, secondary to an inadvertent

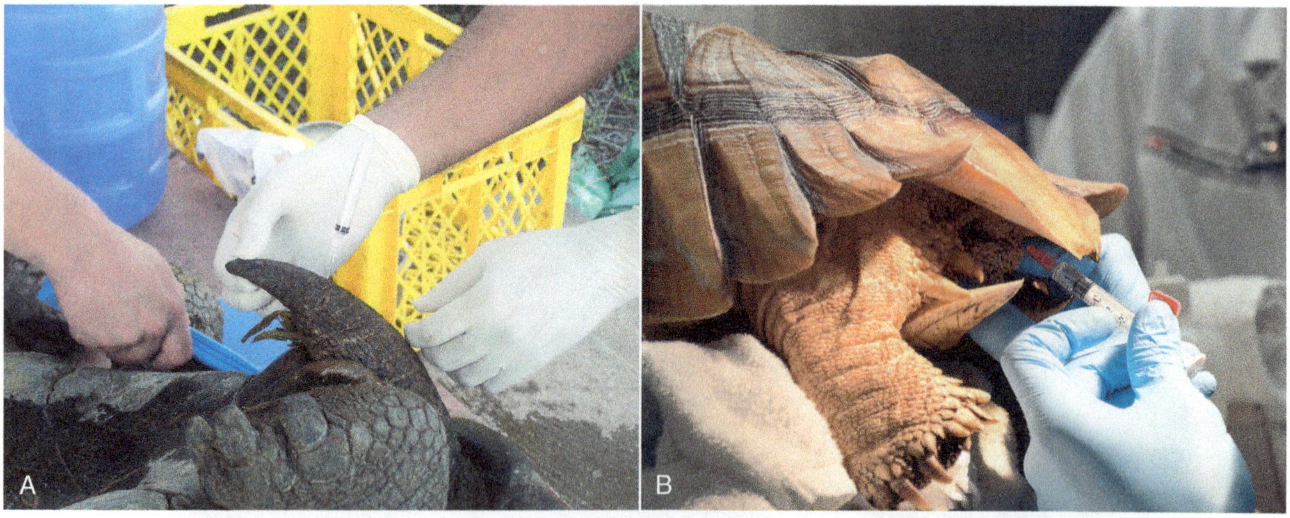

FIGURE 12-4 Spinal anesthesia in tortoises. **A,** Intrathecal injection of lidocaine in a conscious male Galapagos Tortoise *(Chelonoidis [Geochelone] nigra)* in dorsal recumbency before phallectomy. The needle is placed in the intervertebral space at the distal third of the tail. *(Image courtesy of S. Rivera.)* **B,** Intrathecal injection of lidocaine at the proximal tail in a sedated female African Spurred Tortoise *(Centrochelys sulcata)* before prefemoral cystostomy.

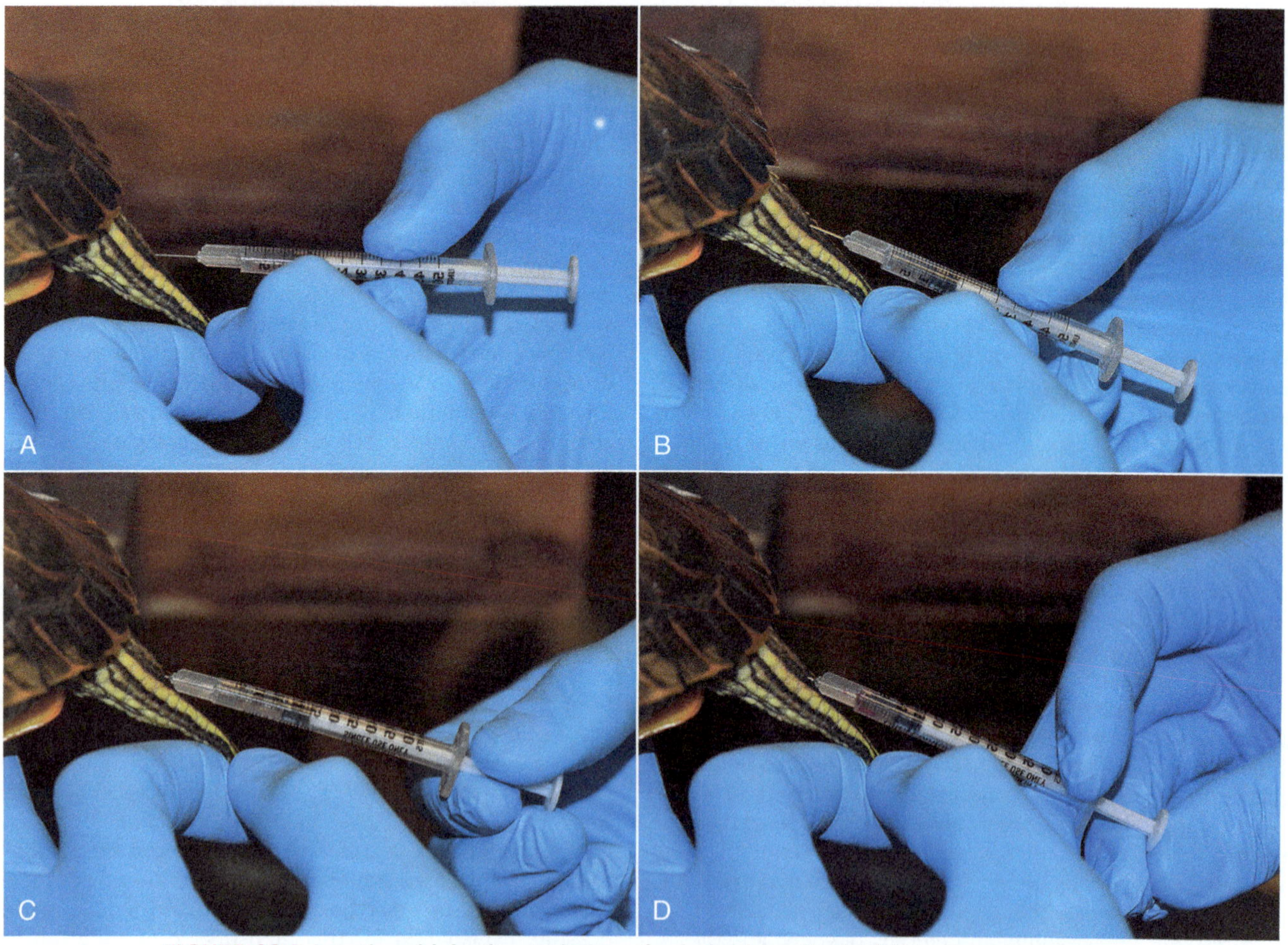

FIGURE 12-5 Intrathecal injection technique for induction of spinal (intrathecal) anesthesia and analgesia in a female Red-eared Slider *(Trachemys scripta elegans).* **A,** Penetration of the skin and neural arch with the needle at an approximately 45-degree angle. **B,** Advancement of the needle into the spinal canal at an approximately 20-degree angle. **C,** Aspiration is performed to ensure correct placement in the intrathecal place. If an excessive amount of blood is aspirated, the needle is repositioned until no further blood is aspirated. **D,** Injection of the drug into the intrathecal space over 5 to 10 seconds.

IV injection into the intravertebral venous plexus. Consequently, care should be taken with needle placement within the intrathecal space by means of repeated aspiration before and during intrathecal injection.

In addition to the injection of anesthetic drugs, drugs with primary analgesic properties can also be injected intrathecally for provision of long-term spinal analgesia. Intrathecally administered morphine relieves somatic and visceral pain by selectively blocking nociceptive impulses without interfering with sensory and motor function or causing sympathetic nervous system blockade leading to hypotension. Morphine is a highly hydrophilic drug that tends to induce long duration of action after intrathecal administration because of delayed systemic absorption and longer maintenance in the spinal cord.[30,31] In male Red-eared Slider Turtles, intrathecal administration of morphine (0.1 to 0.2 mg/kg, 4 mg/mL, preservative-free) and lidocaine (4 mg/kg, 2%) resulted in thermal antinociception of the hindlimbs for up to 48 hours.[24] No sedation was noted in any of the animals after intrathecal morphine administration. Therefore this combination of drugs should be considered so that short-term spinal anesthesia and concurrently long-lasting spinal analgesia can be achieved; if the analgesic effects last throughout the immediate postsurgical period, then the need for systemic opioid analgesic drugs is potentially reduced. It is currently unknown if intrathecal morphine has a potential respiratory effect in turtles, as has been documented for systemically administered morphine.[14]

In summary, spinal anesthesia and analgesia are clinically feasible techniques in chelonia. However, significant anatomic differences exist, particularly the presence of a prominent intravertebral venous plexus in Red-eared Slider Turtles. This makes general recommendations regarding technique and doses across chelonian species challenging. Furthermore, the amount of drug injected intrathecally will affect the extent of the sensory or motor block. Therefore different procedures will require different amounts of anesthetics and analgesics to be injected intrathecally. This technique may have to be repeated depending on the outcome. Currently, no studies have systematically evaluated the long-term effects and safety of intrathecal injections in chelonia. Strict aseptic techniques should be used to avoid iatrogenic complications, and only preservative-free drugs should be injected into the intrathecal space so that spinal toxicity and secondary neurologic complications are avoided. In contrast to mammals, in which the spinal cord terminates in the distal lumbar or lumbosacral region, the spinal cord in chelonia extends caudal to the last coccygeal vertebrae, and a cauda equina is not developed in chelonians.[32] Therefore intrathecal needle placement in chelonia can potentially lead to iatrogenic mechanical trauma of the spinal cord in the coccygeal area and neurologic deficits. Sedation before intrathecal injection is recommended so that the tail is sufficiently restrained and immobilized and the caudal scratch/kick reflex is reduced; otherwise the reflex makes intrathecal injections in conscious turtles and tortoises challenging. In contrast, in male Galapagos tortoises, intrathecal injections were successfully performed without the use of sedation.[25]

ANESTHETIC AGENTS

Before administration of any anesthetic or sedative drugs, reptiles should be maintained within their preferred optimal temperature zone (POTZ), and the core body temperature should be monitored throughout the chemical restraint period. A variety of agents representing different classes of drugs are often used either alone or in combination, depending on the desired level of sedation or anesthesia. Preference should be given to agents that have a specific antagonist available so that recovery time is reduced and the patient is returned as quickly as possible to the preanesthetic state. Similar drugs and drug combinations can also be chosen for premedication before induction of general anesthesia. If the patient is scheduled for a painful procedure, it is recommended that an analgesic agent such as an opioid be included in the preanesthetic protocol.

Most injectable protocols in reptiles include the administration of the dissociative anesthetic agent ketamine in combination with synergistic agents such as midazolam, opioid agents, and alpha-2 agonists (e.g., dexmedetomidine). The addition of synergistic agents such as an alpha-2 agonist will reduce the amount of ketamine required to induce sedation and immobilization. Therefore recovery times after administration of a specific alpha-2 antagonist (e.g., atipamezole) or benzodiazepine antagonists (e.g., flumazenil) will be greatly reduced. Although injectable agents alone can be used to facilitate short, minor procedures, induction and maintenance of a surgical plane of anesthesia for prolonged, invasive procedures is often based on administration of an inhalational agent such as isoflurane or sevoflurane.

Ketamine, a dissociative agent with dose-dependent anesthetic, sedative, and analgesic properties, is frequently used in reptile anesthesia. However, when administered alone, muscle relaxation is considered inadequate and recoveries excessively prolonged, especially when high dosages are used. Administering an alpha-2-adrenergic agonist (e.g., dexmedetomidine) or a benzodiazepine (e.g., midazolam) along with ketamine allows for reduction of the dose of ketamine administered and provides the benefit of partial reversibility of these protocols, leading to more rapid recoveries and increased safety. Even at lower subanesthetic dosages (less than 5 mg/kg), ketamine can provide additional sedation and analgesia if combined with other anesthetic drugs.[24,33]

Tiletamine/zolazepam (Telazol, Fort Dodge Laboratories, Fort Dodge, Iowa) is a commercially available drug combination composed of a dissociative anesthetic (tiletamine) and a benzodiazepine (zolazepam). Dosages of 2 to 10 mg/kg have been recommended for sedation, induction of general anesthesia, or facilitation of intubation.[5,6,20] The anesthetic efficacy of tiletamine/zolazepam can be unpredictable, and recovery may be prolonged. In dehydrated patients or in those with underlying renal or metabolic disorders, the use of this drug combination is contraindicated.[20] Tiletamine/zolazepam is also useful in large or dangerous species (e.g., crocodilians and large monitor lizards), and although not recommended for routine use in most reptiles, some have reported consistently good results (Mader DR: Pers. com., Feb, 2013).

Alpha-2-adrenergic agonists, such as medetomidine and dexmedetomidine, provide sedation, muscle relaxation, and possibly, analgesia in reptiles. Dose-dependent cardiovascular depression has been documented in reptiles after medetomidine administration.[19,34,35] Alpha-2-adrenergic agonists are commonly used in combination with ketamine, especially in chelonian species, for safe, reliable, and reversible sedation but can also be combined with benzodiazepines for procedural sedation.[36-41] Combining ketamine with medetomidine or dexmedetomidine allows reduction of both drug dosages, and reversibility of the alpha-2-adrenergic agonists with atipamezole will lead to faster and more predictable recoveries. Morphine or hydromorphone can be added to alpha-2 adrenergic-agonist-plus-ketamine protocols in cases in which analgesia is needed.[37] If morphine or hydromorphone are used, reversal with naloxone (0.04 to 0.2 mg/kg, subcutaneously [SC]) should be considered after termination of the anesthetic procedure, particularly in freshwater turtles, if respiratory depression is profound or if prolonged recoveries or renarcotization are to be avoided.[37]

Benzodiazepines, such as midazolam and diazepam, have sedative and muscle relaxant properties. Midazolam is water soluble, can be administered SC, IM, and IV, and is considered a more appropriate choice than diazepam, which is not recommended for IM or SC injection.[4] Midazolam, used alone, provides mild but highly variable sedation, which may be sufficient for minor clinical procedures.[16,17] Midazolam, combined with ketamine or an alpha-2-adrenergic agonist, reduces all drug dosages and attenuates the dose-dependent cardiovascular depressant effects and prolonged recoveries commonly observed with high dosages of ketamine. The effects of benzodiazepines can be antagonized with the use of flumazenil (0.05 mg/kg, SC), which shortens recovery from sedation or anesthesia.[41]

Propofol, a short-acting nonbarbiturate anesthetic agent, can be administered IV or IO to provide short-term anesthesia, facilitating procedures such as placement of an esophagostomy tube or abscess debridement, or to induce general anesthesia and allow for endotracheal intubation and maintenance of anesthesia with an inhalational anesthetic agent. Respiratory depression is more profound when propofol is administered rapidly.[20,42] Because propofol does not accumulate in tissues and is rapidly metabolized, complete recovery can be expected with assisted ventilation in cases of overdose. Propofol requires intravascular administration, which can be challenging in some species. Recently, published articles have described complications secondary to accidental extravascular injection of propofol intrathecally and into the subcarapacial sinus or the coccygeal vein of chelonian species.[43-45] Complications associated with intrathecal propofol injection included forelimb and hindlimb paralysis, coma, and spinal necrosis.[43-45] In addition, complications with propofol in sea turtles have been reported and include respiratory arrest and death several hours postanesthesia (Mader DR: Pers. com., Feb 2013).

Alfaxalone is a short-acting steroid anesthetic due for commercial release in the United States in 2013 that has a long history of use in other countries for induction of sedation or anesthesia. Alfaxalone is rapidly cleared and its metabolism is independent of organ function. Similar to propofol administration, alfaxalone administration is associated with smooth and rapid recoveries and dose-dependent cardiovascular and respiratory depression in mammals.[46-48] One major advantage of alfaxalone is that it can be administered IM as well as IV.[46,49-52] However, dose volumes are often large and may need to be divided between injection sites; thus the cost may be prohibitive in larger patients.

The IV administration of alfaxalone in Green Iguanas (*Iguana iguana*) (10 mg/kg) resulted in rapid induction of light anesthesia, which allowed endotracheal intubation.[52,53] The effects of IM administration of alfaxalone have been investigated in Red-eared Sliders, Horsfield's tortoises (*Agrionemys horsfieldii*) and Green Iguanas.[49-51] At a dose of 10 mg/kg IM light-to-moderate sedation, suitable for minor nonpainful procedures such as blood collection and physical examination was induced. At 20 mg/kg, light anesthesia was induced and allowed for endotracheal intubation in all Red-eared Sliders and Green Iguanas, but only in about half of the Horsfield's tortoises, which were moderately to deeply sedated. The administration of 30 mg/kg in Green Iguanas resulted in surgical anesthesia for up to 40 minutes.[50] The induction times after IM alfaxalone administration in Green Iguanas were short (approximately 5 to 10 minutes at 24°C to 27°C), and recovery was smooth. The induction, duration, and recovery times after alfaxalone administration were significantly shorter at 35°C compared with 20°C in Red-eared Slider Turtles.[49] At 20 mg/kg IM, the induction times were 19 ± 6 (20°C) and 7 ± 5 minutes (35°C), and the plateau phase lasted 28 ± 13 (20°C) or 8 ± 5 (35°C) minutes.[49]

Inhalational agents such as isoflurane and sevoflurane can be used for both induction and maintenance of anesthesia in many reptiles (but often not chelonians and crocodilians due to breath holding). Both agents offer the advantages of relatively fast induction and recovery times as well as limited organ toxicity, especially in patients with renal or hepatic impairment. Sevoflurane is commonly used in human and domestic animal anesthesia and has a low blood solubility. A rapid increase in alveolar concentration can be seen during induction with this agent. The low blood solubility allows for rapid changes in anesthetic depth. Investigations of the use of sevoflurane in various reptile species have shown variable results in that some species have not achieved a surgical plane of anesthesia. Few studies have investigated comparative cardiopulmonary effects of sevoflurane versus isoflurane in reptiles.[14] Administration of inhalational agents follows similar principles as those established for domestic animal anesthesia. After induction of anesthesia, the trachea should be intubated with an appropriately sized endotracheal tube, which should be connected to a non–rebreathing (body weight, less than 10 kg) or rebreathing system. IPPV should be performed in all reptiles. The concentration of the inhalational agent necessary to maintain a surgical plane of anesthesia depends on the health status of the patient. Minimum anesthetic concentrations (MAC) of isoflurane and sevoflurane have been determined in Green Iguanas and are 1.8% to 2.1% and 2.1% to 4.1%, respectively.[54,55] Maintenance requirements for a surgical plane of anesthesia have been reported to be 2% to 3% for isoflurane and 3.5% to 4.5% for sevoflurane.[5] Like all anesthetic agents, both isoflurane and sevoflurane will cause cardiopulmonary depression as shown in Green Iguanas, in which isoflurane at 3% induced severe hypotension.[56] Therefore the concentrations of both agents would have to be reduced in debilitated patients. A study in Green Iguanas has shown that cardiopulmonary effects of both inhalational agents are similar; however, sevoflurane will produce faster induction and recovery times.[1]

ROUTES OF ADMINISTRATION

Most commonly, the IM route of drug administration is chosen in reptiles. In snakes, the epaxial muscles are used, whereas in lizards and chelonians, muscles of the front limbs are a common injection site. Intramuscular injection of anesthetics results in quicker and less variable onset times compared with SC injection.[57] However, in Red-eared Slider Turtles administered dexmedetomidine–ketamine, the depth of anesthesia was not significantly different by 45 minutes after either IM or SC injection.[57] Further, SC opioid absorption has been shown to be rapid in Red-eared Slider Turtles. Therefore the SC administration of anesthetic and analgesic drugs offers several advantages over IM injection, including access to a variety of SC sites requiring minimal manual restraint or patient manipulation and the capability of administering larger volumes in a single location.

In lizards, IV injections are most commonly given into the coccygeal vein. Injections into the ventral abdominal vein should only be made through an IV catheter. The jugular vein, subcarapacial sinus, brachial plexus, and dorsal coccygeal vein are the most commonly used sites for IV drug administration in chelonians. Accidental administration of anesthetic agents into the subdural space during attempted coccygeal vein or subcarapacial injection can occur, usually leading to severe complications.[43-45] IV injection sites in snakes are limited to the coccygeal vein and the jugular vein after a cut-down procedure. Intracardiac administration of propofol has also been reported in snakes in a controlled study[58] and results in rapid onset with no significant complications reported. However, cardiac tamponade after cardiocentesis in snakes has been reported, and the increased risk of intracardiac injections should be considered.[59]

Intranasal administration of anesthetic agents has been investigated in chelonians.[57,60,61] Intranasal administration of dexmedetomidine (0.2 mg/kg) and ketamine (10 mg/kg) only induced mild-to-moderate sedation in Yellow-bellied Sliders (*Trachemys scripta scripta*) at doses that would result in surgical anesthesia if administered IM or SC.[62] In Red-eared Sliders, the intranasal complete delivery of dexmedetomidine (0.1 mg/kg) and ketamine (10 mg/kg) was not possible due to the exhibited defense behavior of the turtles, and no anesthesia was induced, in contrast to IM or SC injection of the same doses of drugs.[57] However, for administration of atipamezole in anesthetized Red-eared Sliders, the intranasal route has been shown to be as effective as the IM or SC route.[57] In large chelonians in particular, large volumes of the anesthetic agent are a limiting factor.

Administration in the caudal half of the body can significantly affect drug plasma levels and therefore the efficacy of anesthetic and analgesic drugs in reptiles. In Red-eared Sliders, plasma levels of buprenorphine after SC hindlimb injection were significantly lower compared with forelimb injection.[62] These differences were attributed to a hepatic first-pass effect after hindlimb administration. Furthermore, the administration of dexmedetomidine–ketamine into the hindlimbs of Red-eared Sliders failed to induce anesthesia, whereas the same dose administered in the forelimb induced anesthesia.[57] Therefore the current recommendation is to avoid administration of drugs into the caudal half of the body, the hindlimbs, and/or tail because of more rapid clearance and lower plasma levels compared with administration into the cranial half of the body.[63,64]

GENERAL ANESTHESIA

Induction

Induction of anesthesia can be accomplished with injectable or inhalational agents. In patients with established vascular access, slow administration of propofol (3 to 10 mg/kg IV or IO) or alfaxalone (10 mg/kg IV, 20 mg/kg IM) will induce rapid induction of anesthesia. Alternately, IM administration of alfaxalone, combinations of ketamine, midazolam, alpha-2-agents, and/or opioids will produce a light plane of anesthesia adequate for endotracheal intubation and maintenance with an inhalational agent. Mask or chamber induction with an inhalational agent alone may be prolonged because of most reptiles' ability to breathhold. Aquatic species in particular are capable of converting to anaerobic metabolism and may hold their breath for extended periods of time. However, in snakes and lizards, chamber induction is effective and frequently used, particularly in venomous species (Figure 12-6).

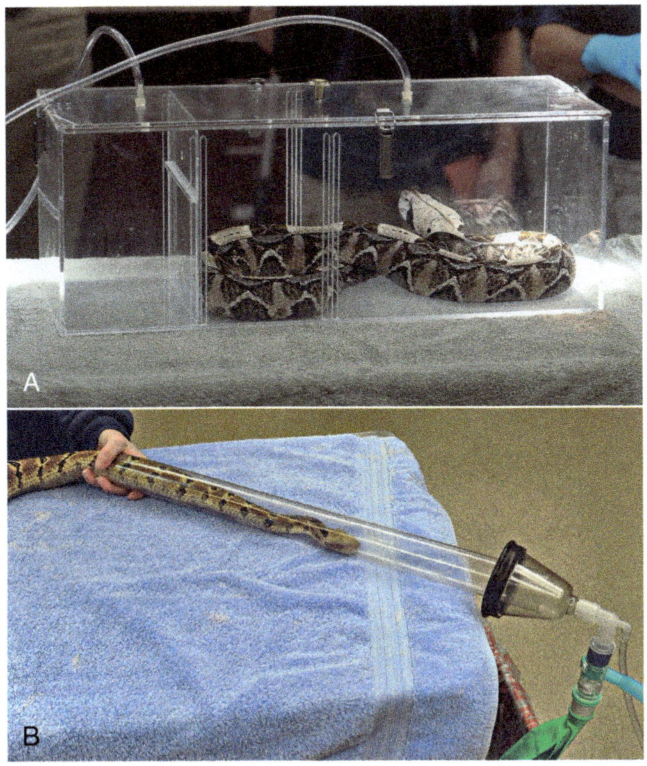

FIGURE 12-6 Anesthetic chamber induction of snakes. **A,** Induction of a Gaboon Viper *(Bitis gabonica)* in an induction chamber. **B,** Induction of an Eastern Massasauga Rattlesnake *(Sistrurus catenatus catenatus)* in a snake tube.

Endotracheal intubation is relatively easy to perform in most snakes and lizards. In these species, the glottis is located rostrally, and the trachea can be intubated with an appropriately sized endotracheal tube (Figure 12-7). Most chelonians have a fleshy tongue and the glottis is located at the base of the tongue, thus making visualization difficult (see Figure 12-7, *A*). Good muscle relaxation is necessary for opening the mouth wide enough to visualize the glottis and intubate the trachea. Care should be taken not to intubate the left or right primary bronchus because the tracheal bifurcation is cranial in most chelonians. In some species, a mouth gag should be used to protect the endotracheal tube and facilitate placement of monitoring devices (e.g., pulse oximeter probe). The trachea in chelonians has closed cartilaginous rings, whereas in lizards and snakes the cartilaginous rings are incomplete. Uncuffed endotracheal tubes are used in chelonians and in small lizards and snakes (see Figure 12-7, *B*). In larger squamates, cuffed tubes can be used instead (Figure 12-8).

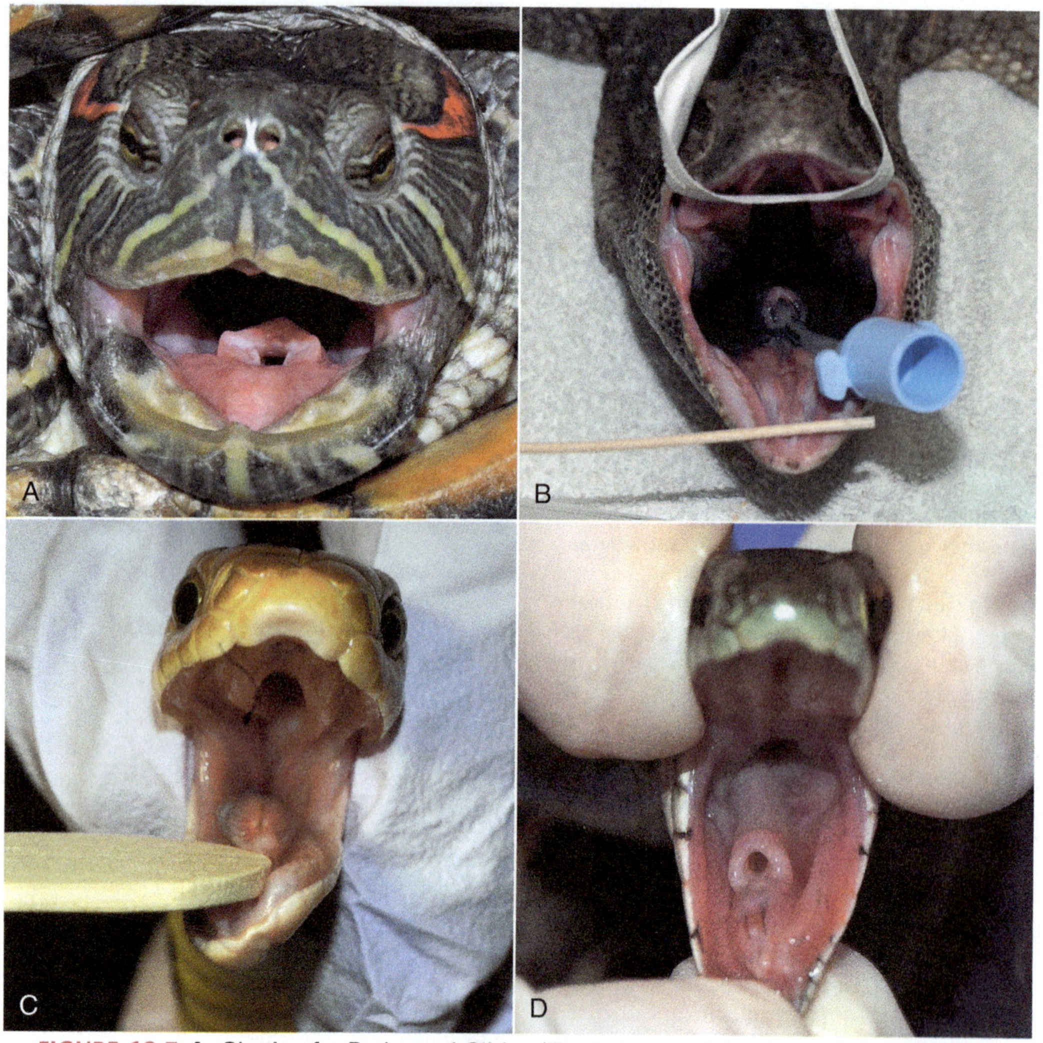

FIGURE 12-7 **A,** Glottis of a Red-eared Slider *(Trachemys scripta elegans).* **B,** Intubation of a Savannah Monitor *(Varanus exanthematicus)* with an uncuffed endotracheal tube. **C** and **D,** Glottis of snakes in closed **(C)** and open position **(D).**

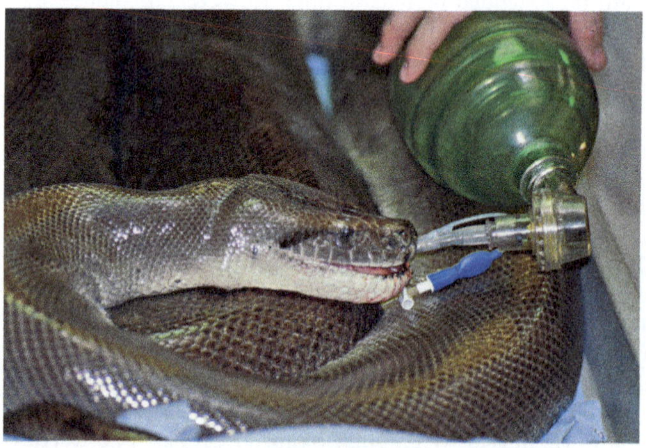

FIGURE 12-8 Papuan python *(Apodora papuana)* recovering from anesthesia. The patient is intubated with a cuffed endotracheal tube and ventilation is assisted by means of a bag-valve mask (Ambubag).

MAINTENANCE

During maintenance of anesthesia, the patient should be monitored regularly for depth of anesthesia, cardiopulmonary performance, and evidence of pain. If indicated, the anesthetic level needs to be adjusted, and additional analgesic therapy may be warranted. Similar to domestic animals, reptiles show dose-dependent cardiopulmonary depression; thus a decrease in heart rate and arterial blood pressure will be seen, although blood pressure monitoring is difficult and often impractical. Throughout the preanesthetic, intraanesthetic, and postanesthetic periods, the patient should be maintained within the POTZ of the species.

All reptiles require IPPV at a surgical plane of anesthesia, which can be performed manually or more accurately with a mechanical ventilator. Pressure-driven ventilators are commercially available and will accurately ventilate even small reptilian patients. Overinflation of the lungs and air sacs will be avoided if the inspiratory pressure does not exceed 12 cm H_2O. It has been recommended anecdotally that the anesthetized reptile receive ventilation at four to six breaths per minute, but the rate of IPPV needs to be adjusted for each patient based on the preanesthetic examination and end-tidal carbon dioxide ($EtCO_2$) values. For example, in anesthetized South American Rattlesnakes *(Crotalus durissus),* five breaths per minute led to respiratory alkalosis and was considered excessive, whereas 0.67 breaths per minute led to mild hypercapnia and mild respiratory acidosis. Therefore a respiratory rate of one to two breaths per minute was recommended for this species.[65]

Depth of Anesthesia

Depth of anesthesia should be evaluated regularly, and adjustments need to be made if the depth is determined to be too deep or too light. If a response to a painful stimulus such as movement or an increase in heart rate occurs, the concentration of the anesthetic agent should be increased; additional systemic or regional analgesic therapy may also be indicated.

Body Temperature

Before induction of anesthesia, the patient should be maintained in the POTZ for the species. Response to anesthetic and analgesic agents is dictated by body temperature, and the reptile should be maintained within the preferred temperature range before, during, and after anesthesia.[49] A hypothermic reptile will have compromised metabolic function, and induction as well as recovery from the anesthetic event will be delayed.[49,66] It has been shown in several studies that body temperature has a profound effect on respiration, blood gas, and acid–base status in reptiles.[67,68] In freshwater turtles such as the painted turtle *(Chrysemys picta bellii),* oxygen uptake increased disproportionately as compared with pulmonary ventilation with increasing temperatures.[67] Body temperature should be measured and recorded with an esophageal or cloacal temperature probe. Every effort should be made to prevent hypothermia during anesthesia and the recovery period. Heat lamps, circulating water blankets, and other equipment should be available to ensure euthermia.

MONITORING TECHNIQUES

Accurate monitoring of anesthetic variables is essential for safely and effectively anesthetizing the reptilian patient. An accurate anesthesia record including preanesthetic findings, anesthetic techniques and drugs, cardiopulmonary variables, and recovery data should be completed (Figure 12-9). Application and interpretation of many monitoring techniques in reptiles is in its infancy, and some devices and techniques may only be of limited value.[69] Monitoring of cardiopulmonary performance in the anesthetized reptilian patient presents challenges, and further work is needed to establish reference data for common reptile species. One should be familiar with the applications and limitations of various monitoring devices developed for human and veterinary anesthesia. Anesthesia monitoring techniques such as pulse oximetry, arterial blood gas analysis, and capnography are commonly used in human and veterinary anesthesia, but few have been validated for use in reptiles. In addition, reference values for common reptile species and common anesthetic protocols are scant. Therefore knowledge of the anatomy, physiology, and pathophysiology of the species to be anesthetized is essential. In addition, the pharmacology of sedative and anesthetic agents being used, as well as their effects on cardiopulmonary performance and organ function, needs to be known. The accurate interpretation of cardiopulmonary performance requires knowledge of normal values in reptiles that are awake; however, few studies have investigated normal cardiopulmonary variables in awake, nonanesthetized reptiles. Most published articles have collected data on cardiopulmonary function from anesthetized animals. Comparison of data requires consideration of the different effects of the anesthetic agent used. A study in Green Iguanas has determined selected cardiopulmonary values in conscious animals including respiratory rate, heart rate, direct arterial blood pressures, and arterial and venous blood gas variables.[70]In addition, the effects of 100% oxygen inspiration were measured. Comparison was also made between arterial blood gas analysis and pulse oximetry readings in conscious Green Iguanas. It was shown that oxygen saturation as measured by pulse oximetry underestimated saturation calculated by arterial blood gas analysis.[70]

Reflexes

In reptiles, determination of the degree of sedation and depth of anesthesia is commonly performed by assessment of the presence or absence of reflexes such as head or limb withdrawal, righting reflex, palpebral and corneal reflexes, toe/tail pinch reflexes, and cloacal tone. However, in some cases, results may be erroneous, and the depth of anesthesia is determined inaccurately. In general, a surgical plane of anesthesia including effective analgesia is present when there is no response to a painful stimulus such as a skin incision and, consequently, no changes in cardiopulmonary variables such as tachycardia, hypertension, or an increase in respiratory rate. The absence of some reflexes, such as the tongue withdrawal reflex, may also indicate too deep of a plane of anesthesia. At present, a classification system to determine anesthetic depth has not been established in reptiles.

Bispectral Index Monitors

Although determination of cardiopulmonary variables such as heart rate and respiratory rate are helpful in the assessment of the patient's overall status, assessment of the depth of anesthesia is challenging.[71] In mammals, measurement of the depth of anesthesia and awareness is difficult at best, and it is almost impossible to assess in reptiles. In human anesthesia, monitors are available that will process the level of corticocerebral activation measured by electroencephalography into a signal, which will reflect the depth of anesthesia. Bispectral index monitors are routinely used in human subjects and have been investigated for use in domestic animals. However, in veterinary anesthesia, species differences and the effects of a multitude of drug combinations affecting bispectral index monitoring need to be taken into consideration. A comprehensive review of bispectral index monitoring and the potential applications and limitations in zoologic medicine has been reported recently.[71] In reptiles, application of bispectral index monitoring is challenging. Studies in chelonians have shown that intraoperative recordings of the electrical activity of the cortex resulted in varying patterns of deep suppression and cortex activation. However, studies in snakes and lizards have demonstrated that bispectral index monitoring may be more useful in these species when compared with chelonians.[71] At present, trends in bispectral index values are more useful than assessment of absolute numbers because of pronounced

Reptile/Amphibian Anesthesia Record

Surgery date:____________ Table time:____________
Estimated time required:________________________
Location of procedure: Hospital ____ Field ____ Other _____
Clinician:________________________________
Technician:__________ Student:________________

PATIENT INFO

PREANESTHESIA

Physical examination:☐ Owner signed consent:☐
Checked previous anesthesia/medical history: ☐
Previous endotracheal tube size:____________
Weight: ________g/kg Code status: R☐ Y☐ G☐
Fast Y☐N☐ for _____hrs, food/water pulled at ______ am/pm
Clin. Path.: CBC ☐ Biochem☐ QUADS☐ UA☐
Risks/concerns?________________________________

Premedications Dose, mg/kg ⇨ mg ⇨ mL Time
1. ______________________
2. ______________________
3. ______________________
4. ______________________

Induction/gas Dose, mg/kg ⇨ mg ⇨ mL Time
1. ______________________
2. ______________________
3. ______________________

Reversal/recovery Dose, mg/kg ⇨ mg ⇨ mL Time
1. ______________________
2. ______________________
3. ______________________

Emergency drugs: sheet printed ☐ drugs drawn-up ☐

ANESTHESIA SETUP

Fluids ☐: Type: ______________ Qty: ________ mL
Catheter setup: IV☐ IO☐ (SQ☐, IP/ICe☐)
Syringe pump: ☐ Rate _______________ mL/hr
ET intubation:☐ Tube size(s):________________
Facemask:☐ Sizes:____________________
Nasal intubation:☐
Ventilation: Y☐N☐ Vetronics☐ Manual☐
Monitoring: Pulse ox ☐ Probe, rectal ☐ Tongue ☐
Thermometer☐ Heated table☐ Bair Hugger ☐
Doppler☐ Stethoscope☐ ECG☐ BP☐
Capnography ☐ Pediatric☐ Adult☐

PROCEDURES TO BE PERFORMED

☐Detailed physical examination
☐Radiography ☐Ultrasonography ☐CT ☐MRI
☐Blood draw ____ml (max: ___ml)
Collection site : ________________
☐Beak/nail trim
☐Endoscopy : ________________
☐Dentistry : ________________
☐Wound management/bandaging
☐Feeding tube (esophagostomy tube)
☐Tattoo/Microchip
Location : ________________
☐Misc surgery : ________________
☐Other ________________

ANESTHETIC SUMMARY

To be completed at end of procedure
Premedication:________________
Induction:________________
Recovery:________________
Additional comments:________________

VERIFICATION

Student/Tech signature:

Miscellaneous Items/Comments

FIGURE 12-9 Recording sheet for use in reptile anesthesia. *(Courtesy Dr. Stephen J. Divers, University of Georgia, Athens, Ga.)*

Reptile/Amphibian Anesthesia Record

Abbreviations												
Time		0	15	30	45	60	15	30	45	60		Anesth. induct.
O_2 flow L/min												Gas started
Vaporizer %												Surgery start
Inspiratory gas %												Surgery end
End-tidal gas %												Anesth. end
Inspiratory O_2												
End-tidal CO_2												
SpO_2												
HR ●	85										400	Extubation
Ventilation ○	80										380	
S Spontaneous												
C Controlled	75										360	
Arterial pressure	70										340	
∇ Systolic												
X Mean	65										320	
△ Diastolic												
	60										300	
	55										280	
	50										260	
	45										240	
	40										220	
	35										200	
	30										180	
	25										160	
	20										140	
	15										120	
	10										100	
	5										80	
	0										0	
Temperature												
CRT/MM												
Fluids												

Detailed comments:____

FIGURE 12-9, cont'd

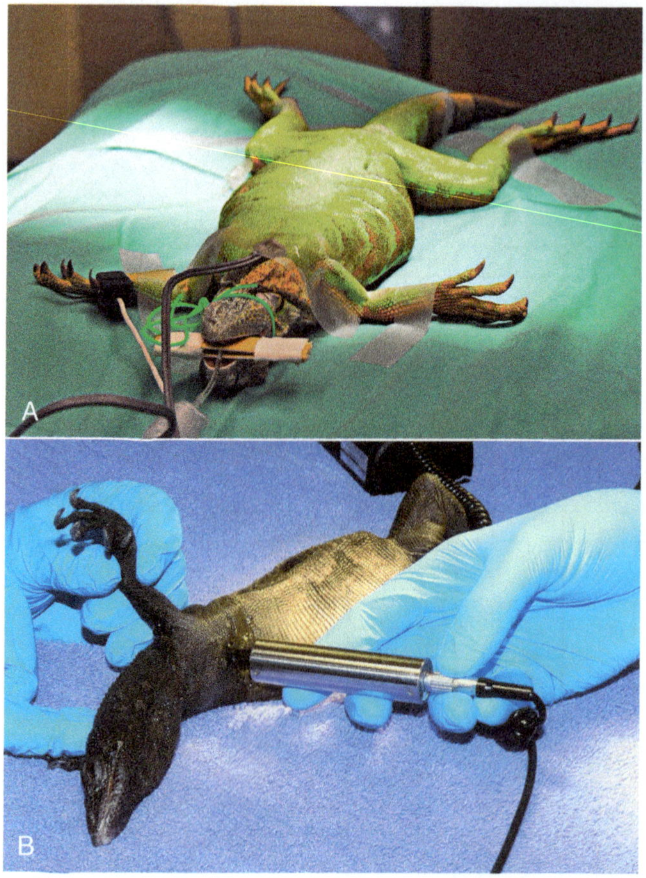

FIGURE 12-10 Placement of an ultrasonic Doppler flow device at the level of the heart in an anesthetized Green Iguana *(Iguana iguana)* **(A)** and a Black Tree Monitor *(Varanus beccarii)* **(B)**. Note that in monitor lizards the heart is located more caudally compared with other lizards. Therefore the Doppler probes are placed at different levels in these two animals. A pulse oximeter probe has also been placed on the left forelimb of the Green Iguana **(A)**.

species and drug variability. Future work is necessary to clearly define the accuracy of this monitoring tool for reptilian patients.

CARDIOVASCULAR PERFORMANCE

In reptiles, monitoring of cardiovascular performance is challenging. Many variables commonly recorded in mammalian species are either impractical to determine in reptiles or reference values have not been established. Assessment of mucous membrane color and capillary perfusion time is inaccurate in reptiles, and measurement of cardiac output has limited clinical applications in reptile anesthesia. The most accurate assessment of cardiac output in reptiles is determination of the heart rate. An esophageal stethoscope can be used in most reptiles for direct auscultation of the heart under anesthesia. Both tachycardia and bradycardia can decrease cardiac output and reduce the flow of blood to peripheral tissues. A baroreceptor reflex has been demonstrated in conscious Green Iguanas.[70]

Ultrasonic Doppler flow devices are the most useful and reliable monitoring devices in reptile anesthesia and allow for noninvasive recording of heart rate and rhythm in both conscious and anesthetized animals. Values derived from the conscious patient before induction of anesthesia should be used as reference values during anesthesia. Depending on the species, the probe can be placed directly over the level of the heart (snakes and lizards; Figure12-10) or over the carotid artery (lizards and chelonians). In chelonians, a pencil probe can be placed on the lateral side of the neck at the level of the carotid artery. For small patients, a pediatric probe can be used because its sensitivity in detecting blood flow in small vessels is higher.

Electrocardiography (ECG) can be performed to monitor cardiac function in the patient (Figure 12-11).[11] Unfortunately, limited data have been published to establish reference variables in commonly kept reptile species. The reptilian ECG is similar to a mammalian ECG with a P, QRS, and T wave, and in some species, an SV wave is present before the P wave. Low

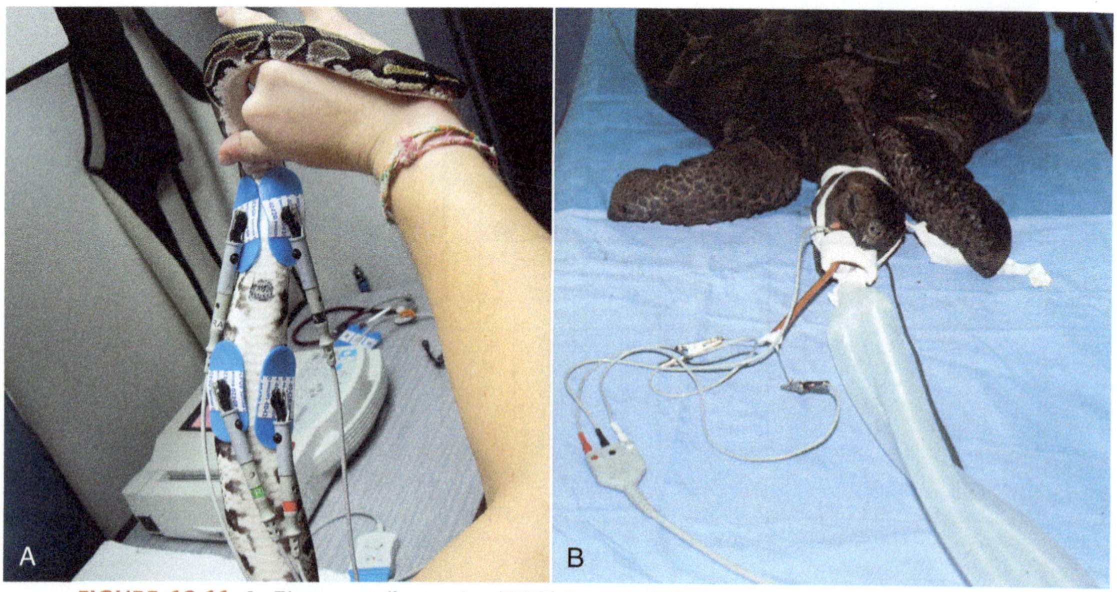

FIGURE 12-11 A, Electrocardiography (ECG) in a Ball Python *(Python regius)* *(Courtesy Dr. Douglas R. Mader, Marathon Veterinary Hospital, Marathon, FL.)* **B,** Placement of an esophageal ECG in an anesthetized Galapagos Tortoise *(Chelonoidis [Geochelone] nigra)*.

electrical amplitudes may make interpretation of a reptilian ECG challenging. An ECG can be performed in all reptiles, and electrodes should be attached in snakes two heart-lengths cranial and caudal to the heart. In lizards and chelonians, electrodes should be placed in the cervical region instead of the front limbs.[10] In larger species, an esophageal ECG can be placed (Figure 12-11, *B*). Factors influencing heart rate, such as environmental temperature and painful stimuli, should be considered when interpreting a reptilian ECG. However, persistent baseline ECG and heart rate can also be detected in reptiles after central nervous system death; therefore ECG as a monitor of cardiac activity for anesthetized reptiles is of limited value.

Indirect blood pressure measurements are possible in many species of reptiles but have poor correlation with values obtained via direct blood pressure measurements.[56,72] Arterial blood pressure is a function of heart rate, blood volume, stroke volume, and arterial compliance. All anesthetic agents will compromise cardiovascular homeostasis to varying degrees. Direct arterial blood pressure measurements have been reported in both conscious and anesthetized reptiles. Baseline arterial pressures have been established in conscious Green Iguanas and Grey Ratsnakes.[70,73] Green Iguanas had lower baseline arterial blood pressures (systolic arterial pressure, 69 ± 10 mm Hg; mean arterial pressure, 62 ± 12 mm Hg; diastolic arterial pressure, 56 ± 13 mm Hg) than those reported for mammals. The baseline peripheral pulse pressure in Green Iguanas was 14 ± 7 mm Hg, which is lower than reported human values (approximately 40 mm Hg). Direct arterial blood pressure measurements require surgical exposure, catheterization of a peripheral artery, and availability of a suitable monitoring device (Figure 12-12). In most reptiles, catheterization of an artery such as the carotid artery in chelonians, snakes, and lizards requires a cut-down procedure. Once established, continuous monitoring of heart rate and direct arterial blood pressures can be accomplished. An added advantage of an arterial catheter is access to arterial blood samples for determination of arterial blood gas variables such as arterial blood oxygen saturation, pH, and partial pressures of oxygen and carbon dioxide. Arterial catheterization for direct blood pressure monitoring and blood gas evaluation is time-consuming and largely impractical for clinical practice; however, these techniques are certainly of value for research purposes.

RESPIRATORY PERFORMANCE

Determination of respiratory rate and effort before administration of sedative agents or induction of anesthesia will give valuable information on the respiratory status of the patient, evidence of underlying respiratory disease processes, and baseline values for the rate of ventilation during anesthesia. The baseline respiratory rate of healthy Green Iguanas is 28 ± 6 breaths/min.[70] Supportive measures such as administration of antimicrobial agents, tracheal suctioning, and administration of oxygen should be initiated before anesthesia. Once the reptile is anesthetized, monitoring of respiratory performance is limited to pulse oximetry, arterial blood gas analysis, and capnography. Unfortunately, most devices have not been validated for reptiles; however, they do give valuable information on trends in the respiratory and metabolic status of the patient. Pulse oximetry has been validated in Green Iguanas.[70,74] The respiratory rate and effort cannot be determined because all reptiles require assisted ventilation during anesthesia, either by means of manual ventilation or use of a mechanical ventilator. Although the accuracy of these monitoring modalities have yet to be validated in reptile anesthesia, investigations have been performed in some reptile species (mainly Green Iguanas) to determine the usefulness and accuracy in reptile anesthesia.[71]

Pulse oximetry is routinely used in mammalian patients to calculate relative arterial oxygen hemoglobin saturation (SpO_2). The accuracy of pulse oximetry is influenced by poor tissue perfusion as well as pigmentation of the skin. In reptile anesthesia, the use of pulse oximetry is associated with several concerns and potential erroneous readings (see Figure 12-10, *A* and Figure 12-13). Pulse oximeters are calibrated based on the human oxygen hemoglobin dissociation curve, and SpO_2 values are calculated. High levels of methemoglobin have been reported for reptiles and will also affect pulse oximeter readings. A further concern is pronounced differences in respiratory physiology and function among reptile species. Therefore a reference value derived from one taxa may not be accurate in other taxa. An unpublished thesis in Green Iguanas has shown that there was a strong correlation between arterial oxygen saturation values derived from pulse oximetry and arterial blood gas analysis.[74] It is a noninvasive technique; however, access to a peripheral artery may be challenging and clinically impractical. Reflectance pulse oximeter probes are most useful and can be placed into the esophagus at the level of the carotid artery or in the evacuated cloaca to provide continuous monitoring of arterial blood oxygen saturation and heart rate. In sevoflurane or isoflurane anesthetized Green Iguanas, a comparison of arterial blood oxygen saturation as determined by pulse oximetry (SpO_2) versus arterial blood gas analysis (SaO_2) showed no significant differences between the two monitoring modalities over time. Although not significant, SpO_2 values were lower than SaO_2 values at all points in isoflurane anesthetized iguanas.[75] A study in conscious Green Iguanas showed that oxygen saturation calculated by pulse oximetry (86 ± 6%) was lower than the SaO_2 (92 ± 5%) indicated by arterial blood gas analysis.[71] Baseline SaO_2 values in conscious iguanas were reported to be greater than 90%.[71]

Blood Gas Analysis

It has been well-established in human and veterinary anesthesia that arterial blood gas analysis allows for accurate assessment of pulmonary function including ventilation, oxygenation, and acid-base status. Venous blood gas values will give an assessment of metabolic status. Venous blood gas values are affected by local tissue metabolism and low blood flow, but in humans, venous blood gas analysis can predict arterial blood gas values for pH, PCO_2, and bicarbonate concentrations. Baseline venous blood gas values in Green Iguanas are similar to those reported in humans and domestic animals.[70] In reptiles, interpretation of arterial blood gas variables is challenging because of the lack of normal reference values and physiologic features such as intracardiac shunting, the ability to tolerate varying degrees of hypoxia, and the capability to convert to anaerobic metabolism. Intrapulmonary shunts will bypass gas exchange in the lungs. In reptiles, many factors will influence arterial blood gas composition, including taxonomic differences (e.g., aquatic versus terrestrial species), inspired concentration of oxygen, and temperature. At present,

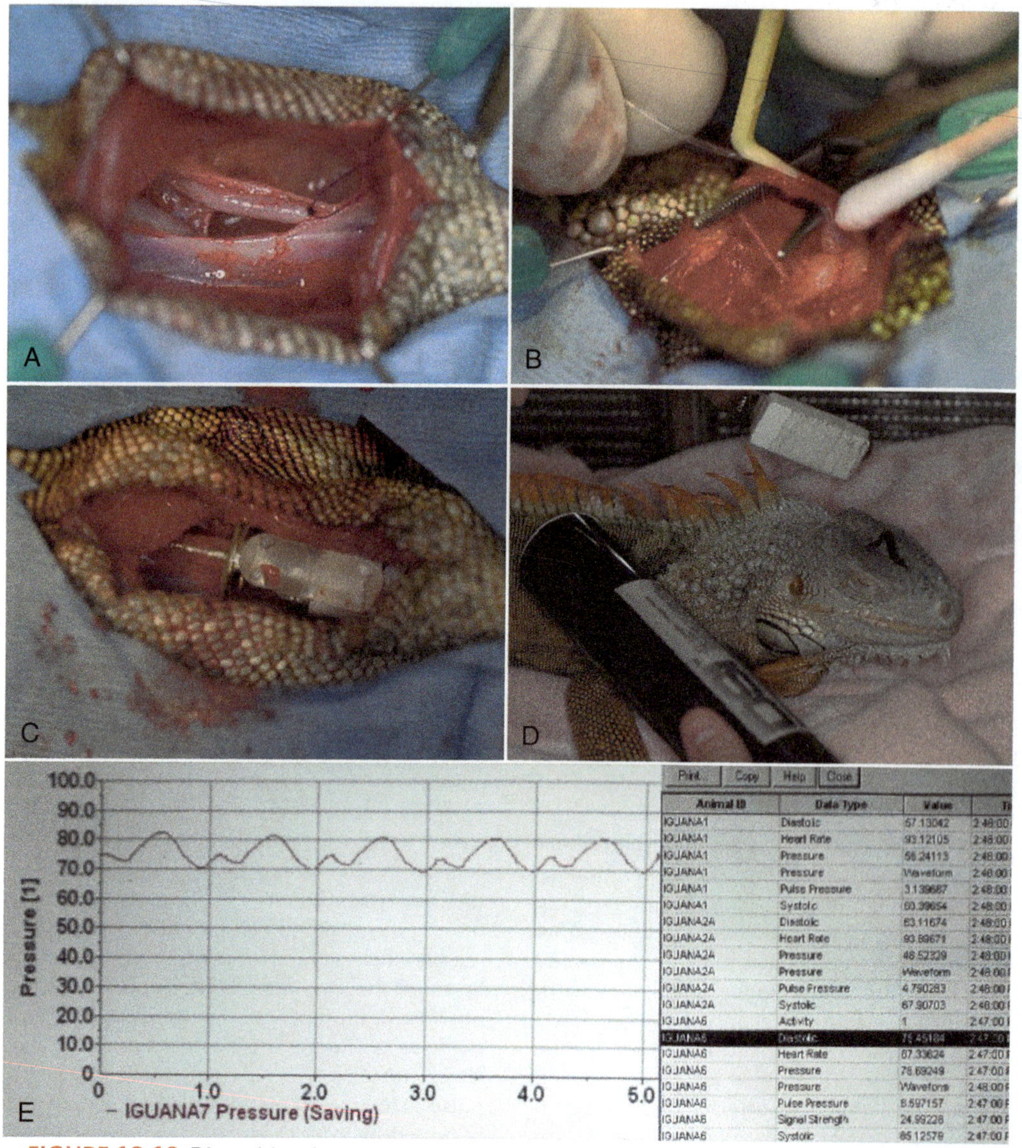

FIGURE 12-12 Direct blood pressure recording in research Green Iguanas *(Iguana iguana)*. **A,** Surgical isolation of the common carotid artery using suture. **B,** An arterial pick being used to facilitate the insertion of the blood pressure telemetry catheter through a small incision in the artery. **C,** Subcutaneous placement of the telemetry blood pressure transmitter. **D,** The blood pressure transmitter is turned on and off using a magnet *(white)*, while a telemetry receiver *(black)* picks up the signal. **E,** Direct blood pressure recording from a conscious green iguana indicating a systolic pressure of 82 and diastolic of 70 mm Hg. *(Courtesy Dr. Stephen J. Divers, University of Georgia, Athens Ga.)*

application of mammalian arterial blood gas values to reptiles is considered inaccurate because reptiles have been shown to be more tolerant to changes in arterial partial pressures of oxygen and carbon dioxide. As previously mentioned, intracardiac shunting and ventilation/perfusion mismatching in reptiles may also result in inaccurate interpretation of arterial blood gas values. In Green Iguanas premedicated with butorphanol and maintained with sevoflurane or isoflurane, arterial blood oxygen saturation as determined by arterial blood gas analysis was greater than 90% throughout the anesthetic event.[75] In the same study, significant decreases in pH values were seen over time. A study in conscious Green Iguanas demonstrated that $PaCO_2$ values (32 ± 7 mm Hg) were similar to those reported in mammalian species.[71] Arterial blood gas values were similar to mammalian species; however, baseline SaO_2 values were lower than in Grey Ratsnakes in a similar study.[73] Circadian changes in arterial PO_2 and SaO_2 have been reported in Green Iguanas: values were significantly lower in the morning than in the afternoon. In most studies, blood gas values are determined at 37°C and corrected for the body temperature of the reptile.[70]

Capnography is used in mammals as a noninvasive tool to determine concentrations of CO_2 in expired air and to assess ventilation (see Figure 12-13). In reptiles, capnography is associated with several limitations that may provide erroneous results. End-tidal CO_2 concentrations will provide an estimate of arterial CO_2 tension; however, this technique needs to be

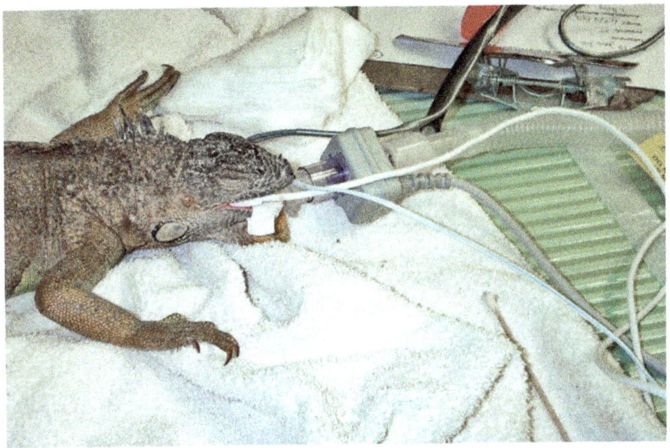

FIGURE 12-13 Anesthetized Green Iguana *(Iguana iguana)* with placement of an esophageal pulse oximeter probe connected to a pediatric mainstream capnography device.

validated for reptiles.[75] Right-to-left intracardiac shunts make this monitoring modality difficult to interpret in aquatic reptiles. Another concern in small reptiles relates to the use of sidestream units with high sampling rates in that they are likely to produce inaccurate results (see Figure12-12). Portable sidestream capnography units are available with low sampling rates adequate for even small patients, whereas pediatric mainstream units avoid the complication of sidestream dilution altogether. In butorphanol premedicated Green Iguanas maintained with either sevoflurane or isoflurane, $EtCO_2$ decreased over time but no differences were seen between groups.[75] $EtCO_2$ concentrations in both isoflurane and sevoflurane anesthetized Green Iguanas reflected $PaCO_2$ values at the beginning (10 minutes) of the anesthetic event; however, over time, $PaCO_2$ values were significantly higher than $EtCO_2$ concentrations. Therefore $ETCO_2$ appears to underestimate $PaCO_2$ but is a useful tool for monitoring trends in arterial CO_2 tension.[56]

Further studies are indicated to validate these monitoring modalities in other reptile species. In the meantime, it is recommended that values obtained with the use of pulse oximetry, arterial blood gas analysis, and capnography be interpreted with caution. Techniques for cardiovascular and pulmonary support have been reported.[76] However, all the above-mentioned techniques will give useful information on trends in respiratory and metabolic performance so corrective and supportive measures can be initiated.

ANESTHETIC EMERGENCIES

The principles and techniques established in domestic animal medicine also apply to reptiles. While topics such as effective fluid therapy, cardiopulmonary support techniques, and administration and selection of emergency drugs have been reported for reptiles, currently there is still a need for further investigations into effective drugs and dosages. Excellent reviews of the principles and techniques of reptile emergency treatment and critical care have been published previously.[77,78]

The need for effective cardiopulmonary resuscitation may arise in any anesthetized reptilian patient, especially in critically sick animals undergoing diagnostic or surgical procedures. The same concepts established for domestic animals apply, and the reptile should be assessed for respiratory status and cardiovascular status. The principles of airway (A), breathing (B), and circulation (C) also apply to reptiles. An airway should be established immediately, and respiratory support should be provided either by manual ventilation or a mechanical ventilator. Devices to monitor cardiac and circulatory function should be used, including ECG and Doppler flow devices, and vascular access should be (re)established. If venous access is not possible, an IO catheter can be placed to administer emergency drugs and fluids. Unfortunately, little information is available on effective dosages of emergency drugs commonly used in mammalian species. Atropine is indicated during episodes of severe bradycardia and should be administered IV or IO. Doxapram is a respiratory stimulant that should be administered via the IV or IO route to be most effective. In the rare case of true cardiac arrest, epinephrine is the drug of choice and can be administered either IV, IO, or diluted with sterile saline via the endotracheal tube. Supportive measures such as effective fluid therapy, provision of heat, and oxygen should accompany resuscitation efforts.

RECOVERY

During recovery, the patient should be kept in a temperature-controlled environment. For most reptilian patients, small animal incubators are ideal for this purpose because they are designed to set the temperature at the patients' POTZ. It is not recommended to raise the temperature above the range recommended for a particular species because this will result in an increased metabolic rate and increased demand by organs and tissues for oxygen. Reptiles recovering from general anesthesia will be in a state of respiratory compromise, and it may be difficult to meet the increased demand of oxygen by the tissues. During the recovery period, it is essential to assess the respiratory status of the patient and continue assisted ventilation until the patient is breathing spontaneously, has regained its reflexes, and can be extubated. Room air for ventilation during recovery is preferred over oxygen, as high oxygen concentrations in the lungs have been shown to significantly delay the return of spontaneous respiration in recovering Green Iguanas.[5] In Green Iguanas, administration of 100% inspired oxygen will increase PaO_2 but will not change respiratory and heart rates.[69] Administration of room air with a bag-valve mask will assist ventilation (Figure 12-8).[73] As is standard protocol for domestic animals, fluid therapy and pain management should be provided during the recovery period, as well as additional analgesia, if indicated. Body and limb massage may help improve venous circulation and drug mobilization.

REFERENCES

1. Sladky KK, Mans C. Clinical analgesia in reptiles. *J Exot Pet Med* 2012;21:158-167.
2. Sladky KK, Mans C. Clinical anesthesia in reptiles. *J Exot Pet Med* 2012;21:17-31.
3. Murray MJ. Cardiopulmonary anatomy and physiology. In: Mader DR, ed. *Reptile medicine and surgery*. St. Louis: Elsevier, 2006;124-134.
4. Mosley CAE. Anesthesia and analgesia in reptiles. *Semin Avian Exot Pet Med* 2005;14:243-262.
5. Schumacher J, Yelen T. Anesthesia and analgesia. In: Mader DR, ed. *Reptile medicine and surgery*. St. Louis: Elsevier, 2006;442-452.

6. Bertelsen MF. Squamates (lizards and snakes). In: West G, Heard D, Caulkett N, eds. *Zoo animal and wildlife immobilization and anesthesia.* Aimes, Iowa: Blackwell, 2007;233-244.
7. Fleming GJ. Crocodilians (crocodiles, alligators, caimans, gharial). In: West G, Heard D, Caulkett N, eds. *Zoo animal and wildlife immobilization and anesthesia.* Aimes, Iowa: Blackwell, 2007;223-231.
8. Schumacher J. Chelonians (turtles, tortoises and terrapins). In: West G, Heard D, Caulkett N, eds. *Zoo animal and wildlife immobilization and anesthesia.* Aimes, Iowa: Blackwell, 2007;259-266.
9. Schumacher J. Respiratory medicine of reptiles. *Vet Clin North Am Exot Anim Pract* 2011;14:207-224.
10. Kik MJL, Mitchell MA. Reptile cardiology: a review of anatomy and physiology, diagnostic approaches, and clinical disease. *Semin Avian Exot Pet Med* 2005;14:52-60.
11. Mitchell MA. Reptile cardiology. *Vet Clin North Am Exot Anim Pract* 2009;12:65-79, vi.
12. Mosley C. Pain and nociception in reptiles. *Vet Clin North Am Exot Anim Pract* 2011;14:45-60.
13. Mans C, Lahner LL, Baker BB, et al. Antinociceptive efficacy of buprenorphine and hydromorphone in red-eared slider turtles *(Trachemys scripta elegans). J Zoo Wildl Med* 2012;43:662-665.
14. Sladky KK, Miletic V, Paul-Murphy J, et al. Analgesic efficacy and respiratory effects of butorphanol and morphine in turtles. *J Am Vet Med Assoc* 2007;230:1356-1362.
15. Coulthard P. Conscious sedation guidance. *Evid Based Dent* 2006; 7:90-91.
16. Bienzle D, Boyd CJ. Sedative effects of ketamine and midazolam in snapping turtles *(Chelydra serpentina). J Zoo Wildl Med* 1992;23: 201-204.
17. Oppenheim YC, Moon PF. Sedative effects of midazolam in red-eared slider turtles *(Trachemys scripta elegans). J Zoo Wildl Med* 1995;26:409-413.
18. Santos ALQ, Hirano LQL, Pereira PC, et al. Anaesthesia of Geoffroy's side-necked turtle *Phrynops geoffroanus Schweigger*, 1812 (Testudines) with the association of midazolam and propofol. *Acta Scientiarum Biol Sci* 2009;31(3):317-321.
19. Sleeman JM, Gaynor J. Sedative and cardiopulmonary effects of medetomidine and reversal with atipamezole in desert tortoises *(Gopherus agassizii). J Zoo Wildl Med* 2000;31:28-35.
20. Redrobe S. Anesthesia and analgesia. In: Girling SJ, Raiti P, eds. *BSAVA Manual of Reptiles.* Gloucester, England: British Small Animal Veterinary Association, 2004;131-146.
21. Di Cianni S, Rossi M, Casati A, et al. Spinal anesthesia: an evergreen technique. *Acta Biomed* 2008;79:9-17.
22. Valverde A. Epidural analgesia and anesthesia in dogs and cats. *Vet Clin North Am Small Anim Pract* 2008;38:1205-1230, v.
23. Mans C, Lahner LL, Steagall P, et al. Feasibility, efficacy and inter-operator variability of spinal anaesthesia in female red-eared slider turtles *(Trachemys scripta elegans)*, in *Proceedings.* 1st Int Conf Avian, Herpetol Exot Anim Med 2013, Wiesbaden, Germany.
24. Mans C, Steagall P, Lahner LL, et al. Efficacy of intrathecal lidocaine, bupivacaine, and morphine for spinal anesthesia and analgesia in red-eared slider turtles *(Trachemys scripta elegans)*, in *Proceedings.* Am Assoc Zoo Vet 2011, Kansas City, Mo.
25. Rivera S, Divers SJ, Knafo SE, et al. Sterilisation of hybrid Galapagos tortoises *(Geochelone nigra)* for island restoration. Part 2: phallectomy of males under intrathecal anaesthesia with lidocaine. *Vet Rec* 2011;168:78.
26. Aitken-Palmer C, Heard D, Jacobson ER, et al. Clinical management of cloacal prolapse in an adult Galapagos tortoise *(Geochelone nigra)*, in *Proceedings.* Assoc Reptile Amphib Vet 2010, South Padre Island, Tex.
27. Wyneken J. Reptilian neurology: anatomy and function. *Vet Clin North Am Exot Anim Pract* 2007;10:837-853, vi.
28. Bojanus LH. *Anatome Testudinis Europaeae.* Vilnius, Lithuania: Typographi Universitis, 1821.
29. Wyneken J. *Anatomy of the sea turtle.* Miami, Fla: National Marine Fisheries Service, U.S. Department of Commerce, 2001.
30. Pascoe PJ, Dyson DH. Analgesia after lateral thoracotomy in dogs. Epidural morphine vs. intercostal bupivacaine. *Vet Surg* 1993;22:141–147.
31. Valverde A, Conlon PD, Dyson DH, et al. Cisternal CSF and serum concentrations of morphine following epidural administration in the dog. *J Vet Pharmacol Ther* 1992;15:91-95.
32. Stark D. Cranio-cerebral relations in recent reptiles. In: Gans C, ed. *Biology of reptilia.* New York: Academic Press, 1979;1-36.
33. Mans C, Drees R, Sladky KK, et al. Effect of body position, leg and neck extension, and sedation on lung volume in red-eared slider turtles *(Trachemys scripta elegans)*, in *Proceedings.* Am Assoc Zoo Vet 2011, Kansas City, Mo.
34. Heaton-Jones TG, Ko JC, Heaton-Jones DL. Evaluation of medetomidine-ketamine anesthesia with atipamezole reversal in American alligators *(Alligator mississippiensis). J Zoo Wildl Med* 2002;33:36-44.
35. Dennis PM, Heard DJ. Cardiopulmonary effects of a medetomidine-ketamine combination administered intravenously in gopher tortoises. *J Am Vet Med Assoc* 2002;220:1516-1519.
36. Greer LL, Jenne KJ, Diggs HE. Medetomidine-ketamine anesthesia in red-eared slider turtles *(Trachemys scripta elegans). Contemp Top Lab Anim Sci* 2001;40:9-11.
37. Hernandez-Divers SM, Stahl S, Sladky KK, et al. Safety, utility and efficacy of intramuscular administration of ketamine/medetomidine/morphine combinations for immobilization of aquatic chelonians, in *Proceedings.* Am Assoc Zoo Vet 2007, Knoxville, Tenn.
38. Hernandez-Divers SJ, Stahl SJ, Farrell R. An endoscopic method for identifying sex of hatchling Chinese box turtles and comparison of general versus local anesthesia for coelioscopy. *J Am Vet Med Assoc* 2009;234:800-804.
39. Hernandez-Divers SJ, Hensel P, Gladden J, et al. Investigation of shell disease in map turtles *(Graptemys spp.). J Wildl Dis* 2009;45:637-652.
40. Knafo SE, Divers SJ, Rivera S, et al. Sterilisation of hybrid Galapagos tortoises *(Geochelone nigra)* for island restoration. Part 1: endoscopic oophorectomy of females under ketamine-medetomidine anaesthesia. *Vet Rec* 2011;168:47.
41. Mans C, Sladky KK. Endoscopically guided cloacal calculi removal in three African spurred tortoises *(Geochelone sulcata). J Am Vet Med Assoc* 2012;240:869-875.
42. Ziolo MS, Bertelsen MF. Effects of propofol administered via the supravertebral sinus in red-eared sliders. *J Am Vet Med Assoc* 2009;234:390-393.
43. Quesada RJ, Aitken-Palmer C, Conley K, et al. Accidental submeningeal injection of propofol in gopher tortoises *(Gopherus polyphemus). Vet Rec* 2010;167:494-495.
44. Innis CJ, DeVoe R, Mylniczenko N, et al. A call for additional study on the safety of subcarapacial venipuncture in chelonians, in *Proceedings.* Assoc Reptile Amphib Vet 2010, South Padre Island, Tex.
45. Hernandez SM, Tuberville TD, Frank P, et al. Health and reproductive assessment of a free-ranging gopher tortoise *(Gopherus polyphemus)* population following translocation. *J Herpetol Med Surg* 2010;20:84-93.
46. Ramsey I. *Small animal formulary.* 6th ed. Gloucester, England: British Small Animal Veterinary Association, 2008.
47. Ambros B, Duke-Novakovski T, Pasloske KS. Comparison of the anesthetic efficacy and cardiopulmonary effects of continuous rate infusions of alfaxalone-2-hydroxypropyl-beta-cyclodextrin and propofol in dogs. *Am J Vet Res* 2008;69:1391-1398.
48. Muir W, Lerche P, Wiese A, et al. Cardiorespiratory and anesthetic effects of clinical and supraclinical doses of alfaxalone in dogs. *Vet Anaesth Analg* 2008;35:451-462.
49. Kischinovsky M, Duse A, Wang T, et al. Intramuscular administration of alfaxalone in red-eared sliders *(Trachemys scripta elegans)*—effects of dose and body temperature. *Vet Anaesth Analg* 2013; 40:13-20.
50. Bertelsen MF, Sauer CD. Alfaxalone anaesthesia in the green iguana *(Iguana iguana). Vet Anaesth Analg* 2011;38:461-466.
51. Hansen LL, Bertelsen MF. Assessment of the effects of intramuscular administration of alfaxalone with and without medetomidine in

Horsfield's tortoises *(Agrionemys horsfieldii)*. *Vet Anaesth Analg* 2013. Epub ahead of print.

52. Scheelings TF, Baker RT, Hammersley G, et al. A preliminary investigation into the chemical restraint with alfaxalone of selected Australian squamate species. *J Herpetol Med Surg* 2011;21:63-67.
53. Knotek Z, Hrda S, Trnkova S. Alfaxalone anesthesia in green iguanas *(iguana iguana)*, in *Proceedings*. 1st Scientif Meet Eur Coll Zoo Med 2011, Madrid, Spain.
54. Barter LS, Hawkins MG, Brosnan RJ, et al. Median effective dose of isoflurane, sevoflurane, and desflurane in green iguanas. *Am J Vet Res* 2006;67:392-397.
55. Mosley CA, Dyson D, Smith DA. Minimum alveolar concentration of isoflurane in green iguanas and the effect of butorphanol on minimum alveolar concentration. *J Am Vet Med Assoc* 2003;222:1559-1564.
56. Chinnadurai SK, DeVoe R, Koenig A, et al. Comparison of an implantable telemetry device and an oscillometric monitor for measurement of blood pressure in anaesthetized and unrestrained green iguanas *(Iguana iguana)*. *Vet Anaesth Analg* 2010;37:434-439.
57. Lahner LL, Mans C, Sladky KK. Comparison of anesthetic induction and recovery times after intramuscular, subcutaneous or intranasal dexmedetomidine-ketamine administration in red-eared slider turtles *(Trachemys scripta elegans)*, in *Proceedings*. Am Assoc Zoo Vet 2011, Kansas City, Mo.
58. McFadden MS, Bennett RA, Reavill DR, et al. Clinical and histologic effects of intracardiac administration of propofol for induction of anesthesia in ball pythons *(Python regius)*. *J Am Vet Med Assoc* 2011;239:803-807.
59. Selleri P, Di Girolamo N. Cardiac tamponade following cardiocentesis in a cardiopathic boa constrictor imperator *(Boa constrictor imperator)*. *J Small Anim Pract* 2012;53:487.
60. Schnellbacher R, Hernandez SM, Tuberville T, et al. Effects of intranasal administration of dexmedetomidine and ketamine on the yellow-bellied slider *(Trachemys scripta scripta)*, in *Proceedings*. Am Assoc Zoo Vet 2012.
61. Emery L, Parsons G, Gerhardt L, et al. Sedative effects of intranasal midazolam and dexmedetomidine in two species of tortoises, in *Proceedings*. 33rd Annu Conf Expo Assoc Avian Vet 2012;17, Louisville, Ky.
62. Kummrow MS, Tseng F, Hesse L, et al. Pharmacokinetics of buprenorphine after single-dose subcutaneous administration in red-eared sliders *(Trachemys scripta elegans)*. *J Zoo Wildl Med* 2008;39:590-595.
63. Holz P, Barker IK, Burger JP, et al. The effect of the renal portal system on pharmacokinetic parameters in the red-eared slider *(Trachemys scripta elegans)*. *J Zoo Wildl Med* 1997;28:386-393.
64. Holz P, Barker IK, Crawshaw GJ, et al. The anatomy and perfusion of the renal portal system in the red-eared slider *(Trachemys scripta elegans)*. *J Zoo Wildl Med* 1997;28:378-385.
65. Bertelsen MF, Buchanan R, Jensen JM, et al. Ventilating anaesthetized snakes—how much is enough? in *Proceedings*. Int Conf Dis Zoo Wild Anim 2012, Bussolengo, Italy.
66. Olsson A, Phalen D. The effects of decreased body temperature on the onset, duration and action of medetomidine and its antagonist atipamezole in juvenile farmed estuarine crocodiles (Crocodylus porosus). *Vet Anaesth Analg* 2013;40:272-279.
67. Glass ML, Boutilier RG, Heisler N. Effects of temperature on respiration, blood gases and acid-base status in the turtle *Chrysemys picta bellii*. *J Exp Biol* 1985;114:37-51.
68. Ackerman RA, White FN. The effects of temperature on acid-base balance and ventilation of the marine iguana. *Respir Physiol* 1980;39: 133-147.
69. Heard DJ. Monitoring. In: West G, Heard D, Caulkett N, eds. *Zoo animal and wildlife immobilization and anesthesia*. Aimes, Iowa: Blackwell, 2007; 83-91.
70. Hernandez SM, Schumacher J, Lewis SJ, et al. Selected cardiopulmonary values and baroreceptor reflex in conscious green iguanas *(Iguana iguana)*. *Am J Vet Res* 2011;72:1519-1526.
71. Hatt JM, Jurado OM. Depth of anesthesia monitoring by bispectral analysis in zoo animals. In: Miller RE, Fowler M, eds. *Fowler's zoo and wild animal medicine, current therapy*. St. Louis: Elsevier, 2012;147-152.
72. Chinnadurai SK, Wrenn A, DeVoe RS. Evaluation of noninvasive oscillometric blood pressure monitoring in anesthetized boid snakes. *J Am Vet Med Assoc* 2009;234:625-630.
73. Schumacher J, Lillywhite HB, Norman WM, et al. Effects of ketamine HCl on cardiopulmonary function in snakes. *Copeia* 1997;1997:395-400.
74. Diethelm G. The effect of oxygen content on inspiratory air (FIO_2) on recovery times in the green iguana *(Iguana iguana)*. Dissertation. University of Zurich, Switzerland, 2001.
75. Hernandez-Divers SM, Schumacher J, Stahl S, et al. Comparison of isoflurane and sevoflurane anesthesia after premedication with butorphanol in the green iguana *(Iguana iguana)*. *J Zoo Wildl Med* 2005;36:169-175.
76. Mosley CA, Gunkel C. Cardiovascular and pulmonary support. In: West G, Heard D, Caulkett N, eds. *Zoo animal and wildlife immobilization and anesthesia*. Aimes, Iowa: Blackwell, 2007;93-102.
77. Mader DR, Rudloff E. Emergency and critical care. In: Mader DR, ed. *Reptile medicine and surgery*. St. Louis: Elsevier, 2006;533-548.
78. Martinez-Jimenez D, Hernandez-Divers SJ. Emergency care of reptiles. *Vet Clin North Am Exot Anim Pract* 2007;10:557-585.
79. Bennett RA, Schumacher J, Hedjazi-Haring K, et al. Cardiopulmonary and anesthetic effects of propofol administered intraosseously to green iguanas. *J Am Vet Med Assoc* 1998;212:93-98.

CHAPTER 13

Diagnostic Endoscopy

Stephen J. Divers

A definitive diagnosis is important in maximizing treatment success, but reptile cases are frequently mismanaged simply because of a failure to identify the specific problem. Definitive diagnosis relies on the direct visualization of a lesion or the demonstration of a host pathologic response (by histopathologic examination, less reliably by cytologic analysis, or with the use of paired rising antibody titers), as well as identification of the causative agent (by microbiologic, parasitologic, or toxicologic analysis). Few reliable serologic tests are available for reptiles, and those that are available require a minimum of 6 to 9 weeks to demonstrate the necessary twofold increase in titers. It is therefore clear that tissue samples offer the most expedient means to a diagnosis, and endoscopy offers a visually accurate, minimally invasive, antemortem method to collect such material. Previously plagued by vague medical histories, nonpathognomonic physical examinations, indistinct diagnostic images, and less than conclusive clinical pathology results, many clinicians have discovered that diagnostic endoscopy offers an unparalleled ability to facilitate antemortem diagnosis and maximize treatment success.

Before the 1990s, there were only sporadic reports of reptile endoscopy. The majority of earlier reports described the use of endoscopy to examine or retrieve foreign objects from the gastrointestinal tract, along with case descriptions of coelioscopy, bronchoscopy, and urogenital endoscopy.[1-11] More recently, there has been further development and reviews of single-entry and multiple-entry techniques that have expanded endoscopic applications in the class Reptilia.[12-15] In particular, validation of endoscopy procedures in lizards (e.g., liver and renal biopsy in iguanas), chelonians (e.g., renal biopsy in various species and neonate gender identification), and snakes (e.g., pulmonoscopy in Royal Pythons) have helped confirm its safety and diagnostic value.[7-11,16] Given the often small and fragile nature of reptile pets, the continued development of minimally invasive endoscopy appears assured in these taxa.

Since Taylor's original chapter on reptile endoscopy was published in the second edition,[17] the 2.7-mm telescope system has continued to gain popularity as an invaluable diagnostic tool in reptile practice. Endoscopy has continued to grow and evolve with multiple journal articles published and proceedings papers presented since the last edition. Indeed, the latest reference cited in the original chapter was from 2001; therefore attempts have been made to cover the past decade of improvements and refinements in this edition. Nevertheless, most if not all of the information that appeared in the second edition is still just as relevant today, and although this is a stand-alone chapter, it would be wise to read it in conjunction with Taylor's original chapter in the earlier edition.

RIGID ENDOSCOPY EQUIPMENT

Despite the advances in flexible endoscopy equipment, rigid endoscopy still maintains its central role in reptile diagnostics largely because of its abilities to gain access to most areas of interest in most reptiles. However, given the variation in reptile size, species-specific anatomy, and variety of procedures that may be performed, a selection of different endoscopes and instruments is recommended, which can then be tailored to suit individual practice needs (Table 13-1). The following equipment descriptions are restricted to Karl Storz simply because that is what is known and used by the author, who receives no salary or consultancy fees from Karl Storz Endoscopy. Other manufacturers may be able to supply similar equipment.

Telescopes and Sheaths

The 2.7-mm telescope system, first championed by Taylor, still remains the workhorse in exotic animal practice because of its versatility and ability to be expanded as individual practice caseload dictates.[18-20] At time of press, a new 2.7 mm telescope with a significantly larger image size was released. The 2.7-mm Hopkins telescope can be used with a 3.5-mm protection sheath or with a 4.8-mm operating sheath that possesses ports for gas or fluid infusion and an operating channel for the introduction of 1.7-mm (5F) instruments (Figure 13-1). A smaller 1.9-mm telescope with an integrated sheath (3.2 mm) that can accommodate introduction of 1-mm (3F) instruments and a 1.0-mm semirigid (fiberoptic) miniature straight endoscope are particularly useful for small species (Figure 13-2).

Flexible Endoscopes

There are two main classifications of flexible endoscope: the fiberscope, which transmits the image via a bundle of fiberoptic fibers, and the video endoscope, which transmits the image electronically from a charge-coupled device (CCD) stationed at the distal tip. Fiberscopes are less expensive and are available in smaller diameters but have the disadvantages of pixilation and poorer image quality compared with video

TABLE 13-1

Endoscopic Instrumentation for Reptiles

Equipment Description	Primary Indications
VISUALIZATION AND DOCUMENTATION	
Endovideo camera and monitor Xenon light source and light guide cable Digital capture device (e.g., AIDA-DVD)	Required for all endoscopy procedures
RIGID TELESCOPES AND ENDOSCOPES	
1-mm × 20-cm semirigid miniscope, 0°	Stomatoscopy, tracheoscopy in animals up to 500 g
1.9-mm × 18.5-cm telescope, 30° oblique, with integrated 3.3-mm operating sheath	Stomatoscopy, rhinoscopy, tracheoscopy, gastroscopy, colonoscopy, cloacoscopy, and coelioscopy in animals up to 2 to 3 kg
2.7-mm × 18-cm telescope, 30° oblique, 4.8-mm operating sheath	Stomatoscopy, rhinoscopy, tracheoscopy, gastroscopy, colonoscopy, cloacoscopy, and coelioscopy in animals between 100 g and 20 kg
5-mm × 29-cm telescope, 0°, with 6-mm × 6.5-cm Ternamian EndoTip cannula	Coelioscopy of animals more than 20 kg
5-mm × 29-cm telescope, 30° oblique, with 6-mm × 6.5-cm Ternamian EndoTip cannula	Coelioscopy of animals, especially chelonians, more than 20 kg
5-mm × 8.5-cm otoendoscope, 0°, with integrated operating sheath	Stomatoscopy in animals between 1 and 50 kg
FLEXIBLE INSTRUMENTS FOR USE WITH RIGID TELESCOPES AND OPERATING SHEATHS	
1-mm biopsy forceps 1-mm grasping forceps	For use with 1.9-mm telescope and integrated sheath
1.7-mm biopsy forceps 1.7-mm single-action scissors 1.7-mm remote injection needle 1.7-mm grasping/retrieval forceps 1.7-mm wire basket retrieval 1.7-mm needle end radiosurgery electrode 1.7-mm polypectomy snare	For use with 2.7-mm telescope and 4.8-mm operating sheath
INSUFFLATION	
Dedicated CO_2 insufflator, capable of insufflation pressures as low as 3 mm Hg and flow rates as low as 0.1 L/min; CO_2 compressed gas with regulator; silicone supply tubing to endoscopy equipment	Used for insufflation during reptile coelioscopy
Sterile saline suspended above endoscopy table with intravenous drip line to a port on the operating sheath	Used for sterile saline infusion for cystoscopy, cloacoscopy, coelioscopy
FLEXIBLE ENDOSCOPES	
Fiberscope, 2.5-mm × 100-cm working length, 1.2-mm instrument channel, 2-way tip deflection	Respiratory and gastrointestinal evaluations
Video bronchoscope, 5.9-mm × 61-cm working length, 2.2-mm instrument channel, 4-way tip deflection, suction, and irrigation	Respiratory and gastro-intestinal evaluations
Video gastroscope, 9 mm x 140 cm working length, 2.2 mm working channel, 4 way tip deflection, suction, insufflation and irrigation	Gastrointestinal evaluations in large reptiles
INSTRUMENTS FOR USE WITH FLEXIBLE ENDOSCOPES	
Grasping forceps, 1 mm × 120 cm Biopsy forceps, 1 mm × 120 cm	For 2.5-mm fiberscope
Biopsy forceps, round cupped jaws, diameter 1.7 mm, working length 120 cm Grasping forceps, alligator jaws, 1.7 mm × 120 cm	For 5.9-mm video bronchoscope
Biopsy forceps, round cupped jaws, diameter 1.8 mm, working length 180 cm Grasping forceps, alligator jaws, 1.8 mm × 180 cm	For 9.0-mm video gastroscope

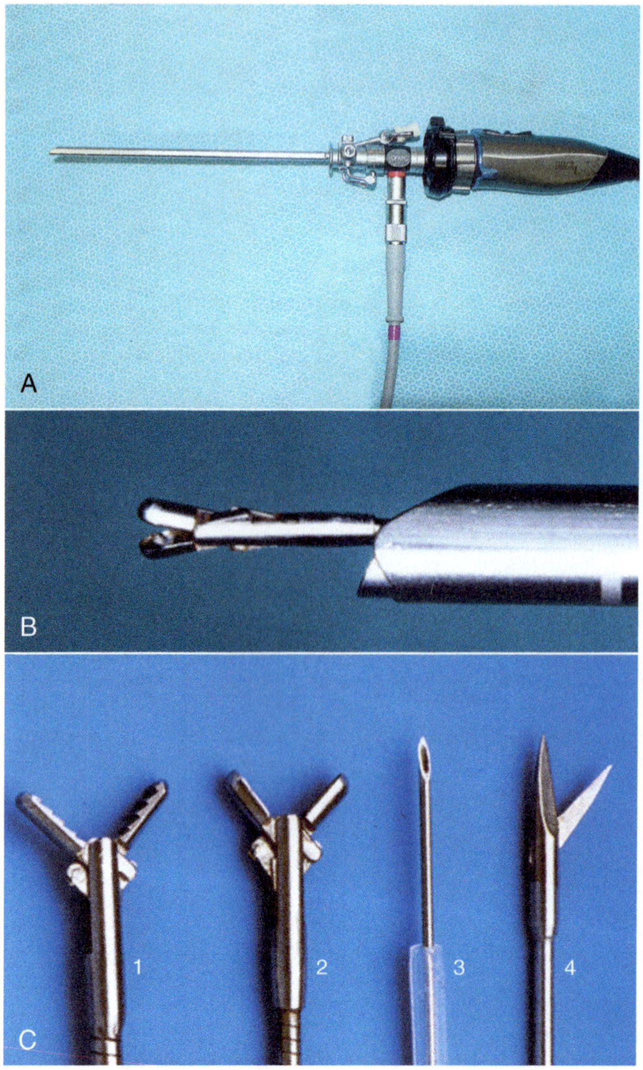

FIGURE 13-1 A 2.7-mm telescope system. **A,** 2.7-mm telescope housed within a 4.8-mm operating sheath, connected to a light cable and an endovideo camera. **B,** A 1.7-mm biopsy forceps inserted down the instrument channel and emerging directly in front of the telescope. **C,** A variety of 1.7-mm instruments can be used through the operating channel, including retrieval forceps *(1)*, biopsy forceps *(2)*, remote injection/aspiration needle *(3)*, and single-action scissors *(4)*. *(Courtesy Dr. Stephen J. Divers, University of Georgia, Athens, Ga.)*

endoscopes (Figure 13-3). Video endoscopes tend to be larger in diameter because of the need to accommodate the terminal CCD chip, and their initial purchase costs have been considerably higher. Furthermore, until relatively recently, flexible and rigid endoscopy light sources and cameras were generally incompatible, which necessitated separate rigid and flexible tower systems. This undoubtedly forced practitioners to purchase one or the other. Fortunately, the advent of modern cameras and light sources now enables practitioners to invest in just one endoscopy tower that can be used with both rigid and flexible endoscopes.

Flexible endoscopes vary from 14 mm to less than 1 mm in diameter, and those greater than 2 mm often possess a working channel (for instruments) and tip deflection. Larger flexible scopes greater than about 7.8 mm often have four-way

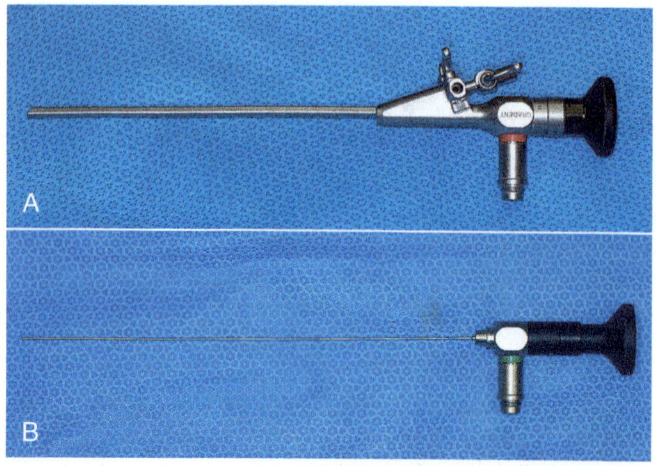

FIGURE 13-2 A, A 1.9-mm telescope with integrated operating sheath. **B,** A 1.0-mm semirigid miniature straight endoscope. *(Courtesy Dr. Stephen J. Divers, University of Georgia, Athens, Ga.)*

tip deflection, working channels, and air insufflation and suction (Figure 13-4). Current technology limits the smallest video endoscope to 3.8 mm although future improvements are expected; therefore smaller fiberscopes (0.5 to 2.5 mm) maybe more useful in small reptiles. However, these smaller fiberscopes often have just one-way or two-way tip deflection and smaller working channels (Figure 13-5).

Light Sources

The telescope is connected via a fiberoptic light guide cable to a light source (Figure 13-6, *A*). Halogen light sources are less expensive and are effective for small animals less than 2 kg, but xenon light sources provide better quality light and an intensity that can illuminate the body cavities of large animals. The hybrid xenon light source of the mobile Karl Storz Telepak is only 25 watts but has been used to perform coelioscopy in giant tortoises up to 100 kg.

Cameras

An endovideo camera connected to the eyepiece of the telescope, although once considered a luxury addition, is an integral part of the endoscopy system and greatly facilitates the surgeon's performance (see Figure 13-6, *A*). Cameras, available in both European PAL and American NTSC formats, can vary dramatically in cost from budget single-chip cameras to three-chip digital high-definition (HD) models. The traditional video system provided a resolution of 720 × 480 pixels; therefore it inevitably led to some cropping of the image for display on a traditional 4:3 aspect monitor. The advent of HD systems has increased the video size to 1920 × 1080 pixels. In addition, the new 16:9 aspect ratio provides a 33% wider field of view while progressive (as opposed to interlaced) scanning produces improved resolution, color clarity, and refresh rates. Operating room setup is important: the monitor should be positioned directly in front of the endoscopist, and instruments should be within easy reach (Figure 13-6, *B*). In summary, the fact remains that any camera will greatly improve performance compared with just the use of an eyepiece and will also facilitate photodocumentation.

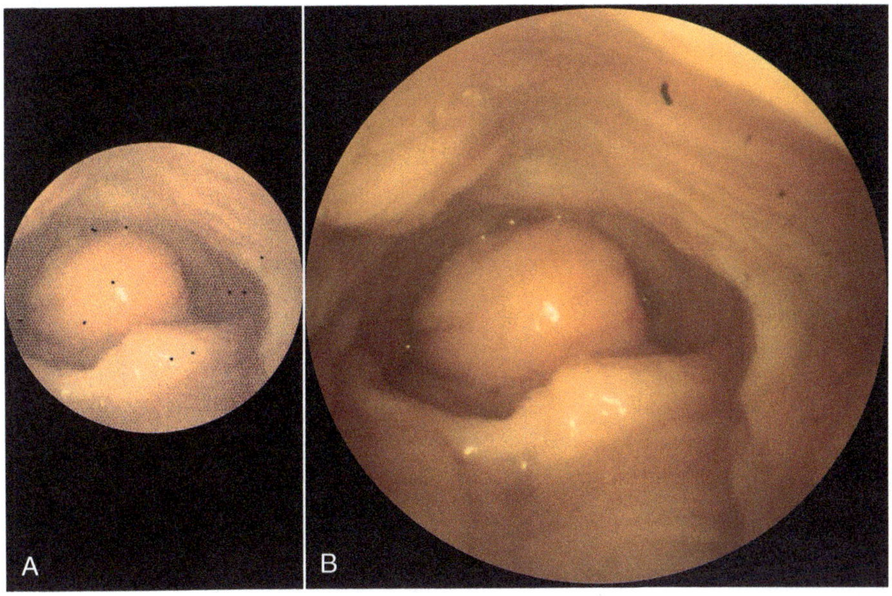

FIGURE 13-3 Relative comparison in endoscopic views of a snake's stomach using a 2.5-mm fiberscope **(A)** and 5.9-mm video bronchoscope **(B)**. Note the smaller image, increased pixilation, and *black dots* (broken fibers) associated with the fiberscope. *(Courtesy Dr. Stephen J. Divers, University of Georgia, Athens, Ga.)*

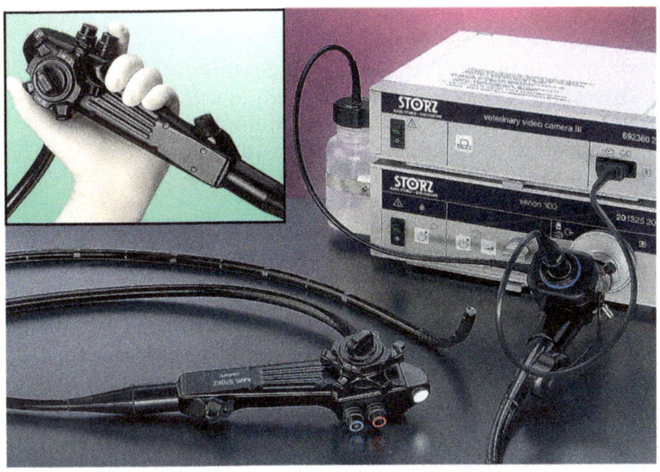

FIGURE 13-4 A 9-mm × 140-cm video gastroscope with 2.2-mm working channel attached to a xenon light source and endovideo camera. *Insert,* Handling technique that permits the endoscopist to control four-way tip deflection using thumb while first finger operates the two buttons that control air insufflation, suction, and fluid irrigation. *(Courtesy KARL STORZ GmbH & Co. KG.)*

PHOTODOCUMENTATION

The ability to record still photographs and video of procedures is becoming increasingly important for maintaining accurate medical records, as well as for generating pictures for brochures, presentations, or scientific publications. Most camera systems generate s-video or digital outputs that can be connected to a myriad of nonprofessional, commercial recording devices (e.g., laptops and DVD recorders) that can ultimately save material in various formats to digital media. Professional-grade devices, although more expensive, provide dedicated functions that are important in medicine (Figure 13-7). For example, most professional endoscopy recording devices will support still images (TIFF, bitmap, JPEG), and video (MPEG2) with audio voiceover (WAV). Modern systems can also provide network and web-based storage and file sharing,

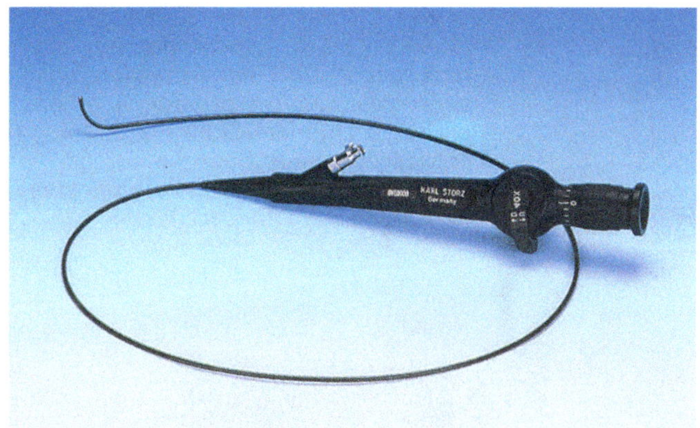

FIGURE 13-5 A 2.5-mm × 100-cm fiberscope with 1.2-mm instrument channel and two-way tip deflection. *(Courtesy KARL STORZ GmbH & Co. KG.)*

including industry-standard Digital Imaging and Communications in Medicine (DICOM) support.

MOBILE UNITS

The Tele Pack Vet system (Karl Storz Veterinary Endoscopy Goleta, Calif) combines a hybrid xenon light source, endovideo camera, 12-inch color liquid crystal display, with digital image and video capture and storage into a portable unit that is well-suited for veterinarians working in the field (Figure 13-8). An even more mobile option is the EndoGo camera and battery-powered light (Envisionier Medical Technologies Inc., Woodstock, Ga), which provides real "pocket-sized mobility", with reductions in light intensity and quality (Figure 13-9).[21]

SALINE AND CO_2 INSUFFLATION

Some form of insufflation is required for most coelioscopy, urogenital, or gastrointestinal procedures. For coelioscopy, medical grade CO_2 gas delivered by a dedicated endoflator is preferred (Figure 13-10), but air delivered by syringe or a

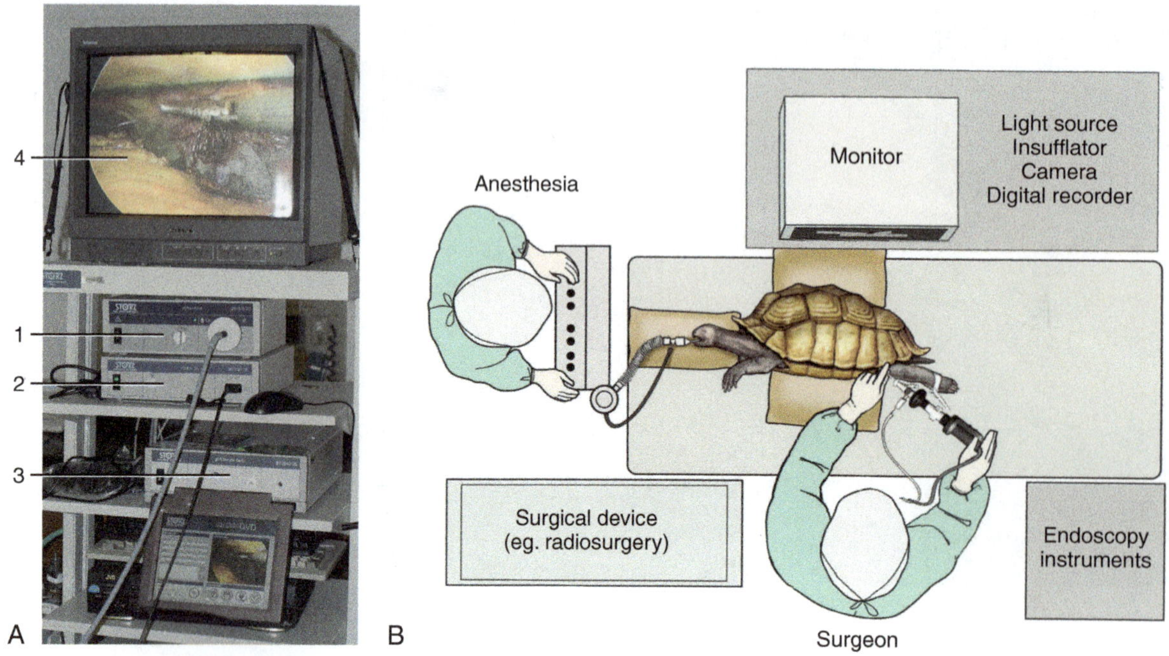

FIGURE 13-6 **A,** Rigid endoscopy tower with xenon light source *(1),* endovideo camera base unit *(2),* DVD digital capture device *(3),* and monitor display *(4). (Courtesy Dr. Stephen J. Divers, University of Georgia, Athens, Ga.)* **B,** Operating room layout demonstrating the preferred ergonomics and positioning for a right-handed surgeon performing chelonian coelioscopy. Note how the surgeon is facing the monitor and endoscopy instruments are within easy reach on the right side. *(Art by Kip Carter [UGA], © University of Georgia Research Foundation, Inc.)*

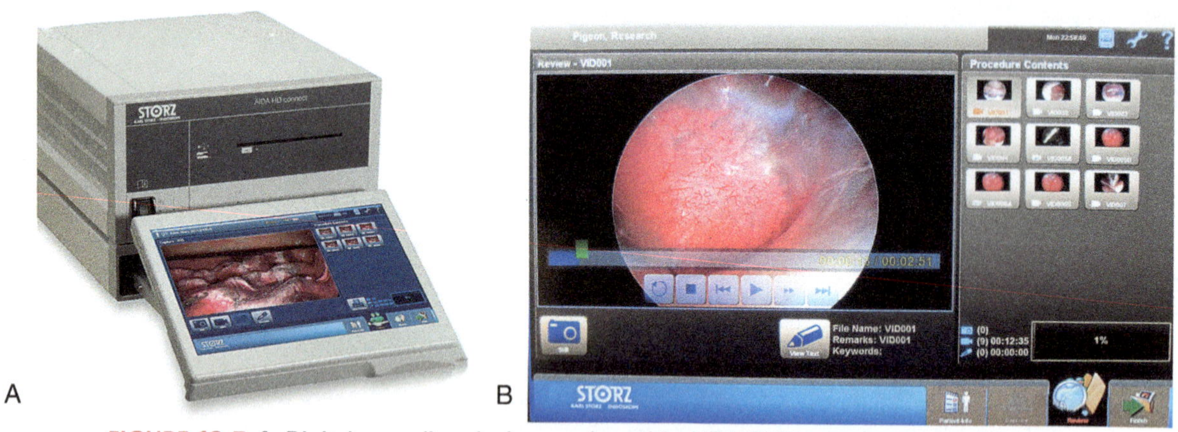

FIGURE 13-7 **A,** Digital recording devices such as this AIDA DVD system can record video (MPEG2) and photographs (.bmp, .jpg, .tiff) and export them to a CD, DVD, or USB stick. **B,** Close-up of the interactive display. *(Courtesy KARL STORZ GmbH & Co. KG.)*

small aquarium air pump has been used with limited success. The risk associated with the use of air, specifically air emboli, is rare but must not be ignored. Dedicated endoflators precisely maintain the set insufflation pressure within the coelom by matching gas in-flow with any leakage.

In some situations, the use of sterile saline can be especially helpful for creating mild distension. Saline infusion is particularly useful when dealing with a hollow viscus (e.g., gastrointestinal tract, bladder, and cloaca) or when coelioscopy is performed in small reptiles (e.g., neonate chelonian gender identification). Saline infusion may also be preferred for coelioscopy of certain aquatic reptiles in which potential ill effects of residual insufflation gas on postoperative buoyancy may occur (Figure 13-11).

HAND INSTRUMENTATION

Rigid Endoscopy

The basic and most frequently used instruments include biopsy forceps, retrieval forceps, scissors, and needle (Figure 13-1, *C*). The 1.0-mm and 1.7-mm (3F and 5F) grasping forceps are useful for manipulating tissues, debriding, and retrieving foreign objects or parasites. The fine aspiration/injection needle

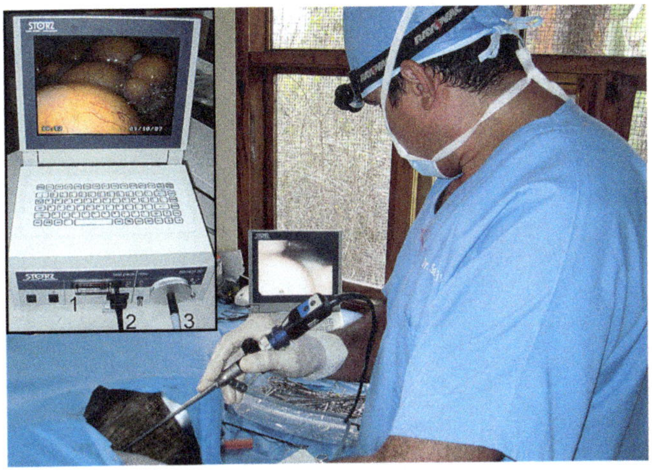

FIGURE 13-8 The Tele Pack (Karl Storz Veterinary Endoscopy, Goleta, Calif) is a mobile unit that can be readily transported and used in field situations. Shown is an endoscopist performing coelioscopy in a Galapagos Tortoise *(Chelonoidis [Geochelone] nigra)* at the Charles Darwin Research Station, Santa Cruz Island, Galapagos Islands. *Insert,* A close-up of the older Tele Pack indicating the PCMCIA card *(1)* for image storage, camera *(2)*, and light source *(3)* connections. A more modern unit is now available that has a larger screen and both still and video capture. *(Courtesy Dr. Stephen J. Divers, University of Georgia, Athens, Ga.)*

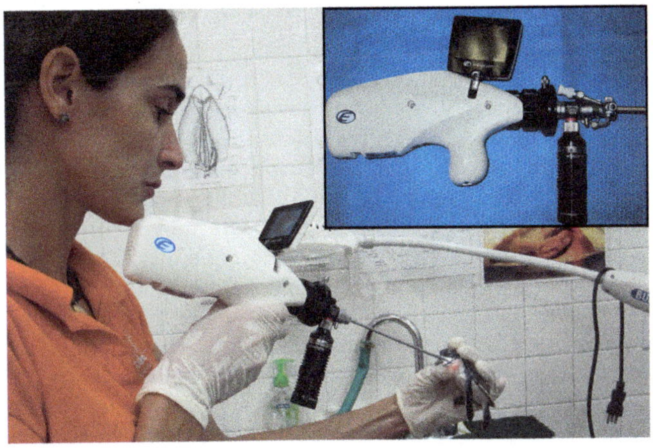

FIGURE 13-9 The EndoGo (Envisionier Medical Technologies Inc., Woodstock, Ga) is a compact, battery-powered endoscopy camera and LED light system that offers true pocket-sized mobility. In this example, the endoscopist is performing an upper gastrointestinal examination in a neonate Green Sea Turtle *(Chelonia mydas)* at the Grand Cayman Turtle Farm, British West Indies. *Insert,* Close-up of the EndoGo camera and E-Zenon LED light source attached to a 2.7-mm telescope. *(Courtesy Dr. Stephen J. Divers, University of Georgia, Athens, Ga.)*

can be used for the aspiration of fluid from cystic structures in cases in which biopsy may be contraindicated because of post-sampling leakage. The needle can also be used for irrigation and drug administration. The 1.0-mm and 1.7-mm flexible biopsy forceps are used to harvest tissue samples for histopathologic and microbiologic analysis in patients as small as 30 g. The small sample size usually permits the collection of several biopsy samples for multiple laboratory tests and serial biopsies to monitor disease progression over time for assessment of a response to treatment. To take a tissue sample, the endoscopist

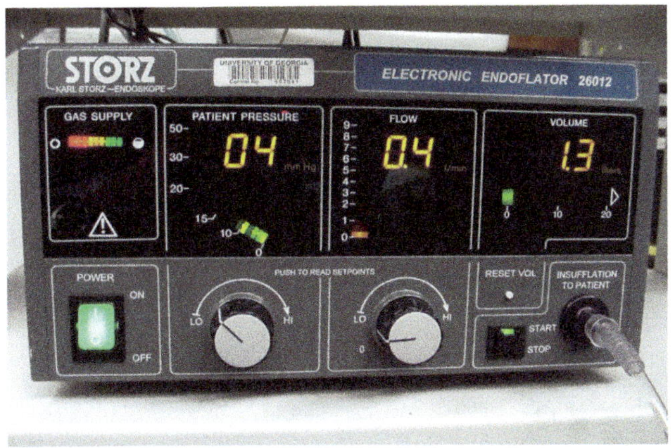

FIGURE 13-10 Electronic endoflator designed to precisely control the delivery of CO_2 for insufflation. In this example, the patient pressure, CO_2 flow rate, and total gas consumption are 4 mm Hg, 0.4 L/min, and 1.3 L, respectively. *(Courtesy Dr. Stephen J. Divers, University of Georgia, Athens, Ga.)*

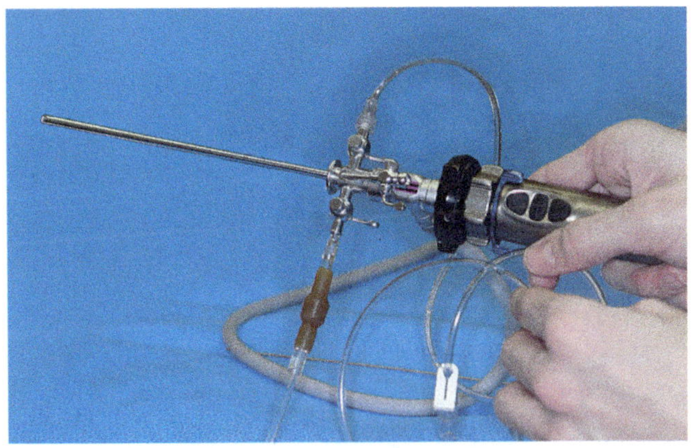

FIGURE 13-11 A simple saline infusion system requires a bag of sterile saline to be suspended above the animal (not shown) and an ingress fluid delivery line attached to one of the ports on the 4.8-mm operating sheath. A second intravenous line is used as an egress and empties into a bucket under the table. By adjusting the sheath ports, the endoscopist can control the rate of fluid entering and leaving an area. Such a system works well for neonate turtle coelioscopy, cloacoscopy, cystoscopy, and gastrointestinal evaluations. The temperature of the saline should be appropriate for the patient so that hypothermia is not induced. *(Courtesy Dr. Stephen J. Divers, University of Georgia, Athens, Ga.)*

inserts the biopsy forceps down the operating channel and into the field of view (Figure 13-12).

It is much easier to advance and manipulate the sheath–telescope–instrument as a single device than to try and keep the sheath–telescope still and independently move the biopsy forceps back and forth. With the biopsy forceps held open, the sheath–telescope–instrument is advanced to the tissue of interest, and when tissue enters the biopsy cup, the handle is released. These instruments are delicate, and the biopsy handle is often only required to open the biopsy jaws. The handle's spring mechanism is usually sufficient to take a soft tissue biopsy sample without additional manual pressure, as long as the instrument is sharp. Clamping down on the handle will damage the forceps and increase biopsy crush artifact.

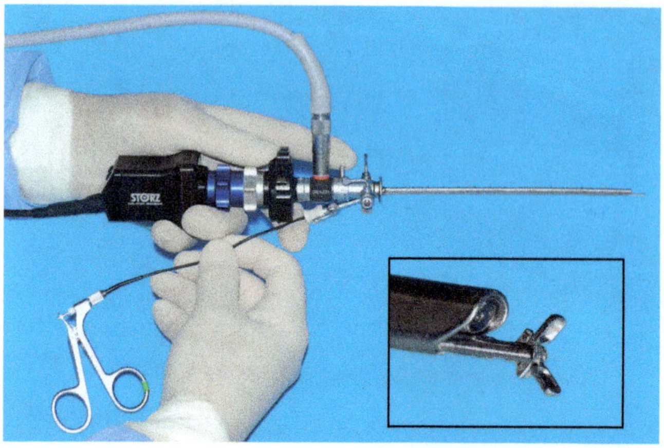

FIGURE 13-12 A 2.7-mm telescope within a 4.8-mm operating sheath with a TriCam three-chip endovideo camera and light guide cable attached (Karl Storz Veterinary Endoscopy, Goleta, Calif). Biopsy forceps (1.7 mm) passed through the working channel emerge in front of the terminal lens *(insert)*. *(© University of Georgia Research Foundation, Inc.)*

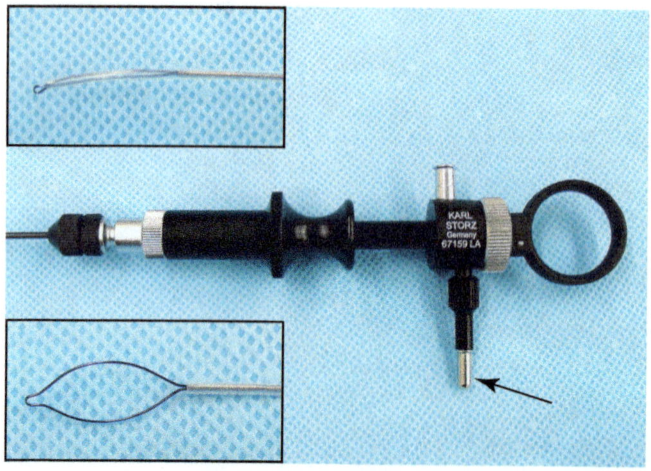

FIGURE 13-14 Polypectomy snare (1.7 mm) with radiosurgical connection *(arrow)* and close-ups of the retracted and extended snare *(inserts)*. *(Courtesy Dr. Stephen J. Divers, University of Georgia, Athens, Ga.)*

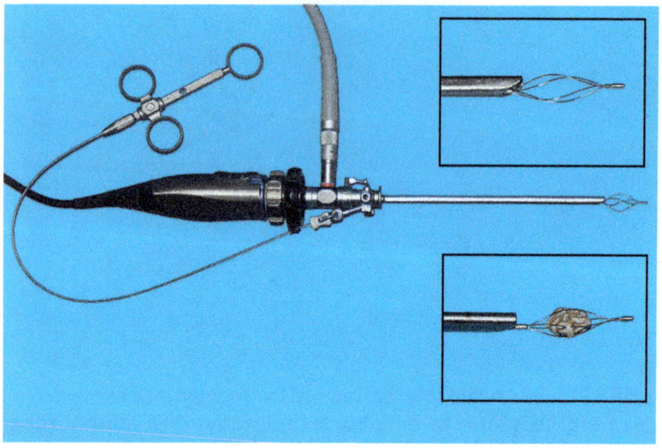

FIGURE 13-13 A 2.7-mm telescope within a 4.8-mm operating sheath with Image-1 endovideo camera and light guide cable attached. Wire-basket retrieval device (1.7 mm) passed through the working channel with close-up views of the device opened and closed around a stone *(inserts)*. *(© University of Georgia Research Foundation, Inc.)*

Some organs may be protected by a more fibrous membrane. The fixed blade of the scissors is inserted at a shallow angle through the membrane, and the sheath–telescope–scissors are advanced as a single unit, cutting the membrane as they proceed. The scissors can then be replaced by the biopsy forceps to take a sample through the capsular incision. Other instruments that can be invaluable in specific situations include a wire basket retrieval device (for removal of fibrous foreign bodies or stones; Figure 13-13), a polypectomy snare (for removal of small growths and polyps; Figure 13-14), and a radiosurgical needle electrode (for pinpoint ablation or coagulation).

EQUIPMENT CLEANING, STERILIZATION, AND STORAGE

Specific and detailed cleaning instructions provided by manufacturers should always be followed. In general, endoscopes are first wiped and flushed to remove gross debris and tissue fluids before being soaked in a neutral pH enzymatic detergent. Ultrasonic cleaners are useful for many endoscopy items but should not be used with any optical equipment. High-level disinfection or sterilization can be achieved with the use of ethylene oxide gas, hydrogen peroxide, or cold sterilization with a 2%, 14-day, low-surfactant glutaraldehyde solution (Cidex or MetriCide; Civco Medical Solutions, Kalona, Iowa). Cold-sterilized equipment must obviously be thoroughly rinsed with sterile water before use. Although most modern telescopes are autoclavable, some optical devices including older endoscopes and camera heads may be irreversible damaged by high pressure, high temperature steam.

Equipment should be stored in a safe and secure manner, and a variety of metal and plastic containers have been designed to purposefully house items and withstand sterilization (Figure 13-15). It can be a disadvantage to store equipment sterilized, as this may dissuade the novice endoscopist from reaching for the endoscope to practice on cadavers.

Rigid Telescope and Instrument Handling

The fact that most pet reptiles weigh less than 2 kg requires careful control of the telescope; the eyepiece and camera should be supported with the superior hand, and the distal shaft of the telescope should be held by thumb and forefinger of the inferior hand (Figure 13-16, *A*). Handling the telescope in this fashion provides fine control without tremors; however, for a single surgeon to be able to use instruments, a modified hold is required. Inserting and manipulating instruments through the operating sheath requires changing from a two-handed to a one-handed technique. The usual thumb and forefinger support of the telescope shaft is now adjusted so that the inferior hand takes the entire weight of the sheath–telescope–camera system. The thumb is slid up the shaft of the sheath, and the fingers are curled over the top to encircle the sheath. Now that the sheath is grasped in a fistlike grip and the sheath is further supported by the thumb to prevent rotation, the superior hand can be removed to pick up and insert an instrument down the operating channel (Figure 13-16, *B*). This can only be performed with a correctly sheathed telescope; damage will occur otherwise.

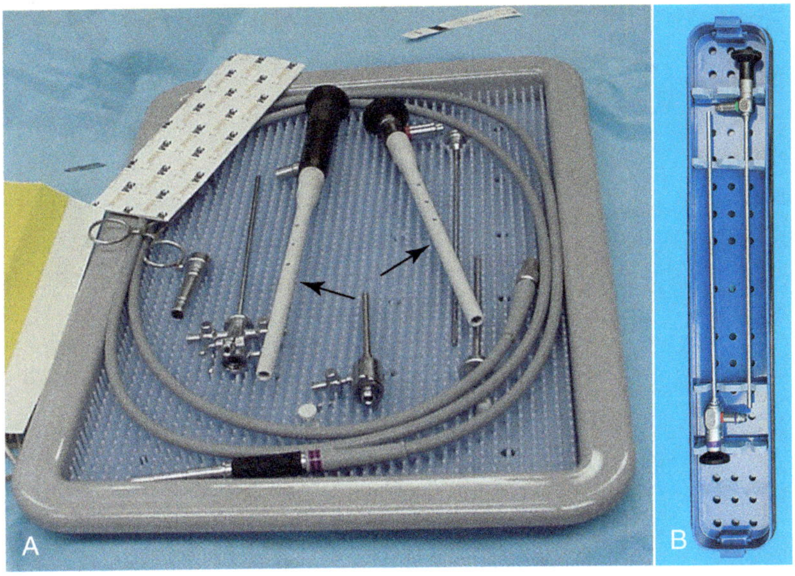

FIGURE 13-15 Dedicated storage and sterilization trays (**A** and **B**) help to protect equipment. Note also the protective plastic sheaths *(arrows)* over the fine diameter telescopes in **(A)**. *(Courtesy Dr. Stephen J. Divers, University of Georgia, Athens, Ga.)*

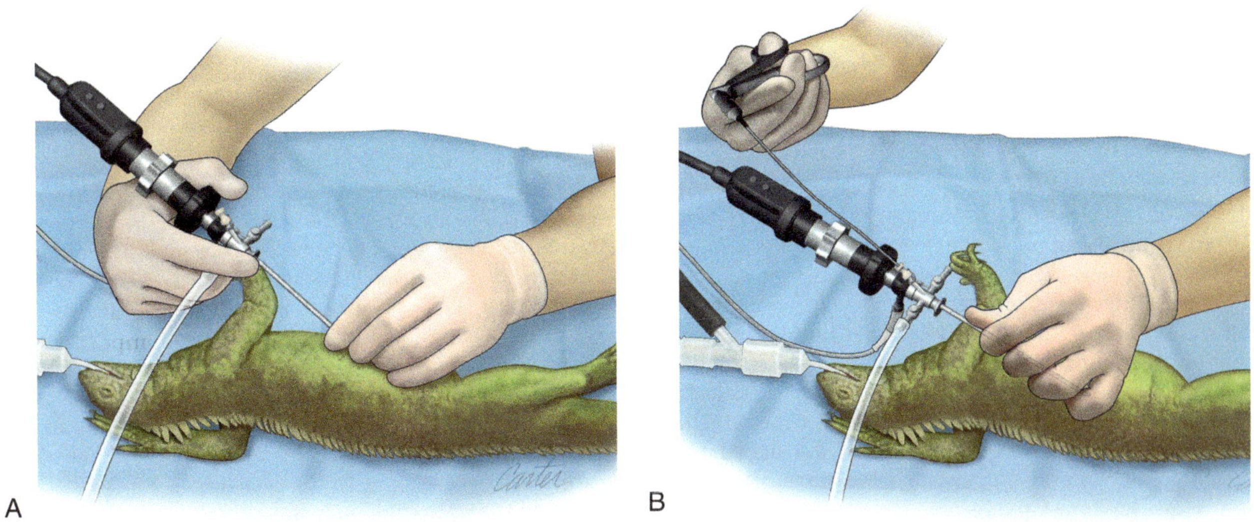

FIGURE 13-16 Correct handling of the 2.7-mm telescope housed within the 4.8-mm operating sheath. **A,** The two-handed technique for general evaluation involves supporting the sheathed telescope and camera with the superior hand while the thumb and forefinger of the inferior hand provide fine motor control and prevents tremor. **B,** The one-handed technique facilitates instrument use by a single surgeon and involves the inferior hand taking the weight of the sheathed telescope and camera by gripping the entire shaft, with the thumb slid up the sheath to prevent rotation. The inferior hand is now free to manipulate an instrument into the operating channel. *(Art by Kip Carter [UGA], © University of Georgia Research Foundation, Inc.)*

Biopsy Care and Handling

It is interesting to note that various studies have concluded that endoscopic biopsy specimens are more diagnostic than ultrasound-guided aspirates or biopsy specimens.[22-24] Endoscopic biopsy specimens are delicate and measure approximately 1 mm^3 when collected with a 1.7-mm forceps. Handling and other histologic artifacts are reduced by gently dislodging the tissue from the biopsy cups into a small volume of sterile saline, then decanting into a biopsy cassette or bag, and submitting in 10% neutral buffered formalin (Figure 13-17, *A*).[11] Picking the biopsy specimen from the instrument with a needle will cause severe damage, and even moistened cotton-tipped applicators have been shown to cause tissue alteration (Figure 13-17, *B, C*). Biopsy samples for microbiologic analysis are best submitted in sterile saline for immediate processing. Alternatively, if mailed to a laboratory, they should be submitted in appropriate transport media. For the submission of samples for toxicologic or parasitologic analysis, it is wise to consult with the laboratory before sample collection.

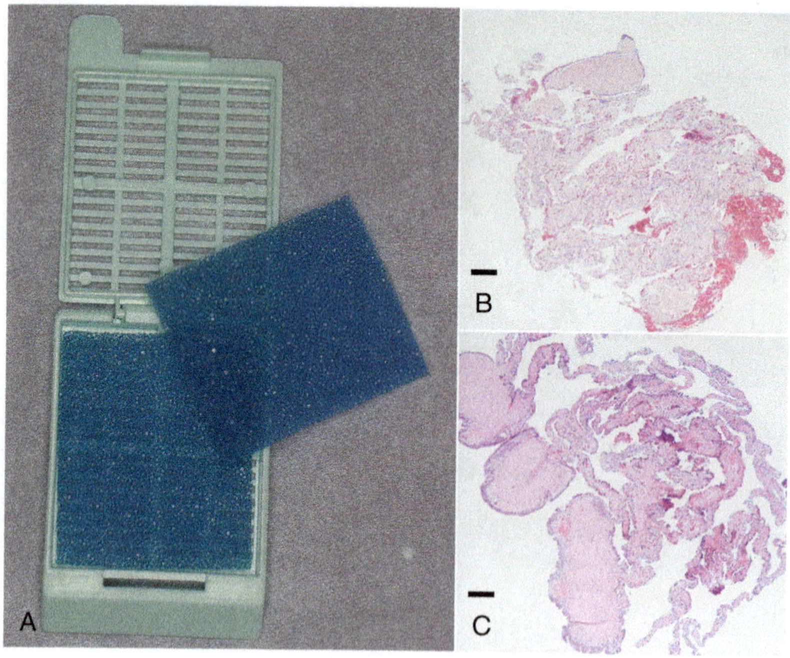

FIGURE 13-17 **A,** Endoscopic biopsy specimens are best sandwiched between foam and secured within a histology cassette. **B,** Crush artifact in a snake lung biopsy sample caused by a cotton-tipped applicator used to transfer the tissue from forceps to histology cassette. **C,** Another snake lung biopsy sample exhibiting reduced artifact because it was shaken from the forceps into sterile saline before being decanted into the histology cassette. *(Courtesy Dr. Stephen J. Divers, University of Georgia, Athens, Ga.)*

PREOPERATIVE EVALUATIONS AND ANESTHESIA

Patient Selection, Evaluation, and Contraindications

Knowledge of species-specific anatomy, physiology, husbandry, and nutritional requirements are vital for properly evaluating the management and medical history of a reptile. Inexperienced clinicians are directed to reviews on the subject and should prepare ahead of time.[25,26] Complete physical examination, including accurate body weight, is essential but may require sedation or anesthesia for aggressive snakes or uncooperative animals, particularly chelonians. Serial clinicopathologic data can be helpful in quantifying dehydration or indicating infection/inflammation, organ damage, or dysfunction. However, most published reference ranges are too broad to be of value unless patient data are severely abnormal. Complete blood counts and biochemistry panels (i.e., total levels of protein, albumin, globulin, aspartate transaminase, bile acids, glucose, creatinine phosphokinase, calcium, phosphorus, sodium, potassium, chloride, uric acid, ammonia, and urea for aquatic species) are recommended, and even in animals less than 100 g, hematocrit, a blood smear for differential white cell counts, and a total protein level can still be obtained.

Reptiles may be seen in a state of advanced, often chronic disease, and it is therefore important to stabilize patients before anesthesia and surgery. In addition to anesthetic complications, small patient size often presents the greatest challenges to the reptile endoscopist. The most common endoscopic procedures performed by the author include coelioscopy, gastroscopy, cloacoscopy, tracheobronchoscopy, and pulmonoscopy. However, most of the procedures described (or necessary modifications thereof) can be undertaken even in smaller reptiles, assuming equipment can be matched to patient size.

Obesity is less of an issue in chelonians and lizards because they store fat in discrete fat bodies rather than diffusely around organs like mammals. Obesity in snakes can still be a significant hindrance during coelioscopy.

Patient Preparation and Anesthesia

When reptile patients that are still feeding need to undergo an operation, fasting should be in accordance with body size and feeding strategy. For example, a 20-kg python would typically be fasted for 3 to 4 weeks, whereas a 50-g gecko would require only 1 to 2 days. Likewise, fasting a carnivorous turtle for 1 to 3 days would reduce the volume of food in the stomach, whereas fasting an herbivorous tortoise for the same period would have little effect, given that the majority of digesta is located within the large intestine. As a general guide, a single feeding cycle should be avoided before anesthesia and surgery.

Fluid therapy is the mainstay of stabilization, and hydration with crystalloids (with an osmolarity of 260 to 290 mOsm/L) at 25 to 45 mL/kg/day is recommended.[27] Fluids may be given intravenously or intraosseously for critical cases, or intracoelomically, subcutaneously, or orally. It is advisable to avoid oral or intracoelomic fluids immediately before gastroscopy or coelioscopy.

Certain examinations (e.g., stomatoscopy and cloacoscopy) may be possible in the conscious or sedated patient with the use of a mouth gag and appropriate restraint, but complete immobilization is preferred so that damage to equipment, patient, or staff is avoided. General anesthesia is recommended for all endoscopy procedures (including oral and cloacal examinations) and is required for any invasive procedures (including coelioscopy).[9,28] Conscious coelioscopic examinations may be acceptable in research or wildlife under an appropriate experimental license, but in clinical practice, analgesia and anesthesia are considered mandatory. Some authors have reported using only local anesthesia for chelonian coelioscopy, but this likely provides inadequate analgesia for more involved coelioscopic procedures.[29] In a recent comparison of local versus general anesthesia for chelonian coelioscopy, anesthetic scores were

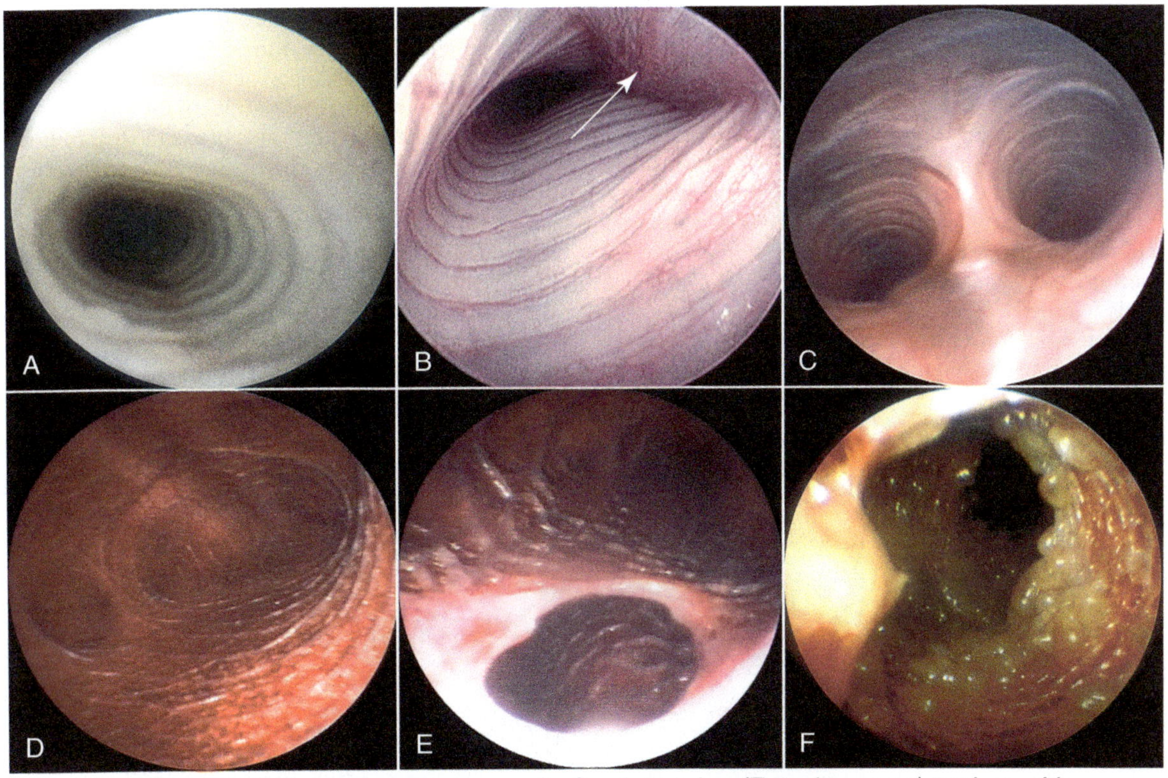

FIGURE 13-18 Tracheobronchoscopy. **A,** Greek tortoise *(Testudo graeca)* trachea with complete tracheal rings. **B,** Ball python *(Python regius)* trachea with obvious dorsal ligament *(arrow)*. **C,** Tracheal bifurcation and primary bronchi in a Green Iguana *(Iguana iguana)*. **D,** Simple saclike lung in a Green Iguana. **E,** Compartmentalized lung in a Panther Chameleon *(Furcifer pardalis)*. **F,** Granulomatous pneumonia due to *Mycobacterium* spp. in a Ball Python. *(Courtesy Dr. Stephen J. Divers, University of Georgia, Athens, Ga.)*

significantly better for procedures conducted under general anesthesia compared with local lidocaine alone.[9] A detailed description of anesthesia is beyond the scope of this chapter, but careful consideration should be given to intubation and adequate ventilation, especially when the coelom is insufflated during coelioscopy. There appear to be taxa-specific effects of opiates in reptiles given morphine (1.5 mg/kg) or hydromorphone (0.5 mg/kg): the dose seems effective in chelonians, whereas very high doses of morphine or butorphanol appear to be required for some lizards and snakes.[30,31] The nonsteroidal antiinflammatory analgesic meloxicam (0.2 mg/kg subcutaneously, intramuscularly, or intravenously) is used routinely in all species and may be repeated after 48 to 72 hours, if necessary.[32]

DIAGNOSTIC ENDOSCOPY PROCEDURES

Tracheoscopy and Pulmonoscopy

Depending on the size of the reptile, a suitably sized rigid or flexible endoscope can be used to examine the glottis and at least part of the anterior trachea of most lizards, chelonians, and snakes (Figure 13-18).[12] It is always preferable to use a protection sheath with the finer telescopes, but the increased diameter may be prohibitive. Rigid scopes of sufficient length can usually be directed into the lungs of lizards by careful manipulation of the lizard's head, neck, and body. It is often beneficial to provide a large breath immediately before inserting the endoscope. For large snakes and chelonians, fine diameter flexible endoscopes or videoscopes will permit a deeper examination into the lungs.[17,33]

The anesthetized reptile is positioned in dorsal or sternal recumbency, with head and neck extended. A mouth gag is recommended to guard against a lightly anesthetized reptile biting down on the endoscope. The endoscope should be inserted through the glottis and gently advanced under direct visual control to avoid damaging the mucosa. Complete tracheal occlusion for several minutes is well-tolerated, and there is no need to provide an alternate airway. The incomplete (Squamata) and complete (Chelonia, Crocodilia) tracheal rings and mucosa can be clearly seen. Parasites, abscesses, granulomas, trauma, and mucosal defects, as well as chondromas and other neoplasms, can be readily appreciated.

A tracheal approach to the chelonian lung is particularly difficult because of the narrow trachea and meandering primary bronchi. It is possible in the largest species (e.g., giant tortoises and sea turtles) with the use of fine flexible endoscopes but not in smaller specimens; therefore two alternative approaches to the chelonian lung have been developed.[12] The first requires a 4-mm temporary osteotomy in the carapace over the suspected lesion that has been pinpointed by diagnostic imaging. The pleuropulmonary membrane is punctured with a trocar or straight hemostats while the animal is held at maximal inspiration. Leakage of anesthetic gases confirms entry into the lung, and additional anesthetic gas scavenging should be positioned close to the surgical site or ventilation should be temporarily suspended during the procedure. The sheathed telescope can then be inserted into the lumen of the lung for examination. It is important to remember that the rigid nature of the shell will restrict telescope movement (Figure 13-19). After endoscopy, the osteotomy can be temporarily maintained with a catheter and injection cap secured within the hole using tissue adhesive or epoxy. This catheter can be used to deliver intrapulmonic drug therapy for days to weeks. Alternatively, the osteotomy can be closed using an epoxy or acrylic compound. The shell typically heals within 12 weeks.

A second method for chelonians involves a prefemoral approach to the lung. This method is most suitable for those species that have a relatively large prefemoral fossa that can facilitate surgical entry into the coelom with identification of the caudolateral aspect of the postpulmonary membrane (septum horizontale) and caudolateral lung. A small (1-cm to 3-cm) craniocaudal incision is made in the craniodorsal aspect of the prefemoral fossa (Figure 13-20, *A*). The coelomic membrane is perforated and opened with hemostats. By frequently and maximally ventilating the chelonian, the endoscopist can readily identify the caudolateral lung. Two stay sutures are placed through the caudoventral border of the lung to elevate the tissue to the level of the skin incision. A stab incision through a thin, avascular portion of the exposed lung provides access for the telescope. Because of the soft tissue nature of

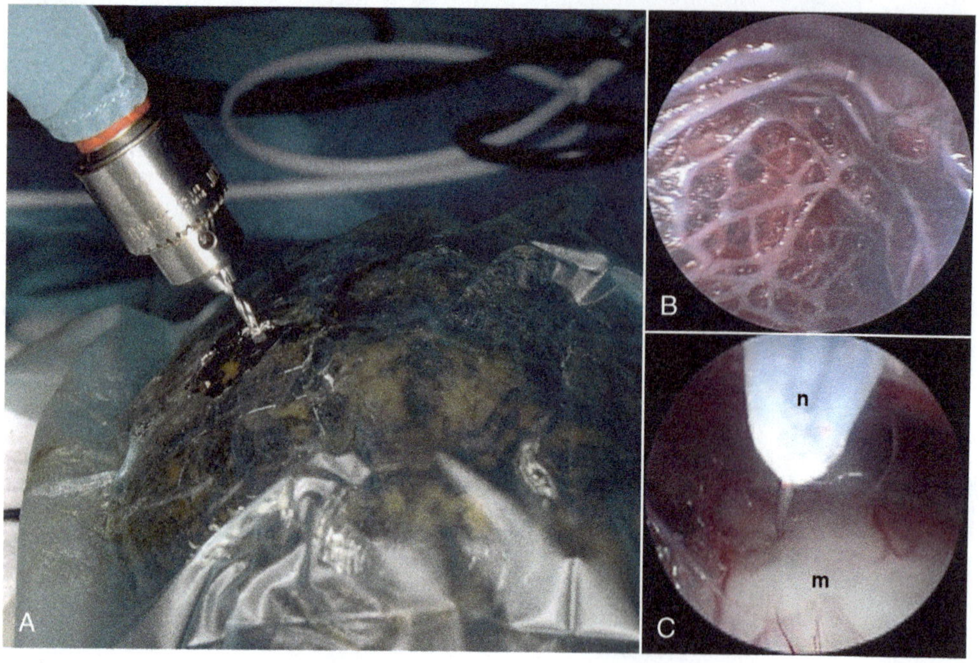

FIGURE 13-19 Chelonian transcarapacial pulmonoscopy. **A,** Drilling a 4-mm temporary osteotomy through the carapace of a Greek tortoise *(Testudo graeca)* to access the lung. **B,** Normal view of the chelonian lung through the temporary osteotomy. **C,** Large mass *(m)* within the lung of a juvenile Loggerhead Sea turtle *(Caretta caretta)* via a temporary carapacial osteotomy. Aspiration is first attempted with an endoscopic needle *(n)*, and, if not fluid-filled, biopsy samples are taken. In this case, the lesion was an encapsulated fungal granuloma. *(Courtesy Dr. Stephen J. Divers, University of Georgia, Athens, Ga.)*

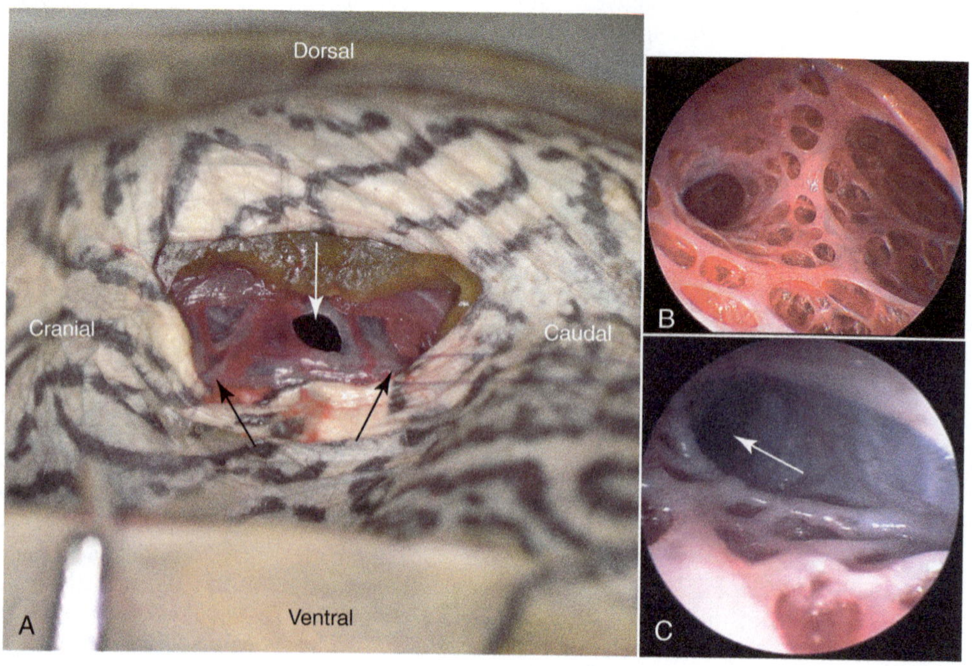

FIGURE 13-20 Chelonian transcutaneous pulmonoscopy. **A,** Surgical view of the prefemoral fossa of a Map Turtle (*Graptemys* sp.) after a minicoeliotomy incision. Two fine stay sutures *(black arrows)* have been placed to elevate the lung to the skin incision, and a small stab incision has been made through an avascular window of the lung *(white arrow)*. **B,** Endoscopic view from within the lung of a Yellow-bellied Slider *(Trachemys scripta scripta)* demonstrating the characteristic edicular nature of the tissue. **C,** Endoscopic view from within the lung of Greek Tortoise *(Testudo graeca)* demonstrating the opening to the left primary bronchus *(arrow)*. *(Courtesy Dr. Stephen J. Divers, University of Georgia, Athens, Ga.)*

this approach, greater endoscope maneuverability is possible and the pulmonary examination can proceed from caudal to cranial; in some species, it is possible to visualize the opening of the primary bronchus (Figure 13-20, *B, C*). On withdrawal of the endoscope, the lung must be closed with fine suture material to avoid postoperative pneumocoelom. Coeliotomy closure is otherwise routine.

A transcutaneous rigid endoscopic approach to the lung of snakes has also been described.[11,34] This involves a minicoeliotomy approach approximately 35% to 45% from snout to vent, on the right side for most snakes (or either left or right side for boas and pythons because they have two lungs). After a 1-cm skin incision and blunt dissection through an intercostal space, the lung is identified as it is ventilated, grasped, secured, and punctured with a scalpel blade before insertion of the telescope. Depending on the size of the snake, this approach can facilitate evaluation of the distal trachea, primary and intrapulmonary bronchus, cranial faveolar lung, transitional zone, and the caudal air sac (Figure 13-21). This technique has been thoroughly evaluated in Ball Pythons *(Python regius)*, in which the surgical approach and visualization of the distal portion of the trachea, primary bronchus, intrapulmonary bronchus, cranial lung lobe, and faveolar, semisaccular, and saccular lung regions were considered excellent.[11] Lung and skin are closed as separate layers with the use of single sutures. This study also evaluated faveolar biopsy specimens collected with 1.7-mm biopsy forceps and concluded that the diagnostic quality of specimens that were shaken from biopsy forceps into physiologic saline solution before fixation in 2% glutaraldehyde or neutral-buffered 10% formalin was considered good to excellent (Fig 13-17, *C*). Reevaluation of the same snakes a year later confirmed complete healing of the previous entry and biopsy sites with no clinically apparent deleterious effects. In larger boids, a flexible endoscope can be inserted below the ventral margin of the rib, just dorsal to the first row of lateral scales, and advanced cranially and caudally to examine most of the unilateral pulmonary system.

Stomatoscopy and Gastroscopy

Ventral or dorsal recumbency of the reptile with head and neck extended is preferred for stomatoscopy and gastroscopy. It is often helpful to have the reptile close to the table edge or positioned on a raised surface. The rigid telescope–sheath system can be used to examine the buccal cavity, esophagus, and stomach of small lizards and chelonians (Figure 13-22). Flexible endoscopes are required to gain access to the stomach for most snakes and larger reptiles of other orders (Figure 13-23). Air insufflation can be used to dilate the tract and provide good exposure for detecting gross lesions and foreign bodies. Warm saline irrigation provides superior clarity, especially when mucosal detail needs to be examined, although tracheal intubation, which ensures a proper seal, is essential for avoiding aspiration. Whether air or saline is used, it is important to gently dilate the tract as the endoscope is advanced to avoid damage and laceration to the wall. Foreign bodies can be readily retrieved, and biopsy collection should be undertaken with

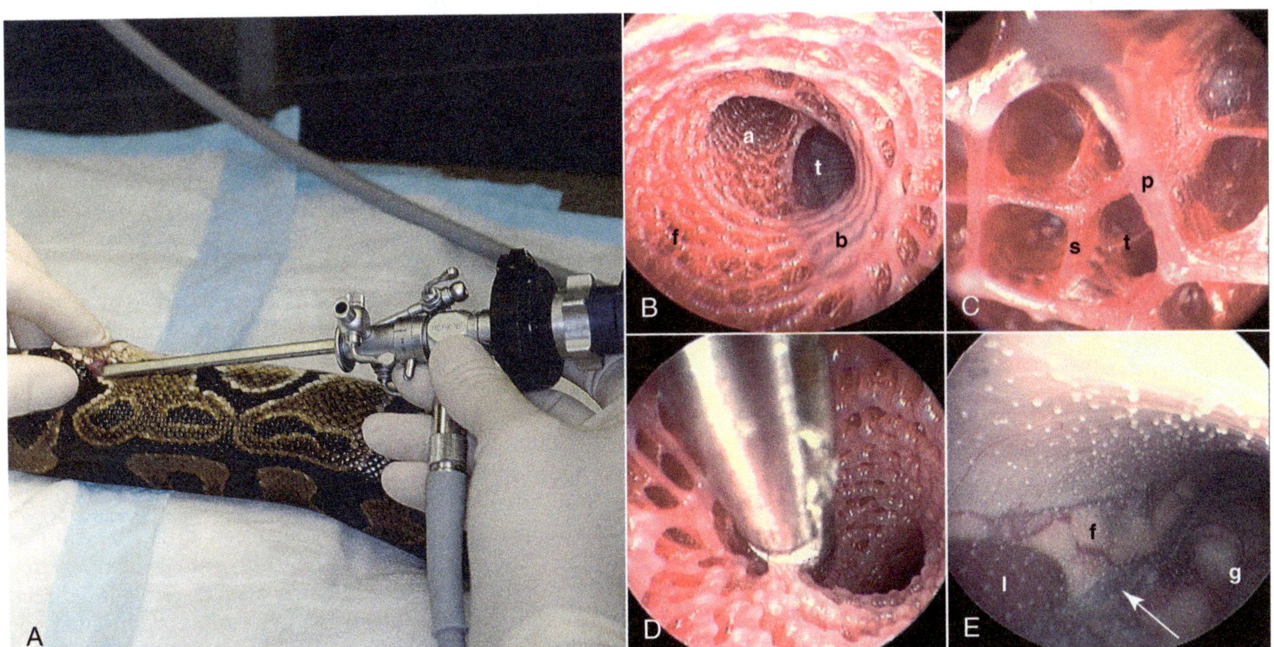

FIGURE 13-21 Ball Python *(Python regius)* transcutaneous pulmonoscopy. **A,** The sheathed 2.7-mm telescope inserted through the lateral body wall and introduced into the cranial lung of a research python that has not been draped to permit visualization of the snake's position and surgical entry site for photography. **B,** View of the cranial lung demonstrating the distal trachea *(t)*, intrapulmonary bronchus *(b)*, anterior lung lobe *(a)*, and the faveolar lung tissue *(f)*. **C,** Close-up view of the faveolar region demonstrating the primary *(p)*, secondary *(s)*, and tertiary *(t)* septae of the anterior vascular lung. **D,** Lung biopsy with the 1.7-mm biopsy forceps. **E,** View of the thin, transparent, caudal air sac through which the caudal edge of the liver *(l)*, fatbody *(f)*, gastrointestinal tract *(g)*, and caudal vena cava *(arrow)* can be seen. *(Courtesy Dr. Stephen J. Divers, University of Georgia, Athens, Ga.)*

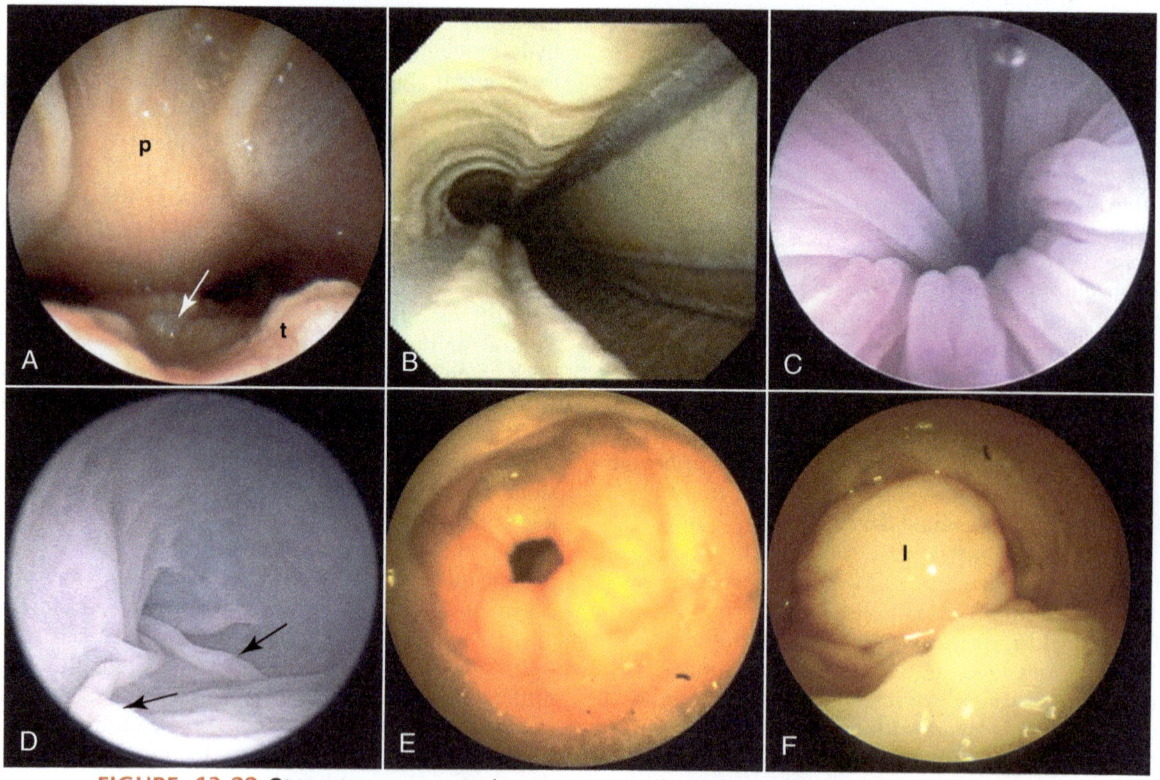

FIGURE 13-22 Stomatoscopy, esophagoscopy, and gastroscopy. **A,** Oral cavity of a Radiated Tortoise *(Astrochelys radiata)* demonstrating the choana and hard palate *(p)*, fleshy tongue *(t)*, and glottis *(arrow)*. **B,** Air-distended esophagus of a Burmese Python *(Python molurus bivittatus)*. **C,** Saline-infusion view of a Green Iguana *(Iguana iguana)* esophagus. **D,** Stomach of a Savannah Monitor *(Varanus exanthematicus)* with normal rugal folds *(arrows)*. **E,** Gastric hypertrophy in a Cornsnake *(Elaphe guttata)* with cryptosporidiosis. **F,** Leiomyoma *(l)* obstructing the pyloric outflow in another Cornsnake that was seen with chronic regurgitation. *(Courtesy Dr. Stephen J. Divers, University of Georgia, Athens, Ga.)*

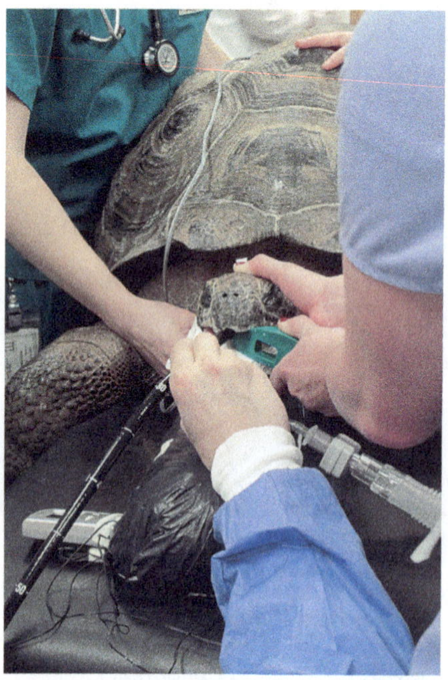

FIGURE 13-23 Gastroscopy in a Galapagos Tortoise *(Chelonoidis [Geochelone] nigra)* with the use of a 9.0-mm Olympus video gastroscope. *(Courtesy Dr. Stephen J. Divers, University of Georgia, Athens, Ga.)*

care to avoid perforation of the alimentary tract, which is more likely in the thin-walled esophagus than in the stomach.

Cloacoscopy

Although snakes can also be positioned in ventral or dorsal recumbency, chelonians and lizards are generally more easily examined in a dorsal position (Figure 13-24). Endoscopy using warm saline irrigation enhances visualization of the proctodeum, urodeum, and coprodeum and allows a detailed appraisal of the distal colon, cloacal mucosa, urogenital papillae, oviductal openings in females, and (when present) the urethral opening and bladder (Figure 13-25).

With practice, the endoscopist can direct the endoscope through the urethra into the thin-walled bladder in chelonians and some lizards. It is also possible to direct the endoscope into the distal oviducts of reproductively active females.

Cloacoscopy has been used to remove shell and egg material from the distal oviducts and bladder and as a guide for resection and for the exteriorization of partially prolapsed tissue. Mucosal biopsy specimens should be taken with care, especially from the colon, because of its thin nature and the risk of perforation. Selleri and colleagues[35] presented a technique for neonate gender identification by observing the gonads through the healthy, diaphanous bladder wall via a cloacoscopic approach. This technique has the advantage of

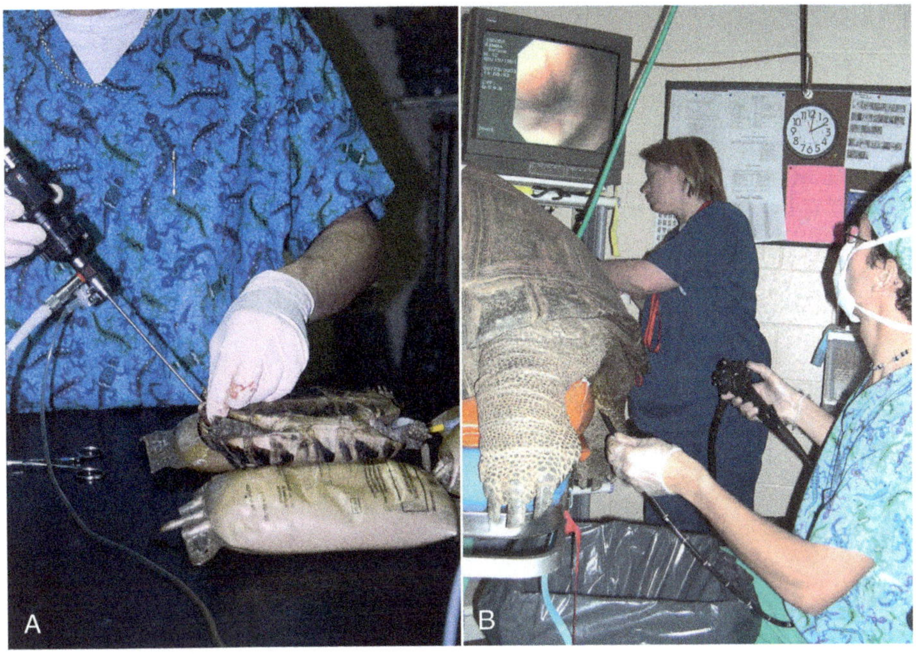

FIGURE 13-24 Chelonian cloacoscopy. **A,** Cloacoscopy using a 2.7-mm telescope and saline infusion in a small tortoise (*Testudo* sp.). **B,** Cloacoscopy using a 9.0-mm video gastroscope in an Aldabra Tortoise *(Aldabrachelys [Geochelone] gigantea). (Courtesy Dr. Stephen J. Divers, University of Georgia, Athens, Ga.)*

avoiding entry into the coelomic cavity but, because examination is through a membrane, may not be as sensitive as direct coelioscopic visualization.

Coelioscopy

Reptiles are coelomates, meaning that they lack a true abdominal cavity, and as a result, the term *coelioscopy* is preferred over laparoscopy. A detailed discussion of generic laparoscopy methodologies can be found elsewhere[36-39]; only reptile specifics will be highlighted here. Laparoscopy has been shown to offer significant advantages over traditional surgical options, both in human and veterinary medicine. In particular, laparoscopy is, with practice, faster, less traumatic, causes less postoperative pain, and is associated with a more rapid return to normal function.[23,24,40-49] Until the advent of 2-mm and 3-mm human pediatric equipment, laparoscopy was limited to a single-entry system with the use of the sheathed telescope; however, multiple-entry techniques are now possible and practical for animals more than 500 g (see Chapter 14).[50]

Precise positioning for coelioscopy depends on the reptile's body shape and conformation, the structure(s) of interest, and the preferences of the endoscopist.[13] The entry site is aseptically prepared and draped, and adhesive clear plastic drapes permit better visualization of the patient. Insufflation is essential for lizards and snakes and, although the shell prevents coelomic collapse, can still be helpful in many chelonians. Typically CO_2 insufflation pressures of 3 to 5 mm Hg are used, which are lower than those recommended for mammals (8 to 12 mm Hg). In some situations, saline infusion may be preferred over gas. This is especially true when dealing with neonates and other very small reptiles or when dealing with aquatic animals, in which residual gas may have a negative effect on postoperative buoyancy. Whatever method of insufflation is used, it is important to appreciate the negative effects on lung ventilation. When a pressure-cycle ventilator is used, it is often possible to overcome increased coelomic pressure by simply increasing the ventilation pressure. However, careful cooperation and communication between the anesthesiologist and surgeon is required at all times. For short periods of up to several minutes, complete lung collapse is well-tolerated; however, for longer endoscopy periods, it will be necessary to temporarily reduce insufflation and permit intermittent ventilation.

LIZARDS

Dorsoventrad compressed lizards (e.g., Bearded Dragons) are often positioned in dorsal recumbency, whereas laterally compressed lizards (e.g., Chameleons) are best placed in lateral recumbency. Round-bodied lizards (e.g., Green Iguanas) can be placed in either lateral or dorsal recumbency, but lateral is generally preferred and allows easier access to both ventral and dorsal structures. Given the relatively small size of most lizards, a single paramedian or paralumbar entry point will usually permit examination of most, if not all, organ systems (Figure 13-26).

Although anatomic differences exist between families, the Green Iguana serves as a useful model for saurian coelioscopy.[7,51] In the iguana, there is no significant difference in visualization of lung, liver, pancreas, small intestine, large intestine, ovary, oviduct, testis, epididymis, vas deferens, bladder, fatbody, or kidney from either left or right approaches. However, a left lateral approach to the heart, stomach, and spleen and a right lateral approach to the gallbladder are preferred.[7] Right-handed surgeons will find that a left paralumbar approach is easier, whereas a left-handed surgeon will prefer a right paralumbar approach. Unless physical examination, diagnostic imaging, or clinicopathologic results suggest an asymmetrical lesion, the endoscopist's preference can prevail (Table 13-2).

The iguana is positioned in lateral recumbency, with the left pelvic limb taped caudad against the tail base. The entry area is bordered craniad by the last rib, dorsad by the spine, caudad by the pelvic limb, and ventrad by the abdominal and pelvic veins (see Figure 13-26). Aseptically, a small skin incision is made in the center of the defined area. The skin

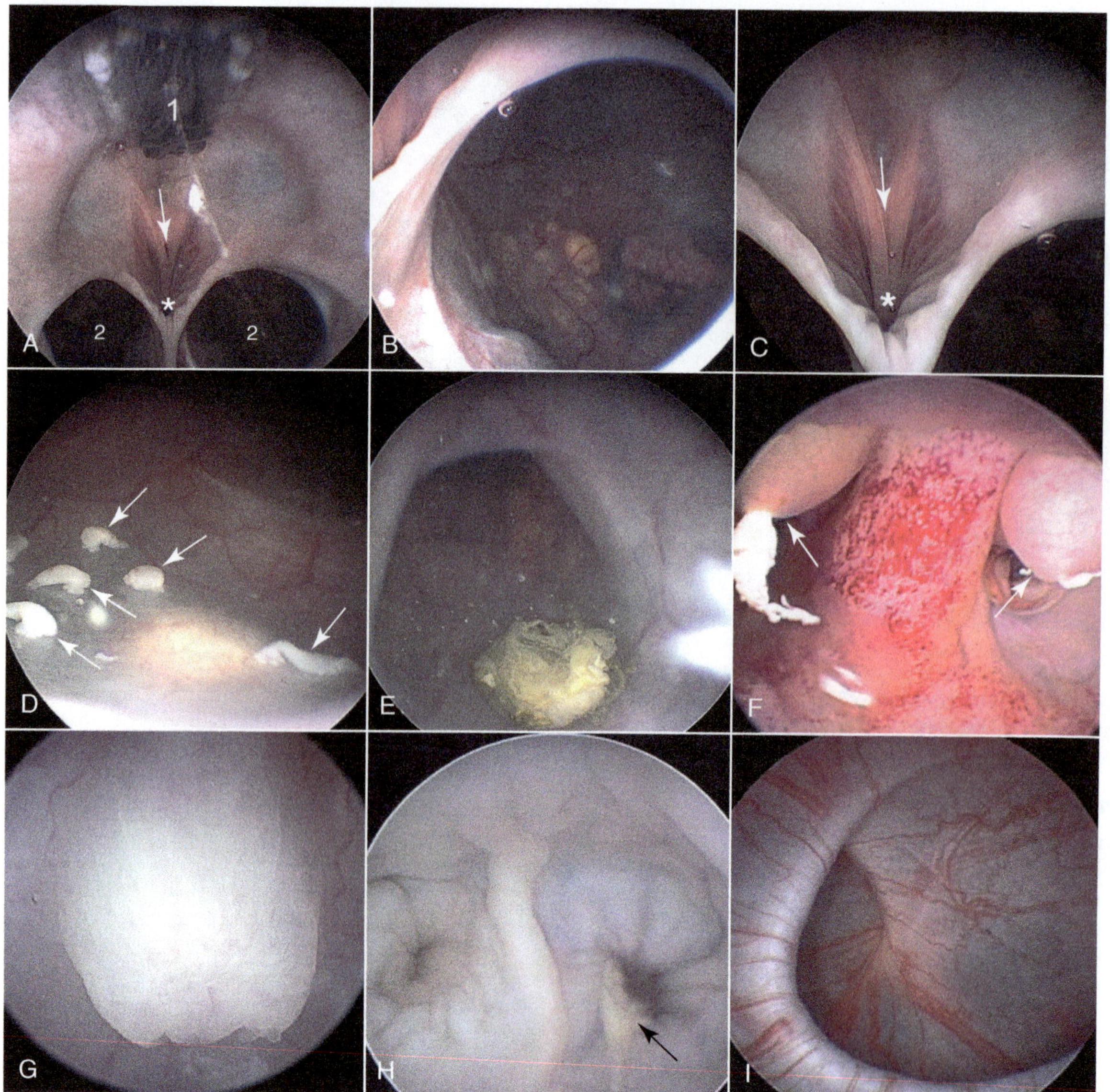

FIGURE 13-25 Cloacoscopy. **A,** Endoscopic view of the cloaca of a female Yellow-bellied Slider *(Trachemys scripta scripta)* demonstrating the clitoris lying on the ventral wall *(1),* bilateral accessory bladders *(2),* and opening to the urethra *(arrow)* and colon *(*)* (dorsal recumbency and the use of saline infusion). **B,** Close-up of one of the accessory bladders. **C,** Close-up of the openings to the urethra *(arrow)* and colon *(*).* **D,** Cystoscopy in a female Yellow-bellied Slider demonstrating several trematode parasites *(arrows)* attached to the bladder wall. **E,** Colonoscopy of a Yellow-bellied Slider with a small fecal mass visible. **F,** View within the urodeum of a Green Iguana *(Iguana iguana)* with uric acid emerging from the urogenital papillae *(arrows). (Courtesy Dr. Scott Stahl.)* **G,** The single urogenital papilla within the urodeum of a Ball Python *(Python regius).* **H,** View within the urodeum of a Hognose snake (*Heterodon nasicus*) demonstrating the oviductal openings. Note the discharge emanating from one of the oviducts *(arrow)* that was associated with retained egg material. *(Courtesy Dr. Scott Stahl.)* **I,** Colonoscopy of a Ball Python demonstrating the normal spiral folds.

and underlying muscle is grasped and elevated away from the coelomic viscera, and the sheath and obturator are gently forced through the coelomic musculature and into the coelomic cavity. It is wise to temporarily cease manual ventilation until the telescope has been introduced into the coelom, thereby reducing the possibility of damage to an inflated lung or viscus. The obturator is replaced by the telescope, and the insufflation line is attached to one of the sheath ports. Making a small skin incision and breach in the muscle ensures that the sheath will be tight fitting and insufflation gas leakage will be minimal. Once a pneumocoelom has been created, it may be necessary to gently touch the tip of the telescope against a coelomic membrane to clean the terminal lens of condensation or tissue fluid. If fat or blood is present on the lens, it is often necessary to remove the telescope from the sheath, clean with gauze moistened with sterile saline, and replace.

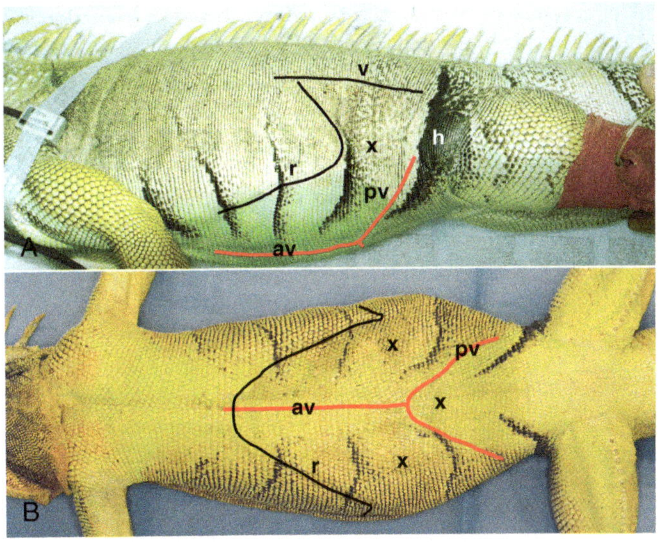

FIGURE 13-26 Telescope entry sites for coelioscopy in lizards. **A,** For a lateral entry into the coelom, the entry point *(x)* is bordered craniad by the last rib *(r)*, dorsad by the lateral processes of the lumbar vertebrae *(v)*, caudad by the musculature of the hindlimb *(h)*, and ventrad by the ventral abdominal *(av)* and pelvic veins *(pv)*. **B,** For a ventral approach to the coelom, insertion points *(x)* may be in the midline, behind the anastomoses of the lateral pelvic veins *(pv)*, or lateral to the ventral abdominal vein *(av)*, caudal to the last rib *(r)*, and cranial to the pelvic veins *(pv)*. *(Courtesy Dr. Stephen J. Divers, University of Georgia, Athens, Ga.)*

On entry via a left paralumbar approach in the iguanid lizard, the first organ to note is the large brown liver lying in the midventral coelom (Figure 13-27, *A*). Advancing the telescope craniad will reveal the heart at the cranioventral extent of the coelom, close to the cranial coelomic inlet (Figure 13-27, *B*). There are no diaphragmatic, postpulmonary, or longitudinal membranes in iguanas. However, these membranes do exist to a greater or lesser extent in tegus, monitors, and certain other saurians (Figure 13-27, *C*). Minor perforation of these membranes by the telescope will not cause any harm, but care is required to avoid perforating the underlying viscera. Dorsal to the heart and extending to midcoelom are the paired lungs (Figure 13-27, *D*). Lung ventilation will be substantially reduced during CO_2 insufflation, and careful communication with the anesthetist is required to balance ventilation and coelomic pressures.

Caudal to the lungs, in the midcoelom, is the stomach with the spleen, an elongated dark red organ in iguanas, situated close behind (Figure 13-27, *E*). Careful examination medial to the stomach and spleen will reveal the splenic limb of the pancreas. The gonads are located just caudal to the spleen, to either side of dorsal midline.

Rigid endoscopy can be used to determine the gender of reptiles, even at a very early age. This is extremely useful in monomorphic species or when one is involved in an endangered species breeding program that requires gender determination in neonates or juveniles.[9] Endoscopy also provides feedback on reproductive activity and disease. The testis is usually ovoid and smooth, and size may vary dramatically with season (see Figure 13-27, *E*). The immature or inactive ovary

TABLE 13-2

Entry Site Preferences for Coelioscopy in Chelonians and Lizards

Reptile	Entry Point	Organ Visualization
Chelonia	Right lateral recumbency: entry through center of left prefemoral fossa	Excellent view of left aspect of heart, left liver lobe, stomach, large intestine, left kidney, left adrenal, left gonad/oviduct, left aspect of bladder Limited view of right gonad/oviduct, small intestine, pancreas Difficult to view spleen, right liver, right lung, right aspect of bladder
	Left lateral recumbency: entry through center of right prefemoral fossa	Excellent view of right aspect of heart, right liver lobe and gallbladder, small intestine, pancreas, right kidney, right adrenal, right gonad/oviduct, right aspect of bladder Limited view of left gonad/oviduct, stomach, spleen Difficult to view left liver lobe, left lung, left aspect of bladder
	Dorsal recumbency: entry through either prefemoral fossa	Excellent view of liver, gallbladder, bladder, and heart Limited view of the gastrointestinal tract and mature ovaries Difficult to view kidneys, testes or immature ovaries, adrenals, lungs, and spleen
Lizards	Right lateral recumbency: left paralumbar entry	Excellent view of left aspect of heart, left liver lobe, left lung, stomach, spleen, small intestine, left kidney, left adrenal, left gonad/oviduct, left aspect of bladder Limited view of large intestine Difficult to view gallbladder, pancreas, right liver lobe, right lung, right aspect of bladder, colon
	Left lateral recumbency: right paralumbar entry	Excellent view of vena cava and right side of heart, right liver lobe and gallbladder, right lung, duodenum, pancreas, right adrenal, right gonad/oviduct, right aspect of bladder, colon Limited view of small intestine Difficult to view stomach, spleen, left liver lobe, left lung, left aspect of bladder
	Dorsal recumbency: caudal paramedian entry	Excellent view of liver, gallbladder, pancreas, bladder Limited view of the heart, lungs, gastrointestinal tract, and mature ovaries Difficult to view kidneys, testes or immature ovaries, adrenals, and spleen

appears as a cluster of small, fluid-filled follicles (Figure 13-27, *F*). As the ovary matures, some of the follicles will enlarge and appear yellow to orange in color as they fill with yolk. Some species of lizards have thin posthepatic and/or postpulmonary membranes that may be pigmented and obscure the gonads. The membrane can be breached to allow better visualization by grasping and tearing with retrieval forceps or incising with scissors. Care must be taken not to damage the follicles because leakage results in coelomitis.

Dorsal to the gonads are the adrenal glands, which lie adjacent to the renal veins (Figure 13-28, *A*). The vas deferens of males and oviducts of females are also visible and can be followed caudad to the pelvic inlet. The kidneys of most lizards are situated in the caudodorsal coelom. Iguanid kidneys are intrapelvic but with precision can still be visualized (Figure 13-28, *B*). Ventrad from the pelvic inlet, the bladder (if present) and fatbody can be seen (Figure 13-28, *C*). A left paralumbar approach will reveal the small intestine and terminal colon; however, a right paralumbar approach will provide access to the gallbladder and cecum (Figure 13-28, *D*). The majority of the pancreas is easier to locate via a right approach, residing caudal to the liver and gallbladder and closely associated with the duodenum (Figure 13-28, *E*). On the right side, the heart is partially obscured by the ascending vena cava (Figure 13-28, *F*).

This approach to saurian coelioscopy has been validated, at least in the Green Iguana and has been found to be both safe and effective.[7] In addition, endoscopic biopsies of liver and kidney have also been demonstrated to be safe and capable of producing samples of diagnostic quality.[10,52]

SNAKES

Snakes are less commonly subjected to coelomic endoscopy because (1) they have more diffuse coelomic fat, (2) it is impossible to examine all the major organs via a single entry point, (3) insufflation is generally more difficult, and (4) targeted coeliotomy can be readily performed along the entire length of the coelom. Nonetheless, if a targeted endoscopic approach to a single coelomic region is required, lateral entry between the ribs in larger snakes and ventrolateral entry just medial to the ribs in smaller snakes are practical options (Figure 13-29, *A*).[13] A recently developed technique for liver biopsy entails access via the pulmonoscopy approach to the serpentine air sac. From within the air sac, it is possible to visualize and sample the liver (Figure 13-29, *B-D*).

CHELONIANS

With the chelonian supported in lateral recumbency, the most useful coelioscopic approach is via the left or right prefemoral fossa (Figures 13-30 and 13-31).[13] Right-handed surgeons will generally find it easier to enter the left prefemoral fossa,

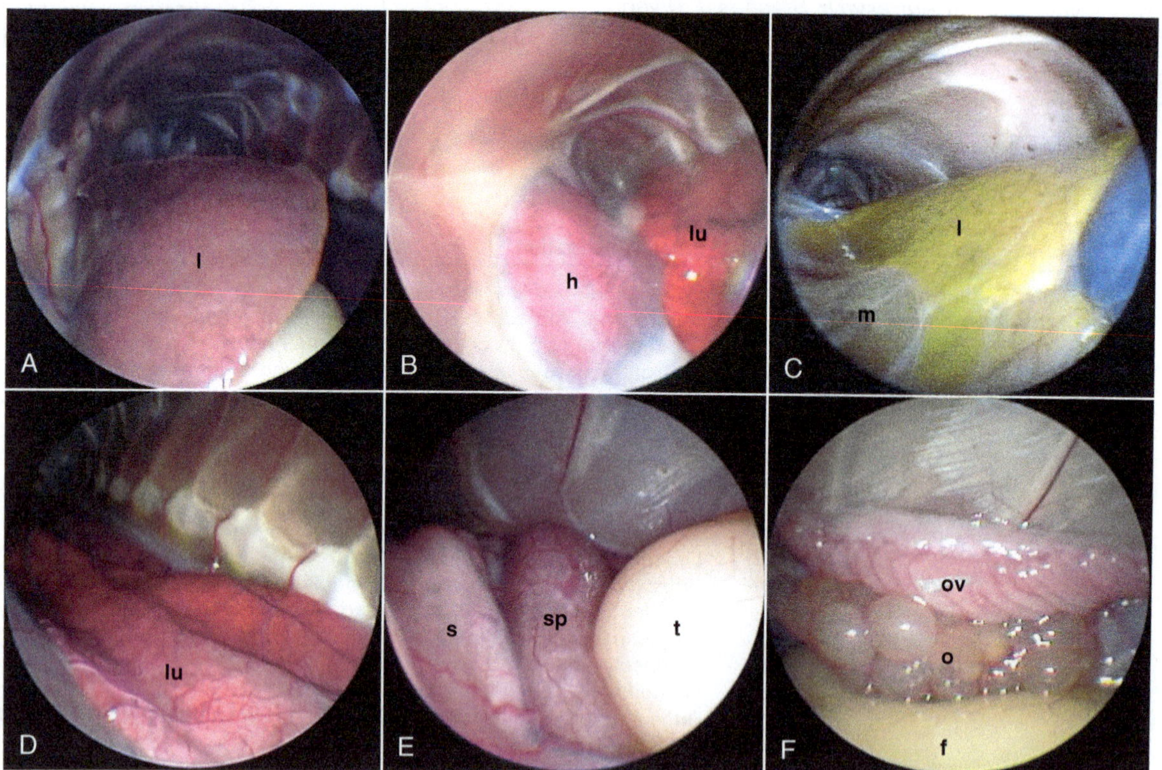

FIGURE 13-27 Lizard coelioscopy. **A,** Left liver lobe *(l)* in an Green Iguana *(Iguana iguana)* (left lateral approach). **B,** Heart *(h)* and lung *(lu)* in a Green Iguana; note the absence of a postpulmonary membrane (left lateral approach). **C,** Left liver lobe *(l)* behind the posthepatic membrane *(m)* in a Monitor Lizard (*Varanus* sp.) (left lateral approach). **D,** Lung *(lu)* in a Green Iguana; note the absence of a postpulmonary membrane in this species (left lateral approach). **E,** Stomach *(s)*, spleen *(sp)*, and testis *(t)* in a Green Iguana (left lateral approach). **F,** Oviduct *(ov)*, ovary *(o)*, and fatbody *(f)* in a Green Iguana (left lateral approach). *(Courtesy Dr. Stephen J. Divers, University of Georgia, Athens, Ga.)*

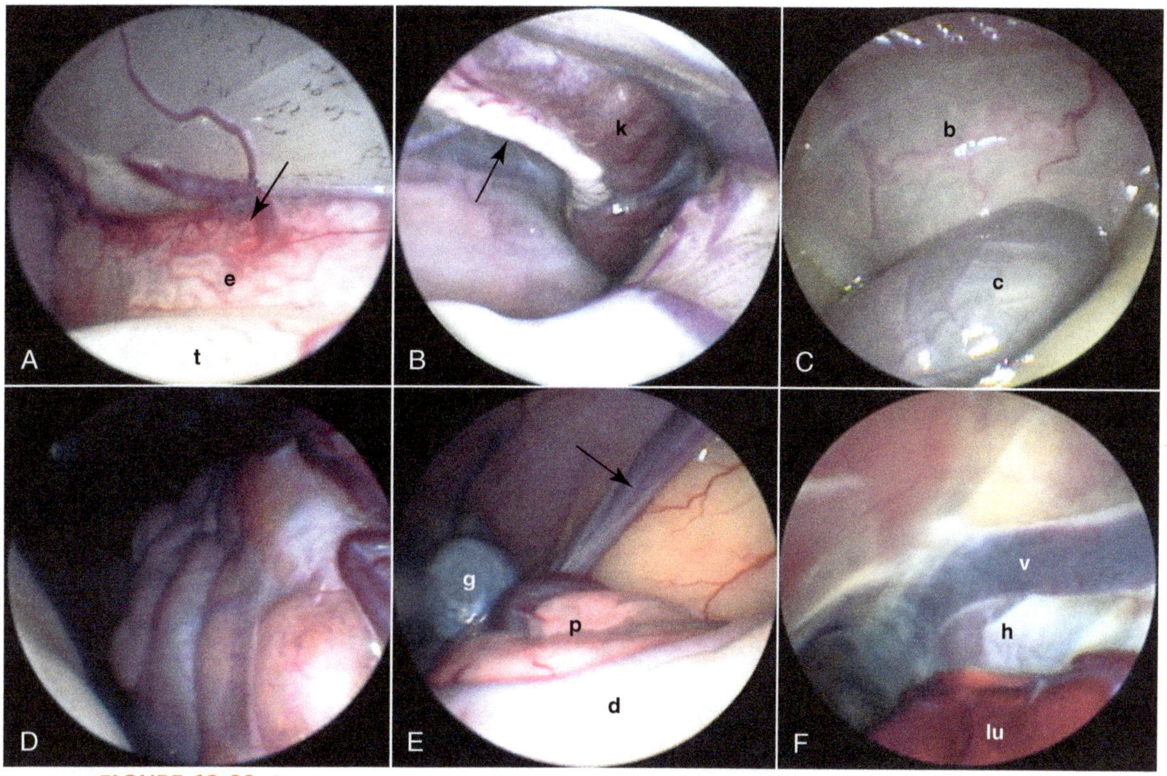

FIGURE 13-28 Green iguana *(Iguana iguana)* coelioscopy. **A,** Epididymis *(e)* and adrenal *(arrow)* lying dorsal to the testis *(t)* in a male (left lateral approach). **B,** Normal vas deferens *(arrow)* and kidney *(k)* emerging from the pelvic inlet (left lateral approach). **C,** Bladder *(b)* and distal colon *(c)* (left lateral approach). **D,** Loops of small bowel (left lateral approach). **E,** Gallbladder *(g)*, pancreas *(p)*, duodenum *(d)*, and ventral abdominal vein *(arrow)* (right lateral approach). **F,** Cranial lung *(lu)* and caudal vena cava *(v)*, partially obscuring the heart *(h)* (right lateral approach). *(Courtesy Dr. Stephen J. Divers, University of Georgia, Athens, Ga.)*

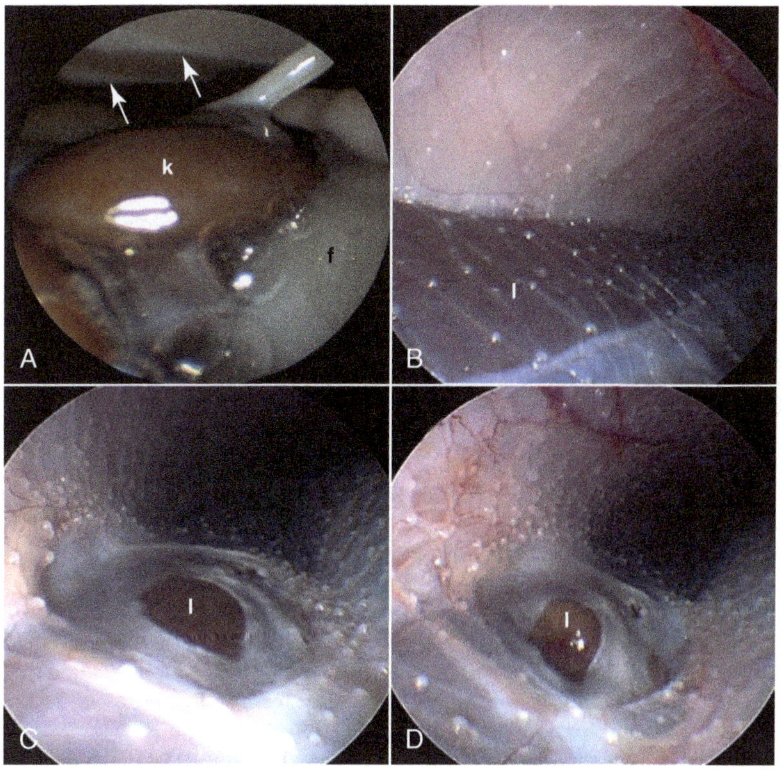

FIGURE 13-29 Snake coelioscopy. **A,** Left lateral approach 82% snout-to-vent revealing the caudal pole of the left kidney *(k)*, fatbody *(f)*, and ribs *(arrows)* in a Boa Constrictor *(Boa constrictor)*. **B,** Ball python *(Python regius)* liver *(l)* viewed from within the air sac of the right lung. **C,** The air sac and serosal membranes have been incised to expose the liver parenchyma *(l)*. **D,** View of the liver *(l)* after biopsy with 1.7-mm forceps. *(Courtesy Dr. Stephen J. Divers, University of Georgia, Athens, Ga.)*

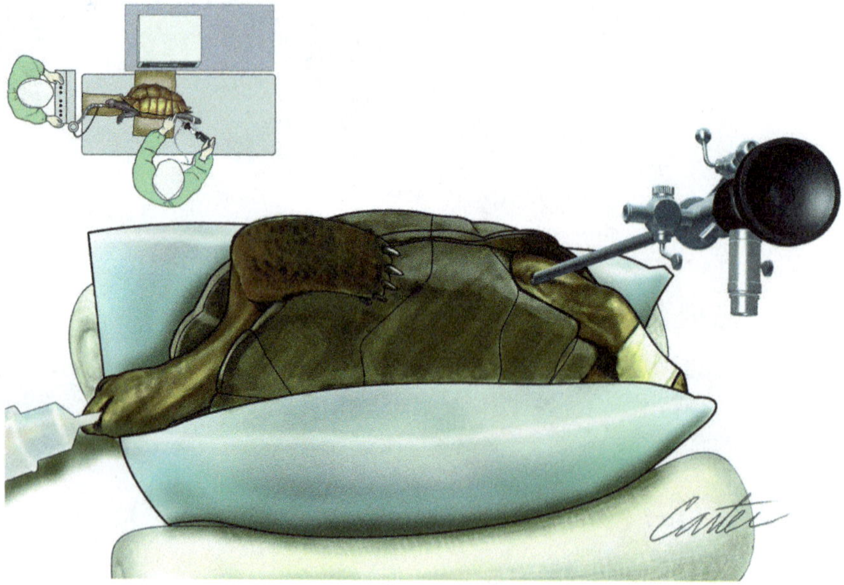

FIGURE 13-30 Operating room layout and positioning for a left prefemoral approach (in front of the left pelvic limb) in order to access the chelonian coelomic cavity. *(Art by Kip Carter [UGA], © University of Georgia Research Foundation, Inc.)*

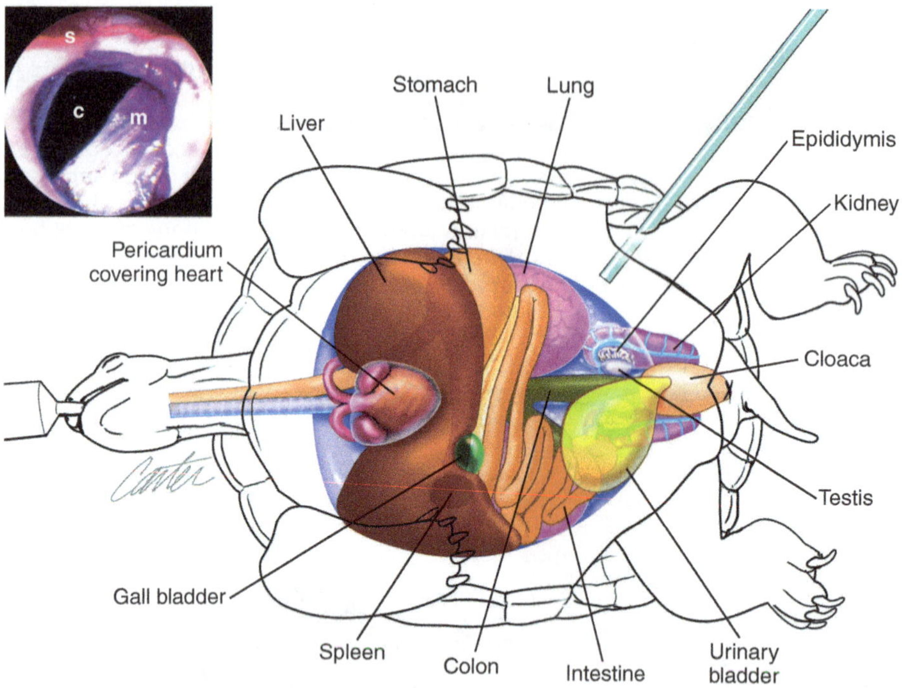

FIGURE 13-31 Diagram to illustrate position and orientation of coelomic viscera inside a male chelonian; note the entry position of the telescope through the prefemoral fossa and the asymmetry of certain organs. *(Art by Kip Carter [UGA], © University of Georgia Research Foundation, Inc.) (Insert)* View through the skin incision *(s)*, showing the coelomic membrane *(m)* and penetration into the coelom *(c)*. *(Courtesy Dr. Stephen J. Divers, University of Georgia, Athens, Ga.)*

and left-handed surgeons the right. Again, unless unilateral pathology exists, the surgeon's preference can prevail. A large bladder can hinder coelioscopy, and chelonians should be encouraged to urinate before surgery. This can be achieved by bathing the animal or by gentle digital stimulation of the cloaca before anesthetic induction.

The pelvic limb is retracted and taped caudad to expose the prefemoral fossa. In chelonians with a well-developed plastron hinge (e.g., Box Turtles), it is wise to place a wedge between the caudal plastron and carapace to maintain exposure. After aseptic preparation, a small (2-mm to 4-mm) craniocaudal skin incision is made in the center of the prefemoral fossa. The subcutaneous fat and connective tissues are bluntly dissected with the use of hemostats down to the coelomic aponeurosis (formed by the broad tendinous portions of the transverse and oblique abdominal muscles) while one is careful to remain cranial to the sartorius muscle and ventral to the iliacus muscle that lies between the femur and ventral surface of the ilium. The coelomic aponeurosis is penetrated by advancing hemostats (or the sheath and obturator) toward the head. Some force is required to breach the coelomic membrane and gain access to the coelomic cavity.

An objective evaluation of coelioscopy in freshwater turtles (*Trachemys scripta* spp) has been published.[53] This study evaluated the ability of the 2.7-mm telescope to visualize the coelomic viscera of Red-eared and Yellow-bellied Sliders and collect diagnostic biopsy specimens from the liver and kidney. Ease of entry and organ visualization was satisfactory to

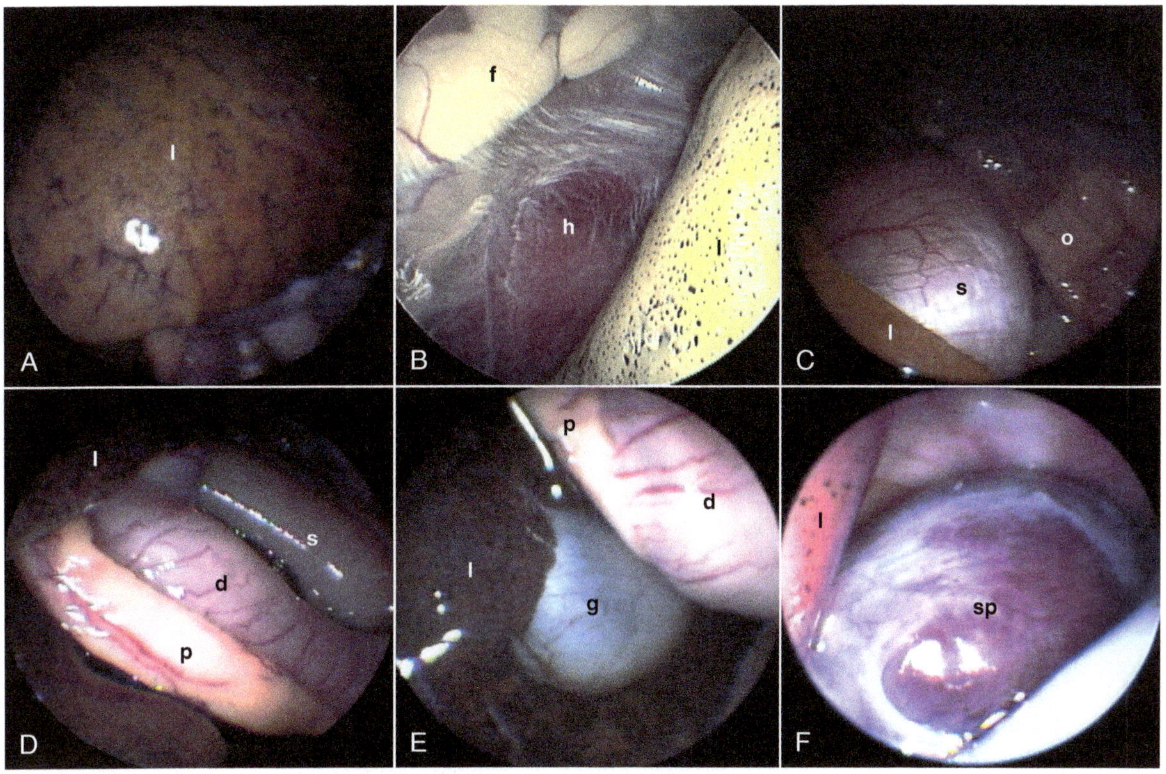

FIGURE 13-32 Chelonian coelioscopy. **A,** Normal liver *(l)* in a Radiated Tortoise *(Astrochelys radiata)* (left prefemoral approach). **B,** Heart *(h)* and pericardial fat *(f)* behind the coelomic membrane of a Yellow-bellied Slider *(Trachemys scripta scripta).* Note the pale liver *(l)* within the coelomic cavity (left prefemoral approach). **C,** Stomach *(s),* liver *(l),* and oviduct *(o)* in a Red-footed Tortoise *(Chelonoidis carbonaria)* (left prefemoral approach). **D,** Liver *(l),* pancreas *(p)* with closely associated duodenum *(d),* and stomach *(s)* in a Red-eared Slider *(Trachemys scripta elegans)* (left prefemoral approach). **E,** Pancreas *(p),* duodenum *(d),* and gallbladder *(g)* embedded within the caudal aspect of the right liver lobe *(l)* in a Red-eared Slider (right prefemoral approach). **F,** Spleen *(sp)* lying under the right liver lobe *(l)* in a Yellow-bellied Slider (right prefemoral approach). *(Courtesy Dr. Stephen J. Divers, University of Georgia, Athens, Ga.)*

excellent for all observed structures, except the spleen, which could only be located from the right side.[16]

The dark red-brown liver is the most obvious organ to use for orientation (Figure 13-32, *A*). The heart is ventral to the liver and partially obscured by a prominent pericardium (Figure 13-32, *B*). The stomach is most prominent on the left (Figure 13-32, *C*), and while potentially seen from either lateral, the pancreas and closely associated duodenum are easier to see from the right (Figure 13-32, *D*). The gallbladder is obvious and associated with the caudal edge of the right liver lobe (Figure 13-32, *E*), but the spleen is often hard to locate under the right liver lobe, close to the duodenum and pancreas (Figure 13-32, *F*). The ventral aspects of the lungs are located dorsad and are most obvious in those species that lack a prominent postpulmonary membrane (Figure 13-33, *A*). The colon, gonads, oviducts (in females), bladder, and kidneys can be viewed from either side. The bladder is situated in the most dependent area, whereas the ovaries and oviducts of reproductively active females can occupy much of the coelom (Figure 13-33, *B, C*). The male testes (cream, yellow, or brown in color) are situated in the caudodorsal coelom and are closely associated with the vasa deferentia, epididymides, adrenal glands, and retrocoelomic kidneys (Figure 13-33, *D*). Recently, coelioscopy using saline-infusion has been shown to be accurate for identifying gender in hatchling and neonate chelonians. A recent study in Chinese Box Turtles *(Cuora flavomarginata)* concluded that gonads could be visualized and sex easily identified in animals as small as 10 g (Figure 13-33, *E, F*).[9]

The kidneys are retrocoelomic, residing behind an often transparent coelomic membrane (Figure 13-34, *A*). When a pigmented coelomic membrane is encountered, the close association with the testis (or immature ovary) can help indicate their location (Figure 13-34, *B*). However, in adult females in which the ovary and suspensory ligament have enlarged and fallen away from the pigmented coelomic membrane, it can be challenging to locate the kidneys unless they are grossly abnormal (Figure 13-34, *C*).[16]

An extracoelomic approach to the chelonian kidney is also possible in those species with a more flattened carapace and negates the need to enter the coelomic cavity. The sheathed endoscope is gently advanced from the same prefemoral skin incision in a caudodorsal direction between the coelomic aponeurosis and the broad iliacus muscle. A combination of gentle lateral movements of the telescope tip and intermittent insufflation are used to further separate the coelomic

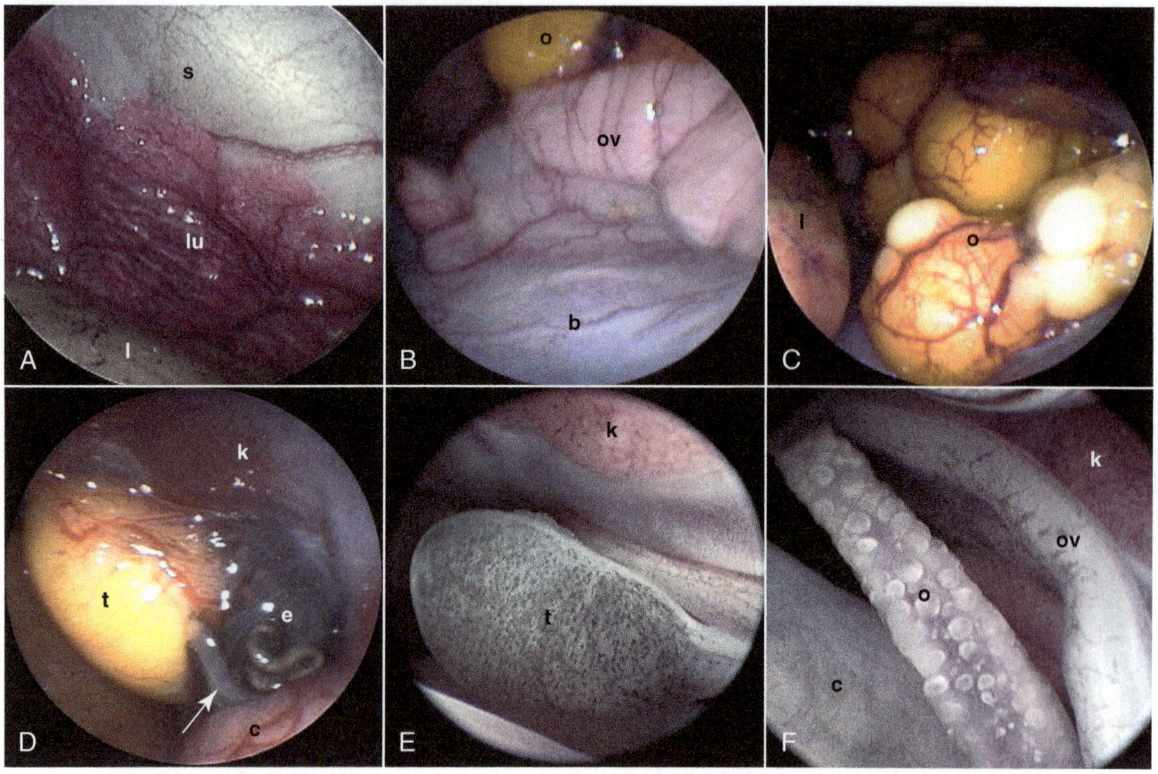

FIGURE 13-33 Chelonian coelioscopy. **A,** View of the serosal surface of the dorsal shell *(s),* left lung *(lu),* and liver *(l)* in a Red-eared Slider *(Trachemys scripta elegans)* (left prefemoral approach). **B,** Urinary bladder *(b),* oviduct *(ov),* and ovary *(o)* in an African Spurred Tortoise *(Geochelone sulcata)* (left prefemoral approach). **C,** Mature ovary *(o)* extending to the caudal edge of the left liver lobe *(l)* in a Hermann's Tortoise *(Testudo hermanni)* (left prefemoral approach). **D,** Testis *(t),* epididymis *(e),* and vas deferens *(arrow)* in the caudodorsal coelom of a Red-eared Slider. Note the closely associated retrocoelomic kidney *(k)* and the distal colon *(c)* (left prefemoral approach). **E,** Immature testis *(t)* closely associated with the kidney *(k)* in a hatchling Chinese Box Turtle *(Cuora flavomarginata)* (left prefemoral approach with saline infusion). **F,** Immature ovary *(o)* and oviduct *(ov)* closely associated with the kidney *(k)* and distal colon *(c)* in a hatchling Chinese Box Turtle (left prefemoral approach with saline infusion). *(Courtesy Dr. Stephen J. Divers, University of Georgia, Athens, Ga.)*

aponeurosis from the adjacent musculature to reveal the kidneys (Figure 13-34, *D*).

NATURAL ORIFICE TRANSLUMINAL ENDOSCOPIC SURGERY

Natural orifice transluminal endoscopic surgery (NOTES) is still largely an experimental surgical technique whereby "scarless" abdominal operations can be performed with an endoscope passed through a natural orifice (e.g., mouth, vagina, or anus) then through an internal incision in the stomach, vagina, bladder, or colon, thus avoiding any external incisions or scars.[54] Nevertheless, an increasing number of clinical procedures have been published in the human literature, and NOTES is considered the next frontier of human endoscopic surgery.[55] To date, the author is unaware of any true NOTES procedures in reptiles. However, there are some examples in chelonians that come close, including the identification of immature gonads through the transparent bladder wall and the endoscopic removal of cystic calculi. Nonetheless, neither technique involves an internal incision.[35,56] The gender identification technique has the advantage of being less invasive (as the coelom is not entered) but does not provide the same degree of visual acuity as direct coelioscopic examination. Therefore, in species in which the immature gonads appear very similar or the bladder wall is less transparent, accuracy may be decreased (Figure 13-35).

PATHOLOGY AND ENDOSCOPIC BIOPSY

In reptiles, a variety of pathologies may be appreciated endoscopically, often with surprisingly few clinicopathologic or discernible radiographic or ultrasonographic changes (Figure 13-36, *A-E*). Tissue samples can be easily harvested from most organs and, in general, any abnormal soft tissue structure. Liver disease may be focal or diffuse, and although the caudal edge is easiest to sample, biopsy specimens can also be taken from the surface by first incising the serosal covering (Figure 13-36, *F*). A variety of renal diseases have also been described (Figure 13-37, *A, B*).[16,57] In lizards and snakes, the lobulated kidney is easy to approach and sample directly (Figure 13-37, *C*). However, in chelonians,

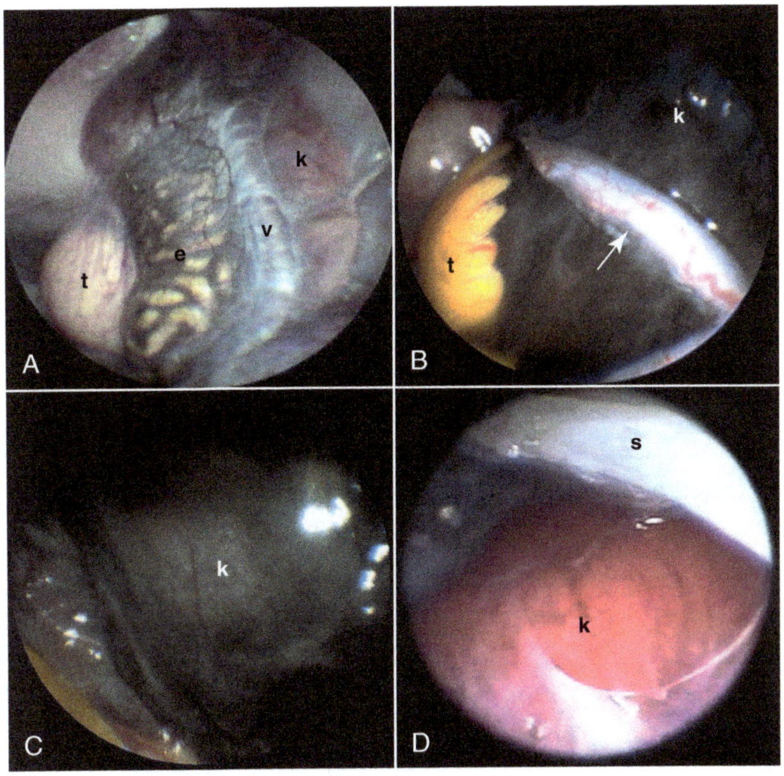

FIGURE 13-34 Chelonian renal examination. **A,** View of the retrocoelomic kidney *(k)*, renal vasculature *(v)*, and closely associated testis *(t)* and epididymis *(e)* in a male Red-eared Slider *(Trachemys scripta elegans)*. Note that renal visualization is possible thanks to the transparent nature of the coelomic membrane (left prefemoral approach). **B,** View of the same caudodorsal region in an adult male Greek Tortoise *(Testudo graeca)*. The retrocoelomic kidney *(k)* is obscured by the pigmented coelomic membrane; however, its position can be determined by the obvious testis *(t)* and vas deferens *(arrow)* (left prefemoral approach). **C,** View of the same caudodorsal region in an adult female Greek Tortoise with the retrocoelomic kidney *(k)* obscured by a pigmented membrane. With no closely associated gonad to indicate the kidney's location, the endoscopist must rely on accurate anatomic knowledge alone (left prefemoral approach). **D,** Direct, extracoelomic view of the kidney *(k)* and internal surface of the caudodorsal carapace *(s)* in a Loggerhead Sea turtle (left prefemoral approach). *(Courtesy Dr. Stephen J. Divers, University of Georgia, Athens, Ga.)*

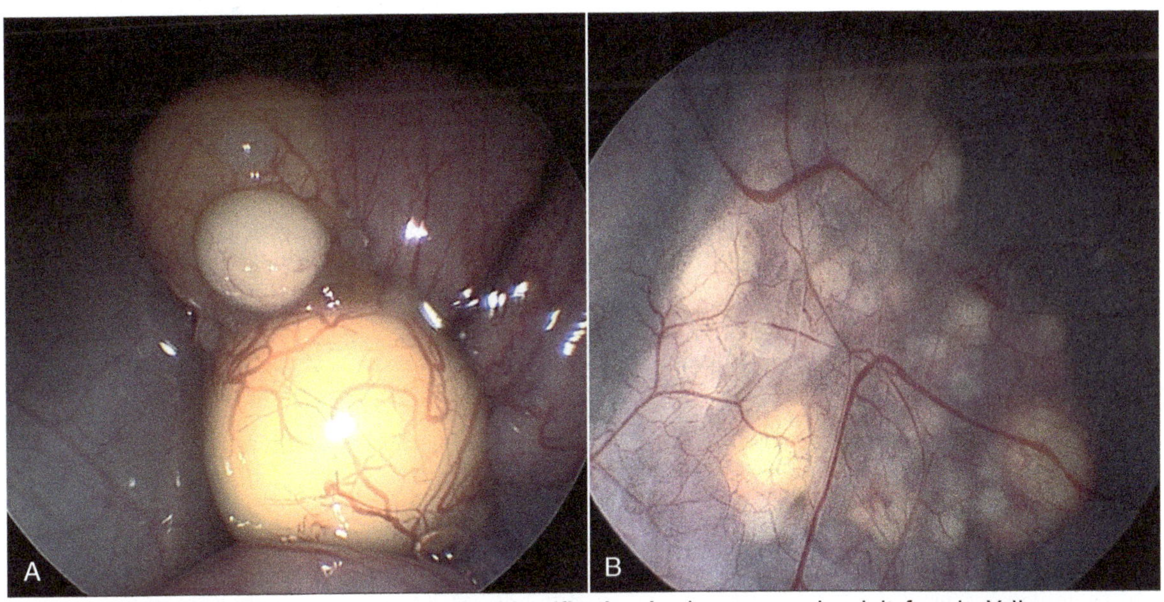

FIGURE 13-35 Endoscopic gender identification in the same sub adult female Yellow-bellied Slider *(Trachemys scripta scripta)*. A comparison between direct examination by coelioscopy using CO_2 insufflation **(A)** and indirect examination using sterile saline and a transluminal technique across the accessory bladder wall **(B)** (natural orifice transluminal endoscopic surgery). Note the reduced clarity of the ovary using the transluminal technique.

its flattened retrocoelomic position first requires incision of the coelomic membrane via a coelioscopic approach (Figure 13-37, *D-F*). Endoscopic liver and kidney biopsies have been objectively assessed in freshwater turtles and Green Iguanas.[10,52,53] These studies have confirmed the ability of the 2.7-mm telescope to visualize the coelomic viscera and harvest samples from liver and kidney with the 1.7-mm biopsy forceps. No significant iatrogenic trauma was reported, and biopsy specimens were consistent with tissues collected at necropsy and were considered acceptable for histologic

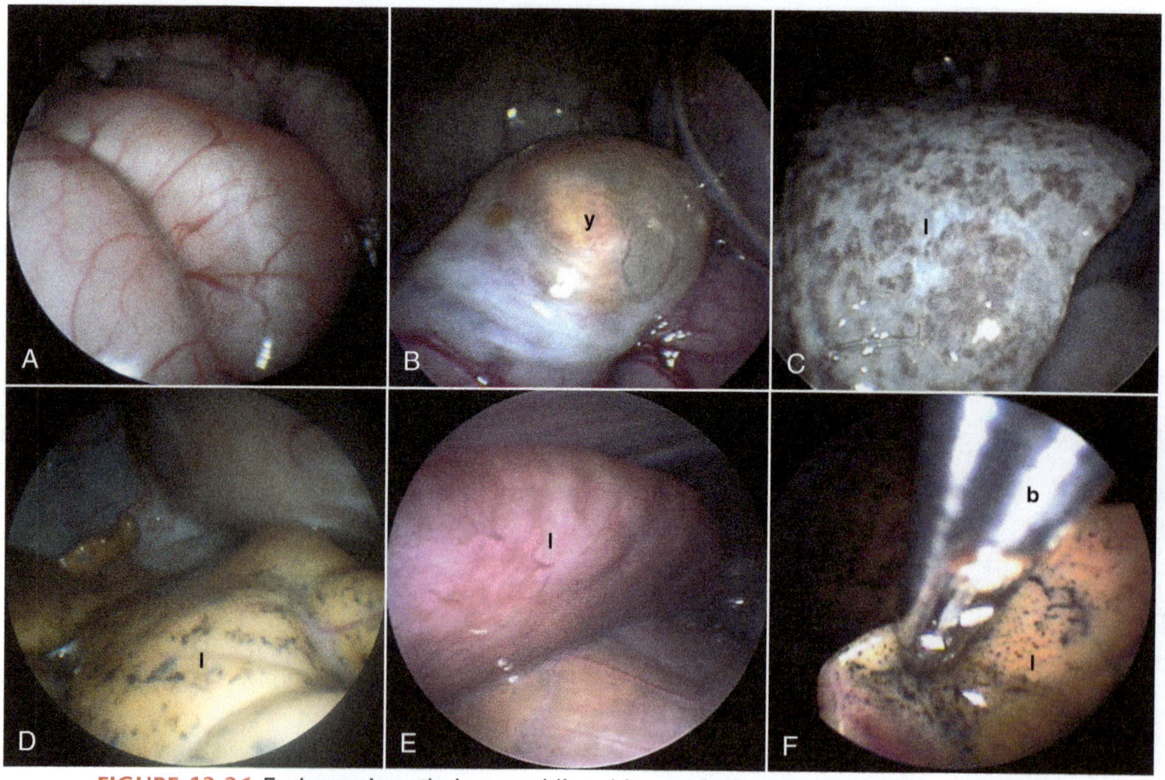

FIGURE 13-36 Endoscopic pathology and liver biopsy. **A,** Grossly distended small intestine in a Russian Tortoise *(Testudo horsfieldii).* This herbivorous tortoise was fed dairy products, which resulted in fermentative enteritis (left prefemoral approach). **B,** Retained, inspissated yolk sac *(y)* in a juvenile Radiated Tortoise *(Astrochelys radiata)* that was seen for intermittent anorexia and poor growth. Clinicopathologic examination and diagnostic imaging were unremarkable, but endoscope-assisted removal proved curative (left prefemoral approach). **C,** Chronic hepatic fibrosis in a Green Iguana *(Iguana iguana)* that was seen for anorexia and occasional regurgitation. Diagnostic imaging was unremarkable, and the only clinicopathologic abnormality was mild elevation of postprandial bile acids. Endoscopic biopsy confirmed the diagnosis of severe hepatic fibrosis with cholestasis (left lateral coelioscopy). **D,** Pale liver *(l)* in an Aldabra Tortoise *(Aldabrachelys [Geochelone] gigantea)* that was seen with intermittent anorexia. All liver variables were unremarkable, but severe hepatic lipidosis was diagnosed after liver biopsy (left prefemoral approach). **E,** Diffuse hepatomegaly *(l)* in a Green Iguana that was seen with lethargy and anorexia. Diagnostic imaging and the liver biochemical profile were unremarkable; however moderate leukocytosis, predominantly heterophilia and azurophilia, was evident. Endoscopic liver biopsy confirmed the diagnosis as bacterial hepatitis caused by *Klebsiella,* and appropriate treatment proved curative (left lateral coelioscopy). **F,** Biopsy from the edge of the chelonian liver *(l)* using 1.7-mm biopsy forceps *(b)* (left prefemoral approach). *(Courtesy Dr. Stephen J. Divers, University of Georgia, Athens, Ga.)*

interpretation. Furthermore, the ability to diagnose renal disease using endoscopic biopsy has also been demonstrated for a variety of chelonian species.[16]

POSTOPERATIVE CARE, COMPLICATIONS, AND OUTCOMES

Reptiles should be closely supervised until ambulatory and be continuously maintained within their species-specific preferred optimum temperature zone. Meloxicam is relied on postoperatively, although opiates and local anesthetics are also useful as part of a balanced approach to analgesia. Continued fluid therapy is critical in the immediate postoperative period, but a return to normal alimentation is the hallmark of recovery. Typically, reptiles return to normal function and behaviors quicker after endoscopic procedures compared with traditional surgeries. kin sutures are removed at 6 to 8 weeks.

The major complications encountered are typically associated with anesthesia and the advanced disease state of many reptile patients. The importance of a thorough preoperative evaluation and stabilization cannot be overemphasized. Ventilation, fluid support, and temperature maintenance are critical. Minor hemorrhaging after tissue biopsy is common but clinically insignificant. Most endoscopy issues are related to operator error until experience and ability have been gained. In general, the ability to examine reptiles internally and collect tissue samples greatly aids diagnosis and improves treatment success. To facilitate the endoscopy caseload without compromising patient welfare, the surgeon should obtain proper training. Reptile (and

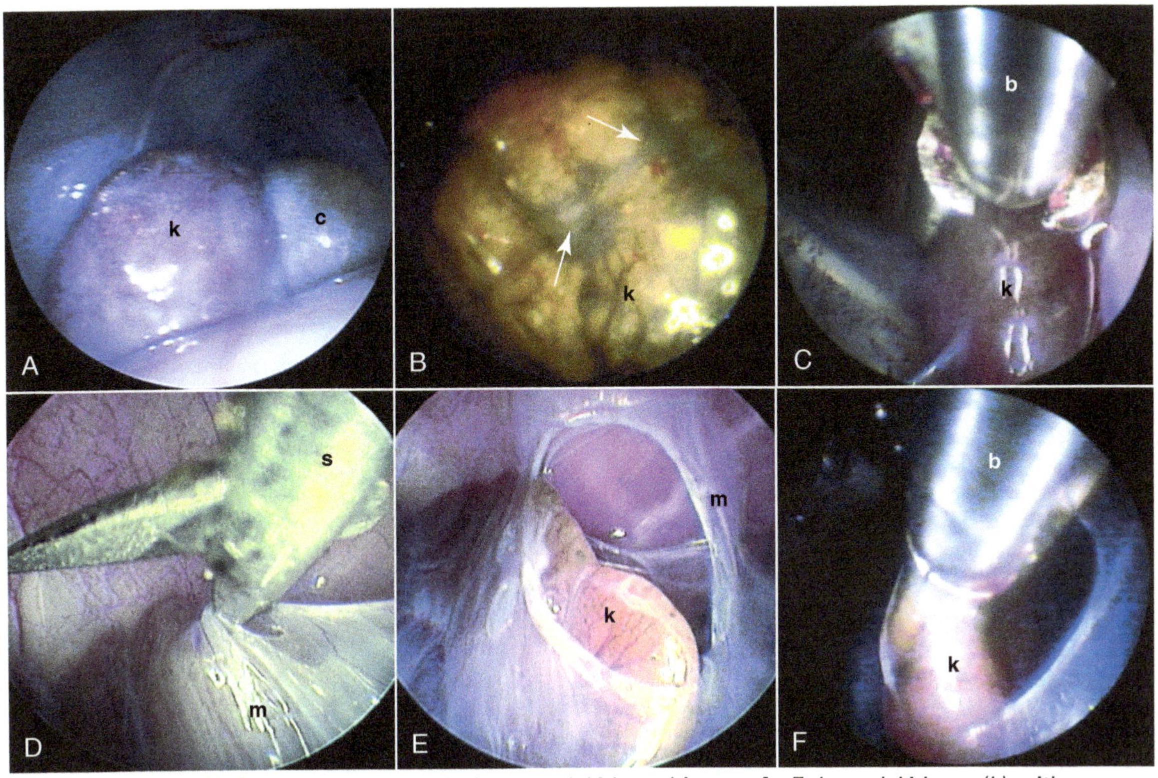

FIGURE 13-37 Endoscopic pathology and kidney biopsy. **A,** Enlarged kidney *(k)* with associated renal cyst *(c)* in a Green Iguana *(Iguana iguana)* that was seen with anorexia and cachexia. Radiography and ultrasonography confirmed renomegaly, while the plasma biochemical profile revealed reversed calcium:phosphorus ratio and elevated uric acid. Endoscopic biopsy confirmed the diagnosis of glomerulonephrosis with renal gout and mineralization (left lateral coelioscopy). **B,** Abnormal kidney *(k)* with fibrous bands *(arrows)* in a female Greek Tortoise *(Testudo graeca)* that was seen with anorexia, lethargy, and polyuria. Diagnostic imaging and clinicopathologic examination were unremarkable; however, renal biopsy confirmed the diagnosis as severe tubulonephrosis (left prefemoral approach). **C,** Biopsy of an iguanid kidney *(k)* using 1.7-mm biopsy forceps *(b)* (right lateral coelioscopy). **D,** Incising the caudodorsal coelomic membrane *(m)* of a Yellow-bellied Slider *(Trachemys scripta scripta)* with the use of 1.7-mm endoscopy scissors *(s)* to gain access to the retrocoelomic kidney (left prefemoral approach). **E,** View of the incised coelomic membrane *(m)* revealing the kidney *(k)* (left prefemoral approach). **F,** Biopsy forceps *(b)* being passed through the incision to collect a biopsy from the kidney *(k)* (left prefemoral approach). *(Courtesy Dr. Stephen J. Divers, University of Georgia, Athens, Ga.)*

other exotic species) endoscopy courses are regularly offered at the University of Georgia (www.vet.uga/edu/ce). It is also imperative that the endoscopist prepare for the option to convert to a traditional surgical approach, if required.

Return to normal behaviors and weight gain are often the most useful indicators of improvement. Serial clinicopathologic examination can also be useful if abnormalities were detected preoperatively. Serial endoscopic evaluations can be used to monitor patients, especially because some diseases (e.g., hepatic lipidosis and glomerulonephrosis) may have a protracted course.

REFERENCES

1. Ackermann J, Carpenter JW. Using endoscopy to remove a gastric foreign body in a python. *Vet Med* 1995;90:761-763.
2. Burrows CF, Heard DJ. Endoscopy in nondomestic species. In: Tams TR, ed. *Small animal endoscopy*. 2nd ed. St. Louis: Mosby, 1999;297-321.
3. Cooper JE. Endoscopy in exotic species. In: Brearley MJ, Cooper JE, Sullivan M, eds. *Color atlas of small animal endoscopy*. 1st ed. St. Louis: Mosby, 1991;111-122.
4. Coppoolse KJ, Zwart P. Cloacoscopy in reptiles. *Vet Q* 1985;7:243-245.
5. Pressler BM, Goodman RA, Harms CA, et al. Endoscopic evaluation of the esophagus and stomach in three loggerhead sea turtles *(Caretta caretta)* and a Malaysian giant turtle *(Orlitia borneensis)*. *J Zoo Wildl Med* 2003;34:88-92.
6. Lafortune M, Göbel T, Jacobson E, et al. Respiratory bronchoscopy of subadult American alligators *(Alligator mississippiensis)* and tracheal wash evaluation. *J Zoo Wildl Med* 2005;36:12-20.
7. Hernandez-Divers SJ, Stahl S, Hernandez-Divers SM, et al. Coelomic endoscopy of the green iguana *(Iguana iguana)*. *J Herpetol Med Surg* 2004;14:10-18.
8. Hernandez-Divers SJ, Stahl S, Stedman NL, et al. Renal evaluation in the green iguana *(Iguana iguana)*: assessment of plasma biochemistry, glomerular filtration rate, and endoscopic biopsy. *J Zoo Wildl Med* 2005;36:155-168.
9. Hernandez-Divers SJ, Stahl SJ, Farrell R. Endoscopic gender identification of hatchling Chinese box turtles *(Cuora flavomarginata)* under local and general anesthesia. *J Am Vet Med Assoc* 2009;234:800-804.

10. Hernandez-Divers SJ, Stahl SJ, McBride M, et al. Evaluation of an endoscopic liver biopsy technique in green iguanas. *J Am Vet Med Assoc* 2007;230:1849-1853.
11. Stahl SJ, Hernandez-Divers SJ, Cooper TL, et al. Evaluation of transcutaneous pulmonoscopy for examination and biopsy of the lungs of ball pythons and determination of preferred biopsy specimen handling and fixation procedures. *J Am Vet Med Assoc* 2008;233:440-445.
12. Hernandez-Divers SJ. Diagnostic and surgical endoscopy. In: Raiti P, Girling S, eds. *Manual of reptiles.* 2nd ed. Cheltenham, England: British Small Animal Veterinary Association, 2004;103-114.
13. Hernandez-Divers SJ, Hernandez-Divers SM, Wilson GH, et al. A review of reptile diagnostic coelioscopy. *J Herpetol Med Surg* 2005;15:16-31.
14. Innis C, Hernandez-Divers SJ, Martinez-Jimenez D. Coelioscopic-assisted prefemoral oophorectomy in chelonians. *J Am Vet Med Assoc* 2007;230:1049-1052.
15. Divers SJ. Reptile diagnostic endoscopy and endosurgery. *Vet Clin North Am Exot Anim Pract* 2010;13:217-242.
16. Hernandez-Divers SJ. Endoscopic renal evaluation and biopsy of Chelonia. *Vet Rec* 2004;154:73-80.
17. Taylor WM. Endoscopy. In: Mader DR, ed. *Reptile medicine and surgery.* 2nd ed. St. Louis: Elsevier, 2006;549-563.
18. Taylor M. Endoscopic examination and biopsy techniques. In: Ritchie BW, Harrison GJ, Harrison LR, eds. *Avian medicine: principles and application.* Fort Worth, Fla: Harrison Bird Diets International, 1994;327-354.
19. Chamness CJ. Introduction to veterinary endoscopy and endoscopic instrumentation. In: McCarthy TC, ed. *Veterinary endoscopy for the small animal practitioner.* St Louis: Elsevier, 2004;1-29.
20. Chamness CJ. Equipment for the avian and exotic endoscopist. *Semin Avian Exot Pet Med* 1999;8:102-106.
21. Divers SJ, Barron GH, Mejia-Fava J, et al. EndoGo mobile endoscopy camera and E-zenon battery powered light source: true mobility for the endoscopist, in *Proceedings.* 31st Annu Conf Assoc Avian Vet 2010;21.
22. Roth L. Comparison of liver cytology and biopsy diagnoses in dogs and cats: 56 cases. *Vet Clin Pathol* 2001;30:35-38.
23. Falcone RE, Wanamaker SR, Barnes F, et al. Laparoscopic vs. open wedge biopsy of the liver. *J Laparoendosc Surg* 1993;3:325-329.
24. Rawlings CA, Diamond H, Howerth EW, et al. Diagnostic quality of percutaneous kidney biopsy specimens obtained with laparoscopy versus ultrasound guidance in dogs. *J Am Vet Med Assoc* 2003;223:317-321.
25. Mader DR. *Reptile medicine and surgery.* 2nd ed. St Louis: Elsevier, 2006.
26. Raiti P, Girling S. *Manual of reptiles.* 2nd ed. Cheltenham, England: British Small Animal Veterinary Association, 2004.
27. Martinez-Jimenez D, Hernandez-Divers SJ. Emergency care of reptiles. *Vet Clin North Am Exot Anim Pract* 2007;10:557-585.
28. Schumacher J, Yelen T. Anesthesia and analgesia. In: Mader DR, ed. *Reptile medicine and surgery.* 2nd ed. St Louis: Elsevier, 2006;442-452.
29. Rostal D, Grumbles J, Lance V, et al. Non-lethal sexing techniques for hatchling and immature desert tortoises *(Gopherus agassizii). Herpetol Monogr* 1994;8:103-116.
30. Sladky KK, Kinney ME, Johnson SM. Analgesic efficacy of butorphanol and morphine in bearded dragons and corn snakes. *J Am Vet Med Assoc* 2008;233:267-273.
31. Sladky KK, Miletic V, Paul-Murphy J, et al. Analgesic efficacy and respiratory effects of butorphanol and morphine in turtles. *J Am Vet Med Assoc* 2007;230:1356-1362.
32. Divers SJ, Papich M, McBride M, et al. Intravenous and oral pharmacokinetics of meloxicam in the green iguana *(Iguana iguana). Am J Vet Res* 2010;71:1277-1283.
33. Hernandez-Divers SJ, Shearer D. Pulmonary mycobacteriosis caused by *Mycobacterium haemophilum* and *M. marinum* in a royal python. *J Am Vet Med Assoc* 2002;220:1661-1663.
34. Jekl V, Knotek Z. Endoscopic examination of snakes by access through an air sac. *Vet Rec* 2006;158:407.
35. Selleri P, Giorgi T, Melidone R, et al. Minimally-invasive endoscopic sex determination technique in juvenile marginated tortoises, *Testudo marginata*, in *Proceedings.* 18th Annu Conf Assoc Reptilian Amphibian Vet 2011;148.
36. Tams TR, Rawlings CA. *Small animal endoscopy.* 3rd ed. St Louis: Elsevier, 2011.
37. McCarthy TC. *Veterinary endoscopy for the small animal practitioner.* St Louis: Elsevier, 2005.
38. Monnet E, Twedt DC. Laparoscopy. *Vet Clin North Am Small Anim Pract* 2003;33:1147-1163.
39. Lhermette P, Sobel D. *BSAVA manual of canine and feline endoscopy and endosurgery.* 1st ed. Cheltenham, England: British Small Animal Veterinary Association, 2008.
40. Golditch IM. Laparoscopy: advances and advantages. *Fertil Steril* 1971;22:306-310.
41. Grauer GF, Twedt DC, Mero KN. Evaluation of laparoscopy for obtaining renal biopsy specimens from dogs and cats. *J Am Vet Med Assoc* 1983;183:677-679.
42. Hancock RB, Lanz OI, Waldron DR, et al. Comparison of postoperative pain after ovariohysterectomy by harmonic scalpel-assisted laparoscopy compared with median celiotomy and ligation in dogs. *Vet Surg* 2005;34:273-282.
43. Kehlet H. Surgical stress response: does endoscopic surgery confer an advantage? *World J Surg* 1999;23:801-807.
44. Lagares-Garcia JA, Bansidhar B, Moore RA. Benefits of laparoscopy in middle-aged patients. *Surg Endosc* 2003;17:68-72.
45. Orlando R, Lirussi F, Okolicsanyi L. Laparoscopy and liver biopsy: further evidence that the two procedures improve the diagnosis of liver cirrhosis. A retrospective study of 1,003 consecutive examinations. *J Clin Gastroenterol* 1990;12:47-52.
46. Reissman P, Gofrit O, Rivkind A. Exploratory laparoscopy: a crucial advantage of laparoscopic over standard appendectomy. *South Med J* 1994;87:576.
47. Vander Velpen GC, Shimi SM, Cuschieri A. Diagnostic yield and management benefit of laparoscopy: a prospective audit. *Gut* 1994;35:1617-1621.
48. Weickert U, Buttmann A, Jakobs R, et al. Diagnosis of liver cirrhosis: a comparison of modified ultrasound and laparoscopy in 100 consecutive patients. *J Clin Gastroenterol* 2005;39:529-532.
49. Yu SY, Chiu JH, Loong CC, et al. Diagnostic laparoscopy: indication and benefit. *Zhonghua Yi Xue Za Zhi (Taipei)* 1997;59:158-163.
50. Hernandez-Divers SJ. Surgery: principles and techniques. In: Raiti P, Girling S, eds. *Manual of reptiles.* 2nd ed. Cheltenham, England: British Small Animal Veterinary Association, 2004;147-167.
51. Divers SJ. Lizard endoscopic techniques with particular regard to the green iguana *(Iguana iguana). Semin Avian Exot Pet Med* 1999;8:122-129.
52. Hernandez-Divers SJ, Stahl SJ, Stedman NL, et al. Renal evaluation in the healthy green iguana *(Iguana iguana)*: assessment of plasma biochemistry, glomerular filtration rate, and endoscopic biopsy. *J Zoo Wildl Med* 2005;36:155-168.
53. Divers SJ, Stahl SJ, Camus A. Evaluation of diagnostic coelioscopy including liver and kidney biopsy in freshwater turtles *(Trachemys scripta). J Zoo Wildl Med* 2010;41:677-687.
54. Tomikawa M, Xu H, Hashizume M. Current status and prerequisites for natural orifice translumenal endoscopic surgery (NOTES). *Surg Today* 2010;40:909-916.
55. Auyang ED, Santos BF, Enter DH, et al. Natural orifice translumenal endoscopic surgery (NOTES): a technical review. *Surg Endosc* 2011;25:3135-3148.
56. Mans C, Sladky KK. Endoscopically guided removal of cloacal calculi in three African spurred tortoises *(Geochelone sulcata). J Am Vet Med Assoc* 2012;240:869-875.
57. Hernandez-Divers SJ, Innis C. Renal disease in reptiles: diagnosis and clinical management. In: Mader DR, ed. *Reptile medicine and surgery.* 2nd ed. St Louis: Elsevier, 2006;878-892.

CHAPTER 14

Endoscope-Assisted and Endoscopic Surgery

Stephen J. Divers

In human medicine, endosurgery has been credited with numerous advantages over traditional open procedures, including reductions in pain, operating time, hospital stay, and convalescence period.[1,2] While such advantages may be less easily quantified or published in veterinary medicine, over the past decade there have, nevertheless, been considerable advances in minimally invasive endosurgery of animals, including reptiles.[3-6] Indeed, considering that most reptiles weigh less than a few kilograms, the development of minimally invasive endosurgery would seem a logical evolution in their surgical care, particularly given the hindrances of the chelonian shell.[7]

The transition from a technique that is purely diagnostic to one that is more complex and capable of surgical manipulation requires additional equipment and, perhaps even more taxing, a considerably more refined surgical skill set. It is no exaggeration to state that the technical difficulty associated with multiple-port endosurgery is a magnitude greater than that required for single-entry diagnostic endoscopy. This chapter is most certainly an extension of the previous chapter and should not be read in isolation. Only additional equipment and supplemental techniques are covered here, and a firm grounding in diagnostic endoscopy is assumed.

ENDOSURGICAL EQUIPMENT

In addition to a telescope, one or more independent instruments must be introduced when the endoscopist operates inside a reptilian coelom.[8] These instruments and the cannulae through which they pass are grouped into various size classes that are often color-coded. For example, 2-mm instruments are used in conjunction with 2.5-mm cannulae, 3-mm instruments with 3.5-mm cannulae, and 5-mm instruments with 6-mm cannulae (Figure 14-1). In addition, the 2.7-mm telescope housed within a 3.5-mm protection sheath will pass through a 3.9-mm cannula. A listing of available equipment is provided in Table 14-1.[8]

Cannulae and Trocars

Cannulae are used to provide additional access ports (Figure 14-2). They are of surgical steel or graphite/plastic construction and have internal leaflet valves and optional insufflation stopcocks for CO_2 delivery. These valves are designed to prevent loss of gas during insufflation. Insufflation stopcocks are optional, but at least one is required for the attachvment of the insufflation line. The metal cannulae are more robust and heavier and therefore are used only for the animals weighing more than 10 kg (i.e., 6-mm cannulae for 5-mm instruments). The plastic/graphite models are extremely light and ideally suited to most small reptiles (i.e., 2.5-mm and 3.5-mm cannulae for 2-mm and 3-mm instruments, respectively). Most cannulae are used in conjunction with trocars. A trocar is a solid, often sharp and pointed, metal rod that is inserted into the cannula to assist with placement. Most are sharp to facilitate perforation of the body wall when axial and penetrative force is applied.

The threaded cannula (e.g., EndoTip) is a recent improvement that has an external screw thread to enable gradual advancement by rotation (see Figure 13-2 *C, D*).[9] These threaded cannulae are available in 3-mm, 3.9-mm, and 5-mm sizes and do not require a trocar or much axial penetrative force for insertion. A telescope positioned inside the cannula provides a magnified view during entry into the coelom. As the cannula is advanced, the fascia and then the muscle fibers

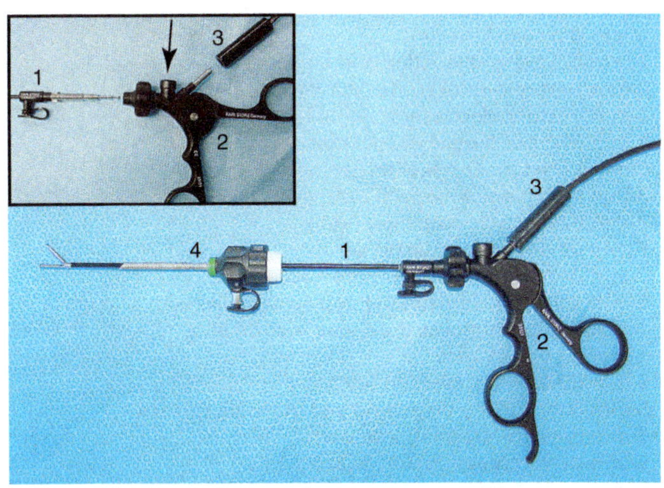

FIGURE 14-1 Human pediatric 3-mm laparoscopy equipment. A 3-mm instrument *(1)* attached to a standard ClickLine handle *(2)*. The instrument, attached to a radiosurgery unit via a connector on the handle (3), has been inserted through a 3.5-mm graphite/plastic cannula *(4)*. *Inset,* Instrument *(1)* and handle *(2)* can be quickly exchanged by pressing on the release button *(arrow)*. The radiosurgical connection is also shown *(3)*. *(Courtesy Dr. Stephen J. Divers, University of Georgia, Athens, Ga.)*

TABLE 14-1

Endoscopic Equipment and Instrumentation Required for Minimally Invasive Endosurgery

EQUIPMENT DESCRIPTION	PRIMARY INDICATIONS
TELESCOPES	
1.9-mm, 30-degree oblique telescope, working length 18.5 cm, with integrated 3.3-mm operating sheath	Endosurgery in reptiles 0.1 to 5 kg
2.7-mm, 30-degree oblique telescope, working length 18 cm, with 3.5-mm protection sheath	Endosurgery in reptiles 0.5 to 10 kg
5-mm, 0-degree telescope, working length 29 cm	Endosurgery in reptiles 10 to 100+ kg
5 mm, 30-degree oblique telescope, working length 29 cm	Endosurgery in reptiles 10 to 100+ kg
VISUALIZATION AND DOCUMENTATION	
Endovideo camera and monitor	Required for all endoscopy procedures
Xenon light source and light guide cable	
Digital capture device (e.g., AIDA-DVD)	
INSUFFLATION	
CO_2 compressed gas with regulator and high-pressure tubing to CO_2 insufflator, and silicone insufflation tubing from insufflator to patient	Essential for endosurgery in snakes and lizards, often useful for chelonians
HANDLES	
Two plastic handles without rackets	These ClickLine handles are interchangeable and can be used with most instruments from 2 mm to 5 mm
One plastic handle with Mahnes-style racket	
One plastic handle with hemostat-style racket	
CANNULAE, TROCARS, AND INSTRUMENTS	
3.9-mm graphite and plastic cannula and trocar, with silicone leaflet valve, and luer-lock insufflation port	Accommodates 2.7-mm telescope and 3.5-mm protection sheath
2.5-mm × 4-cm graphite and plastic threaded cannula and trocar, with silicone leaflet valve, and luer-lock insufflation port (for 2-mm instruments, typically two required)	For endosurgery in animals 0.1 to 5 kg Instruments are all 20 cm in length
2-mm Reddick-Olsen dissecting forceps	
2-mm Metzenbaum scissors	
2-mm Babcock forceps	
3.5-mm graphite and plastic threaded cannula and trocar, with silicone leaflet valve, and luer-lock insufflation port (for 3-mm instruments, typically two required)	For endosurgery in animals 0.5 to 10 kg Instruments are all 20 cm in length
3-mm fenestrated grasping forceps	
3-mm Reddick-Olsen dissecting and grasping forceps	
3-mm short curved Kelly dissecting and grasping forceps	
3-mm atraumatic dissecting and grasping forceps	
3-mm Babcock forceps	
3-mm Blakesley dissecting and biopsy forceps	
3-mm scissors with serrated curved double action jaws	
3-mm microhook scissors, single-action jaws	
3-mm Mahnes bipolar coagulation forceps	
3-mm irrigation and suction cannula	
3-mm palpation probe with centimeter markings	
3-mm distendable palpation probe	
3-mm ultramicro needle holder	
3-mm knot tier for extracorporeal suturing	
6-mm × 5.5-mm Ternamian EndoTip cannula, with silicone leaflet valve and insufflation stopcock (for 5-mm instruments, typically two required)	For endosurgery in animals 10 to 100 kg Instruments can be 36 cm or 43 cm in length
5-mm biopsy forceps	
5-mm Blakesley dissecting forceps	
5-mm curved Kelly dissecting and grasping forceps	
5-mm Babcock grasping forceps	
5-mm curved Metzenbaum scissors	
5-mm suction and irrigation cannula	
5-mm needle holders	
5-mm hook scissors	
5-mm bipolar forceps	

TABLE 14-1

Endoscopic Equipment and Instrumentation Required for Minimally Invasive Endosurgery—cont'd

EQUIPMENT DESCRIPTION	PRIMARY INDICATIONS
HEMOSTASIS EQUIPMENT	
Ellman 3.8 or 4.0 MHz dual radiofrequency unit with foot pedal Karl Storz Autocon 80 unit with foot pedal Monopolar lead to connect to plastic instrument handles Bipolar lead to connect to 3-mm Mahnes bipolar coagulation forceps	Enables many endoscopic instruments to be used as monopolar devices and facilitates bipolar coagulation using bipolar forceps. A wide variety of 2-mm, 3-mm, and 5-mm instruments available
LigaSure ForceTriad energy platform with foot pedal 5-mm x 37-cm LigaSure laparoscopic instrument	Only available in 5-mm or 10-mm instrument sizes but is a useful instrument that combines sealing and cutting. The instruments are disposable human items, but most veterinarians clean and re-use

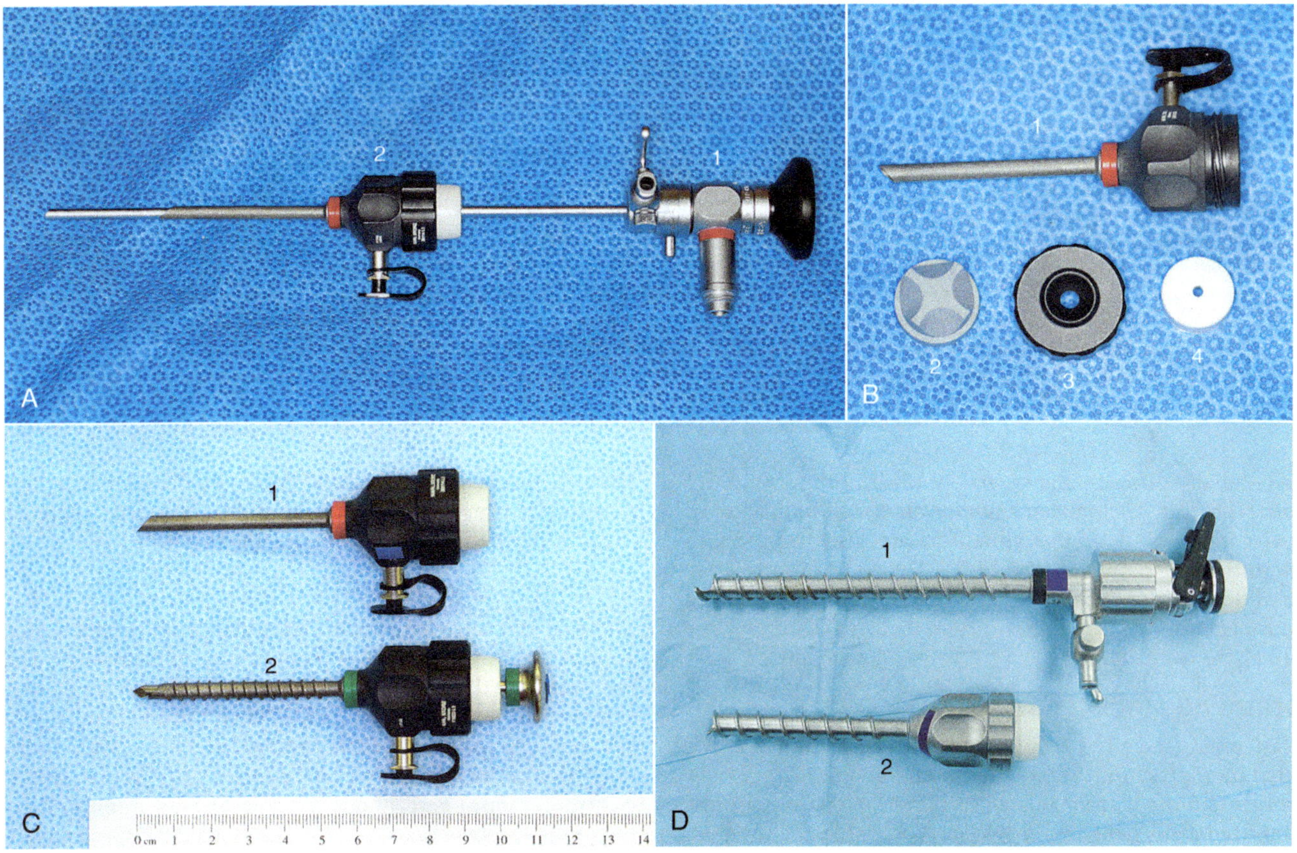

FIGURE 14-2 Cannulae and trocars. **A,** A 2.7-mm telescope within a 3.5-mm protection sheath *(1)* inserted through a 3.9-mm × 10-cm graphite/plastic cannula with insufflation side port *(2)*. **B,** A 3.9-mm × 10-cm graphite/plastic cannula disassembled to illustrate the graphite cannula *(1)*, leaflet valve *(2)*, screw cap *(3)*, and instrument seal *(4)*. **C,** A 3.9-mm × 10-cm graphite/plastic cannula with insufflation side port *(1)* and 3.5-mm × 10-cm threaded cannula with insufflation side port and trocar inserted *(2)*. The 3.9-mm cannula can accommodate the 2.7-mm telescope housed in a 3.5-mm protection sheath, whereas the 3.5-mm cannula can accommodate 3-mm instruments. The threaded design resists dislodgement in small exotic species. **D,** Ternamian EndoTip cannulae; 6-mm × 15-cm with insufflation side port and multifunctional valve *(1)* and 6-mm × 10.5-cm cannula with silicone leaflet valve. These metal cannulae are far heavier and best restricted to animals weighing more than 10 kg. *(Courtesy Dr. Stephen J. Divers, University of Georgia, Athens, Ga.)*

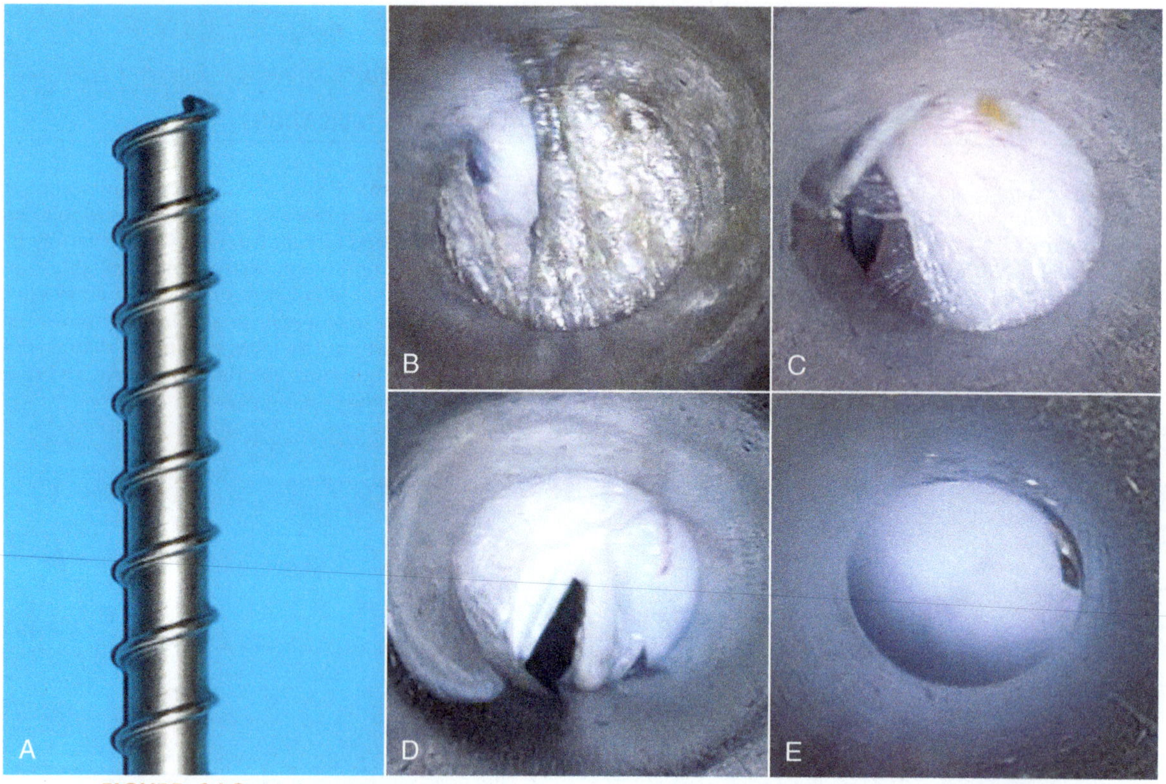

FIGURE 14-3 **A,** A terminal end of a 6-mm threaded cannula. Screwed entry of the threaded cannula through an initial skin incision **(B)**, subcutaneous tissue **(C)**, and finally the coelomic membrane **(D)** before entering the coelomic cavity **(E)**. *(Courtesy Dr. Stephen J. Divers, University of Georgia, Athens, Ga.)*

spread radially and are transposed onto the cannula's outer thread. The thin coelomic membrane is transilluminated so that viscera, vessels, and/or adhesions are visualized before entry into the coelom (Figure 14-3). The risks of iatrogenic visceral damage are therefore greatly reduced. In addition, the threads also provide greater security in that such cannulae are less likely to be dislodged.

Instruments and Handles

At least one, generally two, and rarely three instruments are inserted through cannulae and into the endoscopic field of view. Instruments must be triangulated to bring the instrument tips together (convergence) and enable surgery within the reptilian coelom. A large assortment of 5-mm instruments are available; they were initially developed for humans but are equally applicable for animals more than 10 kg. However, it was not until the development of human pediatric laparoscopy that smaller 2-mm and 3-mm instruments became available and multiple-entry endosurgery became feasible in smaller animals.[10]

Currently, 2-mm instruments are limited to Babcock forceps, dissecting forceps, and scissors. A greater selection of 3-mm instruments are available, including a variety of dissecting forceps, grasping forceps, scissors, biopsy forceps, and palpation and irrigation probes (Figure 14-4). All these instruments have a standard attachment that enables them to be used interchangeably with a selection of ClickLine handles (Figure 14-5). Handles are of plastic or metal construction and may have a radiosurgical connection that enables scissors or forceps to be used as monopolar devices. An optional hemostat, Mahnes, or disengageable-style racket mechanism is available to maintain firm hold of tissue, even if the endoscopist releases the grip on the handle (see Figure 14-5, *B, C, E*).

Surgical Devices and Hemostasis

Effective and safe performance of endoscopic surgery requires accurate hemostasis because the mere act of clamping a bleeding vessel or dabbing with gauze may be impossible. Radiosurgery and laser surgical devices have become available and can facilitate internal incision and debridément while hemorrhaging is controlled. Diode lasers (e.g., AccuVet Lumenis Inc., Norwood, Mass) are, by design, able to pass through flexible fiberoptic probes that can be inserted through instrument channels or cannulae (Figure 14-6).[11,12] A variety of diode laser probes are available; however, 400 to 600 μm conical or flat tips at 2 to 10 watts are generally most useful (SurgiMedics Inc., The Woodlands, Tex). Until recently, CO_2 lasers (AccuVet Lumenis Inc.) could not be used via endoscopic instrument channels because of the inflexible nature of the ceramic delivery probes. The development of a long semirigid probe (AccuVet Lumenis Inc.), however, has enabled the use of the CO_2 laser via the 1.7-mm instrument channel of the 4.8-mm operating sheath. Nonetheless, although it is functional, it is rather cumbersome (Figure 14-7). Probably the most versatile device, especially when using 3-mm or smaller instrumentation systems, is a radiosurgery unit because a wide variety of tools are available for use with foot-pedal activated radiosurgery 3.8 and 4.0 MHz Surgitron, (Ellman International Inc., Oceanside, NY) (Figure 14-8) and electrocautery (Autocon 80, Karl Storz Veterinary

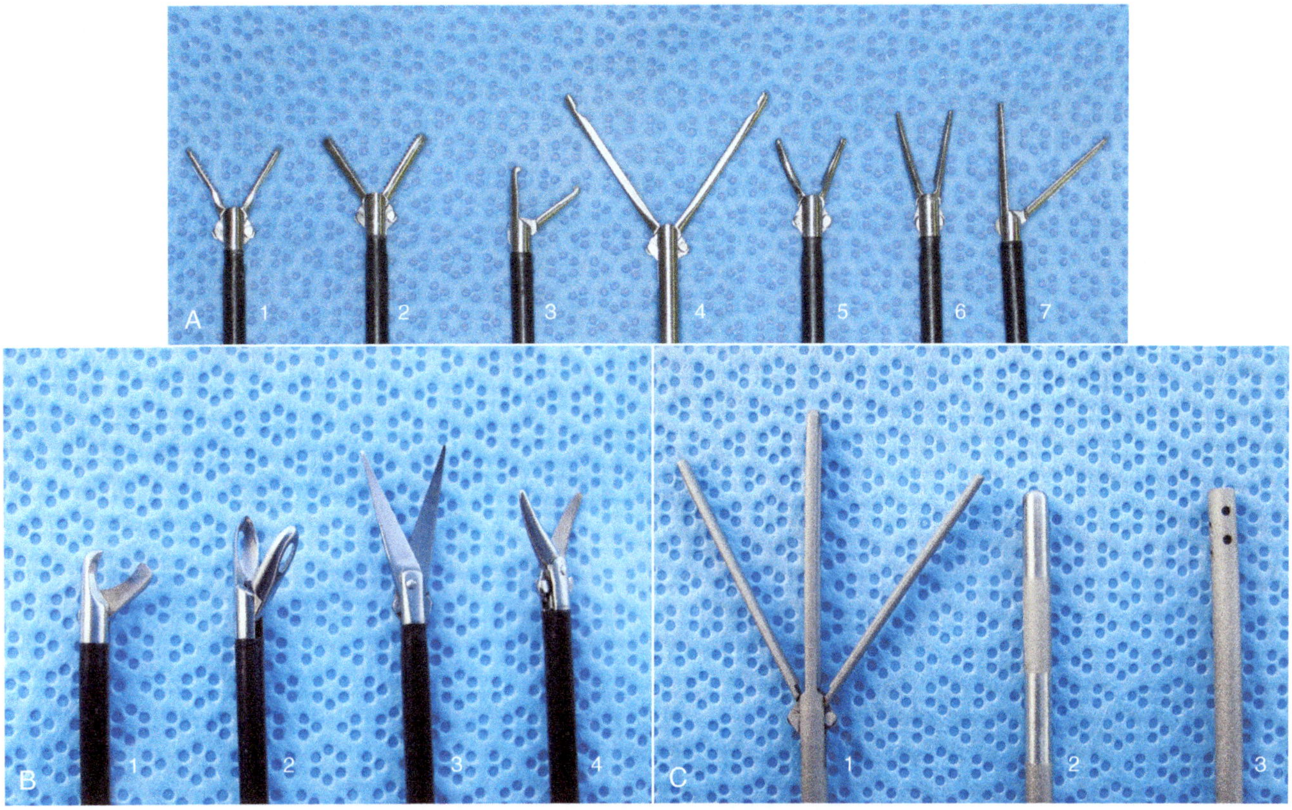

FIGURE 14-4 A selection of 3-mm instruments. **A,** Forceps: fenestrated atraumatic grasping forceps *(1),* Reddick-Olsen dissecting forceps *(2),* small Babcock forceps *(3),* large Babcock forceps *(4),* short curved Kelly dissecting and grasping forceps *(5),* long curved Kelly dissecting and grasping forceps *(6),* and atraumatic dissecting and grasping forceps with single-action jaws *(7).* **B,** Scissors and biopsy instruments: microhook scissors with single action jaws *(1),* Blakesley dissecting and biopsy forceps *(2),* scissors with long sharp curved double action jaws *(3),* and scissors with serrated curved double action jaws *(4).* **C,** Probes: distendable palpation probe *(1),* palpation probe with centimeter markings *(2),* and irrigation and suction cannula *(3). (Courtesy Dr. Stephen J. Divers, University of Georgia, Athens, Ga.)*

Endoscopy, Goleta, Calif) units.[13] The most useful includes various needle electrodes (Ellman International Inc), bipolar forceps, and a retractable polypectomy snare (Karl Storz Veterinary Endoscopy America Inc., Goleta, Calif). The degree of radiosurgical power required during endosurgery varies with operating conditions and the instrument being used, but because of the microsurgical nature of most endosurgical procedures, lower settings are generally required compared with open surgery. Considerable growth in endoscopic radiosurgery has led to the availability of a large number of monopolar and bipolar devices. One particularly favored device among human and veterinary endosurgeons is the LigaSure ForceTriad (Covidien, Boulder, Colo) (Figure 14-9). This system detects the thickness (by measuring the electrical impedance) of tissue to be coagulated and automatically defines the amount of energy required and the delivering time. An acoustic signal informs the surgeon when the vessel obliteration is complete and its division is possible. Unfortunately, endoscopic handpieces smaller than 5 mm are not yet available, limiting its usefulness to 5-mm systems and the largest of reptiles (Figure 14-10).

Another useful item from human and domestic animal laparoscopy is the endoscopic vascular clip applicator (Figure 14-11). These devices contain a cartridge of clips that can be rapidly employed without having to remove the instrument from the patient and reload. Again, the smallest available size is 5 mm, which restricts their use to the largest reptiles.

Endoscopy Tables

In human and domestic animal endosurgery, tilting tables are used to modify patient positioning and create advantageous organ displacement during surgery. Most of the table-mounted configurations used in veterinary medicine are designed for mammals and are incompatible with most reptiles. In addition, joystick-controlled tilting surgery tables (Figure 14-12) are helpful but expensive and likely to be limited to teaching hospitals and other major referral institutions. Most practitioners can probably achieve similar positioning, albeit with less intraoperative versatility, by using towels, sandbags, vacuum pads, tape, and various other positioning aids (Figure 14-13).

Endosurgical Principles and Techniques

As already indicated, endosurgery requires placement of the telescope and triangulation of additional instruments. Advanced endosurgical skills can only be built on a firm foundation in single-entry diagnostic endoscopy. Minor errors or inadequacies that can be tolerated in single-entry procedures

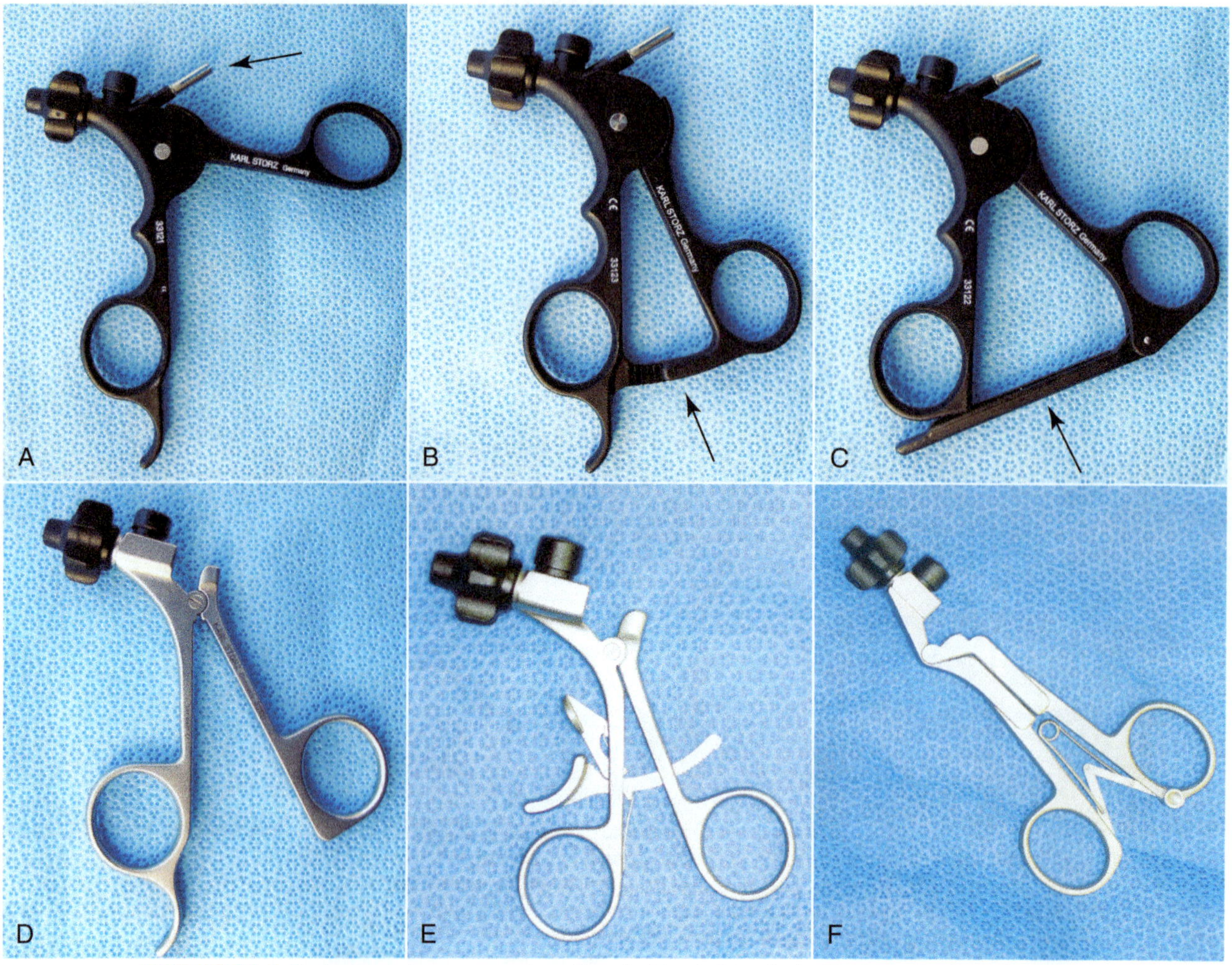

FIGURE 14-5 Endoscopy instrument handles. **A,** Plastic handle (without racket) with radiosurgery connector *(arrow).* **B,** Plastic handle with hemostat-style racket *(arrow).* **C,** Plastic handle with Mahnes-style racket *(arrow).* **D,** Metal handle without racket or radiosurgery connection. **E,** Metal handle with disengageable racket but no radiosurgical connection. **F,** Metal *Y*-handle with spring action. *(Courtesy Dr. Stephen J. Divers, University of Georgia, Athens, Ga.)*

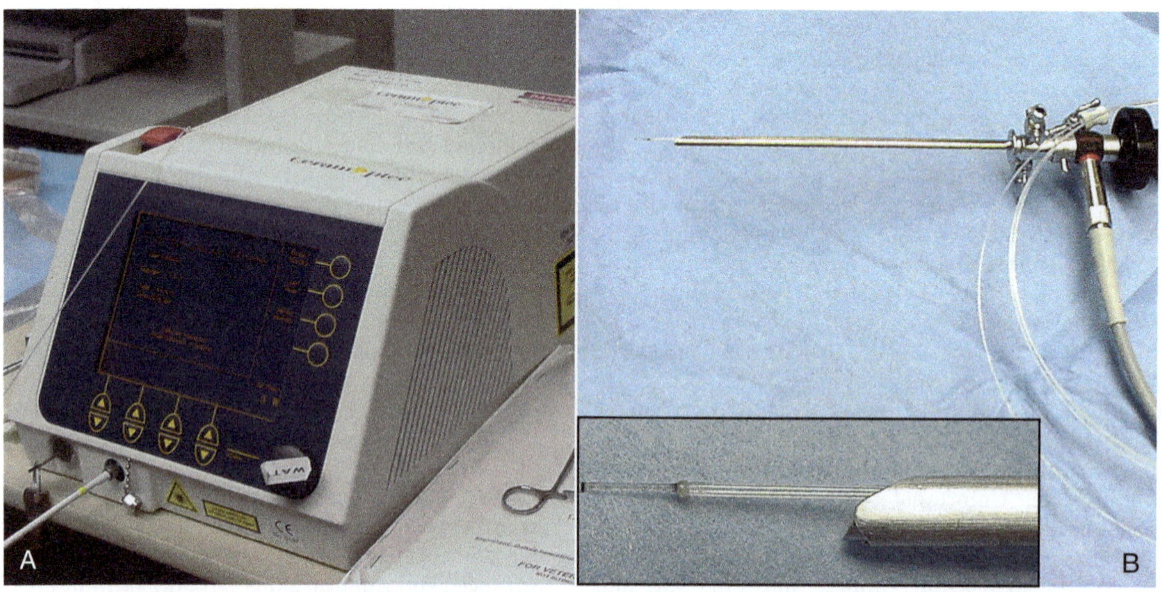

FIGURE 14-6 **A,** A 980-μm diode laser unit. **B,** A 600-μm diode laser fiber inserted down the instrument channel of the 4.8-mm operating sheath and emanating from the terminal end of the sheath in front of the terminal telescope lens *(inset).* *(Courtesy Dr. Stephen J. Divers, University of Georgia, Athens, Ga.)*

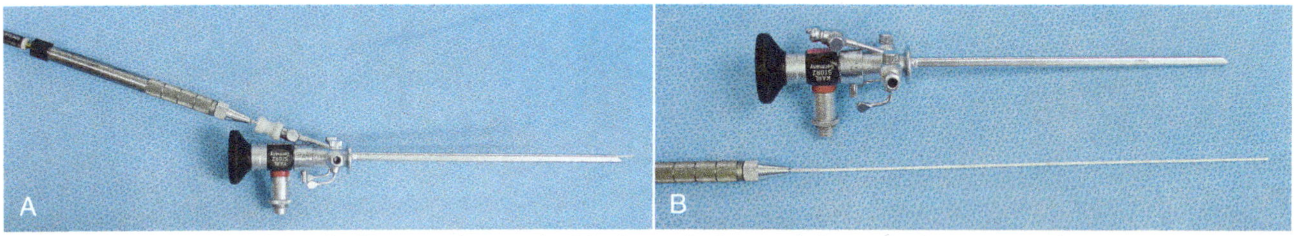

FIGURE 14-7 **A,** Elongated ceramic CO_2 laser tip inserted down the instrument channel of the 4.8-mm operating sheath. **B,** The same ceramic tip alongside the sheath. *(Courtesy Dr. Stephen J. Divers, University of Georgia, Athens, Ga.)*

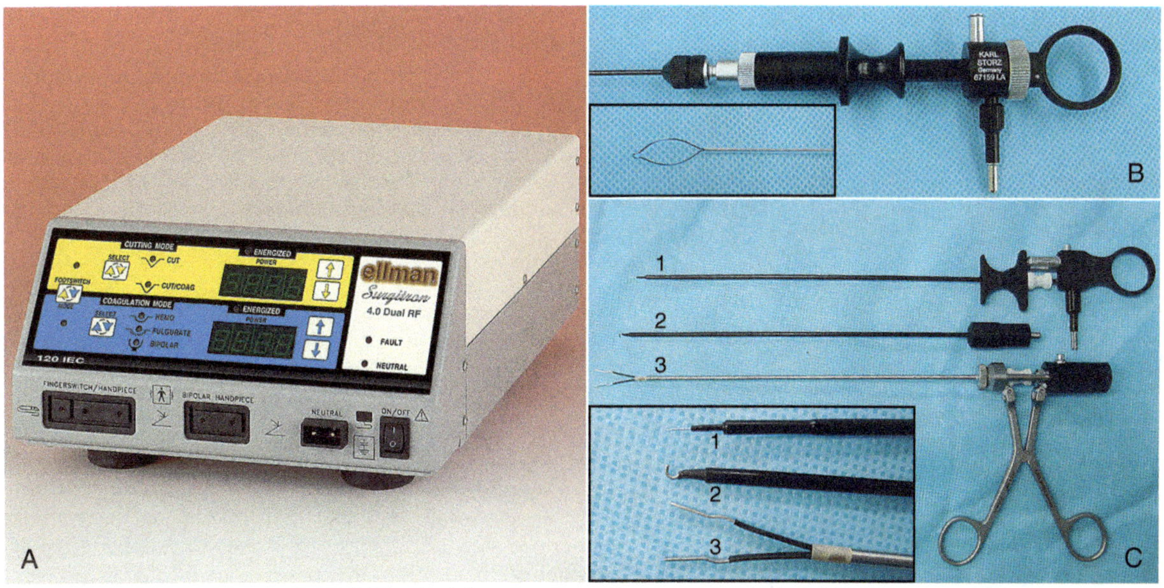

FIGURE 14-8 **A,** A 4.0 MHz dual frequency radiosurgery unit (4.0 MHz Surgitron, Ellman International, Inc.). **B,** Polypectomy snare handpiece with extended end shown *(inset).* **C,** Various radiosurgical endoscopic devices; retractable needle *(1),* dissecting hook *(2),* and bipolar forceps *(3).* Close-up of instrument ends also shown *(inset)* (Karl Storz Veterinary Endoscopy, Goleta, Calif). *(Courtesy Dr. Stephen J. Divers, University of Georgia, Athens, Ga.)*

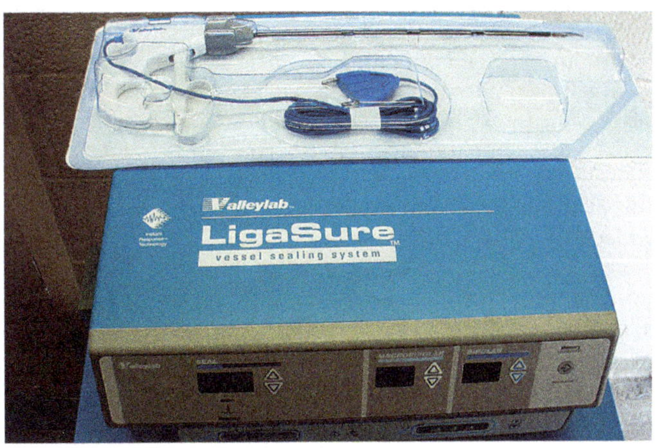

FIGURE 14-9 The LigaSure vessel sealing system and a disposable 5-mm endoscopic sealing and cutting instrument. *(Courtesy Dr. Stephen J. Divers, University of Georgia, Athens, Ga.)*

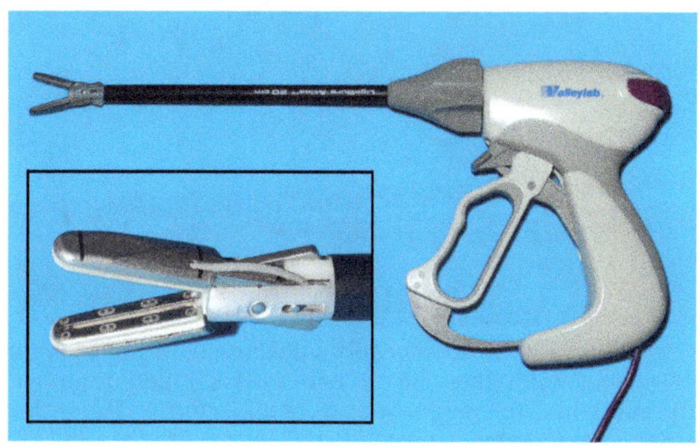

FIGURE 14-10 A LigaSure Atlas handpiece (Covidien, Mansfield, Mass). This 10-mm instrument has a working length of 20 cm and is capable of sealing and transecting vessels up to 7 mm in size. The smallest diameter endoscopic instrument currently available is 5 mm, restricting this device to the largest of reptiles. *(© University of Georgia Research Foundation, Inc.)*

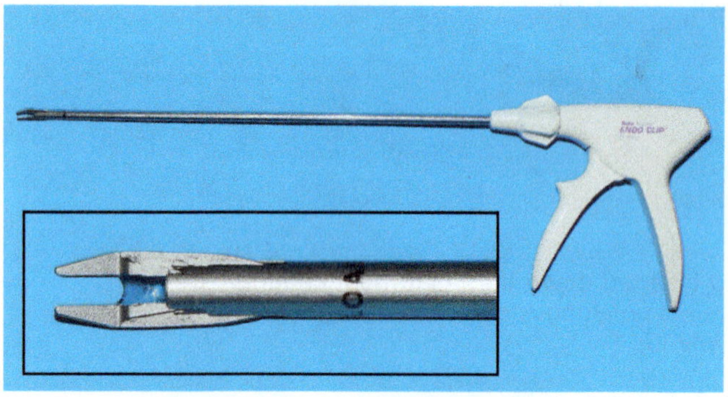

FIGURE 14-11 This 5-mm endoscopic vascular clip has a working length of 28 cm and contains 12 titanium clips. *(© University of Georgia Research Foundation, Inc.)*

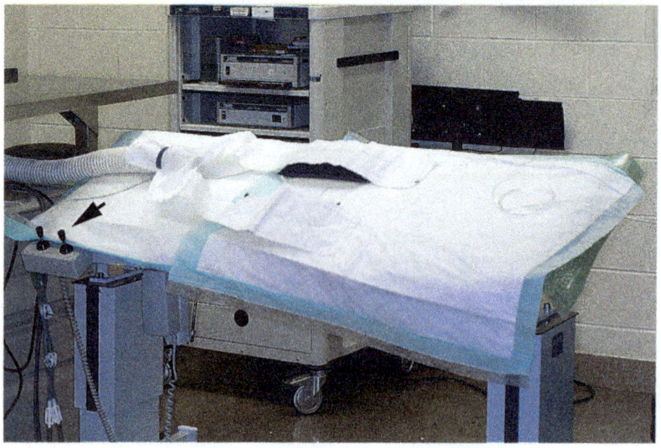

FIGURE 14-12 Electronic tilting table with joy-stick control *(arrow)*. *(Courtesy Dr. Stephen J. Divers, University of Georgia, Athens, Ga.)*

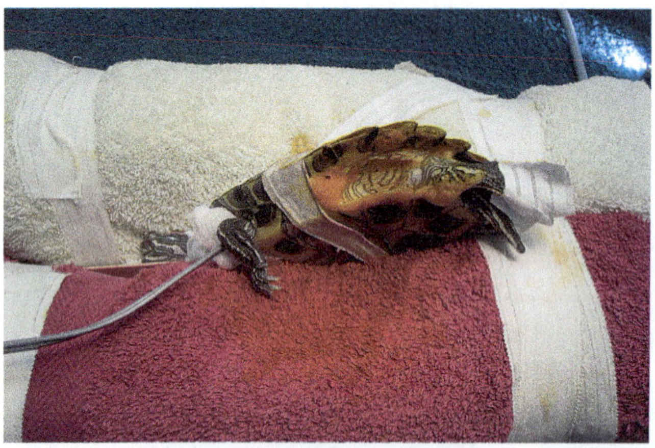

FIGURE 14-13 A freshwater turtle positioned in right lateral recumbency with the use of two towels taped together, in preparation for endosurgical orchidectomy. *(Courtesy Dr. Stephen J. Divers, University of Georgia, Athens, Ga.)*

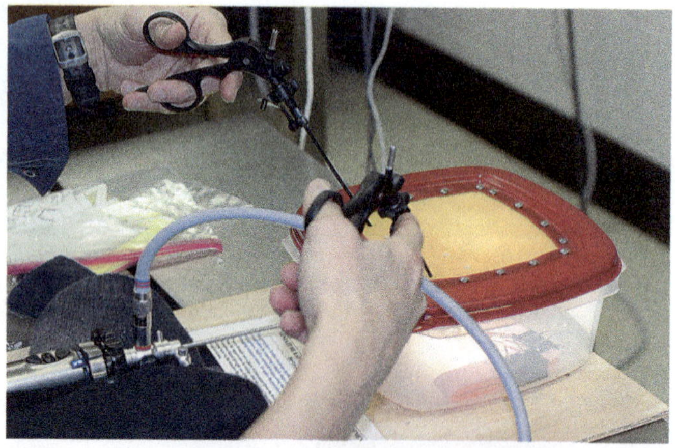

FIGURE 14-14 An endoscopy trainer fashioned from a modified plastic container. Holes at the front permit the introduction of the telescope, which is supported with sandbags. The top has been largely replaced by a sheet of rubber containing several holes for the introduction of instruments. *(Courtesy Dr. Stephen J. Divers, University of Georgia, Athens, Ga.)*

are likely to become magnified and cause serious problems during endosurgery. Well-executed and atraumatic placement of the telescope is essential and can only come from practice. Poor technique will result in tissue damage, increased tissue fluid including blood on the terminal lens, and decreased visibility. The need to practice instrument triangulation and develop fine motor skills with limited tactile feedback in a three-dimensional environment exceeds the endoscopy caseload, at least initially. Therefore the reptile endoscopic surgeon must find additional means to practice and maintain skills. One method is to maintain equipment in a clean yet nonsterile state. This allows and encourages the veterinarian to practice on a cadaver, whereas using instruments that have undergone the entire sterilization process seems to present a barrier to practicing. In addition, inexpensive artificial trainers can be readily made from supplies found at local hobby and home improvement stores. A clear plastic container can serve as the basis for such a trainer. First, a large square hole is cut from the lid and replaced with rubber matting. Several 4-mm holes can be made in the rubber top and in the front of the container to provide a selection of instrument access ports (Figure 14-14). A variety of "endoscopy games" can be devised to be completed inside the box. These can include dissecting a drawn shape on tissue paper, picking up felt disks from one pin and transferring to a second pin, or even endoscopic suturing (Figure 14-15).

Surgeon ergonomics also become increasingly important because fine motor control now becomes more complicated by the need to triangulate and establish a perception of depth with a two-dimensional monitor. The monitor should be directly in front of the surgeon who should be comfortably standing on a padded mat or sitting (Figure 14-16). Finally, the usual degree of tactile feedback experienced when handling tissues with standard instruments is greatly reduced when working with endoscopic instruments at distances of 20 cm or more from the tissues (Figure 14-17).

ENDOSCOPE-ASSISTED PROCEDURES

An endoscope-assisted procedure is a hybrid that combines elements of endoscopy with traditional surgery. In its simplest form, an endoscope-assisted procedure uses endoscopy to identify and grasp an internal structure that is then exteriorized through a miniature coeliotomy incision for completion

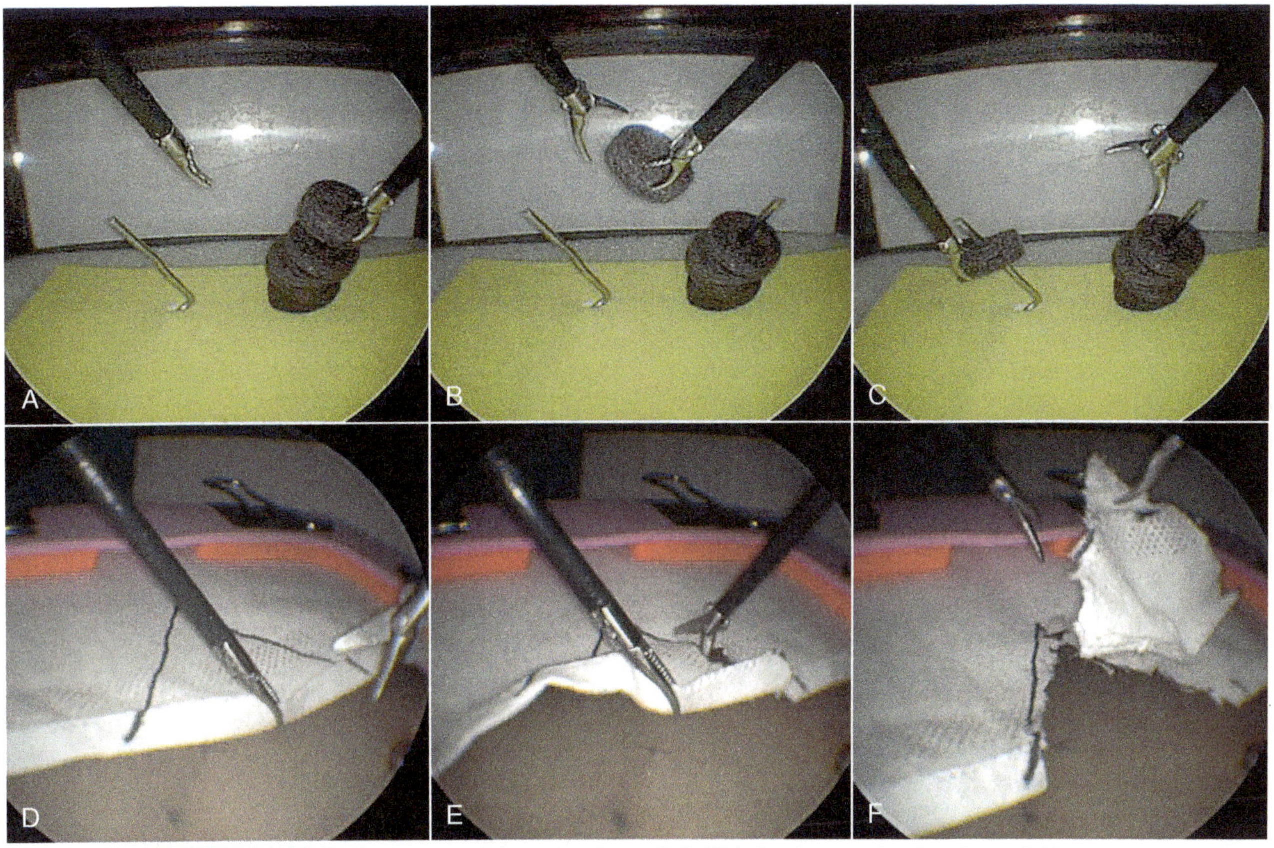

FIGURE 14-15 Endoscopy training exercises. **A-C,** This basic exercise involves picking up a felt ring from one pin with the use of forceps, transferring the ring to a second pair of forceps, and then placing the ring on a second pin. This exercise helps with depth perception, instrument triangulation, and instrument-to-instrument transfer. It can be made more difficult by changing the orientation and direction of the pins. **D-F,** This more difficult exercise involves using forceps and scissors to dissect a shape from a piece of tissue paper. This game helps with depth perception, instrument triangulation, and instrument dexterity. It can be made more difficult by increasing the complexity of the shape and by swapping the scissors and forceps. *(Courtesy Dr. Stephen J. Divers, University of Georgia, Athens, Ga.)*

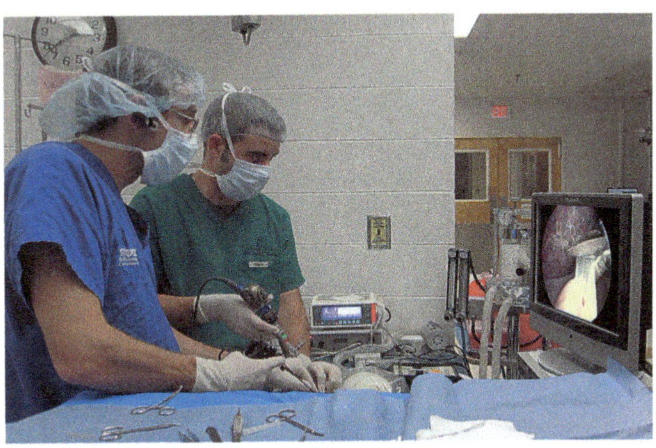

FIGURE 14-16 Proper positioning and orientation of the surgeon(s) to the patient and monitor becomes increasingly critical with endosurgery. In this example, the two surgeons are perpendicular to the monitor while they perform endosurgery in a small chelonian. *(Courtesy Dr. Stephen J. Divers, University of Georgia, Athens, Ga.)*

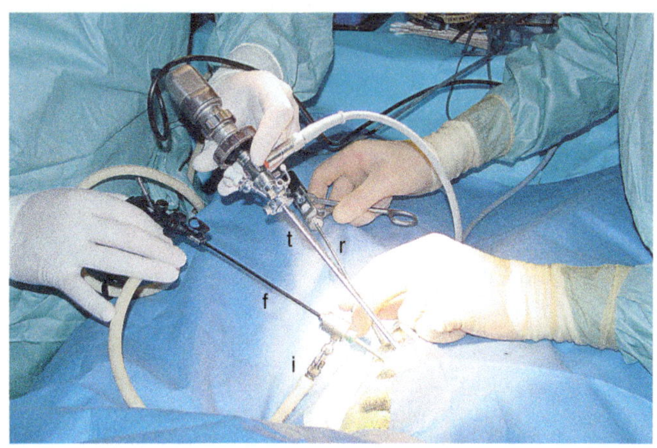

FIGURE 14-17 Tactile feedback and sensation is reduced during endosurgery because tissues are manipulated at a greater distance than with traditional surgery. This photograph also shows the concept of triangulation with the two instruments (bipolar radiosurgery forceps *[r]* and grasping forceps *[f]*) on either side of the camera and telescope *(t)* but converging toward the common endoscopic field of view. The insufflation line *(i)* is also shown connected to a cannula. *(Courtesy Dr. Stephen J. Divers, University of Georgia, Athens, Ga.)*

of the procedure outside the body cavity. The advantages of endoscope-assisted procedures are that they decrease the size of the coeliotomy incision and exposure of internal viscera to the environment. An assortment of endoscope-assisted coelomic procedures including enterotomy, enterectomy, cystotomy, salpingotomy, and salpingohysterectomy are now possible. These techniques rely on the ability to exteriorize the tissue of interest out through a small, targeted coeliotomy incision. If the tissue cannot be exteriorized, then the procedure cannot be completed externally, and a true endosurgical technique is required.

Of particular practical relevance is endoscope-assisted, prefemoral oophorectomy (or ovariectomy) of mature female chelonians that negates the need for a transplastron coeliotomy.[14] With the chelonian in dorsal recumbency, a unilateral, prefemoral coeliotomy is performed, typically 2 to 3 cm in size (large enough to exteriorize the largest follicle). The telescope is inserted through the coeliotomy site and used to identify the ovaries. The telescope guides a pair of atraumatic forceps, the interfollicular tissue is grasped, and the ovary is gently lifted out of the prefemoral incision. Once exteriorized, the ovarian vessels and mesovarian ligament is ligated and the ovary is dissected free. For those species with large prefemoral fossae, it is generally possible to remove the contralateral ovary through the same prefemoral incision. Those species with very small fossae may require a bilateral prefemoral approach.

Similar endoscope-assisted procedures have also been accomplished for the removal of retained eggs, bladder calculi, and gastrointestinal foreign bodies and seem especially beneficial in chelonians. The general technique is similar, and endoscopy skills required are also very similar. First, diagnostic imaging is used to determine which side is favored for the approach. Then after a prefemoral coeliotomy, the telescope is used to identify the structure of interest and guide atraumatic tissue forceps. Any tissue that is due to be resected and removed can be grasped using Kelly or Babcock forceps (or a similar type), but any tissue that is ultimately to be replaced should ideally be handled with atraumatic or fenestrated forceps. This is especially important when the bladder, gastrointestinal or reproductive tracts are handled.

ENDOSURGERY

To date, endosurgery has been more commonly undertaken in chelonians, although endosurgical orchidectomy of iguanids has also been performed. Although established endosurgical dogma dictates that telescopes are often placed through the umbilicus or linea alba and instrument ports are placed far enough apart to facilitate triangulation, reptile anatomy often necessitates a modified approach.

Endosurgical procedures usually commence with the placement of the telescope cannula, and there are two main techniques commonly used. Either the telescope cannula is surgically placed via a minicoeliotomy incision, after which the CO_2 line is attached and the coelom insufflated, or a Veress needle (Figure 14-18), with CO_2 line attached, is blindly inserted into the coelom to facilitate insufflation, after which the telescope cannula can be placed blindly with the use of a trocar to perforate the coelomic wall. Placing the telescope cannula surgically ensures intracoelomic placement and reduces the risk of iatrogenic trauma but requires a mattress suture around the cannula to close the incision to reduce gas leakage. Conversely, using a Veress needle to preinflate allows the telescope cannula to be placed through a smaller, trocar-induced hole without the need for suture but carries increased risks of iatrogenic trauma.

Chelonians

Because of the constraints of the chelonian shell, it is seldom possible to place the telescope and ports where established protocols would suggest. There are two major approaches, depending on the size of the animal. For larger chelonians,

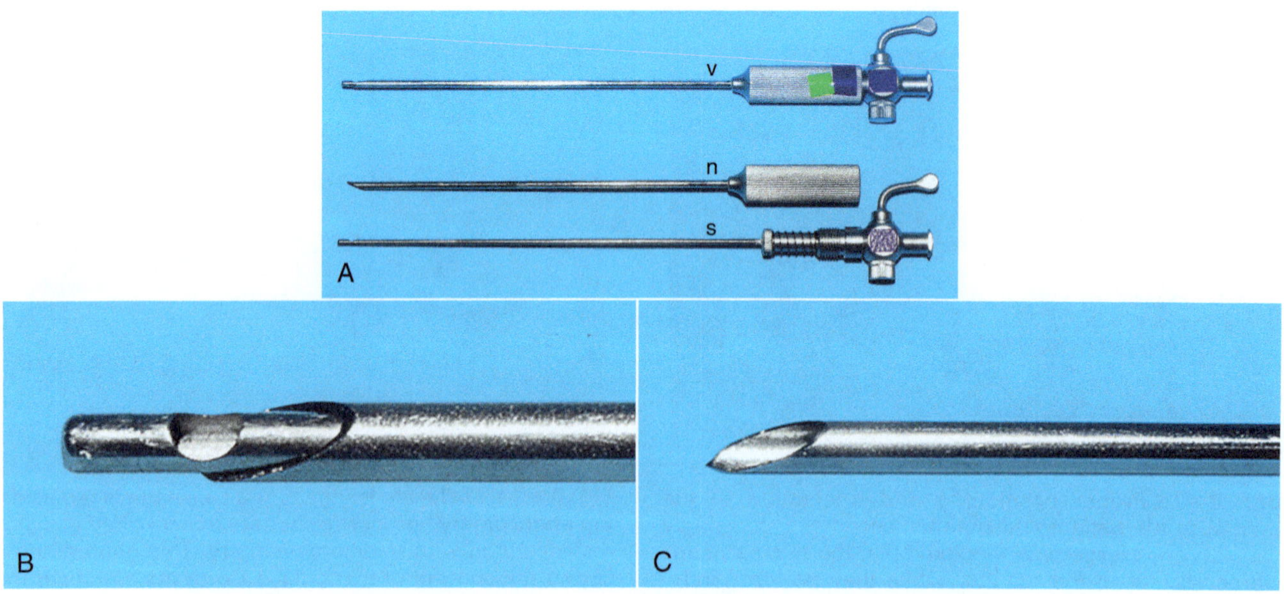

FIGURE 14-18 **A**, A Veress needle *(v)* is composed of an outer sharp needle *(n)* and an inner, spring-action stylet *(s)*. When pressed against a compliant tissue, the stylet is exposed and prevents damage from the needle **(B)**; however, when pressed against a noncompliant linea alba, the stylet is forced into the Veress needle, which exposes the sharp tip that perforates the linea **(C)**. *(© University of Georgia Research Foundation, Inc.)*

the telescope and instruments may all be inserted through one prefemoral fossa (Figure 14-19), whereas in smaller animals, the telescope and instruments may be placed through one or both fossae (Figure 14-20). There are advantages and disadvantages to both approaches. Placing all instrumentation through a single fossa enables the surgeon to control both instruments, even in large animals, but convergence is reduced because of the acute angles involved (often 30 degrees or less): instruments run more parallel, which makes their coordinated use more difficult. Nevertheless, compared with a bilateral fossa technique, a unilateral approach is less invasive in that only a unilateral surgical approach is required; in addition, it enables the animal to be positioned in lateral recumbency, which may aid organ visualization. A single surgeon can use both prefemoral fossae in smaller animals, but here the angle of triangulation is often obtuse (90 degrees to 180 degrees), again making coordinated instrument manipulation more challenging. If the target structure is cranial to the bladder and the chelonian is less than 20 kg, it is often preferable for one instrument and telescope to be inserted through one prefemoral fossa while the second instrument is inserted through the contralateral fossa (see Figure 14-20). For such procedures, the animal is in dorsal recumbency and the advantage is that instruments can be more easily triangulated within the cranial to midcoelom. However, in larger chelonians, it can be difficult to impossible for a single surgeon to operate through both prefemoral fossae simultaneously, and in such cases, a second surgeon is required to operate through one fossa. The endosurgical approach to caudal structures (e.g., bladder, kidney, adrenal, or gonad) is more problematic because it is often difficult to access the same structure simultaneously from both fossae unless a significant angle-deflected endoscope is used (e.g., 90-degree). Therefore where a caudal structure is the focus of the procedure, insertion of telescope and instruments through a single prefemoral fossa may be preferable. In such cases, the chelonian is generally positioned in dorsal or lateral recumbency, which often provides greater accessibility because the intestines and bladder fall to the more dependent areas of the coelom. This approach is easier in those animals with a large prefemoral fossa; nevertheless, the close placement and parallel nature of instrumentation can make triangulation more difficult. In addition, it is often easier (especially in smaller animals) to make a single large prefemoral incision for the insertion of all instruments rather than place three cannulae adjacent to one another (Figure 14-21). Insufflation is seldom essential because of the noncollapsible nature of the chelonian shell; therefore endoscopic devices can still be used through an incision without the need for cannulae.

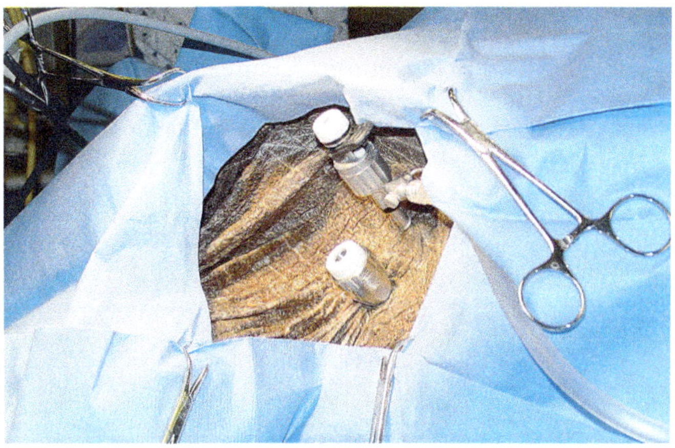

FIGURE 14-19 Two 6-mm threaded cannulae placed through the same prefemoral fossa in an adult Aldabra Tortoise (*Aldabrachelys [Geochelone] gigantea*). The close placement of separate instruments makes triangulation more difficult because of their parallel orientation. *(Courtesy Dr. Stephen J. Divers, University of Georgia, Athens, Ga.)*

Oophorectomy of Immature Females. The only publication to date that describes a truly endosurgical coelioscopic procedure in a reptile involves oophorectomy in immature, hybrid

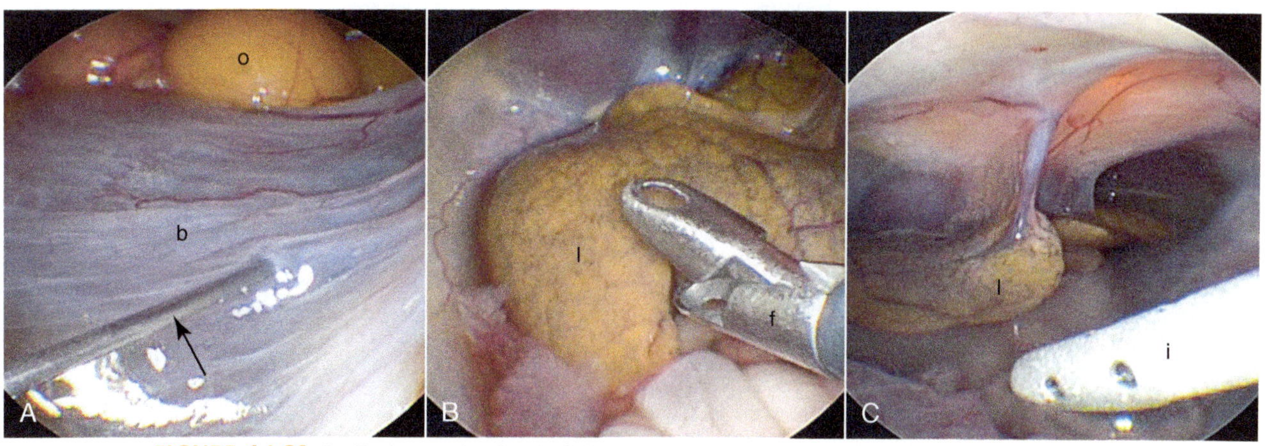

FIGURE 14-20 **A**, Endoscopic view of the caudal coelom demonstrating the bladder *(b)* and right ovary *(o)* as seen through a left prefemoral approach in a Box Turtle *(Terrapene carolina)*. In this example, an aspiration needle *(arrow)* has been placed through the same left fossa and is being used to perform cystocentesis. **B** and **C**, Endoscopic views of the cranial coelom and liver *(l)* of another Box Turtle with ascites, as seen through the left prefemoral fossa. Biopsy forceps *(f)* and irrigation/suction cannula *(i)* have been introduced through the right fossa, which provides greater instrument triangulation. *(Courtesy Dr. Stephen J. Divers, University of Georgia, Athens, Ga.)*

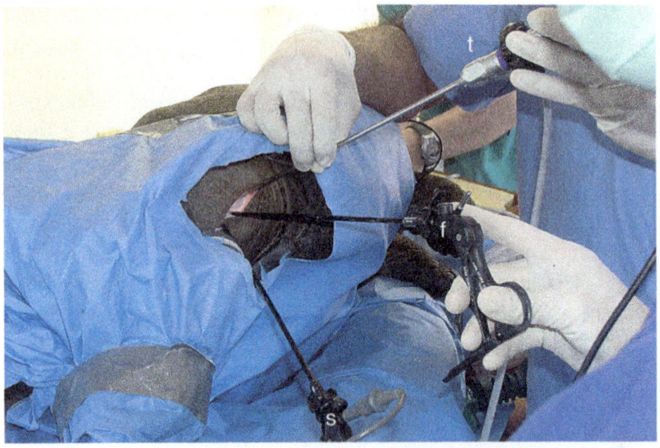

FIGURE 14-21 Surgical view of a juvenile Galapagos Tortoise *(Geochelone [Geochelone] nigra)* undergoing endoscopic oophorectomy. Note that the telescope *(t)*, handled by an assistant, as well as the grasping forceps *(f)* and radiosurgical scissors *(s)*, operated by the primary surgeon, have all been introduced via a single prefemoral incision rather than through separate cannulae. *(Courtesy Dr. Stephen J. Divers, University of Georgia, Athens, Ga.)*

Galapagos Tortoises *(Geochelone [Geochelone] nigra)* with the use of 5-mm instrumentation.[13] However, there is no reason why this same technique could not be applied to smaller chelonians with suitably sized instrumentation. In addition, this technique provides a model for other possible endosurgical procedures. The paired, immature ovaries reside in the caudodorsal coelom, in close association with the retrocoelomic kidney. The bladder obscures the contralateral ovary; thus an endosurgical approach must be repeated on each side, at least in the Galapagos tortoise. With the animal in lateral recumbency, a prefemoral approach to the coelom is made to accommodate the telescope and two instruments via a single incision (see Figure 14-21). Cannulae are generally not helpful because the instruments are so closely aligned and insufflation is not required. The telescope is positioned and held by a surgical assistant so that the view of the ovary is maintained. The immature ovary is lifted away from the serosal surface of the caudodorsal shell and kidney with Babcock or Kelly forceps, and monopolar scissors are used to dissect the ovary free from its mesovarian attachments (Figure 14-22). The prefemoral incision is closed routinely, and the procedure is repeated on the opposite side.

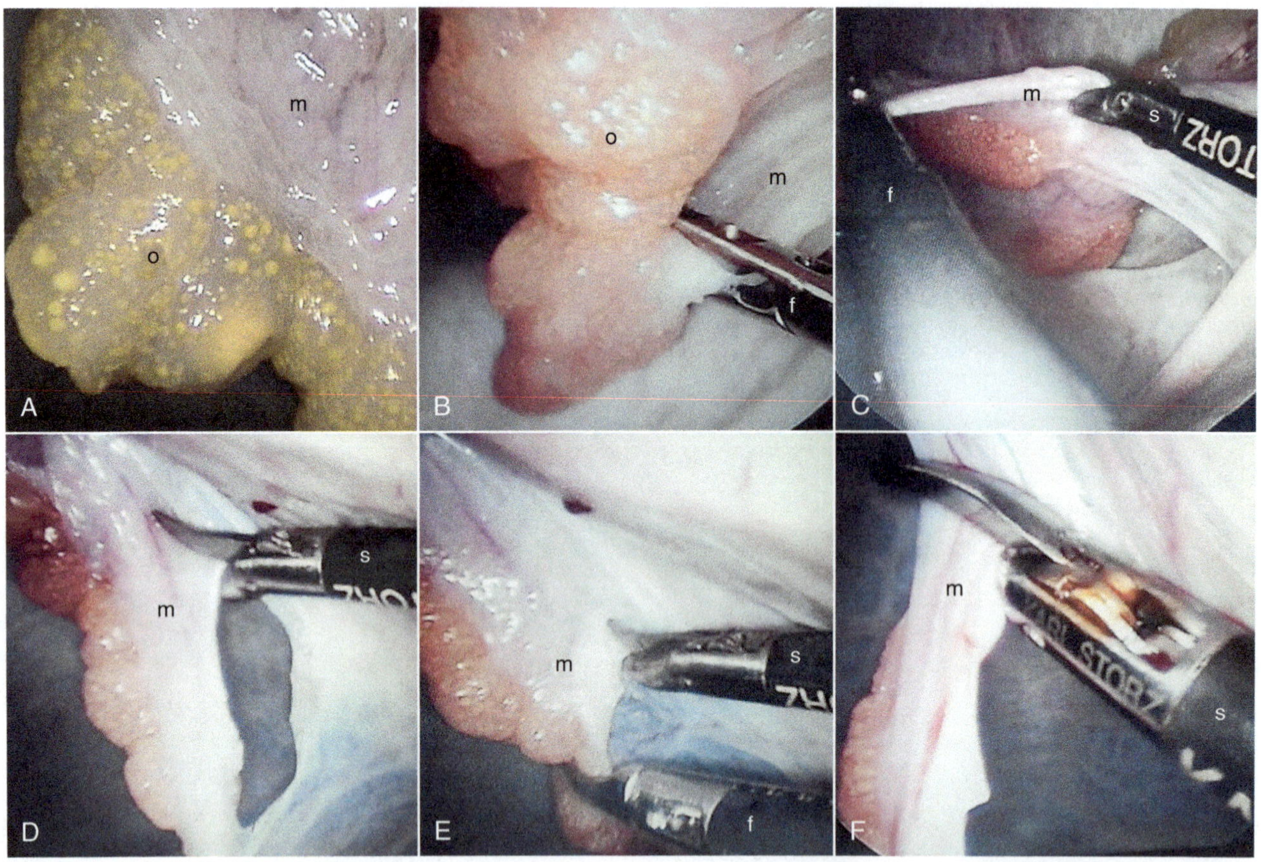

FIGURE 14-22 Endoscopic left oophorectomy in a juvenile Galapagos Tortoise *(Geochelone [Geochelone] nigra)* with all instrumentation inserted through the left prefemoral fossa. **A,** Normal, immature left ovary *(o)* suspended from the caudodorsal body wall by a short mesovarium ligament *(m)*. **B,** Grasping forceps *(f)* are introduced and used to grasp the mesovarium *(m)* but not the friable ovary *(o)*. **C,** The mesovarium *(m)* is stretched by moving the forceps *(f)* cranially, while radiosurgical scissors *(s)* are used to incise through the suspensory ligament. **D-F,** Dissection through the mesovarium *(m)* continues using forceps *(f)* and scissors *(s)* until the ovary is dissected free and can be removed through the prefemoral incision. The incision is closed before the procedure is repeated via the right prefemoral fossa to remove the contralateral ovary. *(Courtesy Dr. Stephen J. Divers, University of Georgia, Athens, Ga.)*

Oophorectomy of Mature Females. By virtue of the extensive mesovarian found in mature females, an endoscope-assisted procedure is practical in animals weighing a few hundred grams to 100 kg or more (Figure 14-23).[13,14] With the chelonian in dorsal recumbency, a unilateral surgical approach to the coelom is made via one prefemoral fossa. The telescope is inserted into the coelom and used to locate the ipsilateral ovary. Then, the telescope is used to guide atraumatic forceps (or even long hemostats in small chelonians) so that the interfollicular tissue is grasped and gently elevated to the skin incision. Once the first follicle is exteriorized, the telescope is no longer required because the ovary is carefully manipulated out of the coelom. Once the entire ovary is exteriorized, oophorectomy proceeds with the use of traditional techniques. The same procedure is repeated for the contralateral ovary, but it is usually not necessary nor recommended to remove the oviducts

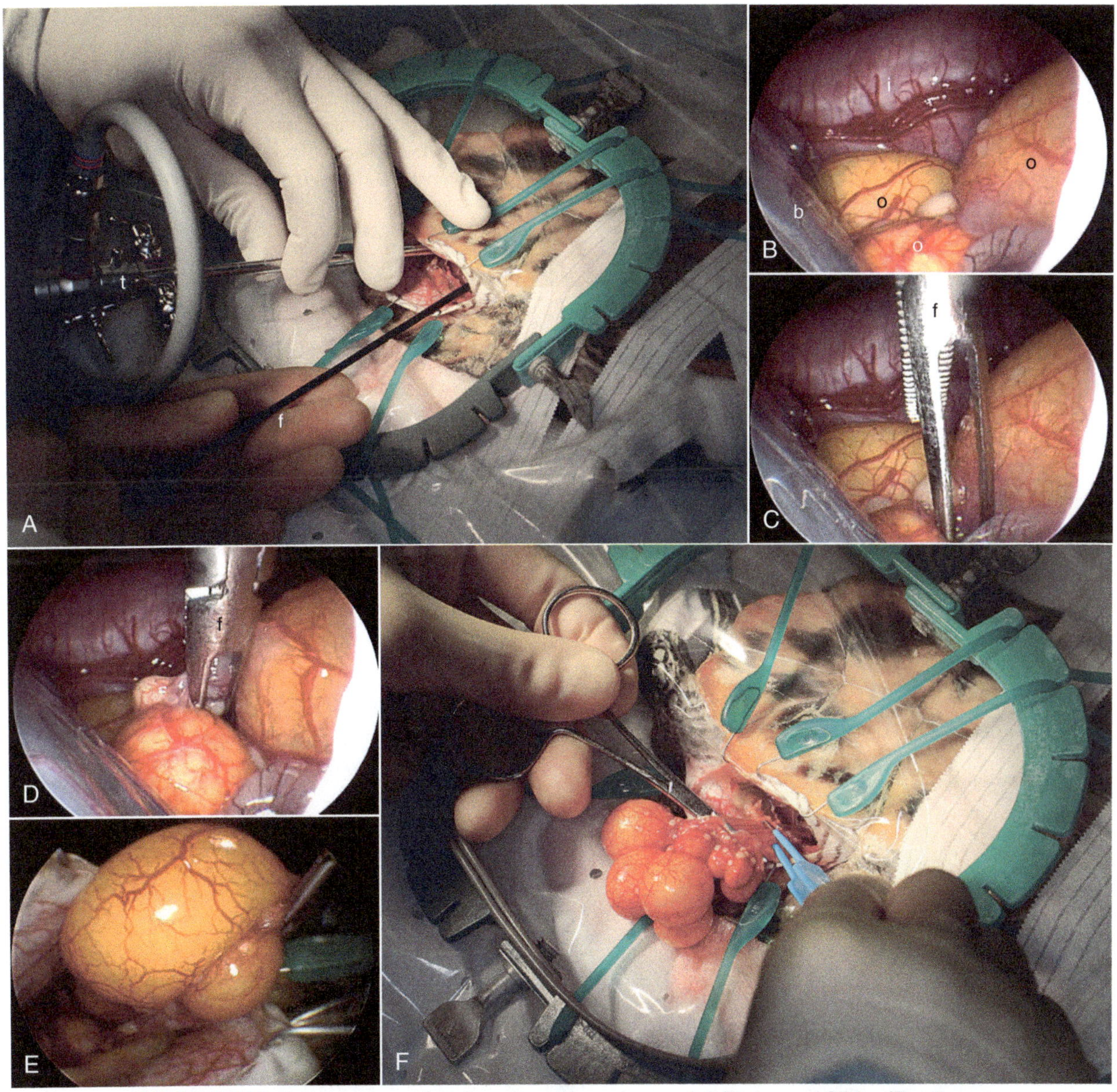

FIGURE 14-23 Endoscope-assisted oophorectomy in an adult Red-eared Slider *(Trachemys scripta elegans)*. **A,** After a prefemoral approach to the coelom, the ipsilateral ovary is located and retracted to the incision with the use of the telescope *(t)* and 3-mm atraumatic forceps *(f)*. **B,** Endoscopic view of the caudal coelom demonstrating the ovary and three large ova *(o)*, closely associated with the bladder *(b)* and intestine *(i)*. **C,** Endoscopic view of 3-mm atraumatic forceps *(f)* being used to grasp the interfollicular tissue. **D,** Endoscopic view of the ovary being gently retracted toward the prefemoral incision. **E,** External view (taken using the telescope) demonstrating the first two follicles of the ovary exteriorized through the prefemoral incision. **F,** Continued manipulation to exteriorize the whole ovary precedes surgical oophorectomy with the use of radiosurgery. In most animals, the contralateral ovary can also be removed through the same prefemoral incision. *(Courtesy Dr. Stephen J. Divers, University of Georgia, Athens, Ga.)*

unless diseased. In most species, both ovaries can be removed from the same incision; however, in some terrestrial tortoises with particularly restrictive prefemoral fossae, it may be necessary to perform a bilateral procedure. The prefemoral approach is closed routinely. This technique has several advantages over traditional plastronectomy, namely, a less invasive soft tissue approach instead of a bony approach, and faster healing.

Orchidectomy. Researchers have developed a similar approach for safe and effective orchidectomy, in red-eared sliders (*Trachemys scripta elegans*) and desert tortoises (*Gopherus agassizii*).[15] The animal is again positioned in lateral recumbency and, after prefemoral coeliotomy, a surgical assistant identifies and maintains a clear view of the testis (Figure 14-24). The endosurgeon then uses Babcock or Kelly forceps to grasp and elevate the testis away from the kidney and epididymis to expose the mesorchium and associated vessels. Both monopolar radiosurgery and vascular clips have been used to ensure hemostasis before scissors are used to dissect the testis free (Figure 14-25). At least in the Red-eared Slider, it is possible to remove both testes via a unilateral prefemoral approach; however, in the desert tortoises a bilateral approach was necessary.

Lizards

The most useful entry points for lizard diagnostic endoscopy also apply when instrument ports are considered. It is particularly important to remember that the standardized placement of cannulae through the linea alba cannot be applied to most lizards caudal to the umbilicus because of the presence of the midline abdominal vein; however, placement of a midline cannula, caudal to the umbilicus, is certainly practical and often preferred, particularly in iguanids (Figures 14-26 and 14-27).

Orchidectomy. With the iguana in right lateral recumbency, the telescope and protection sheath are inserted, just lateral to the ventral midline, close to the anastomosis of the left and right pelvic veins as they form the ventral abdominal vein (see Figure 14-26, *C* and Figure 14-28, *B*). The first cannula is placed cranial to the telescope, just caudal to the last rib, while the second cannula is placed caudal to the anastomosis of the pelvic veins in the ventral midline. Grasping forceps are inserted through one cannula and used to elevate the testis, while scissors (attached to monopolar radiosurgery device) are inserted through the other cannula and used to coagulate and cut through the mesorchium and associated vessels (Figure 14-29). In larger iguanas, bipolar forceps are used to coagulate blood vessels before sharp dissection. The testis is extracted through the forceps cannula hole, which can be enlarged, if necessary. The cannula holes are closed with a single suture or tissue adhesive. The iguana is rotated into left lateral recumbency, and using the same entry sites, the endoscopist repeats the procedure for the second testis.

ENDOSCOPY TRAINING

The ability to perform endosurgery is not innate, and training is certainly required. Fortunately, various continuing education courses offer training in the United States and, less commonly, elsewhere. The Association of Reptilian and Amphibian Veterinarians (www.arav.org) regularly offers a 4-hour introduction to reptile endoscopy at its annual conference. In addition, the University of Georgia offers a 2-day course in reptile/avian, and another in small mammal endoscopy every year, with more advanced endosurgery courses offered intermittently (www.vet.uga.edu/CE/).

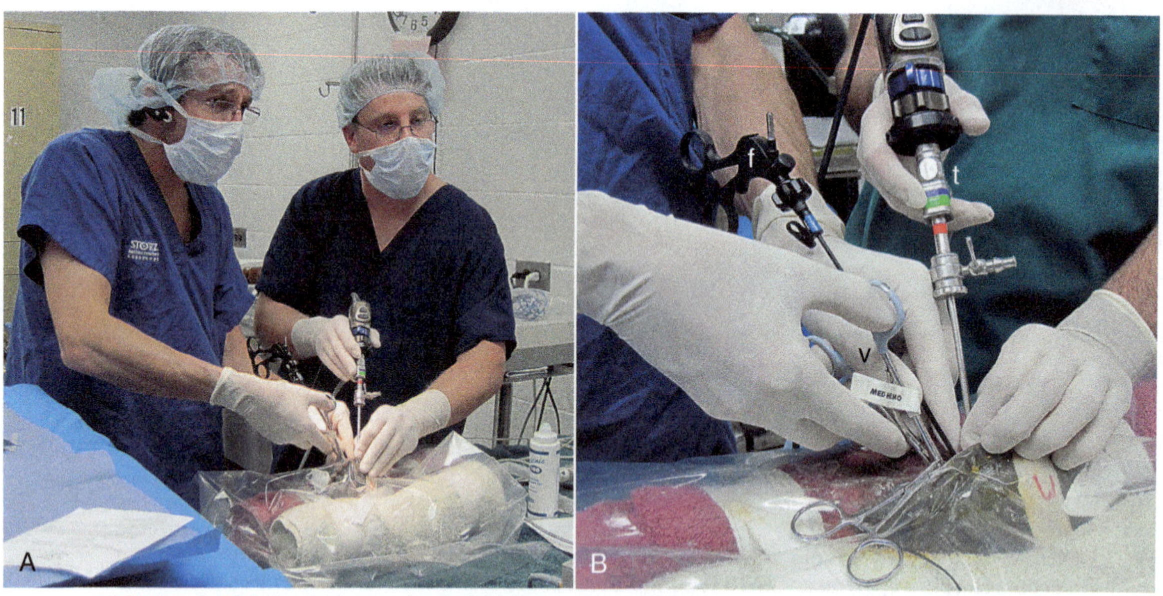

FIGURE 14-24 **A,** Endoscopic orchidectomy in a Red-eared Slider *(Trachemys scripta elegans)*. **B,** Close-up of the surgical site. Note that the assistant controls the camera and telescope *(t)* while the primary surgeon uses 3-mm grasping forceps *(f)* and a vascular clip applicator *(v)* to perform the orchidectomy. *(Courtesy Dr. Stephen J. Divers, University of Georgia, Athens, Ga.)*

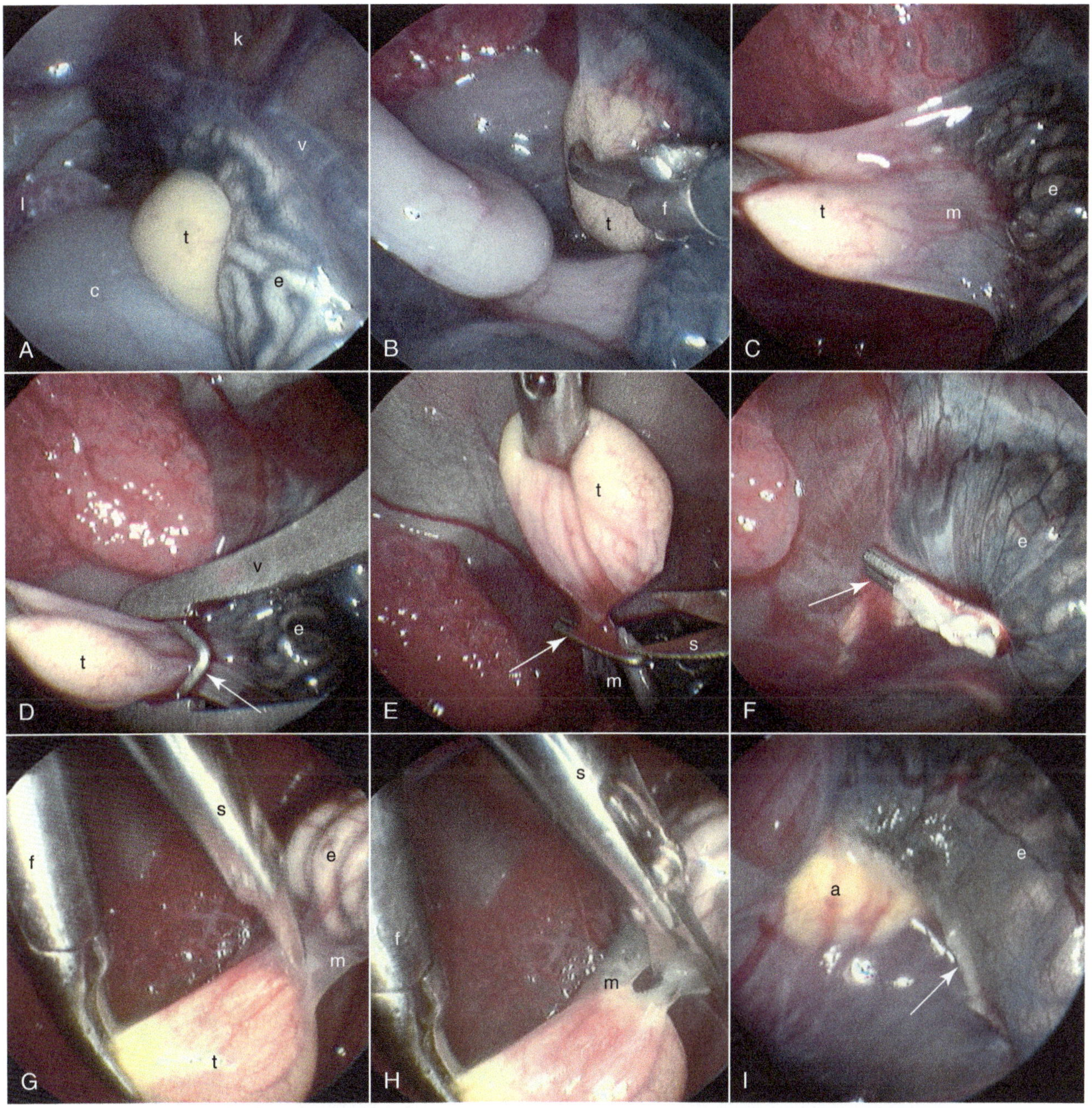

FIGURE 14-25 Endoscopic orchidectomy in the Red-eared Slider *(Trachemys scripta elegans)* via a unilateral prefemoral incision. **A,** View of the left testis *(t)* and epididymis *(e)* closely associated with the kidney *(k)* and renal vein *(v)*. The descending colon *(c)* and caudal lung *(l)* are also visible. **B,** 3-mm Kelly forceps *(f)* are introduced and used to grasp the testis *(t)*. **C,** The forceps are angled to retract the testis *(t)* cranially away from the epididymis *(e)* to expose the mesorchium *(m)* and associated vascular supply. **D-F,** Orchidectomy using vascular clips. A vascular clip applicator *(v)* is introduced and a single clip *(arrow)* is placed across the mesorchium *(m)*, between the testis *(t)* and the epididymis *(e)*, before the testis is dissected free using 3-mm scissors *(s)*. **G-I,** Orchidectomy using radiosurgery. While the testis *(t)* is retracted away from the epididymis *(e)*, monopolar scissors *(s)* are used to coagulate the mesorchial vessels *(m)*, before the testis is dissected free and removed with forceps *(f)*. After orchidectomy, the adrenal gland *(a)* can be seen. *(Courtesy Dr. Stephen J. Divers, University of Georgia, Athens, Ga.)*

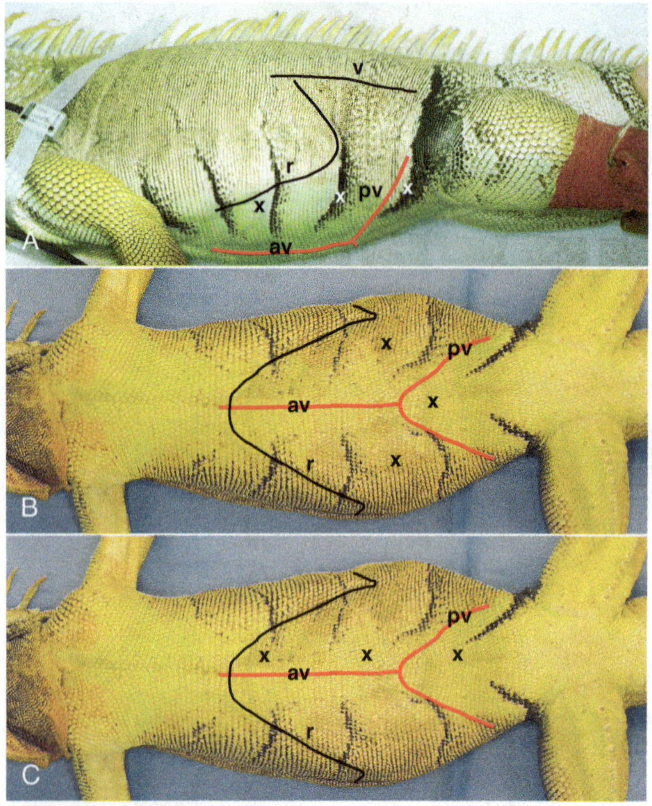

FIGURE 14-26 Lateral **(A)** and ventral **(B, C)** views of an iguanid lizard illustrating the possible cannula insertion points *(x)* for performing multiple-entry endosurgery in lizards. The positions of the vertebral spine *(v)*, last rib *(r)*, ventral abdominal vein *(av)*, and pelvic veins *(pv)* have been shown to indicate anatomic landmarks that should be appreciated. *(Courtesy Dr. Stephen J. Divers, University of Georgia, Athens, Ga.)*

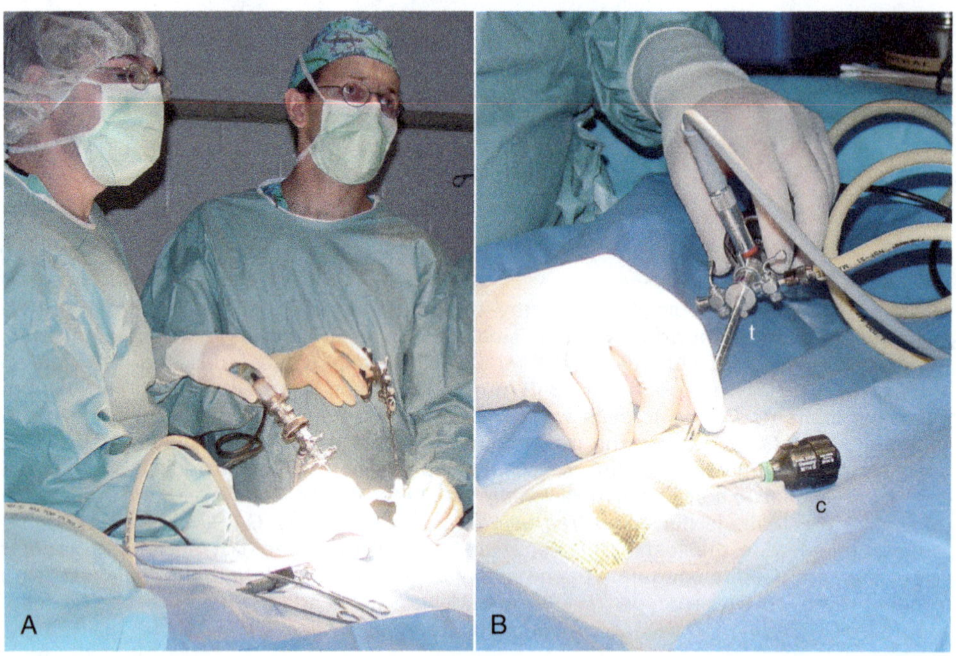

FIGURE 14-27 **A,** A primary surgeon and assistant performing endosurgery in a Green Iguana *(Iguana iguana)*. **B,** Close-up of the surgical site demonstrating the placement of the sheathed telescope with insufflation line attached *(t)* and a 3.5-mm cannula *(c)*. *(Courtesy Dr. Stephen J. Divers, University of Georgia, Athens, Ga.)*

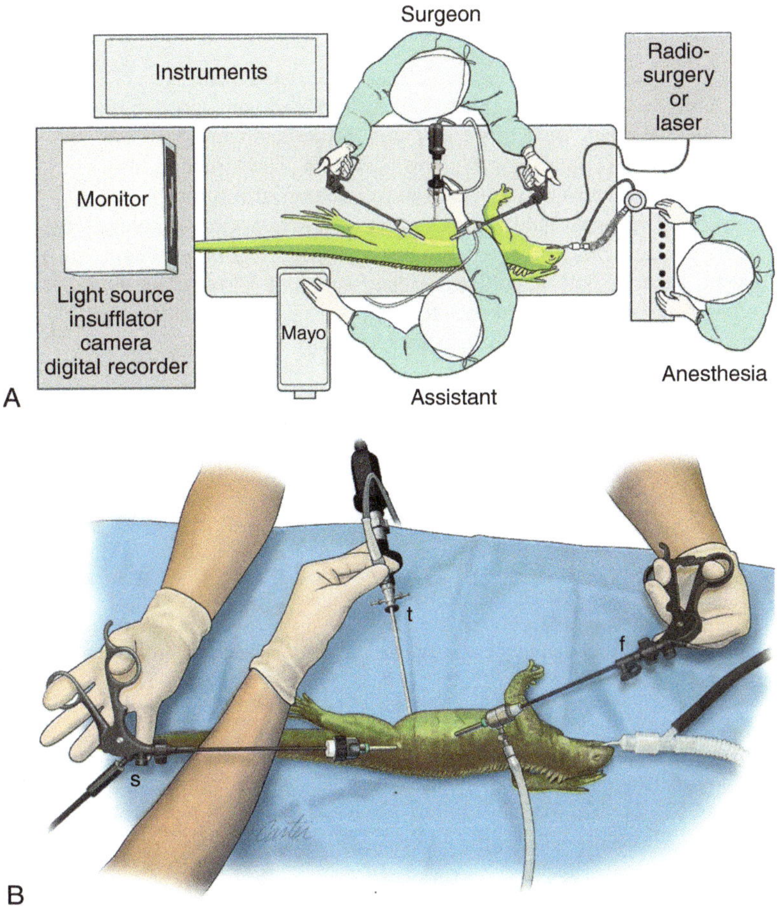

FIGURE 14-28 **A,** General schematic and orientation for performing endosurgical orchidectomy in an iguanid. As an alternative, positioning aids can be used to support the telescope and camera, allowing the monitor to be moved in front of the surgeon. **B,** Diagram illustrating the use of an assistant to support the telescope and camera *(t)*, while the primary (right-handed) surgeon uses forceps *(f)* in the left hand and monopolar scissors *(s)* in the right hand to perform endosurgery within the dorsolateral coelom. *(Art by Kip Carter [UGA], © University of Georgia Research Foundation, Inc.)*

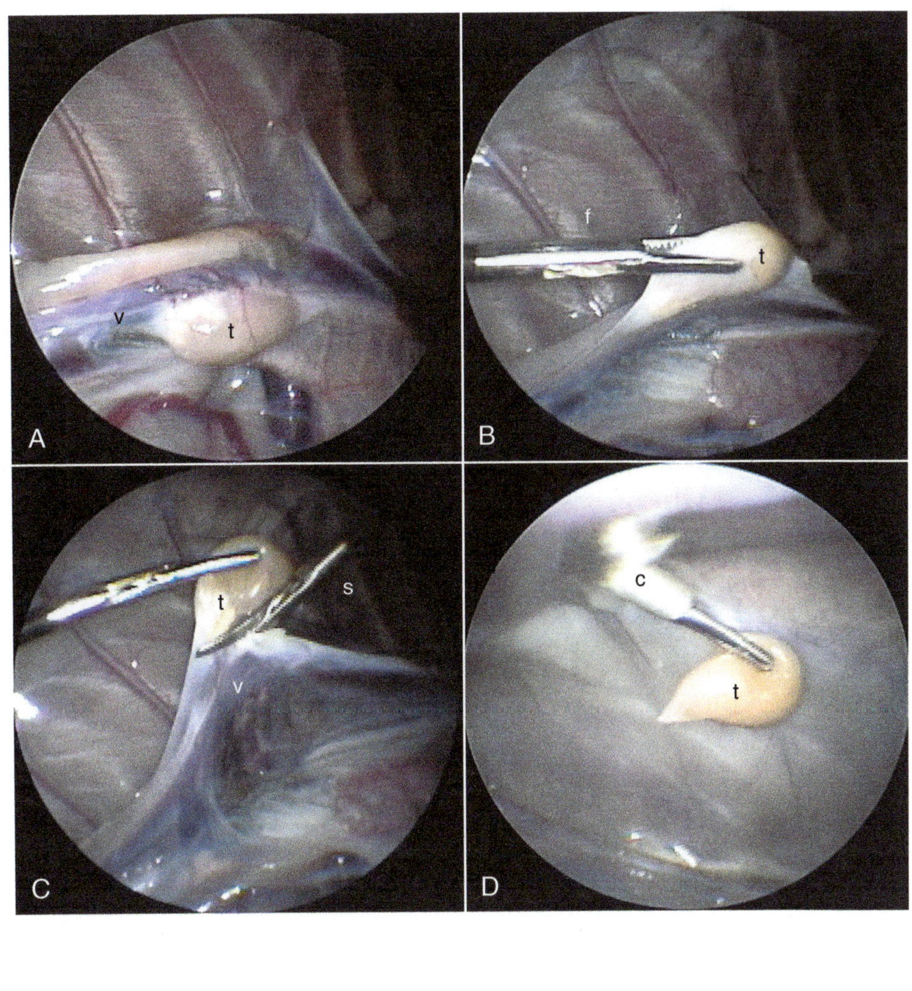

FIGURE 14-29 Endoscopic orchidectomy in a Green Iguana *(Iguana iguana)*. **A,** View of the dorsal coelom showing the right testis *(t)* and closely associated renal vein *(v)*. **B,** Forceps *(f)*, introduced through a caudal cannula, are used to grasp and elevate the testis *(t)* away from the body wall. **C,** With the testis *(t)* elevated away from the renal vein *(v)*, monopolar scissors *(s)* are used to coagulate and cut across the mesorchium. **D,** The freed testis *(t)* is then retracted to the cannula *(c)*, which is slid up the shaft of the forceps before the testis is removed through the cannula hole. If the testis is large, hemostats can be used to temporarily stretch the cannula hole to facilitate removal. *(Courtesy Dr. Stephen J. Divers, University of Georgia, Athens, Ga.)*

ACKNOWLEDGMENTS

The author would like to thank Karl Storz Veterinary Endoscopy and, in particular, Dr. Chris Chamness, Mike Bateman, and Dan McMahon for supporting endoscopy research, development, and training at the University of Georgia. In addition, the author is indebted to Drs. Scott Stahl, Charles Innis, Sam Rivera, Chris Hanley, Jason Norman, Emi Knafo, Randon Feinsod, Justin Oguni, Joe Flannagan, Heather Barron, Johanna Mejia-Fava, Jörg Mayer, Rodney Schnellbacher, and Laila Proenca for their collegiality and assistance in various endoscopic ventures at the University of Georgia.

REFERENCES

1. Lagares-Garcia JA, Bansidhar B, Moore RA. Benefits of laparoscopy in middle-aged patients. *Surg Endosc* 2003;17:68-72.
2. Yu SY, Chiu JH, Loong CC, et al. Diagnostic laparoscopy: indication and benefit. *Zhonghua Yi Xue Za Zhi (Taipei)* 1997;59:158-163.
3. Lhermette P, Sobel D. *BSAVA manual of canine and feline endoscopy and endosurgery*. 1st ed. Cheltenham, England: British Small Animal Veterinary Association, 2008.
4. McCarthy TC. *Veterinary endoscopy for the small animal practitioner*. St Louis: Elsevier, 2005.
5. Tams TR, Rawlings CA. *Small animal endoscopy*. 3rd ed. St Louis: Elsevier, 2011.
6. Divers SJ. Endoscopy and endosurgery. *Vet Clin North Am Exot Anim Pract* 2010;13:171-331.
7. Divers SJ. Reptile diagnostic endoscopy and endosurgery. *Vet Clin North Am Exot Anim Pract* 2010;13:217-242.
8. Divers SJ. Endoscopy equipment and instrumentation for use in exotic animal veterinary medicine. *Vet Clin North Am Exot Anim Pract* 2010;13:171-185.
9. Ternamian AM, Deitel M. Endoscopic threaded imaging port (Endo-TIP) for laparoscopy: experience with different body weights. *Obes Surg* 1999;9:44-47.
10. Hernandez-Divers SJ. Minimally-invasive endoscopic surgery of birds. *J Avian Med Surg* 2005;19:107-120
11. Hernandez-Divers SJ. Endosurgical debridement and diode laser ablation of lung and air sac granulomas in psittacine birds. *J Avian Med Surg* 2002;16:138-145.
12. Hernandez-Divers SJ. Diode laser surgery: principles and application in exotic animals. *Semin Avian Exot Pet Med* 2002;11:208-220.
13. Knafo SE, Divers SJ, Rivera S, et al. Sterilization of hybrid Galapagos tortoises *(Geochelone nigra)* for island restoration: Part 1 female endoscopic oophorectomy under ketamine-medetomidine anaesthesia. *Vet Rec* 2010;168:47-51.
14. Innis C, Hernandez-Divers SJ, Martinez-Jimenez D. Coelioscopic-assisted prefemoral oophorectomy in chelonians. *J Am Vet Med Assoc* 2007;230:1049-1052.
15. Innis CJ, Feinsod R, Hanlon J, et al. Coelioscopic orchiectomy can be effectively and safely accomplished in chelonians. *Vet Rec* 2013; 18;172:526. Epub 2013 Apr 4.

CHAPTER 15

Vacuum-Assisted Wound Closure in Chelonians

Maud L. Marin, Terry M. Norton, and Nancy S. Mettee

WOUND MANAGEMENT

The Vacuum-Assisted Closure (VAC) Therapy system (KCI, San Antonio, Tex) is a noninvasive wound management technique that uses negative pressure wound therapy (NPWT) to accelerate the healing process of difficult wounds.[1] This relatively new technique has been proven successful in small and large mammals (including humans) and reptiles.[1-10] Chelonians are excellent candidates for NPWT because of their unique shell, which allows easy bandage placement, and their tractable nature, as they are not prone to rolling and entangling the vacuum hose. Although this technique requires more equipment compared with traditional wound management, it is relatively simple to apply, and the speed and quality of healing in complicated cases more than outweigh the costs of extended hospitalization (weeks to months).

In chelonian medicine, VAC therapy is used to treat challenging wounds involving carapace and plastron defects and tissue exposure, most often caused by trauma and less frequently by thermal burns or infection. The therapy should be used in the early stages of treatment and can be followed with traditional therapy once wound healing is progressing well with a healthy granulation bed. VAC treatment time for shell injuries in land chelonians has been reported to be from 3 to 43 days, whereas in sea turtles, treatment is generally a few weeks to as long as a year or more, depending on the severity of the wound.[8]

THE THEORY OF VACUUM-ASSISTED CLOSURE THERAPY

NPWT promotes wound healing in several ways: (1) promotes contraction of wound margins to facilitate closure, (2) encourages granulation tissue formation, (3) increases tissue perfusion, (4) removes exudate and (5) reduces edema.[1-3] Reduction of edema that would otherwise accumulate in the wound increases perfusion and provides nutrients, inflammatory cells, oxygen, and growth factors while removing free radicals.[1-3] Severe wounds to the carapace often lead to collapsing of the lung. NPWT has the added benefit of bringing lung tissue back into its original location, favoring a more normal anatomic orientation and preservation of the coelomic space. With NPWT, mechanical force is applied to a wound to promote healing. This is accomplished through two active principles: macrostrain and microstrain. *Macrostrain* is the visible deformation that occurs when negative pressure is exerted on the foam and it collapses. It is a visible, physical response that draws the wound edges closer together, evenly distributes negative pressure, and removes exudate and infectious material. *Microstrain* refers to microdeformation, which leads to cellular stretching. This biologic response occurs at the cellular level to promote perfusion, reduce edema, and promote the rapid formation of granulation tissue. Microstrain facilitates cell migration to the wound, enhancing immune function and increasing the rate of granulocyte cell division.[11]

INDICATIONS AND CONTRAINDICATIONS

In humans, indications for the use of VAC include acute to chronic, traumatic, and dehisced wounds, partial-thickness burns, ulcers, incisions, flaps and grafts, and diabetic wounds.[3] New applications continue to be described, such as spider bite management, osteomyelitis, and exposed bones.[12-14] In chelonians, the main indication for VAC therapy is the treatment of carapace and plastron defects with soft tissue exposure.

Incomplete wound debridement before starting NPWT may result in proliferation of granulation tissues over necrotic tissues and delayed wound healing.[9] Negative pressure should not be used directly over exposed organs, blood vessels, or nerves. If these are present, closed cell foam should be used to protect exposed lungs or other organs. Hemostasis should be verified before application of negative pressure. It should not be used for neoplastic lesions or patients with a bleeding disorder.

EQUIPMENT NEEDED

Basic VAC therapy relies on open-cell foam that is placed into the wound bed, covered by an airtight plastic dressing, and attached to a suction machine by plastic tubing (Figure 15-1). Additional materials such as tape and adhesives have proven useful for the chelonian patient when leaks are present after the initial VAC application and have been included in Table 15-1 (see also Case 15-1). Purpose-made equipment is commercially available at KCI Animal Health (San Antonio, Tex), and clinicians can order wound care kits that fit the needs of a specific patient. Because this treatment can become costly over time, economical alternatives to the VAC components are also included in this chapter.

Nonadherent Barrier

A variety of nonadherent mesh materials or gauze can protect the wound and keep it moist. Nonadherent mesh such as Adaptic (Johnson & Johnson nonstick dressings, Arlington, Tex), Acticoat burn dressing (Smith and Nephew, Largo, Fla), or Silverlon (Argentum Medical, Willowbrook, Ill) can be used with petroleum jelly, saline, or sterile water. This step may not be needed when the wound has a mature granulation bed. Ointments and creams are not recommended because they will be suctioned out quickly.

Foam

Open-cell foam is used on the wound to provide an equal distribution of applied suction to the wound. The most commonly used foam is the standard gray dressing (VAC GranuFoam), but GranuFoam Silver is a newer product that contains microbonded metallic silver and is recommended for use in infected areas. Finally, the VAC WhiteFoam dressing is a thinner but more resilient foam material that is used for undermining wounds and protecting organs and nerves. Alternatively, open-cell foam can be found at home improvement stores (e.g., speaker foam or air conditioning foam) and is inexpensive. The pores should be approximately 400 to 600 μm in diameter, and the foam may be gas sterilized. Complex wounds may require multiple foam pieces. It is vital to have overlap or foam-to-foam connection for uniform suction.

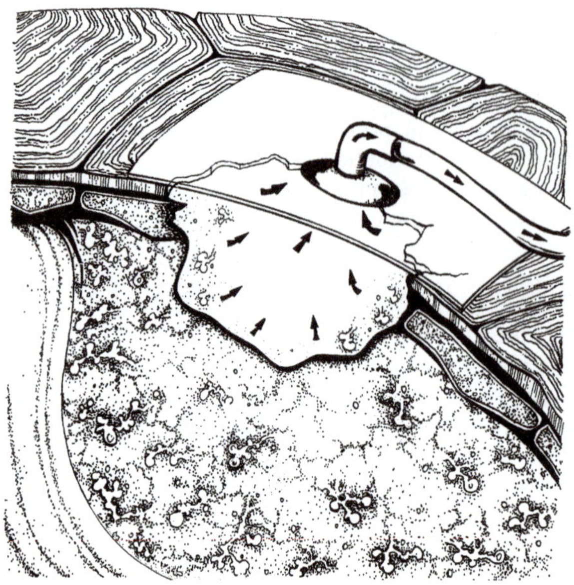

FIGURE 15-1 VAC therapy on a chelonian patient. The foam is placed into the defect and covered with a clear dressing. An egress tube is attached and linked to a suction unit (not shown). *(Drawing courtesy Lori E. Hunt.)*

Adhesive Drape

Several types of occlusive plastic adhesive films can be used and cut to fit. These include VAC adhesive drape (KCI), Steri-drape and Tegaderm (3M, St. Paul, Minn). For large wounds, several drapes may be required and overlapped to cover the foam. Once the vacuum has been applied, leaks may become apparent. Troubleshooting leaks (air or water) can be performed with a variety of techniques and products at the margins of the draped area, including the application of additional adhesive drape material, 100% silicone, or adhesive paste (Stomahesive paste, ConvaTec, Skillman, NJ) (Case 15-2). Bridge defects, especially the ones that connect to the skin from the foreleg or hindleg, can be challenging to drape. Immobilizing the hindleg (in flexion or extension) with gauze and tape can be very helpful in achieving a stable bandage seal.

Tubing

After the dressing is placed over the foam, a slit can be made in the drape over the foam to place the VAC therapy-regulated accurate care (TRAC) pad. This will connect the foam to the suction pump and diffuse the suction across the wound bed. Alternatively, red rubber tubing and suction tubes can be used. They should be fenestrated at the end, cut to fit, and inserted midway through the foam. Extra adherent dressing can be cut and placed over the joint to create a seal. Care must be taken to ensure that the end of the tube is not touching the wound directly but is instead within the foam.

Suction Pump

The purpose-made VAC Freedom suction pump is the apparatus of choice for this treatment. The advantages of the purpose-made pump include quiet operation, a smaller and more portable unit (some are battery operated), accurate pressure

TABLE 15-1

Negative Pressure Therapy: Equipment Needed

Components	Best	Good	Adequate
Nonadherent barrier	Silver-impregnated mesh (Acticoat Silverlon) + saline or petroleum jelly	Adaptic+ saline or petroleum jelly	Telfa gauze + saline
Foam	VAC GranuFoam Standard, Silver or WhiteFoam	Open-cell polyurethane foam (speaker foam at home improvement store)	Loosely placed gauze or laparotomy sponges
Adhesive drape	VAC sterile adhesive drape	Tegaderm, Steri-drape	Food-quality clear plastic wrap with silicone seal on margins
Tubing	Purpose-made pad and tubing (VAC TRAC pad)	Red rubber tube, fenestrated	Any plastic tubing, fenestrated + adaptor
Suction	VAC Freedom Therapy unit	Surgical suction unit	High-volume passive suction grenade

Acticoat burn dressing (Smith and Nephew, Largo, Fla); Silverlon (Argentum Medical, Willowbrook, Ill); Adaptic (Johnson & Johnson Nonstick dressings, Arlington, Tex); VAC products (KCI Animal Health, San Antonio, Tex); Steri-drape and Tegaderm (3M, St. Paul, Minn).

adjustment, and alarm system when the seal is breached. The unit can be either purchased or rented from the manufacturer for the duration of treatment. Continuous or intermittent suction settings are programmed. Intermittent suction has been associated with more rapid cellular division than continuous suction but may create patient discomfort. Therefore it is best to start with the continuous setting until the wound bed is well-developed. The intensity feature addresses how quickly pressure is achieved. Low intensity is recommended for patients new to therapy because the creation of pressure is slower. Higher intensity settings are recommended for larger wounds so that a more rapid seal is obtained. Alternatively, any surgical suction pump or passive suction grenade can be used to generate negative pressure.

CASE 15-1

Aldabra tortoise *(Geochelone [Geochelone] gigantea)* with deep carapace abscess and osteomyelitis[9]

Clinical Application: Treating an Infected Wound

- Pressure setting: continuous at 125 mm Hg
- Nonadherent barrier: Acticoat silver-impregnated mesh
- Foam type: VAC GranuFoam and VAC GranuFoam Silver
- Foam placement: cut to fit and placed over infected area on the carapace
- Adhesive drape: VAC adhesive drape
- Tubing: VAC TRAC pad
- Suction pump: VAC Freedom pump
- Enclosure: small holding area
- Suction unit placement: unit suspended above the animal
- Bandage change regimen: daily initially (4 days) then every 2 days
- Duration of therapy: 55 days of VAC therapy

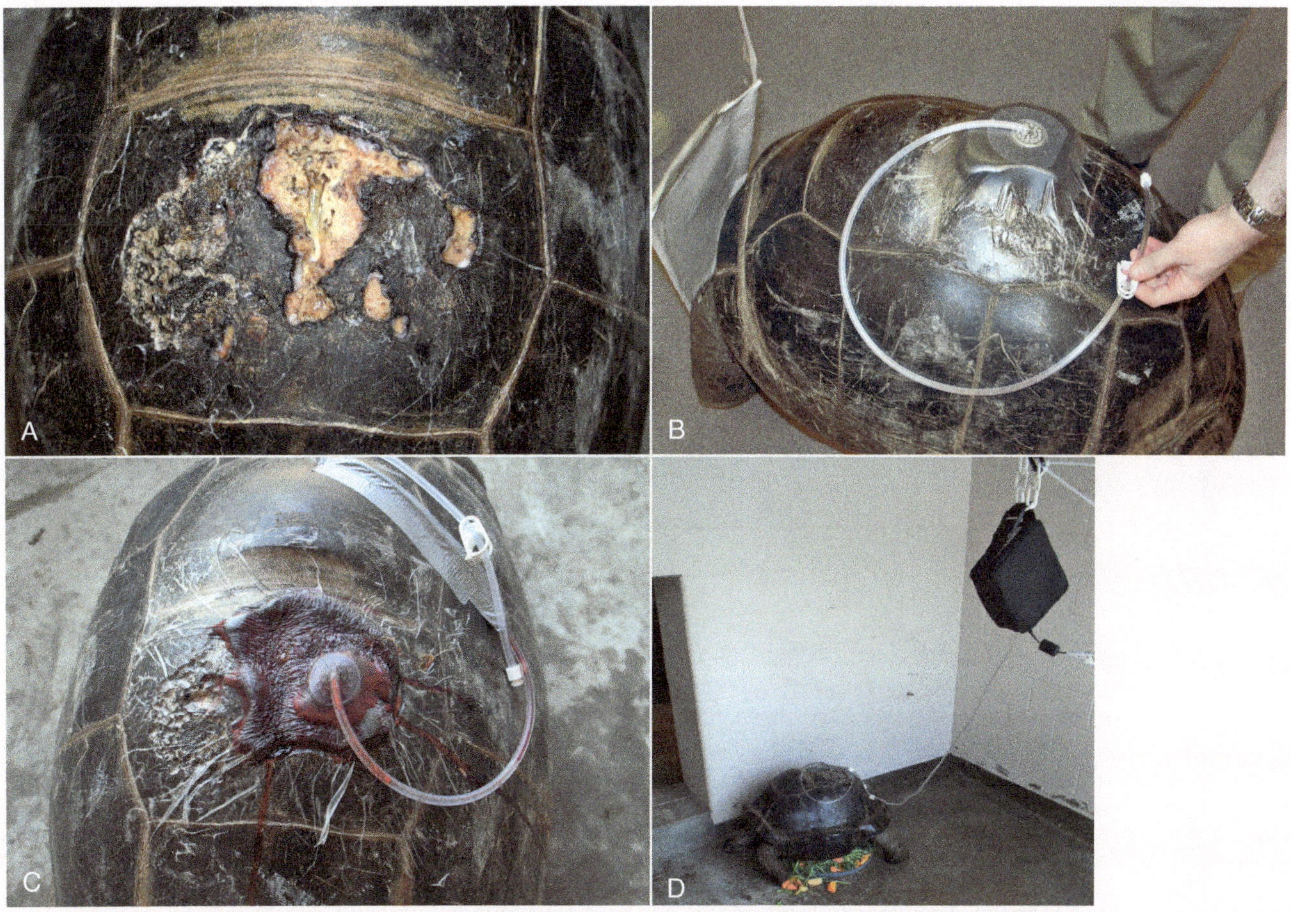

Aldabra tortoise *(Aldabrachelys [Geochelone] gigantea)* seen for focal necrosis of the carapace. **A,** Initial presentation: the wound was debrided surgically before starting the therapy. **B,** The VAC therapy was implemented with the use of a foam pad and occlusive dressing. An adaptor (TRAC pad) and suction tubing was place. Note the foam pad protruding from the shell before suction is applied. **C,** The VAC in place with negative pressure suction turned on; note the shrunken appearance of the foam and the bloody fluid it is removing. **D,** The tortoise with the VAC therapy system in place, with the unit hung in the enclosure. The wound healed after 55 days of treatment. *(Photos courtesy of Michael Adkesson.)*

CASE 15-2

Yellow-bellied slider *(Trachemys scripta scripta)* with shell fracture from vehicular accident[8]

Clinical Application: Treating a Shell Defect After Fracture Reduction; Economical Alternative to Purpose-made Materials

- Fracture stabilization: screws and wire, covered with Elastikon
- Nonadherent barrier: none
- Foam type: open cell foam from hardware store
- Foam placement: cut to fit, placed into defect and flush with the carapace
- Adhesive drape: Steri-drape
- Tubing: available tubing material at the clinic; suction tubing and red rubber catheter
- Suction pump: regular surgery suction pump
- Pressure setting: 100 mm Hg to 120 mm Hg
- Enclosure: small plastic tub
- Suction unit placement: adjacent to the tub
- Bandage change regimen: every day initially (4 to 7 days) then every 2 to 5 days. Animal is left dry-docked during treatment but is allowed into water between bandage changes.
- Duration of therapy: 10 to 40 days of VAC therapy; longer healing time for fractures

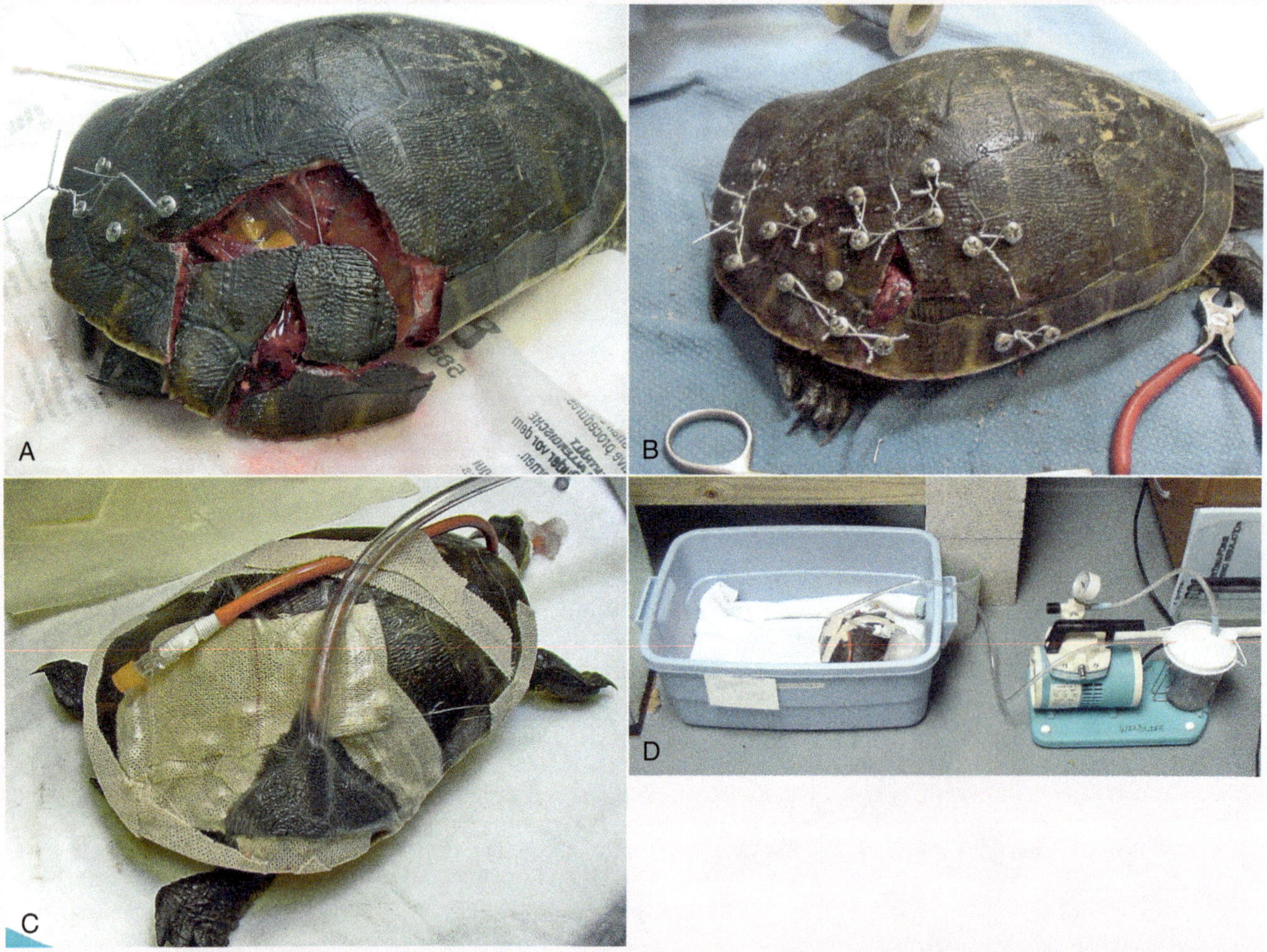

Yellow-bellied slider *(Trachemys scripta scripta)* that was seen with a serious shell fracture after a vehicular accident. **A,** After evaluation, supportive therapy was initiated and the fractures were reduced under anesthesia. **B,** All fractures were reduced, but a shell defect remained on the carapace. **C,** The orthopedic wire is covered with cotton elastic cloth tape, and foam is placed into the defect and covered by clear adhesive film before an egress tube is inserted. Note the esophagostomy tube placed for nutritional support during recovery. **D,** The turtle is placed in a tub for recovery. Larger setups can be used for larger animals. When dry-docking aquatic animals, it is important to monitor fluid balance and let them swim for a few hours between the bandage changes. Alternatively, the bandage can be waterproofed.

TECHNIQUE

General Assessment

Before starting treatment of a shell condition, the patient needs to be examined and the long-term prognosis determined. Baseline evaluation should entail a physical examination including neurologic assessment, body weight and body condition, blood panel values, and survey radiographs (dorsoventral, horizontal beam craniocaudal, and horizontal beam lateral views). Because the spinal cord is closely linked to the carapace, lesions that cross the dorsal midline may entail nerve injury, even in the presence of hindlimb movements.[15] Although certain chelonians with neurologic impairment should be euthanized (such as free-ranging tortoises), captive animals may still remain functional. Multiple considerations must be taken into account while establishing each animal's prognosis.

Basic Wound Management

Once the animal is determined to be a good candidate for treatment, basic wound care is implemented. A bacterial culture can be taken, if appropriate, before the wounds are debrided. All nonviable tissue (including bone) is removed; general anesthesia may be required. Fractures are stabilized, and any sharp edges should be removed.[16-18] Before application of the NPWT, it is important to ensure adequate hemostasis and evaluate any organ exposure. If there will be a delay in applying the NPWT, wet-to-dry bandages or honey dressings can be used and changed daily. Other considerations including appropriate husbandry, pain management, nutritional support (e.g., tube feeding and esophagostomy tube), fluid therapy, and antimicrobials should also be part of the case management.

Applying the Negative Pressure Wound Therapy Dressing

The shell should be dry to permit a strong bond with the adhesive drape. Sterile gauze or mesh wetted with sterile water, saline, or petroleum jelly (Vaseline, Unilever, Greenwich, Conn) can be placed on the wound bed to keep it hydrated. The open-cell foam is cut to size and placed into the defect. Several pieces can be used next or on top of each other, as long as they make contact so that uniform pressure on the wound is achieved.

The chelonian shell is an excellent base for applying an adhesive drape, and often no extra seal is needed. It should extend a few centimeters beyond the edge of the wound to create an air-tight seal. Deep grooves in the scutes can be covered with tape, adhesive materials, or filled in with epoxy. Orthopedic hardware can be covered with adherent bandage material (Elastikon, Johnson & Johnson Medical Inc, Arlington, Tex) before placing the drape. Finally, the purpose-made egress tube and adhesive disk (SensaTRAC) is placed over the adhesive drape, after a small hole is cut at the optimal location. Alternatively, a fenestrated plastic tube or 10F to 14F polyvinyl (red rubber) catheter can be tunneled into the foam or placed between two pieces of foam. The tube should not be in direct contact with the wound bed. Multiple wound areas can be connected with a Y-connector device or bridging technique (see VAC Veterinary User Manual[19] for more information).

Maintenance and Bandage Changes

When suction is applied, the foam should visibly collapse and take on a shrunken appearance beneath the adhesive film. If a leak is found, more dressing can be added to the bandage to create a tighter fit. Negative pressure between 100 mm Hg and 175 mm Hg is used in chelonians. Continuous suction is generally used, and leaving it for 24 hours a day is ideal. If during the treatment, the airtight seal is lost, it needs to be restored by applying more clear adhesive dressing. If it cannot be repaired within 2 hours, the whole dressing should be removed and the wound irrigated and left open until a new bandage can be made. Time off from treatment between bandage changes can be beneficial to some animals and may give an opportunity for aquatic turtles to swim freely. Care must be taken to remove the dressing as soon as the suction is discontinued. Bandages can be changed without sedation or anesthesia, as humans report minimal pain during bandage change or therapy. It is important to monitor fluid loss and hydration status, especially in small patients less than 10 kg. Confinement of the patient will be necessary to prevent entanglement with the tubing. The suction unit needs to be placed to allow the turtle to move about its enclosure.

Combining Other Wound Management Techniques with Negative Pressure Wound Therapy

NPWT has been used extensively in a variety of freshwater turtles, terrapins, and sea turtles. Initially, all patients were dry-docked during the NPWT process; however, although some patients tolerated this well, others became stressed and only tolerated 12 to 24 hours out of the water. At the Georgia Sea Turtle Center, multiple wound care management techniques are often used and rotated on the same patient. For example, NPWT may be used for 12 to 48 hours in a dry-dock situation, and then honey with a waterproof bandage may be used for similar time periods. Sea turtles may be given NPWT at night, and then waterproof bandaging may be placed during the day. NPWT is often used in the initial stages of treatment, especially when the coelomic cavity is open so that a watertight seal and a granulation bed can develop. Other forms of therapy such as honey (Medihoney Derma Sciences Inc, Princeton, NJ), doxycycline gel (Doxirobe Gel, Pharmacia & Upjohn Company, New York, NY), silver sulfadiazine cream and ilex cream combination (iLex Skin Protectant Paste, Medcon Biolab Technologies, Grafton, Mass), and/or bone cement with antibiotics may be used thereafter.

CONCLUSION

NPWT is a useful technique for healing difficult wounds in which a carapace or plastron defect is present. The reduction of healing time is striking in chelonians, saving many months of treatment and hospitalization. VAC therapy has been used successfully in severe wounds in which traditional therapy may not have even been attempted. The technique is relatively simple to use and can be learned rapidly (Cases 15-3 and 15-4).

CASE 15-3

Green Sea Turtle *(Chelonia mydas)* hit by boat

Clinical Application: Treating Large Carapace Defect with Lung Collapse; In-water Use

- Nonadherent barrier: petroleum jelly–soaked Silverlon
- Foam type: VAC GranuFoam Silver
- Foam placement: initially placed inside the carapace to promote debridement; in later stages overlaid above carapace
- Adhesive drape: Steri-drape with additional 5-cm silicone perimeter
- Tubing: KCI tubing
- Suction pump: VAC Freedom pump
- Pressure setting: initial setting was 120 mm Hg continuous for the first 2 months of therapy and was then increased to 175 mm Hg intermittent. Maximum intensity was throughout the treatment.
- Enclosure: dry-docked for 12 hours, then placed in 3-m (8-ft) diameter round fiberglass tank with salt water
- Suction unit placement: a battery-powered VAC suction unit was placed in a waterproof case (pelican-case.com, San Antonio, Tex) with two holes drilled into it to allow tubing and an electric cord to come through. It is best to keep the unit plugged into an electrical source because it will be used for 24 hours a day up to 7 days at a time. The waterproof case was hung from the rafters with a large zip tie and carabiner pulley system. This allowed the turtle to swim freely in the tank.
- Bandage change regimen: every 3 days for first 3 weeks and then up to 7 days or when the water seal was no longer present
- Duration of therapy: 13 months

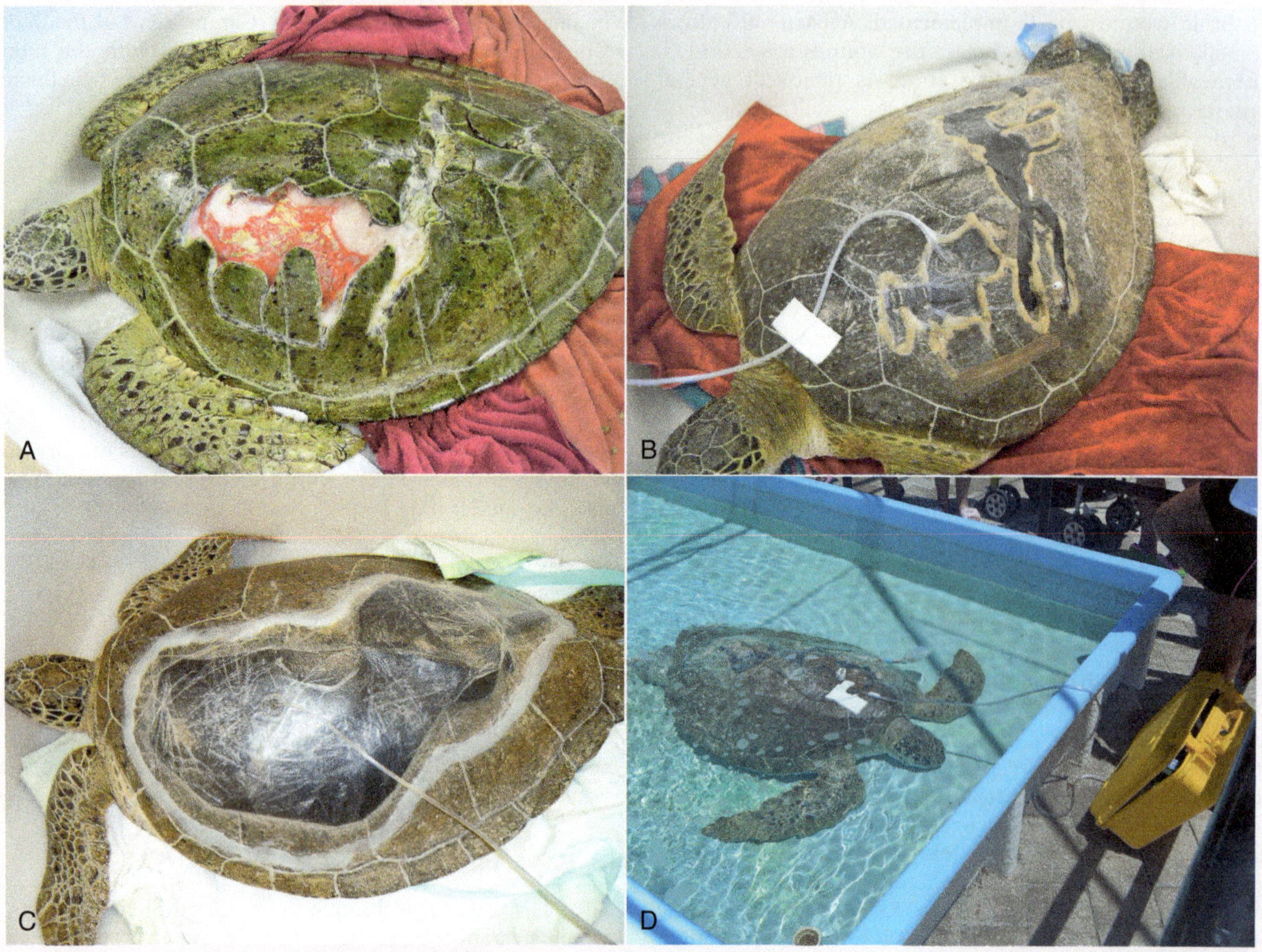

Green Sea Turtle *(Chelonia mydas)* seen with severe propeller wound injuries. **A,** Wound after debridement. **B,** VAC therapy in place. In the early stages when the wound was still grossly contaminated, the gray foam was applied with an underlying technique to facilitate removal of foreign material and exudate. The sharp edges of the fractured carapace were smoothed over with an adhesive paste so that the drape would not be punctured. **C,** As the granulation bed matured, the application of the gray foam was changed to an overlay that allowed further adherence of the soft tissue to the carapace. The addition of the silicone at the margin of the drape created a watertight seal that lasted 5 to 7 days. **D,** In water with portable vacuum therapy unit. The wound healed after 1 year of intensive treatment.

CASE 15-4

Juvenile Green Sea Turtle with boat strike injuries with open coelom. Lung and gastrointestinal tract were visible after initial debridement of dead bone and soft tissue.

Clinical Application: Applying VAC Therapy in Conjunction with Other Therapeutic Modalities

- Nonadherent barrier: saline-soaked Silverlon
- Foam type: VAC GranuFoam Silver
- Foam placement: overlaid above carapace
- Adhesive drape: Tegaderm
- Tubing: KCI tubing
- Suction pump: VAC Freedom pump
- Pressure setting: initial setting was 100 mm Hg continuous for the first week and then was increased to 125 mm Hg thereafter
- Other products used during course of therapy: Medihoney (Derma Sciences Inc., Princeton, NJ) honey and honey comb, antibiotic impregnated bone cement, various types of waterproof bandages with Tegaderm, waterproof tape, and superglue
- Enclosure: dry-docked at night for VAC therapy and then bandaged and placed in 3-m (8-ft) diameter round fiberglass tank with salt water during the day
- Bandage change regimen: every 3 days for first 3 weeks and then up to 7 days or when the water seal was no longer present
- Duration of therapy: VAC therapy was discontinued after approximately 1 month once the coelomic cavity had sealed. Other treatment modalities were used thereafter. Total treatment lasted 11 months

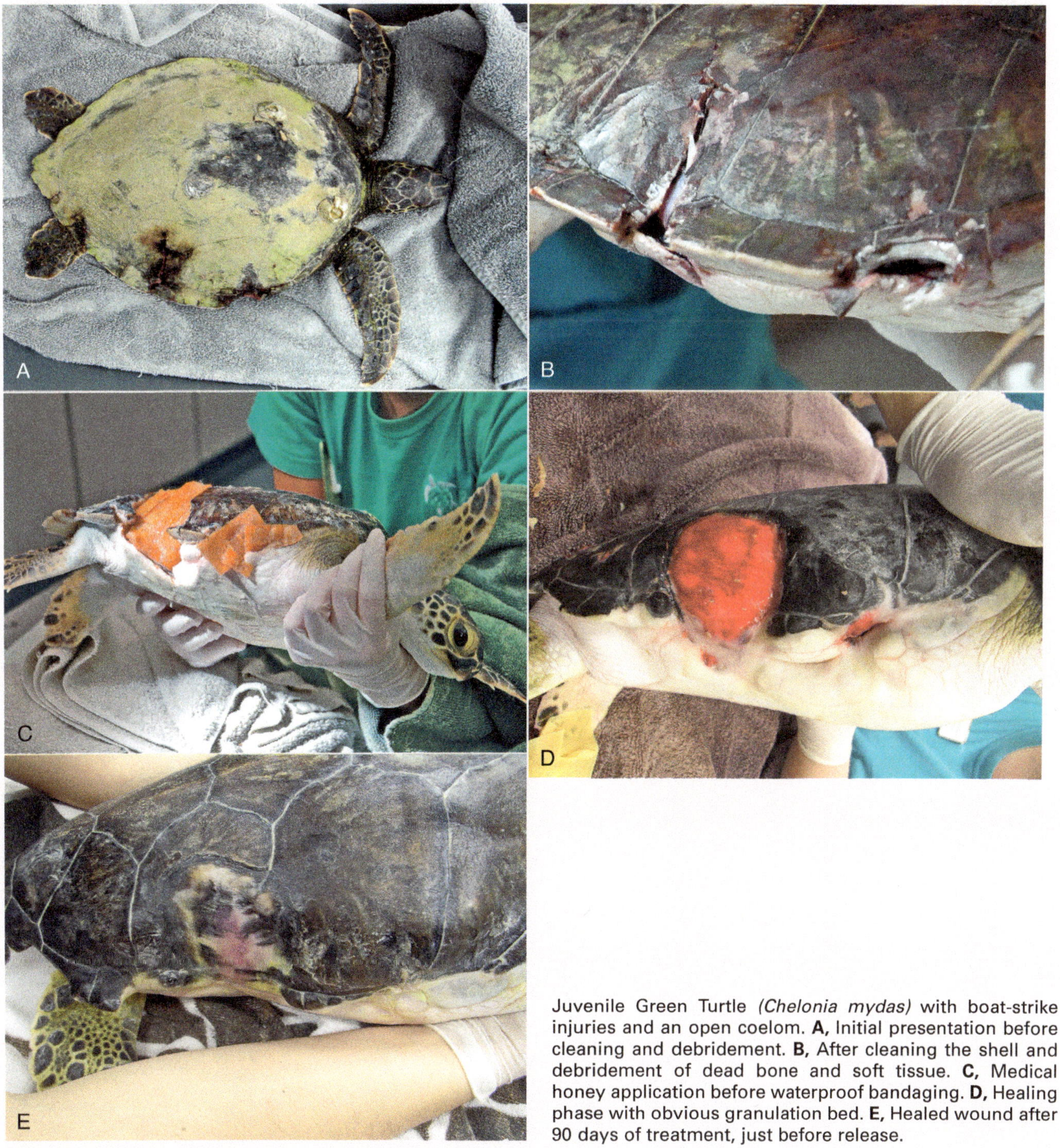

Juvenile Green Turtle *(Chelonia mydas)* with boat-strike injuries and an open coelom. **A,** Initial presentation before cleaning and debridement. **B,** After cleaning the shell and debridement of dead bone and soft tissue. **C,** Medical honey application before waterproof bandaging. **D,** Healing phase with obvious granulation bed. **E,** Healed wound after 90 days of treatment, just before release.

REFERENCES

1. VAC Therapy: Animal Wound Care—Advanced Healing Technology Web Site. Available at: www.kcianimalhealth.com. Accessed May 1, 2013.
2. Morykwas MJ, Argenta LC, Shelton-Brown EI, et al. Vacuum-assisted closure- a new method for wound control and treatment: animal studies and basic foundation. *Ann Plast Surg* 1997;38:553-562.
3. Argenta LC, Morykwas MJ. Vacuum-assisted closure: a new method for wound control and treatment: clinical experience. *Ann Plast Surg* 1997;38:563-576.
4. Kirby KA, Wheeler JL, Farese JP, et al. Surgical views: vacuum-assisted wound closure: clinical applications. *Compend Contin Educ Vet* 2010;32:E1-7.
5. Guille AE, Tseng LW, Orsher RJ. Use of vacuum-assisted closure for management of a large skin wound in a cat. *J Am Vet Med Assoc* 2007;230:1669-1673.
6. Gemeinhardt KD, Molnar JA. Vacuum-assisted closure for management of a traumatic neck wound in a horse. *Equine Vet Educ* 2005;17:27-33.
7. Lafortune M, Fleming GJ, Wheeler JL, et al. Wound management in a juvenile tiger (*Panthera tigris*) with vacuum-assisted closure (V.A.C. Therapy). *J Zoo Wildl Med* 2007;38:341-344.
8. Lafortune M, Wellehan JFX, Heard DJ, et al. Vacuum-assisted closure (Turtle VAC) in the management of traumatic shell defects in chelonians. *J Herpetol Med Surg* 2005;15:4-8.
9. Adkesson MJ, Travis EK, Weber MA, et al. Vacuum-assisted closure for treatment of a deep shell abscess and osteomyelitis in a tortoise. *J Am Vet Med Assoc* 2007;231:1249-1254.
10. Coke RL, Reyes-Fore PA. Treatment of a carapace infection in an Aldabra tortoise, *Geochelone gigantea*, with negative pressure wound therapy. *J Herpetol Med Surg* 2006;16:102-106.
11. Chen CM. Geometric control of cell life and death. *Science* 1997;276:1425-1428.
12. Wong SL, Schneider AM, Argenta LC, et al. Loxoscelism and negative pressure wound therapy (vacuum-assisted closure): an experimental study. *Int Wound J* 2010;7:488-492.
13. Tan Y, Wang X, Li H, et al. The clinical efficacy of the vacuum-assisted closure therapy in the management of adult osteomyelitis. *Arch Orthop Trauma Surg* 2011;131:255-259.
14. DeFranzo AJ, Argenta LC, Marks MW, et al. The use of vacuum-assisted closure therapy for the treatment of lower-extremity wounds with exposed bones. *Plast Reconstr Surg* 2001;108:1184-1191.
15. Chrisman CH, Walsh M, Meeks JC, et al. Neurologic evaluation of sea turtles. *J Am Vet Med Assoc* 1997;211:1043-1047.
16. Richard J. Metal bridges—a new technique of turtle shell repair. *J Herpetol Med Surg* 2001;11:31-34.
17. Barten SL. Shell damage. In: Mader DR, ed. *Reptile medicine and surgery*. 2nd ed. Philadelphia: Elsevier, 2006;893-899.
18. Forrester H, Satta J. Easy shell repair. *Exot DVM* 2005;6:13.
19. *V.A.C. therapy for veterinary use* [user manual]. San Antonio, Texas: KCI, 2011;1-34. Available at www.kcianimalhealth.com.

CHAPTER 16

New Techniques in Chelonian Shell Repair

†Gregory J. Fleming

CHELONIAN SHELL REPAIR

In the past, chelonian shell repair may have resembled crude automobile bodywork. In many cases, the most basic veterinary wound management and fracture fixation principles were not followed. Even though chelonian shell trauma may appear to be foreign to most practitioners, all veterinarians possess the basic skills to successfully treat chelonians with shell injuries.

The ability of the veterinarian to practice shell repair may be due, in part, to the geographic location of the veterinary practice. In areas with an abundance of wild chelonians, the ability to practice shell repair may be greater than in areas with only captive chelonians. This is due to the large number of chelonians that are hit by cars. Other common causes of shell injury in captive chelonians are dog bites, thermal, crush, and fall injuries. This chapter will elaborate on triage, repair, and follow-up of shell trauma in tortoises and turtles.

PHILOSOPHY

In general, wild chelonians appear to sustain more severe injuries than captive chelonians, mainly because of traumatic encounters with humans. With respect to wildlife rehabilitation, the author's philosophy is that if a chelonian can be medically and surgically treated and returned to the wild fully functional, medical intervention will be attempted. If the chelonian cannot be returned to the wild fully functional, it will be humanely euthanized. Determining which injuries are not treatable comes with experience, and triaging patients within the first few hours will determine which chelonians can be successfully treated and which cannot. These decisions are difficult, but with limited time and resources available, it is critical to make this decision quickly to save months of work and emotional energy.

TRIAGE OF SHELL TRAUMA

Developing and following a triage system will assist the clinician in formulating a prognosis and implementing a successful treatment course. The following five categories of prognosis have been developed to assist the clinician in prognosis and treatment outcomes.

Excellent Prognosis

Chelonians seen with a single fracture, hairline fracture, or a fracture that does not involve the spine and those with minor road rash or minor dog bite injuries have the best prognosis for a quick and full recovery. Often these turtles are bright and alert and do not appear to be affected by the injury. Stable fractures have the best prognosis. These wounds will heal quickly and may not need more than a few days of supportive care before the animal is released.

Good Prognosis

Chelonians seen with multiple fractures, unstable fractures, mild open fractures, or dog bites with shell puncture have a good prognosis with treatment. Open fractures are characterized by malunion of a fracture with the bone exposed to the coelom or missing pieces of the bony carapace or plastron. If large pieces of shell are missing, this diagnosis may be, instead, considered a fair prognosis; however, if no penetration of the underlying soft tissue has occurred, the prognosis is still good. These animals will need supportive care, surgical stabilization, and hospitalization for a few months (Figure 16-1).

Fair Prognosis

Chelonians with multiple fractures involving the shoulder or pelvic area or penetrating punctures of the coelom have a fair prognosis (Figure 16-2). Multiple fractures that destabilize the shoulder or pelvis may lead to ambulation difficulties. If the leg cannot be used at all, this would be a grave prognosis; the prognosis increases favorably as the ability to move the leg increases. If a chelonian can move the leg and still walk or has 75% normal range of motion, it may be worth pursuing treatment. Aquatic turtles may have a little more leeway because a water environment is more forgiving. However, the rehabilitation philosophy of the practitioner should ultimately guide the course of treatment.

Guarded Prognosis

Chelonians with open fractures with punctures to the viscera have a guarded or poor prognosis. In some cases, tortoises may be seen with intestines trailing from the fracture or large amounts of debris, dirt, and fly larva in the fracture site or fractured limbs. These cases are difficult to treat successfully. Resection of bowel is possible; however, it is sometimes difficult to diagnosis the extent of the trauma. Further workup may be warranted, but more severe cases of this type of wound fall into the grave prognosis category.

† Deceased.

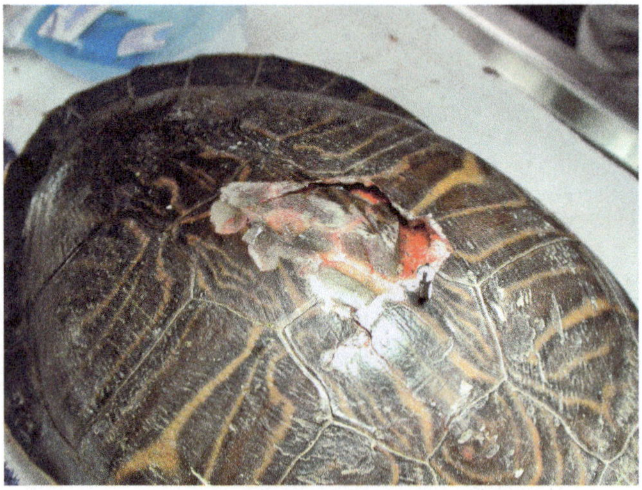

FIGURE 16-1 Good prognosis: image of a Florida Cooter *(Pseudemys floridana)* with a lateral carapace fracture. The fracture is open but not in malunion.

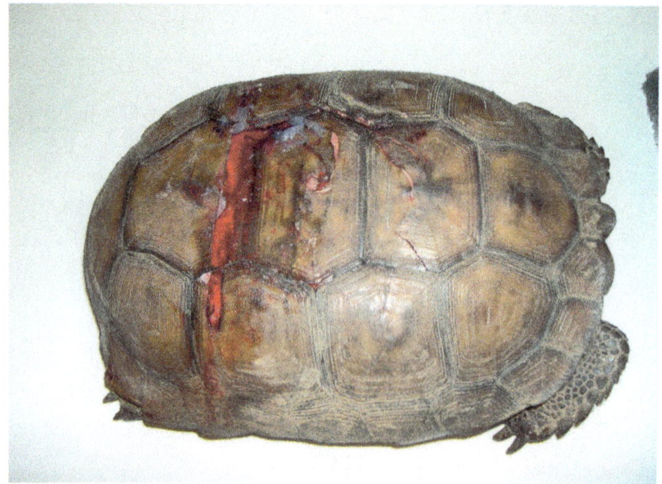

FIGURE 16-3 Grave prognosis: transverse fracture of the dorsal carapace in a Gopher Tortoise *(Gopherus polyphemus)*.

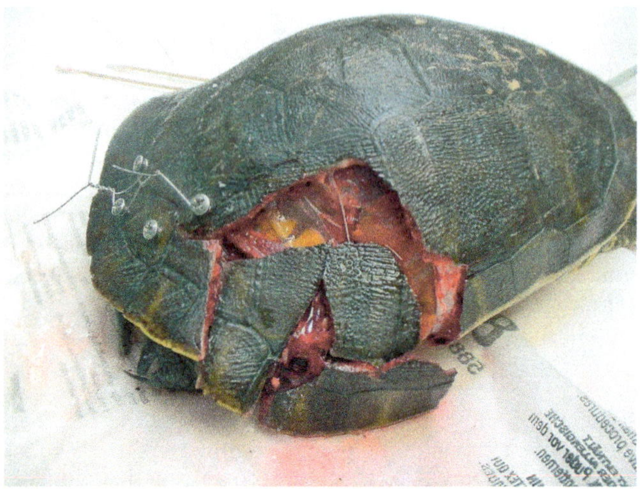

FIGURE 16-2 Fair prognosis: image of a Florida Cooter *(Pseudemys floridana)* with an open, malunion fracture over the right hindleg. Damage to soft tissue around the leg could result in mobility issues with that leg.

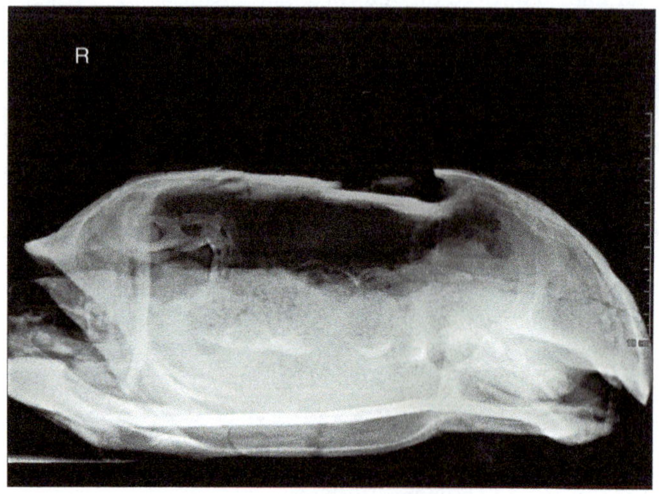

FIGURE 16-4 Lateral radiograph of a Gopher Tortoise *(Gopherus polyphemus)* with a back fracture encompassing the spine.

Grave Prognosis

This group includes chelonians with multiple fractures, internal injuries, head injuries, and, most importantly, fractures incorporating the spine. Spinal injuries are sometimes difficult to assess in tortoises and turtles because of their stoic nature and defensive behaviors. Most spinal injuries in chelonians result in neurologic damage affecting the rear legs. If a fracture can be visualized across the sagittal midline (over the spine) or if the chelonian appears to have neurologic problems, further workup is needed (Figure 16-3). In many cases, even though a fracture may proceed across the spine, it may be difficult to visualize this on radiographs (Figure 16-4). A neuralgic examination, including assessment of sensation and deep pain, may assist in making this diagnosis; however, tortoises are capable of spinal walking, which masks spinal injury. Spinal walking consists of reflexive actions rather than conscious movement. Even if the entire spinal cord is severed, spinal walking is still possible. With spinal injuries, a variety of other problems, such as dennervation of the bladder and lower gastrointestinal tract, are common. In a few of these cases, a tortoise may continue to eat and drink while its urinary bladder and colon enlarges to the point of rupture. If a spinal injury is found, humane euthanasia is suggested. Euthanasia should be completed with euthanasia solution (Beuthanasia-D, Schering-Plough Animal Health, Union, NJ) at 60 to 100 mg/kg. This can be given intravenously, which may prove difficult, or intracoelomically (ICe), which may take up to 12 hours to be completed. An alternative for pet animals is a two-stage euthanasia process, in which the chelonian is anesthetized first and then the euthanasia solution is administered. Intracoelomic injection of barbiturates may adversely affect the histologic features of internal organs.[1]

TRIAGE TREATMENT

Once the chelonian enters the hospital, it should be evaluated immediately for prognosis, and a decision should be made on moving forward with treatment. Once a prognosis has been

TABLE 16-1

Selected Drug Dosages for Chelonians

Drug	Dose	Route	Duration	Comments
Amikacin[10]	5 mg/kg once then 2.5 mg/kg every 72 h	IM	Seven treatments	Not in dehydrated chelonians
Enrofloxacin[10]	5 to10 mg/kg every 72 h	IM or PO	Seven treatments	IM injection may cause pain and inflammation (not recommended)
Ceftazidime[10]	20 mg/kg every 72 h	IM	Seven treatments	Can be stored frozen
Beuthanasia[1]	60 to 100 mg/kg	IV or ICe	Bolus	Euthanasia
Meloxicam[2]	0.1 to 0.4 mg/kg every 24-72 h	IM	3 to 7 days	Analgesia
Tramadol[8]	5 mg/kg every 5 days	PO	Repeat, if needed	Analgesia

ICe, Intracoelomic; *IM*, intramuscular; *IV*, intravenous; *PO*, per os (by mouth).

assigned, analgesics and supportive care should be started immediately.

Analgesia

Although the field of analgesia has been growing over the last 20 years, reptile analgesia has been lagging severely behind mammalian and avian analgesia.[2] Reptiles do not exhibit pain in ways that most veterinarians can recognize; however, it has been shown that many species of reptiles possess antinociception (moving away from a noxious stimulus).[3] For many years, the use of butorphanol was extrapolated because it was shown to have analgesic effects in birds.[4] However, butorphanol has been shown in iguanas and Red-eared Sliders *(Trachemys scripta elegans)* to not be an effective analgesic.[5] Morphine (Baxter Health Care, Deerfield, Ill) (1.5 to 6.5 mg/kg intramuscularly) has produced antinociception in Red-eared Sliders, Freshwater Crocodiles *(Crocodylus johnsoni)*, and *Anolis* lizards.[6-7] Tramadol at 5 mg/kg per os (PO; by mouth), a drug that induces analgesia via both opioid and nonopioid pathways, produced an increase in thermal latency in Red-eared Sliders for 5 days.[8] This is a great way of providing postsurgical analgesia with a single dose. Other drugs such as nonsteroidal antiinflammatories such as meloxicam (Metacam, Boehringer Ingelheim Vetmedica Inc., St. Joseph, Mo) have been developed for analgesia in mammals and have now been used in reptiles.[9] Anecdotal reports that meloxicam is an effective analgesia are widespread. The author has used meloxicam in over 20 species of reptiles at 0.1 to 0.2 mg/kg once daily for 4 to 10 days with positive results. Necropsies by the author on reptiles treated with meloxicam have not shown any secondary kidney effects seen with long-term use of nonsteroidal antiinflammatory drugs in other species but should be considered a complication of treatment.

Fluid Therapy

Most injured chelonians should be considered to be dehydrated from loss of bodily fluids and or lack of fluid intake. This would place them in the mild (<5%) to moderately (7%) dehydrated category.[10] It may be difficult to assess skin tenting in chelonians; however, sunken eyes and changes in packed cell volume (PCV) may be signs of dehydration and and/or blood loss. Reptiles, more so than mammals, can withstand large variations in fluid levels and have developed a larger intracellular fluid volume (48% to 80%) versus extracellular fluid volume (20% to 52%); thus they can withstand longer periods of fluid deficits than mammals.[10]

Nonetheless, fluids should be administered within the first few hours after arrival. For moderate to severe cases of dehydration, parenteral fluid administration is preferred. This can then be followed by oral administration in the days that follow. Fluid maintenance rates for reptiles are less than mammals and range between 10 and 25 mL/kg per day.[10] Fluid selection is also controversial, and long-term use of lactated Ringers may lead to hypokalemia.[11-12] Other fluids such as 0.45% saline with 2.5% dextrose may assist in expanding the intracellular and extracellular spaces, whereas fluids such as Plasma-Lyte and Normosol (Baxter Health Care, Deerfield, Ill) do not contain lactate and have higher levels of potassium.[10-11] In any case, for short-term use (less than 1 week), any of these fluid choices are appropriate and have been used successfully. For chronic disease or longer term administration, please refer to the literature.[10-12]

Antibiotics

The severity of any wound will dictate the use of antibiotics. In most cases, traumatic shell injury warrants the use of antibiotics. In general, antibiotics with a gram-negative spectrum are preferred for reptiles. Chronic wounds and abscesses will need to have culture and sensitivity testing, and the results will then direct the antibiotic choice. A number of different antibiotics from different drug classes can be used; in this chapter, only a few antibiotics are covered (Table 16-1).

Wound Care

Once fluids, antibiotics, and analgesics have been administered, wound care should proceed within the first few hours of presentation. No great differences exist between chelonians—or other reptiles—and mammalian species with respect to wound care. However, a few tricks can assist in treating this unique combination of bony and soft tissue injuries.

Irrigation and Flushing

The basics of irrigation (large volumes of irrigation with a proper pressure) are still applicable. However, with chelonian patients, this may take a team of two people to complete. One person holds the chelonian; they must rotate the chelonian to direct the opening of the wound ventrally to allow for dirt, bone fragments, and other foreign bodies to be flushed from the wound. If the wound is held ventrally, irrigation fluid and debris will not pool inside the coelom of the chelonian. During the first irrigation, a 2% solution

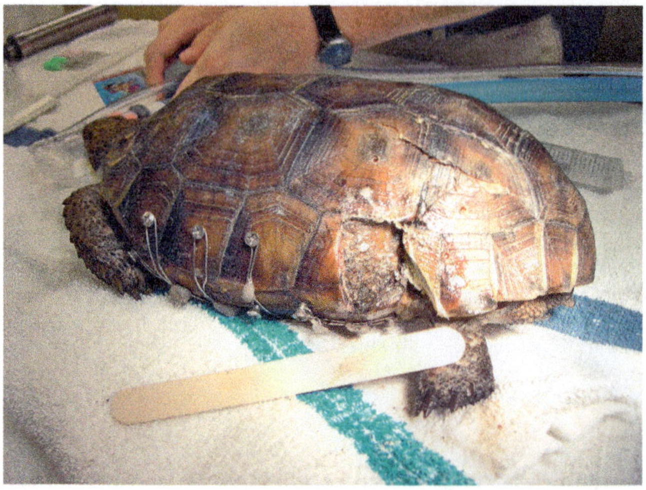

FIGURE 16-5 Mature granulation tissue—brown leatherlike granulation tissue—over an area of missing shell.

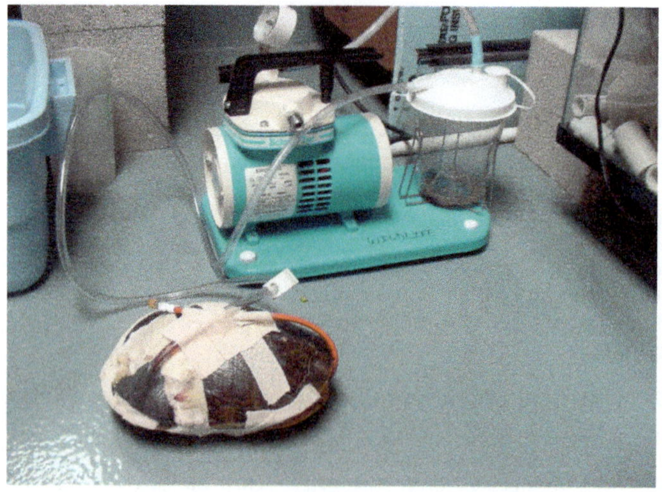

FIGURE 16-6 Vacuum-assisted closure using a suction system.

of chlorhexidine solution (Nolvasan, Fort Dodge, Iowa) is flushed into the wound, followed by sterile saline. This can be completed in a 1:2 ratio (i.e., 1 L 2% chlorhexidine followed by 2 L sterile saline). Depending on the severity of the wound and clinical signs of infection, this may have to be repeated daily (for the first week) and switched to every other day and then weekly, if needed. After the initial flushing, depending on wound conditions, sterile saline should be used alone because chlorhexidine may be cytotoxic to granulation tissues. Avoid using hydrogen peroxide as a flush into wounds or pockets because of the risk of potentially fatal air emboli forming that result from the reaction of the peroxide with the blood and tissues.

Once the wound is irrigated, a wet-to-dry bandage should be applied. Sterile 4 × 4 gauze pads soaked with sterile saline should be applied to the wound, and a layer of dry gauze pads should be laid over the top. This can then be secured to the shell with tape. Elastic tape (Elastikon, Johnson and Johnson) holds to the shell well and allows the wound to breath. This bandage will have to be changed daily. In some cases of severe infection, silver impregnated gauze (Acticoat, Smith and Nephew, Largo, Fla) may be used to reduce infection in open wounds.[12] Wet-to-dry bandages should be replaced daily for the first week because this will reduce contamination and assist with healing. If only closed fractures are present, 1 week of wet-to-dry bandages followed by application of topical silver sulfadiazine (SSD) (Watson Laboratories Inc, Corona, Calif) can be applied to the cracks to assist with pathogen reduction and granulation formation. Wounds can be covered with light bandages to keep additional contamination from occurring.

Open wounds or missing areas of shell will have to be monitored for many months. After the first 2 weeks of wet-to-dry bandaging, the bandages should be changed twice a week. At this point, nonadherent dressing can be applied, followed by gauze and then tape. When the bandage is changed, the wound should be irrigated with saline, as needed. After 1 month, a thick leatherlike granulation bed may form; it may be a brown or gray color but should have no odor (Figure 16-5). Keep this area clean and treat appropriately. By 6 to 8 weeks, the wound may be left unbandaged; however, it should be kept clean with occasional irrigation with saline. Once this thick granulation bed has formed and the surface is dry, the wound does not need bandaging on a daily basis and can be monitored weekly.

Vacuum-Assisted Closure

The use of vacuum-assisted wound management has been described in veterinary medicine (see Chapter 15 for a thorough discussion on vacuum assisted wound closure).[13-14] This technique uses a vacuum to apply constant negative pressure of approximately 125 mm Hg over a wound bed. The negative pressure removes fluid, bacterial load, and other factors that inhibit granulation while stimulating the blood supply in the granulation bed. This technique is best used over missing pieces of shell or severely infected wounds sites.[13] The overall effect of this system is a reduction in the time it takes to heal and a more cosmetic appearance of the wound. Disadvantages include the initial price of the equipment and inexperience of the user, which can be quickly overcome. This system works very well for larger more traumatic wounds or wounds with osteomyelitis and should be considered an excellent treatment choice (Figure 16-6).

AQUATIC TURTLES

The aquatic lifestyle of turtles makes shell wound care more challenging. In general, aquatic turtles can be held out of the water for 10 to 14 days. One case report describes a sea turtle that was dry-docked for over two months while it underwent repair for a large fistula in the plastron.[14] Aquatic turtles must, however, be given fluids PO or ICe and short baths to wet down the shell and skin. Aquatic turtles with simple closed fractures can be kept dry-docked for 7 to 10 days so that wounds can be cleaned and SSD ointment applied. To keep water away from more severe wounds, the veterinarian can apply Ilex ointment (Medcon Biolab Inc, Grafton, Mass), which seals the wound and keeps the water out. This product is available in most pharmacies and is a topical skin cream for infants. When applied over a wound and placed in water, the ointment becomes impervious to the water. It can be applied directly on granulation tissue or mixed with SSD ointment and has no ill effects (Figure 16-7). Ilex can be kept

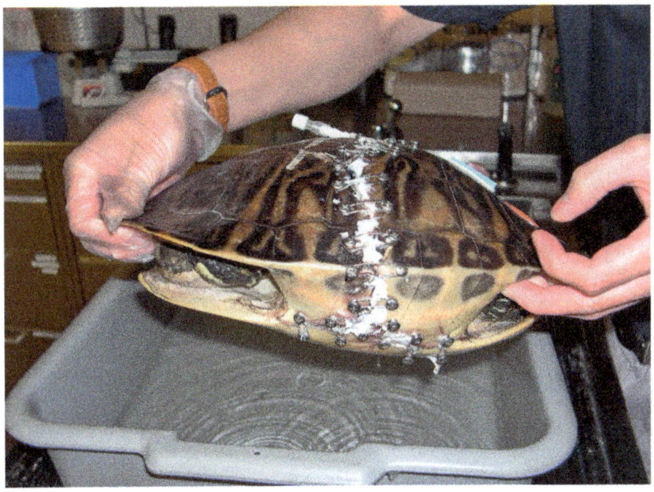

FIGURE 16-7 An aquatic turtle with external fracture fixation with application of a silver sulfadiazine and Ilex mixture over the fracture site.

on large wounds with a piece of transparent wound dressing (Tegaderm, 3M Health, St. Paul, Minn) placed over the Ilex and then glued to the shell with tissue glue. This bandage should be changed, at minimum, every week. Once the thick leatherlike granulation bed is in place, the bandage can be removed and the wound exposed to water. This may change the look of the granulation; however, biweekly flushing with dilute (<2%) chlorhexidine and mild debridement will reduce the pathogen load.

NUTRITIONAL SUPPORT

In most cases, wild chelonians will not eat with any success during their stay the hospital. Wild tortoises may eventually start to eat after 1 month; however, aquatic chelonians rarely will eat while under treatment. To best facilitate enteral nutrition, the placement of a esophagostomy feeding tube is necessary. This is one of the most important tools in supportive care of chelonians and should be completed in every case. In this way, nutritional support, fluids, antibiotics, and analgesics can be given with little handling. It also allows for the chelonian to start eating on its own with the tube in place.

The author has had excellent success using Oxbow Critical Care Herbivore and Carnivore diets (Oxbow Hay Co, Murdock, Nebr). These diets will meet the short-term nutritional needs of both tortoises (herbivore diet) and aquatic turtles (carnivore diet). Both diets are available in a powdered form that mixes easily with water and will pass through the feeding tube without difficulty. Tortoises can be fed 1% to 2% of their body weight every other day, and 1% of their body weight in fluids (water) can alternately be given on opposite days. As the chelonian starts to eat on its own, the feeding schedule can be reduced. Other diets can be prepared in a blender and fed via the feeding tube; however, variations in consistency of the diet fed can block the feeding tube, which may then need to be replaced. In addition, many "homemade diets" are not nutritionally balanced and do not have the caloric density needed for compromised chelonians.

RADIOGRAPHS

Radiographs are important in determining the prognosis of a case. In some cases, fractures to the bony plates of the carapace or plastron may not be visualized because the keratinized epidermal scutes that overlie them may be intact. Thus radiographs will assist in making the diagnosis.

With chelonians, radiographs are taken in three different views. Two of these views are taken with a horizontal beam: craniocaudal (front to back) and lateral. The third view is taken with a vertical beam for a dorsoventral view. These three views allow for the best imaging of a chelonian. The craniocaudal view is useful in assessment of lung fields; however, it can also be used to determine carapace uniformity. In cases of internal injury, the radiographs may also assist in determining the extent of penetration or soft tissue injury (see Figure 16-4).

FRACTURE FIXATION

The current state of shell fracture fixation is continually changing as new techniques and supplies are developed. Many different techniques can be used in part or in combination depending on the situation. The techniques described here have been developed by many individuals and may be used with great success. The use of removable hardware such as screws, bone plates, rods, and wire may be combined with techniques that employ epoxy, hooks, and cable ties (Box 16-1).

Adhesives and Epoxy

The use of epoxy and fiberglass for shell repair in chelonians has been popular for many years. Indeed, for elective plastronotomy closure and nondisplaced fractures, epoxy resin with fiberglass has been the preferred method of closure.[16] However, for traumatic and infected shell injuries, the use of epoxy may not be warranted. Repairing fractured shells with epoxy when a concomitant infected wound is present may result in sealing in the "contamination," resulting in a worse infection and septicemia. Thus fixation with an open system of wires and screws that allows for wound management is preferred. Epoxy putty, cyanoacrylate glue, and two-part epoxy resin have been used successfully in conjunction with bone plates and cable tie attachments to stabilize plastron fractures. The systemic effects of epoxy or fiberglass resin on soft tissues or live bone is not understood and may impede the healing process. The long-term effects on shell growth of chelonians released with epoxy or fiberglass fixation devices is not known, and these adhesives should probably be removed from growing chelonian so as not to impede growth. Nonetheless, epoxy resin is one of many tools that can be used under the correct circumstances for shell fixation.

Fixation with Hardware

For shell fractures that need stabilization, the use of external fixation has provided excellent results. Many of the supplies, such as screws, can be purchased from a home improvement store; however, they should be stainless steel because galvanized screws can release zinc systemically. All fixation devices should be considered contaminated and should be sterilized before use on the chelonian patient.

BOX 16-1 LIST OF EQUIPMENT NEEDED FOR EXTERNAL FIXATION

- Drill, battery operated
- Drill bits, autoclaved or cold sterile prepared
- #6 - ¼-inch flathead Phillips Stainless steel screws (local hardware)
- 18 to 22 gauge stainless wire
- Wire cutters, wire twisters, pliers
- Assortment of rods and plates
- Assortment of hooks, cable ties, and cable tie attachments
- Epoxy putty, two-part epoxy glue, cyanoacrylate glue
- Bandage material
- Silver sulfadiazine ointment, Ilex ointment, sterile saline, chlorhexidine acetate

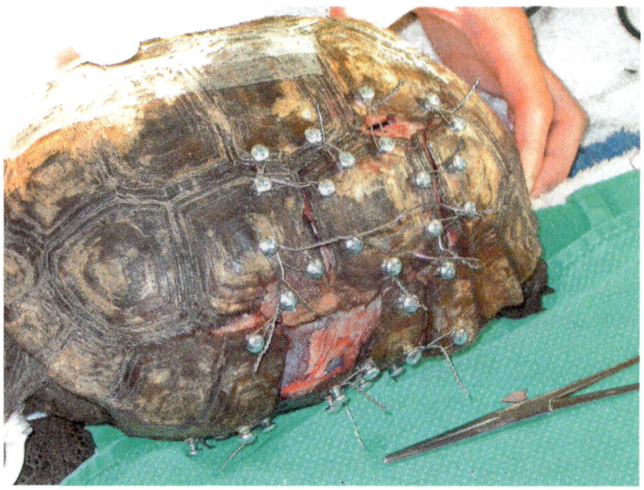

FIGURE 16-8 A Gopher Tortoise *(Gopherus polyphemus)* with a complicated fracture. Multiple wires are being tightened evenly to ensure good shell apposition. A single area of missing shell can be seen in the lateral aspect of the carapace.

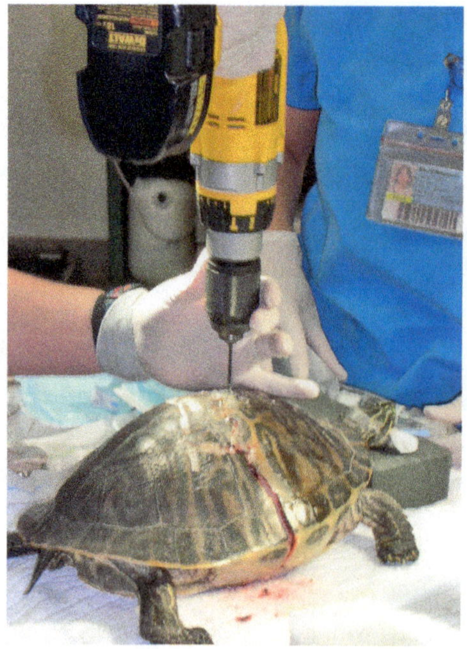

FIGURE 16-9 Use both hands to stabilize the drill when drilling to avoid pushing the drill into the coelomic cavity.

Once the animal is anesthetized, it should be placed on a heated pad while the fixation is performed. In many cases, an assistant may be needed to help position and hold the chelonian while the fixator is being placed. The shell and soft tissue around the fixation area should be surgically prepared. Once the area is prepared and dried, the fixation may take place. Depending on the severity of the fracture, some imagination must be used to piece the shell back together. If there are missing pieces, the surgeon must try to piece the shell together, leaving an open space where the missing piece is (as in a jigsaw puzzle). If the missing pieces total more than 30% of the shell or if the shell cannot be stabilized without the missing pieces, the prognosis is grave. Missing shell fragments are common and occur in about 25% of the cases seen by the author. These fragments vary in size from a ¼ inch to 2 to 3 inches (Figure 16-8).

Screw and Wire Fixation

The screw and wire method of shell fixation may provide the best stabilization in most shell fracture cases. The first step in fixation is to place sterile orthopedic or stainless steel screws where the fixation wire will be attached. First, select a drill bit that is slightly smaller than the screw. Sterilized, Phillips #6 ¼-inch machine stainless steel screws can be used. The machine head looks like a mushroom, and the flat aspect of the ventral screw head provides a secure purchase for holding the wire. When drilling into shell fragments, if possible, stay back at least 0.5 cm from the edge of the fracture to provide proper purchase for the screw and to minimize cracking of the shell. When drilling, be careful not to place too much pressure on the drill as you may sink the bit several centimeters into the coelom and damage the internal organs (see Figure 16-9). Placing a piece of tape around the drill bit at 0.20 cm (⅛ to ¼ inch) of depth will allow for a visual guide to drilling depth. Two hands on the drill with a slow steady force is recommended. Fully penetrating the shell thickness is not a problem as long as trauma to internal organs has not taken place. If drilling is prolonged, heat from the drill may produce necrosis of the tissue. To avoid this, drip sterile saline on the drill bit when engaged. Once a few screws have been placed, the wire should be attached.

To attach the wire, precut a few pieces of wire, 15 cm (6 inches) long (20-gauge stainless steel wire). Wrap the wire around one screw head, cross it over between the screws (like a figure eight), wrap one end around the second screw head, and then wrap the two ends around each other (Figure 16-10). The knot should be between the two screw heads, which allows for the knot to be folded against the shell when completed. At this point, do not tighten the wire with pliers; only hand-tighten it for two to three twists. If a fractured shell fragment is attached to the underlying tissue but not to the rest of the shell, place screws and wires on all sides and then proceed to hand tighten. Tighten alternate sides to make even contact with the surrounding shell. Some small gaps may not close fully but will heal over time. With more severe cases, the entire shell may not stabilize until the last few wires have been tightened. Once tightened, some of the wires may have

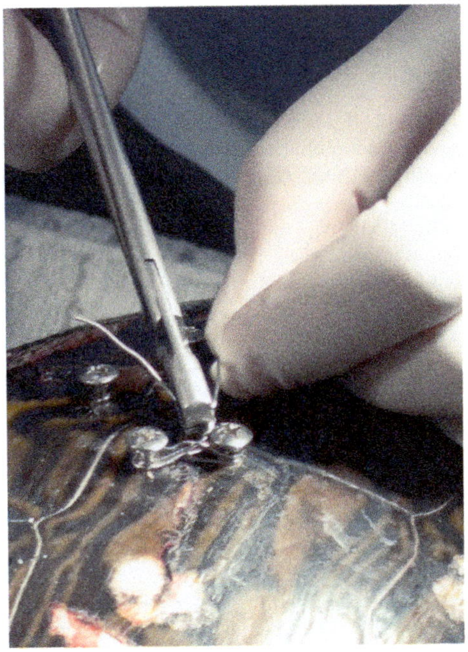

FIGURE 16-10 Stainless steel wire should be placed around the two opposing screw heads in a figure-eight pattern. The knot can then be placed between the two screw caps.

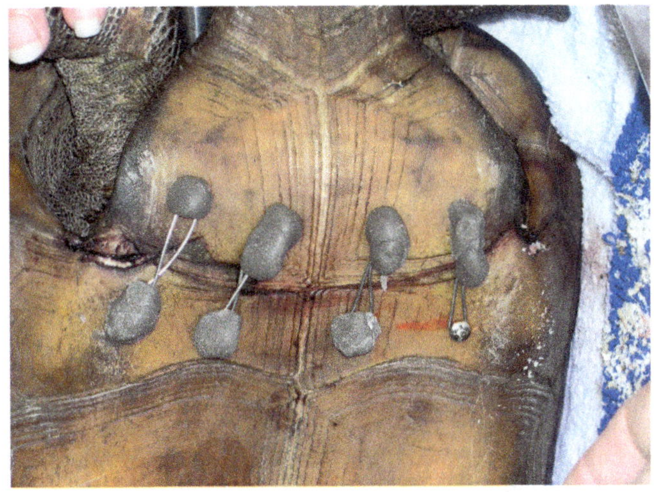

FIGURE 16-11 A small ball of epoxy putty is placed over the twisted wire knot to keep the wire from snagging on substrate.

become loose and should be removed and retightened. When tightening the wire, the surgeon may need to take five to eight twists on the wire; however, do not twist much more or the wire may snap. This takes a little practice. In addition, if the wires are too tight, too much pressure may be placed on the tissue margins, causing pressure necrosis. Once the wires are tightened, use side cutters to remove the twisted knot to the level of four to five twists, and use the pliers to bend the twist down to be parallel with the wire and the shell. In some cases, it may be difficult to flatten the knot against the shell, so a bead of commercial epoxy putty can be used to cover the sharp wire tip (Figure 16-11).

Cable Tie and Hook Fixation

In some cases of nondisplaced shell fractures in which stabilization is needed, an alternate to screw and wire fixation is hook and cable tie attachments (Figure 16-12). This technique is less invasive but, in general, does not provide as much stabilization as the screw and wire method. Plastic grommets or wire hooks are fastened to the shell with glue or epoxy, then wire or cable ties are attached to the grommets/hooks and can be used to stabilize the fracture.[17] For minor fractures or when anesthesia is not available, this technique may be an option and will save time under anesthesia.

Epoxy and Metal Fixation

Plastron fractures are best stabilized with bone plates or flat pieces of metal. In many chelonian species, the plastron is relatively flat, and glue or epoxy can be used to attach a bone plate across the fracture. The low profile of the bone plate will allow for minimal drag when compared with screws and wire, which may become entangled on rough surfaces. Once removed, the bone plate may be resterilized and used for another case.

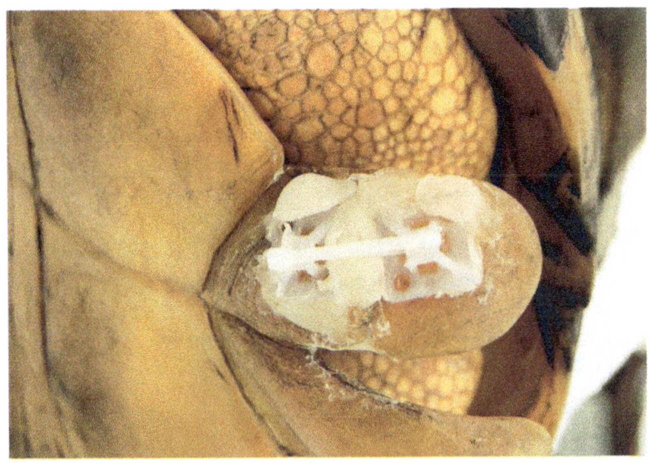

FIGURE 16-12 A gular scute fracture in a Radiated Tortoise *(Astrochelys radiata)*. Cable tie grommets have been adhered to the shell with cyanoacrylate glue, and some epoxy putty has been used around the grommet to smooth the edge down. A cable tie has then been passed through both grommets and tightened to stabilize the fracture site.

Fixation Monitoring and Healing Time

The fixation device should be monitored every few days. Occasionally over time, some of the wires may need some additional tightening. If screws become loose, they should be removed and replaced, if necessary. Healing time should be approximately 4 to 8 weeks, similar to bone in other species. This will depend on the severity of the fracture and the stability of the fixation. Simple closed fractures may have complete bone healing in 4 weeks, whereas more severe cases may take 8 weeks or longer. In more complicated fractures, a staged removal of the screws and wires over 2 to 3 weeks is recommended. Radiographs may be helpful but often do not show callus formation. A better guide to a healed fracture is the stability of the fracture on palpation. If in doubt, leave the fixation device on longer.

Removal of External Fixation

The area of the shell should be prepared just as it would for surgery. This procedure may cause some discomfort but does not require general anesthesia; however, analgesia such as meloxicam or tramadol should be used.[2] Screws may be removed with a screwdriver, and then the holes should be flushed with saline and packed with SSD ointment. This step should be completed twice a week for 2 weeks to ensure that no infection enters the coelom. If the chelonian has more than a few screws, a second 3-week course of antibiotic is indicated (see Table 16-1). Once screws have been removed, the time frame to release could be as little as a week to a month, depending on the number of screw holes present. Epoxy or glues removal may be difficult; thus mineral oil should be applied around the edge of the epoxy and may result in the epoxy popping off the shell. Sometimes the epoxy may have to be ground down; however, care must be taken because the keratin layer on the shell can be easily damaged.

CONCLUSION

Medical and surgical intervention of chelonian shell fractures can be prolonged but rewarding because these reptiles often have life spans greater than 50 years. By rehabilitating an adult chelonian, you are assisting with conservation as well as helping individual animals that are often overlooked.

ACKNOWLEDGMENTS

The author would like to thank the Veterinary Services Department of Disney's Animal Kingdom, including the veterinary technicians, hospital keepers, and wildlife interns who look after the day-to-day needs of these chelonian patients.

REFERENCES

1. Mader DR. Euthanasia. In: Mader DR, ed. *Reptile medicine and surgery*. 2nd ed. St. Louis: Saunders Elsevier, 2006;564–568.
2. Mosley C. Pain and nociception in reptiles. *Vet Clin North Am Exot Anim Pract* 2011;14:45–60.
3. Machin KL. Fish, reptile and amphibian analgesia. *Vet Clin North Am Exot Anim Pract* 2001;4:19–46.
4. Paul-Murphy JR, Brunson DB, Miltec V. Analgesic effects of butorphanol and buprinorphine in conscious African grey parrots (*Psittacus erithacus erithacus* and *Psittacus erithacus timneh*). *Am J Vet Res* 1999;60:1218–1221.
5. Sladky KK, Miletic V, Paul-Murphy JR, et al. Morphine, but not butorphanol, causes analgesia and respiratory depression in the Red-Eared-Slider Turtles (*Trachemys scripta*). *J Am Vet Med Assoc* 2007;230:1356–1362.
6. Kanui TI, Hole K. Morphine and pethidine antinociception in the crocodile. *J Vet Pharmacol Ther* 1992;15:101–103.
7. Mauk MD, Olsen RD, LaHoste GG, et al. Tonic immobility produces hyperalgesia and antagonizes morphine analgesia. *Science* 1981;213:353–354.
8. Baker BB, Sladky KK, Johnson SM. Evaluation of the analgesic effects of oral and subcutaneous tramadol administration in red-eared slider turtles. *J Am Vet Med Assoc* 2011;238:220–227.
9. Read MR. Evaluation of the use of anesthesia and analgesia in reptiles. *J Am Vet Med Assoc* 2004;224:547–552.
10. Mitchel MD. Therapeutics. In: Mader DR, ed. *Reptile medicine and surgery*. 2nd ed. St. Louis: Saunders Elsevier, 2006;631–664.
11. Prezant RM, Jarchow J. Lactated fluid use in the reptile, is there a better solution? in *Proceedings*. 4th Annu Meet Assoc Reptile Amphibian Vet 1997;83–87.
12. Mader DR, Rudloff E. Emergency and critical care. In: Mader DR, ed. *Reptile medicine and surgery*. 2nd ed. St. Louis: Saunders Elsevier, 2006;533–554.
13. Adkesson MJ, Travis EK, Weber MA, et al. Vacuum assisted closure for treatment of a deep shell abscess and osteomyelitis in a tortoise. *J Am Vet Med Assoc* 2007;231:1249–1254.
14. LaFortune M, Wellehan JFX, Heard DJ, et al. Vacuum assisted closure (Turtle VAC) in the management of traumatic shell defects in chelonians. *J Herpetol Med Surg* 2005;15:4–8.
15. Mader DR. The use of a Foretex mesh to repair a traumatic coelomic fistula in a juvenile green sea turtle, Chelonia Mydas. *in Proceedings*. ARAV. Kansas City, MO 1998; 85–86.
16. Mader DR, Bennet RA, Funk RS, et al. Surgery. In: Mader DR, ed. *Reptile medicine and surgery*. 2nd ed. St. Louis: Saunders Elsevier, 2006;581–630.
17. Forrester H, Satta J. Easy shell repair. Available at: http://asianturtlenetwork.org. Accessed 2005.

CHAPTER 17

Video Telescopic Operating Microscope: A Recent Development in Reptile Microsurgery

Stephen J. Divers

THE DEMAND FOR IMPROVED REPTILE SURGERY

High owner expectations, coupled with the fact that most reptile pets weigh less than 2 kg, means that the reptile surgeon has to contend with two major obstacles:

1. A huge diversity in taxa-specific anatomy, physiology, and disease
2. A heavy reliance on magnification for adequate surgical visualization and microsurgical techniques

This need for excellent visualization using a focused light source and magnification have been well-documented and have, in-part, fueled recent developments in minimally invasive endoscopic and endosurgical techniques (see endoscopy chapters).[1-3] Nevertheless, we are far from being able to perform most procedures endoscopically; therefore the need for traditional, open surgical techniques in small reptiles remains of paramount importance.

ILLUMINATION AND MAGNIFICATION: VIDEO TELESCOPIC OPERATING MICROSCOPE

Traditionally, adequate surgical lighting has been achieved by the use of large, focused overhead light units. While magnification can be achieved with the use of operating microscopes, their expense and reduced maneuverability make them less common in most zoologic practices. Instead, headband or frame-mounted operating loupes with a dedicated light source have gained popularity because they are more affordable, versatile, and simpler to operate.

The recent development of a video telescopic operating microscope (VITOM-25, Karl Storz Veterinary Endoscopy America Inc, Goleta, Calif; www.ksvea.com) has provided another option for delivering high-quality focused illumination and magnification. The VITOM uses existing endoscopy equipment, specifically the light source, camera, and documentation hardware that is common in practices, to perform extracorporeal visualization of surgical procedures.

The VITOM 25 system is composed of a 11-cm, zero-degree rod-lens telescope that is held 25 to 60 cm above the surgical site by means of a mechanical arm that clamps to the operating table (Figure 17-1). The system provides a depth of field of 2 to 6 cm and a range of fields of view and magnifications dependent on the distance from the surgical site (Table 17-1). The articulated, mechanical arm has a single lock mechanism that controls all five joint functions, thereby facilitating easy, rapid positioning. A metal clamp holds the telescope and light guide cable in place. Illumination is controlled at the light source, while the surgeon controls zoom, focus, white balance, and photo/video documentation from the camera. The VITOM system is autoclavable and typically sterilized before placement and positioning by sterile surgical staff. The array of potential uses is vast and includes almost any situation in which microsurgery would be an advantage; however, just one example is provided here.

EXPLORATORY COELIOTOMY IN A JUVENILE BEARDED DRAGON

Coeliotomy (laparotomy) is frequently used in reptile medicine and surgery for both diagnosis and treatment.[4-6] Oophorectomy, salpingotomy, salpingectomy, enterotomy, cystotomy, and the collection of visceral biopsy specimens are just some of the reasons for performing coeliotomy. Liver disease is common in reptiles, and although changes in the plasma biochemistry profile may be evident, hepatic biopsy is usually required for a definitive diagnosis.[7,8] Therefore as an illustration of the value of the VITOM in reptile medicine, coeliotomy and liver biopsy in a small Bearded Dragon (*Pogona vitticeps*) are described. The surgical approach to the pet lizard's coelom is complicated, not just by their diminutive size but also by the presence of a significant midline abdominal vein. With the lizard positioned in dorsal recumbency and the VITOM positioned above, a paramedian (or ventral midline) incision is made starting caudal to the umbilicus and extending cranially to the same level as the xiphoid process (Figure 17-2, *A*). Given the paramedian approach, sharp dissection through

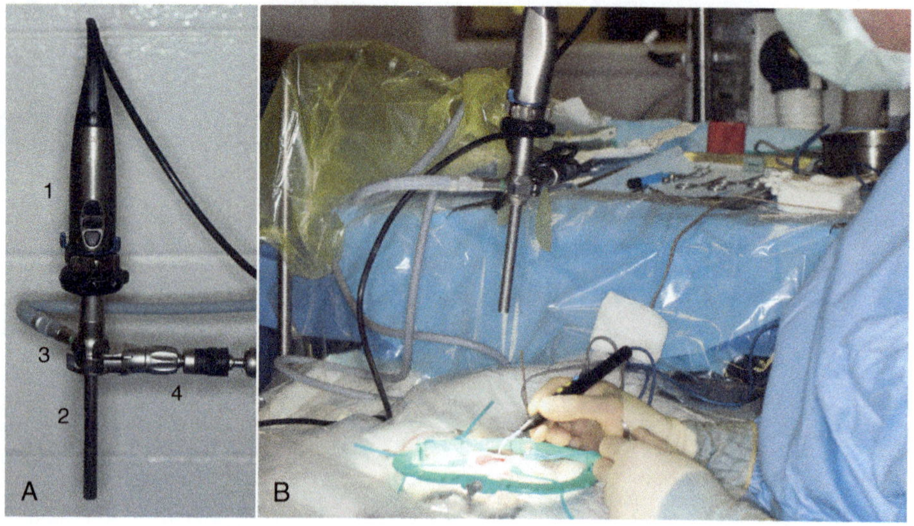

FIGURE 17-1 **A,** Endoscopy camera *(1),* video telescopic operating microscope (VITOM) telescope *(2),* and light-guide cable *(3),* held in place with the clamp and articulated arm *(4).* **B,** Intraoperative view of the VITOM system positioned above the surgical site. *(Photo courtesy Dr. Stephen J. Divers, University of Georgia, Athens, Ga.)*

TABLE 17-1

Specifications of the VITOM System When Used with an Image 1 Camera, Xenon Light Source, and 26-Inch (66 cm) Monitor

	Field of View		Reproduction Scale	
Working distance between telescope and surgical site	Camera zoom ×1	Camera zoom ×2	Camera zoom ×1	Camera zoom ×2
25 cm	5 cm	3.5 cm	8×	16×
50 cm	10 cm	7 cm	4×	8×

VITOM, Video telescopic operating microscope.

muscle causes hemorrhaging; therefore blunt dissection through the rectus abdominis is preferred. An alternative approach through the ventral midline and linea alba has the advantages of less muscle trauma, but greater care may be required to avoid damaging the abdominal vein. Retraction of the skin and muscle with a ring retractor and elastic stays helps expose the coelomic viscera (Figure 17-2, *B*). Given the right paramedian approach, the gallbladder is obvious; however, biopsy from the caudal edge of the right liver lobe is still practical even in small lizards. A single loop of polydioxanone 3/0 suture is placed over the protruding margin of the right liver lobe in for performance of a guillotine biopsy procedure (Figure 17-2, *C*). The suture is tightened to crush the surrounding hepatic tissue (Figure 17-2, *D*) before a scalpel is used to excise the tissue distal to the suture (Figure 17-2, *E*). After hemostasis is ensured, the ventral coelomic musculature is closed in a simple continuous pattern with 5/0 polydioxanone, while the skin is closed with 4/0 polydioxanone in an everting horizontal mattress pattern (Figure 17-2, *F*).

CONCLUSION

The VITOM system uses a practice's existing endoscopy equipment to provide a novel way for performing open microsurgical procedures in an ergonomic manner. The additional costs associated with the VITOM telescope and mechanical arm ($16,000) are 25% higher than those associated with high-quality headband or frame-mounted loupes with xenon light sources and high-definition cameras (e.g., SurgiTel, Ann Arbor, Mich; www.surgitel.com). However, advantages of the VITOM system include the following:

- Utilization of existing endoscopy equipment, including photodocumentation for publications, client education, and practice marketing
- Rapid positioning and ability to quickly reposition and refocus during surgery
- Good ergonomic positioning: the surgeon can sit or stand and face forward instead of down
- Variable magnification with a good depth of field that avoids instrument movements going in and out of focus
- Static positioning advantages:
  - The entire operating room team can follow the procedure
  - High-quality photographs and video can be taken with less image blurring and video editing
  - Avoidance of obstruction of the video field by the surgeon's head (a common complication associated with in-light cameras)
- Advantages to having the entire surgical team observe the procedure from the monitor:
  - Veterinary students, interns, and residents can be taught
  - Assistants can more easily anticipate the surgeon's needs

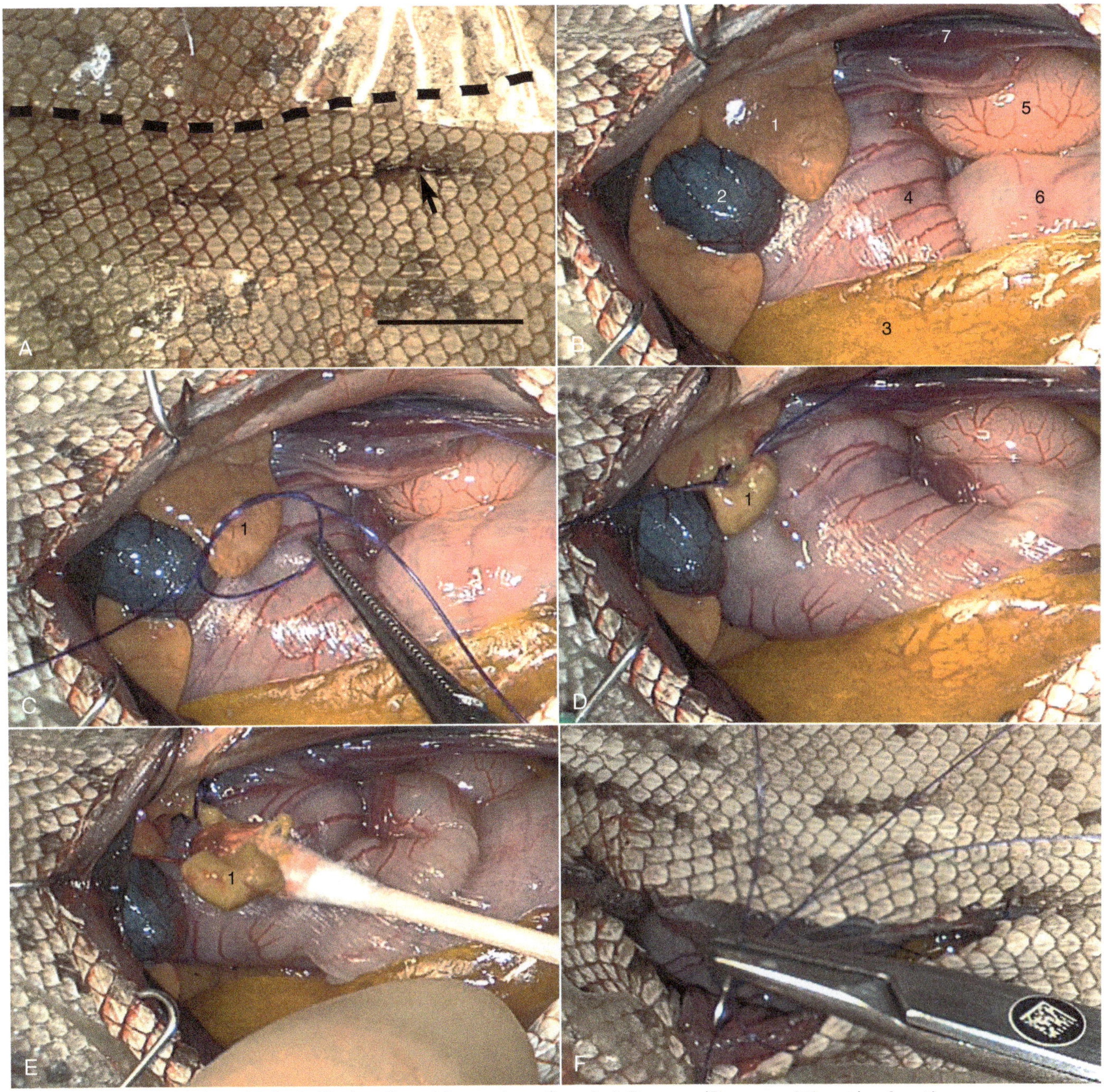

FIGURE 17-2 Guillotine liver biopsy in a Bearded Dragon *(Pogona vitticeps)* using the VITOM system. **A,** View of the ventrum indicating the start of the paramedian coeliotomy incision *(arrow)* and the position of the midline and ventral abdominal vein *(dotted line).* Bar, 10 mm. **B,** View of the exposed coelomic viscera including the liver *(1),* gallbladder *(2),* fatbody *(3),* stomach *(4),* testis *(5),* large intestine *(6),* and ventral abdominal vein *(7).* **C,** Placement of 3/0 polydioxanone suture around the caudal margin of the right liver lobe *(1).* **D,** Tightening the suture to isolate the liver biopsy *(1).* **E,** Removal of the liver biopsy *(1)* after sharp dissection distal to the suture. **F,** Closing the rectus abdominis muscle using 5/0 polydioxanone suture in a continuous pattern. *VITOM,* Video telescopic operating microscope. *(Photo courtesy Dr. Stephen J. Divers, University of Georgia, Athens, Ga.)*

High-quality illumination and magnification require significant capital investment, but poor-quality equipment results in reduced optical quality and suboptimal surgical performance. Veterinarians with existing endoscopy light sources and cameras should consider the VITOM system as a viable alternative to traditional magnification systems.

ACKNOWLEDGMENTS

Thanks goes to Dr. Chris Chamness and Karl Storz Endoscopy for donating the VITOM system to the College of Veterinary Medicine, University of Georgia and for granting permission to reproduce material, written by the author, from a general exotic animal microsurgery article published by Karl Storz Endoscopy.

REFERENCES

1. Divers SJ. Reptile diagnostic endoscopy and endosurgery. *Vet Clin North Am Exot Anim Pract* 2010;13:217-242.
2. Hernandez-Divers SJ. Diagnostic and surgical endoscopy. In: Raiti P, Girling S, eds. *Manual of reptiles*. 2nd ed. Cheltenham, England: British Small Animal Veterinary Association, 2004;103-114.
3. Divers SJ. Exotic pets. In: Tams TR, Rawlings CA, eds. *Small animal endoscopy*. 3rd ed. St. Louis: Elsevier, 2011;623-654.
4. Mader DR, Bennett RA, Funk RS, et al. Surgery. In: Mader DR, ed. *Reptile medicine and surgery*. 2nd ed. St. Louis: Elsevier, 2006;581-630.
5. Hernandez-Divers SJ. Surgery: principles and techniques. In: Raiti P, Girling S, eds. *Manual of reptiles*. 2nd ed. Cheltenham, England: British Small Animal Veterinary Association, 2004;147-167.
6. Hernandez-Divers SJ. Diagnostic techniques. In: Mader DR, ed. *Reptile medicine and surgery*. 2nd ed. St. Louis: Elsevier, 2006;490-532.
7. Divers SJ. Reptilian liver and gastro-intestinal testing. In: Fudge AM, ed. *Laboratory medicine avian and exotic pets*. Philadelphia: WB Saunders, 2000;205-209.
8. Hernandez-Divers SJ, Cooper JE. Hepatic lipidosis. In: Mader DR, ed. *Reptile medicine and surgery*. 2nd ed. St. Louis: Elsevier, 2006;806-813.

CHAPTER 18

Analgesia

Kurt K. Sladky

Veterinary clinical medicine typically lags behind human clinical medicine by several decades. Veterinary analgesia is one such discipline. While the focus in human analgesia is on chronic and neuropathic pain, as well as the molecular mechanisms associated with pain, the focus in veterinary medicine continues to be complications associated with pain measurement, drug efficacy, duration of drug effects, and appropriate routes of administration. Our current understanding of reptile pain and analgesia has advanced within the past 5 years; however, there is much to be learned and some veterinary clinicians continue to debate whether reptiles experience pain.

To put the issue into historical perspective, less than four decades ago, it was routine for human physicians to forego administering analgesic drugs to human infants, even after they had undergone invasive surgical procedures. Before the late 1970s, clinical and empiric research on human pain and pain management focused entirely on adults. Pain management for infants and young children was nonexistent, and surgery was typically performed with only paralytics on board. For example, one of the most common surgical procedures performed on premature babies was thoracotomy for ligation of a patent ductus arteriosus, which most surgeons and anesthesiologists believed was best accomplished with the use of oxygen and pancuronium as the sole anesthetic regimen.[1] At the time, it was hypothesized that human infants had an immature central and peripheral nervous system, which was neither structurally nor functionally capable of receiving and processing noxious stimuli. Because infants are nonverbal, measurement of pain was considered difficult if not impossible. The thinking was that analgesic drugs not only would be ineffective but also would contribute to deleterious physiologic side effects, which would further jeopardize the recovery and, ultimately, the health of the child. During the 1980s and 1990s, clinical analgesia research focusing on human full-term and premature babies blossomed, and we now understand the following: nociceptive neural pathways are fully developed and in place in humans by 22 to 24 weeks' gestation,[2] and nonverbal human infants can respond to pain using vocalizations, facial expressions, body movements, changes in respiratory and heart rate, changes in skin color, and metabolic changes. With this in mind, is it any wonder that we are just beginning to understand nonhuman mammalian pain and analgesia? The acceptance of nonverbal human infants being able to perceive and express pain was a breakthrough and a prelude to a new focus on veterinary analgesia.

Many veterinary clinicians continue to argue that the administration of analgesics is risky to the patient and may mask behavioral signs of pain, which are considered evolutionarily adaptive for survival. This remains particularly true when nonmammalian patients are considered. This issue was expressed in a survey of members of the Association of Reptile and Amphibian Veterinarians.[3] Most respondents (98%) believed that reptiles were capable of experiencing pain, but relatively few clinicians actually administered analgesics to reptiles under conditions in which they would administer analgesics to mammals. The implication from the survey data collected was that there were too many unknowns, recognition of pain was difficult, there was concern about detrimental side effects from analgesic administration, dosages and duration of effect were anecdotal, no pharmacokinetic data were available, and, at the time of the survey, published efficacy data were uncommon. Since that survey, we now recognize that, at some level, reptiles experience pain, and while there is interest in treating pain in reptile patients, we remain unsure if the chosen drugs, dosages, or duration of administration are effective or whether the chosen analgesic will have deleterious consequences. Added to this, the diversity of the class Reptilia makes it difficult to extrapolate analgesic efficacy from one species to the next. Regardless, veterinarians have an ethical obligation to treat painful conditions in all animals because effective pain management reduces stress-induced disruption to homeostatic mechanisms and also decreases morbidity and mortality associated with trauma or surgery. Therefore the primary objective of this chapter is to describe and highlight the most current information with respect to pain and analgesia in reptiles.

REPTILE NOCICEPTION OR PAIN?

Do reptiles feel pain? Can we recognize pain in reptiles? Is the perception of pain by a reptile equivalent to that of a mammal? Does it make anatomic or physiologic sense that the ability to perceive and respond to an aversive stimulus is evolutionarily limited to mammals? We will never be able to objectively answer these questions because reptiles simply cannot tell us. However, like nonverbal human infants or nonhuman mammals, should the inability to communicate dictate whether pain is being perceived or whether an analgesic drug should be administered? I would argue, emphatically, no. By anthropocentric definition, the word *pain* implies higher level cortical processing of information; therefore nociception and antinociception are used when referring to pain and analgesia in most nonmammalian species. This stems from the controversy concerning whether nonmammalian species have the appropriate central and peripheral nervous system structures and pathways capable of "receiving and processing" noxious stimuli and responding appropriately. In other words, can nonmammals "experience" pain, or are they merely capable of demonstrating a "reflexive" response to a noxious stimulus, that is, nociception? Based on published neuroanatomic, neurophysiologic, and behavioral data, reasonable evidence suggests that, structurally and functionally, reptiles have the capacity to experience pain. Therefore, as clinicians, because of limited understanding of pain and analgesia in reptiles, we should err on the side of reptile patient well-being and make the assumption that conditions considered painful in humans and other mammals should be assumed to be painful across all other vertebrate species, including reptiles.

NEUROANATOMIC AND NEUROPHYSIOLOGIC EVIDENCE

Nociceptive Pathways

It is adaptive for all animals to avoid aversive stimuli in the environment as an ultimate mechanism for survival; therefore all vertebrates have specialized sensory receptors, nociceptors that are capable of detecting noxious stimuli (e.g., thermal, mechanical, and chemical receptors), and afferent pathways relaying this information to the central nervous system. Efferent pathways exist to initiate a response, typically a movement away from the noxious stimulus. Therefore for any vertebrate organism to "perceive" a painful stimulus, the following must exist: a peripheral sensory receptor (e.g., nociceptor), a sensory pathway to the spinal cord, initial processing of the painful stimulus within the spinal cord dorsal horn, ascending pathways to the brain, processing of the painful stimulus by the brain, and descending pathways, which exert control over the withdrawal, escape, or defensive or immobile responses. Like mammals, reptiles have all of the anatomic structures considered critical for the recognition of pain: peripheral nociceptors, appropriate central nervous system structures and pathways, opioid receptors and endogenous opioids, reduction of nociceptive response with analgesics (although data are sparse), pain avoidance learning, and suspension of normal behavior with pain.[4-6] Recent research in fish, amphibians, reptiles, and birds has demonstrated the transmission of peripheral sensory signals, via the spinal cord, to midbrain and forebrain regions that are homologous to mammalian cortical and limbic structures.[7-10] Thus the physiologic and anatomic requirements for pain and analgesia appear to be remarkably similar among all vertebrate species.

Nociceptors

Although peripheral nociceptors have not been identified specifically in reptiles, nociceptors are highly conserved across phyla from invertebrates to fish, amphibians, birds, and mammals.[11] Nociceptors have been identified in aquatic and terrestrial invertebrates, teleost fish, amphibians, and birds.[9,10] The only reason nociceptors have not been specifically identified in reptiles is, simply, because nobody has looked.

Functionally, all nociceptors do not respond to the same stimuli. Some may be specifically mechanoreceptors, chemical receptors, or thermoreceptors, and some nociceptors may be multimodal and respond to a variety of different noxious stimuli. Unfortunately, Reptilia are among the least studied taxa with respect to the presence of nociceptors, nociceptive pathways, and central nervous system involvement. In Pit Vipers, touch and thermosensitive and thermomechanosensitive nociceptive neurons were identified in the trigeminal ganglia.[12] Mechanonociceptors were identified in the cutaneous plantar nerve of the American Alligator (*Alligator mississippiensis*) and some of these mechanoreceptors also responded to a noxious thermal stimulus greater than 40°C.[13]

ASCENDING (AFFERENT), CEREBRAL CORTICAL, AND DESCENDING (EFFERENT) PATHWAYS

We know from the mammalian literature that noxious sensory information is initially detected by cutaneous afferents, the cell bodies of which are in the dorsal root ganglia of the spinal cord, and can be separated into two main groups according to axon caliber and myelination: large diameter, myelinated A fibers and small diameter, unmyelinated C fibers.[9] As with mammals, fish, amphibians, and reptiles have myelinated and unmyelinated afferent fibers running together in sensory nerves: large, myelinated A fibers (Aβ); small, myelinated A fibers (Aδ); and small, unmyelinated C fibers (C).[10,14] In amphibians, small, slowly conducting fibers (Aβ and C) transmitted the majority of all impulses induced by noxious heat, pinching, pin pricks, and the application of dilute acetic acid to the skin.[14] Limited published data exist for reptiles. In Pit Vipers, Aβ fibers were shown to respond to nonnoxious mechanical stimuli and to have larger somata, whereas Aδ fibers responding to noxious mechanical stimulation had smaller somata.[12]

Sensory information detected by nociceptors and carried by the cutaneous afferents is transmitted to the dorsal horn of the spinal cord and continues to the brain to activate systems responsible for producing the sensation of pain and the motivational-affective responses that accompany the experience of pain. In mammals, substance P, a peptide that is present in small primary afferents, nerves, and in the dorsal and ventral horns of the spinal cord, is expressed in direct association with painful stimuli. Substance P is highly conserved in mammalian and nonmammalian species, including invertebrates, fish, amphibians, reptiles, and birds. Specifically in reptiles, substance P is present in the nervous system of several turtle species.[15,16]

Transmission of sensory information moves from the spinal cord to the brain. In mammals, pain-related activity detected by the thalamus spreads to the insular cortex, (believed to process the feelings that distinguish, for example, pain from itching) and to the anterior cingulate cortex (believed to control the motivational element of pain). The transmission of nociceptive information from the peripheral to the central nervous system is likely the function of several different ascending pathways originating from neurons located within the spinal cord gray matter. The axons of these neurons travel within the spinal cord white matter, and they terminate in higher centers, including several parts of the thalamus and the brainstem reticular formation.[17] In mammals, the ascending tracts in the anterolateral quadrant of the spinal cord that seem most likely to mediate pain are the spinothalamic, spinoreticular, and spinomesencephalic tracts.[18] Neurons belonging to these pathways project chiefly contralaterally, and recordings in mammalian experiments have demonstrated the presence of nociceptive neurons among the cells of origin of all of these pathways.[18] It was hypothesized that the sensory aspects of pain are mediated primarily by the spinothalamic tract and that the motivational-affective aspects result from activity in all three of these pathways. In reptiles, although the same basic ascending sensory pathways for the visual, auditory, and somatosensory systems are present, they involve fewer cell groups or subdivisions of cell groups in the thalamus and pallium compared with homologous pathways in birds and mammals.[19-23]

The telencephalon of reptiles, birds, and mammals consists of two major subdivisions: the pallium and the subpallium. The subpallium, also called the basal ganglia, is further divided into two main subdivisions: the striatum and pallidum. The striatum and pallidum are also thought to contribute to the septum and subpallial amygdala (central and medial nuclei). The subpallial components are relatively conserved in their organization among amniotes.[24,25] The neocortex of mammals, as a derivative of the dorsal pallium, is homologous as a field only to the hyperpallium of birds and the dorsal cortex of lizards/turtles. The dorsal pallium is present in all amniotes and shares a number of similar cell types and connections across phyla.[26] The organization of the reptile pallium is not yet as well-defined, but it consists of the dorsal cortex and the dorsal ventricular ridge (DVR), as well as olfactory, hippocampal, and pallial amygdala regions. The reptile anterior dorsal ventricular ridge (ADVR) is a large intraventricular protrusion in the reptilian forebrain, which receives information from many different sensory modalities and, in turn, projects massively into the striatum. The ADVR possesses functional similarities to the mammalian isocortex and may perform complex sensory integrations. The ADVR in lizards is composed of three longitudinal zones, which receive visual, somatosensory, and acoustic info. These projections are relayed by the thalamic nuclei.[8] The posterior part of the dorsal ventricular ridge (PDVR) is considered an associative center that projects to the hypothalamus, thus being comparable to the amygdaloid formation. Evidence suggests that the PDVR and neighboring structures constitute the reptilian basolateral amygdala and indicate that an emotional brain was already present in the ancestral amniote.[27]

The descending motor pathways from the hypothalamus and brainstem to the spinal cord in the quadrupedal reptiles studied (turtles [Red-eared Slider, *Trachemys scripta elegans,* and Hermann's Tortoise, *Testudo hermanni*] and lizards [Gold Tegu, *Tupinambis nigropunctatus,* and Savannah Monitor, *Varanus exanthematicus*]) appear to show remarkable similarities to pathways in mammals with regard to their cells of origin and their spinal cord trajectory.[28] In the reptiles studied, the presence of interstitiospinal, vestibulospinal, and reticulospinal pathways could be demonstrated. The crossed reticulospinal tracts regulate the sensitivity of flexor responses to ensure that only noxious stimuli elicit the responses. A crossed rubrospinal tract has been shown in some turtles and lizards but could not be demonstrated in the Python.[29] A small rubrospinal tract was demonstrated in a colubrid snake species (Watersnake, *Nerodia* sp).[30] The nonexistent or reduced rubrospinal tract in snakes is believed to be associated with limblessness. In the Large Psammodromus, efferent fibers from the dorsal cortex reach the rostral midbrain tegmentum, and it was suggested that this was the reptilian representation of the sensorimotor cortex.[31] A similar corticoefferent pathway was described in turtles after lesions in the general cortex.[31] In Tokay Geckos *(Gekko gecko),* anterograde-labeled fibers were observed in the same tegmental area after a tracer injection into different locations of the dorsal cortex.[31] Although axon terminals were not described in the Tokay Gecko midbrain tegmentum, thus far reptile data strongly suggest the presence of a corticoreticulospinal motor pathway. This pathway originates from the rostral dorsal cortex, and it may represent the anatomic substrate for a motor pallium in reptiles, which is comparable to the avian "motor pallium," both topologically and with respect to the organization of efferent pathways.[31] In addition, in Red-eared Sliders, the determination of a descending pathway linking cortical regions with the red nucleus via the hypothalamus suggested indirect cortical control of the reptilian rubrospinal system.[32] Altogether, these findings suggest that the presence of functionally segregated thalamocortical projections is a conserved feature of brain organization among amniotes.

OPIOID RECEPTORS AND ENDOGENOUS OPIOIDS

The opioid receptor gene family is highly conserved across multiple vertebrate orders (e.g., bovids, chickens, bullfrogs, and teleost and elasmobranch fishes),[11] but there is limited information on opioid receptors in reptiles. The three main opioid receptors, μ, δ, and κ, were cloned and sequenced in three nonmammalian vertebrates: the Zebrafish *(Danio rerio),* the Northern Leopard Frog *(Rana pipiens),* and the Rough-skinned Newt *(Taricha granulosa).*[33-35] In aquatic turtles, μ- and δ-opioid receptors are located throughout the brain, and δ-opioid receptors are more abundant than μ-opioid receptors.[36] However, results of the study did not determine the location and distribution of μ- and δ-opioid receptors in the spinal cord (where nociceptive inputs enter the central nervous system) of turtles, nor were κ-opioid receptors examined anywhere in the central nervous system. With respect to endogenous opioid-related neurotransmitters, proenkephalin-derived peptides are present in turtles with a distribution similar to that in mammals and birds.[37] In addition, the reptilian brain (aquatic slider turtles, American Alligators, and anole lizards) was found to contain large quantities of endogenous enkephalins, also known as endorphins (Met-enkephalin, Leu-enkephalin, and Met-enk-Arg-Phe [MERF]).[38]

MEASUREMENT AND QUANTIFICATION OF PAIN AND ANALGESIA IN REPTILES

Measuring pain in any species, particularly reptiles, is the most difficult hurdle in the study of pain and analgesic efficacy. For example, as veterinarians, do we assume that this Bearded Dragon or that sea turtle is experiencing some level of pain and should we attempt to provide an analgesic to make them more comfortable (Figures 18-1 and 18-2)? In mammals, it is well-established that perioperative pain management facilitates recovery and healing, reduces morbidity and mortality, and contributes to more rapid return to normal behavior.[39-41]

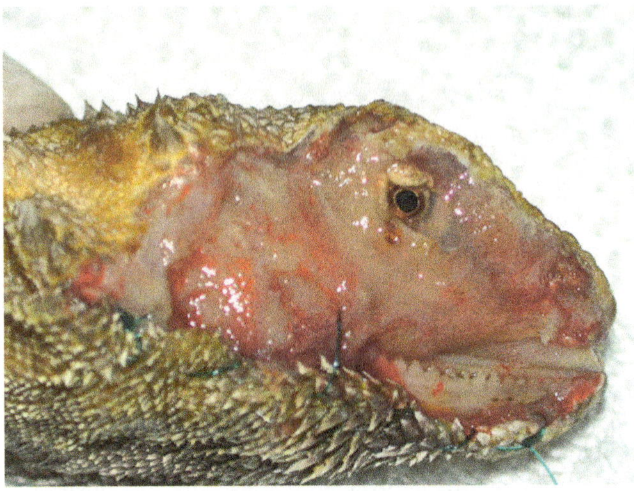

FIGURE 18-1 Bearded Dragon *(Pogona vitticeps)* with complete skin sloughing of the right side of the face due to *Chrysosporium* anamorph of *Nannizziopsis vriesii* (CANV) infection.

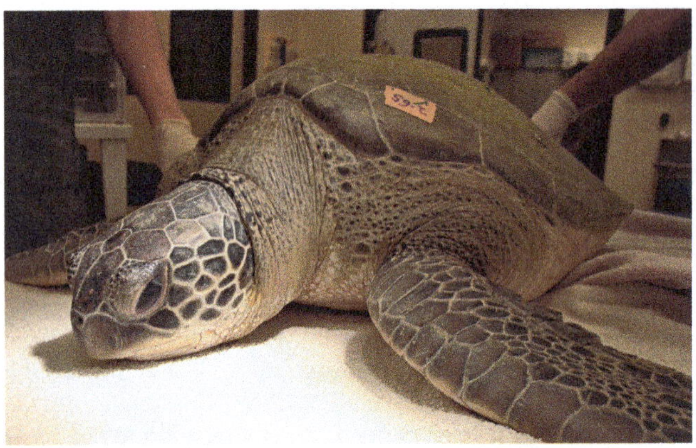

FIGURE 18-2 Green Sea turtle *(Chelonia mydas)* shortly after being struck by a boat propeller; the turtle was being treated at the Georgia Sea Turtle Center, St. Catherines Island, Georgia. *(Courtesy Dr. Terry M. Norton, Georgia Sea Turtle Center, Jekyll Island, Ga.)*

Why not consider this as salient in nonmammalian species? If measuring pain in mammals is challenging, how do we begin to decipher pain-related behavior in reptiles? An objective understanding of normal behavior of a particular species and the ability to differentiate the presence of abnormal behavior indicative of discomfort are critical to the study of pain and analgesia. Therefore one must first have an understanding of normal species-specific behavior within the environmental context in which that behavior is being displayed or observed, to be able to discriminate behavior associated with pain. For example, observing the postovariectomy behavior of an adult female Green Iguana in its own home cage may be different than behavior of the same animal under the same postovariectomy conditions observed in a hospital setting. This is certainly true in some mammalian species.[42] Methods for assessing and measuring pain in reptiles have been described previously.[41] Ideally, a combination of appropriate behavioral and physiologic variables might best be used to measure pain and analgesia in reptiles. Along those same lines, the development of a species- and context-specific ethogram for each species being evaluated would provide the best method for distinguishing normal versus abnormal (e.g., painful) behaviors. Most commonly, animal pain, or lack thereof, is assessed before and after some invasive procedure, such as a surgical procedure. This method requires the development of a behavioral ethogram, which, in turn, requires the observer to become well-versed in subtle behavioral differences through many hours of observation and analysis (videotaped or live observation). Behaviors must be operationally defined, which will provide objectivity and reproducibility (Box 18-1). For example, in a recent study, our laboratory developed a behavioral ethogram to evaluate preoperative and postoperative behavioral responses to food intake, willingness to swim, and breathing in Red-eared Sliders after unilateral orchidectomy.[43] We were able to compare postoperative behavior in turtles with and without analgesic administration of morphine, butorphanol, and saline. Our hypothesis was that preoperative behaviors would return to normal more rapidly in those turtles receiving a μ-opioid receptor agonist analgesic. We demonstrated that those turtles receiving morphine and undergoing unilateral gonadectomy returned to normal preoperative behavior more quickly than those receiving saline or butorphanol. An alternative to studying postsurgical pain is to measure pain under strictly controlled laboratory conditions with the use of established behavioral models during which noxious stimuli (e.g., mechanical, thermal, or chemical) are applied to an anatomic location on the reptile subject.[44-48]

Analgesic drugs can be administered, and the response can be compared with baseline responses. The application of a noxious thermal stimulus provides a well-established behavioral model for assessing pain and analgesia in rodents.[49] In our own studies, we have successfully adapted this classic thermal nociception model developed for use in rodents and determined that reptiles show unambiguous, easily quantifiable withdrawal responses indistinguishable from rodents.[6,44-46] The thermal hindlimb withdrawal latency model uses a noxious thermal stimulus applied to the plantar surface of the hindlimb or the ventral surface of the body (e.g., snake species) of different reptile species (Figures 18-3 and 18-4). A withdrawal latency is automatically determined when the animal withdraws its limb or tail from the noxious stimulus. This model has many advantages over other noxious stimulus paradigms, including rapid application and decay of the noxious stimulus (thereby not causing long-lasting inflammation), instant latency quantification, and unambiguous behavior after stimulus exposure (either the animal does or does not withdraw its limb). Most importantly, the animal can escape the noxious stimulus by simply withdrawing its limb. While some might argue that a withdrawal response to a noxious stimulus is not equivalent to pain, there is evidence in a variety of species that noxious thermal stimulation causes molecular and cellular changes in the central nervous system.[50-52] As a qualification to the noxious thermal stimulus, some have suggested that reptiles are prone to thermal burns; therefore they are less likely to respond to a noxious thermal stimulus. While our understanding of thermal burns in reptiles is inadequate, there is no doubt that all reptile species studied in our laboratory perceive and respond to the focal heat source in an manner identical to that of mammals. In fact, of the hundreds of healthy reptiles across multiple species subjected to a noxious thermal stimulus applied to either the plantar surface of the hindlimb or various areas of the ventral

BOX 18-1 BEHAVIORAL AND PHYSIOLOGIC PARAMETERS ASSOCIATED WITH PAIN IN REPTILES

- Absence of normal behavior
- Hunched posture
- Increased aggression with manual manipulation
- Rubbing affected area (e.g., incision site or wound)
- Skin color changes, especially general darkening
- Head extended away, and ventrally directed, from body; especially obvious in chelonians
- Lameness: graded as 0 (no lameness), 1 (barely perceptible lameness), 2 (lameness always perceptible), and 3 (non-weight-bearing lameness)
- Changes in consumptive behavior (food consumption):
  - Scored as percentage of total food consumed in a 24-hour period
  - Food intake can be quantified based on quantity or weight of food source within a given time limit (e.g., number of pellets consumed/number of pellets offered within 24 hours in aquatic turtles)
- Lack of activity:
  - Duration (in seconds/minutes) of spontaneous and voluntary movement within the tank during each observation period
  - Active versus complete reluctance to move
  - Location within the enclosure during each observation period
- Interactive behavior: immediate response to approaching observer/object
  - Oblivious to environment; nonresponsive to interaction
  - Partial retreat: attempted movement away from observer/object
  - Full retreat: unambiguous movement away from the observer/object
- Rate of respiration: scored as number of breaths per minute at each observation period
- Heart rate: not particularly useful in reptiles. Scored as beats per minute using a stethoscope or Doppler flow probe, although handling may confound the results

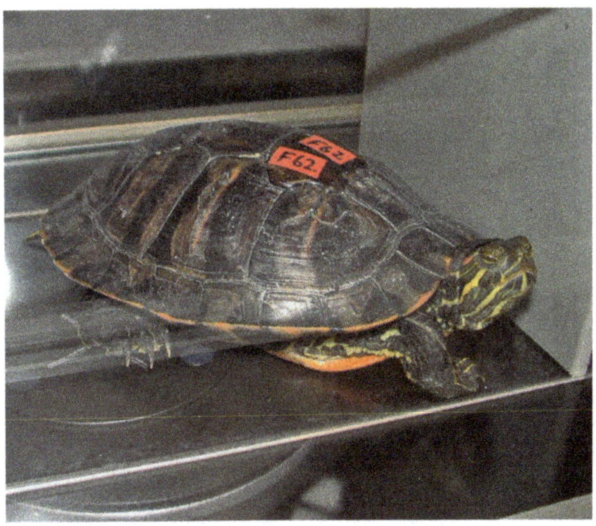

FIGURE 18-3 Red-eared Slider *(Trachemys scripta elegans)* at rest in the Hargreaves apparatus (noxious thermal hindlimb withdrawal apparatus) during research testing of analgesic responses to opioid administration. The turtle has the plantar surface of its right hindlimb placed directly over the infrared heat source.

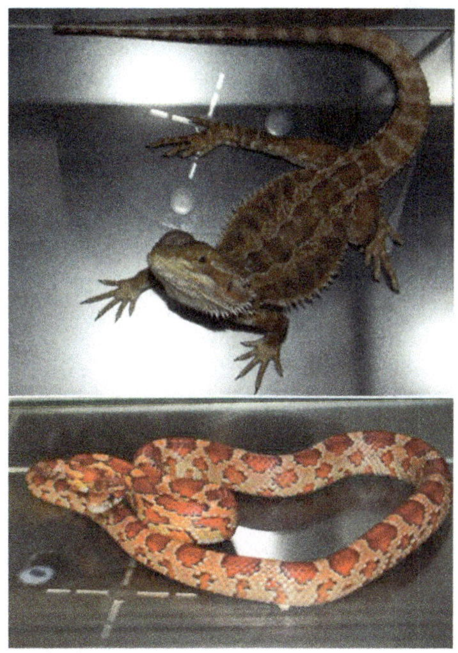

FIGURE 18-4 Bearded Dragon *(Pogona vitticeps; top image)* and Cornsnake *(Elaphe guttata; bottom)* at rest in the Hargreaves apparatus (noxious thermal hindlimb withdrawal apparatus) during research testing of analgesic responses to opioid administration. The Bearded Dragon has the plantar surface of its right hindlimb placed directly over the infrared heat source. Note the circular region at the center of the *X* in the Cornsnake image, just in front of the snake's head, which is the focal infrared heat element.

body surface of limbless snakes in our laboratory, we have observed a 100% response rate to this stimulus paradigm.

Physiologic changes have been used to quantify stress and pain in mammals, and this approach has also been adapted for reptiles.[53]

ANALGESIC DRUGS

Methods of Administration

It is difficult to describe the most appropriate methods for administering analgesic drugs in reptiles because analgesic pharmacokinetic/pharmacodynamic data in reptiles are scarce. Whether an analgesic drug is administered intravenously (IV), intramuscularly (IM), subcutaneously (SC), per os (PO; orally), or transcutaneously (TC) is partially dependent on the size and temperament of the individual reptile. Anatomic location is another consideration because pharmacologic evidence has shown that drug administration to the hindlimbs or tail of a reptile may cause more rapid clearance by the renal portal system or, in the case of opioids, the hepatic first-pass effect.[41,54] However, whether this more rapid clearance has any implication for efficacy remains unknown.

Historically and anecdotally, IM administration was the preferred route for most analgesics and anesthetics in reptiles.[41,55] Many veterinarians believed that the subcutaneous space of reptiles was not well-vascularized and, therefore, drug absorption would be prolonged. However, advantages associated with SC drug administration include access to a variety of subcutaneous sites requiring minimal manual restraint or patient manipulation and, therefore, increased safety and the capability of administering larger volumes in a single location. Currently, there are no published data demonstrating that IM administration results in superior analgesic efficacy compared with SC administration, and results from our laboratory indicate that drug effects can be measured rapidly after SC administration.[56] We determined that meperidine, an opioid analgesic with rapid absorption and excretion in humans, administered SC in Red-eared Sliders causes measurable behavioral changes within 30 minutes.[44] Therefore I routinely administer analgesic drugs and their antagonists SC in chelonians, lizards, and snakes, particularly if larger volumes of anesthetic drugs need to be injected.

Other routes of administration are also useful in reptiles. Transdermal fentanyl patches have been applied to two reptiles species for pharmacokinetic analysis, and plasma concentrations were detectable in both species.[57,58] Recently, our laboratory has evaluated the efficacy of transdermal fentanyl patch (12.5 mcg/h) administration in Ball Pythons and Cornsnakes and determined that fentanyl patches may be the most promising analgesic approach for use in some snake species.[59]

Oral administration is an uncommonly used method for analgesic administration in reptiles because the concern is that a potentially slow gastrointestinal transit time will delay onset, peak efficacy, and clearance. However, we have found just the opposite in our laboratory. Tramadol and metabolite plasma concentrations can be detected within hours of oral administration in Loggerhead Sea turtles,[60] and thermal hindlimb withdrawal latencies increased in Red-eared Sliders within 4 hours of oral tramadol administration.[6] Table 18-1 summarizes commonly used analgesic protocols in reptile species.

Opioids and Opioid-Like Analgesics

Opioids, the most effective drugs for controlling pain in mammals, are classified according to receptor subtypes—mu (μ),kappa (κ), and delta (δ) (Table 18-2). μ-opioid, δ-opioid, and κ-opioid receptors, abbreviated MOR, DOR, and KOR, mediate the analgesic effects of opioids, but the role of the fourth type of opioid receptor, the nociceptin or orphanin FQ receptor (ORL), is less clear.[61,62] For pain management in mammals, many clinicians prefer administering either a μ-opioid receptor agonist (e.g., morphine, fentanyl, or hydromorphone), a partial μ-opioid receptor agonist (e.g., buprenorphine), or a mixed opioid κ-receptor agonist–μ-receptor antagonist (e.g., butorphanol). For exogenous opioids to be effective analgesics in reptiles, opioid receptors must be present. The gene family for opioid receptors (μ,κ, and δ) is highly conserved across multiple vertebrate orders.[11] Two snake species have endogenous brain opiates[63] and Red-eared Sliders have both proencephalin-derived peptides and functional μ- and δ-opioid receptors in the brain.[36,37]

Although opioid receptors are expressed in reptiles, we are just beginning to understand the efficacy of commonly used opioid drugs. Butorphanol tartrate was considered to be the most commonly administered analgesic drug in reptiles.[3] In a published survey of veterinary medical clinicians, the applied reptile dosage range for butorphanol varied from 0.02 mg/kg to 25 mg/kg.[3] However, no clinical data were available to substantiate that butorphanol was an effective analgesic drug in reptiles. Butorphanol was, and is still, being used as a primary analgesic in reptiles because everyone was reporting that it worked. In 2005, our laboratory began to ask the first question: how do we know that butorphanol has analgesic properties in reptiles? Using our own noxious thermal stimulus paradigm and through a series of controlled experiments, we determined that butorphanol had no analgesic efficacy in Red-eared Sliders when administered at dosages of 2.8 or 28 mg/kg SC or in Bearded Dragons when administered at dosages of 2 or 20 mg/kg SC.[44-46] Our butorphanol data in Cornsnakes was too variable to make any firm conclusions; however, an unfortunate consequence of that publication[46] was that several clinicians decided to administer butorphanol (20 mg/kg) to debilitated snakes, and fatal consequences occurred in some cases. Consistent with our turtle and Bearded Dragon data, butorphanol administered IM at a dosage of 1 mg/kg had no analgesic efficacy (determined by use of a thermal noxious stimulus method)[48] and no isoflurane-sparing effect in Green Iguanas.[64] In Ball Pythons, butorphanol administered at 5 mg/kg IM had no effect on physiologic variables compared with saline.[65] Conversely, one study demonstrated that butorphanol may provide analgesia in Green Iguanas exposed to a noxious electrical stimulus.[47] On the other hand, morphine sulfate was an effective analgesic in Bearded Dragons (1 and 5 mg/kg) and in turtles (1.5 and 6.5 mg/kg), as determined with the use of the thermal noxious stimulus method, but data were not as clear in Cornsnakes, even when they were administered morphine at a dosage of 40 mg/kg.[46] Similarly, morphine (5, 7.5, 10, and 20 mg/kg) and meperidine (pethidine) (10, 20, and 50 mg/kg) provided analgesia in Speke's Hinge-back Tortoises *(Kinixys spekii)* exposed to formalin administered into a limb, which was reversible after naloxone administration.[66] In further support of morphine analgesic efficacy in reptiles, morphine increased limb withdrawal latencies in crocodiles[67,68] and increased tail flick latencies in anole lizards.[69]

Fentanyl is a μ-opioid receptor agonist, with 75 to 100 times the potency of morphine, which can be administered either TC as an impregnated patch or IV. A recently completed study in our laboratory evaluated the efficacy of transdermal fentanyl patch (12.5 mcg/h) administration in Ball Pythons and Cornsnakes.[59] The results demonstrated that the mean latency associated with withdrawal from a noxious thermal stimulus increased significantly with fentanyl patch (12.5 mcg/h) administration for 24 hours in Ball Pythons and for 8 hours in Cornsnakes. Two separate studies have evaluated the pharmacokinetics of fentanyl in two reptile species. In Ball Pythons, fentanyl plasma concentrations reached 1 ng/mL within 4 hours of application of a transdermal fentanyl patch (12.5 mcg/h)[58] and were detectable by 4 to 6 hours and for greater than 72 hours in the plasma of Prehensile-tailed Skinks (fentanyl dose was applied at 10% exposure of total surface area of a 25 mcg/h patch for 72 hours).[57] It remains unclear whether these plasma fentanyl concentrations have

TABLE 18-1

Analgesic Protocols for Use in Reptiles

	Dosage [mg/kg]	Route	Frequency	Comments	Ref.
OPIOIDS					
Buprenorphine	0.075-0.1 0.02-0.1	SC, IM	q24h	No evidence of analgesic efficacy; Plasma concentrations equivalent to those effective for analgesia in mammals; Respiratory depression not studied	47,54,70
Butorphanol	1.0-20.0 0.4-8.0	SC, IM	NDA	Analgesic efficacy questionable; Significant respiratory depression in RES (**> 10 mg/kg NOT RECOMMENDED**)	43,45,46,47,48,64,65
Hydromorphone	0.5-1.0	SC, IM	q24h	Good analgesic efficacy in RES; Respiratory depression not studied	70
Fentanyl	12.5 mcg/h 2.5 mcg/h	TC	One patch for 24 to 72 h	Transdermal patch; Provided antinociception in Ball Pythons and Cornsnakes; Plasma concentrations detected in Ball Pythons and Prehensile-tailed Skinks	57,58,59
Meperidine (pethidine)	1.0-5.0 10.0-50.0	SC, IM	q2-4h	Analgesic efficacy short-lived in RES; Respiratory depression not studied	66,67,91
Methadone	3.0-5.0	SC, IM	q24h	Good analgesic efficacy in RES; Anecdotal evidence in lizards species; Respiratory depression not studied	86
Morphine	1.0-40.0	SC, IM, IT	q24h	Good analgesic efficacy in RES and Bearded Dragons; Unknown efficacy in snakes; Significant respiratory depression (**> 5 mg/kg NOT RECOMMENDED**)	43-47, 66-69
Tramadol	5.0-10.0	PO	q48-72h	Good analgesic efficacy with relatively long duration when administered PO in chelonians; Less respiratory depression than other opioids in RES. In Loggerhead Sea turtles 10 mg/kg PO q48-96h	6,60
NSAIDS					
Carprofen	1.0-4.0	SC, IM	NDA	No evidence of analgesic efficacy; Presumed antiinflammatory efficacy	5,41,90
Ketoprofen	2.0	IV	NDA	Pharmacokinetics only; no efficacy data	87
Meloxicam	0.2-0.3	IV, SC, IM, PO	NDA	No evidence of analgesic efficacy; Presumed antiinflammatory efficacy; No physiologic changes in Ball Pythons administered postoperatively	80,81,85,86,92
LOCAL ANESTHETICS					
Lidocaine (1% or 2%)	1-2 (keep <5.0) 4.0	SC, IM IT	NDA	No systematic data published. May be a good focal nerve block and effective IT in RES and Galapagos tortoises; Less effective alone, but more effective when combined with general anesthesia in Asian Box Turtles undergoing coelioscopy	81,83
Bupivacaine (0.5%)	1.0 (keep <2.0) 1.0	SC, IM IT	NDA	No systematic data published but appears to be a good focal nerve block and effective IT in RES	82
Mepivacaine (2%)	1.0	SC	NDA	Used as a mandibular nerve block in alligators	13
OTHER ANESTHETICS					
Medetomidine/ Dexmedetomidine	0.05-0.3 0.1-0.2	SC, IM	NDA	No evidence of analgesic efficacy; Frequently combined with ketamine, midazolam, or an opioid in sedation/anesthesia protocols	41,77,78
Ketamine	2	SC, IM, IV	NDA	No evidence of analgesic efficacy; Low dose as an analgesic is extrapolated from the mammalian literature; Frequently combined with an alpha-2, benzodiazepine or an opioid in sedation/anesthesia protocols	77,79,80
Midazolam	1.0-2.0	SC, IM	NDA	No evidence of analgesic efficacy; Frequently combined with an alpha-2, ketamine or an opioid. Enhances analgesic properties of dexmedetomidine in rats	79,93,94

IM, Intramuscular; *IT*, intrathecal; *IV*, intravenous; *NDA*, no data available; *NSAIDs*, nonsteroidal antiinflammatory drugs; *PO*, by mouth; *q*, every; *RES*, Red-eared Sliders; *SC*, subcutaneous; *TC*, transcutaneous.

TABLE 18-2

Opioid Receptor Subtypes: Exogenous and Endogenous Opioids

Receptor Subtype	Exogenous Opioid Agonist	Endogenous Opioid Agonist	Exogenous Antagonist
mu (μ)-Opioid receptor (MOR) agonists	Morphine, hydromorphone, fentanyl methadone, oxymorphone, experimental drugs (DAMGO)	Endorphins (enkephalins), endomorphins	Naloxone, naltrexone
kappa (κ)-Opioid receptor (KOR) agonists	Butorphanol (κ -agonist/μ-antagonist), nalbuphine (κ agonist/partial μ antagonist), experimental drugs (U50488, U69593)	Dynorphin A	Naloxone, naltrexone
delta (δ)-Opioid receptor (DOR) agonists	Only experimental drugs (DADLE, DPDPE, deltorphan II)	Endorphins (enkephalins)	Naltrindole, naloxone, naltrexone

DADLE, [D-Ala2, D-leu5] enkephalin; *DAMGO,* [D-Ala2, MePhe 4, Gly(ol) 5]enkephalin; *DPDPE,* [D-Pen2, D-Pen5]enkephalin; *U50488,* trans-(-)-3,4-dichloro-N-methyl-N-[2-(1-pyrrolidinyl)cyclohexyl]benzeneacetamide hydrochloride; *U69593,* N-methyl-2-phenyl-N-[(5R,7S,8S)-7-(pyrrolidin-1-yl)-1-oxaspiro[4.5]dec-8-yl]acetamide.

any biological significance. While a final verdict is not definitive, combined, these data suggest that the fentanyl patch may be the most promising analgesic choice for snakes.

Buprenorphine is an effective analgesic in many mammalian species and is used extensively because of its longer duration of action compared with other opioids. Buprenorphine has partial agonist activity at the μ-opioid receptor, partial or full agonist activity at the δ-opioid receptor, and antagonist activity at the κ-opioid receptor. With only a single published study evaluating analgesic efficacy, buprenorphine did not alter responses to an electrical stimulus in Green Iguanas.[47] Similarly, in our laboratory, buprenorphine (0.5 and 1.0 mg/kg, SC) provided no analgesic efficacy in Red-eared Sliders exposed to a noxious thermal stimulus.[70] Buprenorphine pharmacokinetics in reptiles were determined after SC administration in Red-eared Sliders, and effective dosages ranged from 0.075 to 0.1 mg/kg, which provided plasma concentrations associated with analgesic efficacy in humans for approximately 24 hours.[54] Interestingly, plasma concentrations of buprenorphine were reduced by approximately 70% when the drug was administered in the hindlimb compared with the forelimb, the significance of which is unknown.

Tramadol has become a widely used analgesic alternative to other opioids in veterinary medicine because it is administered orally and is currently not considered a controlled substance. Tramadol and its active metabolite, O-desmethyltramadol, produce analgesia in mammals by activating μ-opioid receptors and by inhibiting central serotonin and norepinephrine reuptake.[71,72] Parent tramadol has μ-opioid activity, but O-desmethyltramadol has up to 200 times greater affinity for μ-opioid receptors.[73] Overall, tramadol binds μ-opioid receptors with 6000 times less affinity than morphine,[73] thus having the potential for producing fewer μ-opioid–induced side effects. In fact, tramadol does not appear to alter breathing in humans[74] and produces significantly less respiratory depression than morphine in cats and dogs.[75,76]

In mammals, the analgesic effects of tramadol typically begin within 30 minutes and last for 6 hours. In contrast, tramadol (5.0 mg/kg, PO) administered to turtles significantly increased withdrawal latencies for 12 to 24 hours and 6 to 96 hours after administration of the higher tramadol dosages (10 or 25 mg/kg, PO).[6] Plasma concentrations of tramadol and O-desmethyltramadol remained 100 ng/mL or greater for at least 48 hours and perhaps as long as 96 hours when tramadol was administered at 10 mg/kg in Loggerhead Sea turtle.[60]

With respect to deleterious side effects, respiratory depression associated with tramadol administration in Red-eared Sliders was approximately 50% less than that measured after morphine administration.[6] Therefore tramadol appears to be a promising analgesic alternative to traditional opioids in reptiles. As mentioned, one of the significant deleterious side effects associated with tramadol and all opioid drug administration in mammals is respiratory depression. This problem is paralleled in reptile studies. Our laboratory determined that both butorphanol and morphine caused profound respiratory depression in turtles,[45] whereas respiratory depression was significantly less when turtles were administered tramadol. The bottom line is that it is imperative that clinicians continue to monitor respiration during and after procedures in which any opioid drugs are administered to reptiles.

Parenteral Anesthetics

Ketamine administered at low dosages is commonly used as an analgesic in mammals. However, no data are available to substantiate this finding in reptiles. Combining ketamine with an alpha-2-adrenergic agonist (e.g., medetomidine or dexmedetomidine) increases the level of sedation in reptiles, as in mammals.[77-80] Although such combinations provide analgesia in mammals, it can only be speculated that the same is true in reptiles because no data are available.

Local Anesthetics as Analgesics

Local anesthetics (e.g., lidocaine, bupivacaine, and mepivacaine) are commonly used to block peripheral nerve transmission when mammals or reptiles are exposed to procedures considered minimally painful. However, only two reptile studies have been published. Mepivacaine was used effectively as a mandibular nerve block in an alligator, and a nerve locator was used to facilitate the procedure.[13] In the second study, lidocaine was administered in the prefemoral region of hatchling Chinese Box Turtles *(Cuora flavomarginata)* before endoscopic gender determination.[81] However, lidocaine administered without general anesthesia was insufficient for celioscopy. The limitations associated with local anesthetic administration include a focal nerve block and short duration of action. Local anesthetics, as well as opioids (e.g., preservative-free morphine), can be administered intrathecally into the coccygeal region of chelonians.[82,83] Intrathecal morphine causes antinociception to thermal noxious stimulation of the hindlimbs for more than 24 hours after administration in male Red-eared Sliders.[82]

Nonsteroidal Antiinflammatory Drugs

While not as potent as the opioids, nonsteroidal antiinflammatory drugs (NSAIDs) are used widely in reptile clinical practice as analgesics and for their antiinflammatory properties. NSAIDs provide analgesia in mammals by blocking the binding of arachidonic acid to cyclooxygenase (COX) enzyme, which prevents the conversion of thromboxane A2 to thromboxane B2 (TBX), thus preventing production of prostaglandins, potent mediators of inflammation.[79] NSAIDs are often classified based on their relative specificity. There are two COX enzymes, COX-1 and COX-2, and they participate in renal and gastric protection and inflammation, respectively.[84] The NSAID ketoprofen is equipotent against both isoenzymes, whereas carprofen is slightly more COX-2 specific and meloxicam is COX-2 specific.[84] Therefore the degree of efficacy and side effects may vary with each of the three NSAIDs selected. Although many NSAIDs appear to be relatively safe when used in reptiles, only one study has been published on analgesic efficacy.[85] Ball Pythons administered meloxicam (0.3 mg/kg, IM) before a surgical placement of an arterial catheter showed no physiologic changes (e.g., heart rate, blood pressure, and plasma epinephrine and cortisol levels) indicative of analgesia. With respect to the pharmacokinetics of NSAIDs in reptile species, plasma concentrations of meloxicam (0.2 mg/kg, PO) administered as a single dose to Green Iguanas were at levels considered analgesic in mammals, and these levels were measureable up to 24 hours after administration.[86] In this same study, histopathologic changes were not observed in gastric, hepatic, or renal tissues associated with daily administration of meloxicam for a total of 12 days.[86] Ketoprofen (2 mg/kg, IV), administered to Green Iguanas, had a long half-life (31 hours) compared with ketoprofen pharmacokinetics in mammals, but the bioavailability after IM administration was only 78% with a relatively short half-life (8.3 hours).[87] Because there are no efficacy data and few pharmacokinetics data on NSAID administration in reptiles, appropriate dosages and frequency of administration can only be extrapolated. Additionally, clinicians should be aware of the potential for deleterious side effects documented in avian and mammalian species (e.g., renal impairment, gastrointestinal ulceration/inflammation, and hematologic abnormalities); therefore these drugs should be used with caution.

Acupuncture

While acupuncture has been used as an analgesic across a variety of domestic species, including equine, canine, and rodent patients, systematically derived data collected under controlled conditions have not been described. The analgesic efficacy of acupuncture applied to nondomestic species has not been well-documented. In the second edition of *Reptile Medicine and Surgery*, Ferguson and O'Leary describe their clinical experience with acupuncture in treating reptiles for various conditions.[87a] Electroacupuncture involves application of an electrical stimulus to peripheral nerves via acupuncture needles applied to specific acupuncture points.[88] Electroacupuncture-induced analgesia is attributable to stimulation of μ, κ, and δ receptors in rats.[88] However, little to nothing is known about the efficacy of electroacupuncture as an analgesic in reptiles. One study effectively transposed canine acupuncture points to a Red-footed Tortoise (*Chelonoidis carbonaria*) for successfully treatment of a locomotor disability associated with an injury.[89] In Bearded Dragons, morphine is considered to be the most effective antinociceptive agent, and μ-opioid agonists appear to be the most effective antinociceptive agents across many reptile species.[44,46] Because electroacupuncture also acts on μ-opioid receptors, electroacupuncture may be a promising method for providing analgesia (i.e., antinociception) to Bearded Dragons. The Chi Institute of Traditional Chinese Veterinary Medicine in Florida has effectively treated Bearded Dragons for a variety of ailments such as malnutrition and anorexia with electroacupuncture. In our laboratory, we recently completed a study in which Bearded Dragons were subjected to electroacupuncture, followed by application of a thermal noxious stimulus to determine whether electroacupuncture provided thermal antinociception (Figure 18-5; Conway, et. al., unpublished data). Preliminary data suggest that the Bearded Dragons relaxed under the influence of electroacupuncture and demonstrated a trend toward delayed limb withdrawal after exposure to a thermal noxious stimulus. However, the data are not statistically different from controls. Our future research will include concurrent acupuncture and opioid drug administration for comparison.

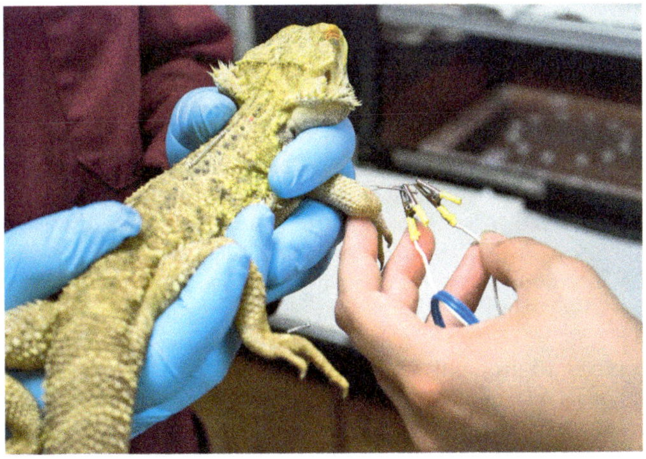

FIGURE 18-5 Bearded Dragon *(Pogona vitticeps)* undergoing electroacupuncture. Needle placement sites were extrapolated from the veterinary mammalian literature. *(Courtesy of D. Conway.)*

MULTIMODAL ANALGESIC APPROACHES

In reptiles, multimodal drug paradigms may be the best approach for managing pain. Multimodal analgesia refers to the administration of multiple drugs that have analgesic efficacy at different levels in the central and peripheral nervous system. For example, opioids will have greatest efficacy at opioid receptors in the central and peripheral nervous, whereas NSAIDs administered at the same time as the opioids will have greatest efficacy as antiinflammatory agents at the peripheral tissues.[90] Local anesthetics can enhance multimodal analgesic protocols by blocking the initial pain cascade at the peripheral level. In concert, all of these drugs have the potential to minimize transmission of pain signals to the brain, especially when administered before a potentially painful procedure is established.

CONCLUSION

Our understanding of reptile pain and analgesia has advanced significantly during the past 5 years; however, there is a great deal of theoretical and clinical research still to conduct, and our ability to extrapolate across orders and species remains a major limitation. In other words, an effective analgesic drug administered to a Leopard Tortoise may not have the same efficacy in a Ball Python. Our inability to have a "one-size-fits-all" model for reptile analgesics stems from the fact that the Class Reptilia is incredibly diverse. Continued research focusing on effective analgesic drugs, dose-dependent effects, duration of drug efficacy, interspecies differences, and potential drug-related adverse side effects will advance the field and begin to reinforce or abolish the perpetuation of anecdotal information, which remains pervasive in the reptile clinical medicine literature.[91]

Butorphanol tartrate (a κ-opioid receptor agonist) administered at mammalian-derived dosages was once believed to be the most effective analgesic drug for use in reptiles. More recently, however, we have begun to systematically investigate pain and analgesia in a variety of reptile species, and our data demonstrate that μ-opioid receptor agonists, such as morphine, hydromorphone, fentanyl, or tramadol, provide effective analgesia, while butorphanol appears to be no more effective than saline.[91] Extrapolation of analgesic efficacy across orders and species remains a major limitation, and there is a clear need for evaluation of analgesic drugs across a variety of clinical situations, particularly as they apply to postsurgical pain. Objectively derived methods for evaluation of pain in animals are critical, but these methods must be species- and context-specific. In addition, determining pharmacokinetic variables, duration of drug efficacy, species-specific requirements, and deleterious side effects of opioid drugs in different reptile species remains critical for advances in the field of reptile analgesia.

REFERENCES

1. Chamberlain DB. Babies don't feel pain: a century of denial in medicine, in *Proceedings*. 2nd Int'l Symposium Circumcision, San Francisco, Calif, May 2, 1991;18.
2. Joseph MH, Brill J, Zeltzer LK. Pediatric pain relief in trauma. *Pediatr Rev* 1999;20:75-83.
3. Read MR. Evaluation of the use of anesthesia and analgesia in reptiles. *J Am Vet Med Assoc* 2004;224:547-552.
4. Bateson P. Assessment of pain in animals. *Anim Behav* 1991;42:827-839.
5. Machin KL. Fish, amphibian, and reptile analgesia. *Vet Clin North Am Exot Anim Pract* 2001;4:19-33.
6. Baker BB, Sladky KK, Johnson SM. Evaluation of the analgesic effects of oral and subcutaneous tramadol administration in red-eared slider turtles. *J Am Vet Med Assoc* 2011;238:220-227.
7. ten Donkelaar HJ. Evolution of the red nucleus and rubrospinal tract. *Behav Brain Res* 1988;28:9-20.
8. ten Donkelaar HJ, de Boer-van Huizen R. A possible pain control system in a nonmammalian vertebrate (a lizard, *Gekko gecko*). *Neurosci Lett* 1987;83:65-70.
9. Smith ESJ, Lewin GR. Nociceptors: a phylogenetic view. *J Comp Physiol A* 2009;195:1089-1106.
10. Sneddon LU. Evolution of nociception in vertebrates: comparative analysis of lower vertebrates. *Brain Res Rev* 2004;46:123-130.
11. Li X, Keith DE, Evans CJ. Multiple opioid receptor-like genes are identified in diverse vertebrate phyla. *FEBS Lett* 1996;397:25-29.
12. Liang YF, Terashima S, Zhu AQ. Distinct morphological characteristics of touch, temperature, and mechanical nociceptive neurons in the crotaline trigeminal ganglia. *J Comp Neurol* 1995;60:621-633.
13. Wellehan JFX, Gunkel CI, Kledzik D, et al. Use of a nerve locator to facilitate administration of mandibular nerve blocks in crocodilians. *J Zoo Wildl Med* 2006;37:405-408.
14. Stevens CW. Analgesia in amphibians: preclinical studies and clinical applications. *Vet Clin North Am Exot Anim Pract* 2011;14:33-44.
15. Partata WA, Krepsky AMR, Xavier LL, et al. Substance P immunoreactivity in the lumbar spinal cord of the turtle *Trachemys dorbigni* following peripheral nerve injury. *Braz J Med Biol Res* 2003;36:515-520.
16. Reiner A, Krause JE, Keyser KT, et al. The distribution of substance P in turtle nervous system: a radioimmunoassay and immunohistochemical study. *J Comp Neurol* 1984;226:50-75.
17. Mehler WR. Subcortical afferent connections of the amygdala in the monkey. *J Comp Neurol* 1980;190:733-762.
18. Willis WD. Nociceptive pathways: anatomy and physiology of nociceptive ascending pathways. *Philos Trans R Soc Lond B Biol Sci* 1985;308:253-270.
19. Hall WC, Ebner FF. Thalamotelencephalic projections in the turtle *(Pseudemys scripta)*. *J Comp Neurol* 1970;140:101-122.
20. Bruce LL, Butler AB. Telencephalic connections in lizards. II. Projections to anterior dorsal ventricular ridge. *J Comp Neurol* 1984a;229:602-615.
21. Bruce LL, Butler AB. Telencephalic connections in lizards. I. Projections to cortex. *J Comp Neurol* 1984b;229:585-601.
22. Kenigfest N, Martínez-Marcos A, Belekhova M, et al. A lacertilian dorsal retinorecipient thalamus: a re-investigation in the old-world lizard *Podarcis hispanica*. *Brain Behav Evol* 1997;50:313-334.
23. Butler AB, Manger PR, Lindahl BI, et al. Evolution of the neural basis of consciousness: a bird-mammal comparison. *Bioessays* 2005;27:923-936.
24. Butler AB, Hodos W. Comparative vertebrate neuroanatomy: evolution and adaptation. 2nd ed. Hoboken, NJ: John Wiley & Sons, 2005.
25. Jarvis ED. Evolution of the pallium in birds and reptiles. In: Binder MD, Hirokawa N, Windhorst U, eds. *New encyclopedia of neuroscience*. Berlin: Springer-Verlag GmbH; 2009;1390-1400.
26. Medina L, Abellán A. Development and evolution of the pallium. *Semin Cell Dev Biol* 2009;20:698-711.
27. Novejarque A, Lanuza E, Martínez-García F. Amygdalostriatal projections in reptiles: a tract-tracing study in the lizard *Podarcis hispanica*. *J Comp Neurol* 2004;479:287-308.
28. ten Donkelaar HJ, Kusuma A, de Boer-van Huizen R. Cells of origin of pathways descending to the spinal cord in some quadrupedal reptiles. *J Comp Neurol* 2004;192:827-851.
29. ten Donkelaar HJ. Descending pathways from the brain stem to the spinal cord in some reptiles. *J Comp Neurol* 2004;67:421-442.
30. Cruce WLR, Larson-Prior L, Newman DB. Rubrospinal pathways in a colubrid snake. *Soc Neurosci Abstr* 1983;9:1064.
31. Guirado S, Dávila JC. Thalamo-telencephalic connections: new insights on the cortical organization in reptiles. *Brain Res Bull* 2002;57:451-454.
32. Zhu D, Lustig KH, Bifulco K, et al. Thalamocortical connections in the pond turtle *Pseudemys scripta elegans*. *Brain Behav Evol* 2005;65:278-292.
33. Bradford CS, Walthers EA, Stanley DJ, et al. Delta and mu opioid receptors from the brain of a urodele amphibian, the rough-skinned newt *Taricha granulosa*: cloning, heterologous expression, and pharmacological characterization. *Gen Comp Endocrinol* 2006;146:275-290.
34. Gonzalez-Nunez V, Rodríguez RE. The zebrafish: a model to study the endogenous mechanisms of pain. *ILAR J* 2009;50:373-386.
35. Stevens CW, Brasel CM, Mohan S. Cloning and bioinformatics of amphibian mu, delta, kappa, and nociceptin opioid receptors expressed in brain tissue: evidence for opioid receptor divergence in mammals. *Neurosci Lett* 2007;419:189-194.
36. Xia Y, Haddad GG. Major difference in the expression of delta- and mu-opioid receptors between turtle and rat brain. *J Comp Neurol* 2001;436:202-210.

37. Reiner A. The distribution of proenkephalin-derived peptides in the central nervous system of turtles. *J Comp Neurol* 1987;259:65-91.
38. Lindberg I, White L. Reptilian enkephalins: implications for the evolution of proenkephalin. *Arch Biochem Biophys* 1986;245:1-7.
39. Liles JH, Flecknell PA. The effects of buprenorphine, nalbuphine and butorphanol alone or following halothane anesthesia on food and water-consumption and locomotor movement in rats. *Lab Anim* 1992;26:180-189.
40. Hardie EM, Hansen BD, Carroll GS. Behavior after ovariohysterectomy in the dog: What's normal? *App Anim Behav Sci* 1997;51:111-128.
41. Mosley CA. Anesthesia and analgesia in reptiles. *Semin Avian Exot Pet Med* 2005;14:243-262.
42. Sladky KK, Horne WA, Goodrowe K, et al. Evaluation of epidural morphine for post-surgical analgesia in ferrets (*Mustela putorius furo*). *Contemp Top Lab Anim Sci* 2000;39:33-38.
43. Kinney M, Johnson SM, Sladky KK. Behavioral evaluation of red-eared slider turtles (*Trachemys scripta*) administered either morphine or butorphanol following unilateral gonadectomy. *J Herpetol Med Surg* 2011;21:54-62.
44. Sladky KK, Kinney ME, Johnson SM. Effects of opioid receptor activation on thermal antinociception in red-eared slider turtles (*Trachemys scripta*). *Am J Vet Res* 2009;70:1072-1078.
45. Sladky KK, Miletic V, Paul-Murphy J, et al. Analgesic efficacy and respiratory effects of butorphanol and morphine in turtles. *J Am Vet Med Assoc* 2007;230:1356-1362.
46. Sladky KK, Kinney ME, Johnson SM. Analgesic efficacy of butorphanol and morphine in bearded dragons and corn snakes. *J Am Vet Med Assoc* 2008;233:267-273.
47. Greenacre CB, Schumacher JP, Talke G, et al. Comparative antinociception of morphine, butorphanol, and buprenorphine versus saline in the green iguana, *Iguana iguana*, using electrostimulation. *J Herpetol Med Surg* 2006;16:88-92.
48. Fleming GJ, Robertson SA. Assessments of thermal antinociceptive effects of butorphanol and human observer effect on quantitative evaluation of analgesia in green iguanas (*Iguana iguana*). *Am J Vet Res* 2012;73:1507-1511.
49. Hargreaves K, Dubner R, Brown F, et al. A new and sensitive method for measuring thermal nociception in cutaneous hyperalgesia. *Pain* 1988;32:77-88.
50. Sandkuhler J. Models and mechanisms of hyperalgesia and allodynia. *Physiol Rev* 2009;89:707-758.
51. Latremoliere A, Woolf CJ. Central sensitization: a generator of pain hypersensitivity by central neural plasticity. *J Pain* 2009;10:895-926.
52. Basbaum AI, Bautista DM, Scherrer G, et al. Cellular and molecular mechanisms of pain. *Cell* 2009;139:267-284.
53. Moorea IT, Jessop TS. Stress, reproduction, and adrenocortical modulation in amphibians and reptiles. *Horm Behav* 2003;43:9-47.
54. Kummrow MS, Tseng F, Hesse L, et al. Pharmacokinetics of buprenorphine after single-dose subcutaneous administration in red-eared sliders (*Trachemys scripta elegans*). *J Zoo Wildl Med* 2008;39:590-595.
55. Schumacher J, Yelen T. Anesthesia and analgesia. In: Mader DR, ed. *Reptile medicine and surgery*. 2nd ed. St. Louis: Elsevier, 2006;442-452.
56. Redrobe S. Anesthesia and analgesia. In: Girling SJ, Raiti P, eds. *BSAVA manual of reptiles*. 2nd ed. Glouchester, England: BSAVA, 2004;131-146.
57. Gamble KC. Plasma fentanyl concentrations achieved after transdermal fentanyl patch application in prehensile-tailed skinks, *Corucia zebrata*. *J Herpetol Med Surg* 2008;18:81-85.
58. Darrow BG, Meyers GE, Kukanich B. Fentanyl transdermal therapeutic system pharmacokinetics in ball pythons (*Python regius*), in *Proceedings. Am Assoc Zoo Vet* 2010;238-239.
59. Gutwillig A, Abbott A, Johnson SM, et al. Opioid dependent analgesia in ball pythons (*Python regius*) and corn snakes (*Elaphe guttata*), in *Proceedings. Assoc Reptile Amphibian Vets* 2012;66.
60. Norton TM, Cox S, Kaylor M, et al. Pharmacokinetics of tramadol and o-desmethyltramadol in loggerhead sea turtles (*Caretta caretta*), in *Proceedings. Am Assoc Zoo Vet* 2012;101.
61. Dhawan BN, Cesselin F, Raghubir R, et al. International Union of Pharmacology. XII. Classification of opioid receptors. *Pharmacol Rev* 1996;48:567-592.
62. Johnson SM, Moris CM, Bartman ME, et al. Excitatory and inhibitory effects of opioid agonists on respiratory motor output produced by isolated brainstems from adult turtles (*Trachemys*). *Respir Physiol Neurobiol* 2010;170:5-15.
63. Ng TB, Ng ASL, Wong CC. Adrenocorticotropin-like and beta-endorphin-like substances in brains of the fresh-water snake *Ptyas mucosa*. *Biochem Cell Biol* 1990;68:1012-1018.
64. Mosley CA, Dyson D, Smith DA. Minimum alveolar concentration of isoflurane in green iguanas and the effect of butorphanol on minimum alveolar concentration. *J Am Vet Med Assoc* 2003;222:1559-1564.
65. Olesen MG, Bertelsen MF, Perry SF, et al. Effects of preoperative administration of butorphanol or meloxicam on physiologic responses to surgery in ball pythons. *J Am Vet Med Assoc* 2008;233:1883-1888.
66. Wambugu SN, Towett PK, Kiama SG, et al. Effects of opioids in the formalin test in the Speke's hinged tortoise (*Kinixys spekii*). *J Vet Pharmacol Ther* 2010;33:347-351.
67. Kanui TI, Hole K. Morphine and pethidine antinociception in the crocodile. *J Vet Pharmacol Ther* 1992;15:101-103.
68. Kanui TI, Hole K, Miaron JO. Nociception in crocodiles—capsaicin instillation, formalin and hot plate tests. *Zool Sci* 1990;7:537-540.
69. Mauk MD, Olson RD, Lahoste GJ, et al. Tonic immobility produces hyperalgesia and antagonizes morphine analgesia. *Science* 1981;213:353-354.
70. Mans C, Lahner LL, Baker BB, et al. Antinociceptive efficacy of buprenorphine and hydromorphone in red-eared slider turtles (*Trachemys scripta elegans*). *J Zoo Wildl Med* 2012;43:662-665.
71. Raffa RB, Friderichs E, Reimann W, et al. Opioid and nonopioid components independently contribute to the mechanism of action of tramadol, an atypical opioid analgesic. *J Pharmacol Exp Ther* 1992;260:275-285.
72. Ide S, Minami M, Ishihara K, et al. Mu opioid receptor-dependent and independent components in effects of tramadol. *Neuropharmacology* 2006;51:651-658.
73. Lewis KS, Han NH. Tramadol: a new centrally acting analgesic. *Am J Health Syst Pharm* 1997;54:643-652.
74. Houmes RJM, Voets MA, Verkaaik A, et al. Efficacy and safety of tramadol versus morphine for moderate and severe postoperative pain with special regards to respiratory depression. *Anesth Analg* 1992;74:510-514.
75. Teppema LJ, Nieuwenhuijs D, Olievier CN, et al. Respiratory depression by tramadol in the cat—involvement of opioid receptors. *Anesthesiology* 2003;98:420-427.
76. Mastrocinque S, Fantoni DT. A comparison of preoperative tramadol and morphine for the control of early postoperative pain in canine ovariohysterectomy. *Vet Anaesth Analg* 2003;30:220-228.
77. Sleeman JM, Gaynor J. Sedative and cardiopulmonary effects of medetomidine and reversal with atipamezole in desert tortoises (*Gopherus agassizii*). *J Zoo Wildl Med* 2000;31:28-35.
78. Greer LL, Jenne KJ, Diggs HE. Medetomidine-ketamine anesthesia in red-eared slider turtles (*Trachemys scripta elegans*). *Contemp Top Lab Anim Sci* 2001;40:9-11.
79. Bienzle D, Boyd CJ. Sedative effects of ketamine and midazolam in snapping turtles (*Chelydra serpentina*). *J Zoo Wildl Med* 1992;23:201-204.
80. Mans C, Sladky KK. Endoscopically guided removal of cloacal calculi in three African spurred tortoises (*Geochelone sulcata*). *J Am Vet Med Assoc* 2012;240:869-875.
81. Hernandez-Divers SJ, Stahl SJ, Farrell R. An endoscopic method for identifying sex of hatchling Chinese box turtles and comparison of general versus local anesthesia for coelioscopy. *J Am Vet Med Assoc* 2009;234:800-804.
82. Mans C, Steagall PVM, Lahner LL, et al. Efficacy of intrathecal lidocaine, bupivacaine, and morphine for spinal anesthesia and analgesia in red-eared slider turtles (*Trachemys scripta elegans*), in *Proceedings*. Am Assoc Zoo Vet 2011;135.

83. Rivera S, Divers SJ, Knafo SE, et al. Sterilisation of hybrid Galapagos tortoises *(Geochelone nigra)* for island restoration. Part 2: phallectomy of males under intrathecal anaesthesia with lidocaine. *Vet Rec* 2011;168:78.
84. Budsberg SC. Nonsteroidal anti-inflammatory drugs. In: Gaynor J, Muir WW, eds. *Handbook of veterinary pain management* 2nd ed. Toronto: Mosby, 2009;183-239.
85. Olesen MG, Bertelsen MF, Perry SF, et al. Effects of preoperative administration of butorphanol or meloxicam on physiologic responses to surgery in ball pythons. *J Am Vet Med Assoc* 2008;233:1883-1888.
86. Divers SJ, Papich M, McBride M, et al. Pharmacokinetics of meloxicam following intravenous and oral administration in green iguanas *(Iguana iguana)*. *Am J Vet Res* 2010;71:1277-1283.
87. Tuttle AD, Papich M, Lewbart GA, et al. Pharmacokinetics of ketoprofen in the green iguana *(Iguana iguana)* following single intravenous and intramuscular injections. *J Zoo Wildl Med* 2006;37:567-570.
87a. Ferguson B, O'Leary N. Alternative and complimentary veterinary therapies. In: Mader DR, ed. *Reptile medicine and surgery* 2nd ed. St Louis: Elsevier, 2006;428-441.
88. Taguchi R, Taguchi T, Kitakoji H. Involvement of peripheral opioid receptors in electroacupuncture analgesia for carrageenan-induced hyperalgesia. *Brain Res* 2010;1355:97-103.
89. Scognamillo-Szabo MVR, Santos ALQ, Olegario MMM, et al. Acupuncture for locomotor disabilities in a South American red-footed tortoise *(Geochelone carbonaria)*—a case report. *Acupunct Med* 2008;26:243-247.
90. Dzikiti TB, Joubert KE, Venter LJ, et al. Comparison of morphine and carprofen administered alone or in combination for analgesia in dogs undergoing ovariohysterectomy. *J S Afr Vet Assoc* 2006;77:120-126.
91. Sladky KK, Johnson SM. Current understanding of analgesic efficacy and associated side effects in reptiles, in *Proceedings. Am Assoc Zoo Vet* 2008;116-117.
92. Trnkova S, Knotkova Z, Hrda A, et al. Effect of non-steroidal anti-inflammatory drugs on the blood profile in the green iguana *(Iguana iguana)*. *Vet Med Czech* 2007;52:507-511.
93. Oppenheim YC, Moon PF. Sedative effects of midazolam in red-eared slider turtles *(Trachemys scripta elegans)*. *J Zoo Wildl Med* 1995;26:409-413.
94. Quagliatto Santos AL, Luz Hirano LQ, Pereira PC, et al. Anaesthesia of Geoffroy's side-necked turtle *Phrynops geoffroanus Schweigger*, 1812 (Testudines) with the association of midazolam and propofol. *Acta Sci Biol Sci* 2009;31:317-321.

SECTION III

ADVANCES IN AMPHIBIAN MEDICINE

CHAPTER 19

A New Era of Amphibian Taxonomy

Jennifer B. Pramuk and Joseph R. Mendelson III

The more than 7000 species of amphibians represent a monophyletic group (i.e., sharing a common ancestor) that is both highly successful and geographically widespread. The earliest amphibians, of which the fossils of *Ichthyostega* and *Elginerpeton* are representatives, date from the Late Devonian, more than 360 million years ago. These fossil forms represent the earliest known ancestors to all extant tetrapods, which include amphibians, birds, reptiles, and mammals. Amphibians were the first vertebrates to hunt, vocalize, and breed on land, and their basic body plan has changed little since the Jurassic period. Because of their highly permeable skin, amphibians are usually intolerant of saltwater; therefore, their wide present-day distribution is largely the result of deeper lineages predating the split of continental landmasses—today, they are present on all continents except Antarctica.

Because closely related organisms are expected to function similarly, understanding taxonomy and phylogeny might yield clues to their physiology and natural history. In most cases, all but the most commonly kept amphibian species have little to nothing about them in the literature regarding their medical treatment or husbandry. A fundamental understanding of the evolutionary relationships or phylogeny of the amphibians is therefore integral to an understanding of their biology, captivity, and medical care. For example, if one is treating a member of a poorly known taxon, such as a leaf frog in the genus *Phasmahyla,* clues to its captive management (e.g., sensitivities to a particular medication or susceptibility to diseases such as *Batrachochytrium dendrobatidis* [amphibian chytrid fungus]) might be revealed by researching literature on its most widely studied sister taxon, in this case, the Red-eyed Tree frog (*Agalychnis callidryas*).

It is ironic that the notion of stability is so entrenched in the concept of taxonomy that the very system of names designed to allow communication across cultural and language barriers cannot itself be changed without reactionary outbursts from the greater community of biologists, land managers, veterinarians, and even the taxonomists themselves. It is as if some feel that taxonomic stability (tradition) is more important than the development of knowledge of biodiversity (progress). Is one not supposed to learn and move forward in understanding of biodiversity? To witness the reaction some have to proposed taxonomic changes, one would infer not! Taxonomic stability is a good thing to have but only if the taxonomy in use adequately communicates both the diversity and evolutionary history of the group of organisms in question.

In the case of amphibians, a stable taxonomy is elusive in part because knowledge of amphibian diversity is still growing at an astonishing rate. Compared with the largely stable taxonomies for mammals or birds, new major lineages (e.g., genera or even families) of amphibians are still being discovered regularly. To put this into perspective, approximately one quarter of all known amphibian diversity has been described in the past 20 years, and the rate of species discovery has not yet plateaued. To confound matters, the last century had been spent tolerating a flawed traditional taxonomy that used useless names for artificial and large groups of animals, such as "Leptodactylidae," a catchall group of neotropical frogs that was far from phylogenetically accurate. The new, molecular data–based phylogenies have revealed that the vast age of amphibians and the phenomenon in many groups in which larval characteristics are retained in adults (i.e., neoteny) have led to repeated appearances and reversals of morphologic traits that were formerly considered to be reliable indicators of shared ancestry. These results have confounded or completely revised earlier morphologic-based phylogenies and classifications. Presented herein are resources for understanding not only current amphibian taxonomy but also the challenges of relying on a stable taxonomy that is undergoing constant flux.

From activities ranging from teaching to veterinary practice, a taxonomy should accurately communicate the state of the art in knowledge related to both actual biodiversity and the phylogenetic relationships among species and groups (e.g., genera). A recent pulse of activity in amphibian systematics, spurred largely by technologic improvements in collecting and analyzing massive molecular data sets, has greatly increased the understanding of the relationships among and within the major groups; this new information has appropriately spurred efforts to revise the antiquated, misleading taxonomy of the last century or so. Given that novel taxonomic arrangements for long-familiar groups can be confusing and frustrating, this chapter endeavors to summarize in a user-friendly fashion the most recent taxonomic changes, especially as they relate to groups likely to be encountered by readers of this chapter. Ideally a taxonomy should reflect the phylogeny—the actual evolutionary history—of the creatures under consideration. Thus, this summary will hopefully be useful for keepers, curators, and veterinarians working with species that are poorly known or with which they are simply unfamiliar. Importantly, knowledge of the phylogenetic position of a species may allow one to extrapolate information relevant to other closely related species, genera, or from another family.

Because taxonomic monographs and treatments include exhaustive citations of all relevant literature and complete reviews of taxonomic changes and synonymies, those efforts will not be duplicated here and readers are referred to the original monographs. The current renaissance in amphibian taxonomy was spurred by a series of three monographs published by the American Museum of Natural History.[1-3] *The Amphibian Tree of Life*[3] was especially influential because it represented the first modern attempt to consider amphibian phylogeny in its entirety. Never claiming to be the last word on knowledge of amphibian phylogeny or taxonomy, it did proceed to frame and encourage a flood of subsequent articles that, considered together, have greatly increased knowledge of the history of Amphibia and represent major steps toward producing a taxonomy that is consistent with their history. Some important recent articles include treatments of the phyllomedusine frogs,[4] hemiphractid frogs (formerly part of Hylidae),[5] microhylid frogs,[6] glass frogs,[7] ranid frogs,[8] bufonid frogs,[9-12] and the terraranan frogs (the so-called eleutherodactylines, formerly included in Leptodactylidae).[13] Additional recent efforts have informed the understanding of the broader groups such as caecilians[14-16] and salamanders.[17-19] Recently, Pyron and Wiens[20] assembled virtually all of the molecular data produced by the mentioned series of articles (plus others not here listed) into a single massive analysis. Their study largely confirmed these previous more focused efforts and added some refinements to the ever-problematic assemblage of South American frogs formerly referred to "Leptodactylidae." However, relationships within the large superfamily Hyloidea (including many families widely kept in captivity, such as the hylid tree frogs) were mostly poorly supported. Moreover, their phylogeny inexplicably retained an untenable nonmonophyletic taxonomy for Bufonidae and Ranidae. Table 19-1 lists a taxonomic summary of generally recognized families of amphibians, including approximate information on species-level diversity within each and geographic distribution.

Current generic-level taxonomy has not been emphasized nor summarized in this chapter because generic limits and species allocations are in constant flux, and, in the case of amphibians, considerable changes at this level can be anticipated in the upcoming years. For current information regarding generic allocations, the reader is referred to these frequently updated online references: The American Museum of Natural History's Amphibian Species of the World at http://research.amnh.org/herpetology/amphibia/index.php and The University of California's Amphibiaweb at http://www.amphibiaweb.org/.

For species occurring in North America, the standard English and scientific names list cosponsored by all four of the major herpetological societies based in the United States is recommended.[21] The most recent edition is available for free download by the Society for the Study of Amphibians and Reptiles at http://www.ssarherps.org/pages/comm_names/Index.php.

Readers working in institutions accredited by the Association of Zoos and Aquariums (AZA) should note that AZA follows the taxonomy of *Amphibian Species of the World* Web site[22]; however, this Web site is updated frequently, and it has not been standard for AZA institutions to update their records accordingly. The International Species Information System (ISIS) record-keeping system officially lists Frost[23] plus the addendum by Duellman[24] as their taxonomic standard. However, because both of those sources are quite outdated, it can be assumed that they now refer to the continuation of that same project, which now exists online in the form of *Amphibian Species of the World.*[22] An additional useful Web site is the International Union for Conservation of Nature (IUCN) Red List (http://www.iucnredlist.org/initiatives/amphibians), which provides detailed information for every known species of amphibian regarding distribution, conservation status, and more, although this particular database is not intended to be a source of the most current taxonomic status of any species or group.

PHYLOGENY AND TAXONOMY OF AMPHIBIANS

Amphibians are a distinct group of tetrapod vertebrates, and despite centuries of communications to the opposite, they are in no way "transitional" between fishes and other groups of tetrapods (e.g., reptiles). For the most part, referring a specimen in hand to one of the three major groups of amphibians (i.e., caecilians, frogs, and salamanders) has never been problematic. However, reconciling the relationships among these three groups has never been intuitive. This is because frogs and caecilians both have highly derived body forms while salamanders remain with what is frequently considered to be the generic tetrapod body plan. Some debate has occurred regarding the relationships among these three groups,[25] but the arrangement shown in Figure 19-1 is now generally accepted.

Taxonomically, or in terms of nomenclature, this arrangement can be summarized as follows:

Class **Amphibia:** amphibians
Order **Gymnophiona:** caecilians
Infraclass **Batrachia:** frogs and salamanders
Order **Caudata:** salamanders
Order **Anura:** frogs

Currently, 7170 species of amphibians are known, and the majority of those are anurans (note: the homepage for amphibiaweb.org includes a convenient daily update of the number of recognized species). Frost et al[3] characterize amphibians as having, among many other unique features, loss of several bones in the typical tetrapod skull (e.g., supratemporal, jugal, postorbital bones, Figure 19-2, *A*), biscuspid, pedicellate teeth (Figure 19-2, *B*), a unique papilla amphibiorum in the ear associated with the and opercular element (Figure 19-2, *C*), glandular skin (Figure 19-2, *D*), gonadal fatbodies, and a lack of epidermal scales.

PHYLOGENY AND TAXONOMY OF CAECILIANS

The caecilians, or Gymnophiona, are the most geographically restricted (limited in distribution to tropical South America, Asia, and Africa but absent from Madagascar) and secretive of all amphibian orders. As with all aspects of caecilian biology, their true species-level diversity is poorly known. Nonetheless, known taxa are commonly referred to 10 families (Figure 19-3), and approximately 192 species are currently recognized. Future taxonomic changes are to be expected

TABLE 19-1

A Taxonomic Summary of Generally Recognized Families of Amphibians*

Taxon	English Name	Approximate Number of Species	General Distribution
GYMNOPHIONA	**CAECILIANS**	**192**	**PANTROPICAL**
Caeciliidae	N/A	42	South and Central America
Chikilidae	N/A	1	India
Dermophiidae	N/A	14	Central and South America and Africa
Herpelidae	N/A	9	Africa
Ichthyophiidae	N/A	53	South and Southeast Asia
Indotyphlidae	Including yellow-banded caecilians	20	India, Africa and the Seychelles
Rhinatrematidae	N/A	11	South America
Scolecomorphidae	N/A	6	Africa
Siphonopidae	N/A	23	South America
Typhlonectidae	Aquatic caecilians	13	northern South America
CAUDATA	**SALAMANDERS**	**648**	**EURASIA AND AMERICAS**
Ambystomatidae	Mole salamanders	32	North America
Amphiumidae	Amphiumas	3	North America
Cryptobranchidae	Giant salamanders and hellbenders	3	Asia and North America
Dicamptontidae	Pacific giant salamanders	4	North America
Hynobiidae	Asian salamanders	59	Asia
Plethodontidae	Lungless salamanders	435	Asia, Europe, and Americas
Proteidae	Muduppies and waterdogs	6	Europe and North America
Rhyacotritonidae	Torrent salamanders	4	North America
Salamandridae	"True" salamanders	98	Eurasia and North America
Sirenidae	Sirens	4	North America
ANURA	**FROGS**	**6289**	**COSMOPOLITAN, EXCEPT ANTARCTICA**
Allophrynidae	N/A, but including Tukeit-hill frog	2	South America
Alsodidae	N/A	30	South America
Alytidae	Midwife toads	5	Europe and North Africa
Arthroleptidae	N/A, but including Hairy frogs	147	Sub-Saharan Africa
Ascaphidae	Tailed frogs	2	Northwestern United States and Canada
Batrachylidae	N/A	15	Argentina and Chile
Bombinatoridae	Fire-bellied toads	10	Eurasia and Southeast Asia
Brachycephalidae	N/A	52	South America
Brevicipitidae	N/A, but including rain frogs	34	Sub-Saharan Africa
Bufonidae	"True" toads	585	Cosmopolitan, except Australo-Papua, Oceania and Madagascar
Calyptocephalellidae	N/A, but including the Helmeted Water toad	4	South America
Centrolenidae	Glass frogs	152	Mesoamerica and South America
Ceratobatrachidae	N/A	86	Southeast Asia
Ceratophryidae	Including Budgett's and Horned frogs	12	South America
Ceuthomantidae	N/A	4	South America
Conrauidae	N/A, but including the Goliath frog	6	Equatorial Africa
Craugastoridae	Stream frogs	115	Mesoamerica and South America
Cycloramphidae	N/A	34	South America
Dendrobatidae	Poison frogs	293	Central and South America
Dicroglossidae	N/A	185	Africa and Asia
Discoglossidae	Painted frogs	6	Europe and northern Africa
Eleutherodactylidae	Rain frogs	206	Americas, including Caribbean
Heleophrynidae	Ghost frogs	6	South Africa
Hemiphractidae	Marsupial frogs	101	Central and South America
Hemisotidae	Shovel-nosed frogs	9	Sub-Saharan Africa
Hylidae	Tree frogs	929	Eurasia, Australo-Papua, and Americas
Hylodidae	N/A	42	South America
Hyperoliidae	Reed frogs	223	Africa and Madagascar
Leiopelmatidae	New Zealand frogs	4	North America and New Zealand
Leptodactylidae	Southern frogs	200	Mesoamerica and South America
Mantellidae	Mantellas	205	Madagascar
Megophryidae	N/A but including Horned frogs and Toothed toads	174	Southeast Asia
Micrixalidae	N/A	11	India

Continued

TABLE 19-1

A Taxonomic Summary of Generally Recognized Families of Amphibians—cont'd

Taxon	English Name	Approximate Number of Species	General Distribution
Microhylidae	Narrow-mouthed toads	525	Americas, Africa, Southeast Asia, and Australo-Papua
Myobatrachidae	Australian ground and water frogs	131	Australo-Papua
Nasikabatrachidae	Purple frog	1	India
Nycibatrachidae	N/A	28	India
Odontophrynidae	Includes Horned frogs	41	South America
Pelobatidae	Spadefoot toads	4	Eurasia and North Africa
Pelodytidae	Parsley frogs	3	Europe
Petropedetidae	N/A	12	Sub-Saharan Africa
Phrynobatrachidae	N/A	86	Sub-Saharan Africa
Pipidae	Clawed frogs and Surinam toads	33	Central and South America and sub-Saharan Africa
Ptychadenidae	Rocket frogs	51	Sub-Saharan Africa
Pyxicephalidae	N/A, including African Bullfrogs	73	Sub-Saharan Africa
Ranidae	"True" frogs	362	Cosmopolitan
Ranixalidae	N/A	10	India
Rhacophoridae	N/A, but including foam-nesting and flying frogs	361	Sub-Saharan Africa and Asia
Rhinodermatidae	Darwin's frogs	3	Chile
Rhinophrynidae	Mexican Burrowing toad	1	Mesoamerica
Scaphiopodidae	American Spadefoot toads	7	North America, including Mexico
Sooglossidae	Seychelles frogs	4	Seychelles
Strabomantidae	Rain frogs	603	Central and South America
Telmatobiidae	Includes water frogs	61	South America

*Based on Frost DR, Grant T, Faivovich J, et al. The amphibian tree of life. *Bull Am Museum Nat Hist* 2006;297:1-370; Pyron RA, Wiens JJ. A large-scale phylogeny of Amphibia including over 2800 species, and a revised classification of extant frogs, salamanders, and caecilians. *Mol Phylogenet Evol* 2011;61:543-583; and Frost DR. Amphibian species of the world: an online reference. Version 5.5. Electronic database available at http://research.amnh.org/vz/herpetology/amphibia/. Accessed January 31, 2011. Approximate numbers of species in each group and a very general description of geographic distribution are also presented (species counts are from Amphibiaweb.org).

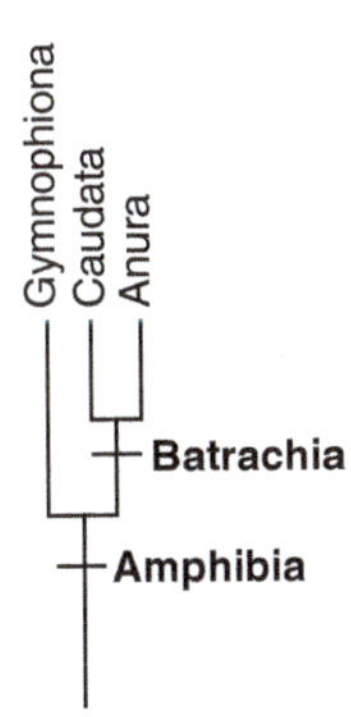

FIGURE 19-1 Relationships among the three major groups of amphibians: Gymnophiona (caecilians), Anura (frogs), and Caudata (salamanders). *(Adapted from Frost DR, Grant T, Faivovich J, et al. The amphibian tree of life.* Bull Am Museum Nat Hist *2006;297:1-370.)*

in this group as additional material for study, discoveries of new species, and studies are forthcoming. For example, Kamei et al[26] recently discovered a new major lineage (family Chikilidae) and suggest that it contains numerous yet unnamed species.

Caecilians, superficially resembling earthworms or snakes in general appearance, share a suite of morphologic features, including a heavily ossified skull that makes them highly adapted to a fossorial or burrowing lifestyle. Frost et al[3] characterize the gymnophionans as being legless amphibians that lack both limbs and girdles (but one fossil taxon is known to have had four limbs) and having a unique dual jaw-closing mechanism, an eversible male intromittent organ (the phallodeum), dermal annuli that encircle the body, and unique paired sensory tentacles on the snout. With the exception of one species *(Atretochoana eiselti)*, all caecilians have lungs, but often the left lung is reduced in size, which is an adaptation for an elongate body shape, much as in snakes. Some species also have dermal calcite scales and are the only living amphibians known to possess them.

PHYLOGENY AND TAXONOMY OF SALAMANDERS

The salamanders represent a moderately speciose group (approximately 648 species) distributed primarily in North America, Central America, northern South America, and Eurasia. Recent efforts in the systematics of salamanders did not greatly modify the understanding of the relationships among the major groups (and Figure 19-4) nor their family-level taxonomy. Readers should be aware that some continuing controversy exists regarding subfamilial classification of salamanders and should consult the Web sites of Amphibiaweb

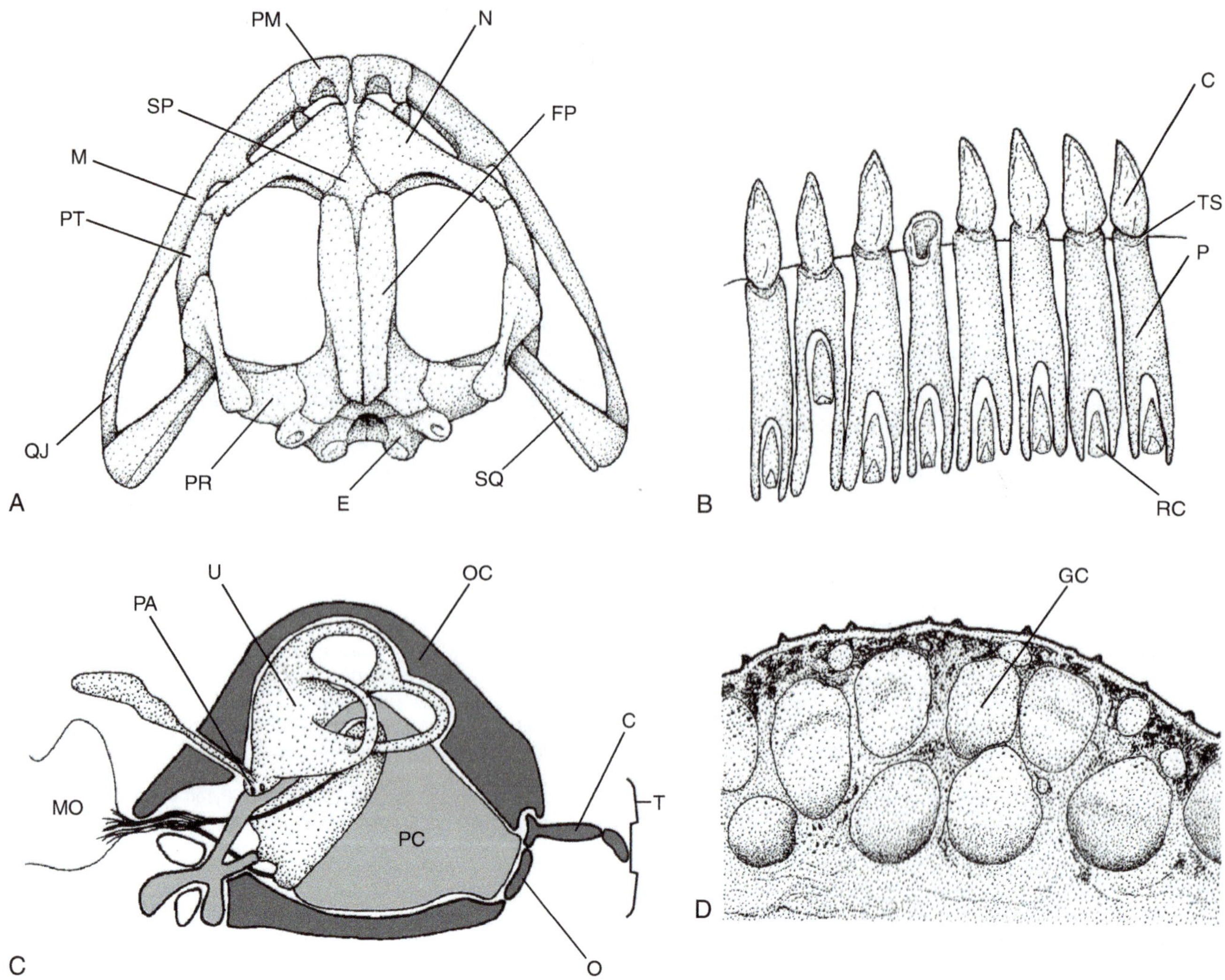

FIGURE 19-2 Amphibians are characterized as having several synapomorphies (i.e., unique, shared, derived characteristics) some of which are illustrated here. **A,** Amphibian evolution includes the loss of several bones found in the typical tetrapod skull (e.g., supratemporal, jugal, postorbital bones) through the fusion of elements such as the frontal and parietal (frontoparietal). Dorsal view of the skull of the North American bullfrog *Lithobates catesbeianus. E,* Exoccipital; *FP,* frontoparietal; *M,* maxilla; *N,* nasal; *PR,* prootic; *PM,* premaxilla, *PT,* pterygoid; *QJ,* quadratojugal; *SP,* sphenethmoid; *SQ,* squamosal. *(Drawing made from the DigiMorph online catalog of CT scans: http://www.digimorph.org/specimens/Rana_catesbeiana//.)* **B,** Lingual view of the biscuspid, pedicellate teeth of the anuran *Calyptocephalella caudiverbera. C,* Crown; *P,* pedicel; *RC,* replacement crown; *TS,* transverse suture. *(Drawing adapted from Parsons TS, Williams EE. The teeth of Amphibia and their relation to amphibian phylogeny.* J Morphol *1962;110:375-389.)* **C,** The inner ear of *Lithobates catesbeianus* illustrating the papilla amphibiorum *(PA),* as well as the opercular element *(O)* and the columella *(C). MO,* Medulla oblongata; *OC,* otic capsule; *PC,* perilymphatic cistern; *T,* tympanum; *U,* utriculus. *(Drawing adapted from Duellman WE, Trueb L.* Biology of Amphibians. *Baltimore: The John Hopkins University Press, 1994.)* **D,** Cross section of the skin of the poisonous toad *Melanophryniscus montevidensis* illustrating granular glands. *(Drawing adapted from Mebs D, Pogoda W, Maneyro R, et al. Studies on the poisonous skin secretion of individual red bellied toads,* Melanophryniscus montevidensis *[Anura, Bufonidae], from Uruguay.* Toxicon *2005;46:641-650.)*

and Amphibian Species of the World to consider current perspectives; this controversy does not, however, greatly affect familial or generic level classifications. Salamanders have always been difficult to characterize in terms of unique morphologic aspects because most persons assume that they have simply retained the primitive ancestral tetrapod body plan. This is an overstatement in many senses, and Frost et al[3] characterize the caudatans as being unique among amphibians by having both forelimbs and a tail and an incomplete maxillary arcade (upper jaw). Additionally, salamanders are unique

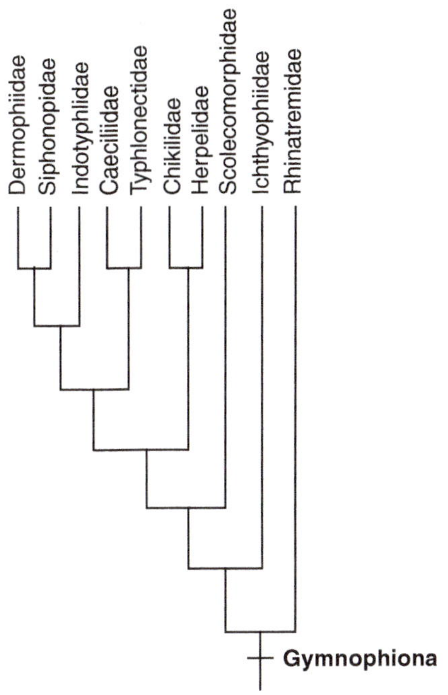

FIGURE 19-3 Relationships among the major clades (families) of caecilians. *(Adapted from Kamei RG, Mauro DS, Gower DJ, et al. Discovery of a new family of amphibians from northeast India with ancient links to Africa.* Proc Biol Sci *2012;279:2396-2401.)*

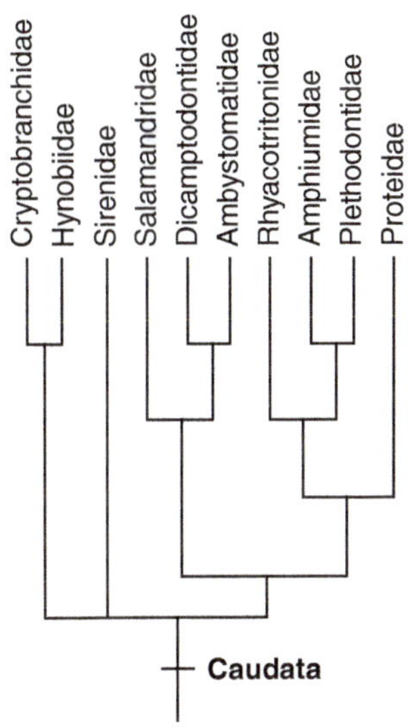

FIGURE 19-4 Consensus of phylogenetic relationships among the major clades (families) of salamanders. *(Adapted from Zhang P, Wake DB. Higher-level salamander relationships and divergence dates inferred from complete mitochondrial genomes.* Mol Phylogenet Evol *2009;53:492-508 and Pyron RA, Wiens JJ. A large-scale phylogeny of Amphibia including over 2800 species, and a revised classification of extant frogs, salamanders, and caecilians.* Mol Phylogenet Evol *2011;61:543-583.)*

in that many species, or entire groups, retain various aspects of the larval morphology into sexual maturity (a phenomenon known as neoteny). Salamanders usually do not vocalize as most anurans do; thus they rely on pheromones and courtship displays to locate and attract a mate.

PHYLOGENY AND TAXONOMY OF FROGS

Frogs, represented by more than 6289 species, have always represented a great challenge to systematists, as their evolutionary history evidently includes explosive radiations, along with high levels of both convergence and extreme morphologic derivation. Because attempts to recover the phylogeny of frogs with morphologic data alone have generally failed, molecular data have been crucial in shaping our understanding of this complex phylogeny. Building on the foundation of the efforts by Frost et al,[3] numerous studies have been produced[11,20] and are greatly increasing the knowledge about this vast and taxonomically difficult group. As soon as an agreement on a phylogeny of frogs is reached, numerous taxonomic changes will be forthcoming. Some stakeholders have expressed frustration about changes already proposed, such as when long-familiar species such as *Rana catesbeiana* and *Bufo americanus* suddenly appeared as *Lithobates catesbeianus* and *Anaxyrus americanus.* Simply put, such changes are necessary and important so that a taxonomy that is both informative and internally consistent can be used when communicating about amphibians. Figure 19-5 summarizes the agreement among recent studies on frog phylogeny. Polytomies, or unresolved branches, represent areas of the tree where recent analyses have produced conflicting results or poor statistical support; in this sense, the phylogeny shown here is conservative.

Anurans are perhaps the most familiar amphibians to most people, and indeed, their unique body plan, adapted largely for saltatorial locomotion (e.g., elongate hindlimbs), makes all but the most bizarre species instantly recognizable to layperson as *frogs.* The many unique features of this group that Frost et al[3] listed as characteristic include the following: reduction of vertebral number to nine or fewer; fusion of the caudal vertebrae to form the bony urostyle; hindlimbs significantly longer than forelimbs (with a few exceptions), produced, in part, by the elongation of the ankle bones; fusion of the radius and ulna of the forelimb and fusion of the tibia and fibula of the hindlimb; presence of keratinous jaw sheaths and keratodonts on larval mouthparts (with some exceptions); skin with large subcutaneous lymph spaces; and during mating, a unique clasping behavior (amplexus) common to most species.

CONCLUSION

Tremendous growth in knowledge of the phylogeny of amphibians has occurred in the last few years. This knowledge is crucial for informing the study of all aspects of their biology, as well as their husbandry and veterinary care, and for pressing conservation concerns. However, more work remains to be done, and changes in the trees presented here are anticipated. Certainly, still more taxonomic changes will accompany increased knowledge of the evolution of amphibians. The regularly updated *Amphibian Species of the World*[22] is recommended as a standard reference for amphibian taxonomy, but the primary literature should be the source for the most recent information on amphibian phylogeny.

ACKNOWLEDGMENTS

The authors would like to thank Darrel Frost for providing information on the latest version of the Amphibian Species of the World Taxonomy.

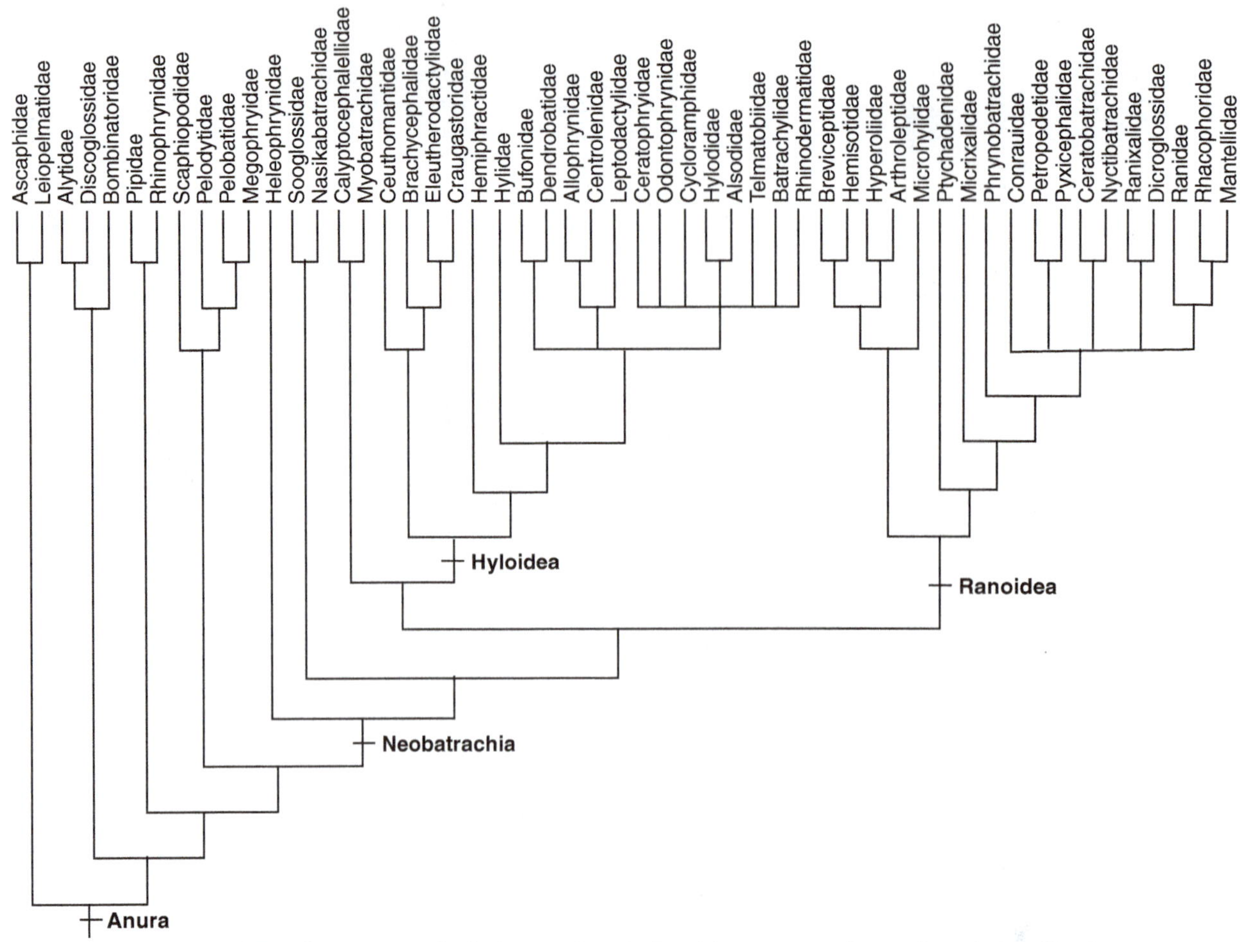

FIGURE 19-5 Consensus of phylogenetic relationships among the major clades (families) of anurans or frogs. *(Adapted from Pyron RA, Wiens JJ. A large-scale phylogeny of Amphibia including over 2800 species, and a revised classification of extant frogs, salamanders, and caecilians.* Mol Phylogenet Evol *2011;61:543-583.)*

REFERENCES

1. Faivovich JCF, Haddad B, Garcia PCA, et al. Systematic review of the frog family Hylidae, with special reference to Hylinae: phylogenetic analysis and taxonomic revision. *Bull Am Museum Nat Hist* 2005;294:1-240.
2. Grant T, Frost DR, Caldwell JP, et al. Phylogenetic systematics of the dart-poison frogs and their relatives (Amphibia: Athesphatanura: Dendrobatidae). *Bull Am Museum Nat Hist* 2006;299:1-262.
3. Frost DR, Grant T, Faivovich J, et al. The amphibian tree of life. *Bull Am Museum Nat Hist* 2006;297:1-370.
4. Faivovich JCF, Haddad B, Baeta D, et al. The phylogenetic relationships of the charismatic poster frogs, Phyllomedusinae (Anura, Hylidae). *Cladistics* 2010;26:227-261.
5. Wiens JJ, Kuczynski CA, Duellman WE, et al. Loss and revolution of complex life cycles in marsupial frogs: does ancestral trait reconstruction mislead? *Evolution* 2007;61:1886-1899.
6. Van der Meijden A, Vences M, Hoegg S, et al. Nuclear gene phylogeny of narrow-mouthed toads (Family: Microhylidae) and a discussion of competing hypotheses concerning their biogeographical origins. *Mol Phylogenet Evol* 2007;44:1017-1030.
7. Guayasamin JM, Castroviejo-Fisher S, Trueb L, et al. Phylogenetic systematics of Glassfrogs (Amphibia: Centrolenidae) and their sister taxon *Allophryne ruthveni*. *Zootaxa* 2009;2100:1-97.
8. Bossuyt F, Brown RM, Hillis DM, et al. Phylogeny and biogeography of a cosmopolitan frog radiation: late Cretaceous diversification resulted in continent-scale endemism in the family Ranidae. *Syst Biol* 2006;55:579-594.
9. Pauly GB, Hillis DM, Cannatella DC. The history of a nearctic colonization: molecular phylogenetics and biogeography of the nearctic toads *(Bufo)*. *Evolution* 2004;58:2517-2535.
10. Pramuk JB, Robertson T, Sites JW Jr, et al. Around the world in 10 million years: biogeography of the nearly cosmopolitan true toads (Anura: Bufonidae). *Global Ecol Biogeogr* 2008;17:72-83.
11. Van Bocxlaer I, Loader SP, Roelants K, et al. Gradual adaptation toward a range-expansion phenotype initiated the global radiation of toads. *Science* 2010;327:679-682.
12. Mendelson JRIII, Mulcahy DG, Williams TS, et al. A phylogeny and evolutionary natural history of mesoamerican toads (Anura: Bufonidae: *Incilius*) based on morphology, life history, and molecular data. *Zootaxa* 2011;3138:1-34.
13. Hedges SB, Duellman WE, Heinicke MP. New world direct-developing frogs (Anura: Terrarana): molecular phylogeny, classification, biogeography, and conservation. *Zootaxa* 2008;1737:1-182.
14. Mauro DS, Gower DJ, Massingham T, et al. Experimental design in caecilian systematics: phylogenetic information of mitochondrial genomes and nuclear RAG1. *Syst Biol* 2009;58:425-438.
15. Wilkinson M, Mauro DS, Sherratt E, et al. A nine-family classification of caecilians (Amphibia: Gymnophiona). *Zootaxa* 2011;2874:41-64.
16. Zhang P, Wake MH. A mitogenomic perspective on the phylogeny and biogeography of living caecilians (Amphibia: Gymnophiona). *Mol Phylogenet Evol* 2009;53:479-491.
17. Kozak KH, Mendyk RW, Wiens JJ. Can parallel diversification occur in sympatry? Repeated patterns of body-size evolution in co-existing clades of North American salamanders. *Evolution* 2009;63:1769-1784.

18. Vieites DR, Roman SR, Wake MH, et al. A multigenic perspective on phylogenetic relationships in the largest family of salamanders, the Plethodontidae. *Mol Phylogenet Evol* 2011;59:623-635.
19. Zhang P, Wake DB. Higher-level salamander relationships and divergence dates inferred from complete mitochondrial genomes. *Mol Phylogenet Evol* 2009;53:492-508.
20. Pyron RA, Wiens JJ. A large-scale phylogeny of Amphibia including over 2800 species, and a revised classification of extant frogs, salamanders, and caecilians. *Mol Phylogenet Evol* 2011;61:543-583.
21. Crother BI, ed. Scientific and standard English names of amphibians and reptiles of North America north of Mexico, with comments regarding confidence in our understanding. 7th ed. *SSAR Herpetol Circ* 37.Retrieved from http?//www.ssarherps.org/pages/comm._names.php 16 May 2013.
22. Frost DR. Amphibian species of the world: an online reference. Version 5.5. Electronic database available at http://research.amnh.org/vz/herpetology/amphibia/. Accessed January 31, 2011.
23. Frost DR, ed. *Amphibian species of the world: a taxonomic and geographic reference.* Lawrence, Kansas: Allen Press and Association of Systematics Collections, 1985.
24. Duellman WE. Amphibian species of the world: additions and corrections. Lawrence, KS: University of Kansas Publications, Museum of Natural History Special Publications 1993;21:1-372
25. Trueb L, Cloutier R. Toward an understanding of the amphibians: two centuries of systematic history. In: Schultze HP, Trueb L, eds. *Origins of the higher groups of tetrapods: controversy and consensus.* Ithaca, NY: Comstock Publishing Associates, 1991;175-193.
26. Kamei RG, Mauro DS, Gower DJ, et al. Discovery of a new family of amphibians from northeast India with ancient links to Africa. *Proc Biol Sci* 2012;279:2396-2401.

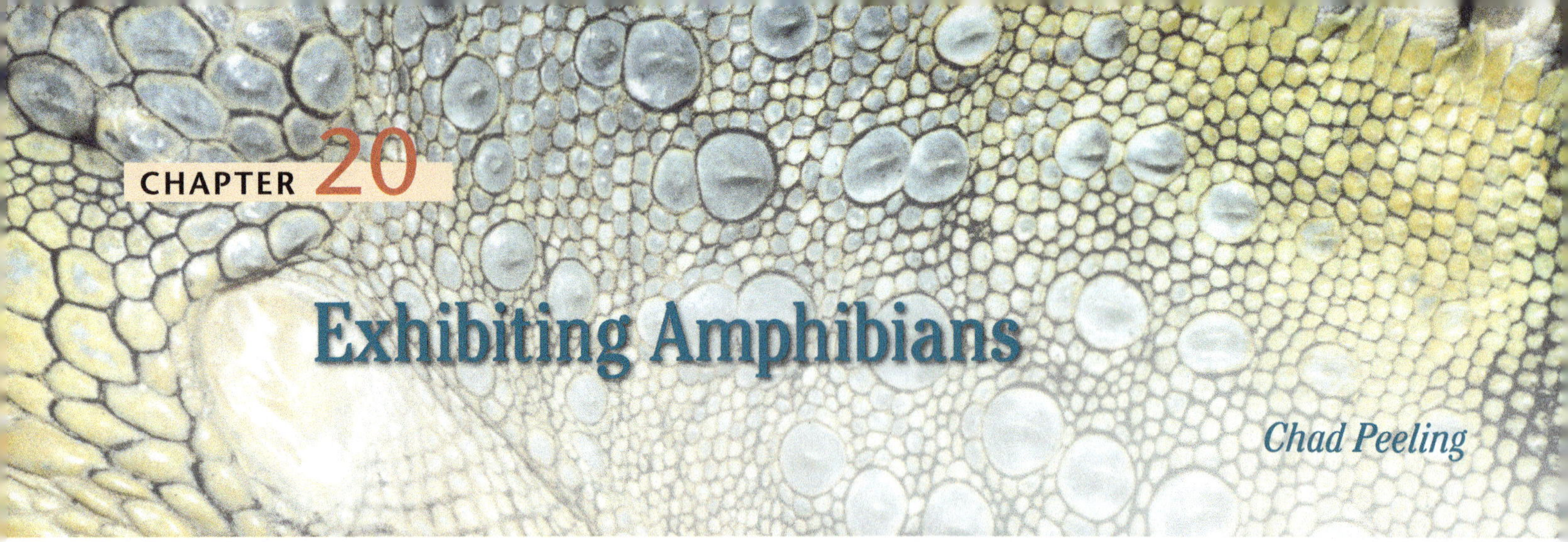

CHAPTER 20

Exhibiting Amphibians

Chad Peeling

Many people underestimate the difficulties in creating successful amphibian exhibits, assuming it is merely a matter of understanding amphibian husbandry. However, exhibiting anything is more challenging than maintaining it off-display, and this is especially true of amphibians. Many species are delicate and shy, and balancing their needs with the needs of the visiting public is both an art and a science. There are at least four major challenges to overcome: keeping the animals visible; keeping the animals comfortable; buffering the internal environment against rapid changes, and making the exhibit easy for keepers to maintain. Failing to meet any of these challenges can be a recipe for disaster.

Good exhibit design is largely a matter of predicting the behaviors and needs of the animals, the visiting public, and the exhibit keepers. One must approach it with a realistic mindset. Hoping that visitors will take time to search for hidden amphibians is naïve. Assuming that keepers will consistently attend to every husbandry detail is dangerous. Successful exhibit designs anticipate likely problems and mitigate human errors. They usually include a good deal of hidden infrastructure and a great deal of hidden planning.

In 2001, *Peeling Productions,* the exhibit arm of Clyde Peeling's Reptiland, a zoologic park in Allenwood, Pennsylvania accredited by the Association of Zoos and Aquariums (AZA), began planning a large-scale traveling exhibition called *Frogs—A Chorus of Colors*. Having exhibited amphibians on a small scale at our permanent facility in Pennsylvania, we knew that a big, complex project would require forethought. We began by visiting public and private amphibian facilities to learn from the experiences of others. Our goal was to emulate the successful aspects of existing exhibits and improve on their weaknesses. Over the next 2 years our exhibit team designed, prototyped, and fabricated the exhibition at our production facility in Pennsylvania, learning along the way. The finished exhibition premiered in 2003 and has been on a nationwide tour of museums, zoos, and science centers ever since (Figure 20-1). Building *Frogs—A Chorus of Colors* affected the trajectory and interests of our company. We created a second copy of the exhibition in 2005 and have since built a series of custom amphibian exhibits for other clients. Each of these projects has left us with strong opinions about what works and what does not. While this chapter is primarily about creating public exhibits, the principles can be applied to amphibian displays of any kind.

WHAT TO AVOID

The most common mistake in public amphibian exhibits is over planting. It is tempting to create a beautiful, lush habitat that closely mimics an animal's native environment and call it an exhibit, but planting with abandon ensures that the subjects of the exhibit—the amphibians—will rarely be seen. Nothing frustrates visitors more than an animal exhibit without animals, even if it is a stunning botanical display. Of course, the solution to overplanting is not to eliminate the plants; there is no reason to sacrifice aesthetics or naturalism. However, planting, arranging props, and all other aspects of decorating an exhibit must be done strategically to keep the animals in view (Figure 20-2).

Another common misstep is selecting species that interest keepers or curators but do not exhibit well. The most obvious example of this is the iconic Red-eyed tree frog (*Agalychnis callidryas*). While stunningly beautiful when active, these frogs are strictly nocturnal. They perch on glass or under leaves by day with their eyes closed and all of their colorful parts tucked beneath their green bodies. From a visitor's perspective they look like small green blobs stuck to various surfaces. Although it is possible to exhibit Red-eyed Tree frogs under reversed lighting conditions, their splendid colors cannot be appreciated in dim or blue light. This is not to suggest that exhibitors avoid experimenting with difficult species but only that some species lend themselves to exhibits far more than others. Amphibians are charming animals, and people are captivated by the chance to see one up close. Displaying dormant or hidden specimens wastes an opportunity to captivate an audience. Save the ultra-shy species for backroom collections and stick with those that are engaging to watch.

The third mistake common to many amphibian exhibits is a labor-intensive design. It is easy to make an exhibit look pretty for opening day, but keeping it beautiful over the long term depends on functionality. Many exhibit designers are out of touch with the needs of keepers and the realities of daily maintenance. Exhibits with limited access, inadequate filtration, or minimal automation are difficult to care for and usually suffer neglect over time. Ease of maintenance should be a design imperative on par with aesthetics, durability, and cost.

ONE APPROACH TO EXHIBIT DESIGN

Species Selection

The natural starting point for designing an amphibian exhibit is species selection, and the range of possible species is often

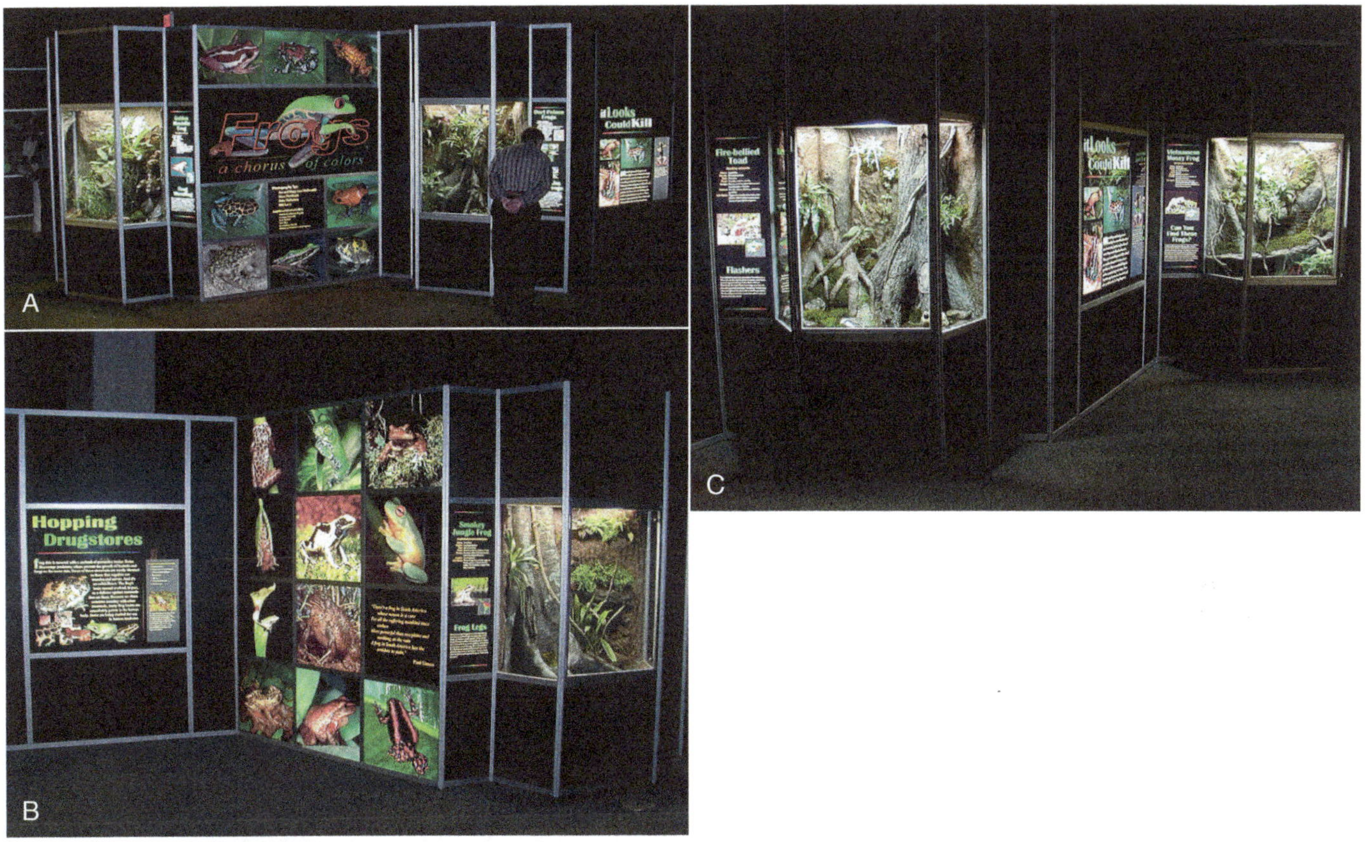

FIGURE 20-1 **A-C,** *Frogs—A Chorus of Colors* is a large traveling exhibition that began a tour of museums, zoos, and science centers in 2003. The exhibition has been hosted by prestigious institutions throughout the United States and Canada. Exhibited well, frogs have an enduring charisma in public exhibits.

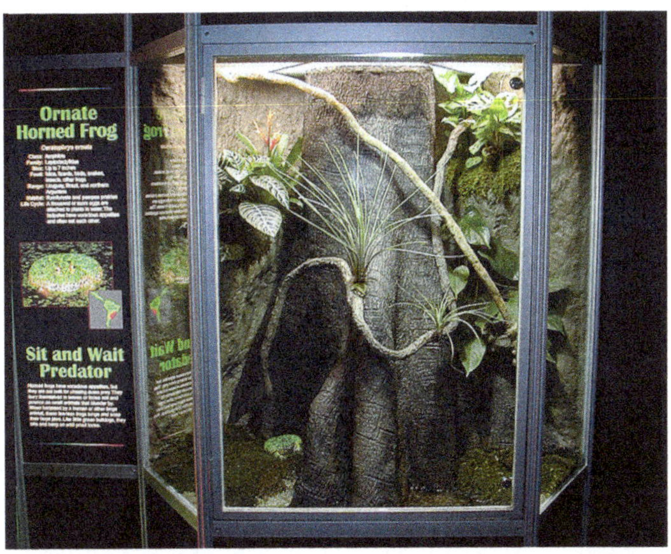

FIGURE 20-2 Keeping exhibit animals visible is a paradigm of good exhibit design. Plants and other décor should be arranged strategically.

dictated by the overarching message or theme of the project. Whatever the theme is, choosing a species that will engage visitors should be a priority. Otherwise, why bother with an exhibit? Defining the qualities of a good exhibit species is subjective, but a few basic questions are worth asking. Is the species nocturnal or diurnal? Does it perch in the open or prefer to stay hidden? Is it colorful or unusual enough to catch a layperson's eye? Is there an interesting or important story to tell? How large is it? Can multiple specimens be kept together? Has anyone else exhibited it successfully?

Practical concerns should also temper species choices. Some of the most spectacular amphibians, like West African Goliath Frogs (*Conraua goliath*), are unavailable or very difficult to maintain. Weigh the skill of exhibit keepers against committing to fragile species or those with unknown husbandry requirements. Consider whether the species is available now and likely to be available in the foreseeable future. Is it being bred in captivity or is it only available through importation? Does it have unusual or costly dietary requirements? Are specimens expensive to replace?

One of the hidden costs of exhibiting amphibians is maintaining a backup colony. Most species are sensitive to subtle environmental changes and can decline quickly if something goes wrong. In addition, the potential for introduced epidemic diseases like chytridiomycosis and ranavirus can quickly ravage a colony or an entire collection. Sooner or later, some specimens will probably need to be removed from exhibit because of illness, social stress, or death. It can be difficult to find replacements in a pinch because many species are only available seasonally. Furthermore, adult specimens of many species come at a premium, if breeders are willing to give them up at all. The obvious solution is to raise backups. Exhibiting amphibians requires allocating space, staff, and budget to

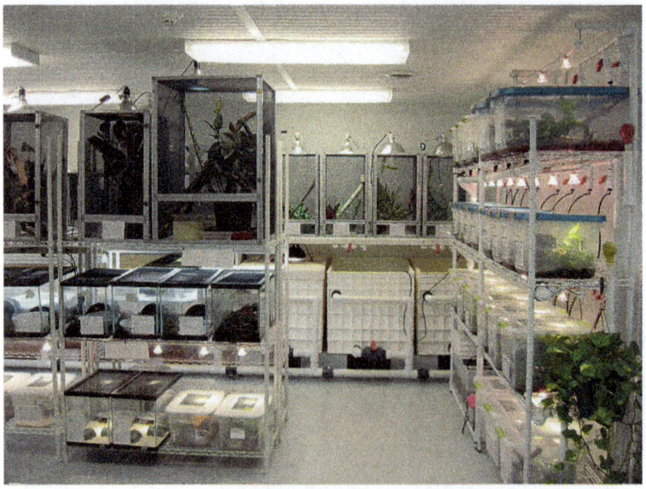

FIGURE 20-3 Off-exhibit holding areas are needed to rear and maintain backup exhibit animals.

continually maintain at least as many animals off display as needed on exhibit. We maintain 400 amphibian specimens off exhibit at Reptiland to support approximately 200 display animals in our various exhibitions (Figure 20-3). Of course, quarantine of newly acquired specimens takes even more space and time.

Research

Exhibit designs need to accommodate the biological and social needs of the inhabitants and strategically address their behavioral patterns. There is no shortcut to research, and we routinely spend days on it before designing anything. Consider where the species lives in the wild. Determine its basic physical needs: temperature, space, and humidity. Think about its typical behaviors: degree and timing of activity, percentage of time spent in water, ability to climb or dig, and the need for cover. Read accounts of care in captivity, looking for common social, physical, or disease-related problems. The results of good research determine the basic structure of the exhibit: size, shape, slopes, plateaus, branches, rocks, water features, and the number and size of plantings.

Enclosures

The outer structure, or tank, that contains an amphibian exhibit may be invisible to the viewing public, but everything inside the exhibit depends on it. The tank must be waterproof and durable and sturdy enough to support the weight of the internal components. Off-the-shelf glass aquaria are the least expensive option, but they are fragile, heavy, difficult to modify, and often the wrong shapes and sizes for functional amphibian exhibits. Custom-built tanks allow the exhibit to be designed around the animals, keepers, and visitors. A variety of materials are commonly used in constructing exhibit tanks including glass, epoxy-covered wood, acrylic, polyethylene, polypropylene, and fiberglass-reinforced plastics (FRP).

Each of these materials has its place, and choosing one depends on the overall scope of the project. In general, glass is the most desirable viewing surface because acrylic and similar transparent plastics scratch and warp over time. However, glass is too heavy and fragile for use in the overall structure. Plywood is probably the most versatile material for hidden structures, but it takes skill and care to properly envelop the wood in a reliable epoxy coating. Plastic shops can quickly fabricate acrylic tanks in nearly any shape and size, and they are relatively lightweight. Acrylic is fragile: the surface scratches under normal wear, and stress cracks often form where fasteners penetrate it. Polypropylene and polyethylene are available in sheets (typically opaque white) that can be heat-welded into watertight containers with specialized equipment. These plastics are rugged and easy to machine, but they are relatively costly and do not accept adhesives well (i.e., to bond glass or interior décor). FRP is available in sheet form, or it can be built up by hand by laying resin-impregnated fiberglass sheets over a removable form. FRP is incredibly strong, lightweight, and versatile, but the resins are toxic when uncured and require a good deal of safety equipment and skill to use.

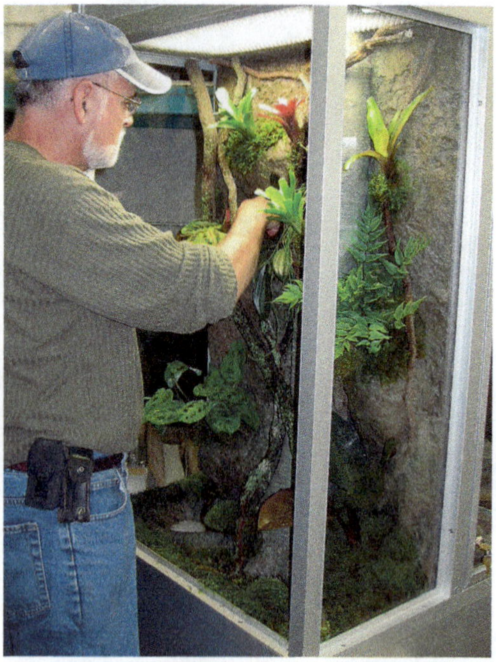

FIGURE 20-4 Front access doors allow keepers to see an exhibit from the public's perspective while cleaning.

Exhibit enclosures should be proportional in shape and size to the species and number of specimens they will house. Bigger is not always better. Most amphibians are secretive and will stay in the farthest corners of an enclosure if given the option. It is usually better to provide adequate living space and security with complex interior terrain rather than a large footprint. In general, limit the depth of enclosures to keep animals relatively close to viewing surfaces, creating cover with gentle cutbacks and careful plantings. Of course, the raw enclosure must be large enough to accommodate the interior décor while still leaving enough room for the animals.

One of the most important considerations in enclosure design is keeper access. It is tempting to think that tall enclosures can be serviced from above or that keepers can reach through small openings to provide care. The reality is that tanks that are difficult to enter will not be cared for as well as those that have easy access. Make doors large enough to allow an adult person to lean inside and locate doors so that shorter people can reach all corners of the enclosure. Consider how difficult it will be to reach around branches and other obstructions to clean glass or tend plants. If possible, include front access to enclosures, so keepers can see the exhibit from a visitor's perspective while cleaning—working in reverse is far more difficult (Figure 20-4). All doors should be designed to

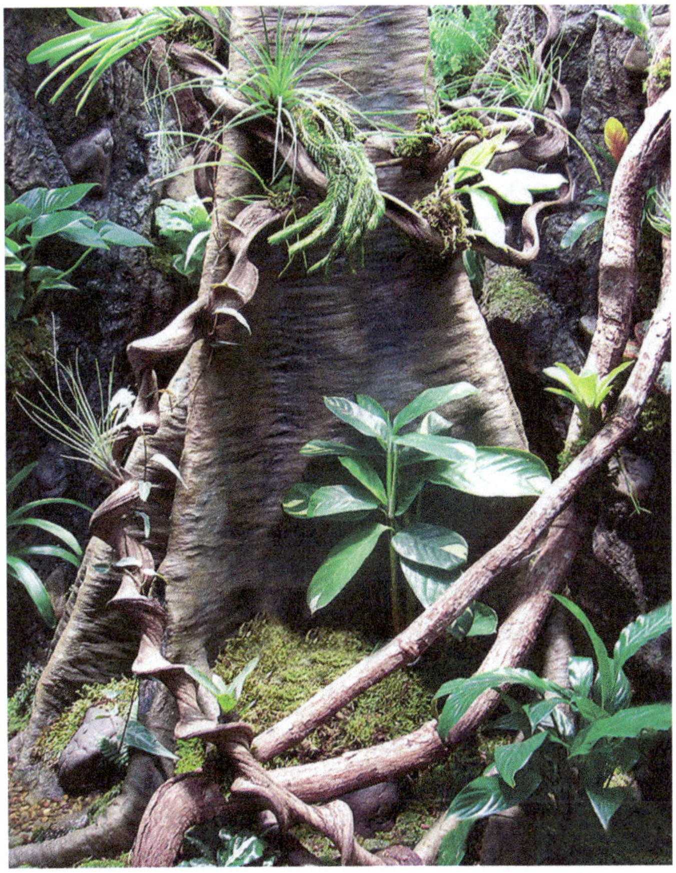

FIGURE 20-5 Natural-looking scenes fabricated with concrete or resins allow designers to re-create a slice of nature, disguise the infrastructure of the tank, and reduce maintenance requirements.

avoid accidentally squashing an amphibian when closing, and perimeter gaps should be small enough to limit insect escapes.

Do not skimp on hardware associated with the exhibit. Anything metallic (i.e. hinges, latches, or wire screens) should be aluminum or stainless steel. Moisture quickly leads to corrosion of ferric metals, even plated or galvanized versions, and the initial cost savings is offset over time by the need for replacements. Metallic structures directly exposed to tank water should be high-grade stainless steel. Other noncorrosive metals (e.g., brass, copper, and bronze) may leach into water and become toxic to amphibians.

Interior Landscapes

Interior decor puts exhibit animals in context and provides a visual backdrop. Its complexity depends on the project's scope and budget. Low cost scenes can be constructed with the use of real rocks, substrates, and branches. Completely "naturalistic" scenes, cast in concrete or resins, are much more costly but provide the illusion of a "slice of nature" (Figure 20-5). Well-designed fabricated interiors are also lower maintenance and can include hidden infrastructure such as contained planting pockets, plumbing, and conduit for electric cables.

Beautiful exhibits can be created with real rocks and branches. However, keeping the animals visible can be tricky if voids are not carefully filled. Any gap between rocks or space behind a branch is likely to become a hiding spot. Filling voids with organic soil mixes or live moss can mitigate this as long as the exhibited species is not a digger. In general, natural materials work better for small species like Poison Dart Frogs (family Dendrobatidae) and Mantella Frogs (*Mantella* sp.) (Figure 20-6). Larger amphibians are often strong enough to dislodge loosely stacked décor, and their larger waste volumes can seep into hidden areas and foul natural substrates.

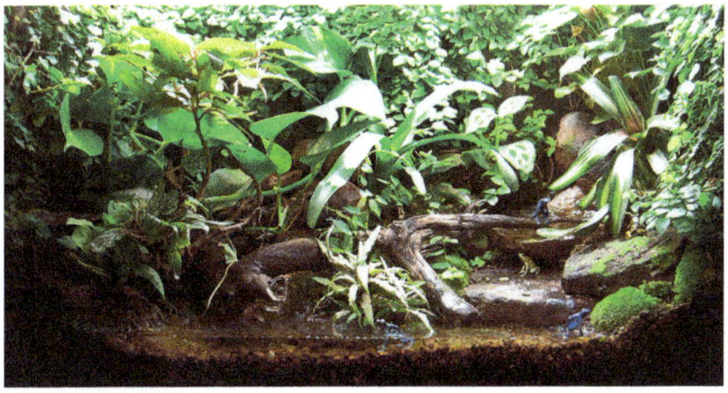

FIGURE 20-6 Decorating exhibits with real rocks and branches is inexpensive, but these habitats are time-consuming to maintain and best suited to small species.

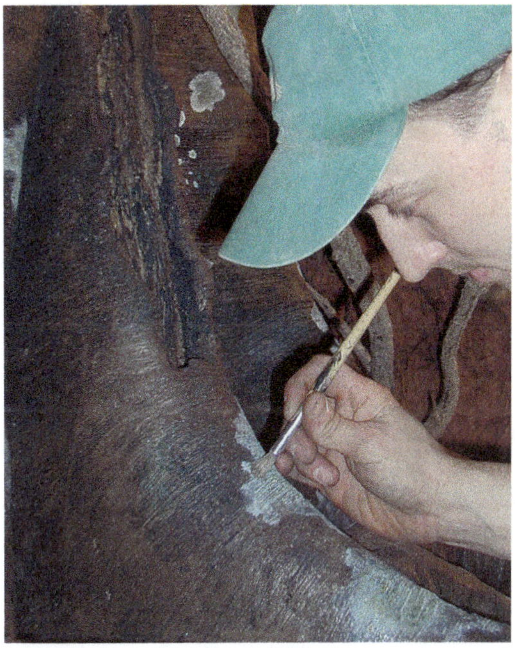

FIGURE 20-7 Fabricating high-fidelity natural scenes is an art that begins with careful observations of nature.

We generally prefer to decorate amphibian exhibits with recreations of nature, cast in concrete or plastic resins. Creating realistic habitat scenes is an art that springs from keen observations of nature, and it takes time and practice to master (Figure 20-7). The best examples capture the flavor of a real habitat and reflect authentic geology, growth habits of trees, and erosive patterns in topography. The goal is to create a strategically shaped scene that controls visibility and disguises the bowels of the tank while still looking natural (Figure 20-8). The specific techniques of fabricating with concrete and resins are beyond the scope of this chapter, but a summary of the materials used and their characteristics is worth mentioning.

Mortar or concrete (mortar with an aggregate) is inexpensive, requires no special equipment, and, when cured, it has

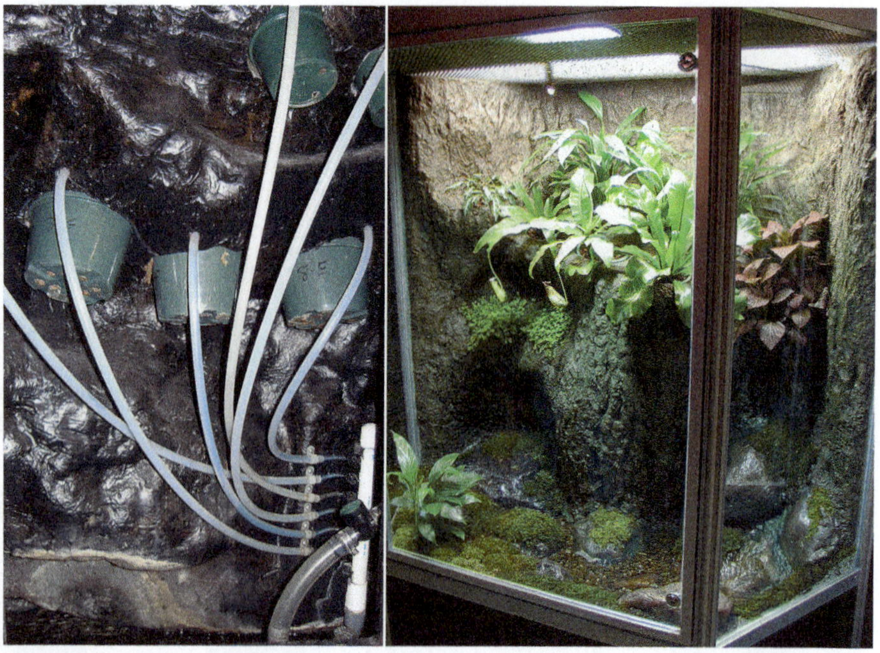

FIGURE 20-8 Strategically designed exhibition hides the internal plumbing of the tank (left), while still looking natural (right).

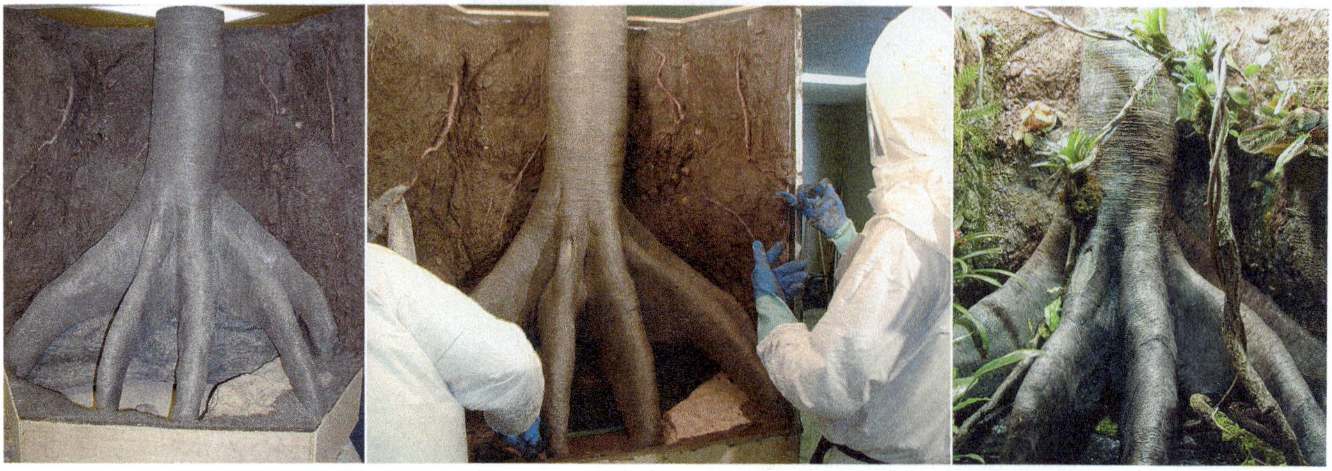

FIGURE 20-9 Fiberglass-reinforced polyester resin is among the most versatile and durable materials for creating artificial habitats, but using it requires protective equipment and a skilled workforce.

a gritty rocklike texture that easily absorbs paints and stains. Adding water to a bag of mortar mix and creating a shape is fairly easy, but producing a strong and durable finished product requires knowledge of mix theory (a discipline in its own right), proper curing techniques, and how to deal with "cold joints." Hastily done concrete fabrications often crumble over time. Because it is heavy and brittle, concrete is generally a poor choice for exhibits that must move. Concrete is relatively inert when cured, but it is composed largely of limestone and, when immersed in water, acts as an alkaline buffer that may skew pH.

Glass fiber-reinforced polyester resin (often referred to simply as *fiberglass*) is probably the most versatile, lightweight, and durable material used in habitat fabrication. However, uncured polyester resin is extremely toxic, and working with it requires protective equipment and a skilled workforce (Figure 20-9). Polyester systems typically consist of one-part resin to which small quantities of catalyst are added. This allows precise control over set times and creative mix effects. It also means that mix ratios are fairly forgiving, and even an undercatalyzed batch will eventually cure completely. Achieving a full cure with polyester is important for limiting off-gassing and potential leaching of toxins into tank water. The key to rapid curing is heat, and we routinely bake polyester fabrications in a large industrial oven. If not overcoated with a thin waterproof layer, polyester will turn white where exposed to standing water.

Epoxy resins are similar to polyester but somewhat less forgiving and much more costly. They have inflexible set times and require precise measurement and mixing. Epoxies are far less toxic to work with than polyester, although a few people develop sensitivity to them over time. They are two-part mixes (typically labeled *A* and *B*), which, when combined in appropriate proportions, bind with each other and harden. Properly mixed epoxies are inert when cured, but errors in measurement (even minor ones) or incomplete mixing may leave uncured residues of one or both components, which are then difficult to remove and potentially toxic to amphibians.

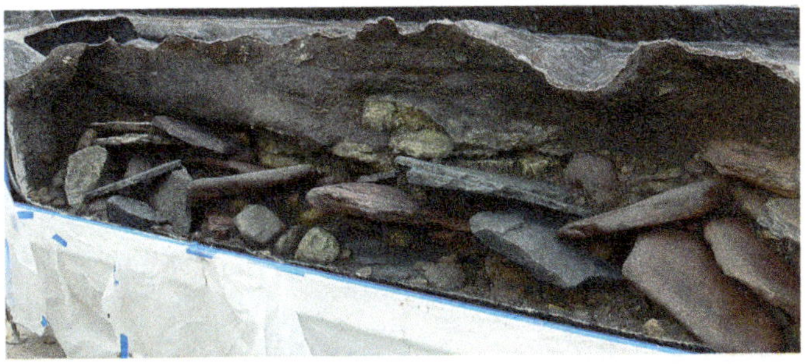

FIGURE 20-10 Exhibits for secretive animals, like this Hellbender habitat, require strategic placement of hiding spots to provide adequate cover, while keeping the animals visible. This often means filling and reshaping until all parts of the finished habitat are visible from at least one viewing angle.

Regardless of whether artificial or natural materials are used, strategic decorating is critical to keeping animals visible. We begin the process of creating artificial scenes by roughing out a shape with wire mesh, wood, or carved foam and overcoating it with resin or concrete. It is important to remove the forming materials afterward to avoid burying metallic or water-absorbing structures in the fabrication. This initial shape defines the details of topography, including overhangs and cutbacks. Then we examine the shape carefully from all viewing angles, looking for spots where amphibians could completely disappear from view. We fill or reshape areas of concern until we can be sure that all parts of the exhibit can be seen from at least one viewing angle (Figure 20-10). Branches and three-dimensional tree trunks are particularly problematic for tree frogs, which can disappear in plain view by perching on the backsides of limbs. We try to choose branches that are proportional in size to the species—big enough for comfortable perching but not so large as to completely hide an animal—and position them at angles that allow visitors to see as much of the backside as possible (Figure 20-11). Surfaces amphibians are likely to come in contact with should be free of sharp projections and smooth enough to prevent skin injuries.

Pools and Water Features

Water is central to the lives of most amphibians, and the vast majority of species need a constant source of it. Nothing animates an exhibit like moving water, and we include trickling or seeping water features in nearly all designs. Running water helps maintain relative humidity and keeps pools from stagnating and accumulating surface films. It is important that each water feature be independently controlled with flow valves, particularly those that originate high in the tank. If the flow cannot be attenuated, water may spill out of the intended path and splash the exhibit glass, creating visibility problems. If a single pump feeds more than one water feature, some degree of balancing will also be necessary to prevent uneven flows.

The size and depth of pools should match the species' needs. Tiny frogs can drown in deep water, whereas aquatic frogs, like Surinam Toads *(Pipa pipa)*, need deep water to adopt natural postures and perform courtship rituals. The walls of pools must be smooth enough to avoid injuring the skins of active swimmers. In deeper pools it is important to produce some movement throughout the water column to prevent wastes from accumulating in dead spots. This can often be accomplished by returning a percentage of the filtered water to the pool below the surface.

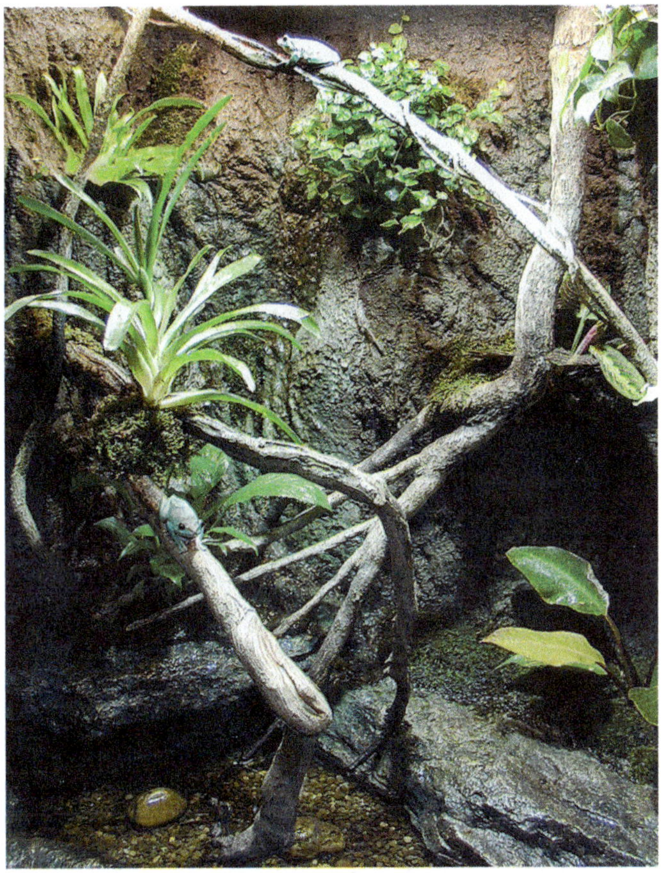

FIGURE 20-11 Carefully sized and positioned branches allow tree frogs to perch comfortably without disappearing entirely from view.

Evaporative water loss is a function of surface area of exposed water and ambient relative humidity. In a closed plumbing system (one in which water is sucked out and returned to the tank under pressure), evaporation can cause dramatic drops in water level, even over a 24-hour period, regardless of the total water volume in the system. If the water is not topped off regularly, a shallow pool can run dry in a few days, which would leave the amphibians without standing water. We prefer to design open flow filtration systems that buffer water levels in the exhibit. We include hidden standpipes in most amphibian exhibits, which passively drain water from the tank into an external reservoir as it spills into the top of the pipe. The height of the standpipe dictates the water level in the exhibit, ensuring that evaporative loss does not affect pools in the exhibit; only the water level in the external reservoir varies.

Substrates

There are several valid approaches to covering the floor of an amphibian exhibit. Gravel beds covered in sheet moss work well for species that do not dig. Organic soil mixes covered in a thin layer of leaf litter can be used with very small species and can double as a planting substrate. Our preference, however, is to cover the dry portions of the exhibit floor with fabricated earthen or rock textures. This gives a solid, cleanable foundation onto which we can add thin layers of sheet moss, leaf litter, or planting mix. It also affords us the freedom to terrace the floor of the habitat.

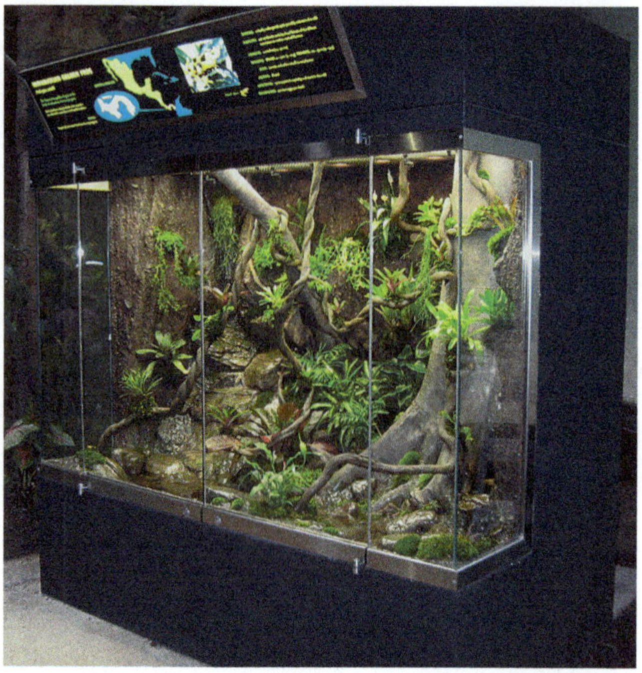

FIGURE 20-12 Striking a balance between overplanting and underplanting requires some trial and error. Regular pruning is needed to keep the plants in check and the animals in view.

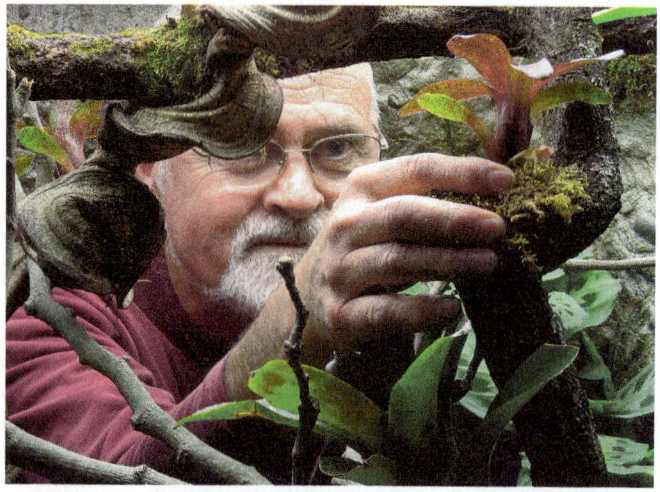

FIGURE 20-13 Epiphytes and other plants should be kept in scale with the exhibit and positioned to offer cover without opportunities for the amphibians to hide completely.

It is self-evident that burrowing species cannot be exhibited in tanks with deep substrate, yet many exhibitors have tried it. The only hope of seeing a digger is to provide very thin substrate and make up for the lack of security with creatively designed landscape cover. For all species, we prefer to limit deep substrates to contained planting areas rather than create a soil bed throughout the enclosure.

Gravel is the most widely used substrate in pool bottoms. It lasts indefinitely, is easy to clean, looks attractive if used properly, and, if water is pulled through it, aids in filtration. Gravels usually look most natural when a variety of sizes are mixed and some small pebbles are included. Some amphibian species, like Budgett's Frogs (*Lepidobatrachus laevis*), are prone to ingesting gravel while eating or, apparently in a few cases, may intentionally seek it out. Small gravel, relative to body size, usually passes through the digestive tract, but larger pebbles can lodge in the stomach. Selecting pebbles that are small enough to pass or too big to be eaten is the obvious solution.

Planting

Plants are key to amphibian exhibits: they enrich the scene aesthetically, help maintain relative humidity, and assist in removing nitrogenous wastes from the water supply. Striking a balance between overplanting and underplanting requires some trial and error. As always, the goal is to provide adequate cover while keeping the animals in view (Figure 20-12).

Try to find plants that fit the scale of the exhibit and represent the natural environment of the amphibian as closely as possible. Sometimes plant species that are found in a particular region are unavailable, but one can usually come close by selecting related or analogous plants from other regions. Choose plants with growth habits that provide cover without allowing animals to completely disappear. For terrestrial amphibians, we often use tall, long stemmed plants on the floor of the exhibit and fill the upper reaches (where the animals cannot venture) with bushy plants and vines. Epiphytes, or air plants, are useful for filling the higher reaches of an exhibit and provide wonderful microhabitats for climbing amphibians (Figure 20-13).

We buy plants from big box stores, greenhouses, and specialty botanical suppliers. Most nursery plants are grown in potting mixes that contain filler materials (i.e., Styrofoam balls) and slow-release fertilizers. Filler materials look unnatural and may be accidentally ingested by foraging amphibians, and fertilizers can play havoc with water quality. We have recorded nitrate spikes in amphibian exhibits just after plant watering because a single slow-release fertilizer pellet was left in one plant. Nursery plants may also have pesticide residue on leaves that needs to be washed off. Despite the pesticides, many plants come with hefty infestations of botanical parasites including thrips (order Thysanoptera), mealy bugs (family Pseudococcidae), scale insects (order Homoptera), and various species of mites. Although we have only circumstantial evidence, we suspect that the fungus *Batrachochytrium dendrobatidis* (Bd) has also entered our collection via nursery plants on several occasions.

To mitigate all of these risks, we repot and pretreat all plants before introduction into amphibian exhibits. The first step is to examine the leaves and stems for parasites. Most can be squashed with a finger, rinsed away under running water, or swabbed with rubbing alcohol. Next, we remove all of the nursery soil from the root ball by teasing it out with fingers or rinsing it off with water. This is traumatic for the plant and must be done delicately. When the roots are completely naked, we wash the entire plant under running water, then briefly immerse it in dilute itraconazole (Sporanox, Janssen Pharmaceutical) as a prophylactic treatment for Bd. Finally, we repot it in organic potting mix and water thoroughly. Many plants are setback briefly by this assault, but most recover in short order.

Plant care is mainly a matter of watering, fertilization, and pruning. Manual watering is a reasonable approach if you have a small number of plants, but automating the process can reduce maintenance time dramatically for larger exhibits. We install timed watering systems with independent flow control for each plant in most of our exhibits. Many fertilizers are not safe to use with amphibians, but Dyna-Gro Nutrition Solutions (Richmond, Calif) produces a series that is. We fertilize once per week by spraying diluted fertilizer directly into each planting pocket. Plant shapes and sizes need to be maintained by constant pruning. Pruning is an art and requires an eye for aesthetics. Simply mowing off leaves and stems that overgrow creates a sculpted, unnatural look reminiscent of a bad hedgerow. Removing whole stems or sections of stems cut back to branch points is a better solution. Because plant growth is slow and steady, many keepers fail to notice that an exhibit is becoming overgrown until someone who has not seen the tank in a while points it out.

Filtration

Water quality is a limiting factor in amphibian husbandry: if it declines, so too will the animals. Although it is certainly possible to create amphibian exhibits with a very simple setup (i.e., shallow pools that are drained and filled daily), the success of the exhibit will be dependent on absolutely consistent keeper care. Water quality and water levels may vary daily. We prefer to design habitats that buffer these important variables to stabilize the experience for the inhabitants, and this requires filtration.

The most overlooked aspect of filtration in amphibian exhibits is total water volume. Many species need small shallow pools, and the visible water volume in an entire exhibit may only amount to a few gallons. Small volumes of water are subject to rapid contamination when animals excrete wastes, and filtration, particularly biological filtration, cannot keep pace. This often leads to spikes in ammonia or nitrite, which can be disastrous. Larger water volumes dilute wastes and other contaminants, allowing time for the filtration system to break them down or remove them. The easiest solution to adding water volume without making exhibit pools deeper is an external reservoir—a container that receives water from the tank or the filter and from which water is returned to the tank.

The variety of filtration designs available is almost endless, and there are many valid approaches. Fundamentally, filtration can be broken down into three types: mechanical, chemical, and biological. Mechanical filtration uses some kind of sieve to capture suspended particles from the water and may include floss, filter pads, cartridges, bags, or sleeves. Chemical filtration involves binding dissolved contaminants in the water by adsorbing them on a surface or precipitating them into aggregates that can be captured by mechanical filters. Chemical filters include activated carbon, polyfilters, flocking agents, and various resins. Biological filtration uses communities of living microorganisms to naturally metabolize animal wastes and is probably the most important category of filtration for amphibians.

Most mechanical and chemical filtration is done in a filter chamber where water is forced over or through the filter media. Biological filtration, however, can occur on any surface that is sufficiently wet and well-oxygenated, inside the tank or out. Gravel beds through which water is drawn provide a growing medium for beneficial bacteria in the exhibit, but objects with far more surface area, like commercially available bio-balls or wheels, can support huge bacterial colonies in the filter chamber. Because these bacteria use oxygen to breakdown wastes, they need water that is well-aerated. A properly designed system will eventually support colonies of *Nitrosomonas* bacteria that break down ammonia into nitrite and *Nitrobacter* bacteria that further metabolize nitrite into nitrate. Live plants in the exhibit absorb and metabolize some nitrate from the water, and whatever fraction remains is easily removed via periodic partial water changes.

Plumbing systems that transport water between tank and filter come in two broad categories: open-loop and closed-loop. Open-loop systems include an open chamber somewhere in the water path and often depend on gravity to carry tank water through a skimmer or standpipe to the open chamber. Filtration can be incorporated into the chamber by allowing the water to cascade through a series of media layers as it falls. A pump then returns the filtered water from the open chamber to the tank under pressure. Open-loop systems are relatively simple and reliable; however, the filter chamber must be lower in elevation than the water level in the tank, and the filter chambers are often bulky. Closed-loop systems are closed with the plumbing, pumps, and various chambers that communicate water from tank to filter and back again sealed, and the water moving through the whole path under pressure. In closed-loop systems, the filter chamber can be located above or below the tank water level, and because it operates under pressure, the filter itself can be small. Closed-loop systems are, however, more difficult to service and more likely to leak if someone improperly seats an O-ring or fails to retighten a plumbing connection.

Whatever filtration and plumbing system is chosen, make ease of maintenance a priority. If you the exhibit is designed for the laziest keeper you can imagine, average and highly motivated keepers will thrive. Make access doors to the filter cabinet as large as possible, and leave plenty of room around components to ease plumbing repairs. Make sure the area around the filter is waterproof because spills are inevitable during routine maintenance.

Humidity and Ventilation

Although it is true that many amphibians live in habitats with high relative humidity, it is also true that humidity varies in most natural environments, both over time and over small distances. A common misconception is that uniformly high humidity is desirable, and some exhibit designs limit ventilation to trap moisture. In our experience this is not the answer. Ventilation is necessary to prevent viewing glass from fogging and accumulating condensation. Most plants also need ventilation to periodically dry off their leaves. In addition, without adequate air exchange, damp substrates grow mold. We prefer to build exhibits with completely open tops, covered in woven mesh. Passive air exchange is enough for most exhibits, but for very tall tanks we use small fans to force air movement to the bottom of the tank. Finding the right amount of air movement to prevent molding without desiccating plants and animals requires experimentation and tweaking.

In our experience the keys to humidity are providing a physical mosaic of moist and dry areas in the exhibit and varying overall humidity over time. As long as standing and running water are always available, most amphibians appear to be capable of regulating themselves by moving in and out of moist areas. For many species, a once-daily hand misting of the animals and plants is the only spike in overall humidity we provide. In situations in which very high humidity is needed—montane species that need to be bathed in fog or rainforest species that benefit from regular misting—we use automated misters and foggers in concert with small equipment cooling fans. After a mist or fog cycle ends, the fans force room air into the exhibit to remove excess moisture by ventilation. If the fans are aimed at the viewing glass, fogging and splashed water quickly evaporate. To avoid mineral spotting on the glass and prolong the life of the equipment, use distilled or reverse osmosis filtered water in misters and foggers.

Lighting

Lighting is a field in and of itself, and a dizzying array of variables needs to be considered in choosing fixtures and lamp types. Plants generally need far more intense light levels than amphibians. As a rule of thumb most low-light plants can eke out an existence between 100 and 150 footcandles. Vigorous growth requires 200 or more footcandles, and flowering for most species requires at least 500 footcandles. The problem with light intensity is that it decreases as the square of the distance from its source. If a light fixture produces 200 footcandles on a surface 2 feet away, it will produce only 50 footcandles at a distance of 4 feet. This precipitous drop-off means that it is much more difficult to light tall enclosures than shorter ones.

In addition to light intensity, exhibit designers must consider color temperature (the dominant wavelengths emitted by the lamp) and color-rendering index (how naturally the lamp reproduces the colors in objects it illuminates). Badly selected lamps can give an entire exhibit a color-shifted cast. The heat produced by a lamp, measured in watts, is of particular importance for amphibians because a dense bank of fixtures can quickly warm an enclosure to dangerous levels. For this reason, fluorescent light fixtures are usually the first choice for lighting amphibian exhibits. Fluorescents produce less heat than most other fixture types, are relatively inexpensive, and lamps are available in a variety of color temperatures with high color-rendering indices. Fluorescent fixtures, however, produce diffuse light and do not penetrate well in tall enclosures.

We often supplement fluorescents with low wattage halogen spotlights or light-emitting diode (LED) fixtures to get adequate intensity on the floor of the tank. Halogen lamps produce intense focused heat and must be positioned carefully to avoid scorching amphibians or burning combustibles. LED fixtures produce far less heat per unit of light (i.e., they are energy efficient), are available in a variety of color temperatures, and offer adjustable beam spreads (by changing plastic lenses that mount over the diodes). Although currently more expensive than halogen or fluorescent fixtures, LEDs will likely become more affordable for general tank lighting in time.

Although most amphibians are adapted to relatively cool environments, many species will bask if given the opportunity. We have recently begun using small halogen light fixtures to produce focused basking areas for all but the most secretive species. We have observed basking in various tree frogs (*Polypedates* sp., *Theloderma corticale, Leptopelis vermiculatus, Phyllomedusa* sp.), Poison Dart Frogs (*Dendrobates* sp., *Phyllobates* sp.), true frogs (*Leptodactylus pentadactylus, Lithobates catesbeianus*), and true toads (*Chaunus marinus, Rhaebo guttatus*). The important thing about basking sites is that they be easy to get away from and not too hot. Like any other aspect of the captive environment, providing a thermal mosaic from which the animals can choose is probably the safest approach.

CONCLUSION

To those who have never tried it, exhibiting amphibians looks easy—the sort of thing almost anyone ought to be able to handle. However, this hubris quickly disappears with experience; amphibians can be downright humbling. In many ways, their captive needs are more like fish than reptiles, and aquarists are sometimes better prepared to accommodate those needs than herpetologists.

Exhibiting these delicate animals requires thinking in terms of systems. While it is certainly possible to maintain every aspect of the internal environment manually, it leaves the exhibit very susceptible to human error. Automating filtration, light cycles, temperature, humidity, and ventilation stabilizes the internal environment and reduces risk. Tank automation is analogous to autopilot in commercial jets; it turns the attention of keepers to managing systems rather than tiny details and prevents minor mistakes from having devastating consequences.

The field of amphibian exhibition is relatively young, and plenty of room for new ideas exists. If one is willing to invest oneself in a project—to approach it thoughtfully, to experiment, and to acknowledge errors—the experience can be rewarding. A well-done exhibit changes people, revealing an aspect of the world they did not know existed. Surely no group of animals is more charismatic as a terrarium subject and has a better story to tell than amphibians.

ACKNOWLEDGMENTS

The information and experiences described in this chapter represent collective knowledge hard-won by our exhibits team. Elliot Peeling has been the driving force behind enclosure design and continually refines our fabrication standards. John Tolbert provided a wealth of experience in filtration, horticulture, and amphibian behavioral observation.

CHAPTER 21

Infectious Diseases of Amphibians: It Isn't Just Redleg Anymore

Allan P. Pessier

Some infectious diseases such as chytridiomycosis and *Ranavirus* infection have been the focus of intensive research efforts to understand their potential role in the global decline of amphibian species.[1] The emergence of these diseases in the last decade has led to the recognition that the knowledge base for amphibian infectious diseases is limited but has also increased the interest in comprehensively investigating and describing amphibian mortality events.

As an example, in the recent past, it was acceptable to give any amphibian with red skin a diagnosis of *redleg syndrome,* which was a result of a gram-negative bacterial infection (bacterial dermatosepticemia), but it is now known that a variety of infectious diseases including ranaviruses, chytridiomycosis, fungal infections, and chlamydophilosis, among others, can result in similar clinical syndromes that are indistinguishable without ancillary diagnostic testing. In retrospect, it is likely that many amphibian mortality events attributed to *redleg syndrome* were, in fact, misdiagnosed because of the gross appearance of their lesions and bacterial culture of *Aeromonas hydrophila,* which is easily isolated from animals dying of other diseases.[2-4] This example emphasizes the need for careful and complete investigation of amphibian infectious diseases.

This chapter provides an update on amphibian infectious and parasitic diseases other than chytridiomycosis and *Ranavirus* infection. Some have been previously described but have new information to be disseminated, and others are newly recognized and often incompletely described. The aim of this chapter is to emphasize the spectrum of infectious diseases being recognized in amphibian submissions to veterinary pathologists. It is hoped that this information will be helpful to those new to amphibian medicine and pathology, will serve as an update for experienced amphibian clinicians, and will encourage comprehensive investigation of amphibian mortality events while discouraging a new trend of relying entirely on molecular diagnostic tests for *Batrachochytrium* (cause of chytridiomycosis) or ranaviruses when these events are investigated. Only by comprehensive investigation that includes necropsy and histopathologic examination of dead animals with ancillary testing that includes traditional techniques such as bacterial culture and virus isolation as well as modern molecular techniques will we develop a complete and accurate understanding of the role of infectious diseases in amphibian ecology and captive management.

BACTERIAL DISEASES

Chlamydophilosis

Infections with obligate intracellular bacteria in the family Chlamydiaceae in captive African Clawed Frogs (*Xenopus* sp.) were first described in the 1980s.[5,6] Although *Chlamydophila psittaci* was identified in early cases, subsequent reports of chlamydophilosis in amphibians have implicated *Chlamydophila pneumoniae,* best known as a common respiratory pathogen in humans. These reports have included an observation of disease in a free-ranging Giant Barred Frog from Australia, suggesting that chlamydophilosis may not simply be a disease of captivity.[7-10] A survey of tissues from both captive and wild frogs in Switzerland revealed by immunohistochemical analysis and molecular methods evidence of a variety of chlamydiae including *C. pneumoniae, Chlamydia suis,* and *Chlamydophila abortus.*[11] No lesions of chlamydophilosis were observed in the Swiss frogs, which suggests that amphibians could be a previously unrecognized reservoir for chlamydial organisms. This author has identified infections with *C. pneumoniae* in critically endangered Wyoming Toads (*Anaxyrus [Bufo] baxteri*), demonstrating that infections can be a concern in programs rearing amphibians for reintroduction into the wild.

Clinically, chlamydophilosis can have a variety of presentations including sudden death, nonspecific clinical signs such as lethargy, and a resemblance to redleg syndrome. Histologic lesions also vary and can include hepatic necrosis, interstitial pneumonia, interstitial nephritis, epicarditis, and myocarditis. Inflammatory cell infiltrates have been described as nonsuppurative, mononuclear, or lymphohistiocytic. In most cases, affected cells such as hepatocytes and macrophages are observed to contain fine granular basophilic cytoplasmic inclusions suggestive of chlamydial infection (Figure 21-1). Recently, definitive diagnosis and classification of chlamydophilosis at necropsy of amphibians has been aided by the use of immunohistochemical analysis with Chlamydiaceae family–specific anti-LPS monoclonal antibodies and by polymerase chain reaction (PCR) and DNA sequencing of chlamydial 16sRNA and *ompA* genes. Diagnostic tests for chlamydial infection in clinically ill amphibians could include PCR; however, the clinician should be aware that these tests have not been validated for this purpose. Treatment with tetracycline group antibiotics has been suggested.[12]

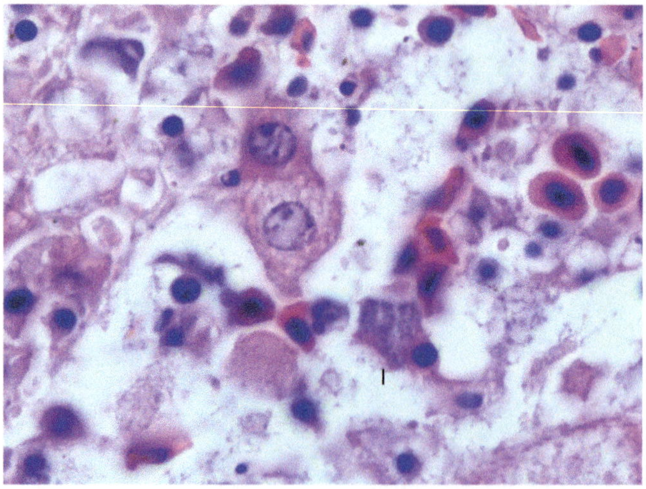

FIGURE 21-1 Histologic section of liver from a Wyoming Toad *(Bufo baxteri)* with necrotizing hepatitis attributed to *Chlamydophila pneumoniae*. Some necrotic hepatocytes have cytoplasmic basophilic granular material suggestive of chlamydial inclusions (I) (×100).

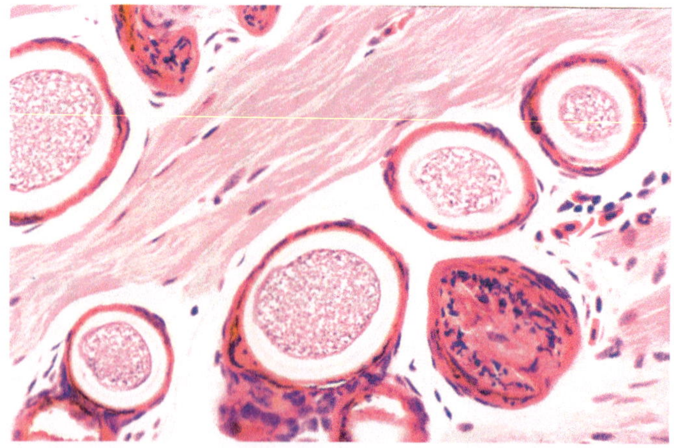

FIGURE 21-2 Histologic section of skeletal muscle from a Red-spotted Newt *(Notophthalmus viridescens)* with granulomatous myositis due to an *Ichthyophonus*-like organism. Five passive spores with a thick refractile wall are demonstrated and are surrounded by attenuated (flattened) macrophages (×20).

Ochrobactrum anthropi-Associated Spinal Arthropathy

A case series of Australian Cane Toads *(Chaunus [Bufo] marinus)* with pyogranulomatous vertebral osteomyelitis and arthritis has recently been reported.[13] Pure cultures of *O. anthropi*, a gram-negative bacterium found in soil and related to organisms in the *Brucella* group, were obtained from some of the affected animals. This is the first published report of an infectious spinal arthropathy in amphibians. The author has observed histologically similar lesions in the spine of Wyoming Toads and Mountain Yellow-legged Frogs *(Rana muscosa)* with mycobacteriosis; routine staining of pyogranulomatous spinal lesions with Fite's acid-fast stain is suggested.

PROTOZOAL AND PROTOZOAL-LIKE DISEASES

Mesomycetozoal Diseases

Protozoa in the Phylum Neomonada, Class Mesomycetozoea have been recognized as pathogens of aquatic animals for some time but had been difficult to classify definitively as either protozoa or fungi. Based on molecular phylogeny, organisms in the Mesomycetozoea are now considered to be protozoa arising from near the animal–fungal divergence. Pathogens within the class include *Dermocystidium* and *Ichthyophonus* and *Ichthyophonus*-like organisms in fish and amphibians, *Psorospermium* in crayfish, and *Rhinosporidium seeberi* in mammals and birds.[14]

Mesomycetozoal organisms in the genera *Dermocystidium, Dermosporidium,* and *Dermomycoides* cause spherical to U-shaped raised skin lesions in a variety of amphibians and especially anurans in the genera *Rana* and *Bufo*. Histologically, lesions consist of dermal cystlike lesions containing myriad spherical 7 μm to 12 μm endospores that are sometimes associated with a granulomatous inflammatory response. Infections have not been associated with mortality. Recent molecular and morphologic studies have suggested that enough differences exist between the better studied *Dermocystidium* of fish and the organisms observed in amphibians to place the amphibian organisms into the new genera *Amphibiocystidium* and *Amphibiothecum*.[15-17]

Organisms that morphologically resemble *Ichthyophonus hoferi* in fish are best known for causing granulomatous myositis with associated body swellings and occasionally cutaneous ulceration in Red-spotted Newts *(Notophthalmus viridescens)* (Figure 21-2). Similar organisms and lesions are increasingly recognized in frogs including American Bullfrogs *(Rana catesbeiana)*, Green Frogs *(Rana clamitans)*, Wood Frogs *(Rana sylvatica)*, Pickerel Frogs *(Rana palustris)*, and Spring Peepers *(Pseudacris crucifer)*. Infections are frequently an incidental finding; however, heavy infections can result in death of individual animals and sometimes have been associated with mortality events.[3] Clinical signs in lethally infected frogs include lethargy, poor response to prodding, and thin body condition without the prominent caudal body swellings observed in newts.[3] Histologically, the skeletal muscle of affected animals contains spherical to elongate spores that vary between 40 μm and more than 200 μm in diameter. Both active and passive spores are described, and passive spores possess a thick (up to 12-μm) triple-contoured wall. Unlike *Ichthyophonus* in fish, infections in amphibians seem to be limited to skeletal muscle, and disseminated systemic infections have not been reported. The life cycle is unknown; however, an association with the leech *Placobella picta* has been proposed and needs experimental support.[18] Additional experimental studies of life cycle and molecular phylogeny are required for the *Ichthyophonus*-like organisms in amphibians.

Alveolate Protozoal Disease

A newly identified organism identified by 18S rRNA sequencing as being most closely related to unspecified alveolate protozoa from freshwater lakes and marine hydrothermal vents and has been associated with mass die-offs of ranid tadpoles in the United States.[19-21] Species affected include Southern Leopard Frogs *(Rana sphenocephala)*, Mink Frogs *(Rana septentrionalis)*, Green Frogs, Mississippi Gopher Frogs *(Rana sevosa)*, and American Bullfrogs. Disease has only rarely been reported from postmetamorphic animals.[22] Clinically affected Southern

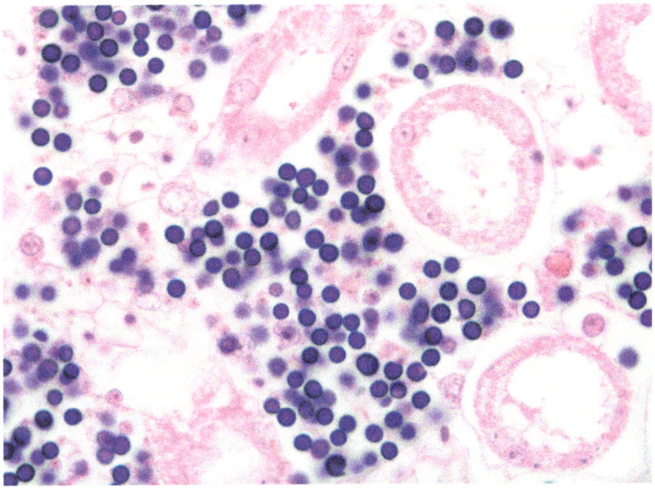

FIGURE 21-3 Histologic section of kidney from a Mississippi Gopher Frog tadpole *(Rana sevosa)* infected with a *Perkinsus*-like protozoan. There is no appreciable inflammatory response to the myriad spherical basophilic organisms that infiltrate the renal interstitium (×40).

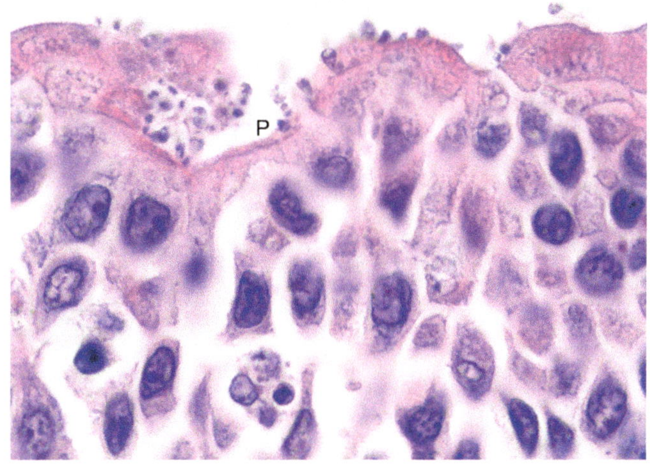

FIGURE 21-4 Histologic section showing the ventral tongue of a Wyoming Toad *(Anaxyrus [Bufo] baxteri)* showing small protozoal organisms *(P)* attached to the mucosal surface that were subsequently identified as a probable *Cryptosporidium* sp (×40).

Leopard Frogs have enlarged abdomens, swim erratically, and can be easily captured by hand.[20] Gross findings in affected tadpoles include white discoloration and enlargement of the liver, spleen, and kidneys. Histologically, organs are infiltrated by large numbers of spherical, 6-μm to 9 μm-diameter, basophilic organisms, and minimal or no evidence of a host inflammatory response is present (Figure 21-3). The organisms morphologically resemble mesomycetozoan organisms and were originally described as *Dermocystidium*-like.[3] Diagnosis is by observation of organisms on organ impression smears or by histopathologic examination. Molecular diagnostic methods may be available through individual researchers but are not commercially obtainable at this time.

Cryptosporidiosis

Coccidian parasites in the genus *Cryptosporidium* are important pathogens of mammals, birds, reptiles, and fish, but until a recent case report in a captive African Clawed Frog *(Xenopus laevis)*, clinically significant infections had not been well-documented in amphibians. The affected frog was seen with a history of chronic weight loss and emaciation and on histologic examination was found to have a proliferative gastritis associated with large numbers of superficial 0.5-μm to 3-μm spherical protozoal organisms.[23] Characteristic features of the genus *Cryptosporidium* were observed by transmission electron microscopy and confirmed the diagnosis. The specific species of *Cryptosporidium* was not determined. Experimental attempts to infect some amphibians with *Cryptosporidium parvum* and *Cryptosporidium serpentis* have been unsuccessful .[24] *Cryptosporidium fragile* has recently been described from the stomach of Black-Spined Toads (*Duttaphrynus melanostictus* imported from Malaysia.[25] The author has observed an unidentified *Cryptosporidium* (confirmed by transmission electron microscopy) infecting the ventral ciliated epithelium of the tongue in captive Wyoming Toads without apparent clinical signs (Figure 21-4). Additional surveys are required to determine the distribution and significance of cryptosporidial infections in amphibians.

Ciliate Protozoal Diseases

Intravascular ciliate protozoa have recently been reported as a major cause of death in captive specimens of the critically endangered Kihansi Spray Toad *(Nectophrynoides asperginis)*.[26] Lesions in affected animals included lymphatic obstruction and lymphangectasia with regional edema and cellulitis, obstruction of hepatic sinusoids by protozoa with associated hepatitis, and obstruction of glomerular capillaries by protozoa. The species of ciliate involved was not reported, and although a cutaneous route of infection was suspected, this could not be confirmed.

Infections with tissue-invasive ciliate protozoa such as *Tetrahymena corlissi* have been mentioned to occur in amphibians, but lesions are not as well-documented as they are in fish.[27] Ciliate protozoa tentatively identified as a *Tetrahymena* sp. have recently been observed in association with necrotizing kidney lesions in Panamanian Golden Frogs *(Atelopus zeteki)* from this author's institution (Figure 21-5). Presumptively, most of these infections represent opportunistic invasion by free-living environmental protozoa. It is important to note that ciliate and opalinid (can morphologically resemble ciliates) protozoa are frequent components of the normal intestinal fauna of many amphibian species.[28,29] Treatment is not usually indicated for protozoa observed on routine fecal screening for parasites.

Microsporidiosis

The microsporidia have traditionally been classified as protozoa, but recent work in molecular phylogeny seems to place them within the Kingdom Fungi.[30] Microsporidial infections in amphibians have been described as far back as the 1920s and are best known for causing myositis in toads (*Pleistophora myotrophica* in common toads, *Bufo bufo*) or as incidental findings in Bidder's organ or ovary.[29,31]

Some observations suggest that microsporidial diseases may be more common or of greater clinical importance in amphibians than might be expected from the literature. Infection with *Alloglugea bufonis* in the Cane Toad tadpoles and recent

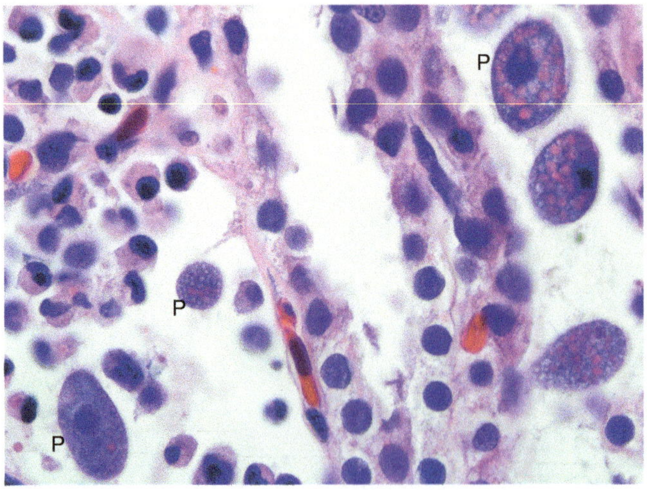

FIGURE 21-5 Histologic section showing the kidney of a Panamanian Golden Frog *(Atelopus zeteki)* with invasive ciliate protozoa *(P)*. Many of the protozoa have a prominent macronucleus (×40).

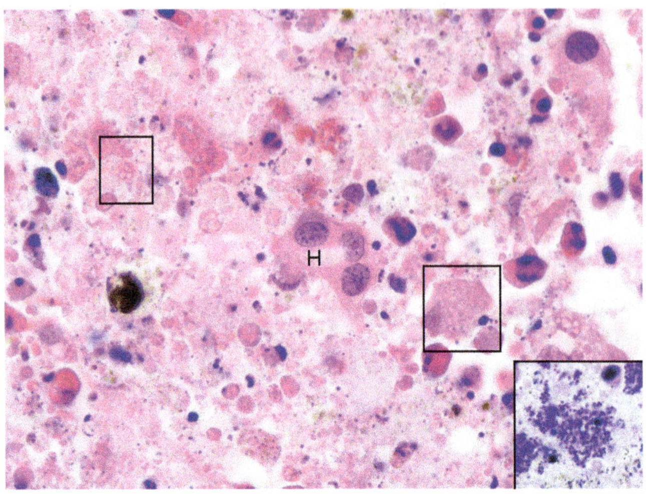

FIGURE 21-6 Histologic section of the liver from a Mountain Yellow-legged Frog tadpole *(Rana muscosa)* with necrotizing hepatitis associated with an unidentified microsporidian parasite. Necrotic hepatocytes *(in boxes)* have faint cytoplasmic vacuoles that were demonstrated to be microsporidial spores using a tissue Gram stain *(inset)*. There are occasional remaining non-necrotic hepatocytes (*H*) (×40).

metamorphs was associated with large xenomas (hypertrophied host cells containing large numbers of microsporidial spores) in the intestinal wall as well as within macrophages in visceral organs such as the spleen and kidney.[32] On gross examination, white nodules were observed in tissues with heaviest levels of infection. Infected tadpoles had no apparent clinical signs and successfully completed metamorphosis. Transmission of infection was thought to be by spores emitted from dead animals or by cannibalism. A fatal wasting syndrome was observed in 18 individual frogs of unspecified species associated with heavy infections of an unidentified microsporidian.[33] Lesions included intestinal xenomas as well as organisms within the liver and kidney. In the same report, metamorphs of the Kunapalari Frog *(Neobatrachus kunapalari)*

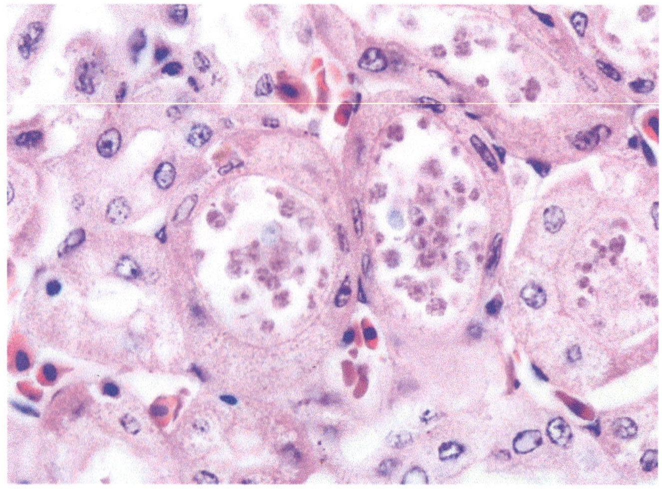

FIGURE 21-7 Histologic section of kidney from an *Eleutherodactylus podi-noblei* frog showing spores of an unidentified myxozoan within renal tubules. There is no appreciable associated inflammatory response (×40).

were described that had skeletal muscle and liver lesions associated with another unidentified microsporidian. Kyphosis and epaxial myositis were associated with infection with a *Pleistophora*-like microsporidian in San Marcos Salamanders *(Eurycea nana)*.[34] This author has observed necrotizing hepatitis due to infection with an unidentified microsporidian in tadpoles of the endangered Mountain Yellow-legged Frog (Figure 21-6).

Diagnosis of microsporidial infection is by observation of characteristic gram-positive spores in histologic section; organisms are not easily observed on routine hematoxylin and eosin–stained sections (see Figure 21-7). Attempts to speciate amphibian microsporidia using combinations of transmission electron microscopy and molecular techniques such as PCR and sequencing of positive bands is encouraged to better define the spectrum of microsporidia affecting amphibians.[35]

Myxozoanosis

The Myxozoa are a phylum of metazoan organisms related to the cnidarians that usually have been classified and studied as protozoans. Until recently, most myxozoal infections in amphibians have been considered to be interesting incidental findings of minimal clinical significance[28] (Figure 21-8). The lifecycle of many myxozoan species is unknown; however, several do use an invertebrate intermediate host.

Infection with a *Myxidium* sp. has been associated with significant periportal fibrosis, biliary hyperplasia, and lymphocytic hepatitis in free-ranging White's Tree Frogs *(Litoria caerulea)* and Green and Golden Bell Frogs *(Litoria aurea)*[36,37] Trophozooites in these cases were observed in the gallbladder and intrahepatic bile ducts. In the affected Bell Frogs, developmental stages of myxozoa were also observed in the central nervous system in association with a nonsuppurative meningoencephalitis. A variety of *Myxidium* sp. (now *Cystodiscus* sp.) are described from the gallbladder of both anurans and caudates worldwide and are not always associated with disease.[38, 39]

Infections with myxozoa have recently been described as a cause of clinically significant kidney disease in two species of anurans. A *Chloromyxum* sp. was associated with tubular dilation and necrosis as well as mild to severe nonsuppurative

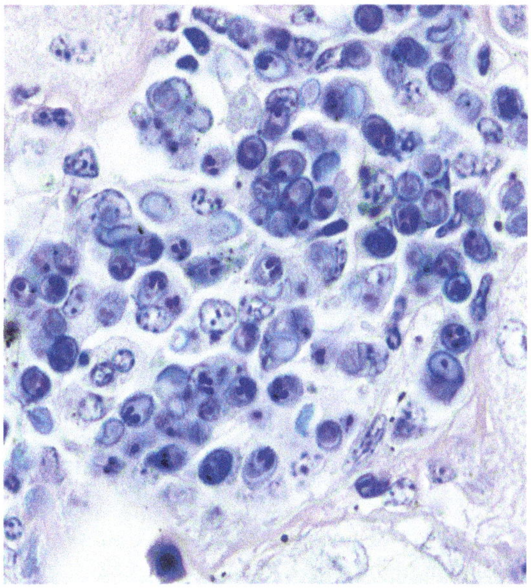

FIGURE 21-8 Histologic section of kidney from an *Eleutherodactylus podi-noblei* frog stained with Giemsa. This stain highlights the polar capsules of myxozoa, which appear as dark blue-purple teardrop-shaped structures (×40).

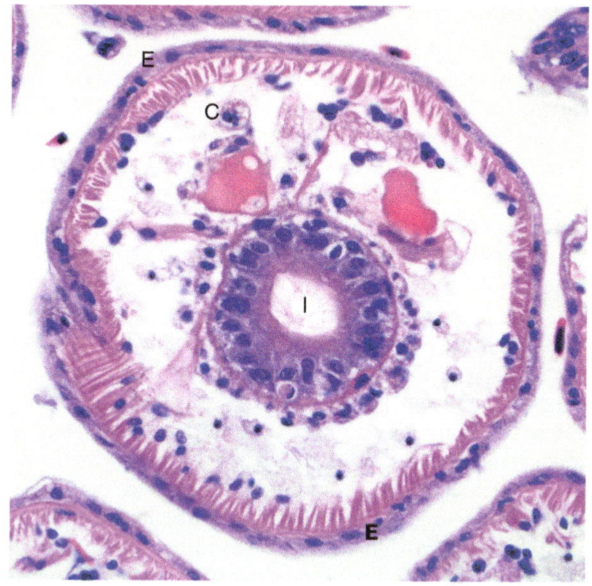

FIGURE 21-9 Transverse histologic section of an oligochaete worm in the cloaca of a Poison Dart Frog (*Dendrobates* sp.). Features include a cellular epidermis *(E)*, foamy cells in the coelomic cavity (coelomic corpuscles), and a central intestine (I) (×40).

tubulointerstitial nephritis in captive Asian Horned Frogs (*Megophrys nasuta*).[40] Plasmodia were observed in affected renal tubules and within the urinary space of glomeruli and contained spherical to pyriform 6-μm to 8-μm spores with four polar capsules. A proliferative and polycystic kidney disease ("frog kidney enlargement disease") was reported in recently imported African Reed Frogs (*Hyperolius* sp.) and associated with intralesional plasmodia and spores of a new species, *Hofferellus anurae*.[41] In both reports, wet mounts and/or impression smears of the kidney were useful for demonstrating organisms and extruded polar filaments.

METAZOAN PARASITES

Oligochaete Worms

Reports of presumably free-living oligochaete worms (Phylum Annelida; Family Naididae) colonizing the cloaca, urinary bladder, and Wolffian duct (ureter), as well as the eye and Harderian gland of frogs, are distributed throughout the parasitology literature.[42,43] Most of the worms infecting the genitourinary tract have been identified as belonging to the genus *Dero (Allodero)*. These were not associated with disease until a brief abstract described peritonitis associated with rupture of ureteral oligochaetes into the coelomic cavity of Harlequin Poison Frogs (*Dendrobates histrionicus*).[44] Dilatation of the Wolffian ducts as a result of oligochaete infection was described in White's Tree Frogs that were euthanized because of myxosporidial hepatitis.[36]

This author has sporadically observed these parasites in dendrobatid and hylid frogs from both private and zoologic collections. Most often these were incidental findings; however, in some cases, the worms extended into the kidney tubules and were associated with an interstitial nephritis. Clinically, oligochaetes are most likely to be identified on histopathologic examination of necropsy samples. These worms can present a diagnostic dilemma because criteria for identifying

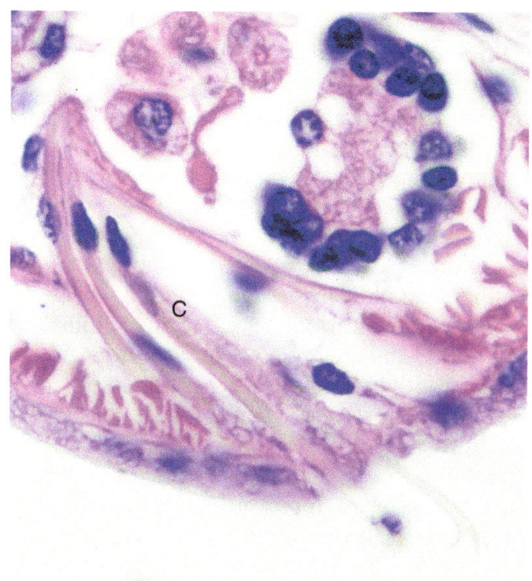

FIGURE 21-10 Transverse histologic section of an oligochaete worm in the cloaca of a Poison Dart Frog (*Dendrobates* sp.) showing the characteristic hairlike chaetae *(C)* exiting the body wall (×100).

oligochaetes in tissue section are not readily available to veterinary pathologists. Features helpful for identification include the hairlike chaetae and cells within the coelomic cavity, termed *coelomic corpuscles* (Figures 21-9 and 21-10). The source of infection is unknown; however, many oligochaetes in the genus *Dero* have been documented as inhabitants of water collected within bromeliads, and frogs have been shown to act as vehicles for dispersion of these worms.[45,46] Both praziquantel and ivermectin were shown to be effective at killing free-living stages of these oligochaetes.[44]

Trematode Parasites and Limb Deformities

The occurrence of limb malformations in anurans including polymelia, ectromelia, amelia, and polydactyly, among others, has attracted a great deal of public and scientific attention since the mid-1990s.[47,48] The cause of these malformations has been the subject of extensive debate and study, and differentials have included exposure to agricultural chemicals, parasites, and UV light. Although identification of a single cause of amphibian limb malformations is unlikely, there is evidence that the digenetic trematode *Ribeiroia ondatrae* can encyst and disrupt developing limb buds of tadpoles with subsequent limb malformation.[49,50] *Ribeiroia* has an indirect life cycle, and amphibians serve as second intermediate hosts. Although malformations attributed to trematode infection have been documented as far back as the 1940s, qualitative evidence suggests that the frequency of malformations has increased. The possibility has been proposed that environmental factors, such as pesticide exposure, agricultural nutrient runoff, and introduced fish, may alter habitats in ways that promote trematodes, hence increasing the frequency of malformations.[51,52] Although limb malformations may affect the survival of individual animals, a role for malformations in amphibian population declines has not been demonstrated. While *Ribeiroia* metacercariae can be observed in histologic sections, techniques such as skeletal clearing and staining may provide more information on the relationship of the trematode to the deformed limb.

Rhabditiform Nematodes

Infection with the rhabditiform nematode *Rhabdias* (the amphibian "lungworm") is commonly reported in wild and captive amphibians.[29,53] The related nematode *Strongyloides* sp. has also been observed in wild amphibians and only recently reported as a potential pathogen.[54-56] These nematodes have a direct life cycle and can have both free-living and parasitic forms; amphibians become infected when third-stage larvae penetrate the skin. Infections in wild animals are usually at a low-level and are not associated with a significant host response. In captivity, conditions may allow environmental buildup of infective larvae, leading to clinically significant superinfections.[27]

The rhabditiform nematodes have been emerging as a potential limiting factor for captive amphibian species conservation programs such as the one developed for the Kihansi Spray Toad, which has experienced significant losses due to *Rhabdias*-like nematode.[57] This author has observed several outbreaks of *Strongyloides* sp. infection associated with mortality in recently imported anurans and deaths attributed to *Rhabdias* sp. in wild frogs brought into captive survival assurance colonies in Central America (Figures 21-11 and 21-12). This author has also seen clinically significant enteritis and intestinal mucosal hyperplasia in a moribund free-ranging tree frog *(Hyla colymba)* from Panama, suggesting that some animals may come into captivity with debilitating parasite loads. Although elimination of natural host–parasite fauna may not always be desirable—especially in animals destined for reintroduction to the wild because of the need to maintain adaptations that may help keep parasite burdens under control[58]—consideration may need to be given to the use of anthelminthics to control rhabditiform nematodes in amphibians brought into high-density captive situations from the wild.

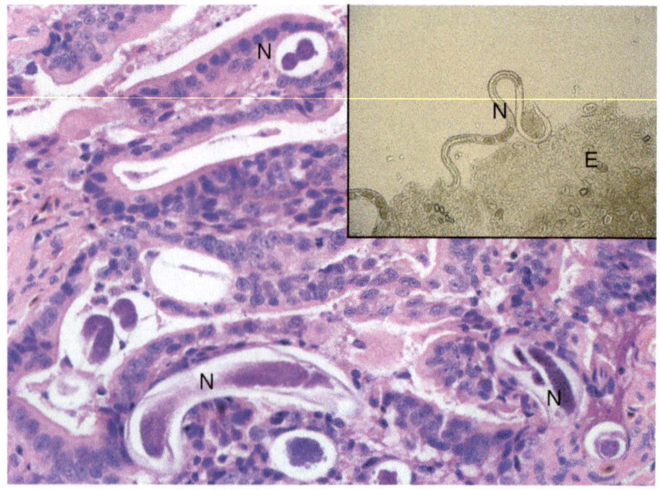

FIGURE 21-11 Histologic section of small intestine from a milky tree frog *(Phrynohyas resinifictrix)* showing numerous intraepithelial nematodes *(N)* identified as a *Strongyloides* sp. The *inset* is of a wet mount of feces from this frog and shows an adult worm *(N)*, as well as larvated eggs (E) (×40).

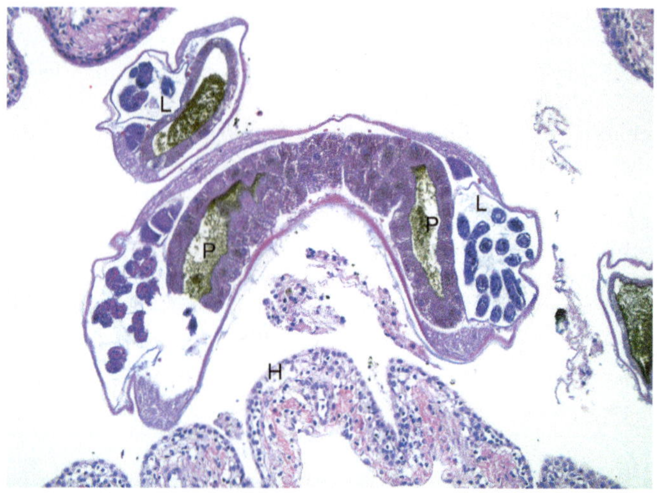

FIGURE 21-12 A histologic section of lung from a tree frog *(Hyla palmeri)* infected with a *Rhabdias* sp. nematode. Some features include larvae *(L)* within the uterus and pigmented material *(P)* within the intestine. The lung is lined by type II pneumocytes *(H)*, which suggests pulmonary injury or irritation as the result of the nematode infection (×20).

VIRAL DISEASES

Inclusion Body Myositis

Degeneration and necrosis of striated muscle in the tongue and panniculus associated with eosinophilic intranuclear inclusion bodies were described in two captive Spring Peepers.[59] Transmission electron microscopy demonstrated 19.6- to 24.5-nm, nonenveloped, icosahedral viruslike particles that were interpreted as being consistent with a parvovirus. Clinical signs in one affected animal included anorexia and lethargy; however, this individual also had concurrent cutaneous chytridiomycosis.

Herpesvirus Infections

The best-documented disease of amphibians caused by a herpesvirus is Lucke's renal adenocarcinoma in Leopard Frogs *(Rana pipiens)* caused by Ranid herpesvirus 1 (RaHV-1).[60,61] RaHV-1 and a second ranid herpesvirus (RaHV-2) of unknown clinical significance are most closely related to the fish virus Ictalurid herpesvirus 1.[4] Other than reports on Lucke's renal adenocarcinoma, there are occasional brief reports of disease associated with herpesvirus-like viral particles on examination by electron microscopy; however, in none of these cases was the virus isolated or characterized by molecular methods. In the Agile Frog *(Rana dalmatina)*, a skin disease associated with white to dark, 1-mm to 3-mm vesicles was noted on the dorsum and, less commonly, on the flanks and abdomen.[62] Histologically, lesions were characterized by epidermal hyperplasia and basal cell degeneration and necrosis, as well as karyomegaly with amphophilic intranuclear inclusions. No mention of systemic disease was mentioned in this article. In Mexican Leaf Frogs *(Pachymedusa dacnicolor)*, affected animals were found dead or moribund and had histologic evidence of necrosis in multiple organs including liver, pancreas, heart, kidney, and skin with occasional intranuclear inclusion bodies.[63] Additional investigation of future putative cases of herpesviral disease in amphibians, perhaps with the use of PCR methods designed to amplify fish herpesviruses, would be of value.

Adenovirus Infection

A frog adenovirus has been described and characterized by molecular methods but is of unknown clinical significance.[64]

REFERENCES

1. Daszak P, Cunningham AA, Hyatt AD. Infectious disease and amphibian population declines. *Divers Distrib* 2003;9:141-150.
2. Carey C, Cohen N, Rollins-Smith L. Amphibian declines: an immunological perspective. *Dev Comp Immunol* 1999;23:459-472.
3. Green DE, Converse KA, Schrader AK. Epizootiology of sixty-four amphibian mortality events in the USA, 1996-2001. *Ann N Y Acad Sci* 2002;969: 323-339.
4. Davison AJ, Cunningham C, Sauerbier W, et al. Genome sequences of two frog herpesviruses. *J Gen Virol* 2006;87:3509-3514.
5. Newcomer CE, Anver MR, Simmons JL, et al. Spontaneous and experimental infections of *Xenopus laevis* with *Chlamydia psittaci*. *Lab Anim Med* 1982;32:680-686.
6. Howerth EW. Pathology of naturally occurring chlamydiosis in African clawed frogs *(Xenopus laevis)*. Vet Pathol 1984;21:28-32.
7. Berger L, Volp K, Mathews S, et al. *Chlamydia pneumoniae* in a free-ranging giant barred frog *(Mixophyes iteratus)* from Australia. *J Clin Microbiol* 1999;37: 2378-2380.
8. Reed KD, Ruth GR, Meyer JA et al. *Chlamydia pneumoniae* infection in a breeding colony of African clawed frogs *(Xenopus tropicalis)*. *Emerg Infect Dis* 2000; 6: 196-199.
9. Bodetti TJ, Jacobson E, Wan C, et al. Molecular evidence to support the expansion of the host range of *Chlamydophila pneumoniae* to include reptiles as well as humans, horses, koalas and amphibians. *Syst Appl Microbiol* 2002;25:146-152.
10. Corsaro D, Venditti D. Emerging chlamydial infections. *Crit Rev Microbiol* 2004;30:75-106.
11. Blumer C, Zimmermann DR, Weilenmann R, et al. Chlamydiae in free-ranging and captive frogs in Switzerland. *Vet Pathol* 2007;44:144-150.
12. Taylor SK, Green DE, Wright KM, et al. Bacterial diseases. In: Wright KM, Whitaker BR, eds. *Amphibian medicine and captive husbandry*. Malabar, Fla: Krieger Publishing Co, 2001;159-179.
13. Shilton CM, Brown GP, Benedict S, et al. Spinal arthropathy associated with *Ochrobactrum anthropi* in free-ranging Cane toads *(Chaunus [Bufo] marinus)* in Australia. *Vet Pathol* 2008;45:85-94.
14. Mendoza L, Taylor JW, Ajello L. The class Mesomycetozoea: a heterogenous group of microorganisms at the animal-fungal boundary. *Ann Rev Microbiol* 2002;56:315-344.
15. Pascolini R, Daszak P, Cunningham AA, et al. Parasitism by *Dermocystidium ranae* in a population of *Rana esculenta* complex in Central Italy and description of *Amphibiocystidium* n. gen. *Dis Aquat Organisms* 2003;56:65-74.
16. Pereira CN, Di Rosa I, Fagotti A, et al. The pathogen of frogs *Amphibiocystidium ranae* is a member of the Order Dermocystida in the Class Mesomycetozoea. *J Clin Microbiol* 2005;43:192-198.
17. Feldman SH, Wimsatt JH, Green DE. Phylogenetic classification of the frog pathogen *Amphibiothecum (Dermosporidium) penneri* based on small ribosomal subunit sequencing. *J Wildl Dis* 2005;41:701-706.
18. Raffel TR, Dillard JR, Hudson PJ. Field evidence for leech-bourne transmission of amphibian *Ichthyophonus* sp. *J Parasitol* 2006;92:1256-1264.
19. Green DE, Feldman SH, Wimsatt J. Emergence of a *Perkinsus*-like agent in anuran liver during die-offs of local populations: PCR detection and phylogenetic characterization. in Proceedings. *Am Assoc Zoo Vet* 2003;120-121.
20. Davis AK, Yabsley MJ, Keel MK, et al. Discovery of a novel alveolate pathogen affecting southern leopard frogs in Georgia: description of the disease and host effects. *EcoHealth* 2007;4:310-317.
21. Cook JO. Transmission and occurrence of *Dermomycoides* sp. in *Rana sevosa* and other ranids in the North Central Gulf of Mexico States. MS thesis, University of Southern Mississippi, Hattiesburg, Miss, 2008.
22. Jones MEB, Armien AG, Rothermel BB, et al. Granulomatous myositis associated with a novel alveolate pathogen in an adult southern leopard frog *(Lithobates sphenocephalus)*. *Dis Aquat Org* 2012;102:163-167.
23. Green SL, Bouley DM, Josling CA, et al. Cryptosporidiosis associated with emaciation and proliferative gastritis in a laboratory-reared South African clawed frog *(Xenopus laevis)*. *Comp Med* 2003;53:81-84.
24. Graczyk TK, Cranfield MR, Geitner ME. Multiple *Cryptosporidium serpentis* oocyst isolates from captive snakes are not transmissible to amphibians. *J Parasitol* 1998;84:1298-1300.
25. Jirku M, Valigurova A, Koudela B, et al. New species of *Cryptosporidium* Tyzzer 1907 (Apicomplexa) from amphibian host: morphology, biology and phylogeny. *Folia Parasitol (Praha)* 2008;55:81-94.
26. Garner MM, Raymond JT, Shellabarger W, et al. Intravascular ciliated protozoa: an important cause of mortality in captive reared Kihansi spray toads *(Nectophrynoides asperginis)*, in Proceedings. Am Assoc Zoo Vet, Am Assoc Wildl Vet, and the Am Zoo Aquarium Assoc Nutr Advis Group 2005;274-275.
27. Noga EJ. *Fish disease, diagnosis and treatment*. St. Louis: Mosby, 1996;104-105.
28. Poynton SL, Whitaker BR. Protozoa in poison dart frogs (Dendrobatidae): clinical assessment and identification. *J Zoo Wildl Med* 1994;25:29-39.
29. Poynton SL, Whitaker BR. Protozoa and metazoa infecting amphibians. In: Wright KM, Whitaker BR, eds. *Amphibian medicine and captive husbandry*. Malabar, Fla: Krieger Publishing Co, 2001;193-221.
30. Hibbett DS, Binder M, Bischoff JF, et al. A higher-level phylogenetic classification of the fungi. *Mycol Res* 2007;111:509-547.
31. Green DE. Pathology of amphibia. In: Wright KM, Whitaker BR, eds. *Amphibian medicine and captive husbandry*. Malabar, Fla: Krieger Publishing Co, 2001;401-485.
32. Paperna I, Lainson R. *Alloglugea bufonis* nov. gen., nov. sp. (Microsporea: Glugeidae), a microsporidian of *Bufo marinus* tadpoles and metamorphosing toads (Amphibia: Anura) from Amazonian Brazil. *Dis Aquat Organisms* 1995;23:7-16.
33. Mutschmann F, Berger L, Marantelli G, et al. Microsporidia in amphibians, occurrence and pathology, in *Proceedings*. 6th Int Symp Pathol Reptiles Amphibians 2002;153-158.
34. Gamble KC, Garner MM, West G, et al. Kyphosis associated with microsporidial myositis in San Marcos salamanders, *Eurycea nana*. *J Herpetol Med Surg* 2005;15:14-17.

35. Weber R, Schwartz DA, Deplazes P. Laboratory diagnosis of microsporidiosis. In: Wittner M, Weiss LM, eds. *The microsporidia and microsporidiosis*. Washington, DC: American Society for Microbiology Press, 1999;315-362.
36. Hill BD, Green PE, Lucke HA. Hepatitis in the green tree frog (*Litoria caerulea*) associated with infection by a species of *Myxidium*. *Aust Vet J* 1997;75:910-911.
37. Hartigan A, Fiala I, Dykova I, et al. A suspected parasite spill-back of two novel *Myxidium* spp. (Myxosporea) causing disease in Australian endemic frogs found in the invasive cane toad. *PLoS One* 2011;6:e18871.
38. Hartigan A, Fiala I, Dykova I, et al. New species of Myxosporea from frogs and resurrection of the genus *Cystodiscus* Lutz, 1889 for species with myxospores in gallbladders of amphibians. *Parasitol* 2012;139:478-496.
39. Jirku M, Bolek MG, Whipps CM, et al. A new species of *Myxidium* (Myxosporea: Myxidiidae), from the western chorus frog, *Pseudacris triseriata triseriata*, and Blanchard's cricket frog, *Acris crepitans blanchardi* (Hylidae), from eastern Nebraska: morphology, phylogeny, and critical comments on amphibian *Myxidium* taxonomy. *J Parasitol* 2006;92:611-619.
40. Duncan AE, Garner MM, Bartholomew JL, et al. Renal myxosporidiasis in Asian horned frogs (*Megophrys nasuta*). *J Zoo Wildl Med* 2004;35:381-386.
41. Mutschmann F. Pathological changes in African hyperoliid frogs due to a myxosporidian infection with a new species of *Hoferellus* (Myxozoa). *Dis Aquat Org* 2004;60:215-222.
42. Goodchild CG. A new endoparasitic oligochaete (Naididae) from a North American tree-toad, *Hyla squirella*, Latrreille, 1802. *J Parasitol* 1951;37:205-211.
43. Harman WJ, Lawler AR. *Dero (Allodero) hylae*, an oligochaete symbiont in hylid frogs in Mississippi. *Trans Am Microsc Soc* 1975;94:38-42.
44. Frenkel JK, Harman WJ. *Allodera hylae*, an endoparasitic worm (Naididae, Oligochaeta, Annelida) from a Coloumbian poison dart frog, *Dendrobates histtrionicus*, ureteral and cloacal habitat and visceral migration, in *Proceedings*. Annu Meet Am Soc Parasitology 1985;36, Abstract 58.
45. Lopez LCS, Rodrigues PJFP, Rios RI. Frogs and snakes as phoretic dispersal agents of bromeliad ostracods (Limnocytheridae: *Elpidium*) and annelids (Naididae: *Dero*). *Biotropica* 1999;31:705-708.
46. Lopez LCS, Filizola B, Deiss I, et al. Phoretic behaviour of bromeliad annelids (*Dero*) and ostracods (*Elpidium*) using frogs and lizards as dispersal vectors. *Hydrobiologia* 2005;549:15-22.
47. Meteyer CU, Loeffler IK, Fallon JF, et al. Hind limb malformations in free-living northern leopard frogs (*Rana pipiens*) from Maine, Minnesota, and Vermont suggest multiple etiologies. *Teratology* 2000;62:151-171.
48. Loeffler IK, Stocum DL, Fallon JF, et al. Leaping lopsided: a review of the current hypotheses regarding etiologies of limb malformations in frogs. *Anat Rec* 2001;265:228-245.
49. Johnson PTJ, Lunde KB, Zelmer DA, et al. Limb deformities as an emerging parasitic disease in amphibians: evidence from museum specimens and resurvey data. *Conserv Biol* 2003;17:1724-1737.
50. Johnson PTJ, Sutherland DR. Amphibian deformities and *Ribeiroria* infection: an emerging helminthiasis. *Trends Parasitol* 2003;19:332-335.
51. Johnson PTJ, Preu ER, Sutherland DR, et al. Adding insult to injury: synergistic effects of predation and parasitism on amphibian malformations. *Ecology* 2006;87:2227-2235.
52. Johnson PTJ, Chase JM, Dosch KL, et al. Aquatic eutrophication promotes pathogenic infection in amphibians. *Proc Natl Acad Sci U S A* 2007;104:15781-15786.
53. Kuzmin Y, Tkach VV, Brooks DR. Two new species of *Rhabdias* (Nematoda: Rhabdiasidae) from the marine toad, *Bufo marinus* (L.) (Lissamphibia: Anura: Bufonidae), in Central America. *J Parasitol* 2007;93:159-165.
54. Little MD. Seven new species of *Strongyloides* (Nematoda) from Louisiana. *J Parasitol* 1966;52: 85-97.
55. Schmidt GD, Whittaker FH. Nematode parasites of Puerto Rican tree frogs, *Eleutherodactylus* spp: two new species and a proposal of *Poekilostrongylus* gen. nov. (Trichostrongylidae). *Parasitology* 1975;70:287-294.
56. Patterson-Kane JC, Eckerlin RP, Lyons ET, et al. Strongyloidiasis in a Cope's grey tree frog (*Hyla chrysoscelis*). *J Zoo Wildl Med* 2001;32:106-110.
57. Lee S, Zippel K, Ramos L, et al. Captive breeding programme for the Kihansi spray toad at the Wildlife Conservation Society, Bronx, New York. *Int Zoo Yearbook* 2006;40:241-253.
58. Cunningham AA. Disease risks of wildlife translocations. *Conserv Biol* 1996;10:349-353.
59. Raymond JT, Reichard T, Shellabarger W, et al. Inclusion body myositis in spring peepers (*Pseudacris crucifer*). *J Vet Diagn Invest* 2002;14:501-503.
60. McKinnell RG, Carlson DL. Lucke renal adenocarcinoma, an anuran neoplasm: studies at the interface of pathology, virology, and differentiation competence. *J Cell Physiol* 1997;173:115-118.
61. Stacy BA, Parker JM. Amphibian oncology. *Vet Clin N Am Exot Anim Pract* 2004;7:673-695.
62. Bennati R, Bonetti M, Lavazza A, et al. Skin lesions associated with herpesvirus-like particles in frogs (*Rana dalmatina*). *Vet Rec* 1994;135:625-626.
63. Garner MM, Collins D, Joslin J, et al. Fatal systemic herpesvirus infection in three Mexican giant tree frogs (*Pachymedusa dacnicolor*), in *Proceedings*. Assoc Reptilian Amphibian Vet 2000;7.
64. Davison AJ, Wright KM, Harrach B. DNA sequence of frog adenovirus. *J Gen Virol* 2000;81:2431-2439.

CHAPTER 22

Chytridiomycosis

Allan P. Pessier

The emerging amphibian skin disease chytridiomycosis was first described in the late 1990s from both captive and free-ranging frogs[1-3] and has rapidly become one of the most studied amphibian diseases. The causative agent, *Batrachochytrium dendrobatidis* (Bd), is a chytrid fungus with very low host specificity, as demonstrated by identification in more than 200 species and 20 families representing both anurans and caudates (www.bd-maps.net). Chytridiomycosis causes die-offs and population declines of free-ranging amphibians, and is a significant cause of disease and management concern in captive amphibian collections.[4,5]

Although commonly associated with aquatic environments, the chytrids (fungi in the Phylum Chytridiomycota) are environmentally ubiquitous, and many are involved in the degradation of plant and animal matter such as cellulose, chitin, and keratin.[6,7] Before the description of Bd in amphibians, parasitic or pathogenic chytrids were recognized only in algae, fungi, invertebrate animals, and plants. Features of most chytrid fungi include a simple thallus (fungal body) in which the cytoplasm cleaves to form distinctive motile uniflagellate zoospores during asexual reproduction (Figure 22-1). Of all the chytrid fungi, only *Batrachochytrium* has been associated with amphibian disease, and Koch's postulates have been fulfilled by experimental infection.[8] Before the definitive descriptions of chytridiomycosis, Bd was observed by pathologists and variably reported to be a protozoan, aquatic fungal-like protist, or a clinical manifestation of infection with the fungus *Basidiobolus ranarum*.[9-12]

CHYTRIDIOMYCOSIS AND AMPHIBIAN POPULATION DECLINES

Amphibian populations worldwide are in decline, and the International Union for Conservation of Nature (IUCN) Global Amphibian Assessment has estimated that 32.5% of all amphibian species are threatened and more than 400 species may be on the brink of extinction.[13] Chytridiomycosis has been identified as a major contributory factor in many of these declines.[4,5,13-16] Published reports of Bd infection have come from Africa, Australia, Europe, North, Central, and South America, the Caribbean, and New Zealand.[1,13,17-27] Many of the best-documented declines due to chytridiomycosis have been reported from stream-dwelling species at high elevations in Central America and Australia.[28,29] In these cases, chytridiomycosis-associated declines progressed in a predictable geographic pattern suggestive of a recently introduced pathogen.[1,15] In Central America, a long-term study has clearly documented loss of amphibian biodiversity only after arrival of Bd at a new location.[23]

There continues to be debate about whether Bd is truly an introduced novel pathogen or an endemic parasite that has increased in virulence or now causes disease secondary to environmental or other cofactors.[4,16,30] Supporting the novel pathogen hypothesis are initial Bd genetic studies that showed minimal genetic variation between North American, African, and Australian Bd isolates consistent with a clonal population.[31] More recent genetic studies are beginning to show more discrimination between geographically distinct isolates of Bd, including the possible emergence of a hypervirulent recombinant lineage.[32-34]

A leading hypothesis for international dissemination of Bd focuses on the African Clawed Frog *(Xenopus laevis)*, which was extensively exported beginning in the 1930s for use in human pregnancy diagnosis.[21] The earliest known case of Bd infection (1938) was found in the African Clawed Frog, and the prevalence of Bd infection (2.7%) in African populations has remained unchanged over many decades, which

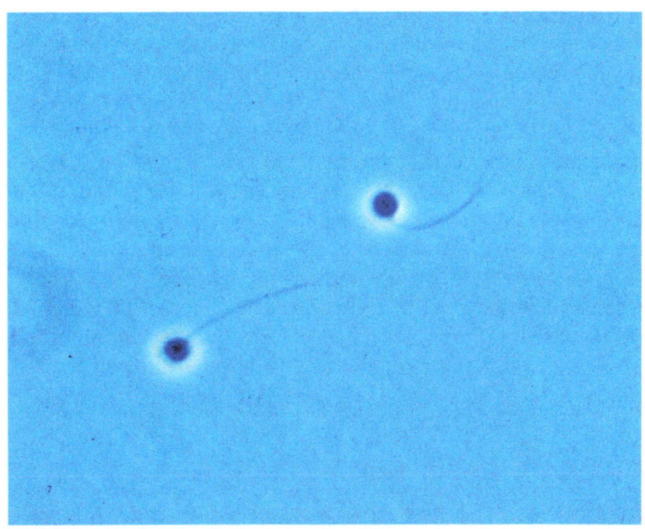

FIGURE 22-1 Zoospores of *Batrachochytrium dendrobatidis* as viewed by phase-contrast microscopy. The single posterior flagellum is characteristic the Phylum Chytridiomycota (×40). *(Photo courtesy Dr. Joyce Longcore, The University of Maine, Orono, Me.)*

suggests endemic rather than introduced infections. In addition to the African Clawed Frog, another species that has been widely introduced worldwide and is a good potential reservoir host for Bd is the American Bullfrog (*Lithobates catesbeianus*).[20,22,33,35] Concerns that international trade in amphibians for food, research, exhibition, teaching, and pets continues to contribute to the introduction of Bd to new areas have led to calls for national risk abatement plans and listing of Bd infection as notifiable under the Aquatic Animal Health Code of the World Organisation for Animal Health (OIE).[36,37] Listing by the OIE will eventually require that amphibians moved in international trade be free of Bd infection or held in biosecure conditions to prevent introduction of Bd or virulent Bd strains to new locations.

There is great interest in the potential role of environmental cofactors in determining the outcome and significance of Bd infection in free-ranging amphibian populations. Climate-related cofactors have received the most attention because maximal growth of Bd occurs in a specific temperature range of 17°C to 25°C.[38] To this end, seasonal variations with higher prevalence and severity of Bd infection in cooler times of the year (winter and spring) have been reported for some species of Australian anurans.[29,39] In another article, thermal springs with water temperatures exceeding 30°C were postulated to provide refugia from Bd infection.[40] The use of ecologic niche modeling has predicted that up to half of all amphibian species live in regions optimal for Bd.[41] Paradoxic relationships between chytridiomycosis-associated declines and changes in microclimate associated with global warming toward those favorable for Bd have been suggested but are controversial.[4,42-45] The recent report of chytridiomycosis in Andean frogs that have recently migrated to higher elevations as the result of deglaciation from environmental change represent the highest elevation and lowest temperatures from which Bd has been observed.[27] Additional research is required to determine what relationships, if any, exist between the emergence of chytridiomycosis and climate change.

Interestingly, some amphibian populations that have experienced chytridiomycosis-associated declines may partially recover and persist with endemic Bd infection.[40,46,47] Other amphibian populations such as those in the northeastern United States and the St. Lawrence River Valley of Quebec, Canada, show evidence of endemic Bd infection without associated declines.[48,49] Because so many amphibian populations are experiencing devastating declines associated with Bd, the hope from these observations is that other populations will be able to develop similar resistance. The possibility of acquisition of resistance to Bd by either natural selection or selective captive breeding provides support for the development of captive survival assurance colonies for species affected by Bd-associated declines.[50,51]

PATHOLOGY AND HOST DEFENSE

Infection with Bd is limited to areas of keratinizing stratified squamous epithelium in the oral disk (jaw sheaths and tooth rows) of tadpoles and the skin of postmetamorphic animals. The skin of tadpoles is nonkeratinizing and the transition to a keratinizing epidermis occurs during metamorphosis. As tadpoles undergo metamorphosis, Bd infection moves from the oral disk onto the skin with subsequent development of clinically significant disease.[52-54]

Invasion of Bd into deeper portions of the skin or dissemination to the visceral organs has not been observed. The primary lesion of chytridiomycosis in postmetamorphic animals is hyperkeratosis and epidermal hyperplasia (Figure 22-2). Thalli (fungal bodies) of Bd are observed in skin cell (keratinocyte) cytoplasm and are most abundant in the keratinized layers (stratum corneum) (Figure 22-3). Infiltrates of inflammatory cells or other epidermal changes such as necrosis and ulceration are inconsistently observed and are more

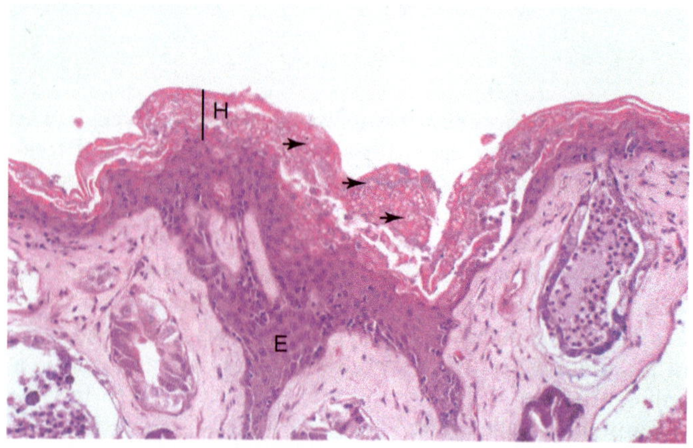

FIGURE 22-2 Lesions of severe chytridiomycosis in a White's Tree Frog *(Litoria caerulea)*. There is marked epidermal hyperplasia *(E)* and hyperkeratosis *(H)* with myriad thalli of *Batrachochytrium dendrobatidis* in the keratinized layers of the skin *(arrows; ×10)*.

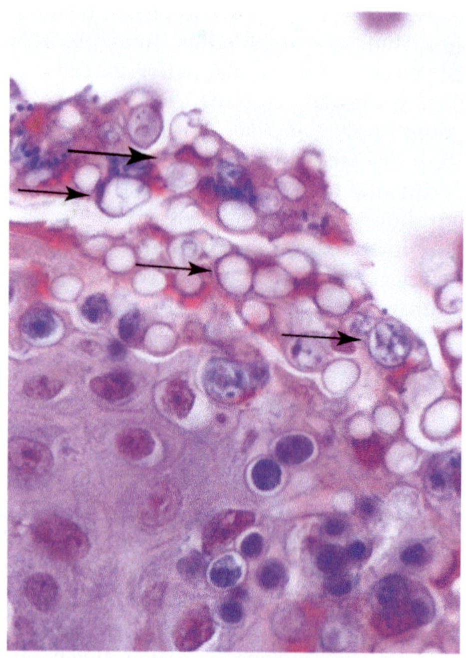

FIGURE 22-3 Chytridiomycosis in a Smoky Jungle Frog (*Leptodactylus pentadactylus*). There are numerous empty and developing thalli of *Batrachochytrium dendrobatidis* in the keratinized skin layers *(arrows)*. In addition, there is secondary colonization of the skin with a small unidentified yeast *(large arrow; ×60)*.

frequently found in cases with secondary bacterial, fungal, or Oomycete (water mold) infections (see Figure 22-3). Such secondary infections are common and may occur because empty Bd thalli (those that have discharged zoospores) and the accumulated keratin layers trap environmental microorganisms.

The mechanism by which chytridiomycosis causes death in susceptible animals has been thought to result from disruption of normal skin function or, alternatively, from exposure to a mycotoxin produced by Bd.[1,2] Unlike other vertebrates, the skin of amphibians has important physiologic functions that include water absorption, osmoregulation, and, in some species, respiration. Studies in White's Tree Frogs *(Litoria caerulea)* with experimentally induced chytridiomycosis demonstrated reduced plasma osmolality, hyponatremia, hypokalemia, hypomagnesemia, and hypochloridemia when compared with uninfected control animals.[55,56] No significant differences were found in hematocrit, albumin, or urea levels, which suggests that disease interfered with mechanisms for cutaneous electrolyte transport but not with hydration status. A limited hematologic evaluation of chorus frogs *(Pseudacris maculata)* with naturally acquired chytridiomycosis demonstrated some evidence of hemoconcentration (suggestive of dehydration) when compared with uninfected frogs; however, results were not statistically significant and the authors felt that additional studies were required.[57] At this time there is no definitive experimental evidence for the role of a mycotoxin in the pathogenesis of chytridiomycosis; however, one hypothesis for the electrolyte depletion observed in experimentally infected White's Tree Frogs is toxin-associated disruption of cutaneous sodium channels.[55] A report of rapid death in Western Toad *(Anaxyrus boreas)* tadpoles after inoculation with cultures of Bd was interpreted to be consistent with toxin exposure; however, a specific mycotoxin was not described.[58] When Bd and chytridiomycosis were first identified, there was concern that lethal effects would be observed in all or most species that became infected. It is now known that a wide range of amphibian species—and probably most species—can become *infected* with Bd, however, not all species are equally susceptible to developing clinically significant chytridiomycosis, the *disease* caused by Bd. For instance, the Tiger Salamander *(Ambystoma tigrinum)*, American Bullfrog, and some African Clawed Frogs become subclinically infected with Bd and may be sources of infection for other species but rarely, under both natural and experimental conditions, develop severe chytridiomycosis.[20,21,35,59] Similarly, tadpoles are usually subclinically infected with Bd and are implicated as reservoirs of infection for postmetamorphic animals.[1,54] Compared with animals with clinically significant chytridiomycosis, subclinically infected animals usually have minimal histologic lesions consisting of small multifocal areas of hyperkeratosis with few Bd thalli (Figure 22-4).[20]

Host factors that influence species susceptibility and the severity of chytridiomycosis in individuals may include aspects of innate and acquired immunity, differences in host skin flora, and aspects of host behavior and biology. Because Bd infection is limited to the superficial (keratinized) layers of the skin and evidence of a significant host inflammatory response is an inconsistent finding, it has been thought less likely that cellular components of innate immune response, such as phagocytic cells (neutrophils and macrophages) or adaptive immune responses (humoral or cell-mediated immunity), play a significant role in protection against Bd. However, recent studies have demonstrated evidence of specific MHC genotypes associated with increased survival of some Bd-infected animals and Bd-specific immunoglobulins in skin mucus.[51,60] Not yet explored are possible roles for cytokines produced by keratinocytes or resident lymphocytes and dendritic cells that could influence keratinocyte proliferation and turnover with subsequent effects on the ability to effectively shed Bd-infected cells. Antimicrobial peptides secreted by granular glands in the skin are potentially important components of innate immunity against Bd infection.[61] There are species-specific differences in the types and mixtures of peptides produced, and these differences in some instances may predict apparent resistance or susceptibility to developing severe chytridiomycosis.[47,62] Complementing work on antimicrobial peptides are observations that specific symbiotic bacteria isolated from the skin of plethodontid salamanders *(Plethodon cinereus* and *Hemidactylium scutatum)* and the Mountain Yellow-legged Frog *(Rana muscosa)* inhibit the growth of Bd in culture and may contribute to survival of Bd-infected frogs.[63,64] Finally, host behavioral factors can influence transmission of Bd and the outcome of Bd infection, and these include the frequency of frog-to-frog contact and contact with water.[28,65]

Nonhost factors such as environmental temperature and virulence of individual isolates (sometimes referred to as strains) of Bd may influence the severity of chytridiomycosis. Low-to-moderate environmental temperatures optimal to the growth of Bd in culture are associated with increased virulence in experimental infection studies.[39,66] Furthermore, environmental temperatures higher than 27°C can result in reduced virulence and even elimination of Bd infection.[39,67] A study in Panamanian Golden Frogs *(Atelopus zeteki)* demonstrated that thermoregulatory behavior of individual frogs influenced the likelihood of Bd infection.[68] Experimental studies in Green Tree Frogs *(Litoria caerulea)* and Western Chorus Frogs *(Pseudacris triseriata)* demonstrated differences between isolates of Bd from different locations in the time to death after exposure and in the numbers of frogs killed by exposure.[69,70] It has been suggested that these observations could represent variation in

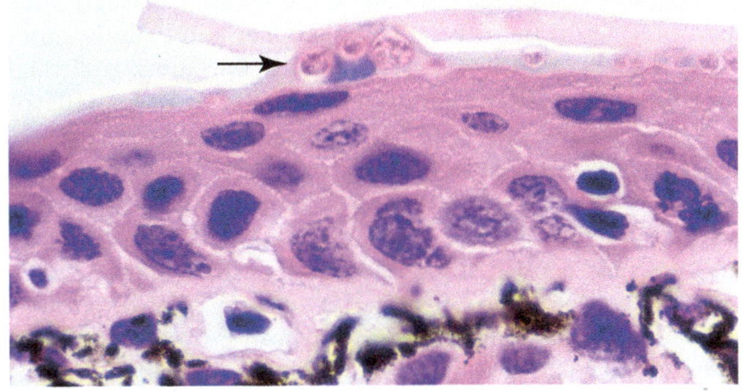

FIGURE 22-4 Subclinical infection with *Batrachochytrium dendrobatidis* in a Tiger Salamander *(Ambystoma tigrinum)*. There is minimal hyperkeratosis, and superficial skin cells contain small numbers of Bd thalli *(arrow; ×40)*.

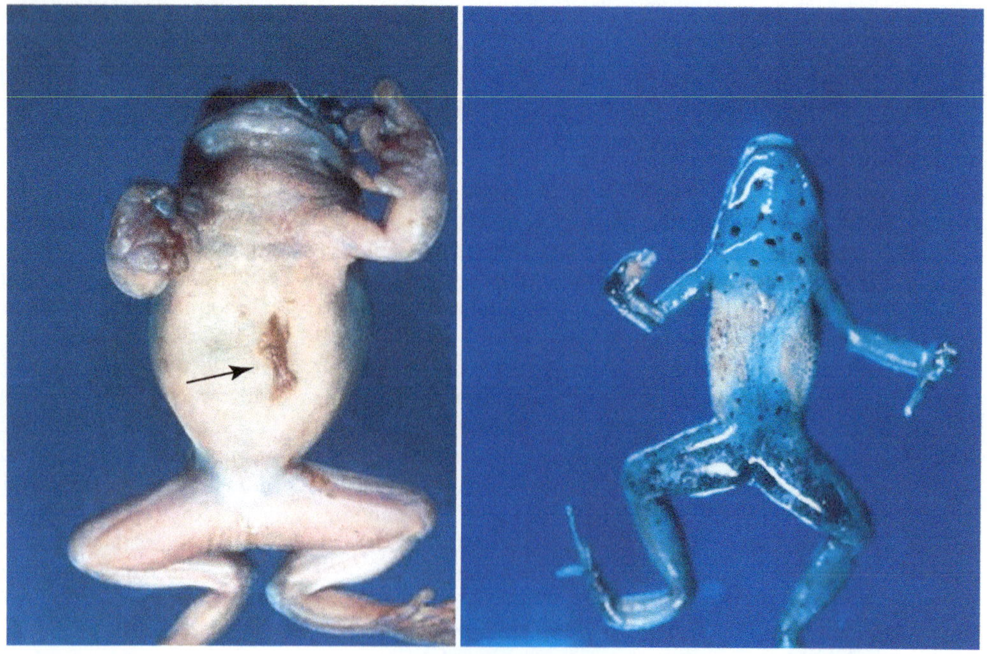

FIGURE 22-5 Gross lesions of chytridiomycosis in a White's Tree Frog (*Litoria caerulea*) and Blue Poison Dart Frog (*Dendrobates azureus*). The White's Tree Frog has mild hyperemia (reddening) of the ventral skin and excessive amounts of brown shedding skin *(arrow)*. The Poison Dart Frog *(right)* has focally extensive areas of brown granular discoloration of the ventral skin.

virulence between Bd strains. Finally, recent genetic evidence suggests that a globalized Bd lineage may be "hypervirulent" compared with other lineages.[34]

CLINICAL SIGNS

The spectrum of clinical signs observed in individual animals infected with Bd can vary from none in animals with low-level infections (subclinical or carrier animals) to grossly evident skin disease. Death without premonitory signs is observed in some animals with heavy infections, and the lack of grossly visible skin lesions should not be used to exclude a diagnosis of chytridiomycosis. Nonspecific clinical signs of anorexia or lethargy are common in severely affected animals. Weight loss has been observed in some experimental infection studies[70]; however, naturally infected animals are often in good nutritional condition. In some cases postural or behavioral changes are observed, such as reluctance to place the ventral body surface in contact with substrate or changes in (increased or decreased) desire for contact with water. Neurologic signs such as a loss of righting reflex are occasionally present.

If grossly visible skin lesions are observed, they are most often present on the ventral body and feet and include excessive skin shedding (dysecdysis), skin discoloration, and rough or granular changes in skin texture (Figure 22-5). Skin discoloration is usually brown to red and can be confused with the "redleg syndrome" (bacterial dermatosepticemia) traditionally associated with gram-negative bacteria such as *Aeromonas hydrophila* (Figure 22-6). Often, cases with significant cutaneous hyperemia are complicated by secondary infections. In addition to excessively shedding skin, black-pigmented spots on the ventral abdomen and dorsal head [59] or in the region around the vent were present on Tiger Salamanders and a plethodontid salamander (*Plethodon neomexicanus*) infected with Bd.[71] In other salamanders infected with Bd, autotomization of the tail has been reported; however, the pathogenesis of this observation is uncertain.[72]

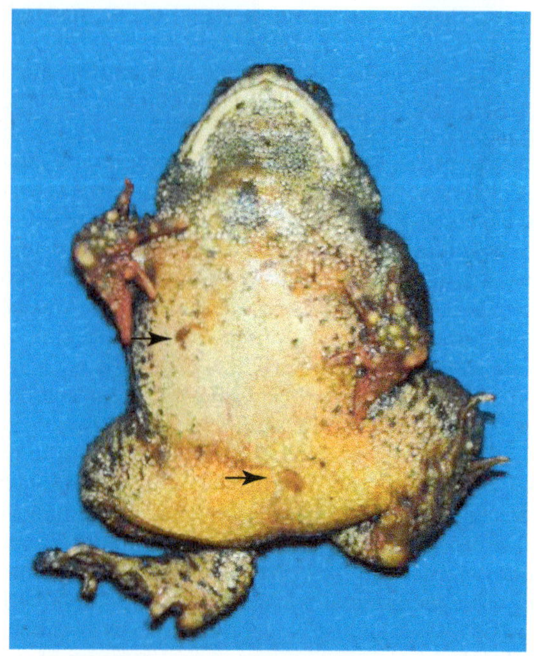

FIGURE 22-6 Gross lesions of chytridiomycosis in a Wyoming Toad (*Anaxyrus [Bufo] baxteri*). There are excessive amounts of brown shedding skin *(arrows)* and marked hyperemia (reddening) of the toes that may be confused with the ubiquitous "redleg syndrome" of captive amphibians.

Infection with Bd in tadpoles (larvae) is usually subclinical; however, grossly apparent depigmentation of portions of the oral disk have been widely reported in infected animals.[54,73-75] Reduced body mass has been observed in infected tadpoles under some experimental conditions,[76,77] but no evidence of decreased growth was noted in a field study of African tadpoles.[78] Death was observed in Western Toad tadpoles shortly after exposure to laboratory cultures of Bd but not in tadpoles of American

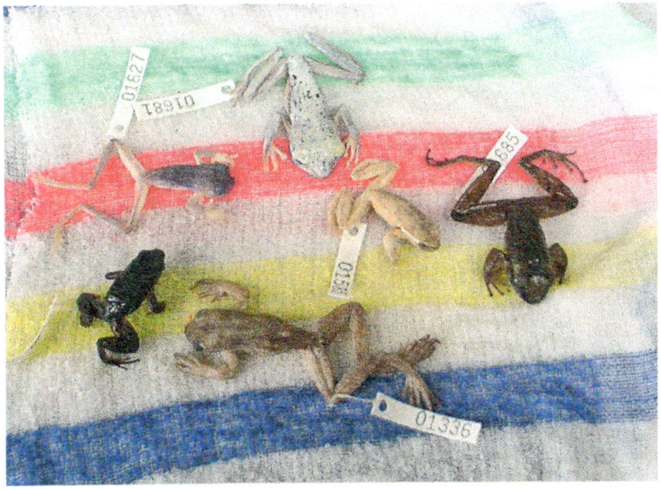

FIGURE 22-7 Panamanian frogs that died during an outbreak of chytridiomycosis and were subsequently submitted for necropsy examination. *(Photo courtesy Dr. Karen Lips, The University of Maryland, College Park, Md.)*

Bullfrogs, Cascades Frogs *(Rana cascadae)*, or Pacific Tree Frogs *(Hyla regilla)*.[58] In free-ranging amphibian populations, chytridiomycosis has had presentations that vary from insidious, in which small numbers of deaths are observed over a period of time with gradual, but significant, loss of population numbers,[79] to dramatic, with large numbers of dead animals and rapid loss of regional amphibian diversity[23] (Figure 22-7). All reported chytridiomycosis-associated mortality events have affected postmetamorphic animals, and die-offs that include large numbers of larval amphibians are likely due to other infectious agents such as *Ranavirus* infection, even if Bd is identified in the course of the diagnostic investigation. Because the clinical signs in individual animals with chytridiomycosis may overlap with a variety of other diseases, complete investigation of all amphibian mortality events, including histopathologic examination, bacterial and virus isolation, and molecular diagnostics (e.g., polymerase chain reaction [PCR] for Bd and ranaviruses), is encouraged.

LIFE CYCLE

The infective stage of Bd to amphibians is the motile flagellated zoospore[8,66] (Figure 22-8). Zoospores are released from mature zoosporangia that have been established within amphibian keratinocytes (skin of postmetamorphic animals or oral disk of tadpoles); they then swim in the environment before reencysting. Under experimental conditions, zoospores swim very short distances (<2 cm) before encysting, and this tendency likely promotes autoinfection of host animal skin and amphibian-to-amphibian contact as mechanisms of Bd transmission.[38] Dispersion of zoospores by water currents and other vectors such as bird feathers and moist substrates are also a consideration.[81] Experimentally, zoospores can persist in sterilized pond water containing organic materials for as long as 7 weeks, up to 3 hours on bird feathers, and at least 12 weeks in sterilized creek bed sand.[80,81] A report of freshwater shrimp as a possible reservoir host for Bd was later retracted.[82] Determination of the importance of reservoirs for Bd outside of an amphibian host is the subject of active ongoing research and will be aided by PCR techniques that detect Bd in environmental samples.[83,84]

The use of mathematical models has suggested that the ability of Bd to persist outside of an amphibian host may increase the probability of driving host animals toward extinction.[85] Unlike some other chytrid fungi, a resting spore that could be involved in long-term environmental persistence or long distance dispersal has not been identified for Bd. However, the recent observation of probable sexual reproduction raises the possibility that a resting spore may occur under some circumstances.[32] Approaches to the identification of subclinically infected amphibians that may serve as reservoir hosts are discussed in the sections on Morphologic Methods of Diagnosis and Molecular Methods of Diagnosis.

DIAGNOSIS AND TREATMENT

Transmission and Disinfection

In captive situations it has been possible to house Bd-infected animals adjacent to noninfected animals as long as special care is taken to avoid transfer of animals, water, substrates, or cage decorations (including plants) between enclosures.[8,86] Protocols that include disinfection of instruments and wearing of gloves (or hand washing) between servicing different enclosures should be incorporated into the standard operating procedures of amphibian collections. Most of the common disinfectants used in captive collections and veterinary hospitals, as well as heat and complete drying (desiccation), have been shown experimentally to kill Bd[38,86, 87-89] (Table 22-1). Ultraviolet light has been shown to be ineffective against cultures of Bd in the laboratory.[87] Before disinfection, enclosures and instruments should always be thoroughly cleaned to remove organic materials that will inactivate most chemical disinfectants. Disinfectant concentrations and application times beyond the minimum suggested by the experimental data are given. In addition to disinfection of equipment and enclosures, consideration should be given to treatment of waste water and substrates used in amphibian collections to minimize the risk of introducing Bd (or other pathogens) to free-ranging amphibian populations.

Sodium hypochlorite in the form of household bleach or that labeled for use in swimming pools is commonly used in zoologic institutions and for the disinfection of field equipment. Concentrations of sodium hypochlorite vary significantly in commercial products (e.g., 3% to 6% in household bleach and 12.5% in liquid products for swimming pools), and users should base dilutions to achieve working disinfectant solutions on the final concentration of hypochlorite (e.g., a 1% solution of sodium hypochlorite rather than a 1:100 dilution ["1%"] of the household bleach product).

Heat and complete drying of surfaces may be most useful in real-world settings when used together or in combination with a chemical disinfection method. For instance, enclosures can be thoroughly cleaned with hot water, disinfected with an appropriate chemical, rinsed thoroughly to eliminate chemical residues, and then set out to dry in a warm place or room (at least 4 hours at 37°C or 98.6°F). Heating of wastewater, wet substrates, and plants before disposal (or before use of heat tolerant plants or substrates that may have been exposed to potentially infected amphibians) is a potentially environmentally friendly approach to disinfection of these items.

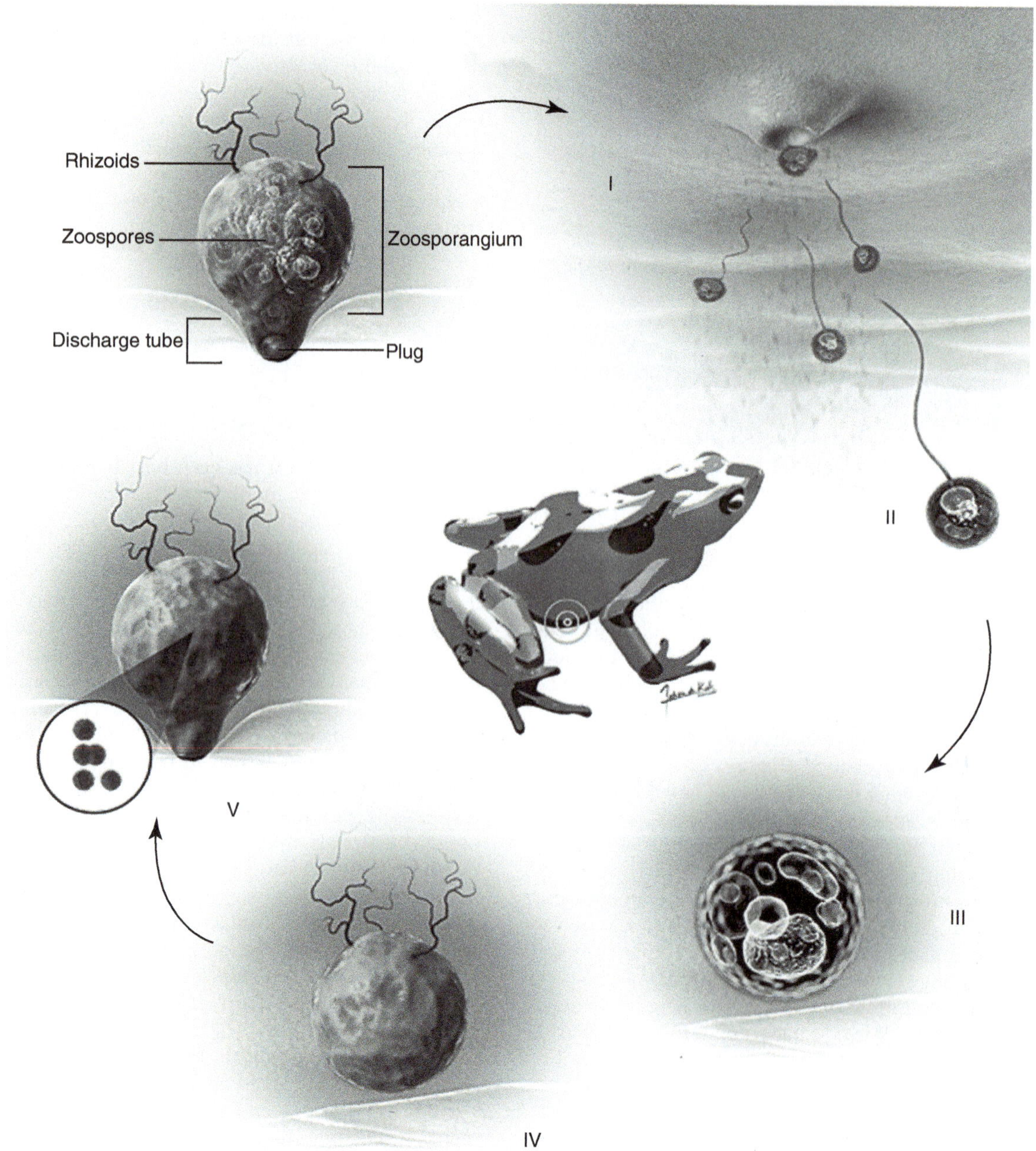

FIGURE 22-8 The life cycle of *Batrachochytrium dendrobatidis* (Bd) in an amphibian host. **I,** A mature thallus (zoosporangium) of Bd inside an amphibian skin cell (keratinocyte) releases uniflagellate zoospores through a discharge tube oriented toward the environment. **II,** Zoospores swim a short distance or may be carried by water currents. **III** and **IV,** The zoospore encounters a new amphibian keratinocyte on the same or different animal and begins to develop a new thallus within the cell cytoplasm. **V,** The cytoplasm of the thallus cleaves to form discrete zoospores culminating in a new zoosporangium to begin the cycle anew. *(Courtesy Fabian de Kok-Mercado, CMI, Johns Hopkins University, Baltimore, Md.)*

Disinfection of items used in amphibian field research programs is an important approach to limiting movement of Bd (or other amphibian pathogens not yet identified) from a location with infected animals to a naïve location that has not yet encountered this organism. Suggested protocols for disinfection of field equipment are available online at the Amphibian Diseases Homepage (http://www.jcu.edu.au/school/phtm/PHTM/frogs/ampdis.htm). Similar to enclosures or equipment used in captive management of amphibians, field equipment should be thoroughly cleaned of dirt or other organic material before disinfection. It has been suggested that at least twice the experimentally effective concentration of disinfectant should be used.[88]

DIAGNOSIS

A variety of morphologic and molecular techniques have been described to diagnose chytridiomycosis or to detect Bd infection in amphibians. The choice of a diagnostic method depends on

TABLE 22-1

Chemical and Physical Methods for Elimination of *Batrachochytrium dendrobatidis* on Surfaces

Chemical or Method	Effective Concentration and Duration of Application
Sodium hypochlorite (NaH):	
1. *Household Bleach* (5% to 6% NaH)	1% to 4% NaH effective at 30 sec of application[87]
2. *Swimming pool disinfectant* (12.5% NaH)	0.01% to 0.2% NaH effective at 10 min of application[87]
Quaternary ammonium compounds:	
1. *Didecyl dimethyl ammonium chloride* (DDAC)	
Roccal-D (9.2% DDAC)	1:1000 dilution of 7.68% and 12% DDAC products at 30 sec of application[87]
Path-X (12% DDAC)	
2. *Benzalkonium chloride*	1 mg/mL effective at 20 sec of application[87]
Ethanol (95%)	70% ethanol effective at 20 sec of application[87]
Trigene	1:5000 dilution effective at 1 min of application[86,88]
Virkon	1 mg/mL effective at 20 sec of application
Heat	47°C (116.6°F) effective at 30 min of application[87]
	37°C (98.6°F) effective at 4 hr of application[87]
	32°C (89.6°F) effective at 96 hr of exposure[87]
Desiccation (complete drying)	Effective at a minimum of 3 hr of exposure[87]

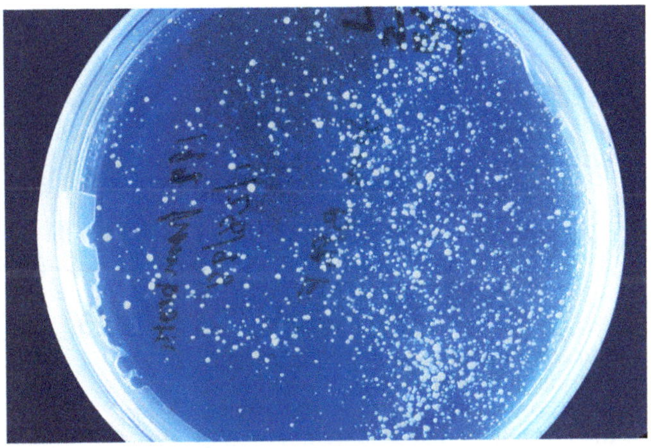

FIGURE 22-9 A pure culture of *Batrachochytrium dendrobatidis* (Bd) on a TGhL agar plate. Culture of Bd is not used for routine diagnosis because isolation requires specialized techniques and media.

factors that include the purpose of the examination, the type of sample available for analysis, and access to specific equipment or reference laboratories.[89] For diagnostic testing, it is important to distinguish between clinical disease or death due to Bd infection (chytridiomycosis) and subclinical infection with Bd. In general, morphologic methods such as wet mounts, cytology, and histopathology are most useful for diagnosing clinically significant Bd infections that have high numbers of organisms present in the skin. In contrast, molecular methods (conventional or Taqman PCR) are considerably more sensitive and have clinical applications that include confirming clinical diagnoses, detecting subclinical infections in quarantine, and performing surveys to detect the presence or prevalence of Bd infection in captive or wild populations.[90,91] Routine fungal culture is not useful for diagnosis because Bd requires specific isolation techniques and media[3,38] (Figure 22-9).

Morphologic Methods of Diagnosis (Wet Mount, Cytology, and Histopathology)

Specific diagnosis of chytridiomycosis with the use of morphologic methods requires identification of the characteristic thalli of Bd within the cytoplasm of skin cells (keratinocytes).[2,3,92] Thalli of Bd range from approximately 7 µm to 20 µm in histologic section, and three forms can be routinely identified: a uninucleate stage with homogenous basophilic cytoplasm, a multinucleate form with stippled to microvacuolated cytoplasm, and the mature zoosporangium that contains multiple discrete 2-µm to 3-µm basophilic spherical zoospores (Figure 22-10). Mature zoosporangia should not be confused with life stages of a protozoal organism. Features that are most useful for definitive diagnosis are thalli with discharge papillae (discharge tubes) that give the thallus a flasklike appearance and colonial thalli that have evidence of fine internal septation (Figure 22-10). Colonial thalli are best observed in zoosporangia that have previously discharged their zoospores (empty thalli). Empty thalli are common and, in some cases, may comprise the majority of organisms visible in histologic section. Additional and diagnostically useful features of Bd thalli are the rhizoids, which are thin, rootlike extensions from thalli that are sometimes visible in silver-stained (Grocott-Gomori's methenamine silver or Steiner's) histologic sections (see Figure 22-10).

For rapid diagnosis of chytridiomycosis, wet mounts or cytologic examination of shedding skin, shed skin recovered from the enclosure, or skin obtained by gentle skin scraping are sometimes useful (Figure 22-11 and Figure 22-12). Wet mounts can be made with the use of distilled water or normal saline, although the addition of dyes such as Congo Red can aid in identifying characteristic features of Bd thalli.[50,93] For cytology, skin samples are flattened onto the glass slides, air-dried, and routinely stained with hematologic dyes such as Wright's or Wright-Giemsa. Immature or degenerate Bd thalli can be difficult to distinguish from yeasts or some stages of Oomycete water molds (see Figure 22-12). Overgrowth of Oomycetes and other organisms is of particular concern when shed skin obtained from enclosures is used for examination.[94] Unless unequivocal Bd thalli are observed, confirmation of the diagnosis by other methods such as PCR (see Molecular Methods of Diagnosis) or histopathology is suggested.

Diagnosis by histopathology is most applicable to necropsy samples, although histology can also be used for clinical samples and in retrospective surveys for Bd in preserved

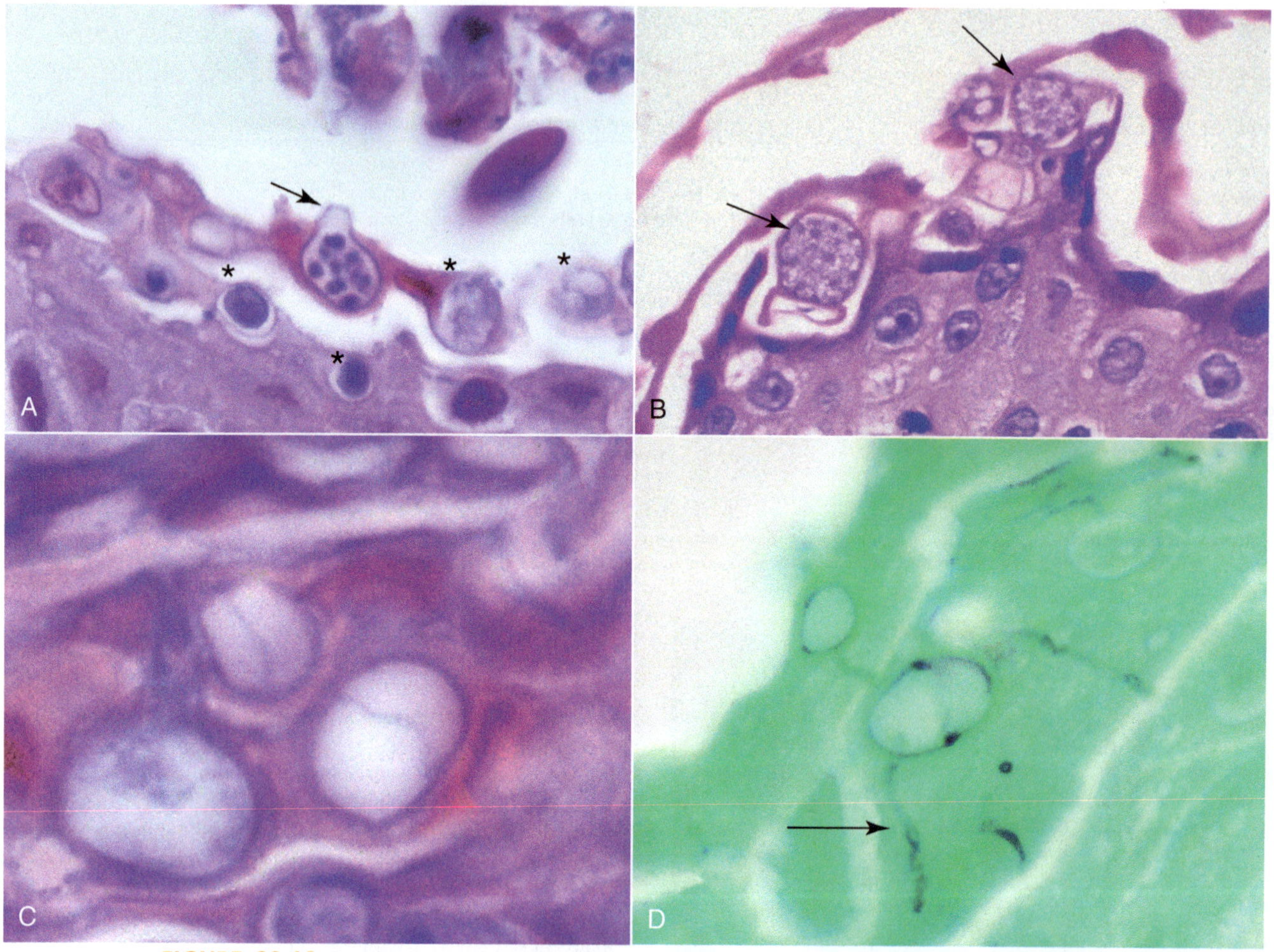

FIGURE 22-10 Detailed morphologic features of *Batrachochytrium dendrobatidis* thalli useful for histopathologic diagnosis. **A,** Mature zoosporangium with discrete basophilic zoospores and a discharge tube *(arrow)*. There are also several uninucleate developing thalli *(asterisk; ×60)*. **B,** Developing multinucleated thalli *(arrows; ×60)*. **C,** Three "empty" thalli that have previously discharged their zoospores. The thalli in the center are "colonial" thalli as indicated by fine internal septation that appears to divide the thallus in half (×100). **D,** A Grocott-Gomori's methenamine silver (GMS)-stained section demonstrating the rhizoids *(arrow),* which are thin rootlike projections from the thallus that are intermittently observed in silver stained histologic sections (×100).

amphibians from museum collections. For a description of the histopathologic lesions associated with chytridiomycosis, see the section on Pathology and Host Defense. Necropsy samples for histopathology should include multiple sections of skin from the ventral body including the pelvic region ("drink patch"), legs, and feet. For small animals (<5 g), submission of the entire carcass for histopathologic examination followed by demineralization and processing of multiple sections (including feet) for histologic examination is adequate. A noninvasive diagnostic method for living animals involves submission of fragments of shed skin in formalin for histopathologic examination. This method can provide better detail of Bd thalli than that obtained by cytologic examination, especially of empty thalli that are common in diagnostic specimens (Figure 22-13).

Occasionally, even animals with severe chytridiomycosis will have few or no detectable Bd thalli on histopathologic examination, and this can result in missed diagnoses (Figure 22-14). Most likely, this relates to recent shedding of heavily infected layers of the stratum corneum.[95,96] As noted earlier, histopathology is not an ideal method for surveying amphibian populations for the presence of Bd infection, and large numbers of skin sections may be required to reach reasonable confidence that subclinical infections have been detected.[90,91,97] Methods to improve the ability to detect Bd in histologic sections include immunohistochemical analysis for Bd and the use of keratin stains to determine the suitability of histologic sections, but these are not required for definitive diagnosis in most cases.[91,95,98]

Molecular Methods of Diagnosis (Polymerase Chain Reaction)

The development of PCR-based tests for the detection of Bd DNA has been an important addition to the diagnostic tools available for diagnosis of infection and for management of amphibian collections. Both conventional and real-time

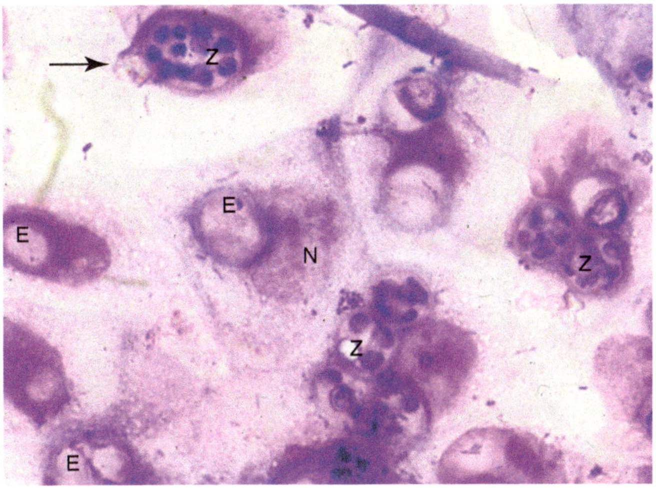

FIGURE 22-11 A sheet of shed skin from a Green And Black Poison Dart Frog with experimentally induced chytridiomycosis. The skin was flattened on a microscope slide, air-dried, and stained for cytology. There are numerous spherical intracellular thalli of *Batrachochytrium dendrobatidis*. Many thalli (zoosporangia) have discrete zoospores *(Z)* while others are empty, having previously expelled zoospores *(E)*. One zoosporangium has an identifiable discharge tube *(arrow; ×100).(Photomicrograph reprinted with permission from Pessier AP. Cytologic diagnosis of disease in amphibians.* Vet Clin N Am Exot Anim Pract *2007;10:187-206)*

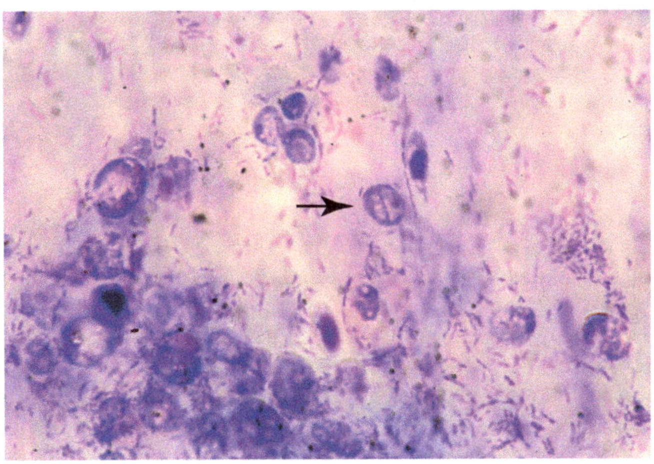

FIGURE 22-12 A skin scraping from a Blue Poison Dart Frog *(Dendrobates azureus)* with naturally acquired chytridiomycosis. There are numerous developing and degenerating thalli of *Batrachochytrium dendrobatidis*. One thallus has evidence of internal septation consistent with a characteristic "colonial thallus" *(arrow; ×100)*.

(Taqman) PCR techniques are described.[33,91,99,100] In the United States, PCR for Bd has been commercially available from Pisces Molecular (www.pisces-molecular.com), Zoologix Laboratories (www.zoologix.com), and, for zoos and aquariums, the Amphibian Disease Laboratory of the San Diego Zoo (www.sandiegozooglobal.org/News/Amphibian_Disease_Laboratory/). PCR is the diagnostic method of choice for quarantine screening of new animals, screening of animals before reintroduction or translocation, surveys of captive and free-ranging populations for the presence and prevalence of Bd infection, and confirmation of positive results from clinical

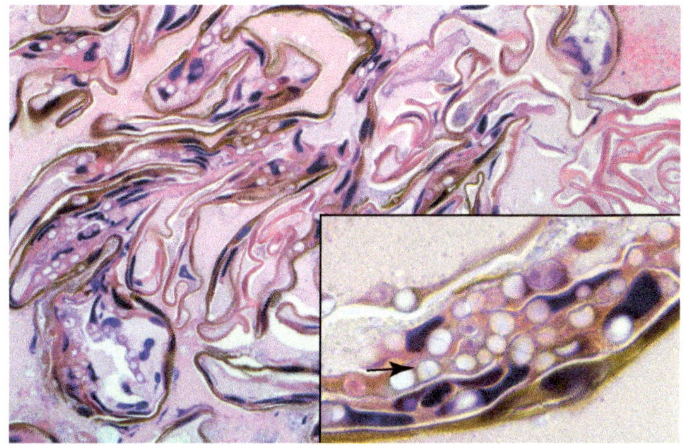

FIGURE 22-13 Shed skin from a plethodontid salamander that has been fixed in formalin and processed for histopathologic examination. There are numerous thalli of *Batrachochytrium dendrobatidis* within skin cells (×20). The *inset (×60)* shows these thalli in greater detail, including many empty thalli that have evidence of internal septation (colonial thalli). Histopathologic examination of shed skin fragments can sometimes be a useful diagnostic procedure for living animals with chytridiomycosis, especially if there is limited access to molecular diagnostic tests such as polymerase chain reaction.

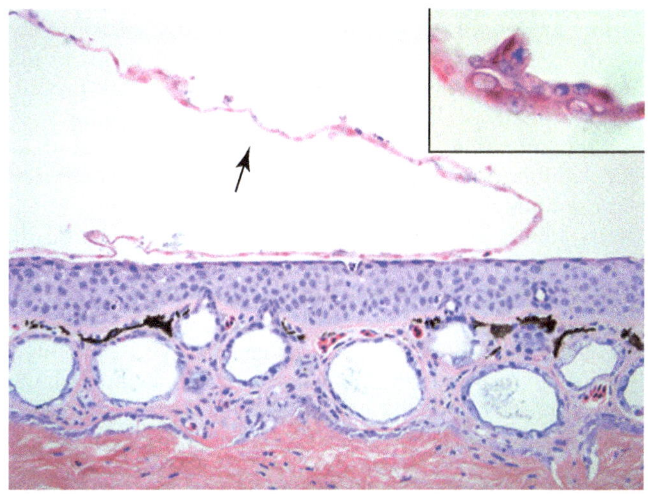

FIGURE 22-14 A histologic section of skin from a Rio Grande Leopard Frog *(Lithobates [Rana] berlandieri)* with chytridiomycosis (×20). In this case, there has been recent shedding of the external keratinized layers of the skin and only low numbers of *Batrachochytrium dendrobatidis* thalli are observed *(inset; ×60)*.

wet mount or cytologic examinations. PCR methods are very sensitive, and the real-time method can experimentally detect as little as a single Bd zoospore.[100] Because of this exquisite sensitivity, a positive PCR result means only that an animal is infected with Bd and does not distinguish between a subclinical infection and a clinically significant infection (chytridiomycosis). This distinction is especially important when amphibian mortality events are investigated, where it should be recognized that positive Bd PCR results alone cannot prove that chytridiomycosis was the cause of an observed die-off.

The real-time (Taqman) PCR technique has significant advantages over the conventional PCR method. These include

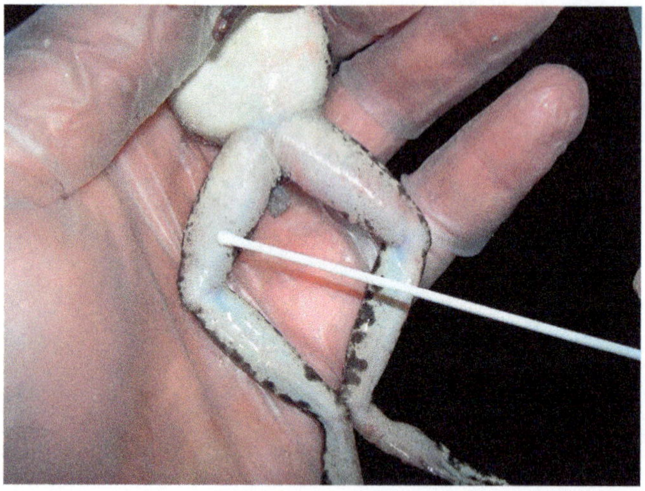

FIGURE 22-15 Collection of a skin swab sample for *Batrachochytrium dendrobatidis* polymerase chain reaction. The swab is applied to multiple areas of the ventral body, legs, and feet. *(Courtesy Jeffery M. Lemm, San Diego Zoo, San Diego, Calif.)*

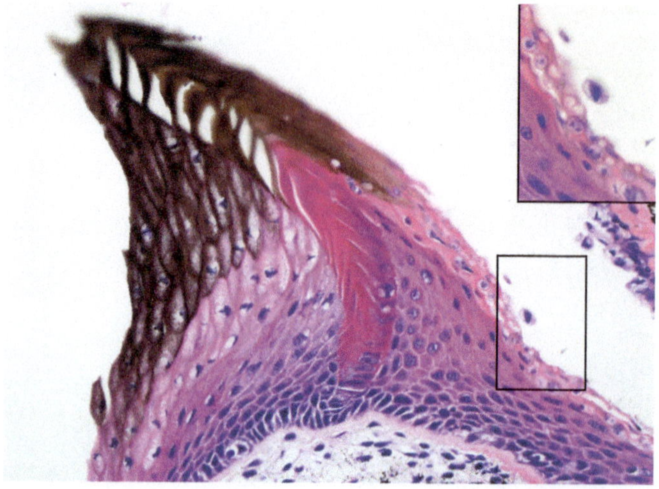

FIGURE 22-16 Infection with *Batrachochytrium dendrobatidis* (Bd) in the jaw sheath of a tadpole (×20). The *inset (×60)* shows detail of the Bd thalli. Note that the pigmented keratinized layers are not yet affected; therefore this tadpole may not show the grossly visible mouthpart depigmentation described for chytridiomycosis.

increased sensitivity (experimental detection of 1 zoospore genome equivalent compared with 10 zoospores with conventional PCR); a reduced potential for cross-contamination during processing (resulting in false-positive tests); use of specific probes for product detection that eliminate the need to confirm positive results by DNA sequencing of PCR products (not routinely performed in many diagnostic laboratories); and incorporation of internal positive controls that detect PCR inhibitors. Detection of PCR inhibitors is important because amphibian skin swab samples submitted for Bd PCR are frequently contaminated with dirt or plant material that are good sources of such inhibitors. Without internal controls for inhibitors, some samples positive for Bd may be reported as negative (false-negative tests). Disadvantages of the real-time PCR method are higher costs and limited availability of specialized real-time PCR equipment when compared with conventional PCR.

In postmetamorphic animals, the preferred samples for both conventional and real-time PCR for Bd are swabs of the ventral skin. Sampling from the dorsal skin is not recommended, as most chytrid thalli (and DNA) will be present on the ventrum. Other samples such as tissue (toe clips) can be used but have lesser sensitivity.[91] For the real-time PCR technique, samples are obtained by rubbing a fine-tipped rayon swab (e.g., Dryswab Fine Tip, MW113, Medical Wire and Equipment Company, www.mwe-usa.com) on the skin of the ventral pelvic region, ventral legs, and feet (including toes) approximately three to five times in each area[89,91] (Figure 22-15). Details of the swabbing technique, including video clips, are available online at http://amphibiaweb.org/chytrid/swab_protocol.html or http://www.amphibianark.org/chytrid.htm. After collection, the swabs are briefly air-dried, and the tip of the swab is broken off into a 1.5-mL microcentrifuge tube. Swabs prepared in this manner have been shown to have stable Bd DNA for 18 months at room temperature (23°C). Storage of swabs in a freezer may be helpful if analyses cannot be performed immediately. For tropical fieldwork with humid and very hot conditions, storage of swabs in 95% ethanol has been suggested (http://amphibiaweb.org/chytrid/swab_protocol.html). Samples for conventional PCR are routinely preserved in 95% ethanol after collection. For both conventional and Taqman PCR, a variety of different swab types have been used successfully; however, the plastic-handled fine rayon-tipped swabs already mentioned have advantages that include reduced consumption of laboratory reagents and elimination of concerns about PCR inhibitors that may be present in wood-handled swabs.

Diagnosis in Tadpoles

Surveillance for the presence of Bd in amphibian populations may use larvae (tadpoles) because of the ease in obtaining samples and meaningful sample numbers. Observation of grossly visible depigmentation of the oral disk has been described as an initial screening method of detecting Bd infection[74,75] but may not be effective in all species or circumstances.[101] Because not all infected tadpoles will show depigmentation and because depigmentation can be associated with other circumstances such as chemical exposure and low environmental temperatures,[54] confirmation of the diagnosis by other means such as histopathology, PCR, or both is required (Figure 22-16 and Figure 22-17). For histopathology, the head of the tadpole (or oral disk dissected from the head) is bisected sagittally through the center of the oral disk, and both halves are processed routinely for histologic examination. When histopathology is used to detect Bd in tadpoles, selection of larger individuals or those at more advanced developmental stages increases the likelihood of finding infected individuals.[74,75] PCR (as already described) using swabs of the oral disk or excised oral disk tissue is an alternative to histopathologic examination, and swabs have the advantage of allowing for nonlethal sampling.[91,101]

Determination of Sample Size for Population Surveys

To determine the temporal, regional, and worldwide distribution of Bd, amphibian biologists are increasingly performing

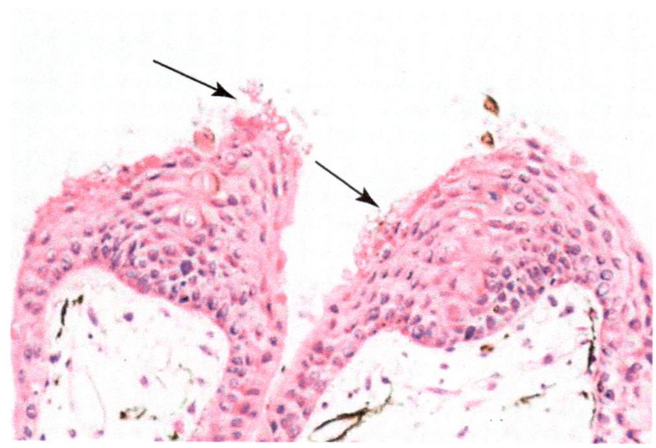

FIGURE 22-17 Infection with *Batrachochytrium dendrobatidis* in the jaw sheath and tooth rows of a tadpole. The pigmented keratinized layers are heavily infected *(arrows)*, and grossly visible depigmentation of the mouthparts was observed. Compare with Figure 22-16 (×20).

surveys of wild amphibian populations and preserved museum samples for evidence of infection. A common question in the design of these surveys is the number of samples required from a region or time period to determine, with a reasonable degree of confidence, whether Bd is present or absent in a population. Methods for calculating the sample sizes required for these kinds of surveys can be found in standard veterinary epidemiology texts.[102] In general, formulas for these calculations require data inputs such as population size and estimates of the minimum prevalence of infection in the population. Prevalence estimates of Bd infection from other amphibian populations that can aid in sample size calculations are increasingly available in the literature. Although greatly simplified approaches to determining sample size for infectious disease surveys[103] can be useful in some circumstances, investigators should be keenly aware that these methods assume a 100% sensitivity and specificity for the chosen diagnostic test. This level of test performance has not been established for available Bd diagnostic methods (especially histology) under field conditions and may significantly affect the conclusions that can be drawn from a survey effort. Additional information on sampling for population surveys can be found in the literature.[104]

TREATMENT

Overview

A variety of chemical and physical methods have been described to treat Bd infection in captive amphibians, and these have recently been reviewed.[89,105] Although a single therapeutic protocol that is effective in eliminating infection in all amphibian species and life stages (especially tadpoles) has not been identified, it is possible to successfully treat and clear Bd infection in many instances.[86] Ongoing experimental trials that identify new treatment methods or that refine and improve existing treatment protocols are in progress. Studies that look at the combination of treatment types (e.g., an antifungal drug combined with elevated temperature) may be especially useful. The type of treatment used may depend on a variety of factors, including cost, availability of specific drugs, the number of animals to be treated, and the anticipated tolerance of more sensitive species to treatments such as elevated environmental temperature. In addition, there may be significant species or life stage differences in the ability to tolerate some drugs. In groups of valuable animals for which there is no experience with a specific medication, it is advisable to first treat a small subset of individuals to evaluate safety before treating the group as a whole.

As noted earlier, frogs with chytridiomycosis can have significant electrolyte imbalances; therefore, in addition to antifungal treatment, affected animals may benefit from fluid and electrolyte therapy. Approaches to amphibian fluid therapy have been reviewed elsewhere.[106] For mildly to moderately affected animals, electrolyte baths, such as amphibian Ringer's solution applied continuously for aquatic species or supplied as a water source for terrestrial species, may be adequate. For depressed or moribund animals, intracoelomic administration of balanced (nonlactated) electrolyte solutions diluted 1:1 or 2:1 with 5% dextrose may be necessary. Because secondary bacterial infections are common, a broad-spectrum antibiotic is also useful in the supportive care of animals with chytridiomycosis.

In most cases, treatments are applied topically because of the superficial location of Bd infection on the skin. For bath treatments, it is important to periodically agitate the treatment solution to ensure contact of the medication with the entirety of the animal's skin. Equally important after each topical treatment, animals should be transferred to a clean enclosure to eliminate the possibility of reinfection from environmental contamination. Many treatment failures can be attributed to one or both of these common mistakes.

Because treatment protocols for Bd infection are not uniformly effective, the use of posttreatment PCR testing to evaluate animals for treatment failure is suggested. Testing should begin at least 2 weeks after the end of treatment, and 2 to 3 posttreatment PCR tests may be required .[89] If positive PCR reactions are obtained after an initial course of treatment, a second round of treatment with the same or different drug or method (e.g., heat) is necessary to ensure clearance of Bd infection.

Itraconazole and Other Azole-type Antifungals

Antifungal drugs in the azole family are commonly used in veterinary medicine, are relatively safe, and act by inhibiting the synthesis of ergosterol, a major component of fungal cell membranes.[107] The most common azole used in amphibian conservation programs is itraconazole supplied as a 1% (10 mg/mL) oral solution for human use (Sporanox Oral Solution, Ortho Biotech, Raritan, NJ). Itraconazole has a theoretical advantage over other azoles for treating Bd infections because in mammals it becomes concentrated and persists in keratinizing tissues such as the skin for weeks after treatment cessation. Although some azole-type drugs may decrease synthesis of steroid hormones such as testosterone or corticosteroids, these effects are minimal in mammals treated with itraconazole. Possible effects on amphibian steroid synthesis have not been reported.

For treatment, a protocol diluting the 1% itraconazole oral solution in amphibian Ringer's solution (25 g NaCl, 0.57 g KCl, 0.57 g $CaCl_2$, and 0.76 g $NaHCO_3$ in 1 gallon of water)

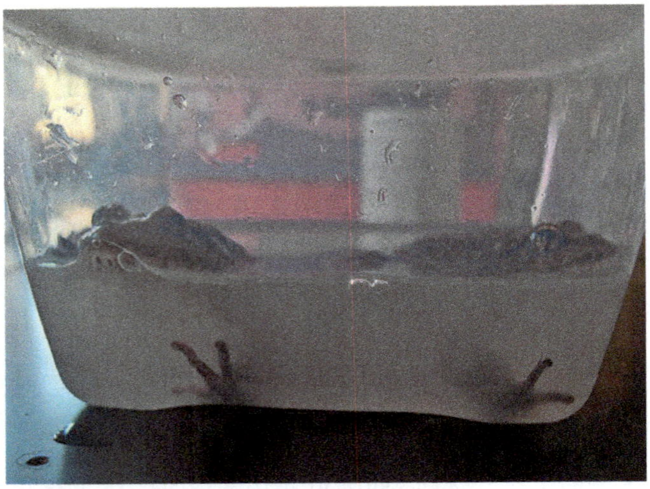

FIGURE 22-18 Mountain Yellow-legged Frogs *(Rana muscosa)* receiving a bath treatment of 0.01% itraconazole for chytridiomycosis. The bath should be periodically agitated to ensure that all skin surfaces are exposed to the medication. *(Courtesy Jeffery M. Lemm, San Diego Zoo, San Diego, Calif).*

or 0.6% saline to a concentration of 0.01% (100 mg/L) has been commonly used in zoos and amphibian conservation programs.[52,108-110] Although well-tolerated by many species, there have been anecdotal reports of treatment-associated side effects and death, and the use of lower itraconazole concentrations (50 mg/L or less) has recently been advocated.[89,111,112] Animals are soaked in a shallow bath for 5 minutes daily for a total of 10 to 11 days (Figure 22-18). The 0.01% itraconazole bath should absolutely be avoided for treatment of tadpoles or very small postmetamorphic animals as deaths have been observed in both Australia and the United States. Deaths in these cases may have been due to the low pH of itraconazole solutions (necessary for solubility) or to components of the itraconazole formulation. A preliminary report described successful treatment of Majorcan Midwife Toad *(Alytes muletensis)* tadpoles with low doses of itraconazole (0.5 mg/L) compared with the 0.01% solution (100 mg/L) that has been associated with tadpole deaths.[113] It is unknown whether this significantly lower itraconazole dose is effective for treating postmetamorphic animals, but if broadly applicable, it would be advantageous in terms of treatment cost and reduced potential for treatment-associated side effects.

The use of other azole antifungal drugs has been described with varying success. Miconazole nitrate administered as a 0.01% bath made from the commercially available 1% lotion marketed for companion animals (Conofite Lotion, Schering-Plough Animal Health, Kenilworth, NJ) was effective in clearing Bd infection in dendrobatid frogs but was less well tolerated when compared with itraconazole.[108] Effectiveness and safety of miconazole for tadpoles was not examined in that study. The use of fluconazole (formulation unspecified) at 6.6 mg/L for 6 hours a day for 7 days was apparently safe and moderately reduced the prevalence of—but did not eliminate—Bd infection in Great Barred Frog *(Mixophyes fasciolatus)* tadpoles.[114] Recently, successful treatment of experimentally infected Iberian Midwife Toads *(Alytes cisternasii)* has been reported with once-daily sprays of a 1.25 μg/mL solution of voriconazole in water.[115]

Malachite Green and Formalin

Malachite green is a textile dye that has been used extensively as an antiprotozoal and antifungal medication for fish. A combination of 0.1 mg/L malachite green and 25 parts per million (ppm) formalin administered as a bath for 24 hours every other day for a total of four treatments was effective at treating Western Clawed Frogs *(Xenopus tropicalis)* with Bd infection.[116] Although this treatment protocol could be considered for use in other species, both malachite green and formalin are known to be potentially either teratogenic and/or carcinogenic and are associated with human health concerns.[86,117, 118] Furthermore, not all species will tolerate malachite green or formalin, and treatment should be approached with caution.[106,118]

Benzalkonium Chloride

Benzalkonium chloride (benzalkonium chloride 50% concentrate, National Fish Pharmacy, Tucson, Ariz) is a quaternary ammonium disinfectant occasionally used as an antifungal medication for fish and amphibians. A bath of 2 mg/L benzalkonium chloride applied for 30 minutes on alternate days for a total of three treatments with the cycle repeated once after an 8-day treatment-free interval was used in Western Dwarf Clawed Frogs *(Hymenochirus curtipes)* diagnosed with *Basidiobolus ranarum* infection (subsequently determined to be Bd infection).[9] This treatment reduced the overall number of deaths in affected animals; however, organisms consistent with Bd were still observed on histopathologic examination, suggesting a fungistatic rather than fungicidal effect. Benzalkonium at 1 mg/L reduced the prevalence but did not eliminate Bd infection in Great Barred Frog tadpoles.[114]

Chloramphenicol

The antibiotic chloramphenicol has paradoxically been shown to have both in vitro and in vivo activity against Bd.[119] Initial trials using a continuous bath of 20 ppm (20 mg/L) chloramphenicol (chloramphenicol C0378; Sigma-Adrich, St. Louis, Mo) for 2 to 4 weeks showed its apparent safety and effectiveness in eliminating Bd infection in Southern Bell Frogs *(Litoria raniformis)* and Brown Tree Frogs *(Litoria ewingii)*. A recent experimental study demonstrated efficacy of chloramphenicol when combined with electrolyte supplementation in White's Tree Frogs *(Litoria caerulea)*.[120] If, with additional studies, chloramphenicol can be shown to be safe and active against Bd in a wide variety of amphibians, it would be a useful and cost-effective drug for management of infection in captive animals. Chloramphenicol is associated with bone marrow suppression in cats and is rarely associated with aplastic anemia in susceptible humans.[121] The latter is an occupational safety concern, and individuals treating amphibians with chloramphenicol should use precautions to avoid contact with the bath solution. Chloramphenicol derivatives such as florfenicol have fewer human health concerns and need to be evaluated for activity against Bd and safety in amphibian patients.

Terbinafine

The antifungal drug terbinafine hydrochloride has shown recent success in clearing Bd infection in 5 of 13 amphibian species examined in an experimental trial.[122] Treatments used a 1% ethanol-based formulation sold over-the-counter for treatment of athlete's foot in humans (Lamisil AT, Novartis Pharmaceuticals, Basel, Switzerland). Solutions were diluted to 0.01% and 0.005% with distilled water and applied as a 5 minute bath for 5 consecutive days or six treatments spread over 10 days.

Elevated Environmental Temperature

The use of elevated environmental temperature to eliminate Bd infection exploits the preference of Bd for lower temperatures (maximal growth at 17°C to 25°C).[38] In a pilot study, juvenile Red-eyed Tree Frogs (*Litoria chloris*) experimentally infected with Bd and held for 16 hours at 37°C were cleared of infection while most animals held at 20°C died of chytridiomycosis.[67] Not all species will tolerate temperatures this high; however, there is some evidence that prolonged exposure to lower temperatures that are still above the maximal growth range for Bd may also aid in clearing of infection. For instance, great barred frogs inoculated with Bd and housed at 27°C had no evidence of infection by 98 days postinoculation.[123] A more recent article described successful treatment of American Bullfrogs and Northern Cricket Frogs (*Acris crepitans*) at 30°C for 10 days.[124] When temperature is considered as a treatment method for Bd, it is important to maintain animals at a constant rather than intermittent temperature elevation. As with other treatment methods, temperature elevation has been inconsistently effective between species.[86]

TREATMENT OF LARGE GROUPS AND DEVELOPMENT OF Bd-FREE AMPHIBIAN COLLECTIONS

Treatment of entire groups of amphibians for Bd infection has become more common as infected animals are brought into captivity for use in "survival assurance colonies" or captive breeding programs for endangered species. In other instances, group treatment is initiated because of repeated outbreaks of chytridiomycosis in closed colonies (suggesting the presence of subclinical carrier animals) or in attempts to create colonies of Bd-free amphibians for zoologic collections or for the pet and laboratory animal industry. For creation of Bd-free colonies, all individuals are assumed infected and are treated with an antifungal protocol and disinfection of enclosures as previously described. Treatment is followed by PCR testing of all animals or a representative sample of animals in the colony. If infected animals are identified by PCR, the treatment and testing cycle is repeated until negative results are obtained. Once the colony is PCR negative, long-term surveillance with the use of necropsy and histopathologic examination of all animals that die, as well as periodic PCR testing, is initiated. For captive breeding programs that intend to release animals to the wild, a surveillance period of 1 year with negative necropsy and PCR results is suggested. In addition to ongoing surveillance, a quarantine program should be in place for animals coming into Bd-free collections that includes PCR screening of new animals and necropsy of all animals that die. If infected animals are identified in quarantine, a treat, test, and surveillance program should be initiated before introduction of the new animals to the Bd-free colony.

REFERENCES

1. Berger L, Speare R, Dazsak P, et al. Chytridiomycosis causes amphibian mortality associated with population declines in the rain forests of Australia and Central America. *Proc Natl Acad Sci U S A* 1998;95:9031-9036.
2. Pessier AP, Nichols DK, Longcore JE, et al. Cutaneous chytridiomycosis in poison dart frogs (*Dendrobates* spp.) and White's tree frogs (*Litoria caerulea*). *J Vet Diagn Invest* 1999;11:194-199.
3. Longcore JE, Pessier AP, Nichols DK. *Batrachochytrium dendrobatidis* gen. et sp. nov., a chytrid pathogenic to amphibians. *Mycologia* 1999;91:219-227.
4. Skerratt LF, Berger L, Speare R, et al. Spread of chytridiomycosis has caused the rapid global decline and extinction of frogs. *EcoHealth* 2007;4:125-134.
5. Fisher MC, Garner TWJ, Walker SF. Global emergence of *Batrachochytrium dendrobatidis* and amphibian chytridiomycosis in space, time and host. *Annu Rev Microbiol* 2009;63:291-310.
6. Barr DJS. Phylum Chytridiomycota. In: Margulis L, Corliss JO, Melkonian M, et al, eds. *Handbook of protoctista*. Boston: Jones and Bartlett, 1990;454-466.
7. Powell MJ. Looking at mycology with a Janus face: a glimpse at Chytridiomycetes active in the environment. *Mycologia* 1993;85:1-20.
8. Nichols DK, Lamirande EW, Pessier AP, et al. Experimental transmission of cutaneous chytridiomycosis in dendrobatid frogs. *J Wildl Dis* 2001;37:1-11.
9. Groff JM, Mughannam A, McDowell TS, et al. An epizootic of cutaneous zygomycosis in cultured dwarf African clawed frogs (*Hymenochirus curtipes*) due to *Basidiobolus ranarum*. *J Med Vet Mycol* 1991;29:215-223.
10. Nichols DK, Smith AJ, Gardiner CH. Dermatitis of anurans caused by fungal-like protists, in *Proceedings*. Am Assoc Zoo Vet, 1996;220-221.
11. Taylor SK, Williams ES, Mills KW. Causes of mortality of the Wyoming toad. *J Wildl Dis* 1999;35:49-57.
12. Pessier AP. An overview of amphibian skin disease. *Semin Avian Exot Pet Med* 2002;11:162-174.
13. Stuart SN, Chanson JS, Cox NA, et al. Status and trends of amphibian declines and extinctions worldwide. *Science* 2004;306:1783-1786.
14. Muths E, Corn PS, Pessier AP, et al. Evidence for disease-related amphibian decline in Colorado. *Biol Conserv* 2003;110:357-365.
15. Daszak P, Berger L, Cunningham AA, et al. Emerging infectious diseases and amphibian population declines. *Emerg Infect Dis* 1999;5:735-748.
16. Rachowicz LJ, Hero J, Alford RA, et al. The novel and endemic pathogen hypotheses: competing explanations for the origin of emerging infectious diseases of wildlife. *Conserv Biol* 2005;19:1441-1448.
17. Bosch J, Martinez-Solano I, Garcia-Paris M. Evidence of a chytrid fungus infection involved in the decline of the common midwife toad (*Alytes obstetricans*) in protected areas of central Spain. *Biol Conserv* 2001;97:331-337.
18. Waldman B, Van de Wolfshaar KE, Klena JD, et al. Chytridiomycosis in New Zealand frogs. *Surveillance* 2001;28:9-11.
19. Bradley GA, Rosen PC, Sredl MJ, et al. Chytridiomycosis in native Arizona frogs. *J Wildl Dis* 2002;38:206-212.
20. Hanselmann R, Rodriguez A, Lampo M, et al. Presence of an emerging pathogen of amphibians in introduced bullfrogs (*Rana catesbeiana*) in Venezuela. *Biol Conserv* 2004;120:115-119.
21. Weldon C, du Preez LH, Hyatt AD, et al. Origin of the amphibian chytrid fungus. *Emerg Infect Dis* 2004;10:2100-2105.
22. Garner TWJ, Perkins M, Govindarajulu P, et al. The emerging amphibian pathogen *Batrachochytrium dendrobatidis* globally infects introduced populations of the North American bullfrog (*Rana catesbeiana*). *Biol Lett* 2006;2:455-459.
23. Lips KR, Brem F, Brenes R, et al. Emerging infectious disease and the loss of biodiversity in a Neotropical amphibian community. *Proc Natl Acad Sci U S A* 2006;103:3165-3170.

24. Oliveira de Queiroz Carnaval AC, Puschendorf R, Peixoto OL, et al. Amphibian chytrid fungus broadly distributed in the Brazilian Atlantic rain forest. *EcoHealth* 2006;3:41-48.
25. Rachowicz LJ, Knapp RA, Morgan JA, et al. Emerging infectious disease as a proximate cause of amphibian mass mortality. *Ecology* 2006;87:1671-1683.
26. Diaz LM, Cadiz A, Chong A, et al. First report of chytridiomycosis in a dying toad (Anura: Bufonidae) from Cuba: a new conservation challenge for the island. *EcoHealth* 2007;4:172-175.
27. Seimon TA, Seimon A, Daszak P, et al. Upward range extension of Andean anurans and chytridiomycosis to extreme elevations in response to tropical deglaciation. *Global Change Biol* 2007;13:288-299.
28. Lips KR, Reeve JD, Witters LR. Ecological traits predicting amphibian population declines in Central America. *Conserv Biol* 2003;17:1078-1088.
29. Woodhams DC, Alford RA. Ecology of chytridiomycosis in rainforest stream frog assemblages of tropical Queensland. *Conserv Biol* 2005;19:1449-1459.
30. McCallum H. Inconclusiveness of chytridiomycosis as the agent in widespread frog declines. *Conserv Biol* 2005;19:1421-1430.
31. Morehouse EA, James TY, Ganley ARD, et al. Multilocus sequence typing suggests the chytrid pathogen of amphibians is a recently emerged clone. *Mol Ecol* 2003;12:395-403.
32. Morgan JAT, Vrendenberg VT, Rachowicz LJ, et al. Population genetics of the frog-killing fungus *Batrachochytrium dendrobatidis*. *Proc Natl Acad Sci U S A* 2007;104:13845-13850.
33. Goka K, Yokoyama J, Une Y, et al. Amphibian chytridiomycosis in Japan: distribution, haplotypes, and possible route of entry into Japan. *Mol Ecol* 2009;18:4757-4774.
34. Farrer RA, Weinert LA, Bielby J, et al. Multiple emergences of genetically diverse amphibian infecting chytrids include a globalized hypervirulent recombinant lineage. *Proc Natl Acad Sci U S A* 2011;108:18732-18736.
35. Daszak P, Strieby A, Cunningham AA, et al. Experimental evidence that the bullfrog *(Rana catesbeiana)* is a potential carrier of chytridiomycosis, an emerging fungal disease of amphibians. *Herpetol J* 2004;14:201-207.
36. Fisher M, Garner TWJ. The relationship between the emergence of *Batrachochytrium dendrobatidis*, the international trade in amphibians and introduced amphibian species. *Fung Biol Rev* 2007;21:2-9.
37. Schloegel LM, Daszak P, Cunningham AA, et al. Two amphibian diseases, chytridiomycosis and ranaviral disease, are now globally notifiable to the World Organization for Animal Health (OIE): An assessment. *Dis Aquat Org* 2010; 92: 101-108.
38. Piotrowski JS, Annis SL, Longcore JE. Physiology of *Batrachochytrium dendrobatidis*, a chytrid pathogen of amphibians. *Mycologia* 2004;96:9-15.
39. Kriger KM, Hero JM. Large-scale seasonal variation in the prevalence and severity of chytridiomycosis. *J Zool* 2007;271:352-359.
40. Schlaepfer MA, Sredl MJ, Rosen PC, et al. High prevalence of *Batrachochytrium dendrobatidis* in wild populations of lowland leopard frogs *Rana yavapaiensis* in Arizona. *EcoHealth* 2007;4:421-427.
41. Ron SR. Predicting the distribution of the amphibian pathogen *Batrachochytrium dendrobatidis* in the new world. *Biotropica* 2005;37:209-221.
42. Pounds JA, Bustamante MR, Coloma LA, et al. Widespread amphibian from epidemic disease driven by global warming. *Nature* 2006; 439:161-167.
43. Alford RA, Bradford KS, Richards SJ. Ecology: global warming and amphibian losses. *Nature* 2007;447:E3-E4.
44. Bosch J, Carrascal LM, Duran L, et al. Climate change and outbreaks of amphibian chytridiomycosis in a montane area of central Spain; is there a link? *Proc R Soc B* 2007;274:253-260.
45. Lips KR, Diffendorfer J, Mendelson JR, et al. Riding the wave: reconciling the roles of disease and climate change in amphibian declines. *PloS Biol* 2008;6:e72.
46. Retallick RWR, McCallum H, Speare R. Endemic infection of the amphibian chytrid fungus in a frog community post-decline. *PloS Biol* 2004;2:1965-1971.
47. Woodhams DC, Ardipradja K, Alford R, et al. Resistance to chytridiomycosis varies among amphibian species and is correlated with skin peptide defenses. *Anim Conserv* 2007;10:409-417.
48. Ouellet M, Mikaelian I, Pauli BD, et al. Historical evidence of widespread chytrid infection in North American amphibian populations. *Conserv Biol* 2005;19:1431-1440.
49. Longcore JR, Longcore JE, Pessier AP, et al. Chytridiomycosis widespread in anurans of northeastern United States. *J Wildl Manag* 2007;71:435-444.
50. Mendelson JR, Lips KR, Gagliardo RW, et al. Confronting amphibian declines and extinctions. *Science* 2006;313:48.
51. Savage AE, Zamudio KR. MHC genotypes associate with resistance to a frog-killing fungus. *Proc Natl Acad Sci U S A* 2011;108:16705-16710.
52. Lamirande EW, Nichols DK. Effects of host age on susceptibility to chytridiomycosis in blue-and-yellow poison dart frogs *(Dendrobates tinctorius)*, in *Proceedings*. 6th Int Symp Pathol Amphibians Reptiles, St. Paul, Minn 2002;3-16.
53. Marantelli G, Berger L, Speare R, et al. Distribution of the amphibian chytrid *Batrachochytrium dendrobatidis* and keratin during tadpole development. *Pacif Conserv Biol* 2004;10:173-179.
54. Rachowicz LJ, Vrendenberg VT. Transmission of *Batrachochytrium dendrobatidis* within and between amphibian life stages. *Dis Aquat Organ* 2004;61:75-83.
55. Voyles J, Berger L, Young S, et al. Electrolyte depletion and osmotic imbalance in amphibians with chytridiomycosis. *Dis Aquat Organ* 2007;77:113-118.
56. Voyles J, Young S, Berger L, et al. Pathogenesis of chytridiomycosis, a cause of catastrophic amphibian declines. *Science* 2009;326:582-585.
57. Green DE, Muths E. Health evaluation of amphibians in and near Rocky Mountain National Park (Colorado, USA). *Alytes* 2005;22:109-129.
58. Blaustein AR, Romansic JM, Scheessele EA, et al. Interspecific variation in susceptibility of frog tadpoles to the pathogenic fungus *Batrachochytrium dendrobatidis*. *Conserv Biol* 2005;19:1460-1468.
59. Davidson EW, Parris M, Collins JP, et al. Pathogenicity and transmission of chytridiomycosis in tiger salamanders *(Ambystoma tigrinum)*. *Copeia* 2003;2003:601-607.
60. Ramsey JP, Reinert LK, Harper LK, et al. Immune defenses against *Batrachochytrium dendrobatidis*, a fungus linked to global amphibian declines in the South African clawed frog, *Xenopus laevis*. *Infect Immun* 2010;78:3981-3992.
61. Rollins-Smith LA, Reinert LK, O'Leary CJ, et al. Antimicrobial peptide defenses in amphibian skin. *Integr Comp Biol* 2005;45:137-142.
62. Woodhams DC, Voyles J, Lips K, et al. Predicted disease susceptibility in a Panamanian amphibian assemblage based on skin peptide defenses. *J Wildl Dis* 2006;42:207-218.
63. Becker MH, Brucker RM, Schwantes CR, et al. The bacterially produced metabolite violacein is associated with the survival of amphibians infected with a lethal fungus. *Appl Environ Microbiol* 2009;75:6635-6638.
64. Harris RN, Brucker RM, Walke JB, et al. Skin microbes on frogs prevent morbidity and mortality caused by a lethal skin fungus. *ISME J* 2009;3:818-824.
65. Rowley JJ, Alford R. Behaviour of Australian rainforest stream frogs may affect the transmission of chytridiomycosis. *Dis Aquat Organ* 2007;77:1-9.
66. Carey C, Bruzgul JE, Livo LJ, et al. Experimental exposures of boreal toads *(Bufo boreas)* to a pathogenic chytrid fungus *(Batrachochytrium dendrobatidis)*. *EcoHealth* 2006;3:5-21.
67. Woodhams DC, Alford RA, Marantelli G. Emerging disease of amphibians cured by elevated body temperature. *Dis Aquat Organ* 2003;55:65-67.
68. Richards-Zawacki C. Thermoregulatory behavior affects prevalence of chytrid fungal infection in a wild population of Panamanian Golden Frogs. *Proc Biol Sci* 2010;277:519-528.

69. Berger L, Marantelli G, Skerratt LF, et al. Virulence of the amphibian chytrid fungus *Batrachochytrium dendrobatidis* varies with the strain. *Dis Aquat Organ* 2005;68:47-50.
70. Retallick RWR, Miera V. Strain differences in the amphibian chytrid *Batrachochytrium dendrobatidis* and non-permanent, sub-lethal effects of infection. *Dis Aquat Organ* 2007;75:201-207.
71. Cummer MR, Green DE, O'Neill EM. Aquatic chytrid pathogen detected in terrestrial plethodontid salamander. *Herpetol Rev* 2005;36:248-249.
72. Pasmans F, Zwart P, Hyatt AD. Chytridiomycosis in the Central American bolitoglossine salamander *(Bolitoglossa dofleini)*. *Vet Rec* 2004;154:153.
73. Fellers GM, Green DE, Longcore JE. Oral chytridiomycosis in the mountain yellow-legged frog *(Rana muscosa)*. *Copeia* 2001;2001:945-953.
74. Knapp RA, Morgan JAT. Tadpole mouthpart depigmentation as an accurate indicator of chytridiomycosis, an emerging disease of amphibians. *Copeia* 2006;2006:188-197.
75. Symonds EP, Hines HB, Bird PS, et al. Surveillance for *Batrachochytrium dendrobatidis* using *Mixophyes* (Anura: Myobatrachidae) larvae. *J Wildl Dis* 2007;43:48-60.
76. Parris MJ, Baud DR. Interactive effects of a heavy metal and chytridiomycosis on gray treefrog larvae *(Hyla chrysoscelis)*. *Copeia* 2004;2004:344-350.
77. Parris MJ, Cornelius TO. Fungal pathogen causes competitive and developmental stress in larval amphibian communities. *Ecology* 2004;85:3385-3395.
78. Smith KG, Weldon C, Conradie W, et al. Relationships among size, development, and *Batrachochytrium dendrobatidis* infection in African tadpoles. *Dis Aquat Organ* 2007;74:159-164.
79. Green DE, Converse KA, Schrader AK. Epizootiology of sixty-four amphibian mortality events in the USA, 1996-2001. *Ann N Y Acad Sci* 2002;969:323-339.
80. Johnson ML, Speare R. Possible modes of dissemination of the amphibian chytrid *Batrachochytrium dendrobatidis* in the environment. *Dis Aquat Organ* 2005;65:181-186.
81. Johnson ML, Speare R. Survival of *Batrachochytrium dendrobatidis* in water: quarantine and disease control implications. *Emerg Infect Dis* 2003;9:922-925.
82. Rowley JJL, Hemingway VA, Alford RA, et al. Experimental infection and repeat survey data indicate the amphibian chytrid *Batrachochytrium dendrobatidis* may not occur on freshwater crustaceans in Northern Queensland, Australia. *EcoHealth* 2007;4:31-36.
83. Kirshtein JD, Anderson CW, Wood J, et al. Quantitative PCR detection of *Batrachochytrium dendrobatidis* DNA from sediments and water. *Dis Aquat Organ* 2007;77:11-15.
84. Walker SF, Baldi Salas M, Jenkins D, et al. Environmental detection of *Batrachochytrium dendrobatidis* in a temperate climate. *Dis Aquat Organ* 2007;77:105-112.
85. Mitchell KM, Churcher TS, Garner TWJ, et al. Persistence of the emerging pathogen *Batrachochytrium dendrobatidis* outside the amphibian host greatly increases the probability of host extinction. *Proc R Soc B* 2007;275:329-334.
86. Young S, Berger L, Speare R. Amphibian chytridiomycosis: strategies for captive management and conservation. *Int Zoo Yearbook* 2007;41:1-11.
87. Johnson ML, Berger L, Phillips L, et al. Fungicidal effects of chemical disinfectants, UV light, desiccation and heat on the amphibian chytrid *Batrachochytrium dendrobatidis*. *Dis Aquat Organ* 2003;57:255-260.
88. Webb R, Mendez D, Berger L, et al. Additional disinfectants effective against the amphibian chytrid fungus *Batrachochytrium dendrobatidis*. *Dis Aquat Organ* 2007;74:13-16.
89. Pessier AP, Mendelson JR, eds. *A manual for control of infectious diseases in amphibian survival assurance colonies and reintroduction programs*. Apple Valley, Minn: IUCN/SSC Conservation Breeding Specialist Group, 2010.
90. Kriger KM, Hines HB, Hyatt AD, et al. Techniques for detecting chytridiomycosis in wild frogs: comparing histology with real-time Taqman PCR. *Dis Aquat Organ* 2006;71:141-148.
91. Hyatt AD, Boyle DG, Olsen V, et al. Diagnostic assays and sampling protocols for the detection of *Batrachochytrium dendrobatidis*. *Dis Aquat Organ* 2007;73:175-192.
92. Berger L, Hyatt AD, Speare R, et al. Life cycle stages of the amphibian chytrid *Batrachochytrium dendrobatidis*. *Dis Aquat Organ* 2005;68:51-63.
93. Briggs C, Burgin S. Congo red, an effective stain for revealing the chytrid fungus, *Batrachochytrium dendrobatidis*, in epidermal skin scrapings from frogs. *Mycologist* 2004;18:98-103.
94. Pessier AP. Cytologic diagnosis of disease in amphibians. *Vet Clin N Am Exot Anim Pract* 2007;10:187-206.
95. Olsen V, Hyatt AD, Boyle DG, et al. Co-localisation of *Batrachochytrium dendrobatidis* and keratin for enhanced diagnosis of chytridiomycosis in frogs. *Dis Aquat Organ* 2004;61:85-88.
96. Berger L, Speare R, Skerratt LF. Distribution of *Batrachochytrium dendrobatidis* and pathology in the skin of green tree frogs *Litoria caerulea* with severe chytridiomycosis. *Dis Aquat Organ* 2005;68:65-70.
97. Puschendorf R, Bolaños F. Detection of *Batrachochytrium dendrobatidis* in *Eleutherodactylus fitzingeri*: effects of skin sample location and histologic stain. *J Wildl Dis* 2006;42:301-306.
98. Van Ells T, Stanton J, Strieby A, et al. Use of immunohistochemistry to diagnose chytridiomycosis in dyeing poison dart frogs *(Dendrobates tinctorius)*. *J Wildl Dis* 2003;39:742-745.
99. Annis SL, Dastoor FP, Ziel H, et al. A DNA-based assay identifies *Batrachochytrium dendrobatidis* in amphibians. *J Wildl Dis* 2004;40:420-428.
100. Boyle DG, Boyle DB, Olsen V, et al. Rapid quantitative detection of chytridiomycosis *(Batrachochytrium dendrobatidis)* in amphibian samples using real-time Taqman PCR assay. *Dis Aquat Organ* 2004;60:141-148.
101. Padgett-Flohr GE, Goble ME. Evaluation of tadpole mouthpart depigmentation as a diagnostic test for infection by *Batrachochytrium dendrobatidis* for four California anurans. *J Wildl Dis* 2007;43:690-699.
102. Thrusfield M. Surveys. In: *Veterinary epidemiology*. 3rd ed. Ames, IA: Blackwell Publishing, 2007;228-246.
103. DiGiacomo RF, Koepsell TD. Sampling for detection of infection or disease in animal populations. *J Am Vet Med Assoc* 1986;189:22-23.
104. Skerratt LF, Berger L, Speare R, et al. Survey protocol for detecting chytridiomycosis in all Australian frog populations. *Dis Aquat Organ* 2008;80:85-94.
105. Berger L, Speare R, Pessier AP, et al. Treatment of chytridiomycosis requires urgent clinical trials. *Dis Aquat Organ* 2010;92:165-174.
106. Wright KM, Whitaker BR. Pharmacotherapeutics. In: Wright KM, Whitaker BR, eds. *Amphibian medicine and captive husbandry*. Malabar, Fla: Kreiger Publishing, 2001;309-330.
107. Papich MG, Heit MC, Riviere JE. Antifungal and antiviral drugs. In: Adams HR, ed. *Veterinary pharmacology and therapeutics*. 8th ed. Ames, IA: Iowa State University Press, 2001;918-946.
108. Nichols DK, Lamirande EW, Pessier AP. Experimental transmission and treatment of cutaneous chytridiomycosis in poison dart frogs (*Dendrobates azureus* and *Dendrobates tinctorius*), in *Joint Proceedings*. Am Assoc Zoo Vet and Int Assoc Aquat Anim Med, New Orleans, La, 2000;42-44.
109. Forzan MJ, Gunn H, Scott P. Chytridiomycosis in an aquarium collection of frogs: diagnosis, treatment and control. *J Zoo Wildl Med* 2008;39:406-411.
110. Gagliardo R, Crump P, Griffiths E, et al. The principles of rapid response for amphibian conservation using the programmes in Panama as an example. *Int Zoo Yrbk* 2008;42: 125-135.
111. Jones MEB, Paddock D, Bender L, et al. Treatment of chytridiomycosis with reduced-dose itraconazole. *Dis Aquat Org* 2012; 99:243-249.
112. Brannelly LA, Richards-Zawacki CL, Pessier AP. Clinical trials with itraconazole for chytrid fungal infections in amphibians. *Dis Aquat Org* 2012;101:95-104.

113. Walker S, Garner TWJ, Bosch J, et al. *Batrachochytrium dendrobatidis* infection of the Red List species *Alytes muletensis* in Mallorca; routes of introduction and establishment of an itraconazole-based protocol for treatment, in *Proceedings*. Amphibian Declines and Chytridiomycosis, Translating Science into Urgent Action Conf, Tempe, Ariz, November 5-7, 2007.
114. Marantelli G, Berger L, McInnes K. Investigations into the treatment of *Batrachochytrium* in frogs and tadpoles, in *Proceedings*. Getting the Jump on Amphibian Disease Conf, Cairns, Australia, 2001;27.
115. Martel A, Van Rooij P, Vercauteren G, et al. Developing a safe antifungal treatment protocol to eliminate *Batrachochytrium dendrobatidis* from amphibians. *Med Mycol* 2011;49:143-149.
116. Parker JM, Mikaelian I, Hahn N, et al. Clinical diagnosis and treatment of epidermal chytridiomycosis in African clawed frogs (*Xenopus tropicalis*). *Comp Med* 2002;52:265-268.
117. Srivastava S, Sinha R, Roy D. Toxicological effects of malachite green. *Aquat Toxicol* 2004;66:319-329.
118. Intorre L, Meucci V, Di Bello D, et al. Tolerance of benzalkonium chloride, formalin, malachite green, and potassium permanganate in goldfish and zebrafish. *J Am Vet Med Assoc* 2007;231:590-595.
119. Poulter RTM, Busby JN, Bishop PJ, et al. Chloramphenicol cures chytridiomycosis, in *Proceedings*. Amphibian Declines and Chytridiomycosis, Translating Science into Urgent Action Conf, Tempe, Ariz, November 5-7, 2007.
120. Young S, Speare R, Berger L, et al. Chloramphenicol with fluid and electrolyte therapy cures terminally ill green tree frogs (*Litoria caerulea*) with chytridiomycosis. *J Zoo Wildl Med* 2012;43:330-337.
121. Papich MG, Riviere JE. Chloramphenicol and derivatives, macrolides, lincosamides, and miscellaneous antimicrobials. In: Adams HR, ed. *Veterinary pharmacology and therapeutics*. 8th ed. Ames, IA: Iowa State University Press, 2001;868-897.
122. Bowerman J, Rombough C, Weinstock SR, et al. Terbinafine hydrochloride in ethanol effectively clears *Batrachochytrium dendrobatidis* in amphibians. *J Herpetol Med Surg* 2010;20:24-28.
123. Berger L, Speare R, Hines HB, et al. Effect of season and temperature on mortality in amphibians due to chytridiomycosis. *Aust Vet J* 2004;73:175-192.
124. Chatfield MWH, Richards-Zawacki C. Elevated temperature as a treatment for *Batrachochytrium dendrobatidis* infection in captive frogs. *Dis Aquat Organ* 2011;94:235-238.

CHAPTER 23

Short Tongue Syndrome and Hypovitaminosis A

Allan P. Pessier

Basic knowledge of amphibian nutrition lags behind that of reptiles and even fish. Awareness of worldwide amphibian population declines and extinctions and subsequent development of a variety of conservation-oriented captive propagation programs, as well as increased interest in amphibians for the pet trade, will increase the demand for improved nutritional management. Because the class Amphibia has such rich species diversity, development of a satisfactory "one size fits all" approach to dietary husbandry is unlikely; approaches that include careful observation of species' natural history and experimental studies as have been described for reptiles will be necessary.[1] Unfortunately, in many cases, advances in amphibian nutrition may come about only after the investigation of disease conditions that have features of nutritional disorders described in other taxonomic groups.

This chapter describes newly recognized conditions in captive amphibians that are suspected to be due to vitamin A deficiency. Vitamin A is a fat-soluble vitamin involved in a diverse variety of physiologic functions that include vision, epithelial cell differentiation, innate and adaptive immune response, reproduction, and bone development.[2,3] Dietary sources of vitamin A include active forms from animal tissues (retinol) and provitamin forms (carotenoids) found in plants that are converted to active vitamin A in the intestinal mucosa. Vitamin A deficiencies are recognized in a variety of animal species, including domestic and nondomestic mammals, birds, reptiles, and fish, but had not been previously recognized in amphibians.[2,4-8] , The histologic finding considered to be characteristic of vitamin A deficiency is squamous metaplasia (SM) in which normal mucus-producing epithelium is replaced by a keratinizing stratified squamous epithelium.

SM of the mucous glands of the tongue was observed in association with a condition coined *short tongue syndrome* (STS) in the critically endangered Wyoming Toad (*Anaxyrus [Bufo] baxteri*).[9] SM was clearly evident in affected toads because, unlike the normal keratinizing stratified squamous epithelium typical of the tongue in birds and mammals, the epithelium of the tongue in amphibians is nonkeratinizing, glandular, and mucus-producing, a feature that aids in capturing prey items[10,11] (Figure 23-1). Subsequent investigation demonstrated that captive Wyoming Toads with SM had significantly lower liver retinol (vitamin A) levels when compared with wild Wyoming Toads, and the combined findings were considered to be highly suggestive of vitamin A deficiency. A review of the literature shows a single previous report of lingual SM in a long-term captive Pig Frog (*Rana grylio*) that was interpreted as a precancerous change or "epithelial malignancy" but, in retrospect, possibly represented a lesion associated with vitamin A deficiency.[12]

SM of the tongue and symptoms of STS have also been observed in a variety of other captive anurans including Grey Foam-Nest Tree Frogs (*Chiromantis xerampelina*), Boreal Toads (*Anaxyrus [Bufo] boreas boreas*), Puerto Rican Crested Toads (*Peltophryne lemur*), Woodhouse's Toads (*Anaxyrus [Bufo] woodhousii*), American Toads (*Anaxyrus [Bufo] americanus*), Panamanian Golden Frogs (*Atelopus zeteki*), and Kihansi Spray Toads (*Nectophrynoides asperginis*).[9,13-15] Periocular and conjunctival swellings responsive to vitamin A supplementation have been observed in ranid and dendrobatid frogs, as well as a Tiger Salamander (*Ambystoma tigrinum*).[16-18]

SIGNALMENT AND CLINICAL SIGNS

In the Wyoming Toad, STS occurs in adults of both sexes, and occasionally in juveniles. The condition is acquired, and toads gradually lose the ability to capture prey items, despite vigorous effort. Severely affected animals usually require hand feeding. The term *STS* originated from early observations that repeated unsuccessful attempts to strike at prey items gave the appearance that the tongue was simply too short. Quantitative assessments of tongue length were considered, but attempts were abandoned out of practicality.

Ranid and dendrobatid frogs and a Tiger Salamander with vitamin A–responsive ocular lesions were seen with unilateral to bilateral opaque white conjunctival to periocular swellings centered on the lower eyelids.

Because of the wide range of physiologic functions associated with vitamin A, it is worthwhile considering the possibility of hypovitaminosis A as a contributory factor in any sick captive amphibian maintained on a predominantly insectivorous diet. Potential clinical indicators at both an individual or population level could include bacterial or fungal infections occurring at levels greater than would be expected with good husbandry practices; poor reproductive success, including reduced egg viability and poor tadpole survival; failure to thrive; and hydrocoelom secondary to renal disease because SM of renal tubules has been observed in some animals with STS.

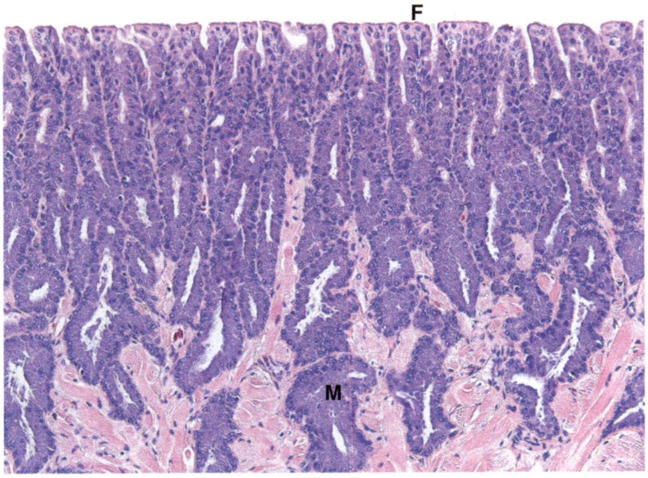

FIGURE 23-1 Histologic section of a normal tongue from a Wyoming Toad *(Anaxyrus [Bufo] baxteri)* (×20). Cells of the mucosal glands *(M)* are packed with a granular purple material (mucus). The dorsal surface has distinct filiform papillae *(F)*.

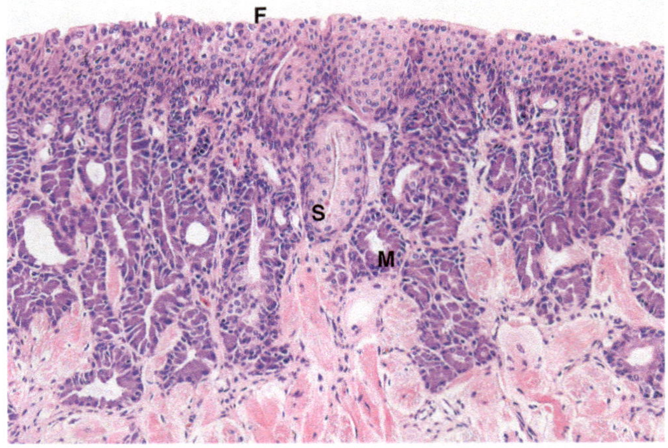

FIGURE 23-2 Histologic section of the tongue from a Wyoming Toad *(Anaxyrus [Bufo] baxteri)* with early squamous metaplasia (×20). Compare with Figure 23-1. Some mucosal glands are lined by large pale-staining squamous epithelial cells *(S)*. Other mucosal glands still contain abundant cytoplasmic mucus *(M)*. The dorsal filiform papillae are indistinct and fused *(F)*.

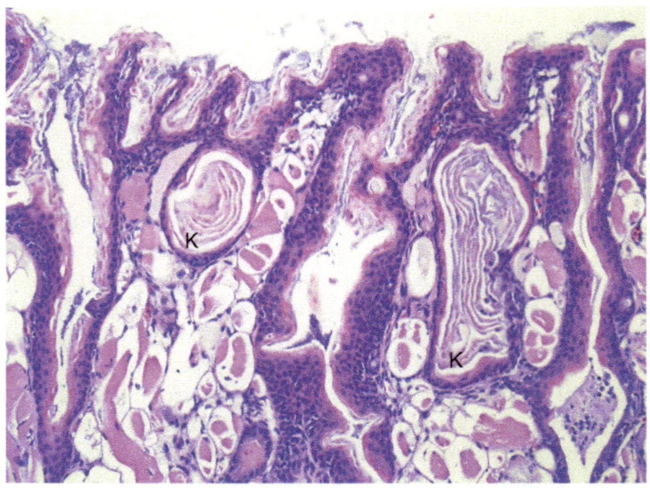

FIGURE 23-3 Histologic section of the tongue from a Wyoming Toad *(Anaxyrus [Bufo] baxteri)* with advanced squamous metaplasia that diffusely affects the mucosal glands (×20). Many glands contain laminated luminal aggregates of keratin *(K)*.

DIAGNOSIS

In most situations, a presumptive diagnosis of hypovitaminosis A in captive amphibians will be based on clinical signs of STS or will be made by clinical suspicion based on the nonspecific signs that may be associated with vitamin A deficiency. Exclusion of other diseases or husbandry-based cofactors (e.g., inappropriate environmental temperatures and overcrowding, among others) that could result in a decreased ability to feed should be attempted, if possible. An observation of empirical resolution or improvement of clinical signs with both vitamin A supplementation and correction of any identified dietary deficiencies can be helpful. In large amphibian collections, routine histopathologic examination of animals that die may reveal SM in tissues such as the tongue, ciliated oral and esophageal mucosa, urinary bladder, or kidney and cloaca, and these observations should raise the index of suspicion for hypovitaminosis A in the remaining collection animals. If feasible, collection of liver or serum samples for determination of retinol levels may also be helpful for confirmation of the diagnosis.

Histopathology

Postmortem histopathologic evaluation for evidence of SM requires that the entire tongue be submitted in formalin and bisected longitudinally (median plane) before histologic processing. Early or mild SM of the lingual epithelium occurs rostrally in the dorsal mucus-producing glands and is observed in more caudal regions as lesions progress. Because of this specific lesion distribution, areas of SM can be easily overlooked if transverse sections from only the middle to caudal portions of the tongue are examined. Areas of SM in lingual glands can range from simple replacement of mucus-producing cells by larger pale-staining squamous epithelial cells to glands that are filled with laminated keratin (Figure 23-2 and Figure 23-3). In advanced lesions, SM can involve the entire dorsal mucous-producing surface of the tongue, as well as the ventral ciliated epithelium (see Figure 23-3). SM may not be observed in all animals with vitamin A deficiency; therefore the presence of this change is interpreted as a possible indicator of deficiency in a population, and the absence of SM should not be used to exclude the possibility of deficiency.[19,20]

Liver, Whole Body, and Serum Retinol Determination

In domestic animals, the liver is the principal site of vitamin A storage and is the preferred sample tissue for evaluation of suspected deficiencies.[2,4] Published information on levels of liver retinol in amphibian species is limited, and interpretation of results for diagnostic purposes is based on comparison of values (if available) in normal free-ranging animals of the same or related species and, to a lesser degree, comparison of values reported for domestic animals.

TABLE 23-1

Liver Retinol in Wild Anuran Amphibians and Reference Ranges for Selected Domestic Animals

Species/Number Examined (n)	Mean liver retinol µg/g (range)
Wyoming Toad (*Anaxyrus baxteri*) n = 10	104.6 wet (44.4-164)*
Southern Toad (*Anaxyrus terrestris*) n = 4	150.3 wet (96.4-242.6)*,†
American Toad (*Anaxyrus americanus*) n = 2	493.5 wet (417.6-569.3)*,‡
Boreal Toad (*Anaxyrus boreas boreas*) n = 1	62.9 wet
American Bullfrog (*Lithobates catesbeiana*) n = 1	12.2 wet*
Domestic cattle	400-700 dry§
Domestic horses	200-500 dry§
Domestic chickens	60-300 wet§,¶

*Analyses performed by Dr. Ellen Dierenfeld, Wildlife Conservation Society.
†Samples provided courtesy of Dan Pearson.
‡Samples provided courtesy of Dr. April Paulman.
§From Puls R. *Vitamin levels in animal health.* Aldergrove, BC, Canada: Sherpa International, 1994;14-30.
¶Values cited as IU/g and converted to µg/g (1 IU = 0.3 µg).

For investigation of STS in Wyoming Toads, liver samples for determination of retinol levels were obtained from a variety of free-ranging toads including Wyoming Toads (available during a natural outbreak of chytridiomycosis), American Toads, Southern Toads (*Anaxyrus [Bufo] terrestris*), and a Boreal Toad (Table 23-1). The mean liver retinol values for 11 Wyoming Toads with STS and histologic evidence of lingual SM were 1.48 µg/g (range, not detectable to 7.3 µg/g) compared with a mean of 104.6 µg/g (range, 44 to 164 µg/g) for 10 free-ranging toads that had histologically normal tongues. In general, samples from all species of normal free-ranging toads examined had lower liver retinol values than ranges expected for domestic animals, but values still significantly exceeded those observed in toads with STS (see Table 23-1). A single free-ranging American Bullfrog (*Lithobates [Rana] catesbeianus*) had a liver retinol level of 12.5 µg/g, and this value is similar to those obtained for free-ranging bullfrogs in Canada (see Table 23-1).[21] Based on limited information, a liver retinol value of less than 40 µg/g has been suggested as being suspicious for vitamin A deficiency, especially for bufonids; however, additional research on hepatic retinol levels in free-ranging amphibians is clearly indicated.[17]

For very small amphibian species in which there is suspicion of vitamin A deficiency, consideration might be given to determination of whole body vitamin A as reported for a small number of free-ranging Green Frogs (*Lithobates [Rana] clamitans*) and Southern Toads. The mean vitamin A levels for these species expressed in International Units (IU) (1 IU is equivalent to 0.3 µg of retinol) were approximately 25,000 and 38,000 IU/kg dry weight, respectively.[22]

Determination of serum or plasma retinol levels has not been reported in animals affected with STS or other manifestations of suspected vitamin A deficiency but may be feasible in larger species from which an adequate sample volume for analysis can be obtained. It should be noted that, in domestic species, serum retinol values often do not decline until after liver retinol has been depleted; low serum retinol values reflect advanced deficiency. As with liver retinol values, results of blood retinol determinations should be viewed with caution because normal values have not been established for amphibians. Serum values reported for wild bullfrogs from Quebec, Canada are similar to those observed in domestic mammals and birds, as well as some free-ranging turtles. A "normal" range of 0.2 to 0.8 µg/mL of retinol may be useful as a starting point for interpretation.[4,23,24] Studies to address normal values of serum retinol for the range of amphibian species housed in captivity would be a useful contribution.

All samples used to determine retinol concentrations should be protected from light and high temperatures after collection because vitamin A degrades rapidly under these conditions. Because many amphibian carcasses submitted for necropsy are significantly autolyzed, samples for retinol determination should be carefully selected to obtain the most meaningful results.

POSSIBLE CAUSES OF HYPOVITAMINOSIS A

Factors that contribute to the development of hypovitaminosis A and STS in amphibians and that may be responsible for a possible overrepresentation of this condition in bufonids have not been completely determined. Suggested areas for prospective research in order of priority include (1) determination of dietary requirements for insectivorous species and the need for nutrient supplementation in captive diets, (2) the role of carotenoids (plant-based provitamin A forms) in amphibian nutrition, and (3) the unlikely potential role of chemical exposures that may interfere with vitamin A metabolism.

Diet and Dietary Supplementation

Most cultured invertebrates fed to captive amphibians, including domestic crickets (*Acheta domestica*), mealworms (*Tenebrio molitor*), superworms (*Zophobas morio*), waxworms (*Galleria mellonella*), fruit flies (*Drosophila melanogaster*), silkworm larvae (*Bombyx mori*), and earthworms (*Lumbricus terrestris*), are poor sources of preformed vitamin A or carotenoids and require supplementation by dusting or gut-loading before use as prey items.[6,25-29] Investigation of STS in toads has revealed instances of inadequate dietary husbandry including feeding of insect-based diets without addition of vitamin supplements; provision of vitamin supplements solely by dusting of prey items, which, if insects are not consumed immediately, has the disadvantage of losing dusting powder by attrition or insect grooming behavior; and use of vitamin supplements that have been improperly stored (e.g., exposure to light or high heat and humidity) or have originated from bulk containers in extended use (more than 4 to 6 months). All of these situations can result in inadequate delivery of preformed vitamin A to captive animals and subsequent development of deficiency-related disease. Given that many captive amphibians are likely fed vitamin A–deficient diets, the frequent recognition of deficiency-associated disease in bufonids could represent high group-specific requirements for vitamin A, vitamin A precursors (carotenoids—see further on), or other nutrients related to vitamin A metabolism.

As noted earlier, very little is known about amphibian nutrition; as a result, captive feeding and nutrient supplementation practices are usually based on institutional preference or habit rather than scientific formulation. Several nutrient interactions might need to be considered when investigating the cause of hypovitaminosis A in captive animals. For example, zinc and vitamin A interact, both in the synthesis of retinol-binding protein required for vitamin A transport and as components of enzymes required for vitamin A metabolism.[2,30] Differences in lipid profiles between naturally consumed insect diets and diets fed in captivity may be important because of roles for fatty acids in absorption and metabolism of vitamin A and carotenoids.[31-34] Interactions between fat-soluble vitamins that might influence the absorption of dietary vitamin A should also be considered. For instance, captive Wyoming toads with lingual SM and low liver retinol levels had higher levels of liver vitamin E (α-tocopherol) when compared with free-ranging toads (49 μg/g wet and 16 μg/g wet, respectively).[9] Finally, other dietary factors can influence vitamin A requirements in domestic animals; these include levels of free nitrate in feed, inadequate dietary protein, and low dietary phosphorus.[2,4]

Carotenoids and Carotenoid Metabolism

Provitamin A carotenoids are important natural sources of vitamin A that insectivorous animals obtain by ingestion of prey items that have consumed a variety of different plants.[29] However, the ability to absorb, accumulate, or metabolize different carotenoids for conversion to active vitamin A in the intestine varies significantly between animal species.[6,35] For example, the Green Iguana *(Iguana iguana)* is a selective accumulator of xanthophylls but not carotenes such as β-carotene.[3,36] Similarly, a recent study has confirmed that the Cane Toad *(Bufo marinus)* and the Cuban Tree Frog *(Osteopilus septentrionalis)* are unable to convert β-carotene to active vitamin A.[37] In contrast, carotenoids, including β-carotene, have been detected in the liver of Leopard Frogs *(Rana pipiens)*; however, little is known about how these carotenoids are utilized.[37] Therefore it is possible that the very low amounts of preformed (active) vitamin A found in captive insect diets combined with a lack of appropriate types of dietary carotenoids may ultimately result in vitamin A deficiency in susceptible amphibian species. As an example, the vitamin A-responsive periocular swellings reported in Chiricahua Leopard Frogs *(Rana chiricahuensis)* were associated with the use of a commercial vitamin supplement that solely utilized β-carotene as a vitamin A source.[16,17]

Exposure to Organochlorine Compounds

Some organochlorine compounds used as agricultural pesticides are known to interfere with vitamin A metabolism and are suspected to cause aural abscesses and SM of the tympanic epithelium in free-ranging Box Turtles *(Terrapene carolina carolina)*.[38,39] Recent investigations have tried to determine whether organochlorines may also have negative effects on retinoid metabolism in free-ranging amphibians; however, histopathologic lesions suggestive of vitamin A deficiency have not been reported.[21,24,40,41] Exposure to environmental organochlorine contaminants is an unlikely explanation for an acquired condition such as STS in captive animals; however, continued research in this area could broaden our overall understanding of vitamin A metabolism in amphibians.

TREATMENT AND DIETARY SUPPLEMENTATION

Lesions of SM associated with vitamin A deficiency are possibly reversible if the deficiency is corrected. For treatment of STS and suspected vitamin A deficiency, injectable, oral, and topical methods of treatment have been suggested or attempted. A recent study in Grey Foam-Nest Tree Frogs compared oral supplementation with vitamin A (added to crickets used as food items) with topical application of water-miscible vitamin A palmitate (Aquasol A, Mayne Pharma, Paramus, NJ). Whole body vitamin A concentrations increased significantly only in frogs that received topical supplementation of approximately 50 IU vitamin A every other day or once weekly.[15]

Commercially available veterinary injectable solutions of vitamin A are too concentrated for safe use in most small captive amphibians. If diluted solutions can be obtained from a compounding pharmacy, intramuscular doses of 2 IU vitamin A/g body weight every 72 hours until resolution of clinical signs has been suggested.[16,17] The same author has suggested oral administration of 1 IU vitamin A/g body weight given daily for 2 weeks or until resolution of clinical signs. Vitamin A for oral use can be prepared from commercially available liquid gel caps—usually 10,000 IU vitamin A each—marketed for human use; capsule contents should be diluted in vegetable oil to achieve a concentration that allows accurate administration to small patients. Finally, a protocol for topical treatment of affected toads has been tried that uses a water-miscible injectable formulation of vitamin A marketed for use in humans (Aquasol A Parenteral, Mayne Pharma, Paramus, NJ) (Armstrong D: Pers. com., Mar 27, 2007). The 50,000 IU/mL solution is diluted with sterile water to 5000 IU/mL, and the dilution is applied directly to the skin. For 15-g to 25-g body weight toads, one drop of the diluted solution is dispensed from a tuberculin syringe without a needle, and for smaller 1-g to 5-g body weight animals, one drop is applied from a tuberculin syringe with a 27-gauge needle attached. Treatments are given daily for up to 2 weeks for severely affected animals and as little as twice weekly for less severely affected individuals.

In addition to direct administration of vitamin A, the diets provided to groups of animals affected with STS should be reviewed. As a standard practice, amphibians fed a predominantly insectivorous diet should have vitamin supplementation of those diets by dusting or gut-loading of prey items (or both) with the use of a supplement that contains preformed (active) vitamin A rather than a single carotenoid such as β-carotene. However, use of prey items (e.g., crickets) that have been gut-loaded with a mixed carotenoid-rich diet of fresh fruit and vegetables may be useful.[29,42] In formulation of gut-loading diets, a suggested concentration of vitamin A has been calculated for adult crickets (8310 μg/kg), cricket nymphs (5270 μg/kg), and mealworms (13,310 μg/kg).[28] Dietary supplements should be stored under cool and dark conditions and used in their entirety within 6 months of opening the container.

HYPERVITAMINOSIS A

To date, the author is not aware of a well-documented case of hypervitaminosis A (vitamin A toxicity) in an amphibian treated for clinical signs of STS; however, this is a significant concern whenever vitamin A supplementation is considered. On the basis of observations in other species, tissues that may show clinical manifestations of hypervitaminosis A include the skin (i.e., increased shedding, vesicles, and/or ulcers); liver (i.e., hepatocellular degeneration and/or fibrosis), and bone (i.e., osteoporosis and/or deformities).[2,7,43] Excess vitamin A may also interfere with the metabolism of other fat-soluble vitamins such as vitamin D, as evidenced by a report of metabolic bone disease (rickets and osteoporosis) in African Clawed Frogs *(Xenopus laevis)* fed a diet containing high levels of vitamin A.[44] For most insectivorous amphibian species, hypervitaminosis A is probably unlikely to occur, except in cases of an extreme error in calculating amounts of vitamin A used for supplementation or treatment.

REFERENCES

1. Oftedal OT, Allen ME. Nutrition as a major facet of reptile conservation. *Zoo Biol* 1996;15:491-497.
2. McDowell LR. Vitamin A. In: *Vitamins in animal and human nutrition.* 2nd ed. Ames, IA: Iowa State University Press, 2000;15-90.
3. Kane AB, Kumar V. Environmental and nutritional pathology. In: Cotran RS, Kumar K, Collins T, eds. *Robbins pathologic basis of disease.* 6th ed. Philadelphia: WB Saunders, 1999;403-457.
4. Puls R. *Vitamin levels in animal health.* Aldergrove, BC, Canada: Sherpa International, 1994;14-30.
5. Elkan E, Zwart P. The ocular disease of young terrapins caused by vitamin A deficiency. *Pathol Vet* 1967;4:201-222.
6. Dierenfeld ES, Norkus EB, Carroll K, et al. Carotenoids, vitamin A, and vitamin E concentrations during egg development in panther chameleons *(Furcifer pardalis)*. *Zoo Biol* 2002;21:295-303.
7. Boyer T. Hypovitaminosis A and hypervitaminosis A. In: Mader D, ed. *Reptile medicine and surgery.* 2nd ed. Philadelphia: Saunders Elsevier, 2006;831-835.
8. Cortes PL, Tiwary AK, Puschner B, et al. Vitamin A deficiency in turkey poults. *J Vet Diagn Invest* 2006;18:489-494.
9. Pessier AP, Linn M, Garner MM, et al. Suspected hypovitaminosis A in captive toads (*Bufo* spp.), in *Proceedings*. Am Assoc Zoo Vet 2005;57.
10. Gonzalez-Elorriaga M. Las glandulas de la mucosa dorso-distaldela lengua del sapo *Bufo marinus* L. (Amphibia: Anura): histologia y ultraestructura. *Acta Cient Venezolana* 2002;53:49-59.
11. Iwasaki S. Evolution of the structure and function of the vertebrate tongue. *J Anat* 2002;201:1-13.
12. Elkan E. Two cases of epithelial malignancy in salientia. *J Pathol Bacteriol* 1968;100:496-499.
13. Lee S, Zippel K, Ramos L, et al. Captive-breeding program for the Kihansi spray toad at the Wildlife Conservation Society, Bronx, New York. *Int Zoo Yearb* 2006;40:241-253.
14. Poole V. *Husbandry manual panamanian golden frog* Atelopus zeteki. Baltimore, Md: National Aquarium in Baltimore, 2006.
15. Sim RR, Sulivan KE, Valdes EV, et al. A comparison of oral and topical vitamin A supplementation in African foam-nesting frogs *(Chiromantis xerampelina)*. *J Zoo Wildl Med* 2010;41:456-460.
16. Wright K. Advances that impact every amphibian patient. *Exot DVM* 2005;7:82-86.
17. Wright K. Overview of amphibian medicine. In: Mader D, ed. *Reptile medicine and surgery.* 2nd ed. Philadelphia: Saunders Elsevier, 2006;941-971.
18. Kummrow M, Tseng F, Pessier AP. What is your diagnosis? *J Herpetol Med Surg* 2006;16:144-146.
19. Honour SM, Trudeau S, Kennedy S, et al. Experimental vitamin A deficiency in mallards *(Anas platyrhynchos)*: lesions and tissue vitamin A levels. *J Wildl Dis* 1995;31:277-288.
20. Aye PP, Morishita TY, Mo Saif Y, et al. Induction of vitamin A deficiency in turkeys. *Avian Dis* 2000;44:809-817.
21. Boily M, Berube VE, Spear P, et al. Hepatic retinoids of bullfrogs in relation to agricultural pesticides. *Environ Toxicol Chem* 2005;24:1099-1106.
22. Schairer ML, Dierenfeld ES, Fitzpatrick MP. Nutrient composition of whole green frogs, *Rana clamitans* and Southern toads, *Bufo terrestris*. *Bull Assoc Rept Amphib Vet* 1998;8:17-20.
23. Dierenfeld ES, Leontyeva OA, Karesh WB, et al. Circulating α-tocopherol and retinol concentrations in free-ranging and zoo turtles and tortoises, in *Proceedings*. Am Assoc Zoo Vet 1999;329-331.
24. Berube VE, Boily MH, DeBlois C, et al. Plasma retinoid values in bullfrogs, *Rana catesbeiana,* in relation to agricultural intensity of sub-watersheds in the Yamaska River drainage basin, Quebec, Canada. *Aquat Toxicol* 2005;71:109-120.
25. Pennino M, Dierenfeld ES, Behler JL. Retinol, α-tocopherol and proximate nutrient composition of invertebrates used as feed. *Int Zoo Yearb* 1991;30:143-149.
26. Barker D, Fitzpatrick MP, Dierenfeld ES. Nutrient composition of selected whole invertebrates. *Zoo Biol* 1998;17:123-134.
27. Finke MD. Complete nutrient composition of commercially raised invertebrates used as food for insectivores. *Zoo Biol* 2002;21:269-285.
28. Finke MD. Gut loading to enhance the nutrient content of insects as food for reptiles: a mathematical approach. *Zoo Biol* 2003;22:147-162.
29. Ogilvy V, Fidgett AL, Presiosi RF. Differences in carotenoid accumulation among three feeder-cricket species: implications for carotenoid delivery to captive insectivores. *Zoo Biol* 2011;30:1-9.
30. Christian P, West KP. Interactions between zinc and vitamin A: an update. *Am J Clin Nutr* 1998;68(suppl):435S-441S.
31. Tso P, Lee T, DeMichele SJ. Randomized structured triglycerides increase lymphatic absorption of tocopherol and retinol compared with the equivalent physical mixture in a rat model of fat malabsorption. *J Nutr* 2001;131:2157-2163.
32. Carta G, Angioni E, Murru E, et al. Modulation of lipid metabolism and vitamin A by conjugated linoleic acid. *Prostaglandins Leukot Essent Fatty Acids* 2002;67:187-191.
33. Wright K. Cholesterol, corneal lipidosis, and xanthomatosis in amphibians. *Vet Clin N Am Exot Anim Pract* 2003;6:155-167.
34. Raju M, Lakshminarayana R, Krishnakantha TP, et al. Micellar oleic and eicosapentaenoic acid but not linoleic acid influences the B-carotene uptake and its cleavage into retinol in rats. *Mol Cell Biochem* 2006;288:7-15.
35. Slifka KA, Bowen PE, Stacewicz-Sapuntzakis M, et al. A survey of serum and dietary carotenoids in captive wild animals. *J Nutr* 1999;129: 380-390.
36. Raila J, Schuhmacher A, Gropp J, et al. Selective absorption of carotenoids in the common green iguana *(Iguana iguana)*. *Comp Biochem Physiol A Mol Integr Physiol* 2002;132:513-518.
37. McComb A. Evaluation of vitamin A supplementations for captive amphibian species. M.S. Thesis, North Carolina State University, Raleigh, NC, 2010.
38. Khachik F, de Moura FF, Zhao D, et al. Transformations of selected carotenoids in plasma, liver, and ocular tissues of humans and in nonprimate animal models. Invest Ophthalmol Vis Sci 2002;43:3383-3392.
39. Holladay SD, Wolf JC, Smith S, et al. Aural abscesses in wild caught box turtles *(Terrapene carolina)*: possible role of organochlorine-induced hypovitaminosis A. *Ecotoxicol Environ Saf* 2001;48:99-106.
40. Brown JD, Richards JM, Robertson J, et al. Pathology of aural abscesses in free-living eastern box turtles *(Terrapene carolina carolina)*. *J Wildl Dis* 2004;40:704-712.
41. Keshavan R, Deshmukh PB. Vitamin A concentrations in liver and serum of the frog *Rana tigrina,* treated with DDT and sevin. *Indian J Comp Anim Physiol* 1984;2:32-36.

42. Leiva-Presa A, Jenssen BM. Effects of p, p′-DDE on retinoid homeostasis and sex hormones of adult male European common frogs *(Rana temporaria)*. *J Toxicol Environ Health A* 2006;69:2051-2062.
43. Li H, Vaughan MJ, Browne RK. A complex enrichment diet improves growth and health in the endangered Wyoming Toad *(Bufo baxteri)*. *Zoo Biol* 2009;28:197-213.
44. Jones TC, Hunt RD, King NW. Nutritional deficiencies. In: *Veterinary pathology.* 6th ed. Baltimore, Md: Williams and Wilkins, 1997;783.

CHAPTER 24

Ranavirus

Debra Lee Miller

Ranaviruses are members of Iridoviridae and are known to cause morbidity and mortality in amphibians, reptiles, and fish. Current research is exploring the mechanism of interclass transmission and variations in host susceptibility, both of which can potentially contribute to mortality events in nature. Given that ranaviruses in reptiles are discussed elsewhere (see Chapter 5) and that fish are not a focus of this book, this chapter will only address ranaviruses in amphibians.

Ranaviruses are globally distributed, having been reported on five continents.[1] Anthropogenic spreading (e.g., from infected animals used as live fishing bait, field and recreational equipment, boots, and import/export of infected animals for food or pets) has resulted in exposure of naïve populations and subsequent mortality events in wild amphibians.[2-4] Ranaviruses have infected 14 families and more than 70 individual species of amphibians and, likely, can infect most if not all amphibian species.[1] Host–pathogen coevolution may have resulted in widespread infection with minimal health effects in intact ecosystems, but these same ranaviruses may be virulent in nonadapted amphibian species or in adapted species that are in degraded environments and subject to stressors.[1,2,5]

Susceptibility to ranaviruses varies by host species, ranavirus isolate, and across phylogenetic lineages.[5,6] Eggs appear to be resistant to infection, likely because of the mechanical protection of the capsule.[7] In general, hatchling and metamorphs are the most susceptible age groups[7]; however, adults are reported most often in die-offs of several European species.[8-10]

Ranaviruses are horizontally transmitted via direct contact, ingestion of virus or infected animals, and water exposure.[11] Vertical transmission is suspected but remains unknown.[11,12] There is evidence for interclass transmission among amphibians, reptiles, and fish.[13-19] Therefore, community composition may play a role in emergence within an ecosystem.

Ranaviruses cause necrosis of many different cell types, leading to organ failure and death in susceptible individuals. Clinical signs include swelling (appendages, body), hemorrhages (especially on the ventrum and legs), ulceration, discoloration of the skin, lethargy, buoyancy problems, and erratic swimming (Figure 24-1).[1] Additional gross lesions noted at necropsy may include hemorrhages of internal organs, tan friable organs, hydrocoelom (edema), and swelling of the lymph sacs (Figure 24-2).[1] Microscopic lesions may include hemorrhage, cellular necrosis (e.g., hematopoietic tissue, hepatocytes, epithelial cells, endothelial cells), and inclusion bodies (intracytoplasmic; however, intranuclear have been reported but are rare [Figure 24-3]).[1] In addition, caudates may develop ulcers on their feet, particularly the toe tips, and white polypoid lesions (noted in experimentally infected tiger salamanders).[20] However, not all individuals will have observable ranaviral lesions, and sudden death may be the only sign. Incubation time remains unknown but may vary by host species, host age group, and virus isolate. The incubation period can be as short as 3 days but may also extend into weeks.[21] In die-offs, ongoing mortality may occur in a population over a span of weeks to months, but later deaths are often attributed

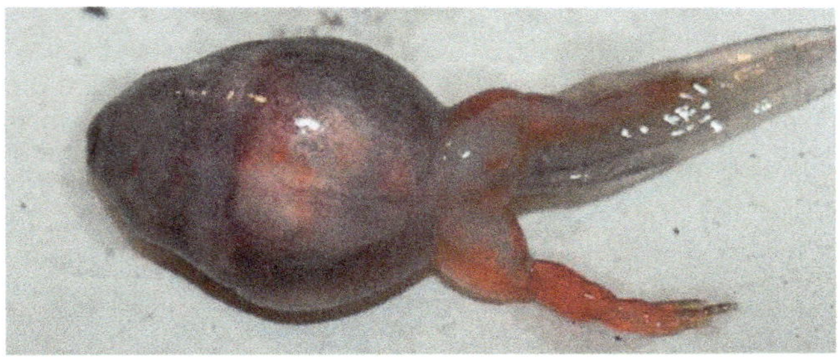

FIGURE 24-1 A Wood Frog *(Lithobates sylvatica)* larva with ranaviral disease has swelling of the body and legs and hemorrhage of the right rear leg.

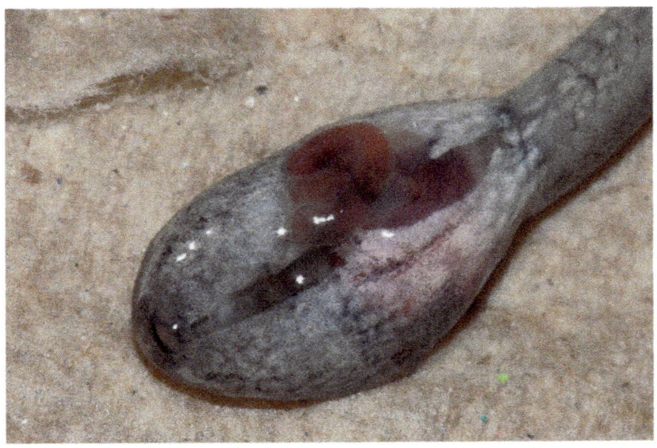

FIGURE 24-2 Internal lesions in ranaviral disease can include hemorrhage and edema as seen in the exposed intestinal tract of this Green Frog *(Lithobates clamitans)* larva. *(Photo courtesy Nathan Haislip, Wetlands Program, The University of Tennessee-Knoxville.)*

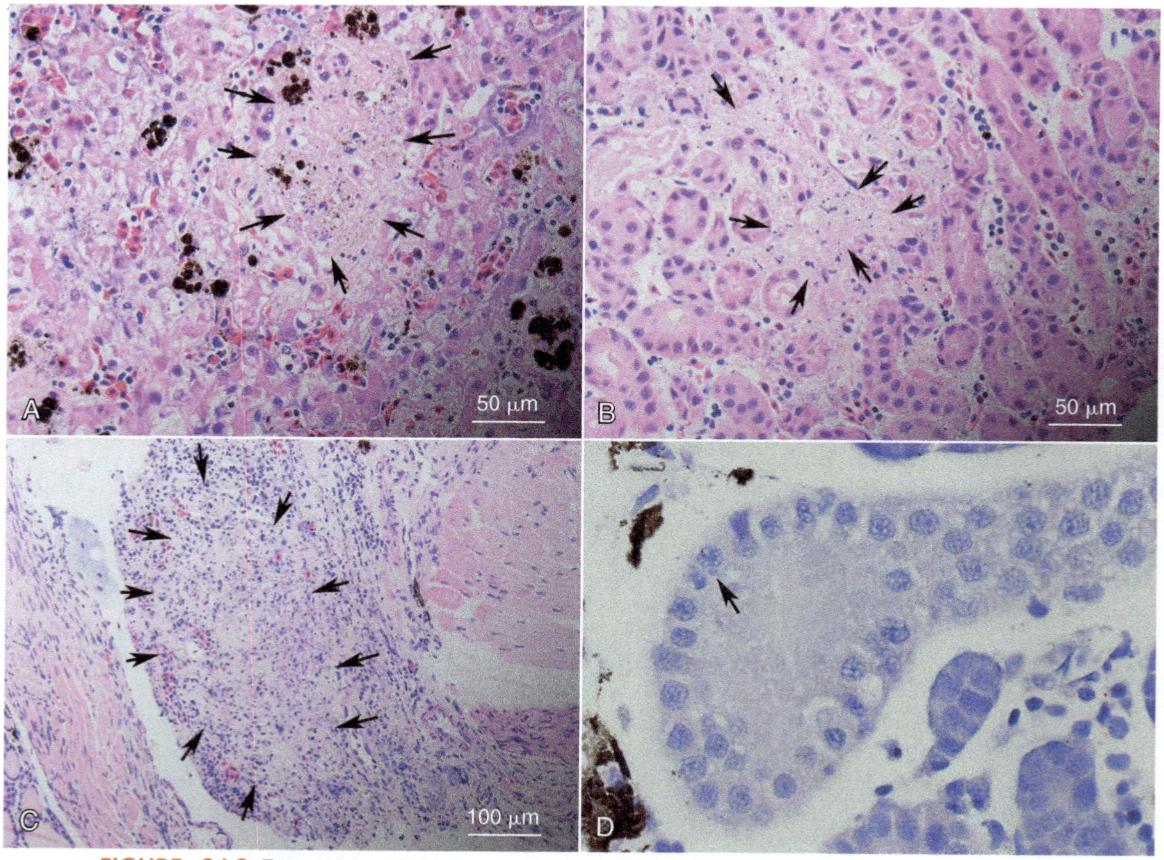

FIGURE 24-3 Examples of histopathologic changes observed in ranaviral disease. Necrosis of multiple organs *(arrows)*, including liver (**A**), mesonephros (**B**), and lymphoid tissue (**C**) was observed in American Bullfrog *(Lithobates catesbeianus)* metamorphs from a die-off event. **D,** Cytoplasmic inclusion bodies *(arrow)* are not consistently seen but were observed within tubule epithelial cells of the mesonephros of an experimentally infected Wood Frog *(Lithobates sylvatica)* larva.

to secondary invaders.[1] Finally, subclinical infection has been detected in wild amphibians[22] and in experimental challenges.[21,23] Individuals that are subclinically infected often have nonspecific histologic changes such as vacuolation of renal tubular epithelium and hepatocytes.

Currently, no treatment exists for ranaviral infection. Therefore ranavirus-positive amphibians should be isolated, provided optimal husbandry conditions, and exposed to minimal stress in order to have the best chance of recovering and developing resistance. Similarly, newly acquired animals should always be isolated and tested (e.g., quantitative polymerase chain reaction analysis on tail or toe clips) for the presence of ranaviruses before being introduced to captive colonies. When ranaviral infection occurs, treatment for secondary invaders and correction of nutritional deficiencies (e.g., hypovitaminosis A, which causes immunosuppression) may limit the severity of the disease. Current studies are investigating whether temperature might be used to control ranaviruses, but these studies are still in their infancy. Likewise, the potential for development of a Ranavirus vaccine is promising, particularly considering that Majji and collegues[24] found that prior infection with FV3 led to enhanced immunity against subsequent ranavirus exposure. The use of a vaccine might have limited field utility, but it could be valuable in captive populations. Although not yet commercially available, an oral formulation of an iridoviral vaccine is being tested for use in fish[25] and may be a starting point for development of a similar vaccine for amphibians.

Water changes may be helpful in controlling ranaviruses in captive amphibians. A complete water change performed daily will reduce the virion load; however, it may result in undo stress on the amphibian(s) inhabiting the tank/enclosure. Even with filtered systems that are equipped with an ultraviolet sterilizer, water changes are necessary because some virions never pass through the sterilizer. However, less dramatic water changes (e.g., 20% volume daily and complete changes every 5 days) may be used in filtered systems (Wright K: Pers. com.,Apr 2, 2012). Regardless, a reservoir of water that is the same temperature as the cage's water and that has a very similar chemical profile is necessary for minimizing stress on the amphibian(s). The chemical profile of the water should be monitored daily to ensure the levels are as follows: dissolved oxygen, >2 mg/L; ammonia, <0.6 mg/L; nitrite, <2 mg/L; and nitrate, <30mg/L (Wright K: Pers. com.,). Water from tanks/enclosures housing infected animals should be disinfected before discarding to inactivate the virus. Likewise, all equipment and surfaces should be disinfected after use. A minimum of 1 minute contact time with greater than 3% bleach, greater than 1% Virkon, or greater than 0.75% Nolvasan will inactivate ranaviruses.[26]

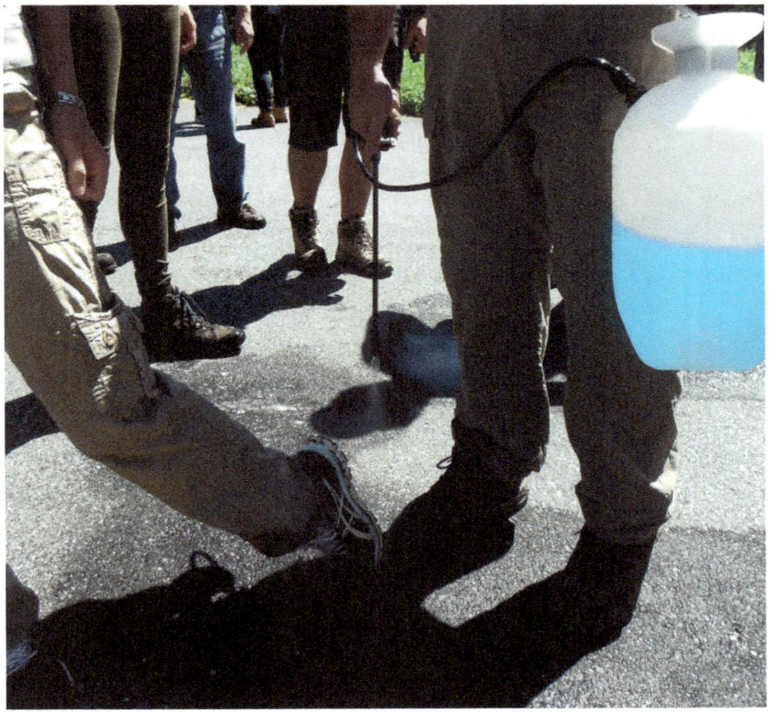

FIGURE 24-4 Footwear is disinfected after removing soil and other debris. It is important to disinfect footwear and equipment before moving to the next field site. *(Photo courtesy Dr. Matthew Gray, University of Tennessee, Knoxville, Tenn.)*

Ranaviruses can have a severe impact on conservation measures. Ranaviruses are not distributed uniformly across the landscape; rather, infection hotspots exist.[27] Therefore these viruses can negatively affect repatriation of endangered species. Rare species that are highly susceptible (e.g., the Gopher Frog [*Lithobates capito*])[5] are at greatest risk. Translocation of animals into environments from where they did not originate should be discouraged; however, relocation and translocation often are the only viable option in conservation efforts. In such cases, only individuals that test negative for ranaviruses should be released, and surveillance of native amphibians, reptiles, and fish should be done to confirm that ranaviruses are not detected. Animals intended for release that test positive will need to be retested. Repeat testing of positive individuals has revealed that ranavirus-positive amphibians may test negative after several weeks, suggesting that viral clearance might be occurring. In the field, disinfection of equipment and boots is mandatory when one travels between field sites to reduce the likelihood of anthropogenic spreading of ranaviruses (Figure 24-4).

REFERENCES

1. Miller DL, Gray MJ, Storfer A. Ecopathology of ranaviruses infecting amphibians. *Viruses* 2011;3:2351-2373.
2. Storfer A, Alfaro ME, Ridenhour BJ, et al. Phylogenetic concordance analysis shows an emerging pathogen is novel and endemic. *Ecol Lett* 2007;10:1075-1083.
3. Picco AM, Collins JP. Amphibian commerce as a likely source of pathogen pollution. *Conserv Biol* 2008;22:1582-1589.
4. Schloegel LM, Picco AM, Kilpatrick AM, et al. Magnitude of the US trade in amphibians and presence of *Batrachochytrium dendrobatidis* and ranavirus infection in imported North American bullfrogs (*Rana catesbeiana*). *Biol Conserv* 2009;142:1420-1426.
5. Hoverman JT, Gray MJ, Haislip JT, et al. Phylogeny, life history, and ecology contribute to differences in amphibian susceptibility to ranaviruses. *Ecohealth* 2011;8:301-319.
6. Schock DM, Bollinger TK, Collins JP. Mortality rates differ among amphibian populations exposed to three strains of a lethal ranavirus. *Ecohealth* 2010;6:438-448.
7. Haislip NA, Gray MJ, Hoverman JT, et al. Development and disease: how susceptibility to an emerging pathogen changes through anuran development. *PLoS ONE* 2011;6:e22307.
8. Ariel E, Kielgast J, Svart HE, et al. Ranavirus in wild edible frogs, *Pelophylax kl. esculentus*, in Denmark. *Dis Aquat Organ* 2009;85:7-14.
9. Balseiro A, Dalton KP, Del Cerro A, et al. Outbreak of common midwife toad virus in alpine newts (*Mesotriton alpestris cyreni*) and common midwife toads (*Alytes obstetricans*) in northern Spain: comparative pathological study of an emerging ranavirus. *Vet J* 2010;186:256-258.
10. Duffus ALJ, Cunningham AA. Major disease threats to European amphibians. *Herpetol J* 2010;20:117-127.
11. Gray MJ, Miller DL, Hoverman JT. Ecology and pathology of amphibian ranaviruses. *Dis Aquat Organ* 2009;87:243-266.
12. Duffus ALJ, Pauli BD, Wozney K, et al. Frog virus 3-like infections in aquatic amphibian communities. *J Wildl Dis* 2008;44:109-120.
13. Moody NJG, Owens L. Experimental demonstration of the pathogenicity of a frog virus, Bohle iridovirus, for a fish species, barramundi, *Lates calcarifer*. *Dis Aquat Organ* 1994;18:95-102.
14. Bang Jensen BB, Ersboll AK, Ariel E. Susceptibility of pike, *Esox lucius*, to a panel of ranavirus isolates. *Dis Aquat Organ* 2009;83:169-179.
15. Gobbo F, Cappellozza E, Pastore MR, et al. Susceptibility of black bullhead, *Ameiurus melas*, to a panel of ranavirus isolates. *Dis Aquat Organ* 2010;90:167-174.
16. Jancovich JK, Bremont M, Touchman JW, et al. Evidence for multiple recent host species shifts among the ranaviruses (Family Iridoviridae). *J Virol* 2010;84:2634-2647.
17. Picco AM, Karam AP, Collins JP. Pathogen host switching in commercial trade with management recommendations. *Ecohealth* 2010;7:252-256.

18. Johnson AJ, Pessier AP, Jacobson ER. Experimental transmission and induction of ranaviral disease in western ornate box turtles (*Terrapene ornate ornate*) and red-eared sliders (*Trachemys scripta elegans*). *Vet Pathol* 2007;44:285-297.
19. Schock DM, Bollinger TK, Chinchar VG, et al. Experimental evidence that amphibian ranaviruses are multi-host pathogens. *Copeia* 2008;1:133-143.
20. Jancovich JK, Davidson EW, Morado JF, et al. Isolation of a lethal virus from the endangered tiger salamander *Ambystoma tigrinum stebbinsi*. *Dis Aquat Organ* 1997;31:161-167.
21. Robert J, George E, De Jesús Andino F, et al. Waterborne infectivity of the ranavirus frog virus 3 in *Xenopus laevis*. *Virology* 2011;2:410-417.
22. Gray MJ, Miller DL, Schmutzer AC, et al. Frog virus 3 prevalence in tadpole populations inhabiting cattle-access and non-access wetlands in Tennessee, U.S.A. *Dis Aquat Organ* 2007;77:97-103.
23. Robert J, Abramowitz L, Gantress J, et al. *Xenopus laevis*: a possible vector of ranavirus infection? *J Wildl Dis* 2007;43:645-652.
24. Majji S, LaPatra S, Long SM, et al. *Rana catesbeiana* virus Z (RCV-Z): a novel pathogenic ranavirus. *Dis Aquat Organ* 2006;73:1-11.
25. Tamaru Y, Ohtsuka M, Kato K, et al. Application of the arming system for the expression of the 380R antigen from red sea bream iridovirus (RSIV) on the surface of yeast cells: a first step for the development of an oral vaccine. *Biotechnol Prog* 2006;22:949-953.
26. Bryan LK, Baldwin CA, Gray MJ, et al. Efficacy of select disinfectants at inactivating Ranavirus. *Dis Aquat Organ* 2009;84:89-94.
27. Hoverman JT, Gray MJ, Miller DL, et al. Widespread occurrence of ranaviruses in pond-breeding amphibian populations. *Ecohealth* 2012;9:36-48.

CHAPTER 25

Amphibian Therapy

†Kevin Wright

It has been over a decade since publication of *Amphibian Medicine and Captive Husbandry* by Wright and Whitaker in 2001. The management of several commonly seen amphibian health conditions has changed in response to the expanding information on amphibians diseases.

RANAVIRUS

Ranavirus is a worldwide viral infection that may cause morbidity and mortality in most, if not all, species of amphibians and is covered elsewhere in detail in this text. It should be part of the differential diagnosis for any amphibian with erythema, petechia, ecchymoses, plaques, punctuate nodules, ulcers, exposed muscle or bones, hydrocoelom, lethargy, inappetence, tremors, seizures, opisthotonos, or sudden death (Figures 25-1, 25-2, and 25-3); in short, almost any ill amphibian should be suspected of having a ranavirus until proven otherwise. From a practical point of view, supportive care should begin while polymerase chain reaction (PCR) and other diagnostic tests are pending. Critical steps in managing a possible ranavirus-infected amphibian include providing a "hot spot" so that the amphibian may thermoregulate to reduce viral replication; a temperature of at least 26°C is needed for infected amphibians to have the highest chance of survival. Providing a localized warmer temperature (30°C to 40°C) may also improve survival chances. Another critical step is preventing fatal electrolyte imbalances with the use of a balanced electrolyte bath such as amphibian Ringer's solution or, if that is not available, 0.6% saline solution (6 g of NaCl in 1 L distilled water). Amphibian Ringer's solution is made by adding 6.6 g NaCl, 0.15 g KCl, 0.15 g $CaCl_2$, and 0.2 g $NaHCO_3$ to 1 L of distilled water. It may be stored for up to 7 days or longer if the solution can be autoclaved and stored in sterile containers. An alternative formulation consists of 6.5 g NaCl, 0.42 g KCl, and 0.25 g $CaCl_2$ to 1 L of distilled water. Up to 10 g glucose may also be added to the solution, but this reduces the shelf life of unsterilized solution to 24 hours. Cutaneous respiration should be supported with an enriched oxygen environment, and secondary infection with bacteria and other pathogens should be prevented. Ulcers and open wounds can be managed with enrofloxacin/ silver sulfadiazine (Baytril Otic) and silver sulfadiazine cream. Compounded doxycycline topical gel has also been used for lesions because of its antibacterial and potential antiinflammatory properties. The goal is to apply 2.5 mg/kg to 5 mg/kg in total volume to the total number of wounds. In practice, many compounding pharmacies will only produce 1%, 2%, or 5% gels, so the dosing is often much larger than the goal. The wound should be patted dry before application, and the amphibian should be maintained on damp paper towels for at least 15 minutes after application of the gel. Provide nutrition via gavage with a highly digestible liquid diet (e.g., LaFeber's Emeraid for Carnivores). The typical volume is 2% of the amphibian's body weight and should be given every 5 days. Underlying malnutrition such a hypovitaminosis A should be addressed and inflammation reduced, but this step is controversial because human literature currently is in flux about the value of nonsteroidal antiinflammatory drugs. Further, not much is known about the COX-1 and COX-2 pathways in amphibians. This author's impression is that meloxicam at 0.4 to 1 mg/kg applied intramuscularly or topically may help. He also administers doxycycline orally at 2.5 mg/kg per os (PO, by mouth) once daily and topically (see previously) for its antiinflammatory properties described in other species. Stocking density should be reduced. Most amphibian patients do best kept alone. Stress may be further reduced with minimal handling or observation other than what is essential for treatment.

There is some evidence that amphibians may acquire immunity to ranavirus (see Chapter 24, Ranaviruses), so culling of known ranavirus-positive amphibians may be counterproductive for managing a healthy captive population.

SUGGESTED READINGS

Grayfer L, De Jesus Andino F, Chen G, et al. Immune evasion strategies of ranaviruses and innate immune responses to these emerging pathogens. *Viruses* 2012;4:1075-1092.

La Fauce K, Ariel E, Munns S, et al. Influence of temperature and exposure time on the infectivity of Bohle iridovirus, a ranavirus. *Aquaculture* 2012;354-355:64-67.

Lesbarrères D, Balseiro A, Brunner J, et al. Ranavirus: past, present and future. *Biol Lett* 2012;8:481-483.

Nazir J, Spengler M, Marschang RE. Environmental persistence of amphibian and reptilian ranaviruses. *Dis Aquat Organ* 2012;98:177-184.

Stöhr AC, Hoffmann A, Papp T, et al. Long-term study of an infection with ranaviruses in a group of edible frogs *(Pelophylax kl. esculentus)* and partial characterization of two viruses based on four genomic regions. Vet J, in press. Available online 25 March 2013, at http://www.sciencedirect.com/science/article/pii/S1090023313000762.

†Deceased.

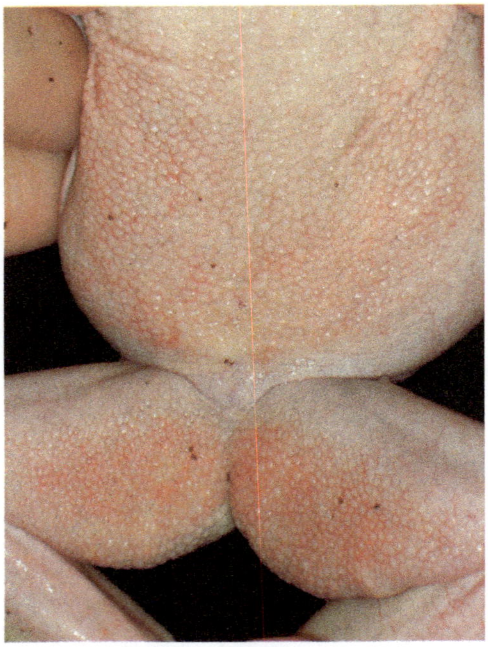

FIGURE 25-1 White's Tree Frog *(Litoria caerulea)* with ventral erythema consistent with ranavirus infection.

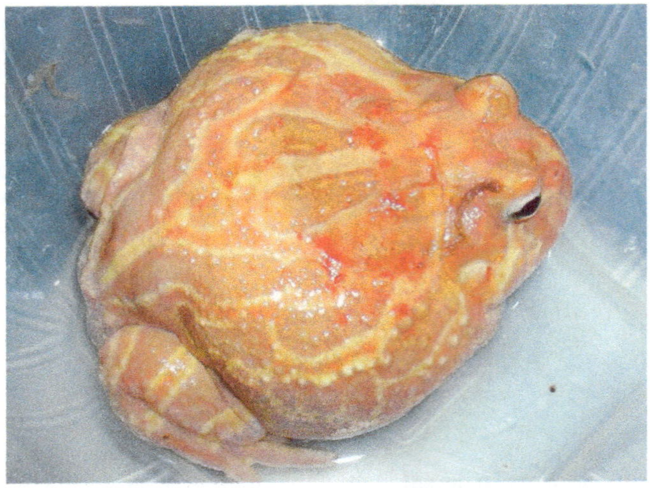

FIGURE 25-2 Albino Horned Frog *(Ceratophrys ornata)* with bleeding ulcers consistent with ranavirus infection.

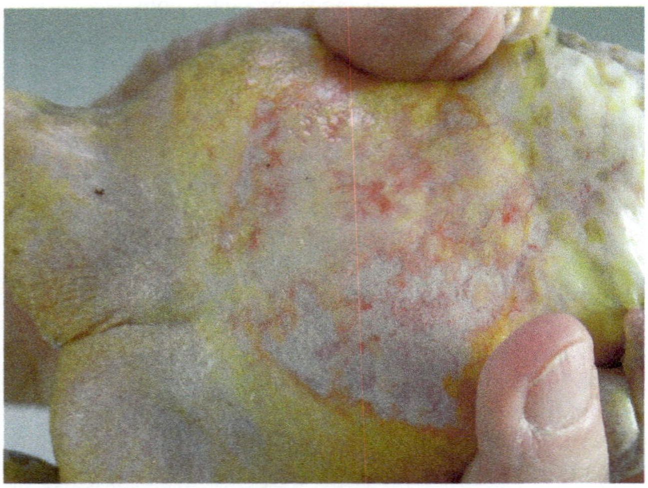

FIGURE 25-3 Petechia and ecchymosis of the same albino Horned Frog *(Ceratophrys ornata)*.

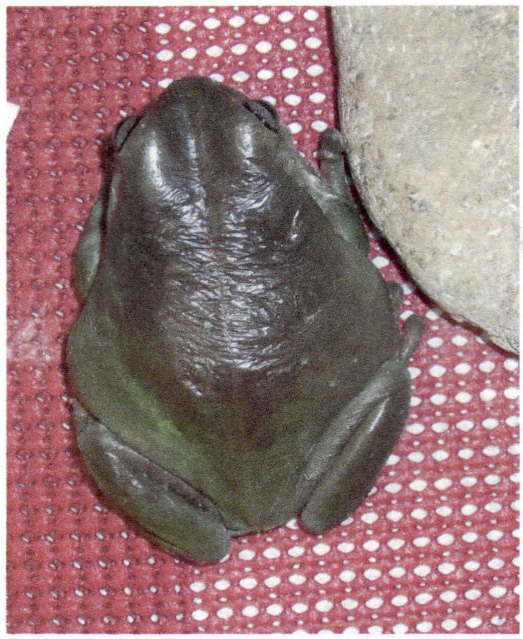

FIGURE 25-4 Hyperkeratosis of a White's Tree Frog *(Litoria caerulea)* infected with chytrid. Note hunched posture.

CHYTRIDIOMYCOSIS

Batrachochytrium dendrobatidis is a major threat to the health of wild and captive amphibians worldwide. This fungus infects the keratinized epidermis of amphibians. Some amphibian species tolerate its presence, betraying little outward sign of infection other than increased frequency of shedding, while others show brown discoloration of the skin, erythema, excess keratinized skin buildup on the toe tips and ventral skin, and a hunched posture (Figures 25-4, 25-5, 25-6, and 25-7). Bufonids may develop erythema of the ventral drink patch and may soak in the water more than normal. Some chytrid-infected amphibians may die without outward signs of illness, which is apparently the result of a fatal electrolyte imbalance (low sodium, potassium, chloride, and magnesium). Known carrier species include African Clawed Frogs *(Xenopus laevis)*, which are the presumptive origin of this disease, American Bullfrogs *(Rana catesbeiana)*, and Tiger Salamanders *(Ambystoma tigrinum)*, but it is likely that many other species are also carriers.

Many captive amphibians develop chytridiomycosis due to an inappropriate thermal environment that lacks opportunities for elevating their body temperatures by basking in a hot white light or absorbing infrared radiation from a warmed surface. If an amphibian reaches a core body temperature of 85°F (27°C) for at least 60 minutes a day, it is less likely to become infected with chytrid. Hypovitaminosis A also increases the risk of infection because it causes hyperkeratosis and immunosuppression.

Real-time PCR is the most sensitive antemortem diagnostic test for chytridiomycosis; other PCR techniques are used in many laboratories but are slightly less sensitive. Light

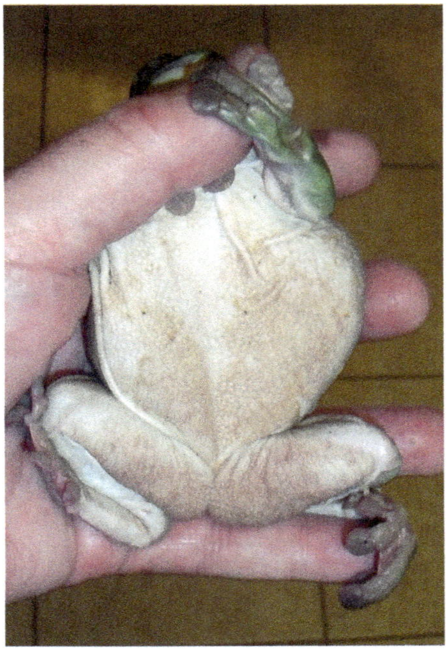

FIGURE 25-5 Brown discoloration of ventral skin due to hyperkeratosis caused by chytrid.

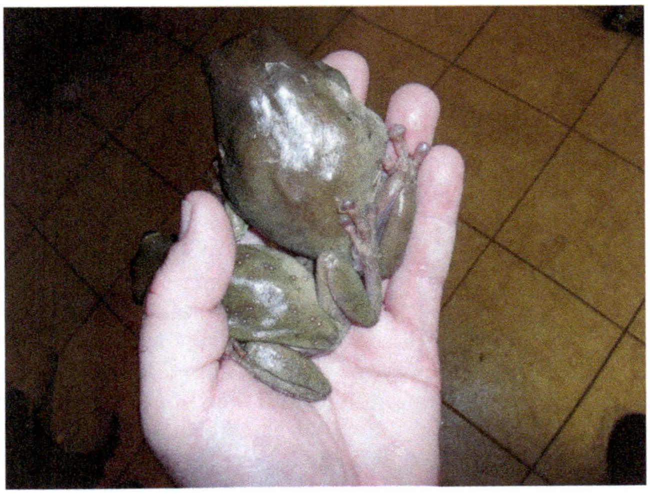

FIGURES 25-6 Excess skin shedding from two chytrid-infected White's Tree Frogs.

microscopy evaluation of biopsy samples and wet mounts of skin scrapes miss all but very advanced infections.

Almost any ill amphibian should be considered a chytridiomycosis suspect until proven otherwise. Supportive care should begin while PCR and other diagnostic tests are pending.

SUGESTIONS FOR ELIMINATING CHYTRID FROM AMPHIBIANS

Provision of a hot spot will allow the amphibian to thermoregulate in order to reduce chytrid replications. A temperature of at least 30°C is needed. Providing a localized warmer temperature (35°C to 37°C) may improve chances of survival.

No single agent has been shown to both completely eliminate chytrid *in vivo* and be safe for use in all life stages of all species of amphibians. Larvae and recent metamorphs may become stunted or die from a treatment regimen that is without clinically detected deleterious effects in older specimens of the same species. Caution is urged when any treatment is administered to a new species or even a new population of a species, as well as when it is applied to a different life stage of a population. Where practical, a treatment should be given to a small subset of the patients from a new population or life stage to ensure its safety before all patients from that same cohort undergo treatment.

BOX 25-1 THERAPEUTIC 0.01% ITRACONAZOLE SOLUTION

- Make 0.6% saline by combining 100 mL 0.9% saline with 50 mL distilled water. Alternatively, 6 g of pure sodium chloride (table salt without iodine) may be dissolved in 1 L distilled water
- Add 1 mL 1% itraconazole solution to 99 mL 0.6% saline. This "therapeutic" solution should be discarded within 24 hours of constitution.
- Various treatment regimens appear effective
  - 5 min bath every 24 h for 11 days
  - 5 min bath every 24 h for 2 days, then every 48 h for 10 days
  - 5 min bath every 48 h for 14 days

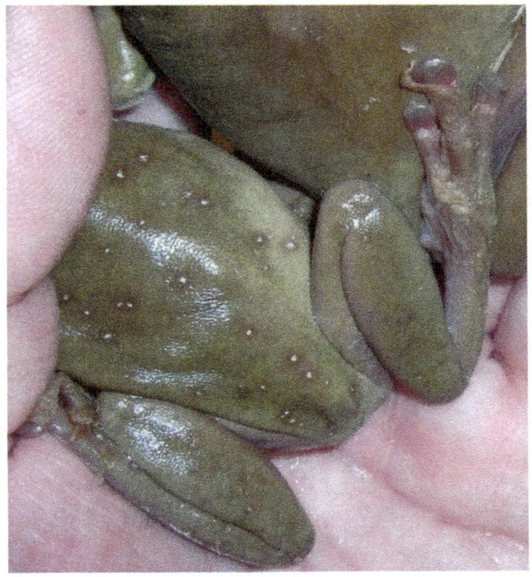

FIGURE 25-7 Close-up view of excess skin shedding from two chytrid-infected White's Tree Frogs from Figure 25-6.

Itraconazole

Itraconazole is effective for juvenile and adult specimens of several species of amphibians, but causes death in larvae and recent metamorphs. Any hospital that treats amphibians should always have unexpired containers of 1% itraconazole (Sporonox) in its pharmacy. While compounded itraconazole has been widely used, there is some question as to its stability and activity between batches and between pharmacies. To make therapeutic 0.01% itraconazole solution, see Box 25-1.

BOX 25-2 THERAPEUTIC 0.01% TERBINAFINE SOLUTION

Option 1

- Add 1 mL terbinafine (Lamisil AT 1% spray) to 99 mL distilled water
- Shake thoroughly and use immediately

Option 2

- Add 1 mL 10 mg/g terbinafine in ethanol to 99 mL distilled water
- Shake thoroughly and use immediately

Treatment Regimen

- 5 min bath every 24 h for 2 days, then every 48 h for 8 days
  Note: 15 min bath for 24 h for 10 days appeared safe and effective

BOX 25-3 THERAPEUTIC 30 PPM CHLORAMPHENICOL SOLUTION

- Add 120 mg chloramphenicol to a 1 gallon (3.8 L) bottle of spring water
- Shake thoroughly
- Make fresh daily

Treatment Regimen

- Use as continuous bath for 30 days

Terbinafine

Terbinafine may be available as an over-the-counter medication to treat athlete's foot in humans (e.g., Lamisil AT 1% spray). It may also be purchased through a compounding pharmacy (i.e., 10 mg/g terbinafine in ethanol). To make the therapeutic 0.01% solution of Terbenafine, see Box 25-2.

Chloramphenicol

Chloramphenicol is rarely used in the United States because of the risk of aplastic anemia developing in people who have contact with even miniscule amounts of this medication. Chloramphenicol appears to be safe and effective for all life stages of some amphibians and has a further advantage of treating some of the common secondary bacterial infections. The pure chloramphenicol powder may be purchased through a compounding pharmacy. Anyone handling the powder or therapeutic solution should wear disposable gloves. To make the therapeutic 30 ppm solution of chloramphenicol, see Box 25-3.

Florfenicol

Florfenicol has effectiveness similar to chloramphenicol but without the proven risk of aplastic anemia. One study demonstrated it was stable for at least 10 days in fresh water. It also concluded that florfenicol at 10 ppm significantly reduced the chytrid load but did not clear chytrid entirely; toxic effects developed at 100 ppm. The author commonly uses it at 30 ppm. It appears to be empirically effective and safe at this concentration; further work should be done to determine whether 30 to 50 ppm is truly safe and effective.

Voriconazole

Voriconazole at 1.25 mcg/mL appeared safe and eliminated chytrid used as a spray on midwife toads and dendrobatid frogs. It also appears to be stable in water for at least 7 days. A 12.5 mcg/mL solution appeared to be safe and effective.

Amphotericin B

Amphotericin B kills chytrid zoospores within 30 min at 0.8 mcg/mL but had toxic side effects in midwife toads.

SUGESTIONS FOR ELIMINATING CHYTRID FROM THE ENVIRONMENT

Disinfectants

Where appropriate, a cage may be broken down and disinfected with many readily available disinfectants (e.g., chlorine bleach or full strength ammonia). Tools should be similarly disinfected between cages. Live plants may be dug up, bare-rooted, and bathed in the same antifungal solutions used for amphibians.

Temperature Elevation

Chytrid is heat sensitive and will not reproduce or survive when the environmental temperature is 27°C to 37°C or higher for 16 hours a day. This is an effective way to treat a cage containing live plants; however, not all plants will tolerate these temperatures. Some amphibian species may be left in their cages during heat treatment and may be cured of their chytrid infections, but others that cannot tolerate the high temperatures should be moved to other cages for medical treatments.

Reintroduction of chytrid should be prevented. New cage furnishings such as rocks, soil, bark, and dead leaves may be heated to temperatures of 45°C for 60 minutes. Live plants should have all soil removed from the roots, and the plants should be rinsed well in fresh water, followed by a bath in the same antifungal solution used for amphibians. Plants species that survive 98°F (37°C) may be kept at that temperature for at least 16 hours in place of antifungal baths.

Many invertebrates such as earthworms, *Daphnia*, springtails, and crickets may briefly carry chytrid spores. Aquatic and semiaquatic invertebrates may be rinsed in fresh water, followed by a bath in the same antifungal solution used for amphibians. Crickets will survive 90°F to 98°F (30°C to 37°C) when provided sufficient drinking water and moist foods. Fruit flies should not need any special treatment if they have been raised on aseptic media. Some invertebrates are difficult to treat because of their size (springtails) or fragility (white worms). It is important to recognize that live food is a potential source of reintroduction of chytrid; therefore long-term monitoring for chytrid is appropriate in large amphibian collections

Prevention of Fatal Electrolyte Imbalance

To prevent fatal electrolyte imbalances (e.g., hyponatremia, hypokalemia, hypochloremia, and hypomagnesemia) or restore levels to normal ranges, see Box 25-4.

BOX 25-4 PREVENTION OF FATAL ELECTROLYTE IMBALANCES

- Place in a continuous bath of modified amphibian Ringer's solution (ARS) with added magnesium.
  - 1 L distilled water with 6.6 g NaCl, 0.42 g KCl, 0.15 g CaCl2, 0.2 g NaHCO3, 0.2 g $MgSO_4$
  - It may be stored for up to 7 days or longer if the solution can be autoclaved and stored in sterile containers.
- Intracoelomic therapy may use the sterilized modified ARS at a rate of 0.05 mL per g body weight daily.
- Amphibians with erythema and hyperkeratosis may need both an enriched oxygen environment to support cutaneous respiration and antibiotics to prevent secondary infection with bacteria and other pathogens.
- Address underlying malnutrition such as hypovitaminosis A. Give vitamin A at a dose of 1 IU/g by mouth daily or intracoelomically for 7 days with adjustment of diet.
- Reduce stocking density. Most amphibian patients do best kept alone. Stress may be further reduced with minimal handling or observation other than what is essential for treatment.

SUGGESTED READINGS

Brannelly LA, Richards-Zawacki CL, Pessier AP. Clinical trials with itraconazole as a treatment for chytrid fungal infections in amphibians. *Dis Aquat Organ* 2012;101:95.

Chatfield M, Richards-Zawacki C. Elevated temperature as a treatment for *Batrachochytrium dendrobatidis* infection in captive frogs. *Dis Aquat Organ* 2011;94:235-238.

Geiger CC, Küpfer E, Schär S, et al. Elevated temperature clears chytrid fungus infections from tadpoles of the midwife toad, *Alytes obstetricans*. *Amphibia-Reptilia* 2011;32:276-280.

Hanlon SM, Kerby JL, Parris MJ. Unlikely remedy: fungicide clears infection from pathogenic fungus in larval southern leopard frogs (*Lithobates sphenocephalus*). *PloS One* 2012;7:e43573.

Jones MEB, Paddock D, Bender L, et al. Treatment of chytridiomycosis with reduced-dose itraconazole. *Dis Aquat Organ* 2012;99:243-249.

Martel A, Van Rooij P, Vercauteren G, et al. Developing a safe antifungal treatment protocol to eliminate *Batrachochytrium dendrobatidis* from amphibians. *Med Mycol* 2011;49:143-149.

Muijsers M, Martel A, Van Rooij P, et al. Antibacterial therapeutics for the treatment of chytrid infection in amphibians: Columbus's egg? *BMC Vet Res* 2012;8:175.

Peterson JD. Physiological effects of chytridiomycosis, a cause of amphibian population declines. Dissertation. Auburn University, Alabama, 2012.

Stockwell MP, Clulow J, Mahony MJ. Sodium chloride inhibits the growth and infective capacity of the amphibian chytrid fungus and increases host survival rates. *PloS One* 2012;7:e36942.

Woodhams DC, Geiger CC, Reinert LK, et al. Treatment of amphibians infected with chytrid fungus: learning from failed trials with itraconazole, antimicrobial peptides, bacteria, and heat therapy. *Dis Aquat Organ* 2012;98:11.

Young S, Speare R, Berger L, et al. Chloramphenicol with fluid and electrolyte therapy cures terminally ill green tree frogs (*Litoria caerulea*) with chytridiomycosis. *J Zoo Wildl Med* 2012;43:330-337.

NEMATODIASIS

Parasitic nematodes are ubiquitous in amphibian collections. It is important that a discussion take place between the veterinarian and the client to understand the purpose of captive amphibians and to develop a preventive health program based on an assessment of the health risk posed by nematodes and the potential impact their presence may have on management (e.g., exchanging specimens with other collections). A particularly thorny issue is the presence of nematodes in amphibians destined for assurance colonies. These amphibians are genetic reservoirs against extinctions in the wild, and they arrive with a spectrum of parasites that they shared with their natural environments. The host–parasite–environment triangle shifts in captivity for a variety of reasons, many of which are incompletely understood. Is it the best management choice to eliminate these parasites in captive specimens, thereby possibly artificially selecting for amphibians that have immune systems that have never encountered these nematodes when their offspring may one day be reintroduced into the wild and have to face these same parasites?

In many cases, amphibians appear to be perfectly healthy despite a high number of nematode ova or larvae being found regularly in their feces (Figures 25-8, 25-9, and 25-10). It is possible that prolonged rigorous anthelmintic treatments and associated sanitation and hygiene management may have caused some amphibians to decline and die.

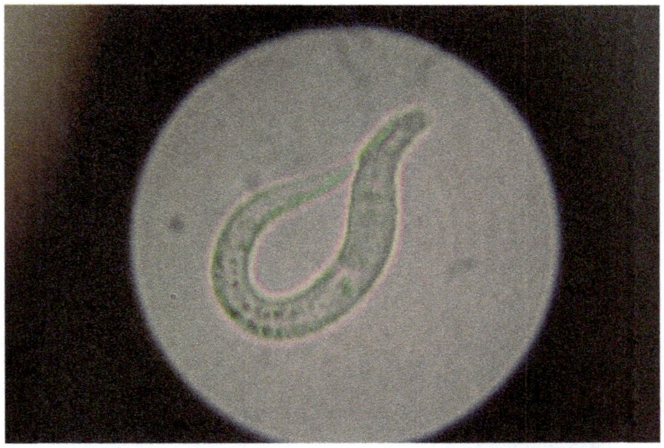

FIGURE 25-8 Strongyle larva from a Fire-bellied Toad *(Bombina bombina)*.

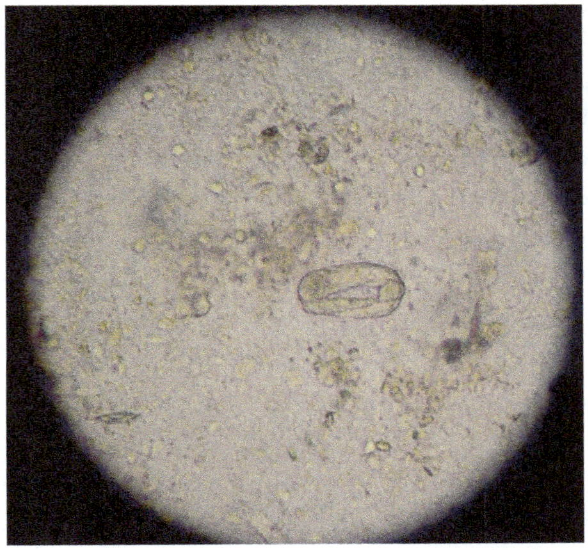

FIGURE 25-9 Embryonated strongyle ovum from a Fire-bellied Toad *(Bombina bombina)*.

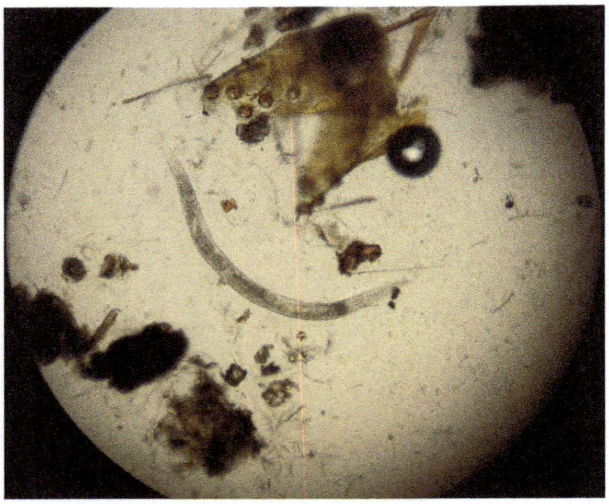

FIGURE 25-10 Gravid female mature strongyle from a White's Tree Frog *(Litoria caerulea)*.

BOX 25-5 MANAGEMENT OF AN AMPHIBIAN WITH AN ACTIVE ILLNESS ASSOCIATED WITH NEMATODIASIS

- Reduce or eliminate the nematode load in the amphibian.
- Provide a "hot spot" so that the amphibian may thermoregulate to optimize its immune response to the nematodes; a temperature of at least 30°C is needed. Providing a localized warmer temperature (35°C to 37°C) may improve chances of survival.
- No single agent has been shown to completely eliminate nematodes in vivo and still be safe for use in all life stages of all species of amphibians. Larvae and recent metamorphs may become stunted or die from a treatment regimen that is without clinically detected deleterious effects in older specimens of the same species. Caution is urged when any treatment is administered in a new species or even a new population of a species, as well as when it is applied to a different life stage of a population. Where practical, a treatment should be given to a small subset of the patients from a new population or life stage to ensure its safety before all patients from that same cohort undergo treatment.

The author does not recommend treatment for amphibians that are apparently healthy, have a healthy body condition score, are eating well and maintaining or gaining weight, and producing normal feces with few nematode ova or larvae per 100× light microscope field on direct or flotation fecal parasite examinations.

The author does recommend treatment if any of the following situations apply: if any amphibians in the collection appear unthrifty or underweight or are losing weight, if mortalities have occurred with nematodes implicated or if otherwise unexplained mortalities have occurred, or if direct fecal parasite examinations reveal more than 5 to 10 red blood cells (RBCs) or 1 to 5 white blood cells (WBCs) per 100× microscope field along with nematode ova or larvae (Box 25-5).

Pyrantel Pamoate

Pyrantel pamoate is an excellent choice for eliminating nematodes if the amphibian may be orally medicated. A typical dose is 5 to 10 mg/kg PO repeated every 7 days for 28 days. A combination of pyrantel pamoate and praziquantel (Drontal) has been used, and the dosage is determined by the amount of pyrantel pamoate.

Ivermectin

Ivermectin may be applied topically or by bath if an amphibian is too small for oral or injectable administration. A topical dose of 4 mg/kg may be given every 7 days for 28 days. A 60-minute bath in a solution containing 10 mg of ivermectin and 1000 mL of water appears to be effective every 7 days for 28 days. Oral and injectable doses are much lower: 0.4 mg/kg every 7 days for 28 days. When ivermectin needs to be delivered to tiny amphibians, a 0.1 mg/mL compounded solution should be considered.

Fenbendazole

Fenbendazole at 25 to 50 mg/kg PO daily for 3 days and repeated in 14 days is also effective but must be given orally. Leukopenia may occur with prolonged treatment or with overdosage.

Levamisole

Levamisole baths, either a continuous bath of 10 mg/L for 3 days repeated every 14 days or a 1 hour bath at 100 mg/L repeated weekly, are effective for many aquatic amphibians. Flaccid paralysis is a risk associated with this bath, so it should be used with caution in unfamiliar species.

Other management techniques focus on reducing or eliminating the nematode load in the environment. Reduced stocking density, that is, fewer amphibians kept in a cage together, decreases the amount of nematode ova and larvae shed. Disinfectants, anthelmintics, and temperature elevation also reduce the nematode load in an amphibian's environment.

Disinfectants

Where appropriate, a cage may be broken down and disinfected with many readily available disinfectants (e.g., chlorine bleach or full strength ammonia). Tools should be similarly disinfected between cages.

Anthelmintics

If a cage cannot be broken down, amphibians may be moved to temporary quarters and the original enclosure drenched once a week in either 10 mg/L ivermectin or 100 mg/L levamisole. One hour after treatment, the cage should be drenched in fresh water several times to remove residue. The amphibians may then be returned after the rinse.

Temperature Elevation

Some nematodes (L3 larval stage) are heat-sensitive and will not survive when the environmental temperature is higher than 45°C for 24 hours. This is an effective way to treat a cage containing live plants, but not all plants will tolerate these temperatures. Reintroduction of nematodes should be prevented. New cage furnishings such as rocks, soil, bark, and dead leaves may be heated to temperatures of 65°C for 60 minutes. Live plants should have all soil removed from their roots, and the plants should be rinsed well in fresh water, followed by a levamisole or ivermectin bath. Plant species that survive 45°C may be kept at that temperature for at least 24 hours in place of anthelmintic baths.

BOX 25-6 MANAGEMENT OF AN AMPHIBIAN WITH AN ACTIVE ILLNESS ASSOCIATED WITH HYPERLIPIDEMIA

- **Reduce caloric intake:** An adult White's Tree Frog *(Litoria caerulea)* needs approximately four to six adult crickets per week to maintain a healthy body condition score. As a general rule, do not feed rodents or goldfish to amphibians. Crickets and mealworms should be maintained on low-fat diets such as vegetables and whole grain products rather than high cholesterol diets such as kibbled dog food.
- **Increase caloric burning:** Provide basking spots that meet or exceed the upper level of POTZ so that the amphibian can reach higher body temperatures that may help mobilize lipid deposits. Provide exercise opportunities. Some frogs and salamanders will use "hamster balls" to walk around a room. Swimming is another useful exercise for some amphibians. However, because amphibians do not have a high aerobic scope, exercise periods must be brief to avoid debilitating fatigue.
- **Reduce inflammation:** NSAIDs such as meloxicam (1 mg/kg PO every 24 h) may reduce inflammation associated with xanthomas.
- **Nutriceuticals:** Vitamin A (1000 IU/kg PO every 7 days) may be appropriate since xanthomas tend to develop in tissue prone to squamous metaplasia. Vitamin E (100 IU/kg PO every 7 days) may reduce the risk of thrombi.
- **Manage quality of life:** It is often difficult to convince a client that it is time to euthanize an amphibian with corneal lipidosis because the animal will still feed, even with both eyes obscured by fat deposits. Some continue to feed with ulcerated bleeding lesions on the surface of the eyes. It is important to emphasize that eating is not a measure of pain for most amphibians. Skin color, posture, and activity better reflect whether an amphibian is in pain. Critical anthropomorphism, in which owners are asked if they would feel comfortable with the same condition, may help some owners come to terms with their amphibian's poor quality of life.

NSAID, Nonsteroidal antiinflammatory drug; *PO,* by mouth; *POTZ,* preferred optimal temperature zone.

It is important to recognize that live food is a potential source of nematode reintroduction; therefore long-term monitoring to detect nematodes is appropriate, even for seemingly healthy amphibians.

The amphibian or cage should be monitored with quarterly direct fecal parasite examinations to detect a shift in cytologic features and fluctuations in nematode ova and larvae. Often, no correlation may exist between a reduction in nematode ova or larvae in feces and an actual reduction in nematode numbers, but improvements in ill amphibians may be seen when the ova or larvae counts decrease and the feces has less than 5 to 10 RBCs/100× field and 1 to 5 WBCs/100× field. The goal is for the amphibian to recover and maintain a healthy weight and body condition score, have normal stool results, and show normal behaviors. With problematic amphibians and their enclosures, more frequent surveillance is appropriate.

SUGGESTED READINGS

Hawley DM, Altizer SM. Disease ecology meets ecological immunology: understanding the links between organismal immunity and infection dynamics in natural populations. *Funct Ecol* 2011;25:48-60.

Kelehear C, Brown GP, Shine R. Influence of lung parasites on the growth rates of free-ranging and captive adult cane toads. *Oecologia* 2011;165:585-592.

Koprivnikar J, Marcogliese DJ, Rohr JR, et al. Macroparasite infections of amphibians: what can they tell us? *Ecohealth* 2012;9:342-360.

Pizzatto L, Shine R. Lungworm infection modifies cardiac response to exercise in cane toads. *J Zool* 2012;287:150-155.

Pizzatto L, Shine R. The effects of experimentally infecting Australian tree frogs with lungworms *(Rhabdias pseudosphaerocephala)* from invasive cane toads. *Int J Parasitol* 2011;41:943-949.

Shaw S, Speare R, Lynn DH, et al. Nematode and ciliate nasal infection in captive Archey's frogs *(Leiopelma archeyi)*. *J Zoo Wildl Med* 2011;42:473-479.

Wiley M, Wu J, Dawson B. A comparison of two treatments for nematode infections in the Túngara frog, *Engystomops pustulosus*. *J Herpetol Med Surg* 2009;19:21-22.

CORNEAL LIPIDOSIS AND HYPERLIPIDEMIA

Captive amphibians may have a lipid storage disorder resulting in hyperlipidemia and some external manifestations such as the accumulation of cholesterol deposits in the corneal tissues. The term *corneal lipidosis* has been used synonymously for the systemic lipid storage disorder called *xanthomatosis,* the deposition of cholesterol-rich deposits in any tissues in the body.

Most amphibians have evolved feeding on prey items with inherently low cholesterol levels. It is likely that the domestic prey species contain higher amounts of cholesterol than wild prey species and may also have a different balance of fatty acids. Amphibians may not be equipped to assimilate and eliminate the excessive levels of lipids of these domestic prey species, so an amphibian that is fed too much (or perhaps the wrong kind of fat) accumulates fat in tissues other than the fatbodies, the normal storage organs for excess fat. With time, calcium deposits may form within these abnormal fat deposits, and inflammation may surround the xanthomas.

Although overfeeding of high-cholesterol items is the obvious trigger for corneal lipidosis, amphibians that are not able to reach the higher temperatures within their preferred optimal temperature zone (POTZ) are also at high risk of corneal lipidosis. Other risk factors include lack of exercise, lack of reproduction, and insufficient turnover of fat stores, either through egg production or mate attracting behaviors. It is possible that hypovitaminosis A may play a role in this disease through its impact on epithelial cell development, but this theory has not been explored. For management of an amphibian with hyperlipidemia, see Box 25-6.

SUGGESTED READINGS

Shilton CM, Smith DA, Crawshaw GJ, et al. Corneal lipid deposition in Cuban tree frogs *(Osteopilus septentrionalis)* and its relationship to serum lipids: an experimental study. *J Zoo Wildl Med* 2001;32:305-319.

Wright K. Cholesterol, corneal lipidosis, and xanthomatosis in amphibians. *Vet Clin North Am Exot Anim Pract* 2003;6:155.

BOX 25-7 MANAGEMENT OF AN AMPHIBIAN WITH PRESUMPTIVE OR CONFIRMED HYPOVITAMINOSIS A

- **Review vitamin supplementation and feeding practices:** This may reveal potential issues, such as offering vitamin-dusted crickets in the day to nocturnally feeding species or holding the vitamins in high humidity or high temperature situations that degrade their potency. The crickets can groom off the vitamins before they are consumed by the amphibians. At present, there is little evidence that adult amphibians have the ability to convert provitamins such as beta-carotene into the active form of vitamin A.
- **Husbandry review with attention to POTZ:** Provide basking spots that meet or exceed the upper level of POTZ so that the amphibian can reach higher body temperatures that may help absorb and utilize lipid-soluble vitamins.
- **Supplement with pure vitamin A:** Natural vitamin A in the form of fresh mouse, rat, or fish liver may be better absorbed than synthetic vitamin A. This may be pureed for assist-feeding if the amphibian cannot be stimulated to eat pieces of the liver. Aquasol A (Mayne Pharma, Paramus, NJ) contains 50,000 USP vitamin A palmitate/mL (which equals 15 mg retinol/mL). Mix 1 mL of this with 9 mL sterile water for a final concentration of 5000 USP units of vitamin A palmitate/mL (or 1.5 mg retinol/mL). Fresh batches should be made daily because it breaks down with warmth and light. A drop, applied topically, from a tuberculin syringe with a 27-gauge needle will contain about 33 IU of vitamin A (or 0.01 mg of retinol). For small amphibians (under 5 g), this gives between 6 and 33 IU vitamin A/g of amphibian per treatment. A drop from a tuberculin syringe with no needle delivers about 200 IU of vitamin A and is recommended for frogs 15 to 30 g of body weight. Severely affected amphibians should be treated daily (1 drop per 10 g body weight) for up to 2 weeks and thereafter every 4 to 7 days. Another possible treatment route is oral administration at a dose not to exceed 1 IU/g orally daily for 2 weeks or until clinical signs resolve. An over-the-counter human grade vitamin A supplement (liquid gel cap) should be used and diluted with liquid vegetable oil to an appropriate concentration; it can be administered orally or topically. The unused diluted vitamin A solution should be discarded, and a fresh batch should be made daily.

POTZ, Preferred optimal temperature zone.

HYPOVITAMINOSIS A

Hypovitaminosis A is an often overlooked disease in captive amphibians. This nutritional disorder was first recognized in captive Wyoming Toads. Many toads raised for release back into the wild appeared unable to prehend their prey. An afflicted toad would sight and target a moving prey animal, such as a live domestic cricket, and then rock forward and flick its tongue out to capture that prey. Often the cricket would walk away from this attack, apparently missed by the tongue flick, something that became known as *short tongue syndrome*. The condition appeared to be acquired (rather than congenital) because clinical signs occurred after the toadlet stage. Juveniles or adult animals slowly worsened over time. Affected toads became completely unable to capture prey.

Pessier (2005) determined that the underlying cause was squamous metaplasia of the mucus glands of the tongue. A healthy toad tongue is coated with a sticky layer of mucus that serves to "glue" a prey item to the tongue and hold the prey as the tongue is retracted into the mouth. Postmortem liver analysis revealed that these toads had low to undetectable levels of vitamin A. Several other amphibians have been noted with lingual squamous metaplasia. Squamous metaplasia has also been noted in the urinary bladder and kidney. Hypovitaminosis A is associated with an impaired immune system and secondary infections.

Leopard Frogs developed opaque white swellings in the lower eyelid associated with a commercial multivitamin supplement that provided only beta-carotene and no vitamin A. The frogs responded to supplementation with vitamin A and antibiotic treatment. It seems possible, if not likely, that the underlying cause of this lesion is hypovitaminosis A. Similar lesions of the eyelid have been noted in dendrobatid frogs that were unresponsive to antibiotic treatments but that resolved after topical treatment with vitamin A. The ability of amphibians to convert carotenoids to vitamin A is uncertain but appears minimal in many species.

Given the findings of squamous metaplasia in the renal tissue in clinically ill amphibians, it seems possible that hypovitaminosis A may be a contributing factor to the development of renal failure–induced hydrocoelom. Hydrocoelom is a very common clinical sign in ill amphibians.

Hypovitaminosis A is known to interfere with reproduction and is likely associated with reproductive problems encountered in captive amphibians, such as reduced egg hatchability and reduced tadpole survival.

Even multivitamin supplements with sufficient vitamin A (provided as vitamin A and not beta-carotene) at the time the container is opened will lose their potency if the supplement is stored in areas that have high humidity, warm temperatures, or both. A multivitamin supplement should be used within 6 months of breaking the seal on the container. If the supplement is stored improperly, it should be replaced more often. See Chapter 23, Short Tongue Syndrome and Hypovitaminosis A, for a more in-depth discussion on hypovitaminosis A and Box 25-7 for steps in managing an amphibian with clinical signs of hypovitaminosis A.

SUGGESTED READINGS

Baruah P, Goswami UC. In vitro metabolism of carotenoids, β-carotene and lutein into retinoids in amphibians. *J Ecobiotechnol* 2012;4:46-50.

McComb A. Evaluation of vitamin a supplementations for captive amphibian species. Thesis. North Carolina State University, Raleigh, 2010. Available at: http://repository.lib.ncsu.edu/ir/bitstream/1840.16/6567/1/etd.pdf

Ogilvy V, Preziosi RF, Fidgett AL. A brighter future for frogs? The influence of carotenoids on the health, development and reproductive success of the red-eye tree frog. *Anim Conserv* 2012;15:480-488.

Ogilvy V, Fidgett AL, Preziosi RF. Differences in carotenoid accumulation among three feeder-cricket species: implications for carotenoid delivery to captive insectivores. *Zoo Biol* 2012;31:470-478.

Pessier AP, Linn M, Garner MM, et al. Suspected hypovitaminosis A in captive toads (*Bufo* spp.), in Proceedings. *Am Assoc Zoo Vet* 2005;57.

Pessier P. Edematous frogs, urinary tract disease, and disorders of fluid balance in amphibians. *J Exot Pet Med* 2009;18:4-13.

Sim RR, Sullivan KE, Valdes EV, et al. A comparison of oral and topical vitamin A supplementation in African foam-nesting frogs (*Chiromantis xerampelina*). *J Zoo Wildl Med* 2010;41:456-460.

SECTION IV

ADVANCES IN BIOLOGY, CONSERVATION, LAW, AND RESEARCH

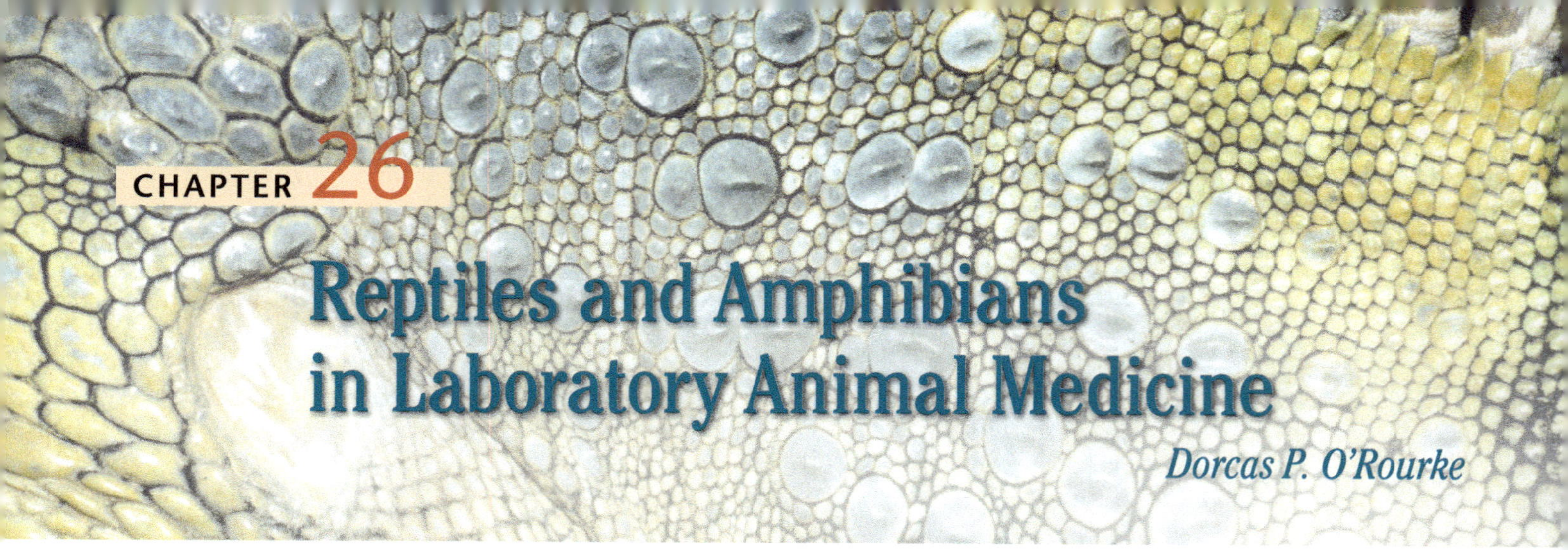

CHAPTER 26

Reptiles and Amphibians in Laboratory Animal Medicine

Dorcas P. O'Rourke

Reptiles and amphibians are found in a wide variety of institutional settings, ranging from corporate biomedical research facilities to veterinary colleges and herpetology teaching collections. Some amphibian species, such as the African Clawed Frog (*Xenopus laevis*) have become so commonplace that entire books are devoted to their husbandry and care in laboratory animal settings.[1] African Clawed Frogs were originally used for pregnancy assays and toxicology research; more recent biomedical uses include oocyte harvesting for molecular biology research and, along with *Xenopus tropicalis*, developmental biology studies. In addition to *Xenopus*, commonly used laboratory species of amphibians include Axolotls (*Ambystoma mexicanum*), American Bullfrogs (*Lithobates catesbeianus*), Leopard Frogs (*Lithobates pipiens*), Tiger Salamanders (*Ambystoma tigrinum*), and Marine Toads (*Bufo marinus*). Axolotls have long been popular as animal models for limb regeneration studies; these have expanded to include cardiac and central nervous system regeneration. Bullfrogs and Leopard Frogs are commonly used in physiology laboratory instruction and in endocrinology, nociception, and infectious disease research. Tiger Salamanders and Marine Toads are used as models for studies involving neurology and ophthalmology. Most recently, wild and captive populations of amphibians have been used in environmental toxicology, endocrine disrupter, and chytridiomycosis investigations.

Reptiles are relatively uncommon in biomedical research institutions but are frequently found in universities. Among reptiles, anoles (Polychrotidae), skinks (Scincidae), and other lizard species are most commonly used for physiology, endocrinology, and behavior studies. Red-eared Sliders (*Trachemys scripta elegans*) and related aquatic species are used in physiology laboratories and for infectious disease research. Snakes are typically found in teaching collections and displays and are also used to study behavior, ecology, and evolution. Biochemistry and medical applications of reptile venom are specific areas of study involving venomous species. Crocodilians are used commonly in biochemistry, physiology, and environmental toxicology research. Both reptiles and amphibians are extensively studied by herpetologists in laboratories and in the field, to better understand their ecology and evolutionary biology.

FUNDING AGENCY REQUIREMENTS

In the 1980s, several federal agencies formed the Interagency Research Animal Committee (IRAC). Members of this group developed and published the U.S. Government Principles for the Utilization and Care of Vertebrate Animals Used in Testing, Research, and Training (U.S. Government Principles). These nine principles address federal laws, research relevance, appropriateness of species and numbers, consideration of alternatives, minimization of pain and distress, appropriate anesthesia, analgesia, and euthanasia, proper housing and veterinary care, personnel qualifications and training, and involvement of an objective body such as an animal care and use committee. Agencies that committed to adhere to these principles when conducting and sponsoring research include the Department of Health and Human Services (including the National Institutes of Health [NIH], Centers for Disease Control [CDC], and Food and Drug Administration [FDA]), the Department of Defense (DoD), Department of Agriculture (USDA), Department of the Interior (DoI), the Environmental Protection Agency (EPA), the National Aeronautics and Space Administration (NASA), and the National Science Foundation (NSF).[2]

Individuals applying for grant funding from NIH and NSF must be from an institution that has a Public Health Service (PHS) Assurance. An institutional PHS Assurance follows the U.S. Government Principles, the Public Health Service Policy on Humane Care and Use of Laboratory Animals (PHS Policy),[3] and the *Guide for the Care and Use of Laboratory Animals* (*Guide*).[4] DoD funding requires compliance with the U.S. Government Principles and the *Guide*; NASA follows NASA Policy, PHS Policy, and the *Guide*; and FDA and EPA require compliance with Good Laboratory Practice regulations for projects focused on drug and product approval. Nonfederal granting agencies may request information on Institutional Animal Care and Use Committee (IACUC) approval or adherence to animal care guidelines on grant applications.[5,6]

Many professional organizations have standards for ethical conduct of research and criteria for publication in scientific journals. The Society for the Study of Amphibians and Reptiles (SSAR) Ethics Statement requires compliance with rules, including obtaining appropriate permits and IACUC approval for publication in the *Journal of Herpetology* and *Herpetological Review*.[7] The American Society of Ichthyologists and Herpetologists requires that IACUC approval be cited in the manuscript when submitting to *Copeia*.[8] The Herpetologists League similarly requires documentation of IACUC approval in the cover letter and manuscript when submitted to *Herpetologica* and *Herpetological Monographs*.[9] All three organizations collaborated on and published guidelines, *Guidelines for Use of Live Amphibians and Reptiles in Field and Laboratory Research*.[10]

Veterinary journals such as the *Journal of the American Veterinary Medical Association*, *American Journal of Veterinary Research*, *Journal of the American Association for Laboratory Animal Science*, and *Comparative Medicine* require compliance with applicable federal regulations and guidelines and evidence of IACUC approval.[11-13] The *Journal of Zoo and Wildlife Medicine* requests a statement of IACUC approval in the cover letter,[14] and the Association of Reptile and Amphibian Veterinarians expects that IACUC approval has been obtained for experimental studies when submitting manuscripts to the *Journal of Herpetological Medicine and Surgery* (Mitchell M: Pers. com., Mar 28, 2012).

If an individual wishes to conduct a study and is not affiliated with a university or other institution, she/he may either be able to obtain an adjunct appointment or collaborate with a faculty member of an institution that has a research program and an IACUC in place.

Regulatory Oversight and Accreditation Guidelines

The USDA requires registration as a research facility if USDA-covered species are used in research and teaching. Registered facilities are subject to at least annual unannounced inspections by veterinary medical officers of the USDA. Significant uncorrected deficiencies in animal care and use programs can ultimately lead to fines and facility closure. At this time, USDA regulations cover only a defined subset of mammals. They are not applicable to reptiles and amphibians and will not be further included in this discussion. The U.S. Government Principles, PHS Policy, and *Guide* are much broader in scope and cover all vertebrate species. A division of NIH, the Office of Laboratory Animal Welfare (OLAW) is charged with overseeing institutional compliance with the U.S. Government Principles, the PHS Policy, and the *Guide*.[15] This is accomplished through several mechanisms, including reviewing and approving an institution's PHS Assurance and conducting visits to the institution, if warranted. Conducting NIH-funded research activities without approval by an IACUC can result in an investigator having to return grant money. In addition to required federal oversight, many universities and research facilities are voluntarily accredited by the Association for the Assessment and Accreditation of Laboratory Animal Care, International (AAALAC). AAALAC requires adherence to all applicable national, regional, and local legislation and uses the *Guide* as one of its three primary resources.[16] AAALAC conducts triennial site visits to accredited institutions to review animal care and use programs.

Federal wildlife and fisheries agencies require permits to conduct research on certain wildlife species; these will be addressed later. State agencies dealing with natural resources, fisheries, and wildlife may also require permits or regulate acquisition and possession of certain species. Local regulations may also apply. When planning research or teaching activities involving reptiles and amphibians, investigators should check federal, state, and local regulatory requirements governing their species of interest.

The Guide for the Care and Use of Laboratory Animals

The *Guide* is used by many institutions when developing and implementing internal policies and procedures for vertebrate animal care and use. Although the term *laboratory animal* appears somewhat misleading, the *Guide* is careful to clearly define laboratory animals as all vertebrates used in research, teaching, and testing.[17] The most recent edition of the *Guide* specifically addresses husbandry and care of aquatic species in research settings. It further explains that while it does not specifically discuss wildlife and aquatic species in natural settings, it does provide ethical considerations and general principles that are equally relevant to these circumstances.[17]

Performance standards are an integral component of the *Guide*. The *Guide* provides basic standards for animal care and use programs and establishes desired outcomes but allows institutions flexibility in how they achieve those outcomes. For example, air exchange rates in animal rooms must be sufficient to prevent accumulation of excess humidity and ammonia, which is a respiratory irritant. Therefore, typical air exchange rates are 10 to 15 air changes per hour. However, species such as reptiles and amphibians with slower metabolic rates and less waste production do not generally require the same rapid turnover of room air; in fact, air exchanges that are too rapid can desiccate species that require high humidity. Consequently, rooms with lower air exchange rates may be preferred for these species and can be appropriately justified through the use of these performance standards.

Institutional Animal Care and Use Committee

The aforementioned regulations and guidelines all require animal care and use program oversight by a body such as an IACUC. For PHS-assured institutions, there must be at least five members on the IACUC. Membership must include a laboratory animal veterinarian, a practicing scientist, a nonscientist, and a community member with no institutional affiliation.[18] Animal care programs with reptiles and amphibians often find it advantageous to appoint IACUC members with experience in these groups of vertebrates. An alternative approach is to utilize consultants with expertise in the species being reviewed; these individuals can often provide valuable information that will enable the IACUC to make sound decisions on proposed animal use.

The IACUC is charged with several important functions, including review of the animal care and use program at least every 6 months.[19] Components of this review include evaluation of the institution's training program for researchers and research staff, animal care personnel, and the IACUC itself; the occupational health and safety program; the veterinary care program; security and disaster plan; deviations from standards in the *Guide*; and mechanisms for reporting concerns about animal welfare.

Collaborations between researchers at institutions are becoming quite common and can create some challenges for IACUCs. Whenever collaborations across institutions occur, there should be a formal written agreement addressing the responsibilities for oversight and IACUC review.[20] These agreements help eliminate ambiguity and reduce redundancy in oversight.

Another IACUC responsibility is inspecting animal facilities and use areas every 6 months. Although inspection of animal housing areas, surgery and procedure areas, and research laboratories is relatively straightforward, accessing remote field stations and research sites can be difficult (Figure 26-1). Accessibility is further complicated by the seasonality of field

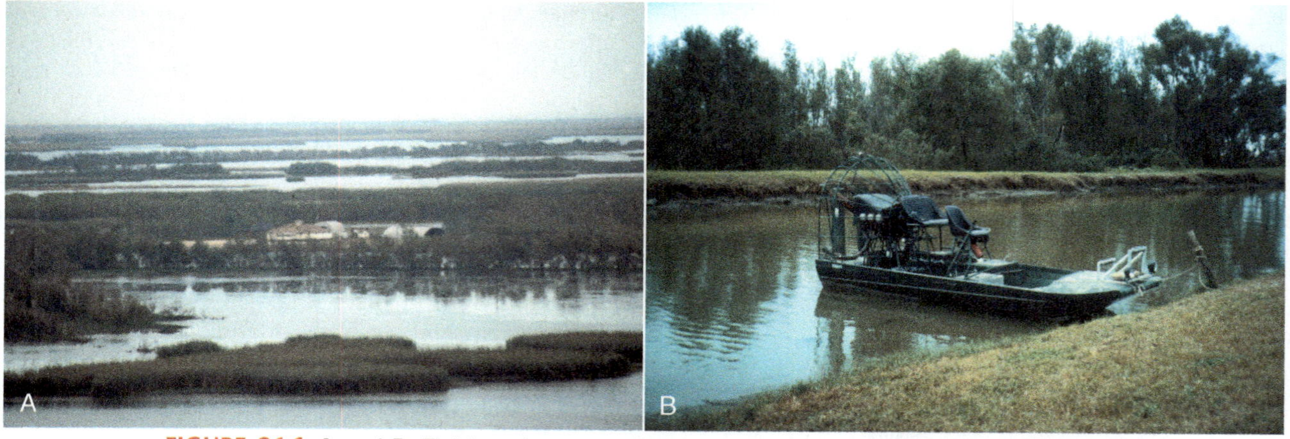

FIGURE 26-1 **A and B, Field stations are often located at remote sites and require specialized transportation, making them difficult for the Institutional Animal Care and Use Committee (IACUC) to access.**

work. One solution for evaluating field research is for the IACUC to request videos or photographs of procedures conducted during the field season.

The IACUC must review all proposals for research, teaching, and testing involving vertebrate animals and also must review any proposed changes to approved ongoing activities. No work may begin until protocols and amendments are fully approved by the IACUC. When submitting protocols for consideration by the IACUC, investigators should realize that the content contained in many of the questions is information required by federal regulations and guidelines. This includes rationale and purpose of the animal use; justification of species and animal numbers (statistically justified if appropriate); consideration of the impact on animal well-being and availability of alternatives; assurance that the work is not unnecessarily duplicative; provision of information confirming appropriate training and experience with proposed procedures and species; identification of hazards and methods to minimize risk; description of animal procedures in nontechnical language; provision of information on atypical housing and husbandry; detailed description of anesthesia, analgesia, surgical and other procedures, and postprocedural care; provision of criteria for intervention and rationale for selected endpoints; and description of euthanasia or other disposition of animals.[21] Euthanasia methods must be consistent with the American Veterinary Medical Association (AVMA) Guidelines for the Euthanasia of Animals.[22] The IACUC is required to carefully consider experimental endpoints and humane endpoints and to determine a method of dealing with unexpected outcomes.[23]

Certain procedures demand intense scrutiny by the IACUC and are typically covered in significant detail in protocols. These include prolonged restraint, multiple survival surgery procedures, food and fluid restriction or regulation, and use of non–pharmaceutical-grade substances.[24] Use of hypothermia as an anesthetic for reptiles and amphibians remains controversial and continues to be discouraged.[25,26]

Investigators should expect and be prepared to provide specific information and rigorous justification if proposing any of these procedures.

Researchers and instructors submitting protocols involving reptiles and amphibians should be aware of additional items for consideration. Although embryos are not typically covered by the PHS policy, larval forms of amphibians and fish are covered and require a protocol. The use of dead animals or their tissues is not covered unless the animals were killed for the purpose of the collection or if the animals were manipulated before death for the purpose of the study. In those cases, a protocol is required.[27]

Field studies can include a wide range of activities, from capture, identification, and release to invasive sample collection and surgery. Manipulation of animals in the field brings new sets of risk and challenges to both animals and personnel, and these must be addressed in the animal care and use protocol. Investigators are encouraged to consult with professional guidelines when planning field studies.[10]

Methods of capture should be described in detail in the protocol. A description of the capture device or method should be provided, so that IACUC members unfamiliar with it can clearly understand its operation. Live traps must be checked frequently enough to minimize stress and risk from predators to the animals, and any items placed in the trap that increase animal well-being should be included in the description. Site selection should take into account protection from the elements, and methods to prevent inadvertent capture of nontarget species should be provided. Expected mortality rates, adverse effects associated with the capture method, and humane endpoints should also be addressed.

Once reptiles and amphibians are captured, they should be processed as soon as feasible so that stress associated with excess handling is minimized. In some cases, processing requires transportation to a research laboratory, field station, or another site. Animals must be transported in secure containers that prevent escape and injury. During transport, vehicles must have adequate climate control to prevent animals from exposure to temperature extremes. Adequate hydration must also be maintained.

Compared with more traditional laboratory animal species, there are significantly less vendors from which to purchase reptiles and amphibians for research and teaching (*Xenopus* is a notable exception). Vendors providing reptiles and amphibians tend to collect from wild populations, and the condition of animals can be quite variable, depending on the season

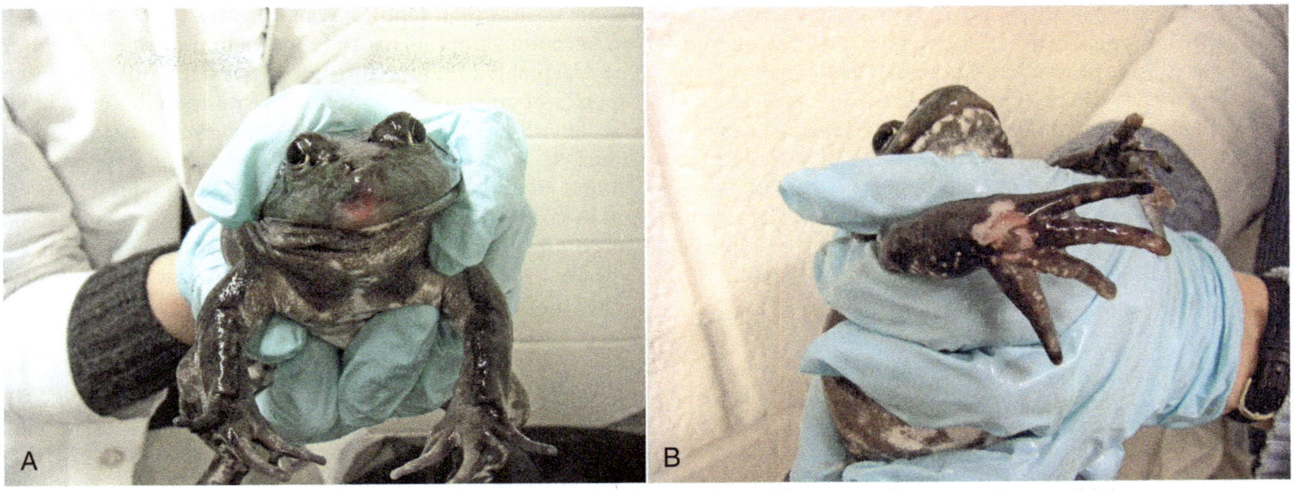

FIGURE 26-2 **A** and **B**, Wild-caught animals purchased from vendors may have widely variable health status.

collected and the holding facilities used (Figure 26-2). If possible, investigators are encouraged to buy purpose-bred animals from reputable vendors, to ensure healthy research subjects and to protect wild populations. If reptiles and amphibians are wild-caught, the investigator is responsible for obtaining all appropriate permits; the IACUC will ask for necessary documentation.

Federal permits may be required for conducting research on reptiles and amphibians. Agencies granting these permits evaluate the risk to the species and population proposed for study and set the criteria for collection, including numbers allowed to be taken. IACUCs may rely on the permitting agency's decision when determining appropriateness of species and numbers. If work is done on federal lands, such as National Park Service land, site-specific permits may be required.[28] Endangered or threatened species of reptiles and amphibians fall under the Endangered Species Act (ESA) and require special permits from the U.S. Fish and Wildlife Service (USFWS); sea turtles require an ESA permit from the National Marine Fisheries Service (NMFS). If endangered species are to be imported or exported, a Convention on International Trade in Endangered Species of Wild Fauna and Flora (CITES) permit is required. CITES permits fall under the authority of the USFWS. State permits may be required in addition to federal permits, and investigators should contact both federal and state agencies for current requirements before protocol preparation and submission.

Occupational health and safety (OHS) concerns must be addressed when research or teaching activities involving reptiles and amphibians is planned. In addition to standard OHS procedures, personnel should be evaluated on the basis of risk and provided appropriate training in relevant zoonoses.[29] They must be instructed in how to correctly use personnel protective equipment when required. Written procedures must be in place for dealing with injuries sustained while handling reptiles and amphibians because bites from large lizards and crocodilians can be severe (Figure 26-3), and toxins secreted from parotid glands of some toad species can be very problematic. Housing and working with venomous reptiles is especially dangerous, and specific standard operating procedures for handling animals and responding to envenomations must be written and followed. Field studies also require attention to incidental hazards, including extreme heat, water, ticks, venomous species, and plant toxins. Investigators should be prepared to respond to IACUC questions regarding both direct and incidental OHS concerns.

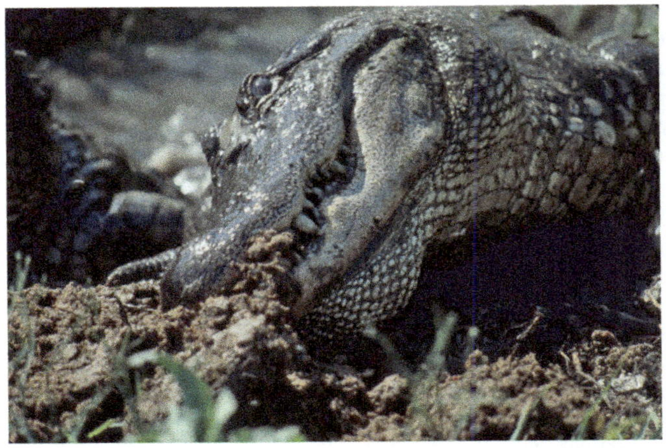

FIGURE 26-3 Bites from large crocodilians can be severe.

Performing procedures in the field brings additional challenges to the researcher. Methods of individual animal identification are more limited than in the laboratory, and some techniques such as toe clipping are controversial.[30,31] Identification methods must be described in detail to the IACUC, and justification must be provided in the protocol for proposed methods that cause pain or impact mobility. Survival surgery must be conducted aseptically; this often requires creative approaches and careful planning when the project is designed. Appropriate anesthesia and analgesia must be provided. Inhalant anesthetic vaporizers designed for laboratory rodents are reasonably easy to transport and set up in field stations. Analgesic selection should be species-appropriate and take into consideration potential drug effects on released animals. Consultation with the institutional veterinarian allows the researcher to plan procedures that address animal welfare in the context of the scientific goals of the study.

Similarly, euthanasia in the field presents a special set of challenges. Drugs typically used for euthanasia such as sodium pentobarbital cannot be used in carcasses left for scavengers. If physical methods such as gunshot are used for large dangerous crocodilians, the investigator must be prepared to provide evidence of both proficiency and safety in use of that method. In addition to the proposed euthanasia method, the investigator must also provide a proposed method for ensuring death. Any deviations from euthanasia methods approved in the AVMA euthanasia guidelines must be rigorously justified to the IACUC in the protocol.

HOUSING AND CARE OF REPTILES AND AMPHIBIANS IN THE LABORATORY ANIMAL FACILITY

The *Guide* contains few specific criteria for housing and caring for reptiles and amphibians. Rather, it relies on the institution's application of performance standards and IACUC approval of those performance standards. Specific information on reptile and amphibian husbandry and care in laboratory animal facilities is available.[32-34] Investigators working with an unfamiliar species should understand the biology and natural history of that species so that they can work with animal care staff to develop appropriate guidelines and provide rationale to justify these care standards to the IACUC.

Reptiles and amphibians should be housed in enclosures that provide a safe, secure, species-appropriate environment (Figure 26-4). Cages should be constructed of materials that are nontoxic and can be sanitized. There must be room enough for the animal to engage in species-appropriate behaviors. Hiding places, visual barriers, and substrates conducive to burrowing are essential for most species, and branches or other perches are required for arboreal animals. Group housing may be appropriate for some species of reptiles and amphibians but contraindicated in territorial or cannibalistic species. Provision of an appropriate humidity level is critical to the health and well-being of the animals. The typical range of 30% to 70% relative humidity maintained in animal facilities may be inappropriate for desert species or tropical rainforest species. Although some amphibians do well in warmer temperatures, many species thrive in much cooler temperatures than reptiles; consequently, it may be ill-advised to keep both amphibians and reptiles in the same room. It may be acceptable to house different species of reptiles or different species of amphibians within the same room because of similar environmental requirements; however, careful attention must be paid to the health status of the animals and availability of satisfactory equipment and techniques to prevent cross-contamination. Provision of thermal gradients, basking sites, and full spectrum lighting may be necessary for some species. Aquatic amphibians require water quality analysis and chlorine and toxin removal, and husbandry records must reflect this. Feed must be used before expiration dates to ensure nutritional quality. If used, live vertebrate prey must be covered in the protocol, and attention must be given to issues of pain, distress, and humane endpoints. For example, the investigator must discuss why humanely euthanized prey cannot be used. Duration of time that the uneaten prey animal is left in the predator's enclosure should be described, as well as disposition of the prey animal once it is removed from the cage. Sanitation methods and intervals will likely differ from the general recommendations in the *Guide*, and the investigator should be able to provide rationale for these variances. Tanks housing aquatic amphibian species with recirculating life support systems and biofilters may require routine partial water changes and excess debris removal but may not require a complete breakdown and sanitation for prolonged periods, provided that appropriate water quality is maintained. Desert species of reptiles that are singly housed may tolerate less frequent cage changes if enclosures do not become excessively soiled. Territorial species of salamanders that scent mark can become stressed if cage changes occur too frequently. In all cases, it is critical to balance the health requirements with the behavioral needs of the species. In semicaptive or outdoor housing, it is important to consider impacts of environmental factors such as temperature excursions and extreme drought or precipitation. Many environments for semicaptive animals provide limited opportunities for escape from inclement weather, and care must be taken to provide extra protection. Similarly, extra effort should be made to exclude predators.

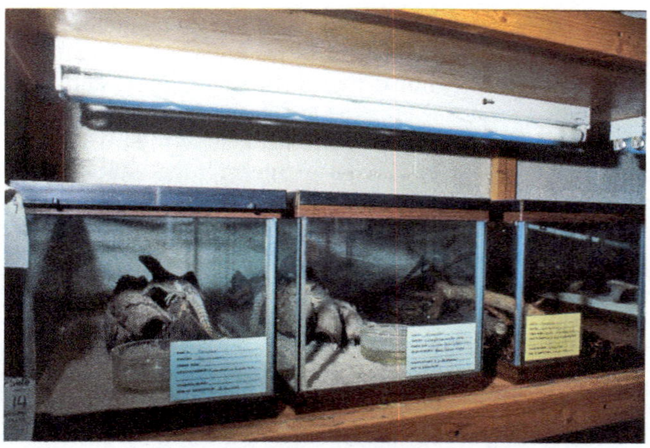

FIGURE 26-4 Reptiles should be housed in a safe, secure, species-appropriate environment.

Institutional veterinarians should have experience with the species housed or must be able to consult specialists who can provide advice and training. There should be appropriate provisions for quarantine of newly arrived animals, isolation of sick animals, routine health surveillance of colonies, facilities and equipment for anesthesia and surgery, and necropsy capabilities. The institutional veterinarian also has responsibility for oversight of other aspects of the program, so researchers should work collaboratively with these individuals when developing and proposing animal care procedures.

CONCLUSION

In summary, investigators interested in submitting proposals for research, teaching, or testing involving reptiles and amphibians should become familiar with federal, state, and institutional requirements, as well as those of granting agencies and professional organizations. Collaborative planning with institutional veterinarians and IACUCs will educate all parties to the species needs and care, as well as the scientific goals, and should facilitate the process of protocol approval.

REFERENCES

1. Green SL. *The laboratory Xenopus sp.* Boca Raton, Fla: CRC Press, 2010.
2. U.S. Interagency Research Animal Committee. US government principles for the utilization and care of vertebrate animals used in testing, research and training. *Fed Reg* 1985;50:97.
3. Office of Laboratory Animal Welfare. *Public health service policy on humane care and use of laboratory animals*. Bethesda, Md: Office of Laboratory Animal Welfare, National Institutes of Health, 2002.
4. Institute for Laboratory Animal Research. *Guide for the care and use of laboratory animals*. 8th ed. Washington, DC: National Academies Press, 2011.
5. Society for the Study of Amphibians and Reptiles Web site. Grants in herpetology guidelines for proposal submission. Available at: http://www.ssarherps.org/pages/GIH.php. Accessed March 27, 2012.
6. Chicago Herpetological Society Web site. Grants. Available at: http://www.chicagoherp.org/index.php?link=grants. Accessed March 27, 2012.
7. Society for the Study of Amphibians and Reptiles Web site. SSAR ethics statement. Available at: http://www.ssarherps.org/pages/ethics.php. Accessed March 27, 2012.
8. American Society of Ichthyology and Herpetology Web site. Instructions to authors. Available at: http://www.asih.org/notice. Accessed March 27, 2012.
9. The Herpetologists' League Web site. Author instructions. Available at: http://www.hljournals.org/page/authors. Accessed March 27, 2012.
10. American Society of Ichthyology and Herpetology Web site. Guidelines for use of live amphibians and reptiles in field and laboratory research. Available at: http://www.asih.org/ASIHLinks. Accessed March 27, 2012.
11. *Journal of the American Veterinary Medical Association* Web site. JAVMA instructions for authors. Available at: https://www.avma.org/News/Journals/Pages/javma-ifa.aspx. Accessed March 27, 2012.
12. *Journal of the American Veterinary Medical Association* Web site. AJVR instructions for authors. Available at: https://www.avma.org/News/Journals/Pages/ajvr-ifa.aspx. Accessed March 27, 2012.
13. American Association for Laboratory Animal Science Web site. AALAS journals info for authors. Available at: http://www.aalas.org/publications/cm_jaalas_info_for_au.aspx. Accessed March 27, 2012.
14. *Journal of Zoo and Wildlife Medicine* Online Submission and Peer Review Web site. Instructions to authors. Available at: http://jzwm.allentrack.net/cgi-bin/main.plex. Accessed March 27, 2012.
15. Office of Laboratory Animal Welfare Web site. Grants and funding. Available at: http://grants.nih.gov/grants/olaw/olaw.htm. Accessed March 29, 2012.
16. Association for the Assessment and Accreditation of Laboratory Animal Care International Web site. Three primary standards. Available at: http://www.aaalac.org/about/guidelines.cfm. Accessed March 29, 2012.
17. Institute for Laboratory Animal Research. *Guide for the care and use of laboratory animals*. 8th ed. Washington, DC: National Academies Press, 2011;2.
18. Office of Laboratory Animal Welfare. *Public health service policy on humane care and use of laboratory animals*. Bethesda, Md: Office of Laboratory Animal Welfare, National Institutes of Health, 2002;11.
19. Office of Laboratory Animal Welfare. *Public health service policy on humane care and use of laboratory animals*. Bethesda, Md: Office of Laboratory Animal Welfare, National Institutes of Health, 2002;12.
20. Institute for Laboratory Animal Research. *Guide for the care and use of laboratory animals*. 8th ed. Washington, DC: National Academies Press, 2011;15.
21. Institute for Laboratory Animal Research. *Guide for the care and use of laboratory animals*. 8th ed. Washington, DC: National Academies Press, 2011;25-26.
22. AVMA Guidelines for the Euthanasia of Animals: 2013 Edition. Available at: www.avma.org/KB/Policies/Documents/euthanasia.pdf. Accessed August 23, 2013.
23. Institute for Laboratory Animal Research. *Guide for the care and use of laboratory animals*. 8th ed. Washington, DC: National Academies Press, 2011;27-29.
24. Institute for Laboratory Animal Research. *Guide for the care and use of laboratory animals*. Eighth ed. Washington, DC: National Academies Press, 2011;29-31.
25. Martin BJ. Evaluation of hypothermia for anesthesia in reptiles and amphibians. *ILAR J* 1995;37:186-190.
26. Green SL. Are post-operative analgesics needed for South African clawed frogs (*Xenopus laevis*) after surgical harvest of oocytes? *Comp Med* 2003;53:12-15.
27. Office of Laboratory Animal Welfare Web site. Frequently asked questions. Available at: http://grants.nih.gov/grants/olaw/faqs.htm. Accessed February 27, 2012.
28. Applied Research Ethics National Association and Office of Laboratory Animal Welfare (OLAW). *Institutional animal care and use committee guidebook*. 2nd ed. Bethesda, Md: OLAW, 2002;199-206.
29. Mitchell MA. Zoonotic diseases associated with reptiles and amphibians: an update. *Vet Clin North Am Exot Anim Pract* 2011;14:439-456.
30. Narayan EJ, Molinia FC, Kindermann C, et al. Urinary corticosterone responses to capture and toe-clipping in the cane toad (*Rhinella marina*) indicate that toe-clipping is a stressor for amphibians. *Gen Comp Endocrinol* 2011;174:238-245.
31. McCarthy MA, Parris KM. Clarifying the effect of toe clipping on frogs with Bayesian statistics. *J Appl Ecol* 2004;41:780-786.
32. O'Rourke DP, Schultz TW. Biology and diseases of amphibians. In: Fox JG, Anderson LC, Loew FM, et al, eds. *Laboratory animal medicine*. 2nd ed. Amsterdam: Academic Press, 2002;793-826.
33. O'Rourke DP, Schumacher J. Biology and diseases of reptiles. In: Fox JG, Anderson LC, Loew FM, et al, eds. *Laboratory animal medicine*. 2nd ed. Amsterdam: Academic Press, 2002;827-861.
34. Association for the Assessment and Accreditation of Laboratory Animal Care International Web site. Council of Europe. Appendix A of the European convention for the protection of vertebrate animals used for experimental and other scientific purposes (ETS NO. 123). Guidelines for accommodation and care of animals (Article 5 of the Convention). 2006. Available at: http://www.aaalac.org/about/guidelines.cfm. Accessed March 30, 2012.

CHAPTER 27

Conservation Issues

Charles J. Innis

VETERINARY CONTRIBUTIONS TO REPTILE CONSERVATION

Veterinarians play an important role in biodiversity conservation.[1] Veterinarians with expertise in the medical management of reptiles have participated in a variety of reptile conservation programs for several decades, and involvement in such programs has increased substantially in the first decade of the twenty-first century. Well-known conservation and recovery programs for species such as Galapagos Tortoises *(Chelonoidis [Geochelone] nigra),* Chinese Alligators *(Alligator sinensis),* and Kemp's Ridley Sea Turtle *(Lepidochelys kempii)* have utilized veterinarians in developing quarantine programs, disease management, pathology investigations, nutritional planning, and more (Figures 27-1 and 27-2).[2-7]

The number of endangered reptile species is increasing, largely because of habitat loss and unsustainable harvesting or incidental mortality associated with human activities.[8-10] In addition, it is likely that for some taxa, climate change, pollution, competition with invasive species, and disease, may also be detrimental.[8] In 2011, the International Union for the Conservation of Nature (IUCN) Red List of Threatened Species categorized 32 turtle species, 6 crocodilian species, and 83 squamate species as critically endangered and 44 turtle species, 1 crocodilian species, and 189 squamate species as endangered.[11] These categories respectively indicate an "extremely high" or "very high" risk of extinction in the wild. Of great concern is the continued decline of many populations despite significant conservation efforts over the past decade.[12] Regardless of numerous conservation activities, threats to many reptile populations remain extremely serious.

BASIC ECOLOGY STUDIES

Implementing effective conservation strategies for any species requires a thorough understanding of its natural history. Data such as population size, home range, fecundity, recruitment, sex ratios, longevity, migratory patterns, and genetic diversity are required. While historically the realm of herpetologists, ecologists, and general biologists, field studies increasingly involve or require veterinary expertise or oversight. Veterinarians have particularly become involved with the surgical implantation or attachment of telemetry devices, passive integrated transponder (PIT or microchip) tagging, laparoscopic reproductive evaluation, oversight of capture events, administration of anesthesia in the field, and assessment of the safety of techniques used by field biologists. Surgical implantation or attachment of radio or satellite transmitters has become a routine part of many reptile ecology studies (Figure 27-3).[13,14] Such transmitters can be used to track the location of the animal over time, and more advanced transmitters can also record temperature or dive depth data. While PIT tags have been used by reptile biologists for some time, recent veterinary observations have led to modification of tag implantation techniques and have highlighted complications seen with PIT tag insertion in certain species and in certain anatomic locations.[15,16] See Chapter 29 for more details.

Laparoscopy and, recently, cystoscopy have been used to determine the sex of immature reptiles so that sex ratios produced under natural or artificial conditions could be assessed (see Chapter 13, Diagnostic Endoscopy.[17-19] This information is especially important for programs that artificially incubate eggs of species that exhibit temperature-dependent sex determination or artificially enhance the survival likelihood of juveniles ("head starting"). Nonlethal early identification of sex may be

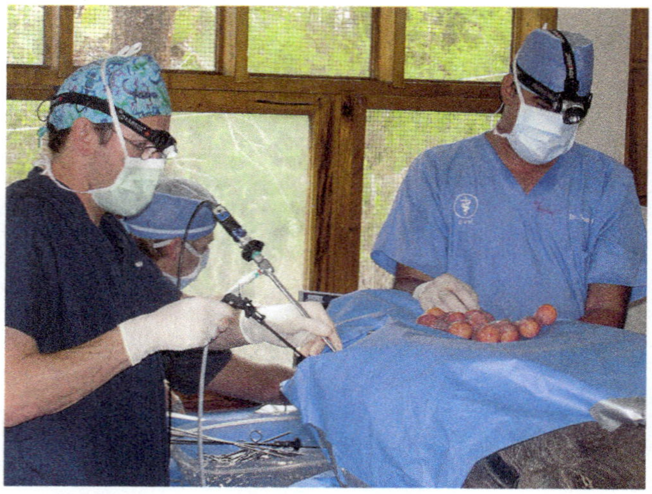

FIGURE 27-1 Drs. Stephen Divers and Sam Rivera performing endoscope-assisted oophroectomy in a Galapagos Tortoise *(Chelonoidis [Geochelone] nigra)* in the Galapagos Islands. This project sterilized genetically hybridized tortoises so that they could be released onto the islands to function as ecologically important large herbivores until genetically pure tortoises can be reestablished. *(Photo courtesy Dr. Joe Flanagan, Houston Zoo, Houston, Tex.)*

important for monitoring the potential effects of global climate change on species for which sex determination is temperature dependent. Laparoscopy has also been used, particularly in sea turtles, for assessment of the reproductive status of subadults and adults as part of population-based reproductive health studies.[20]

Veterinary involvement in field procedures has resulted in the development of safe short-acting anesthetic protocols and has highlighted possible adverse effects of some types of manual restraint.[4,5,21-23] For example, potentially adverse positional effects on intraocular pressures were documented by veterinarians during a Loggerhead Sea Turtle *(Caretta caretta)* laparoscopy study.[23] Blood collection is often required for basic ecology studies, and veterinarians have recently developed position statements on acceptable and unacceptable methods for blood collection from tortoises in the field.[24]

Federal authorities may require a veterinarian to be involved with certain procedures for protected species. For example, in the United States, studies that involve capture and handling of the endangered Leatherback Sea Turtle *(Dermochelys coriacea)* require the presence of a veterinarian for physiological monitoring and emergency resuscitation if adverse events occur (Figure 27-4).[14,25]

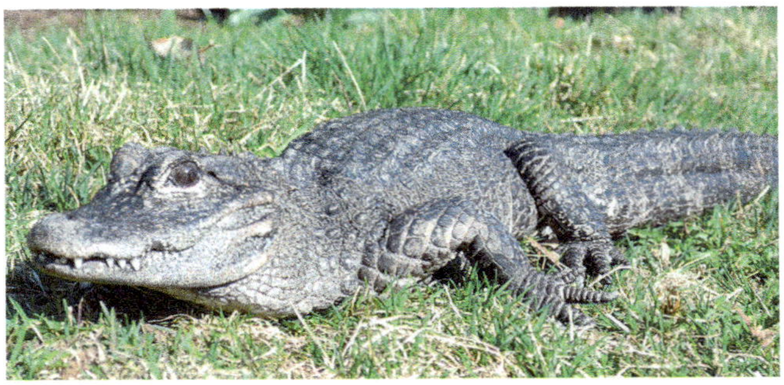

FIGURE 27-2 This Chinese Alligator *(Alligator sinensis)* was hatched as part of a captive breeding program for this rare species. *(Photo courtesy Michael Ralbovsky, Rainforest Reptile Shows, Mass.)*

HEALTH EVALUATION OF REPTILE POPULATIONS

The number of "health assessment" or "health evaluation" studies of "normal" populations of free-ranging reptiles is increasing. It can be debated how to define *normal,* and many reptile populations have already been infiltrated by disease, toxins, and other stressors. Clinical pathologists debate whether these studies are producing baseline data, normal values, reference intervals, or other values. In many cases, the number of animals involved in the study is less than desired for determination of true reference intervals. Nonetheless, these studies seek to characterize various aspects of the health of native reptiles in their natural habitats, often focusing on hematology, plasma biochemistry, fecal parasitology, and serologic evidence of disease exposure. In many cases, these studies provide the only available data for a given species; thus they can be valuable for comparison to clinical data obtained from captive reptiles and for comparison to future data from the same population.[26-31] Health evaluations have highlighted the significant effects of seasonality, sex, age, and stressors on clinical pathology data of reptiles.[14,25,31-33] If free-ranging reptiles are broadly screened, specific abnormalities may be found, which may lead the way to more specific studies.

INFECTIOUS DISEASE RESEARCH

The population decline of North American tortoises of the genus *Gopherus* has been well-documented and is likely due in part to an upper respiratory tract disease caused by *Mycoplasma agassizii.*[34] The identification and characterization of this disease was largely due to the efforts of veterinary professionals and their colleagues.[34] Similarly, much of the characterization of the fibropapilloma syndrome of sea turtles was completed by veterinarians.[33,35] The threat of disease for many reptile populations is unclear, but it is likely that catastrophic population declines could occur due to the introduction of infectious diseases. As such, characterization of infectious diseases of reptiles is critical for reptile conservation, even if only characterized in captive reptiles. Familiarity with etiologic

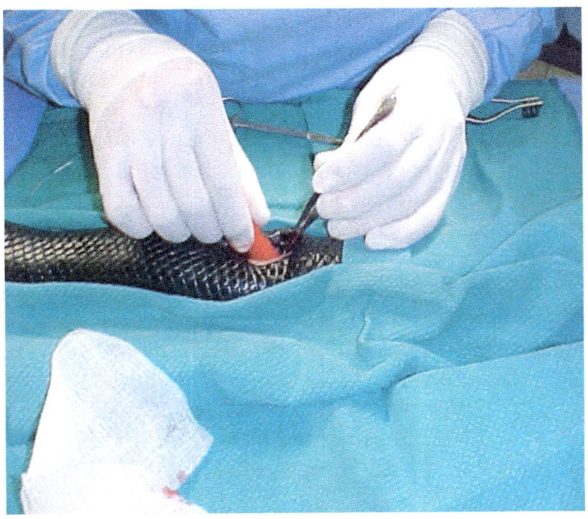

FIGURE 27-3 Radio transmitter implantation into the coelom of an Indigo Snake *(Drymarchon couperi)* in Georgia, United States. *(Photo courtesy Dr. Terry M. Norton, Georgia Sea Turtle Center, Jekyll Island, Ga.)*

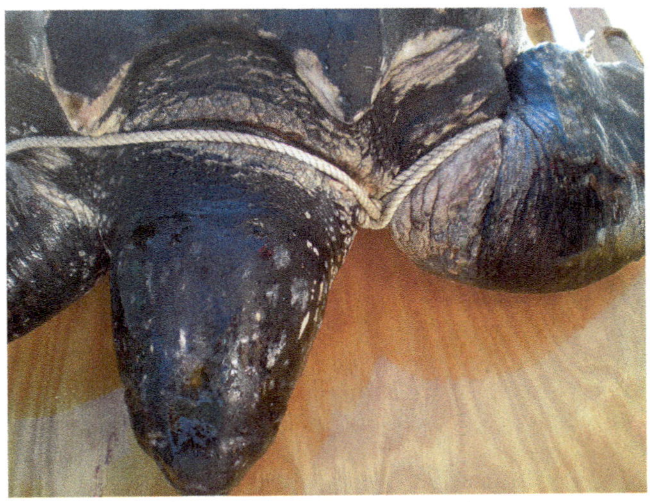

FIGURE 27-4 A live Leatherback Turtle *(Dermochelys coriacea)* evaluated during fisheries gear disentanglement in Massachusetts. *(Photo courtesy Dr. Charles Innis, New England Aquarium, Boston, Mass.)*

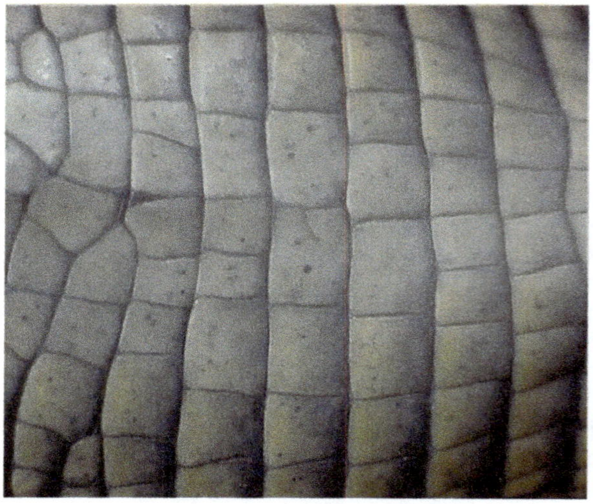

FIGURE 27-5 Typical skin lesions (black dots) seen with West Nile Virus infection of American Alligators *(Alligator mississippiensis). (Photo courtesy Dr. Javier G. Nevarez, Louisiana State University, Baton Rouge, La.)*

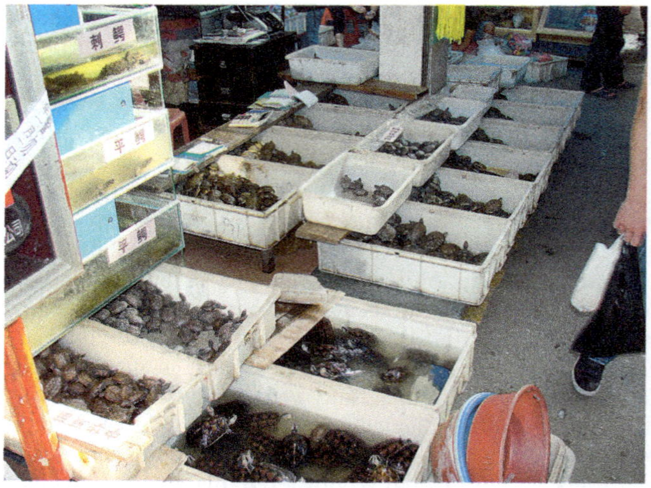

FIGURE 27-6 Live turtle market in Southeast Asia. *(Photo courtesy of Cris Hagen.)*

agents, clinical signs, pathologic lesions, pathogenesis, and diagnostic modalities may expedite the future identification of known pathogens in free-ranging populations and may allow for more rapid characterization of novel pathogens.

In recent years, characterization of iridovirus, adenovirus, herpesvirus, and novel protozoal infections in captive and free-ranging chelonians has provided a great deal of basic data that will be useful for future disease investigations.[36-45] Documentation of West Nile Virus infection in alligators in the United States demonstrated infection of a novel host with an exotic virus (Figure 27-5).[46-48] Such outbreaks should convince those involved with reptile conservation programs that the risk of infectious disease is real, especially for programs involving translocation and repatriation. Animals involved in such programs should be carefully screened for disease by following recommended veterinary protocols.[28,49,50]

ASIAN TURTLE CRISIS

The magnitude of the live turtle trade in Southeast Asia has been widely reported over the past decade.[9] Beginning in the late 1990s, a number of conservation organizations and private individuals began to document the unsustainable consumption of Asian turtles for food and medicinal use. Networks of turtle collectors began to harvest species broadly across Southeast Asia and channel them into large markets in cities such as Hong Kong (Figure 27-6). Among the literally tons of turtles in the trade were a variety of critically endangered species and species previously unknown to science. In some cases, novel species were described from specimens found in food markets, having never been observed in the wild.[51] As species that rely on the longevity of reproductively mature individuals to ensure population survival, turtles are particularly prone to extirpation due to mortality of adults.[52] It became clear that many Asian species were in imminent risk of extinction. In response to this crisis, a number of workshops were held throughout the world, and several alliances and consortiums were created. Since that time, veterinarians have continued to participate in Asian turtle conservation efforts focused on range country programs, ex situ captive breeding, rehabilitation of confiscated specimens, disease description, and education.

Initially, much effort was focused on medical management and rehabilitation of confiscated Asian turtles, for purposes of establishing ex situ "assurance colonies". Many species' husbandry needs were poorly known, and most individuals were seriously ill at the time of confiscation. Attempts to maintain these specimens in captivity often failed because the turtles refused food and succumbed to parasitic and bacterial diseases.[53-56] Soon, however, medical management protocols began to improve the survival rate of these specimens.[53-56] Combined with natural history field studies, this work led to successful treatment, establishment of founder captive populations, and eventual successful breeding of species with historically high mortality rates, such as the Impressed Tortoise *(Manouria impressa)* and the Sulawesi Forest Turtle *(Leucocephalon yuwonoi)* (Figure 27-7).[57-59] Veterinary work with these species also led to descriptions of a number of novel parasites (e.g., *Myxidium hardella*), viral diseases (e.g., Sulawesi tortoise adenovirus-1), and common pathologic findings.[55,56,60,61]

Veterinarians have also helped to establish and implement range country conservation and veterinary education programs in Southeast Asia. These efforts have included provision of clinical care, implementation of quarantine programs, and education of local veterinarians at centers such as Cuc Phuong in Vietnam and Madras Crocodile Bank in India.[62,63] Recently, veterinarians played a critical role in the transport of one of the last living Yangtze Giant Softshell Turtles *(Rafetus swinhoei)* into a captive breeding program in China, and veterinarians continue to be involved in the nutritional, medical, and reproductive management of the last individuals of this species (Figure 27-8).[64,65] Despite these efforts, the outlook for the majority of Asian turtle species is grim. Recent reassessments of these species by the IUCN demonstrate a 90% increase in the number of species listed as Critically Endangered over the past decade.[12]

REPTILES AFFECTED BY OIL SPILLS

In the last 10 years, veterinarians have been involved in medical management of reptiles affected by several major oil

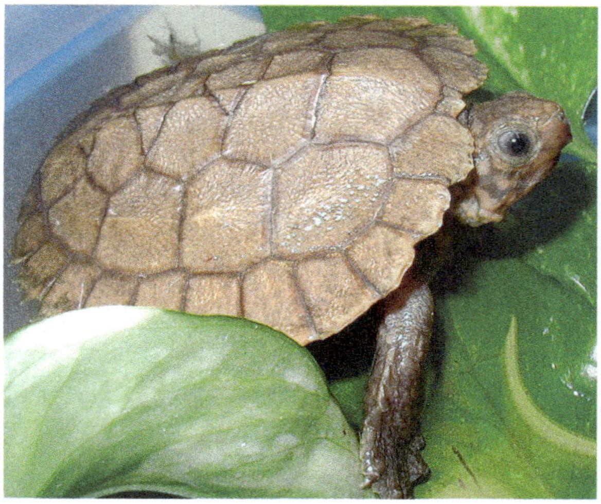

FIGURE 27-7 The first known captive-bred hatchling of the Sulawesi Forest Turtle *(Leucocephalon yuwonoi)*. This hatchling is the offspring of adults salvaged from the Southeast Asian live turtle trade. *(Photo courtesy Dr. Charles Innis, New England Aquarium, Boston, Mass.)*

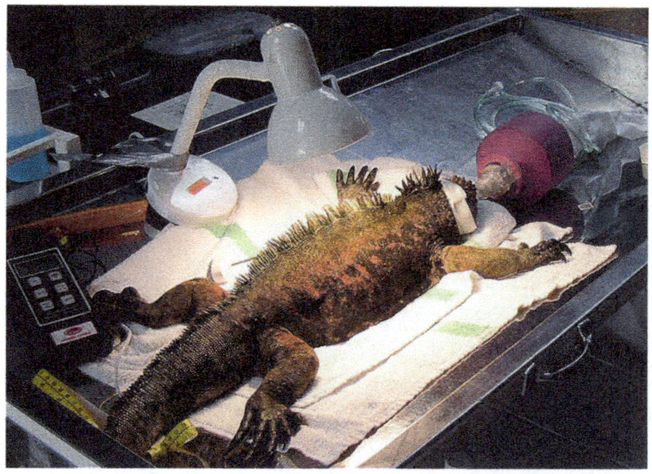

FIGURE 27-9 Galapagos Marine Iguana *(Amblyrhynchus cristatus)* during general anesthesia in the Galapagos Islands. Liver biopsies were performed as part of a post–oil spill health assessment. *(Photo courtesy Dr. Mark Mitchell, University of Illinois, Urbana, Ill.)*

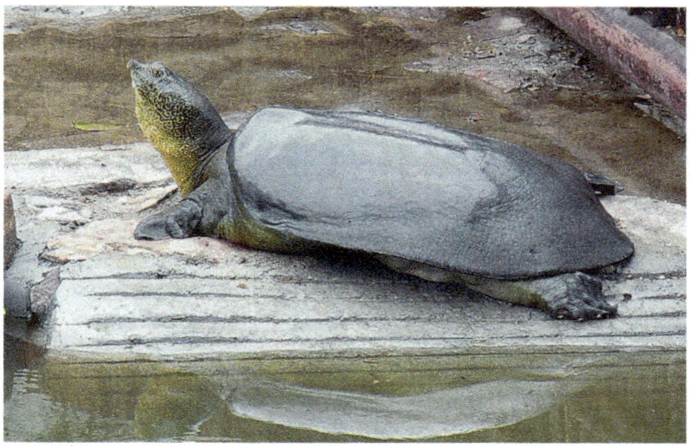

FIGURE 27-8 One of the last living Yangtze Giant Softshell Turtles *(Rafetus swinhoei)*. *(Photo courtesy Dr. Paul P. Calle, Wildlife Conservation Society, Bronx, NY.)*

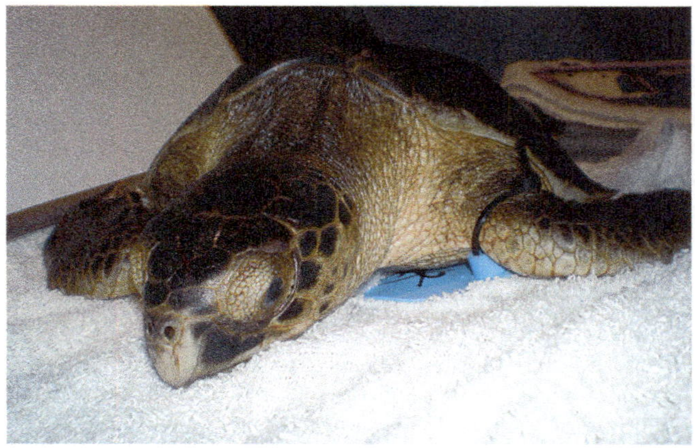

FIGURE 27-10 A Kemp's Ridley Sea Turtle *(Lepidochelys kempii)* undergoing medical evaluation after being recovered at sea during the Deepwater Horizon oil spill in the Gulf of Mexico, 2010. *(Photo courtesy Dr. Charles Innis, New England Aquarium, Boston, Mass.)*

spills. In 2001, a large oil spill in the Galapagos Islands led to the death of 62% of Marine Iguanas *(Amblyrhynchus cristatus)* on one affected island, and veterinarians subsequently became involved with the health assessment of this species (Figure 27-9).[66,67] In 2010, approximately 800,000 gallons of oil were spilled into the Kalamazoo River in Michigan, and approximately 2000 reptiles and amphibians were admitted into rehabilitation.[68] Also in 2010, the massive Deepwater Horizon oil spill in the Gulf of Mexico resulted in contamination of hundreds of endangered sea turtles, including Kemp's Ridley, Loggerhead, Green *(Chelonia mydas)*, and Hawksbill *(Eretmochelys imbricata)* Sea Turtles (Figure 27-10).[69] Although the majority of turtles that were admitted to rehabilitation survived, the number of turtles that died entrapped in oil at sea remains unknown. The most current publicly available data from the Deepwater Horizon oil spill indicate that approximately 90% of turtles that were admitted to rehabilitation were later released.[69] Clinical data obtained by veterinarians during treatment of these oiled turtles are being withheld until legal aspects of the case have been resolved.

COLD-STUNNED SEA TURTLES

Stranding of sea turtles during periods of cold weather *(cold-stunning)* has been reported from several countries.[70-72] In January, 2010, approximately 4500 sea turtles were stranded during a cold-stun event in Florida.[73] While such events inevitably occurred throughout history and may not have represented a threat to large, healthy populations of sea turtles, these events may represent a threat to the depleted sea turtle populations of the twenty-first century. In addition to widespread sea turtle mortality from fishery interactions, nesting beach destruction, harvesting, toxin exposure, and disease, the death of hundreds of sea turtles from cold-stunning likely has a negative impact on the population.

In some geographic areas, cold-stunning events involving the rarest sea turtle species, Kemp's Ridley Sea Turtle, occur annually, often affecting hundreds of turtles and resulting in a more than 50% mortality rate.[70] Over the past 20 years, veterinary protocols for the management of cold-stunned turtles

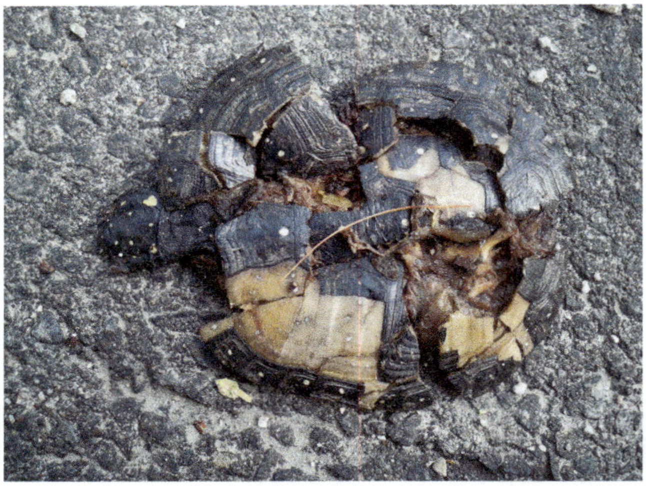

FIGURE 27-11 A Spotted Turtle *(Clemmys guttata)* killed by a vehicle on a Massachusetts road. This once common species has been recently upgraded to Endangered by the International Union for the Conservation of Nature (IUCN). *(Photo courtesy Dr. Charles Innis, New England Aquarium, Boston, Mass.)*

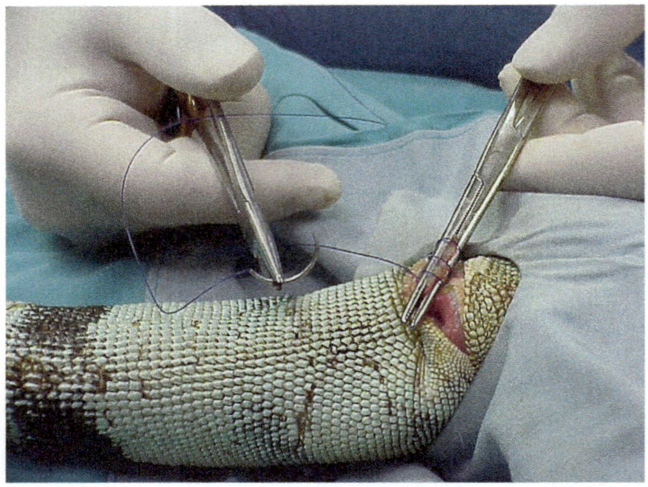

FIGURE 27-12 Phallectomy for sterilization of a feral Green Iguana *(Iguana iguana)* in south Florida. *(Photo courtesy Dr. Douglas R. Mader, Marathon Veterinary Hospital, Marathon, Fla.)*

have emerged, and a relatively high survival rate has been achieved.[74] Data from these events have helped to document the adverse physiologic and common pathologic findings in cold-stunned sea turtles and have provided prognostic information for the assessment of individual animals.[75-81]

WILDLIFE REHABILITATION

Wildlife rehabilitation centers throughout the world provide care for injured reptiles. Although snakes, crocodilians, and lizards are occasionally seen, the majority of reptiles presented to wildlife rehabilitators are turtles. The number of turtles that are injured by vehicles each year globally is beyond estimation. Locally, thousands of turtles and other reptiles can be killed adjacent to a single wetland in a single year (Figure 27-11).[82] Marine turtles are often injured by boats, caught in fishing gear, or affected by neurologic syndromes of unknown etiology.[14,83-86] In some cases, injured and ill reptiles can be successfully treated and released to the wild. A "turtle team" has been established at one U.S. veterinary school to provide students with early exposure to clinical case management of injured native reptiles.[87]

In addition to providing clinical care, wildlife rehabilitation centers can play an important role in reptile conservation through documenting locality data of rare native species, investigating local disease outbreaks, hatching eggs recovered from road-killed females, and educating the public about risks to local native species. Veterinarians with expertise in wildlife rehabilitation have assisted in the development of triage guidelines and injury assessment protocols for several reptile species.[88,89]

INVASIVE SPECIES

Global commerce has led to the purposeful and accidental movement of reptiles to localities far from their native ranges. In some cases, these new localities provide a favorable environment for establishment of breeding populations. Such introductions have been especially damaging for island environments, where native species are often unable to compete with aggressive introduced species. The introduction of the Brown Tree Snake (*Boiga irregularis*) to Guam and other Pacific islands has been devastating for many bird species, as well as native reptiles.[90]

In south Florida, Monitor Lizards, Green Iguanas, pythons, and many other reptiles have been introduced.[91,92] The North American Red-eared Slider (*Trachemys scripta elegans*) has been introduced to many other continents.[93] The impact of these species is not yet well-defined but is subject to heated debate. Veterinarians have become involved in these situations to develop sterilization strategies, provide testimony in legal and political venues, assess disease risk, and determine likelihood of range expansions (Figure 27-12).[94,95] Some studies have demonstrated transmission of parasites between native and invasive reptile species.[93,96] See Chapter 28, Invasive and Introduced Reptiles and Amphibians for more details.

ENVIRONMENTAL TOXICOLOGY

In collaboration with toxicologists, endocrinologists, and other colleagues, veterinarians have demonstrated exposures of free-ranging reptiles to heavy metals, pesticides, and other toxic chemicals. High levels of such contaminants have been found in many species, and recent data demonstrate significant correlations between contaminant concentrations, immune function, and hematologic and biochemical variables.[97-99] Further research is needed to document the mechanisms for these correlations, sources of contaminants, and as yet undescribed effects.

GENERAL VETERINARY MANAGEMENT OF CAPTIVE REPTILES

Although not immediately apparent, general veterinary care for captive reptiles contributes to reptile conservation. In thousands of zoos, aquaria, and nature centers around the world, healthy captive reptiles act as ambassadors for their species.

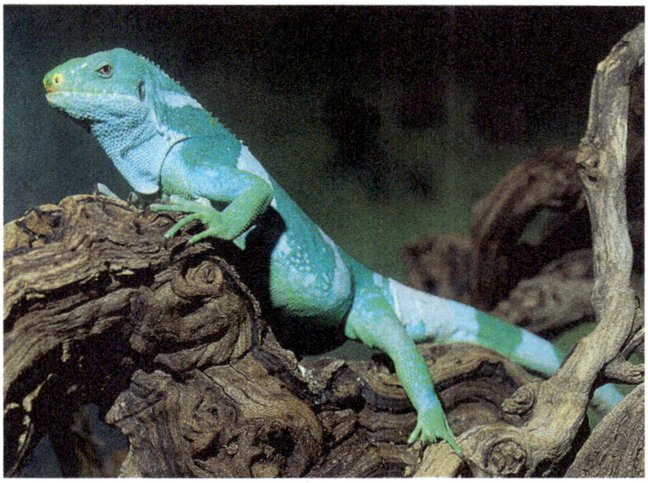

FIGURE 27-13 An endangered Fiji Iguana *(Brachylophus fasciatus)* in a captive breeding facility in the United States. *(Photo courtesy San Diego Zoo Global, San Diego, Calif.)*

In an increasingly urbanized world, these animals may provide the only exposure of humans to live reptiles. Such experiences can be quite profound, and their importance in fostering environmental stewardship, particularly for children, should not be discounted. On a larger scale, veterinary management of captive individuals in zoos and aquaria has been important for the establishment and maintenance of captive breeding programs for endangered species such as the Fiji Banded Iguana (*Brachylophus fasciatus*) (Figure 27-13).[100,101]

ADVERSE EFFECTS OF GOOD INTENTIONS

Well-intentioned programs and well-intentioned individuals can have potential adverse effects. Veterinarians are in a strong position to prevent such problems. By providing leadership in the realms of quarantine and disease risk, veterinarians can reduce the likelihood of adverse effects. Well-intentioned individuals may not, at first, recognize that untreated waste water from an exotic turtle breeding facility could present an infectious disease risk to local native turtles. They may not realize that native snakes for a head start program should not be raised in the same facility as nonnative snakes. It is critical for veterinarians to provide information and advice in such cases.

THE ROLE OF PRIVATE VETERINARY PRACTITIONERS

While often considered the realm of zoo, aquarium, or university veterinarians, reptile conservation can be greatly enhanced by private practitioners. Much of the work cited herein was conducted in part or entirely by private practitioners. It is realistic that a reptile with a previously unknown disease will be seen at any private practice on any given day. It is possible that a turtle presented to a private practice after being found on a local road is, in fact, an endangered species from a previously unknown population. It is possible that veterinary care provided by a private practitioner will allow a local reptile education program to inspire the next generation of reptile conservationists. It is possible that a new technique developed in private practice may have wider application in the realm of reptile conservation. For example, the laparoscopic-assisted oophorectomy technique that was recently used to sterilize hybrid Galapagos Tortoises for an in situ ecologic recovery project was originally developed in private practice for management of pet turtle reproductive disorders.[4,102] It is clear that many of the advances in clinical management of reptiles over the past 40 years were made by private practitioners that took the time to thoroughly document their work, teach veterinary students and other veterinarians, and publish their findings.[103]

REFERENCES

1. Mainka SA. The veterinarian's role in biodiversity conservation. *J Zoo Wildl Med* 2001;32:165-167.
2. Jacobson ER, Rostal DC, Lance VA, et al. Temperature dependent sex determination in chelonians and studies with neonate captive hatched and reared Hood Island Galapagos tortoises, *Geochelone nigra hoodensis*, in *Proceedings*. 6th Annu Conf Assoc Rept Amphib Vet 1999;87-90.
3. Flanagan J. Vets and conservation: helping to restore the balance. *Vet Rec* 2011;168:45-46.
4. Knafo SE, Divers SJ, Rivera S, et al. Sterilisation of hybrid Galapagos tortoises *(Geochelone nigra)* for island restoration. Part 1: endoscopic oophorectomy of females under ketamine-medetomidine anaesthesia. *Vet Rec* 2011;168:47-51.
5. Rivera S, Divers SJ, Knafo SE, et al. Sterilisation of hybrid Galapagos tortoises *(Geochelone nigra)* for island restoration. Part 2: phallectomy of males under intrathecal anaesthesia with lidocaine. *Vet Rec* 2011;168:78-81.
6. Rafael B. Health component of Chinese alligator *(Alligator sinensis)* reintroductions, in *Proceedings*. 13th Annu Conf Assoc Rept Amphib Vet 2006;50-51.
7. Leong JK, Smith DL, Revera DB, et al. Health care and diseases of captive-reared loggerhead and Kemp's ridley sea turtles, in *Proceedings*. 1st Int Symp Kemp's Ridley Sea Turtle Biol Cons Manage 1998;178-201.
8. Whitfield J, Scott DE, Ryan TJ, et al. The global decline of reptiles, déjà vu amphibians. *Bioscience* 2000;50:653-666.
9. Cheung SM, Dudgeon D. Quantifying the Asian turtle crisis: market surveys in southern China, 2000-2003. *Aquat Conserv Marine Freshwat Ecosyst* 2006;16:751-770.
10. Zhou Z, Jiang Z. International trade status and crisis for snake species in China. *Cons Biol* 2004;18:1386-1394
11. IUCN Web site. IUCN red list of threatened species. Version 2011.1. Available at: www.iucnredlist.org. Accessed October 1, 2011.
12. van Dijk PP. IUCN red list documents continuing decline of turtles. *Turtle Survival* 2011:32-33.
13. Hyslop NL, Meyers JM, Cooper RJ, et al. Survival of radio-implanted *Drymarchon couperi* (eastern indigo snake) in relation to body size and sex. *Herpetologica* 2009;65;199-206.
14. Innis C J, Merigo C, Dodge K, et al. Health evaluation of leatherback turtles *(Dermochelys coriacea)* in the northwestern Atlantic during direct capture and fisheries gear disentanglement. *Chelon Cons Biol* 2010;9:205-222.
15. Wyneken J, Epperly SP, Higgins B, et al. PIT tag migration in seaturtle flippers. *Herpetol Rev* 2010;41:448-454.
16. Gál L. Complications of microchip implantation in tortoises. *Emys* 2007;13:6-11.
17. Ligon DB, Lovern MB. Temperature effects during early life stages of the alligator snapping turtle *(Macrochelys temminckii)*. *Chelon Cons Biol* 2009;8:74-83.
18. Hernandez-Divers SJ, Stahl S, Farrell R. An endoscopic method for identifying sex of hatchling Chinese box turtles and comparison of general versus local anesthesia for laparoscopy. *J Am Vet Med Assoc* 2009;234:800-804.

19. Selleri P, DiGirolamo N, Melidone R. Cystoscopic sex identification of posthatchling chelonians. *J Am Vet Med Assoc* 2013;242:1744-1750.
20. Blanvillain G, Pease AP, Segars AL, et al. Comparing methods for the assessment of reproductive activity in adult male loggerhead sea turtles *Caretta caretta* at Cape Canaveral, Florida. *Endang Spec Res* 2008;6:75-85.
21. MacLean RA, Harms CA, Braun-McNeill J. Propofol anesthesia in loggerhead *(Caretta caretta)* sea turtles. *J Wildl Dis* 2008;44:143-150.
22. Harms CA, Eckert SA, Kubis SA, et al. Field anaesthesia of leatherback sea turtles *(Dermochelys coriacea)*. *Vet Rec* 2007;161:15-21
23. Chittick B, Harms C. Intraocular pressure of juvenile loggerhead sea turtles *(Caretta caretta)* held in different positions. *Vet Rec* 2001;149:587-589.
24. Johnson J. Nail trimming for blood collection from desert tortoises, *Gopherus agassizii*: panel summary. *J Herpetol Med Surg* 2006;16: 61-62.
25. Harris HS, Benson SR, Gilardi KV, et al. Comparative health assessment of western Pacific leatherback turtles *(Dermochelys coriacea)* foraging off the coast of California: 2005-2007. *J Wildl Dis* 2011;47:321-337.
26. Espinosa-Aviles D, Salomon-Soto VM, Morales-Martinez S. Hematology, blood chemistry, and bacteriology of the free-ranging Mexican beaded lizard *(Heloderma horridum)*. *J Zoo Wildl Med* 2008;39:21-27.
27. James SB, Iverson J, Greco V, et al. Health assessment of Allen Cays rock iguana, *Cyclura cyclura inornata*. *J Herpetol Med Surg* 2006;16:93-98.
28. Gartrell BD, Jillings E, Adlington BA, et al. Health screening for a translocation of captive-reared tuatara *(Sphenodon punctatus)* to an island refuge. *N Z Vet J* 2006;54:344-349.
29. Deem SL, Dierenfeld ES, Sounguet GS, et al. Blood values in free ranging nesting leatherback sea turtles *(Dermochelys coriacea)* on the coast of the Republic of Gabon. *J Zoo Wildl Med* 2006;37:464-471.
30. Fisse A, Draud M, Raphael B, et al. Differential leukocyte counts of critically endangered Grand Cayman blue iguanas, *Cyclura nubila lewisi*. *J Herpetol Med Surg* 2004;14:19-21.
31. Brenner D, Lewbart G, Stebbins M, et al. Health survey of wild and captive bog turtles *(Clemmys muhlenbergii)* in North Carolina and Virginia. *J Zoo Wildl Med* 2002;33:311-316.
32. Gottdenker NL, Jacobson ER. Effect of venipuncture sites on hematologic and clinical biochemical values in desert tortoises *(Gopherus agassizii)*. *Am J Vet Res* 1995;56:19-21.
33. Aguirre AA, Balazs GH, Spraker TR, et al. Adrenal and hematological responses to stress in juvenile green turtles (*Chelonia mydas*) with and without fibropapillomas. *Physiol Zool* 1995;68:831-854.
34. Brown MB, Schumacher IM, Klein PA, et al. Mycoplasma agassizii causes upper respiratory tract disease in the desert tortoise. *Infect Immun* 1994;62:4580-4586.
35. Herbst LH, Jacobson ER, Klein PA, et al. Comparative pathology and pathogenesis of spontaneous and experimentally induced fibropapillomas of green turtles *(Chelonia mydas)*. *Vet Pathol* 1999;36:551-564.
36. Johnson AJ, Pessier AP, Wellehan JFX, et al. Ranavirus infection of free-ranging and captive box turtles and tortoises in the United States. *J Wildl Dis* 2008;44:851-863.
37. Johnson AJ, Wendland L, Norton TM, et al. Development and use of an indirect enzyme-linked immunosorbent assay for detection of iridovirus exposure in gopher tortoises *(Gopherus polyphemus)* and eastern box turtles *(Terrapene carolina carolina)*. *Vet Microbiol* 2010;142:160-167.
38. Johnson AJ, Pessier AP, Jacobson ER. Experimental transmission and induction of ranaviral disease in western ornate box turtles *(Terrapene ornata ornata)* and red-eared sliders *(Trachemys scripta elegans)*. *Vet Pathol* 2007;44:285-297.
39. Rivera S, Wellehan JFX, McManamon R, et al. Systemic adenovirus infection in Sulawesi tortoises *(Indotestudo forstenii)* caused by a novel siadenovirus. *J Vet Diagn Invest* 2009;21:415-426.
40. Marschang RE, Gravendyck M, Kaleta EF. Herpesviruses in tortoises: investigations into virus isolation and the treatment of viral stomatitis in *Testudo hermanni* and *T. graeca*. *Zentralbl Veterinarmed B* 1997;44:385-394.
41. Origgi FC, Romero CH, Bloom DC, et al. Experimental transmission of a herpesvirus in Greek tortoises *(Testudo graeca)*. *Vet Pathol* 2004;41:50-61.
42. Stacy BA, Wellehan JFX, Foley AM, et al. Two herpesviruses associated with disease in wild Atlantic loggerhead sea turtles *(Caretta caretta)*. *Vet Microbiol* 2008;126:63-73.
43. Garner MM, Gardiner CH, Wellehan JF, et al. Intranuclear coccidiosis in tortoises: nine cases. *Vet Pathol* 2006;43:311-320.
44. Innis CJ, Garner MM, Johnson AJ, et al. Antemortem diagnosis and characterization of nasal intranuclear coccidiosis in tortoises. *J Vet Diagn Invest* 2007;19:660-667.
45. Schmidt V, Dyachenko V, Aupperle H, et al. Case report of systemic coccidiosis in a radiated tortoise *(Geochelone radiata)*. *Parasitol Res* 2008;102:431-436.
46. Miller DL, Mauel MJ, Baldwin C, et al. West Nile virus in farmed alligators. *Emerg Infect Dis* 2003;9:794-799.
47. Jacobson ER, Ginn PE, Troutman JM, et al. West Nile Virus infection in farmed American alligators *(Alligator mississippiensis)* in Florida. *J Wildl Dis* 2004;41:96-106.
48. Nevarez JG, Mitchell MA, Morgan T, et al. Association of West Nile virus with lymphohistiocytic proliferative cutaneous lesions in American alligators (*Alligator mississippiensis*) detected by RT-PCR. *J Zoo Wildl Med* 2008;39:562-566.
49. Jacobson ER, Behler JL, Jarchow J. Health assessment of chelonians and release into the wild. In: Fowler ME, ed. *Zoo and wild animal medicine: current therapy*. 4th ed. Philadelphia: WB Saunders Co, 1999;232-242.
50. Pasmans F, Blahak S, Martel A, et al. Introducing reptiles into a captive collection: the role of the veterinarian. *Vet J* 2008;175:53-68.
51. Lehr E, Fritz U, Obst FJ. *Cuora galbinifrons picturata* subsp. nov., eine Unterart der Hinterindischen Scharnierschildkröte. *Herpetofauna* 1998;20(113):5-11.
52. Congdon JP, Dunham AE, van Loben Sels RC. Delayed sexual maturity and demographics of Blanding's turtles *(Emydoidea blandingii)*: implications for conservation and management of long-lived organisms. *Conserv Biol* 1993;7:826-833.
53. Bonner BB. Chelonian therapeutics. *Vet Clin N Am Exot Anim Pract*. 2000;3(1):257-332.
54. Innis C. Medical issues affecting the rehabilitation of Asian chelonians. *Turtle Tortoise Newslett* 2000;4:14-16.
55. Innis CJ, Garner M, Raymond J. Observations on captive husbandry and pathology of the critically endangered Sulawesi forest turtle, *Leucocephalon yuwonoi*, in *Proceedings*. 9th Annu Conf Assoc Rept Amphib Vet 2002;21-26.
56. Innis C, Garner M, Tabaka C, et al. Gross necropsy and histopathological findings in imported impressed tortoises *(Manouria impressa)*: seventeen cases. *J Herpetol Med Surg* 2006;16:49-52.
57. Rivera S, Crane M, MacManamon R. Medical and surgical treatment of gastric foreign bodies in newly imported impressed tortoises, in *Proceedings*. 13th Annu Conf Assoc Rept Amphib Vet 2006: 78-82.
58. Lawson D. Captive reproduction of the impressed tortoise—sustained success. *Turtle Survival Alliance Newslett* 2008:17.
59. Hagen C, Platt SG, Innis CJ. *Leucocephalon yuwonoi* (McCord, Iverson, and Boeadi 1995)— Sulawesi forest turtle, Kura-Kura Sulawesi. In: Rhodin AGJ, Pritchard PCH, van Dijk PP, et al, eds. *Conservation biology of freshwater turtles and tortoises: a compilation project of the IUCN/SSC Tortoise and Freshwater Turtle Specialist Group. Chelonian research monographs* 5. 2009;039.1-039.7. Available at: http://www.iucn-tftsg.org/cbftt/.
60. Garner MM, Bartholomew JL, Whipps CM, et al. Renal myxozoanosis in crowned river turtles *Hardella thurjii*: description of the putative agent *Myxidium hardella* n. sp. by histopathology, electron microscopy, and DNA sequencing. *Vet Pathol* 2005;42:589-595.
61. Bursey CR, Goldberg SR, Miller CL. Two new species of Falcaustra and comments on helminths of *Norops tropidolepis* (*Sauria: Polychrotidae*) from Costa Rica. *J Parasitol* 2004;90:598-603.

62. Naorem L, Sirsi S, Singh S. Chelonian health management and rehabilitation training workshop for Indian veterinarians. *Turtle Survival* 2011;96.
63. Hendrie D. The Turtle Conservation Center celebrates a banner year. *Turtle Survival Alliance Newslett* 2006;10.
64. Kuchling G. Historic efforts to save the world's rarest turtle. *Turtle Survival Alliance Newslett* 2008:4-7.
65. Kuchling G, Shunqing L, King EH. The fourth year of *Rafetus swinhoei* breeding attempts. *Turtle Survival* 2011:78-79.
66. Wikelski M, Wong V, Chevalier B, et al. Marine iguanas die from trace oil pollution. *Nature* 2002;417:607-608.
67. Mitchell M, Nevarez J, Kim DY, et al. Evaluating the long term health effects of an unnatural oil spill on marine iguanas *(Amblyrhynchus cristatus)*, in *Proceedings*. 10th Annu Conf Assoc Rept Amphib Vet 2003;81-82.
68. Binder Park Zoo Web site. Kalamazoo River animal information. Available at: http://www.binderparkzoo.org/kalamazooriver/index.php. Accessed September 27, 2011.
69. National Marine Fisheries Service Web site. Sea turtles and the Gulf of Mexico oil spill. Available at: http://www.nmfs.noaa.gov/pr/health/oilspill/turtles.htm. Accessed September 30, 2011.
70. Morreale SJ, Meylan A, Sadove SS, et al. Annual occurrence and winter mortality of marine turtles in New York waters. *J Herpetol* 1992;26:301-308.
71. Still BM, Griffin CR, Prescott R. Climatic and oceanographic factors affecting daily patterns of juvenile sea turtle cold-stunning in Cape Cod Bay, Massachusetts. *Chelon Conserv Biol* 2005;4:883-890.
72. Bentivegnal F, Breber P, Hochscheid S. Cold stunned loggerhead turtles in the south Adriatic Sea. *Marine Turtle News* 2000;97:1-3.
73. Metee N. Florida's 2010 cold stunned sea turtles, in *Proceedings*. 17th Annu Conf Assoc Rept Amphib Vet 2010;43.
74. Wyneken J, Mader DR, Weber ES, et al. Medical care of seaturtles. In: Mader D, ed. *Reptile medicine and surgery*. 2nd ed. St. Louis: Elsevier, 2006;972-1007.
75. Carminati C, Gerle E, Kiehn LL, et al. Blood chemistry comparison of healthy vs. hypothermic juvenile Kemp's ridley sea turtles *(Lepidochelys kempii)* in the New York Bight, in *Proceedings*. 14th Ann Symp Sea Turtle Biol and Cons. NOAA Tech Mem NMFS-SEFSC-351, 1994;203-207.
76. Turnbull BS, Smith CR, Stamper MA. Medical implications of hypothermia in threatened loggerhead *(Caretta caretta)* and endangered Kemp's ridley *(Lepidochelys kempii)* and Green *(Chelonia mydas)* sea turtles, in *Proceedings*. Joint Conf Am Assoc Zoo Vet Int Assoc Aquat Anim Med 2000;31-35.
77. Innis C, Tlusty M, Merigo C, et al. Metabolic and respiratory status of cold-stunned Kemp's ridley sea turtles *(Lepidochelys kempii)*. *J Comp Physiol B* 2007;177:623-630.
78. Innis CJ, Ravich JB, Tlusty MF, et al. Hematologic and plasma biochemical findings in cold-stunned Kemp's ridley sea turtles *(Lepidochelys kempii)*: 176 cases (2001-2005). *J Am Vet Med Assoc* 2009;235:426-432.
79. Innis CJ, Nyaoke AC, Williams CR, et al. Pathologic and parasitologic findings of cold-stunned Kemp's ridley sea turtles *(Lepidochelys kempii)* stranded on Cape Cod, Massachusetts, 2001-2006. *J Wildl Dis* 2009;45:594-610.
80. Anderson ET, Harms CA, Stringer EM, et al. Evaluation of hematology and serum biochemistry of cold-stunned green sea turtles *(Chelonia mydas)* in North Carolina, USA. *J Zoo Wildl Med* 2011;42:247-255.
81. Keller KA, Innis CJ, Tlusty MF, et al. Metabolic and respiratory derangements associated with mortality in cold-stunned Kemp's ridley turtles *(Lepidochelys kempii)*: 32 cases (2005-2009). *J Am Vet Med Assoc* 2012;240:317-323.
82. Aresco MJ. Mitigation measures to reduce highway mortality of turtles and other herpetofauna at a North Florida lake. *J Wildl Manage* 2005;69:549-560.
83. Orós J, Torrent A, Calabuig P, et al. Diseases and causes of mortality among sea turtles stranded in the Canary Islands, Spain (1998-2001). *Dis Aquat Organ* 2005;63:13-24.
84. Jacobson ER, Homer BL, Stacy BA, et al. Neurological disease in wild loggerhead sea turtles *Caretta caretta*. *Dis Aquat Organ* 2006;70:139-154.
85. Valente A, Parga M, Velarde R, et al. Fishhook lesions in loggerhead sea turtles. *J Wildl Dis* 2007;43:737-741.
86. Deem SL, Norton TM, Mitchell M, et al. Comparison of blood values in foraging, nesting, and stranded loggerhead turtles *(Caretta caretta)* along the coast of Georgia, USA. *J Wildl Dis* 2009;45:41-56.
87. Lewbart GA, Kishimori J, Christian LS. The North Carolina State University College of Veterinary Medicine Turtle Rescue Team: a model for a successful wild-reptile clinic. *J Vet Med Ed* 2005;32:377-381.
88. Phelan SM, Eckert KL. *Marine turtle trauma response procedures: a field guide*. Beaufort, North Carolina: Wider Caribbean Sea Turtle Conservation Network (WIDECAST), 2006.
89. Upite C. Evaluating sea turtle injuries in northeast fishing gear. US Dept Commerce, Northeast Fish Sci Cent Ref Doc 11-10; 2011. Available at http://www.nefsc.noaa.gov/nefsc/publications. Accessed September 30, 2011.
90. Perry G, Rodda GH, Fritts TH, et al. The lizard fauna of Guam's fringing islets: island biogeography, phylogenetic history, and conservation implications. *Glob Ecol Biogeogr Lett* 1998;7:353-365.
91. Krysko KL, Burgess JP, Rochford MR, et al. Verified non-indigenous amphibians and reptiles in Florida from 1863 through 2010: outlining the invasion process and identifying invasion pathways and stages. *Zootaxa* 2011;3028:1-64.
92. Reed RN, Rodda GH. Giant constrictors: biological and management profiles and an establishment risk assessment for nine species of pythons, anacondas, and the boa constrictor. *USGS Open File Report* 2009;1202.
93. Hidalgo-Vila J, Díaz-Paniagua C, Ribas A, et al. Helminth communities of the exotic introduced turtle *Trachemys scripta elegans* in southwestern Spain: transmission from native turtles. *Res Vet Sci* 2009;86:463-465.
94. Mader D. Methods for altering reproductive status in green iguanas *(Iguana iguana)*, in *Proceedings*. 16th Annu Conf Assoc Rept Amphib Vet 2009;61-62.
95. Jacobson ER. The ability of large constrictors to invade areas of the United Sates beyond southern Florida: fact vs fiction, in *Proceedings*. 17th Annu Conf Assoc Rept Amphib Vet 2010;58-59.
96. Criscione CD, Font WF. The guest playing host: colonization of the introduced Mediterranean gecko, *Hemidactylus turcicus*, by helminth parasites in southeastern Louisiana. *J Parasit* 2001;87:1273-1278.
97. Keller JM, Kucklick JR, Stamper MA, et al. Associations between organochlorine contaminant concentrations and clinical health parameters in loggerhead sea turtles from North Carolina, USA. *Environ Health Perspect* 2004;112:1074-1079.
98. Day RD, Segars AL, Arendt AD, et al. Relationship of blood mercury levels to health parameters in the loggerhead sea turtle *(Caretta caretta)*. *Environ Health Perspect* 2007;115:1421-1428.
99. Innis C, Tlusty M, Perkins C, et al. Trace metal and organochlorine pesticide concentrations in cold-stunned, juvenile Kemp's Ridley sea turtles *(Lepidochelys kempii)* from Cape Cod, Massachusetts, USA. *Chelon Conserv Biol* 2008;7:230-239.
100. Stacy BA, Howard L, Kinkaid J, et al. Yolk coelomitis in Fiji Island banded iguanas *(Brachylophus fasciatus)*. *J Zoo Wildl Med* 2008;39:161-169.
101. Association of Zoos and Aquariums. Aruba Island rattlesnake *(Crotalus unicolor)* SSP master plan. Available at: http://snaketag.org/SSP-PMPs/Unicolor%20files/Uni_Start.html, Accessed June 8, 2013.
102. Innis C, Hernandez-Divers SJ, Martinez-Jimenez D. Coelioscopic-assisted pre-femoral oophorectomy in chelonians. *J Am Vet Med Assoc* 2007;230:1049-1052.
103. Jacobson E, Heard D, Isaza R. Future directions in zoological medical education: expectations, potential, opportunities, and mandates: future directions in reptile medical education. *J Vet Med Ed* 2006;33:373-381.

CHAPTER 28

Invasive and Introduced Reptiles and Amphibians

Robert N. Reed and Kenneth L. Krysko

AMPHIBIANS AND REPTILES

Why is there a section on introduced amphibians and reptiles in this volume, and why should veterinarians care about this issue? Globally, invasive species are a major threat to the stability of native ecosystems,[1,2] and amphibians and reptiles are attracting increased attention as potential invaders. Some introduced amphibians and reptiles have had a major impact (e.g., Brown Tree Snakes *[Boiga irregularis]* wiping out the native birds of Guam[3] or Cane Toads *[Rhinella marina]* poisoning native Australian predators).[4] For the vast majority of species, however, the ecological, economic, and sociopolitical effects of introduced amphibians and reptiles are generally poorly quantified, largely because of a lack of focused research effort rather than because such effects are nonexistent. This trend is alarming given that rates of introduction have increased exponentially in recent decades.[5,6]

The live animal trade is an annual multibillion dollar industry. Millions of amphibians and reptiles from all around the world are imported into the United States each year and sold as pets and food for pets. With such a large number of individual animals being traded, it is inevitable that some will either escape from enclosures or be intentionally introduced into the wild. By no means should all members of the live animal trade be vilified for the irresponsible actions of a minority of importers, breeders, and owners, nor should the reader get the impression that the live animal trade is the only source of introduced herpetofauna (stowaways in cargo and nursery plants are not unheard of, some have escaped from zoos, and some species have been intentionally introduced for biocontrol, food, or other reasons). However, the live animal trade is by far the predominant introduction pathway and must be acknowledged as such if strategies to reduce the rate of introduction are to be identified and populations that are already established are to be controlled.

Not all introduced amphibians and reptiles establish reproducing populations, and few of those that become established have expanded their range widely or result in negative ecological or economic effects or cause harm to human health, thereby achieving the rank of "invasive". When warranted in this chapter, the term *introduced herps* will be used as broadly inclusive of exotic amphibians and reptiles, regardless of invasion stage. The authors' experience in Florida is relied on heavily, but the general themes are applicable to other geographic areas.

The state of Florida has experienced more documented introductions of exotic herps (139 species are known through 2010) and has more established species (57) than anywhere else in the world.[6-8] However, the problem is certainly not limited to Florida: Hawaii has 31 established species of nonnative herps, California has 19 established species, and the magnitude of the problem in the United States (whether measured in the number of species or the geography of introductions) is likely to increase.[5] Many of these numbers are certainly underestimates of the actual number of established species because many introductions are of small and/or secretive species that have yet to be discovered or reported to researchers and a number of challenges are associated with determining when released individuals become a reproducing population. Although most established populations are in the warmest climates of the United States, some species have established in more temperate areas (e.g., European Wall Lizards [*Podarcis* spp.] have established in several northern cities). Furthermore, as international standards of living rise and the demand increases for pets, additional populations of introduced herps can be expected to become established around the globe. As an example, introduced populations of California Kingsnakes (*Lampropeltis californiae*) originating from the pet trade are now widespread on Grand Canary Island and threaten populations of endemic vertebrates[9]; this example is more remarkable for the fact that these snakes are albinos, a recessive phenotypic trait usually thought to be associated with low survival rates because light-colored individuals are detected by predators at much higher rates than are their normally colored conspecifics.

HIGH-PROFILE INTRODUCTIONS IN THE UNITED STATES

Giant Constrictor Snakes

Of all the introduced herps in the continental United States, Burmese Pythons (*Python molurus bivittatus* or *P. bivittatus*) in Florida have attracted the most attention from the media and general public (Figure. 28-1). A large population of pythons (estimates from credible sources start at 10,000 pythons and increase from there) is spread across several thousand square kilometers of the Everglades and adjacent ecosystems,[10,11] and these exotic snakes consume a variety of vertebrates such

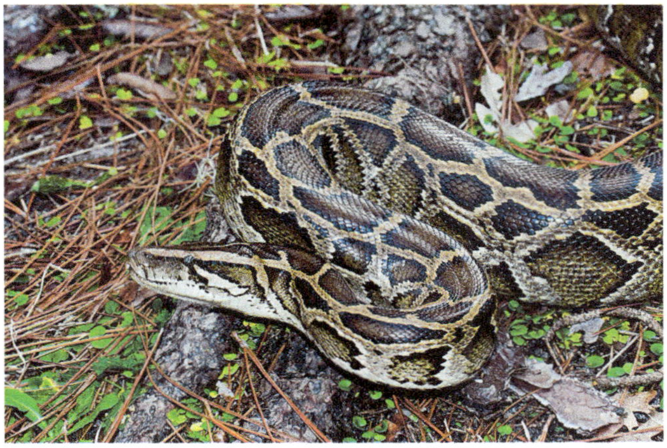

FIGURE 28-1 Now distributed across thousands of square kilometers of southern Florida, the Burmese Python (*Python molurus bivittatus* or *P. bivittatus*) is a true giant among snakes and has been implicated in declines of native mammals in the Everglades.

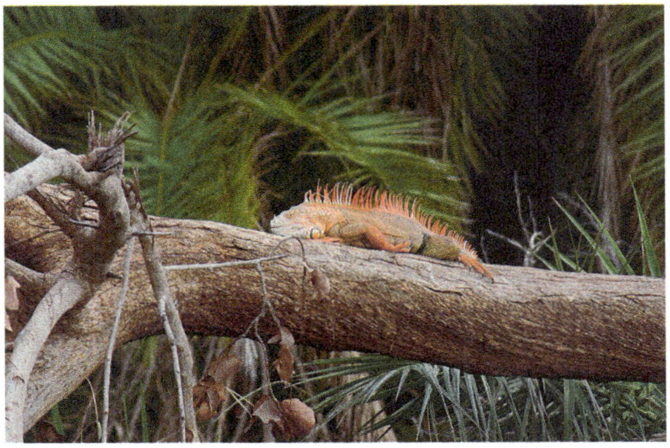

FIGURE 28-2 Despite the color implied by their common name, Green Iguanas (*Iguana iguana*) may exhibit a variety of colors. This is especially true of males such as this bright orange individual.

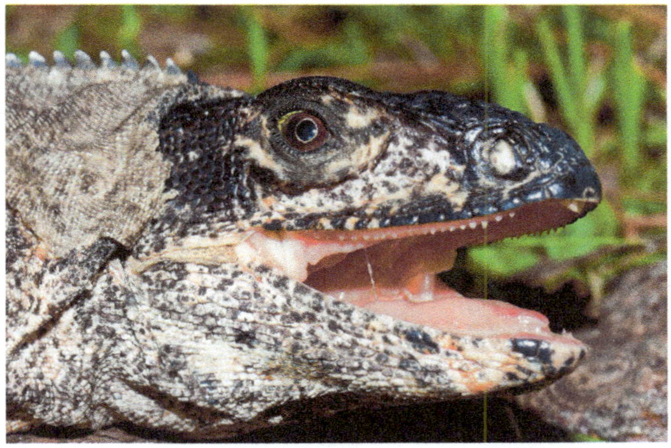

FIGURE 28-3 The Black Spiny-tailed Iguana *(Ctenosaura similis)* is the largest member of its genus, and males can approach 1.5 m in total length.

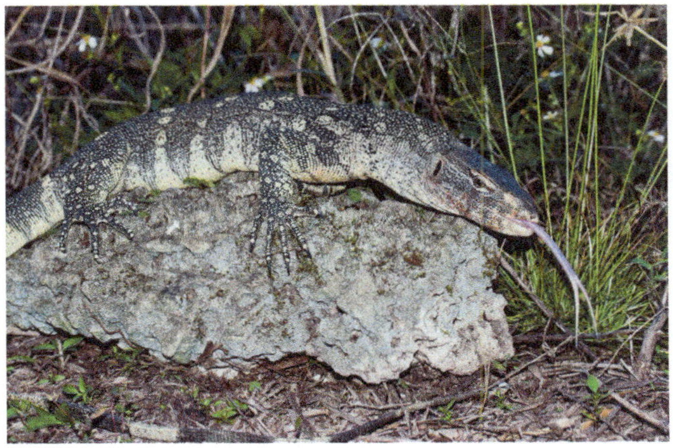

FIGURE 28-4 The Nile Monitor (*Varanus niloticus*) is a large-bodied active predator that consumes a wide range of prey, from fish to nestling birds to turtle eggs.

as mammals (including domestic pets), reptiles, and birds, many of which are species of conservation concern. Effects on native species may be severe.[12] Two additional established species of giant constrictors (Boa Constrictor *[Boa constrictor]* and Northern African Python *[Python sebae]*) are as yet confined to smaller areas.[13,14] The Boa Constrictor is also an established invader on several Caribbean islands.[11] All three exotic snake species were introduced via the pet trade, but only the Burmese Python has been studied enough to be labeled as invasive.

Large Lizards

There are currently at least five species of established large lizards in Florida: Green Iguana (*Iguana iguana*, Figure 28-2), Black Spiny-tailed Iguana (*Ctenosaura similis*, Figure 28-3), Mexican Black Spiny-tailed Iguana *(Ctenosaura pectinata)*, Nile Monitor *(Varanus niloticus*, Figure 28-4), and Argentine Tegu *(Tupinambis merianae)*. All were introduced via the pet trade, and all but the Mexican Black Spiny-tailed Iguana have been studied enough to be labeled as invasive. Iguanas are known to carry and possibly transmit *Salmonella* to humans,[15] the Black Spiny-tailed Iguana has been documented consuming the protected Gopher Tortoise *(Gopherus polyphemus)*,[16] as well as birds and their eggs,[17] and the Nile Monitor is known to consume birds, bird eggs, and crocodile eggs but is large enough to also take domestic pets. The Tegu and Monitor Lizard inhabit relatively temperate climates in their native ranges, which suggests that they may be an establishment risk for other states.

Anoles

There are roughly 60 populations of about 20 species of established introduced anoles worldwide, including at least nine species established in the United States and its insular territories (Figure 28-5).[5,6] While ecological effects have been documented for some species, such as Brown Anoles (*Anolis sagrei*, Figure 28-6) in Florida,[18] most introductions have received little to no ecological attention. In Florida, residents often spray insecticides to control insect pests around their homes—these insecticide applications have been observed

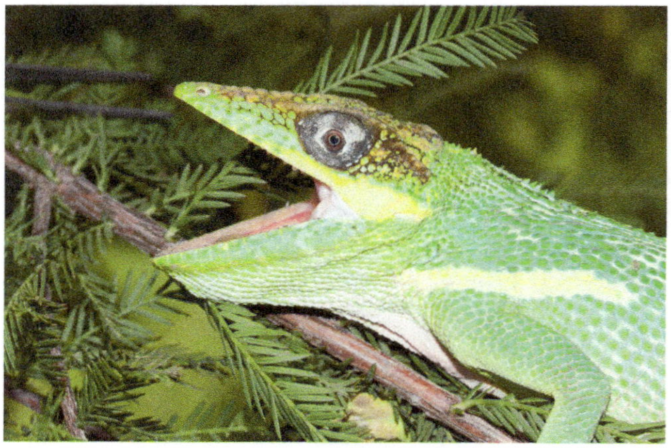

FIGURE 28-5 Among the largest of the species-rich anole clade, the Knight Anole (*Anolis equestris*) is a diurnal predator on invertebrates and small vertebrates. Long-established populations in Florida appear to be sensitive to cold weather, thus restricting their spread northward.

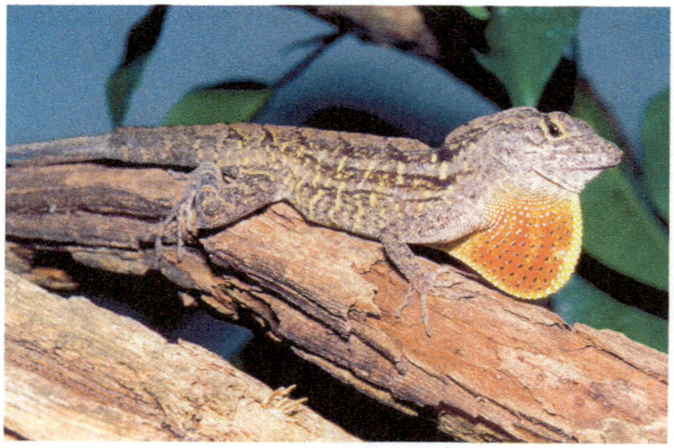

FIGURE 28-6 A male Brown Anole (*Anolis sagrei*) displaying its distinctively colored dewlap.

to occasionally result in the death of domestic cats that have consumed introduced Brown Anoles that in turn had ingested toxic and dying insects (Krysko KL: Pers. com., 1988).

Turtles and Tortoises

The Red-eared Slider (*Trachemys scripta elegans*, Figure 28-7) is established outside of its native range in multiple countries and in the United States, and several other species are established in the United States. Pet sliders are often released into urban and suburban bodies of water; thus this species may be one of the introduced herps most commonly encountered by veterinarians across the country. Turtles are typically introduced via the pet trade and human food pathways. Aquatic turtles are known to carry and possibly transmit *Salmonella* to humans, and Leopard Tortoises (*Stigmochelys pardalis*) in the pet trade have been found infested with African ticks (*Amblyomma* spp.) that carry heartwater disease, which is potentially fatal to ungulates.[19]

Frogs

Relatively few introduced frogs are established in the United States, but two species are of considerable veterinary interest. When stressed or molested, the Cane Toad (Figure 28-8)

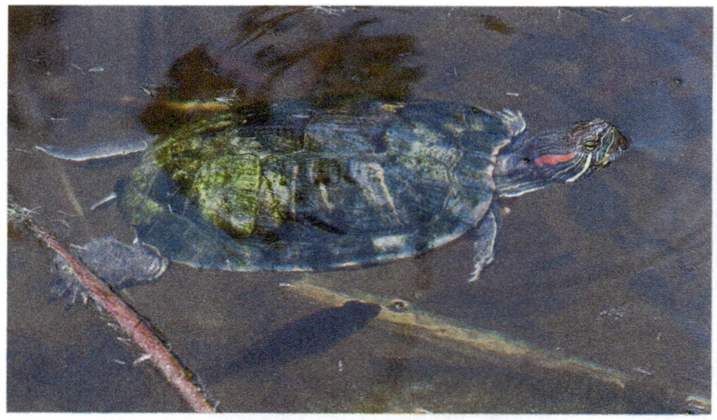

FIGURE 28-7 The Red-eared Slider (*Trachemys scripta elegans*) has been exported from the United States by the tens of millions for the pet and food trades. With invasive populations established on six continents, it is perhaps the most successful herp invader worldwide.

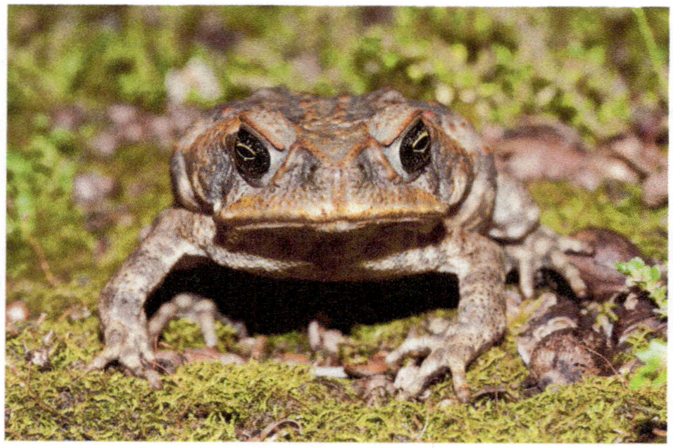

FIGURE 28-8 The Cane Toad (*Rhinella marina*) was widely introduced worldwide in failed attempts to control insect pests, especially in sugarcane fields. Its large poison glands often result in mortality among native animals attempting to eat a toad.

excretes bufotoxin from its large parotid glands, which can cause extreme pain or even death in domestic pets such as cats and dogs by causing a digitalis effect, hallucinations, uncontrollable salivating, coughing, vomiting, and convulsions. Domestic pets frequently attack or consume Cane Toads, especially in southern Florida. While collecting Cane Toads in a remote area near Lake Okeechobee in March 2002, K.L. Krysko observed an adult (approximately 35-kg) Rottweiler swallow a Cane Toad followed by the aforementioned effects for 45 minutes and death of the dog.

With females sometimes exceeding 130 mm snout-vent length, the Cuban Tree Frog (*Osteopilus septentrionalis*, Figure 28-9) far exceeds the length of most native tree frogs in the United States and is known to prey on these and a variety of native vertebrates. This species also excretes toxins from its skin, which can cause extreme irritation to mucous membranes of humans and other animals. Individuals have gone to the hospital for prolonged extreme pain after touching a Cuban Tree Frog then rubbing their eyes, and similar incidents may occur with companion animals.

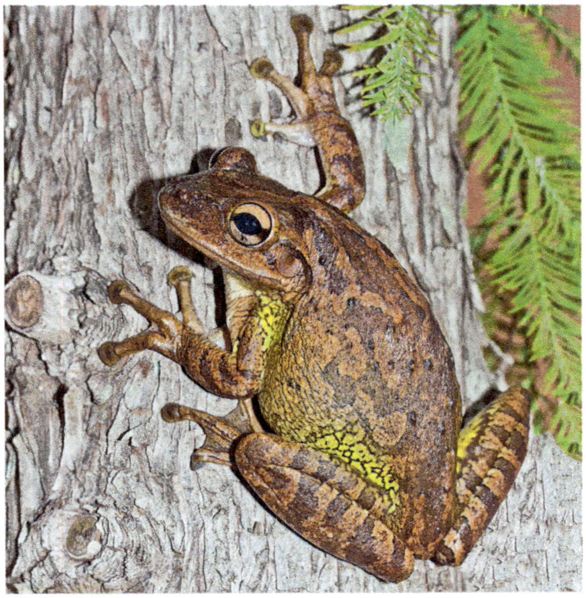

FIGURE 28-9 The Cuban Tree Frog (*Osteopilus septentrionalis*) attains much larger body sizes than most native tree frogs, and regularly preys on native frogs in its introduced range in Florida.

CHALLENGES FOR VETERINARIANS

Veterinarians are often the first point of contact when citizens encounter an introduced herp. An exotic animal may be captured and brought to a veterinarian's office, either for treatment of injury/illness or simply because citizens do not know who else to give it to. Alternatively, citizens may call veterinarians to report sightings of introduced herps. In such situations, a number of possible challenges can be predicted for the veterinarian.

What Is It?

Given the panoply of species in the live animal trade and a relatively large pool of native species in most areas, it can be difficult to determine whether an animal presented to a veterinarian is native or introduced, much less its species identity. A number of means exist by which veterinarians and members of the general public can identify the species of an animal. Field guides to U.S. herps can be helpful for identifying native species and sometimes include identification aids for some known established introduced herps.[20,21] Online resources are available for identifying all native and many introduced herps in some states (e.g., California Herps Web site [www.californiaherps.com] and the Florida Museum of Natural History Web site [http://www.flmnh.ufl.edu/herpetology/herpetology.htm]).[22,23] However, what should be done when these resources are insufficient for identifying an animal? In such cases, consultation with experts may be necessary. Herpetoculturists can sometimes identify species common in the pet trade, but consultation with herpetologists trained in systematics (typically museum, university, or government agency employees) may be more appropriate for some species, especially those that are uncommon in the pet trade or that are visually similar to closely related species. Inquirers should not be satisfied with a response of "I don't know" and the follow-up response should be to request contact information for a suitable expert who can provide positive identification. Note that these guidelines are generally true for both animals in hand and for photographs of animals taken in the field. Sometimes it might be necessary to provide the exotic animal to a museum herpetologist. This is particularly true if a physical voucher specimen is needed to confirm identity and/or document it for scientific purposes.

What Information Should Be Collected?

Veterinarians can be an important conduit for transmitting information on species identification and localities to researchers and centralized databases on introduced species, thus providing resource managers with real-time data on new observations. These data are important for early detection of incipient populations and have implications for successful control efforts because eradication is rarely successful after a population has achieved large size or is established across a large area. The ability to determine whether a given animal is a single released or escaped individual or part of an establishing or established population is largely dependent on timely reporting of observations. Besides providing the specimen and/or digital images, baseline data such as the name of the collector, collection date, and specific locality (preferably including latitude/longitude or UTM coordinates) are vital. Kraus[5] suggested that additional information, when available, can be helpful to managers, including the number of animals seen at the locality, how many introductions were involved, when the introduction may have occurred, identification of introduction pathways and motivations for release; and the status of the population, if established.

Who Should Be Told?

Synthetic assessments of establishment and population trends of introduced herps are dependent on citizen reporting of observations to centralized databases, but unfortunately, no universally adopted reporting system currently exists for herps. The U.S. Geological Survey includes amphibians and reptiles in its online reporting system[24], and the Global Invasive Species Information Network maintains a list of regional, national, and international online databases.[25] The University of Georgia maintains a reporting system and searchable database for vertebrates in Florida[26] that is very easy to use and that could serve as a model for other states. Note that some databases may conceal specific localities from the public to reduce the odds that herp fanciers will trespass on private lands or collect exotic herps in hopes of establishing new populations elsewhere or selling the animals back into the pet trade.

Besides reporting observations to databases, contacting local stakeholders can help spur additional field efforts to determine whether an observation is representative of an established population. Who to contact varies by locale, but the list of potential contacts includes state game and fish agencies, animal control officers, university researchers, museum collections, and local/regional hotlines. Florida has a nonnative species reporting hotline (1-888-I've-Got-1 or 1-888-483-4681).

Because verification of species identification is an important component of maintaining the integrity of the reporting process, it is highly recommend that veterinarians and members of the public send voucher specimens and/or digital images along with all associated data to researchers. In Florida, for example, the Florida Museum of Natural History Web site[22] (http://

www.flmnh.ufl.edu/herpetology/herpetology.htm) is the official repository for specimen records, and specimen information from this and other museums has been provided to create the first Atlas of Amphibians and Reptiles in Florida.[27] Remember that seemingly isolated or trivial observations can help reveal trends when coalesced in a centralized repository, so being proactive about reporting observations is encouraged.

What Are the Legal and Ethical Issues?

Laws on collection and ownership of native and introduced herps are variable between (and even within) each state, and this legal mosaic poses potential problems for veterinarians. For example, many states prohibit release of exotic animals once they have been captured in the wild, yet private citizens may encounter an injured or sick exotic herp and bring it to a veterinarian for treatment with the idea of releasing it afterward. Veterinarians thus need to be aware of local regulations on capture, treatment, and release of both native and introduced herps and must be ready to counsel their clients on this ethical dilemma. Rereleasing introduced herps is illegal and (in the authors' opinion) always unethical; veterinarians can direct clients to online educational materials to help them understand the potential consequences of releases.[28,29]

It is unrealistic to expect a common ethical standard for everyone, and the alternatives to release will depend on the situation. As researchers, the authors' preference is that introduced herps be humanely euthanized and provided as voucher specimens to a credible museum; this option provides the most information and a permanent physical record of the species' presence. Some citizens, however, may insist on keeping the animal as a pet. With the assumption that they meet any legal requirements to own the animal, it is suggested that digital images and associated data be provided to an appropriate repository (mentioned previously) and that the new owner be pointed to a specialty pet store to learn about proper husbandry. Alternatively, regional reptile societies often sponsor adoption networks so that unwanted animals can be provided to responsible, experienced keepers. The authors' least preferred alternative is for the animal to be given or sold back to an animal dealer because this provides an additional opportunity for escape or release if the animal is sold to an uninformed or unprepared new owner.

CONCLUSIONS

Ties between veterinarians and herpetoculturists may generally be stronger than those between veterinarians and herpetologists. Strengthening ties between the latter groups could be beneficial to both, and a number of questions posed by herpetologists studying introduced herps could benefit from veterinary expertise. Examples include

- *Species composition and loads of parasites*—Do introduced herps bring exotic parasites with them?[18] Are these parasites transferred to native species? Conversely, do exotic herps serve as reservoirs for native parasites? What are the zoonotic risks?
- *Pathology of introduced herps*—Most introduced herps found in the wild appear healthy, but on occasion impaired or dead individuals are discovered. Is impairment due to disease, is it environmentally induced (e.g., thermal stress), or is it due to some other proximate stressor? Can necropsy by veterinarians trained in pathology help answer these questions, and can the answers be used to identify vulnerabilities that may assist in control efforts?
- *Humane control of introduced herps*—In some cases, resource managers without specialized training resort to restraint and euthanasia methods that are not considered acceptable by veterinary advisory panels on animal care.[30] We hope that veterinarians can assist with development of guidelines for handling introduced herps to make field procedures more humane. Veterinarians can also assist with review of project proposals to render field methods more palatable to Institutional Animal Care and Use Committees.

These are only a few of the potentially fruitful arenas for collaboration among veterinarians, herpetologists, and invasive species biologists, and it is hoped that teamwork will become more common in the future. Unlike researchers and agency personnel, veterinarians have a presence in virtually every town in the country and can serve as a vital "early warning system" for the presence of introduced herps.

ACKNOWLEDGMENTS

The author's would like to thank Gordon H. Rodda and Tracy Holcombe for helpful reviews of previous versions of this manuscript.

REFERENCES

1. Lockwood J, Hoopes M, Marchetti M. *Invasion ecology*. Hoboken, N.J., Wiley-Blackwell, 2006.
2. Simberloff D, Rejmanek M. *Encyclopedia of biological invasions*. Berkeley, University of California Press, 2010.
3. Savidge, JA. Extinction of an island forest avifauna by an introduced snake. *Ecology* 1987;68:660-668.
4. Shine R. The ecological impact of invasive cane toads *(Bufo marinus)* in Australia. *Q Rev Biol* 2010;85:253-291.
5. Kraus F. *Alien reptiles and amphibians: a scientific compendium and analysis*. New York, Springer, 2009.
6. Krysko KL, Burgess JP, Rochford MR, et al. Verified non-indigenous amphibians and reptiles in Florida from 1863 through 2010: Outlining the invasion process and identifying invasion pathways and stages. *Zootaxa* 2011;3028:1-64.
7. Krysko KL, Somma LA, Rochford MR, et al. Taxonomic corrections of certain verified non-indigenous reptiles from Florida reported by Krysko, et al. (2011). *Zootaxa* 2012;3199:66-68.
8. Ugueto GN, Harvey MB. Revision of *Ameiva ameiva* Linnaeus (Squamata: Teiidae) in Venezuela: Recognition of four species and status of introduced populations in southern Florida, USA. *Herpetol Monogr* 2011;25:113-170.
9. Pether J, Mateo JA. La culebra real *(Lampropeltis getulus)* in Gran Canaria, otro caso preocupante de reptil introducido en el Archipiélago Canario. *Bol Asoc Herpetol España* 2007;18:20-23.
10. Reed RN, Rodda GH. Giant constrictors: biological and management profiles and an establishment risk assessment for nine large species of pythons, anacondas, and the Boa Constrictor. *US Geol Surv Open File Rep* 2009:2009-1202.
11. Reed RN, Rodda GH. Burmese pythons and other giant constrictors. In: Simberloff D, Rejmanek M, eds. *Encyclopedia of invasive introduced species*. Berkeley: University of California Press, 2011.
12. Dorcas ME, Willson JD, Reed RN, et al. Severe mammal declines coincide with proliferation of invasive Burmese pythons in Everglades National Park. *Proc Natl Acad Sci U S A* 2012;109:2418-2422.
13. Reed RN, Krysko KL, Snow RW, et al. Is the Northern African Python *(Python sebae)* established in southern Florida? *IRCF Rept Amphib* 2010;17:52-54.

14. Snow RW, Krysko KL, Enge KM, et al. Introduced populations of *Boa constrictor* (Boidae) and *Python molurus bivittatus* (Pythonidae) in southern Florida. In: Henderson RW, Powell R, eds. *Biology of the boas and pythons*. Eagle Mountain, Utah: Eagle Mountain Publishing, 2007.
15. Krysko KL, Enge KM, Donlan EM, et al. Distribution, natural history, and impacts of the introduced green iguana (*Iguana iguana*) in Florida. *Iguana* 2007;14:142-151.
16. Avery ML, Tillman EA, Krysko KL. *Gopherus polyphemus* (Gopher Tortoise), *Ctenosaura similis* (Gray's Spiny-tailed Iguana). *Predation. Herpetol Rev* 2009;40:435.
17. Krysko KL, Larson KW, Diep D, et al. Diet of the nonindigenous Black Spiny-tailed Iguana, *Ctenosaura similis* (Gray 1831)(Sauria: Iguanidae) in southern Florida. *Florida Sci* 2009;72:48-58.
18. Campbell TS. *Analyses of the effects of an exotic lizard* (Anolis sagrei) *on a native lizard* (Anolis carolinensis) *in Florida, using islands as experimental units*. Knoxville Tenn: University of Tennessee, 2000.
19. Burridge MJ. *Non-native and invasive ticks. Threats to human and animal health in the United States*. Gainesville, Fla: University of Florida Press, 2011.
20. Conant R, Collins JT. *A field guide to reptiles and amphibians: eastern and central North America. Peterson field guide series*. Boston, Mass, Houghton Mifflin, 1998.
21. Powell R, Collins JT, Hooper ED, Jr. *Key to the herpetofauna of the continental United States and Canada*. 2nd ed. Lawrence, Kans., University Press of Kansas, 2012.
22. California Herps Web site. A guide to the amphibians and reptiles of California. Available at: www.californiaherps.com. Accessed December 20, 2011.
23. Florida Museum of Natural History Web site. Division of herpetology. Available at: http://www.flmnh.ufl.edu/herpetology. Accessed Dec 20, 2011.
24. U.S. Geological Survey Web site. Nonindigenous aquatic species. Available at: nas.er.usgs.gov. Accessed Dec 20, 2011.
25. Sellers E, Simpson A, Curd-Hetrick S. Global Invasive Species Information Network Web site. List of invasive alien species (IAS) online information systems. Available at: www.gisinetwork.org/documents/draftiasdbs.pdf. Accessed Dec 20, 2011.
26. University of Georgia Web site. EDDmaps—early detection and distribution mapping system. Available at: eddmaps.org. Accessed Dec 20, 2011.
27. Krysko KL, Enge KM, Moler PE. *Atlas of amphibians and reptiles in Florida. Final report*. Project No. 08013. Tallahassee, Fla: Florida Fish and Wildlife Conservation Commission, 2011.
28. Everglades National Park Web site. Don't let it loose. Available at: www.nps.gov/ever/forteachers/dlil.htm. Accessed Dec 20, 2011.
29. Habitattitude Web site. Habitattitude—protect our environment. Available at: www.habitattitude.net. Accessed Dec 20, 2011.
30. American Veterinary Medical Association. *AVMA guidelines for the euthanasia of animals: 2013 edition*. Schaumburg, Ill: AVMA, 2013.

CHAPTER 29

Techniques for Working with Wild Reptiles

Terry M. Norton, Kimberly M. Andrews, and Lora L. Smith

Capturing wild animals for identification purposes, as well as for radio and satellite telemetry applications, is common in amphibian and reptile research and conservation efforts. In the past, these efforts have been predominantly performed by research biologists with minimal veterinary input. Institutional Animal Care and Use Committees (IACUC) are now required by most research institutions and for publication of research in the peer-reviewed literature. Veterinarians are being asked more frequently for their input, advice, and expertise in areas of infectious disease prevention, aseptic techniques, pain management, anesthesia, and surgery, all of which are critical in the topics discussed in this chapter. The techniques described here are not inclusive but are either commonly used by the authors or important techniques used by the scientific community.

AMPHIBIAN AND REPTILE CAPTURE TECHNIQUES

A variety of techniques are available for capturing amphibians and reptiles. Passive capture methods generally do not restrict an animal's movements; thus they are less likely to result in stress or injury to the animal. Active sampling methods require careful monitoring to prevent injury to animals or mortality but can yield valuable data on population size, individual growth rates, health, reproductive state, and survival. A general overview of commonly used passive and active capture methods for amphibians and reptiles is presented, along with selected references that provide more detail on specific methodologies.

Passive Capture Methods

Cover Objects. Terrestrial amphibians and reptiles can often be captured under natural cover objects such as woody debris and logs, which offer a favorable microclimate. Artificial cover objects can be placed in suitable habitats to attract them so that these species may be systematically sampled. For terrestrial salamanders, "cover boards" consisting of untreated lumber should be placed flush with the soil in shaded or moist conditions (Figure 29-1). Cover boards can be of varying sizes, but relatively small, thick boards are most effective for salamanders.[1] Cover boards should be anchored with a metal stake if they are placed adjacent to a stream or river, where flooding could occur.[2] Tin roofing material or black plastic cover sheets can be used to attract snakes and lizards.[3] These materials should be placed in open sunny areas and checked in the early morning during hot times of the year or in early afternoon in winter. Any type of artificial cover should be left undisturbed for 2 to 4 weeks after placement to allow it to weather and attract target animals. Cover objects can be carefully lifted with a snake hook to check for amphibians and reptiles.

Leaf Litter Bags. Leaf litter offers substrate to larval salamanders and their invertebrate prey but can be a limited resource in many streams. Leaf litter bags made from plastic bird netting (1.9-cm mesh size) and packed with aged leaf litter can be used to attract larval salamanders in streams.[4] Bags can be made by cutting the net into various sized squares (50 × 50 cm to 90 × 90 cm), adding a handful of leaf litter and a few small stones to weight the bag, and pulling the corners of the square together with a plastic zip tie to create a bag.[5] The litter bags should be placed in slow moving pools or meanders within streams and anchored to adjacent vegetation. Researchers can check the bags every 2 to 4 weeks by gently removing them from the stream and placing them directly into a shallow pan along with 3 to 4 cm of stream water. The litter can then be carefully searched for larvae.

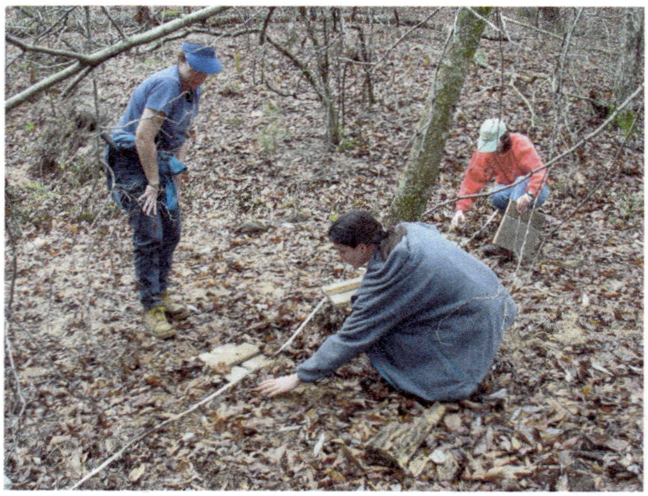

FIGURE 29-1 Field crew installing cover boards along a streamside to attract terrestrial salamanders.

Polyvinylchloride Pipe Refugia. Polyvinylchloride (PVC) pipe or large diameter sections of bamboo can be used to attract tree frogs.[6-8] Pipes or bamboo can be cut into short lengths and can be placed in the ground or hung vertically on a nail placed on the trunk of a tree (Figure 29-2). The diameter of the pipes may affect the number of captures, but generally pipes of ¾″ to 2″ diameter are used.[9,10] Ground pipes should be approximately 1 m long, and one end of the pipe should be cut at an angle so they can easily be inserted upright into the soil. Tree pipes should be hung between 1 and 2 m above ground on large diameter trees. Tree pipes can be 0.60 m in length, and placement of a cap on the bottom allows rainwater to accumulate, which makes the pipe more attractive to frogs. A small drain hole should be drilled into capped pipes about 10 cm above the cap to prevent the pipe from completely filling with water. Pipes can be checked by removing them from the ground or tree and checking for tree frogs (Figure 29-3). Frogs can be coaxed from the pipes with the use of a small diameter wooden dowel with a small circular piece of sponge on one end that serves as a plunger. Nontarget taxa (e.g., flying squirrels) may enter the tree pipes and be unable to escape. Thus a short section of nylon rope tied through a hole at the top of the pipe and dangled into the pipe is recommended to allow squirrels a means of escape.[11]

Active Capture Methods

Netting. A variety of nets and netting techniques are available to capture aquatic amphibians and reptiles; net mesh size and configuration should be based on the size and habit of the species targeted for capture. For most freshwater taxa, sampling with nets should be concentrated in emergent vegetation and other available microhabitats. If netting is conducted systematically, the method can be used to estimate densities of target organisms.[12] Sturdy dip nets with a mesh size of 3 mm or less are effective for capturing amphibian larvae and work best in water that is less than 1 m in depth (Figure 29-4). Dip nets should be dragged along the substrate to dislodge and capture amphibian larvae. Seine nets require at least two people but can be used to capture larger amphibians and reptiles in waist deep water. Seine and trammel nets are frequently used to capture Diamondback Terrapins *(Malaclemys terrapin)* in estuarine systems during mid-ebb through mid-flood tides[13] (Figure 29-5).

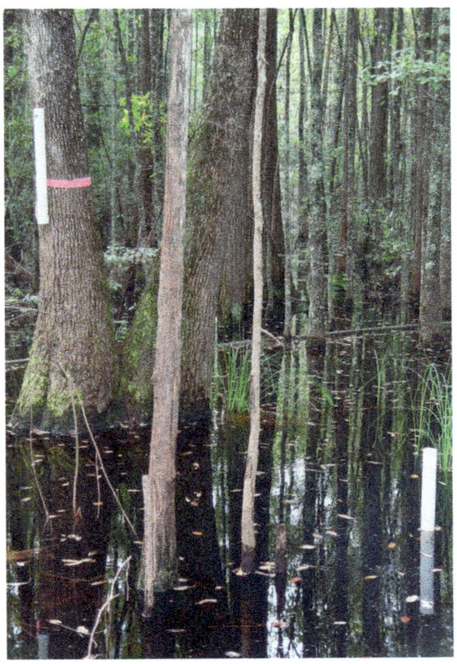

FIGURE 29-2 Polyvinylchloride (PVC) pipes used to attract tree frogs. Pipes can be mounted on tree trunks *(left)* or placed in the ground *(right)*.

Hoop Traps. Baited hoop traps are a common method for capturing freshwater turtle species.[14] Hoop traps consist of two to three large-diameter hoops enclosed in netting (Memphis Net and Twine Co. Inc., Memphis, Tenn), with a closed end that can be secured above water to a stake or tree and an open end with an inverted funnel that can be anchored to the bottom of a stream or wetland (Figure 29-6). In streams, hoop traps are typically set with the opening pointed downstream, which allows the scent of bait to disperse downstream. In ponds or lakes, hoop traps can be set either perpendicular or parallel to

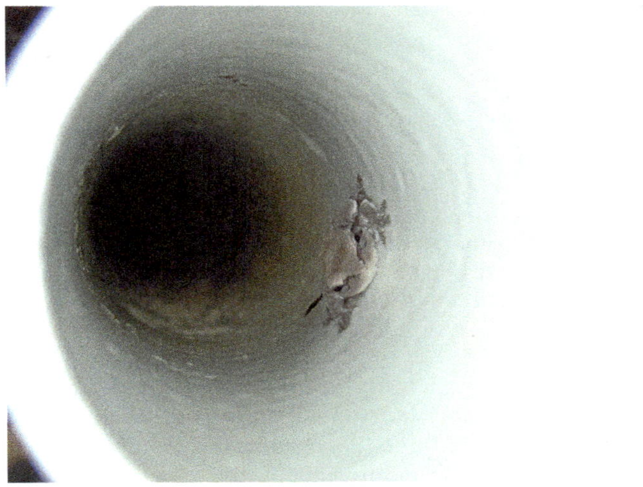

FIGURE 29-3 Pine Woods Tree Frog *(Hyla femoralis)* in a polyvinylchloride (PVC) pipe.

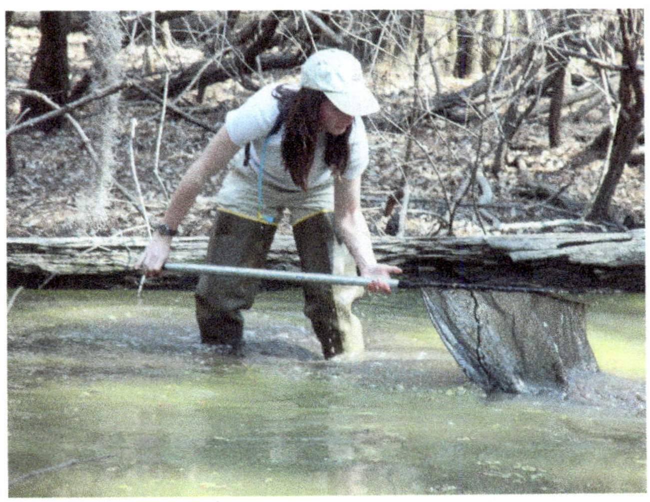

FIGURE 29-4 Dip netting for larval amphibians in a forested wetland.

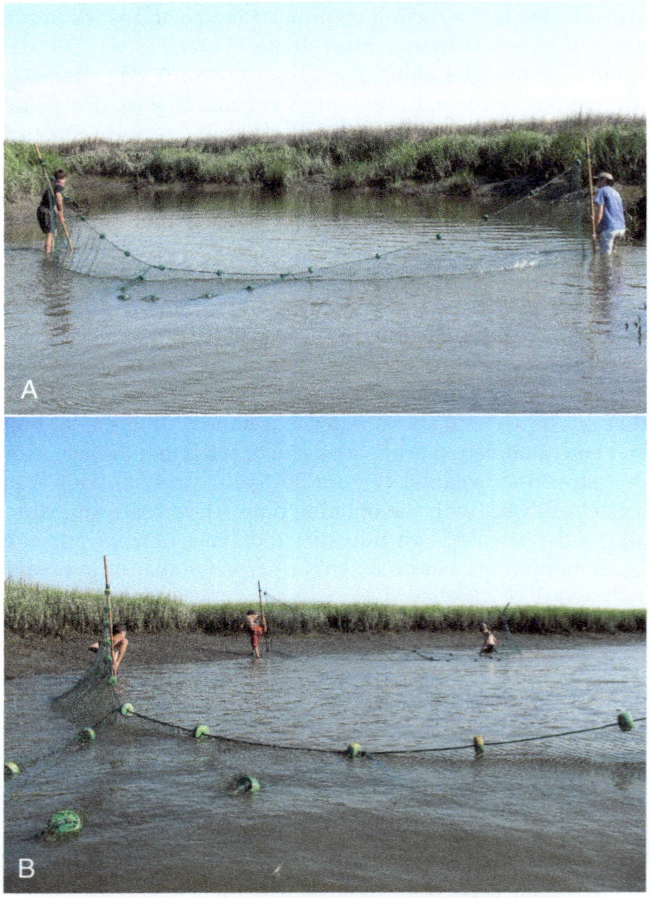

FIGURE 29-5 **A** and **B**, Biologists seining for Diamondback Terrapins *(Malaclemys terrapin)*.

the bank (held in place with two stakes), and the top of the trap should be above water to allow turtles to breathe. A fyke net can be extended from the open end of the hoop trap out into a stream or wetland to guide turtles into the trap. Traps can be baited with chicken livers, sardines, fresh or frozen fish, cat food, canned corn, canned green beans, and watermelon rinds, depending on the diet of the target species.[14-16]

Basking Traps. Freshwater turtles can be captured using basking traps, which consist of either a wire basket anchored to an existing basking log or a floating artificial basking platform with a net in the center that is placed in a wetland or stream so that turtles are attracted to bask on it. In the latter case, a shallow basket (of varying size depending on the target species) can be made with chicken wire and attached to the side of a basking log with the use of a staple gun or zip ties. The chance of success with this method is maximized if appropriate basking logs can be identified in advance with the use of binoculars. Once a suitable log is identified, the trap should be placed on the downstream side of the log to capture turtles as they attempt to jump into the water away from the boat. Artificial basking platforms can be made with a square floating frame with treadles that can tip the turtles into a barrel or net in the center or that simply relies on the turtles falling into the trap when disturbed.[17,18] Artificial basking traps are especially effective when placed amidst floating aquatic vegetation in water bodies with few natural basking sites. Traps can be checked when the sun is high and turtles would be expected to be out basking. Traps should be checked frequently to prevent turtles from overheating.

Drift Fences. A drift fence is a barrier that directs amphibians and reptiles toward traps.[19] Fences may be constructed from aluminum flashing, hardware cloth, or siltation fence, a portion of which is buried below ground to prevent animals from digging under the fence. Drift fences can be placed in specific configurations called arrays or may encircle particular habitats, such as a pond, to capture animals migrating to and from a breeding site[19,20] (Figure 29-7). Traps are generally placed every 5 to 10 m along a fence or at the ends of short sections of fence. Pitfall (bucket) or funnel traps (described further on) are most effective for terrestrial amphibians, small snakes, lizards, and turtles. Wooden box traps[21,22] are effective for capturing large snakes; lizards and terrestrial amphibians can also be captured in box traps along drift fences (Figure 29-8). Traps should be shaded with cover boards, and a wetted sponge or shallow water bowl should be placed in the traps to protect animals from desiccation. This method requires considerable effort to install and maintain, particularly if a wetland is completely encircled. Traps must be checked daily or multiple times a day during migration events and extreme weather conditions (hot or cold) to prevent mortality.

Funnel Traps. Various trap designs with inverted funnels at the openings are highly effective at capturing amphibians and reptiles. For example, commercial minnow traps and crayfish traps can be used to capture large aquatic salamanders (*Siren* spp. and *Amphiuma* spp.), juvenile and small aquatic turtles, and aquatic or semiaquatic snakes.[23] These traps can be placed in standing water with a portion of the trap left above water to allow animals to surface and breathe. Traps should be anchored to a tree or stake so they cannot be dislodged by predators and should be clearly marked so they are easy to find. Several iterations of funnel traps can be made by hand with the use of inexpensive, readily available material. For trapping along a drift fence, funnel traps can be made with the use of aluminum window screen (Figure 29-9). Screen funnel traps can be staked down using a wire pin flag or can be floated in shallow water. A recent variation of a funnel trap is made from a 120-L plastic trash can and funnels made from 6-mm mesh galvanized hardware cloth,[24] which was inexpensive to make and highly successful for capturing sirens, amphiumas, and aquatic snakes.

Hook and Line Noose or Cage Traps. Crocodilians can be captured by a hook and line noose or by cage trapping.[25,26] The use of a hook and line noose requires close access to the alligator and considerable strength to catch the animal and pull it to shore for further restraint. A treble hook and fishing line can be used to snag the animal on the osteoderms or bony scutes of the dorsum. Capturing individuals greater than 1 or 1.5 m in length generally requires a large (7 to 11) gauge treble hook and doubled 30-lb line with a 6 ft leader and a hook secured with a bimini twist (Andrews K: Pers. observation, 2007). When snagged, the animal can be gradually pulled close enough that a noose can be eased over the snout and tightened, after which the animal can be pulled to

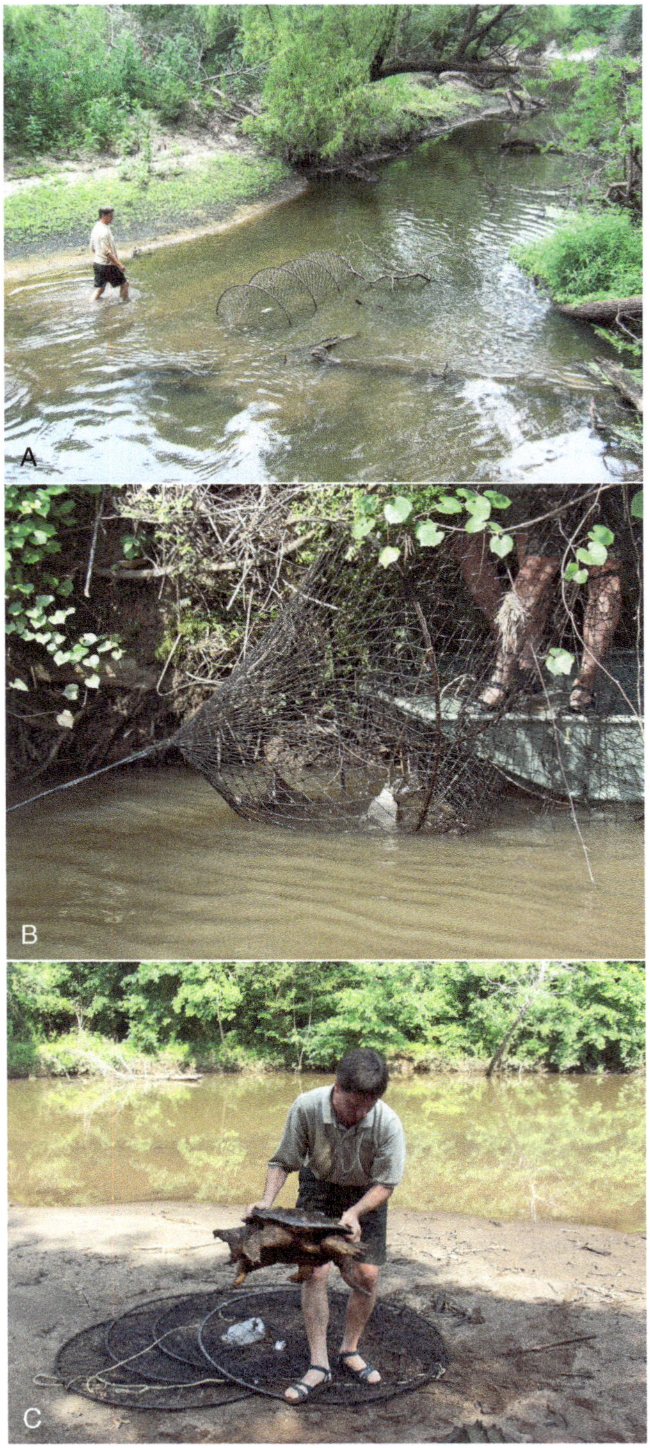

FIGURE 29-6 **A,** Funnel trap set for Alligator Snapping Turtles *(Macrochelys temminckii)* in shallow water in a river in southwest Georgia. **B,** Pulling the funnel trap into the boat for transport to process. **C,** Pulling an Alligator Snapping Turtle out of a trap.

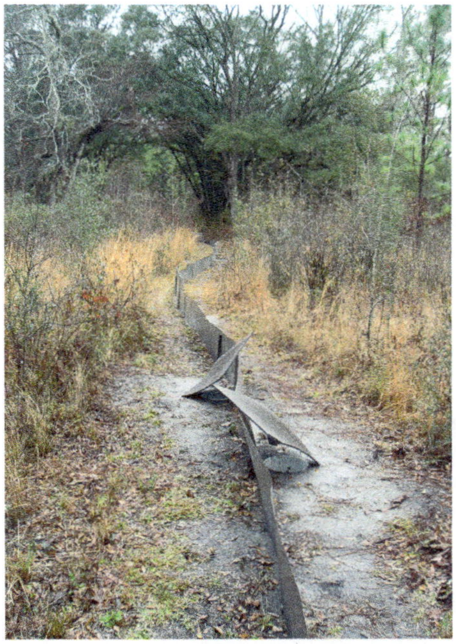

FIGURE 29-7 Drift fence surrounding an isolated wetland in southwestern Georgia. The fence directs amphibians and reptiles toward pitfall traps (19-L plastic buckets) that are shaded and contain a wetted sponge.

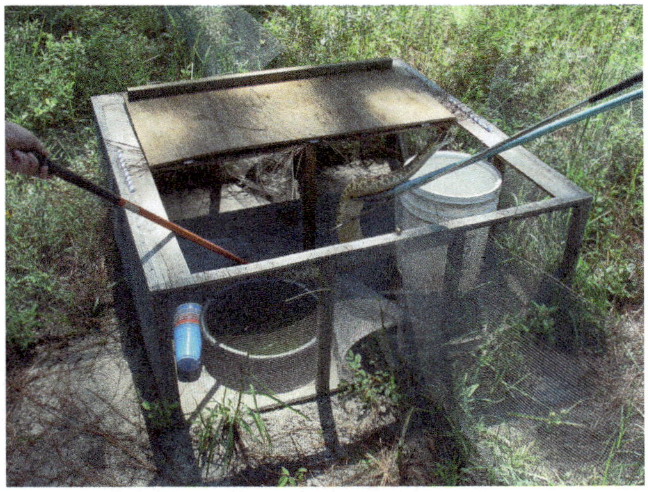

FIGURE 29-8 Researchers are removing an Eastern Diamondback Rattlesnake *(Crotalus adamanteus)* from a box trap associated with drift fences constructed with the use of hardware cloth.

shore. Once on shore, the tail can also be noosed (on larger crocodilians), and the jaws and front and hind legs can be restrained with electrical tape. Hook and line techniques can be time-consuming because multiple throws may be required to properly secure the animal, and it may be necessary to allow the animal to become fatigued. However, this technique is the best approach when capturing animals that are close to shore or in habitats inaccessible by boat (e.g., stormwater lagoons). Elsey and Trosclair[26] describe large steel traps that can be used for crocodilians; smaller wire-cage live traps (Havahart; Woodstream Corp., Lititz, Pa) can be used for small crocodilians.[25]

Hand Capture. A number of amphibians and reptiles can be captured by hand under appropriate conditions. Snakes, salamanders, and frogs are frequently collected on roads at night, particularly during or immediately after rain. Many aquatic species, including snakes, frogs, and alligators, can also be captured in wetlands at night using a bright light or head lamp to detect eyeshine or by homing in on movements or calls. With training, many people can identify frogs by their unique calls. For many species of frogs, it is possible to quietly approach them as they call and catch them by hand or with a dip net. During the day, many frogs can be detected along the margins of wetlands or under natural cover objects such as logs. Scuba, snorkeling, and jump/catch/hand grab techniques have been used for a variety of freshwater turtles, Diamondback Terrapins, and sea turtles.

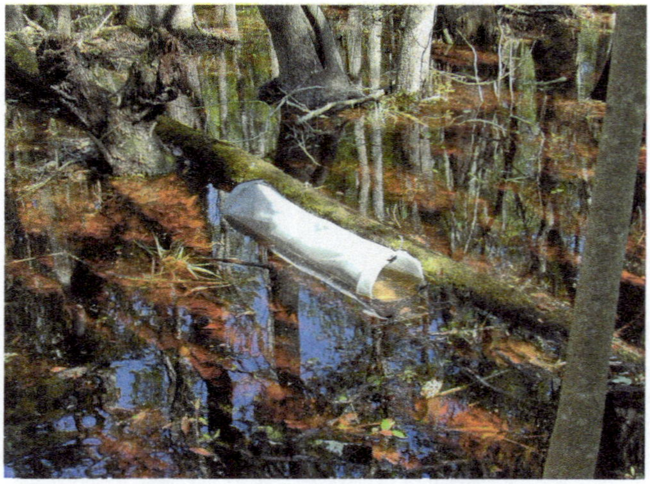

FIGURE 29-9 Funnel trap made from aluminum window screen and used to capture small amphibians and reptiles in a swamp.

Cage Traps/Bucket Traps for Gopher Tortoises. The two most commonly used methods to trap Gopher Tortoises (*Gopherus polyphemus*) are bucket traps[27] (Figure 29-10) and wire-cage, one-door live traps (Havahart; Woodstream Corp., Lititz, Pa)[28] (Figure 29-11). A bucket trap is made with a 5-gallon light-colored plastic bucket with at least ten 0.25″-diameter holes drilled in the bottom. Smaller buckets, or plastic plant pots, can be used to trap juvenile tortoises. The bucket is placed in a hole dug in front of the burrow entrance. Care should be taken when digging the hole because this is typically where female tortoises lay their eggs (eggs may be in the nest from mid-April through October). Newspaper, wax paper, or brown wrapping paper is used to cover the top of the bucket once it has been sunk into the ground. The paper is cut so that it is approximately 2 inches wider on all sides than the diameter of the bucket and secured tightly around the edge of the bucket with a few slits to ensure that it tears as the tortoise steps onto it. A thin layer of sand is placed on the paper to conceal the trap. Shading each bucket trap will prevent trapped tortoises from being exposed to direct sunlight for prolonged periods. Drowning and overheating are the most common problems occurring with this trapping technique. One advantage of this technique over wire-cage traps is that the tortoise can be captured whether it is inside or outside the burrow.

An alternative method is using a wire-cage trap in front of the burrow. The burrow should be scoped to ensure that the tortoise is in the burrow before setting a trap. A major advantage of this method is that a hole does not have to be dug; thus there is no chance of damaging eggs if a nest is present, and it is less stressful to the tortoise. Small wire-cage traps can be used to capture juvenile tortoises. The trap should be well

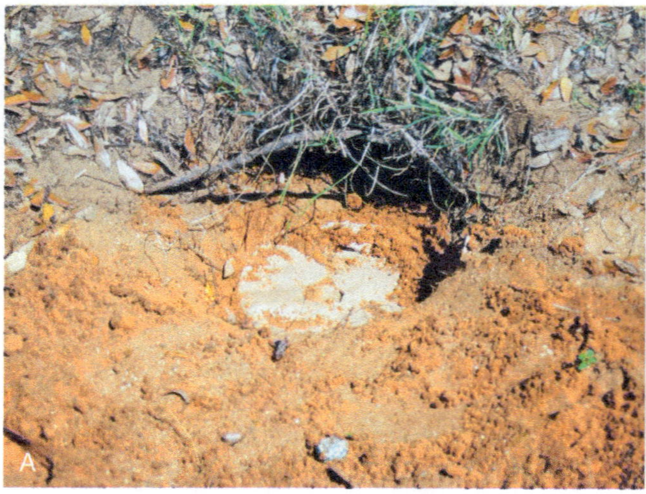

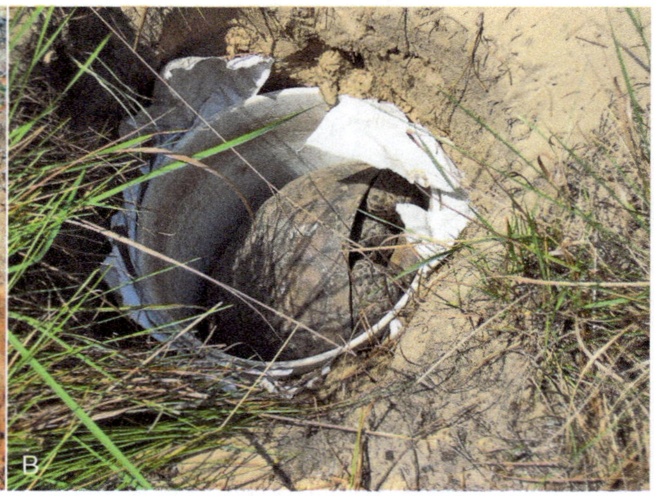

FIGURE 29-10 **A,** Bucket trap set and ready for trapping. **B,** Gopher Tortoise *(Gopherus polyphemus)* caught in a bucket trap. *(Photos courtesy Tracey D. Tuberville, Savannah River Ecology Laboratory, The University of Georgia, Athens, Ga.)*

camouflaged and shaded. It is advisable to check the traps two to three times per day regardless of type. During the colder months of the year (mid-October through mid-April), tortoises may not leave their burrows for extended periods, which makes these techniques less effective. Tortoises generally will not surface to bask until temperatures reach at least 18°C to 21°C (65°F to 70°F).

Shrimp Trawl. Foraging sea turtles can be collected by independent fishery trawlers. Twenty-meter four-seam nets with 20-cm mesh, without turtle excluder devices, are used by one research vessel to capture sea turtles.[29] The trawl duration was limited to 30 minutes (Figure 29-12).

Nesting Beach Encounters. Nesting female sea turtles can be sighted during nightly beach patrols and observed from a distance until they finish nest excavation. Once the turtle starts the process of oviposition, she typically enters a trancelike state and may be safely processed without disrupting normal nesting behavior (Figure 29-13). The turtle should be allowed to complete the nesting process and cover her eggs. Procedures that are more time-consuming, such as satellite tag placement, may require additional restraint. Four slotted boards can be interlocked to create a box around the turtle. Sand can be pushed around the box for further security (Figure 29-14).

Hoop Net and Boat Approach. Foraging Leatherback Sea Turtles *(Dermochelys coriacea)* can be located via aerial surveys and captured from a boat with the use of a 1.5-m diameter breakaway hoop net. Once secured in the net, the turtle is brought aboard the capture boat for processing. Injury to the turtle can be avoided if the boat is equipped with rubberized surfaces and rounded edges, and air-filled plastic or other similar padding should be placed around the turtles to cushion the body. A continuous flow of sea water over the turtle will help keep it cool while on deck (Figure 29-15).

HANDLING

Recommended Precautions to Prevent Disease and Other Health Problems

Infectious diseases can be transmitted within and between amphibian and reptile populations when handled for various procedures by field workers. Some examples of significant

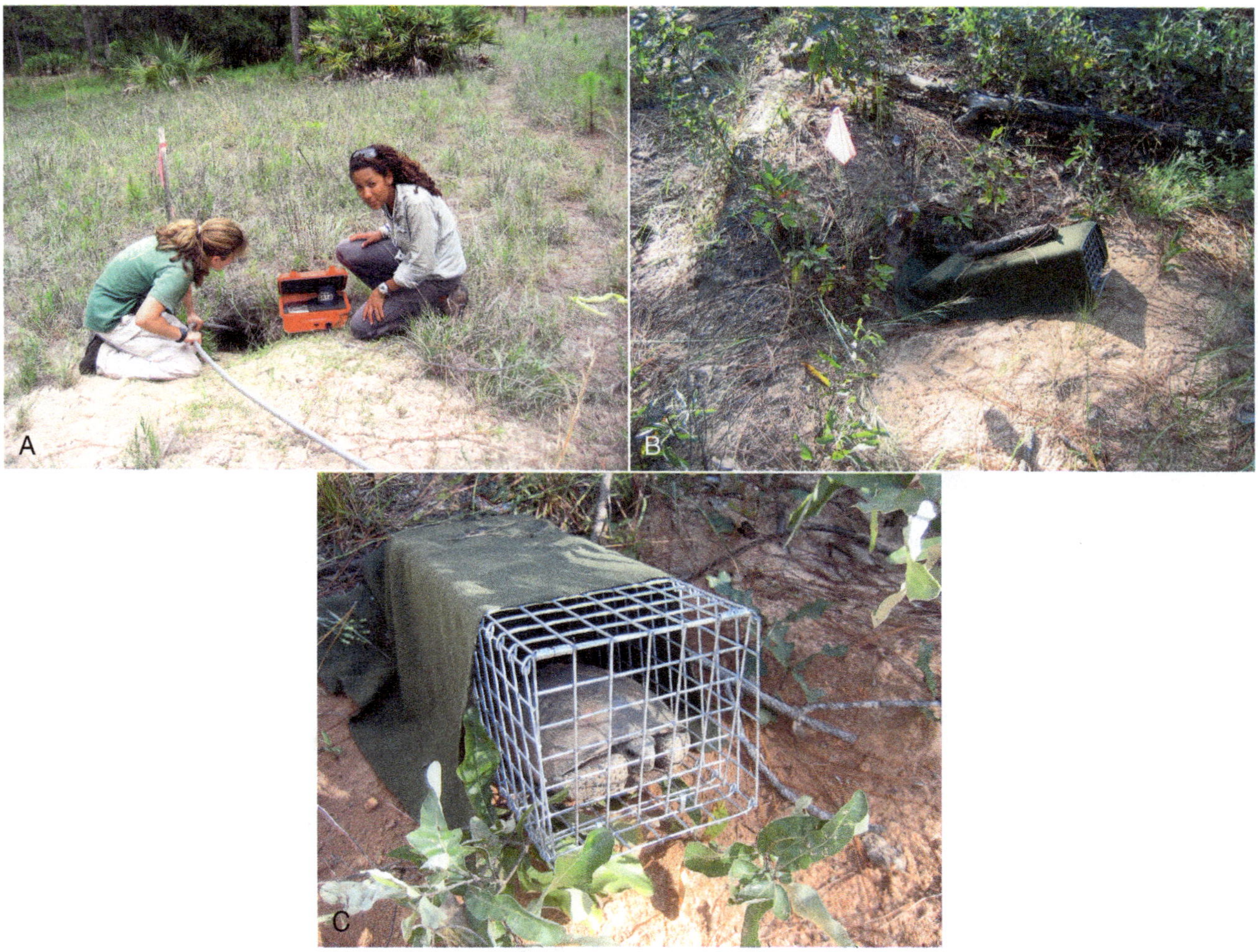

FIGURE 29-11 **A,** Scoping a Gopher Tortoise *(Gopherus polyphemus)* burrow to see if it is inhabited before setting a wire trap. *(Photo courtesy Dr. Terry M. Norton, Georgia Sea Turtle Center, Jekyll Island, Ga.)* **B,** Live wire trap, shaded and set in front of Gopher Tortoise burrow. **C,** Juvenile Gopher Tortoise captured in live wire trap. *(Photos courtesy Tracey D. Tuberville, Savannah River Ecology Laboratory, The University of Georgia, Athens, Ga.)*

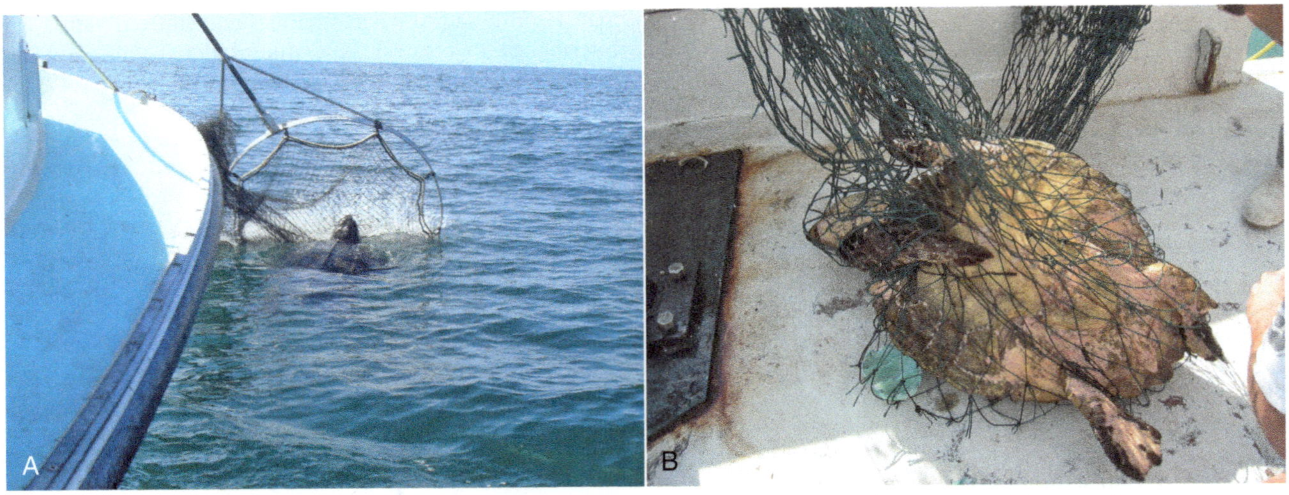

FIGURE 29-12 **A,** Leatherback Sea Turtle *(Dermochelys coriacea)* captured with a quick release hoop net. *(Photo courtesy of Connie Merigo, New England Aquarium, Large Pelagics Research Center, NMFS Permit #1557-3.)* **B,** Leatherback Sea Turtle on board for tagging, health assessment, and satellite transmitter placement. *(Photo courtesy of Kara Dodge, Large Pelagics Research Center, NMFS Permit #1557-3.)*

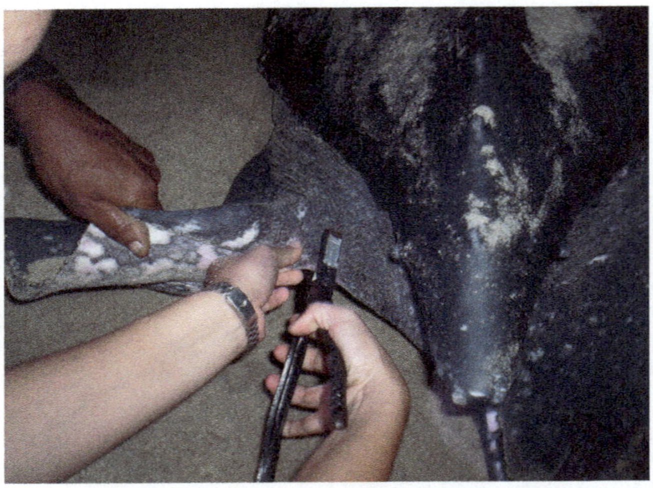

FIGURE 29-13 Female Leatherback Sea Turtle *(Dermochelys coriacea)* being tagged while laying eggs. *(Photo courtesy St. Kitts Sea Turtle Monitoring Network.)*

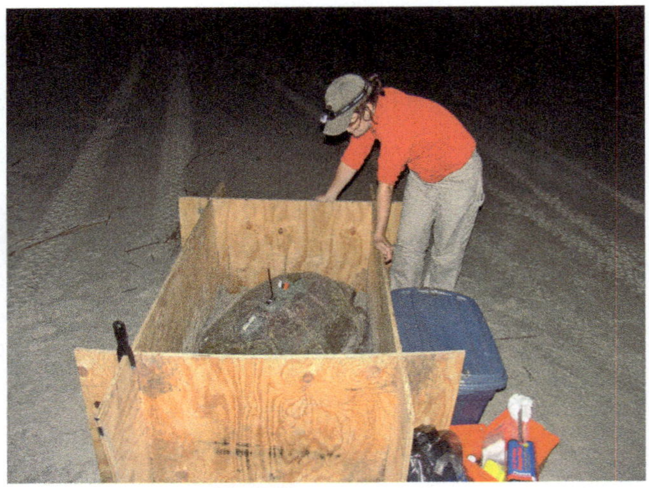

FIGURE 29-14 Loggerhead Sea Turtle *(Caretta caretta)* surrounded by a wooden restraint box for satellite telemetry placement after finishing the nesting process. *(Photo courtesy of Mark Dodd.)*

infectious and parasitic diseases that may be transmitted when appropriate precautions are not taken include chytrid fungus (*Batrachochytrium dendrobatidis*) in amphibians, iridovirus in amphibians and reptiles, *Cryptosporidium serpentis* in snakes, paramyxovirus in snakes, *Entamoeba invadens* in reptiles, *Mycoplasma agassizii* in tortoises, and herpesvirus (fibropapillomatosis) in sea turtles. The following are some general guidelines for handling and manipulating herpetofauna in the field:

- Avoid using insecticides before handling amphibians and reptiles.
- Wash hands with disinfectant hand wash or wear separate disposable examination gloves after handling each animal.
- Clean any handling equipment with an appropriate disinfectant between each animal.
- Use a separate clean, well-ventilated container or bag for each animal if temporary containment or transport is needed.
- Avoid high or low temperatures during transport of the animal.
- Do not handle or transport amphibians and reptiles from different populations at the same time.
- If wild amphibians or reptiles are held in captivity for various procedures such as surgical placement of radio transmitters, each animal should be isolated in a well-ventilated container and kept at its preferred optimal temperature zone with a thermogradient. The enclosure should be easily disinfected. Wood enclosures should be avoided because they cannot be disinfected.

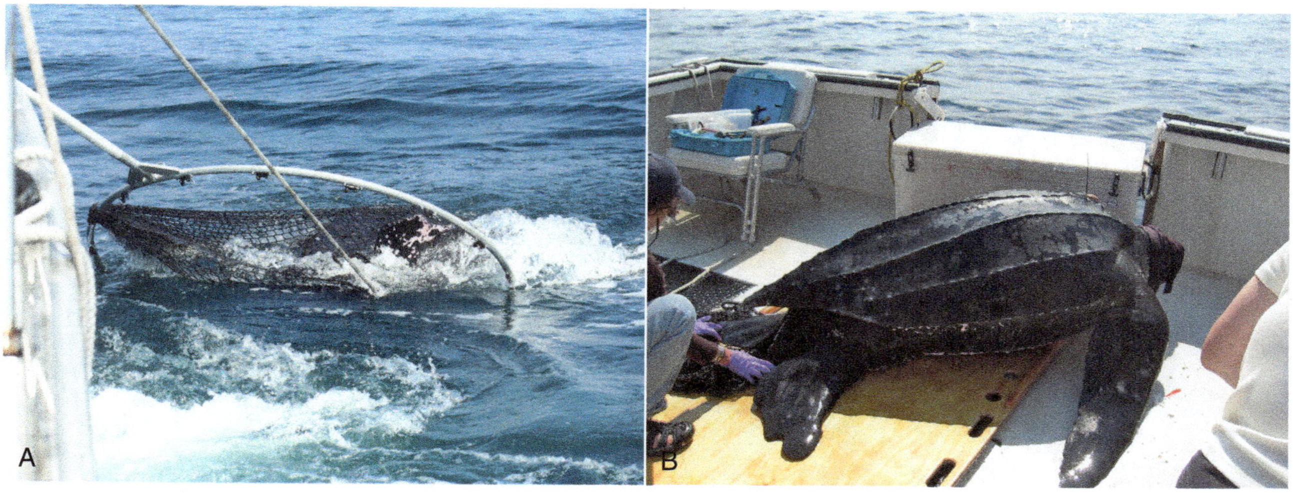

FIGURE 29-15 A, Leatherback sea turtle (*Dermochelys coriacea*) captured with a quick-release hoop net. **B,** Leatherback Sea Turtle on board for tagging, health assessment, and satellite placement. *(Photos courtesy of Kara Dodge, Large Pelagics Research Center, NMFS Permit #1557-3.)*

MARKING

Recommended Precautions to Prevent Disease and Other Health Problems

Field researchers working with amphibians and reptiles should have some basic aseptic technique and disease prevention protocols established for the field site and species under investigation that are practical but effective. Preventing individual animal infections and spreading of disease from one individual to another within a population and, most importantly, preventing population level disease outbreaks should be the ultimate goal. A risk assessment should be conducted for each project that evaluates the appropriate level of precautions that should be taken for that specific situation.

Amphibians. Because of the permeable nature of the amphibian skin, they are very sensitive to many toxins at levels that are well-tolerated without ill effects by reptiles, birds, and mammals. The amphibian skin is very sensitive to human handling. Soaps, lotions, and natural oils can all irritate or damage the skin. Researchers should wear powderless vinyl or plastic gloves when handling amphibians. Many of the common antiseptics and disinfectants are toxic to amphibians (e.g., surgical scrubs with soaps or detergents, iodine products, chlorhexidine, quaternary ammonium compounds, chlorine, alcohol, and ammonia). For these reasons, surgical, injection, and tag sites should be wiped clean of debris and secretions with clean unchlorinated water or saline before the procedure.[30]

Reptiles. Depending on the procedure, the area should be cleaned at least once with a surgical scrub (betadine or chlorhexidine) followed by 70% isopropyl alcohol. For invasive surgical procedures, such as internal placement of radio transmitters, surgical preparation that repeats this aforementioned process four times is recommended. Examination gloves should be worn when minor invasive procedures are performed on reptiles and should be changed between animals. Where feasible, hand washing or an alcohol-based hand disinfectant should be used between animals. Ideally, instruments such as tagging applicators, passive integrated transponder (PIT) tag injectors, and other instruments should be gas sterilized ahead of time or cold sterilized in the field with the use of an appropriate disinfectant such as dilute chlorhexidine solution (2% chlorhexidine gluconate; Phoenix Pharmaceutical, Inc., St. Joseph, Mo) between animals. A review of the advantages and disadvantage of the various antiseptics and disinfectants available can be found in other chapters of this book. For true disinfection of instruments to be achieved, a 30-minute soak time is preferred, but no less than 10 minutes is recommended before use on the next animal. This precaution may not be practical in every situation; thus the researcher will need to establish specific protocols depending on the species, potential for disease transmission, and numbers of animals being processed.

Manual Restraint, Analgesia, and Anesthesia

Many of the procedures discussed in this section can be performed with manual restraint alone. Some procedures, depending on the species, may require local anesthesia, pain management, sedation, or general anesthesia. The research team should consult and collaborate with a veterinarian experienced with amphibians and reptiles when deciding on the implementation of appropriate protocols. Other chapters in this book may be consulted for details in this area.

Temporary or Semipermanent Marking and Identification Methods

Photo Identification. Photographs are frequently taken as a form of identification in amphibians and reptiles and can be particularly useful in the case of a morphologic anomaly or injury. High-resolution digital photographs that clearly show the anomaly, injury, mark, or natural pattern of individuals can be taken each time the animal is captured. Photos can be stored electronically or printed and used in the field. Although noninvasive, this method can be time-consuming for identifying individuals and requires that patterns are stable throughout the life of the animal. Thus photographs are most useful as a

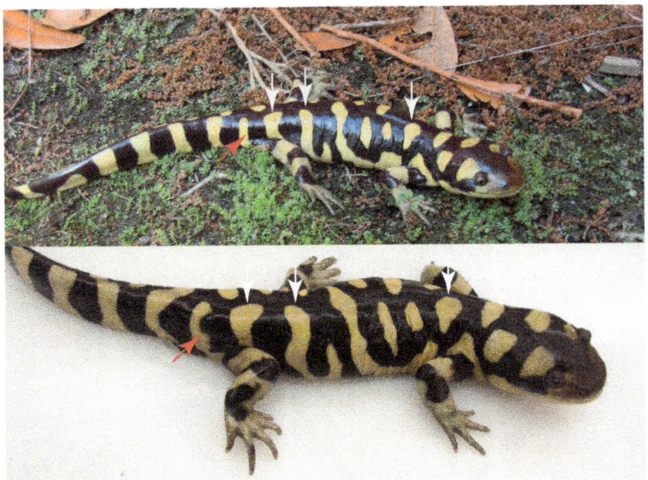

FIGURE 29-16 Spot patterns on the dorsum of an Eastern Tiger Salamander *(Ambystoma tigrinum)*. The *upper* photograph was taken in 2007 and the *lower* photograph was taken in 2011. *White arrows* indicate unique spots that can be used to recognize this individual. The *red arrows* show a slight change in one of the spots over the 5-year period.

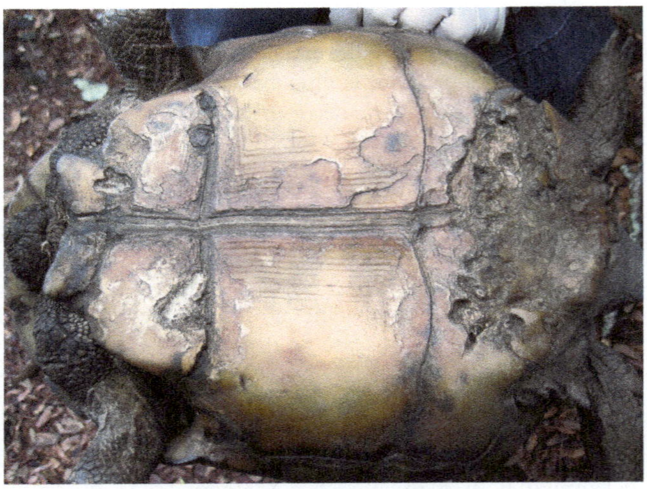

FIGURE 29-17 Gopher Tortoise (*Gopherus polyphemus*) with very distinct, old, healed pitting lesions that have been used for photo identification.

secondary means of identifying individuals. Some amphibians (e.g., Eastern Tiger Salamander, *Ambystoma tigrinum*) do not develop spots until several months after metamorphosis, and spots may change slightly as the animal ages. However, with careful attention, patterns can be clearly recognized even after several years (Figure 29-16). Photo identification also has utility for monitoring freshwater, marine, and terrestrial turtles, in which shell anomalies and injuries are common (Figure 29-17). Photographs of the pineal spot of Leatherback Sea Turtles can be useful for later identification.[31] This technique can also be useful with patterned snakes, such as rattlesnakes, that have variation in the number or shape of dorsal markings.

Paint Marking. Paint marking has been used as a noninvasive means of identifying reptiles. Different color

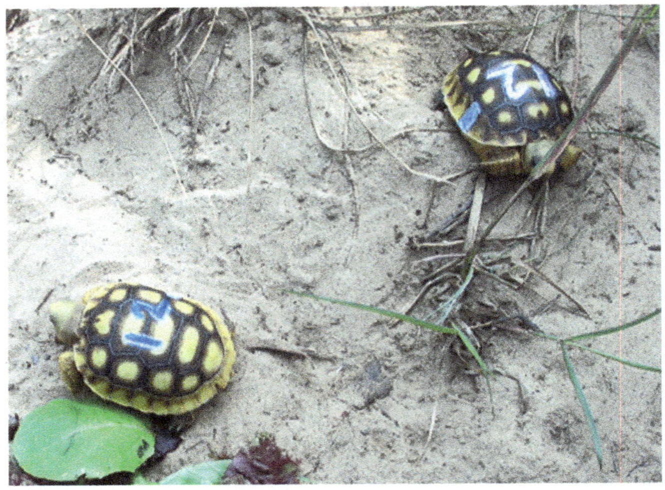

FIGURE 29-18 Gopher Tortoise *(Gopherus polyphemus)* hatchlings marked with a paint pen and nail polish.

combinations and paint locations can yield numerous individual marks. Small daubs of model airplane paint applied to the limbs, base of the tail, and dorsum have been recommended for temporarily marking lizards.[32,33] Data suggest that paint marking did not increase mortality of lizards from predation[34]; however, care should be taken to use the minimum amount of paint necessary to identify the lizard. Paint marking has limited utility for most snake species because recaptures are so infrequent. However, paint has been widely used to temporarily mark the rattles on crotalids.[35] This technique is particularly useful for capture–mark–release programs in which thorough visual searches for snakes are conducted over short time frames. In this case, recently captured individuals can be identified visually without having to have them in hand. An individual marking scheme can be developed based on color and the position of the marks on the rattle, or a common mark can be used for a cohort or population. The mark can be lost completely if the rattles break; therefore this technique is most useful for identifying individuals within an activity season.

Paint pens and nontoxic nail polish have been useful in temporarily marking the carapace of a variety of freshwater aquatic and terrestrial chelonian species (Figure 29-18). One example in which this is particularly useful is for identifying individual Gopher Tortoises in their burrow with a burrow camera scope. If the tortoise had already been processed that season, it had a number on its carapace that was readily visible with the scope. This information is essential when setting traps to capture these tortoises (Figure 29-19).

Paint and other temporary marks have also been applied to sea turtles, but the technique is less common than in freshwater and terrestrial turtles. Because of the wear on the carapace and the corrosive nature of salt water, paints do not last as long as in freshwater. Two-part resins have also been used to temporarily mark sea turtles.[36,37] To further increase retention throughout a nesting season, one can use a Dremel tool to create grooves in scutes that can then be filled with paint.[36] Paint, like other temporary marking techniques, is generally used in conjunction with other more permanent marking techniques.[38]

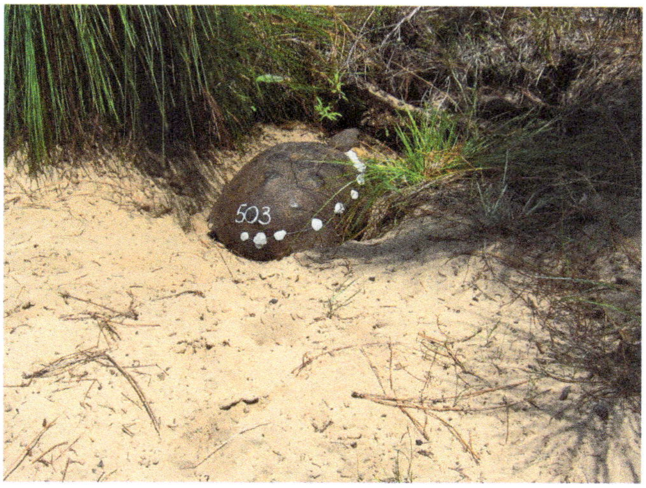

FIGURE 29-19 Adult Gopher Tortoise *(Gopherus polyphemus)* with paint pen number and radio transmitter on carapace going into a burrow.

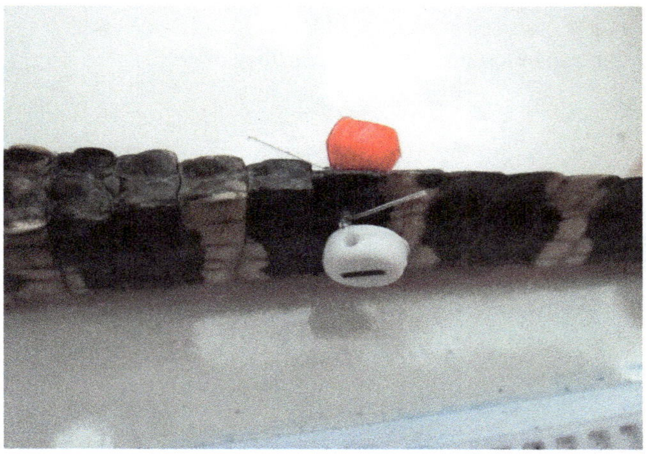

FIGURE 29-20 Photograph of colored and numbered beads used to mark American Alligators *(Alligator mississippiensis)*. *(Photo courtesy Tracey D. Tuberville, Savannah River Ecology Laboratory, The University of Georgia, Athens, Ga.)*

Colored Beads. Small colored and numbered beads have been used to mark American Alligators ([*Alligator mississippiensis*]; Tuberville T: Pers. com., Jan 14, 2012; [Figure 29-20]) and West Indian Rock Iguanas (*Cyclura* spp.; Hudson R: Pers. com.; [Figure 29-21]). In the alligator study, researchers applied two beaded tags on the single row of tail scutes using fishing line. Using two tags that varied in color and number, they were able to identify individuals and to differentiate among experimental groups without having to handle the animals. Marking could involve one to three beads of varying colors and numbers on each individual. Bead retention was sufficiently high in captive animals, but this marking technique would presumably not be viable in the wild where interaction with other animals and habitat debris would decrease retention rates.

Fluorescent Polymers, Pigments, and Tags. Acrylic polymers (also called visible implant elastomers [VIEs]) and fluorescent pigments can be injected into the skin of amphibians in different portions of the body (e.g., the tail of salamanders, sides of the body, and hind legs of frogs). Different injection sites, color combinations, and numbers of marks can allow for large numbers of individuals to be uniquely marked, and marks can be retained for up to 2 years.[39] This technique is one of the few reliable methods for marking larval amphibians; polymers can be injected into the tail fins of larvae.[40]

Small prenumbered fluorescent tags (Figure 29-22); Northwest Marine Technology, Inc., Shaw Island, Wash; Floy Tag, Inc., Seattle, Wash) also can be implanted subcutaneously in frogs and salamanders.[41] These tags come in a variety of colors and sizes and work best in species with lightly pigmented skin. These fluorescent tags can be accurately read using an LED light.[42] Floy tags have been used as tertiary identification in some chelonian research projects. The numbered tags can be secured to the shell with a clear, fast-curing epoxy. As stated earlier, the tags come in a variety of sizes and are small enough to use on juveniles without compromising their growth.

Monel, Inconel, and Cattle Ear Tags. Monel and cattle ear tags are effective and an inexpensive means of marking crocodilians. Monel tags have been attached to the webbing on the rear foot of American Alligators[43]; this technique requires recapturing the animal to read the tag. Monel tags do not corrode as rapidly in freshwater systems as they do in salt water (see further on); thus these tags are effective for most crocodilians. Plastic cattle ear tags have also been used to mark crocodilians. Roto (Sheepman Supply Co., Frederick, Md) and Allflex (Allflex USA, Inc., Dallas, Tex) ear tags, in particular, are inexpensive. These tags experience a higher rate of retention when the scute is pierced on the tail of American Alligators prior to attachment, by using a fine drill bit on the tagging device to facilitate penetration and secure latching of the male and female components of the tag (Andrews K: 2010). However, retention of external tags is generally low in crocodilians because of extensive, aggressive interactions with conspecifics. The use of these tags is beneficial because individuals can be identified from a distance with binoculars when the animal is out of the water.

Both plastic and metal tags are used to mark the flippers of sea turtles. Tags come in varying sizes, and smaller tags should be used on immature turtles. Plastic tags are inexpensive but are susceptible to breakage, wear, and entanglement in nets.[36] Although tags made from metal alloys (Monel, Inconel, and titanium) may last longer than plastic tags, these tags are more expensive than plastic tags and Monel tags can also be susceptible to breakage or corrosion, which can lead to infection at the attachment site.[44] Research entities such as the Archie Carr Center for Sea Turtle Research at the University of Florida and the Wider Caribbean Sea Turtle Network (WIDECAST) work in coordination to facilitate a global database of turtle tags and to reduce potential redundancy in marking. In addition to individual marking codes, contact information can be placed on the back tags to assist with tag recoveries.

In sea turtles, tags are generally attached to the edge of fore flippers, and when they are applied correctly, the risk of infection or injury at the attachment site is generally low. Tags may either be inserted through the keratinized scales on the flippers or in the soft tissue between scales. Although no comparative data are available, tags placed in the middle of the scales have been retained for approximately 20 years in some

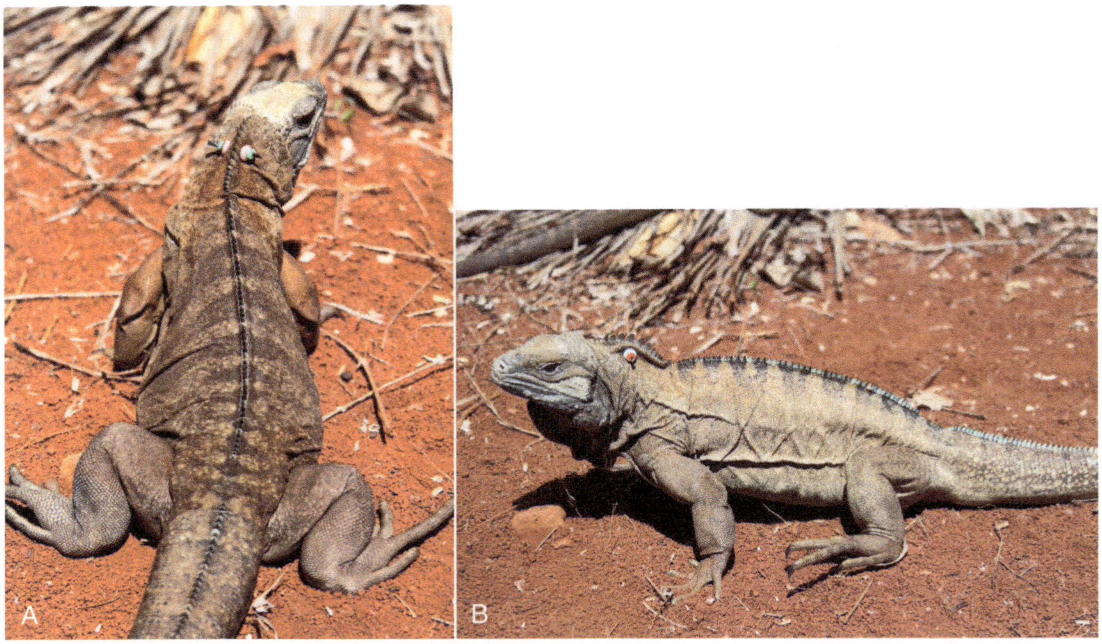

FIGURE 29-21 **A** and **B,** Colored beads to identify Caribbean iguanas. *(Photos courtesy of Rick Van Veen.)*

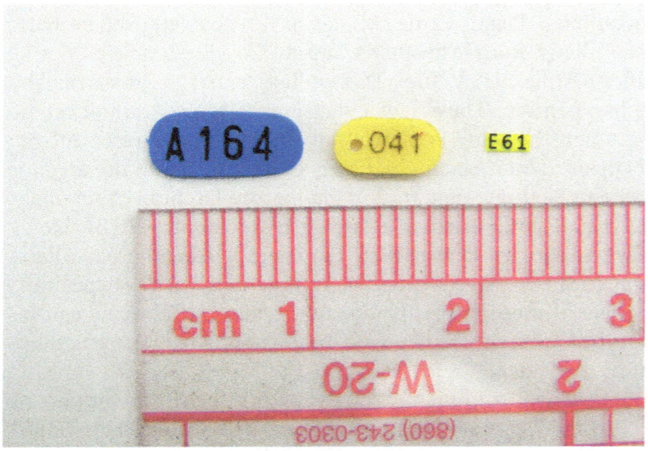

FIGURE 29-22 Alphanumeric tags for marking amphibians. Tags come in a variety of sizes and colors and can be implanted subcutaneously in amphibians via a small incision or with a specially designed syringe.

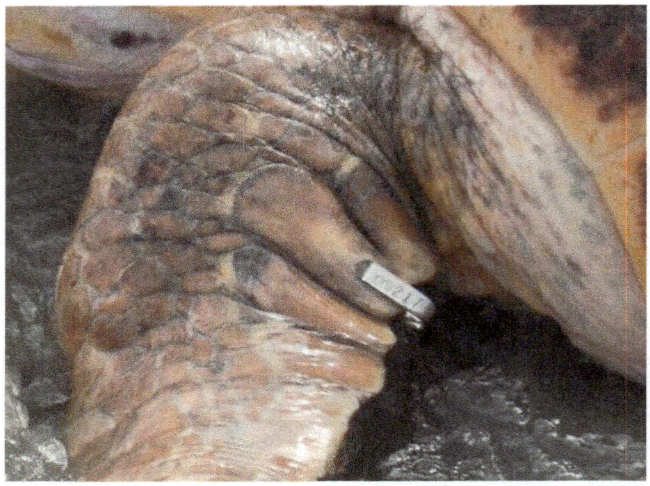

FIGURE 29-23 Placement of metal Inconel flipper tags on proximal pads on the front flipper of a marine turtle; the curved part of the tag allows room between the tag and flipper to reduce risk of constriction. *(Photo courtesy of S. Dilts.)*

individuals.[36,45] Tags are typically placed either in the most proximal pad on the posterior edge of the fore flipper or on the second pad to prevent the turtle from biting the tag[46] and to reduce drag or contact with other animals (Figure 29-23).[47] If the original tag is lost, replacement tags should be placed in a different pad rather than over the scar from the initial tag. Researchers generally tag both foreflippers, but the proximal pad of rear flippers are frequently tagged on juveniles and Leatherback Sea Turtles.[36]

Many of the factors affecting retention are avoidable through proper application and the incorporation of aseptic techniques to reduce risk to turtle health. A common cause of tag loss is failure of the locking mechanism[44]; tags should be double-checked before release and replaced if necessary. Applicators should be cleaned regularly to reduce rust and debris that can impede proper application of the tag, and they should be replaced when necessary to avoid tag loss. Tags may also be lost if they are snagged by debris (e.g., nets)[44] or substrate, as is the case with Hawksbill Sea Turtles *(Eretmochelys imbricata),* which shelter in coral reefs. Tearing generally results in tag scars that are readily visible and provide some information on whether the animal was marked in the past. Flipper tags can also be lost because of tissue necrosis if they are improperly applied. Tags should be placed such that roughly two thirds of the tag covers the flipper and the remaining one third, specifically the curved part, hangs over the edge of the fore flipper so that it does not constrict

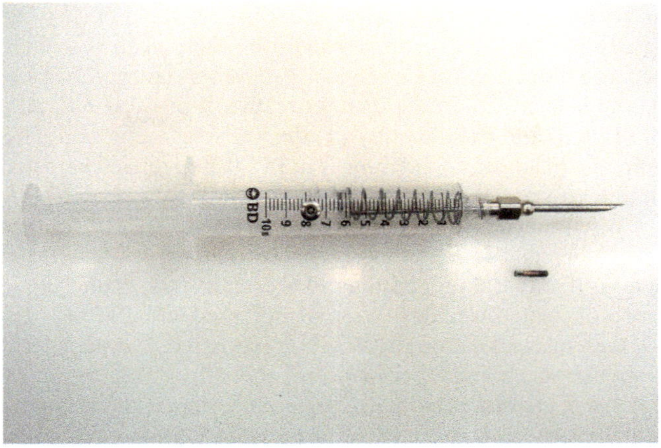

FIGURE 29-24 Syringe and passive integrated transponder (PIT) tag used to mark amphibians and reptiles for individual recognition. Tags are passive (no battery).

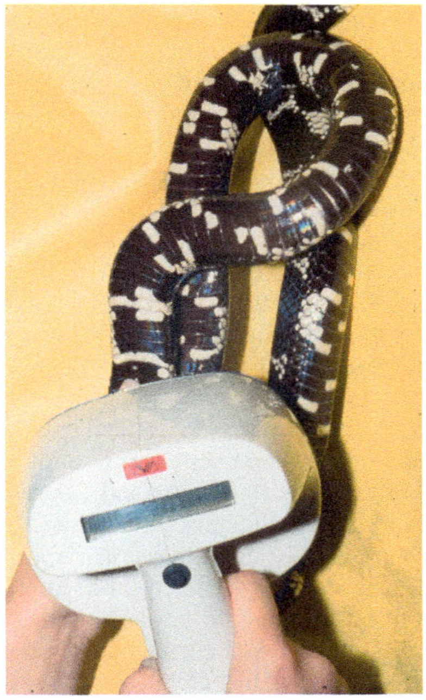

FIGURE 29-25 The unique alphanumeric code of a passive integrated transponder (PIT) tag is activated when scanned by a manufacturer-specific PIT tag reader. *(Photo courtesy of D.E. Scott.)*

circulation or growth. Because of problems with tag retention, biologists regularly tag both fore flippers in addition to using permanent marking methods such as PIT tagging. It is imperative to account for flipper tag loss to avoid overestimation in population abundance and underestimation of survivorship.[48]

Permanent Marking Methods

Passive Integrated Transponder Tags. Passive radio frequency identification (RFID) tags (or PIT tags) are one of the most widely used and reliable tools for marking amphibians and reptiles.[49,50] A PIT tag is an electronic microchip encased in biocompatible glass that ranges in size from 8 to 22 mm long and about 2 mm in diameter; the smallest tags weigh less than 0.10 g (Figure 29-24). Tags are dormant until activated by a handheld reader (Figure 29-25), which generates a close-range, electromagnetic field. Each tag contains a unique alphanumeric code that allows an indefinite number of individuals to be marked. The detection range for PIT tags varies with the size of the tag and type of reader. PIT tags can be expensive when large numbers of individuals are marked but have the benefit of small size and a potentially infinite life span.

There are two mainstream manufacturers of PIT tags: EZid American Veterinary Identification Devices (AVID, Weld, Colo) and Biomark, Inc. (Boise, Idaho), although there are additional manufacturers.[50] Both companies manufacture tags that are reliable and functional for the life of most animals, provided tags are inserted correctly (see further on); however, data on retention in long-lived species are not yet available. Biomark offers waterproof readers that are durable for use in the field. It is best to use one supplier at a field site because some brands are encrypted and cannot be read with the readers of other manufacturers. Further, care should be taken when recording identification codes from the reader because it is easy to accidentally transpose numbers or letters.

In addition to marking individuals, PIT tags can be used to monitor thermoregulatory behavior and movements of animals. BioMedic Data Systems, Inc. (Seaford, Del) produces temperature-sensitive PIT tags that have been used to monitor body temperature in snakes.[51,52] Automated scanning systems placed in areas the animal is expected to cross can be used to track movements of PIT-tagged animals. Scanning systems have been used to monitor migrations of PIT-tagged amphibians to and from breeding ponds or burrows[53-55] and use of passages and culverts under roads by Desert Tortoises *(Gopherus agassizii)*.[56] However, scanning systems are expensive, and the detection range of PIT tags in the field can be very limited.

PIT tags are injected or inserted through a surgical incision, most commonly under the skin, into muscle or the body cavity (Figure 29-26). Application of tissue glue at the insertion site can help with tag retention and can control bleeding (Norton T: Pers. observation, 2011). Tags can be purchased in preloaded sterile syringes or individually and loaded into a sterilized stainless steel syringe for implantation (see Figure 29-24). All PIT tags should be sterilized before insertion if this has not been done by the commercial source. The preferred technique for sterilization is ethylene oxide gas (STERIS Isomedix Services, Mentor, Ohio) or hydrogen peroxide plasma sterilization (Sterrad, Advanced Sterilization Products, Irvine, Calif). Sterility should be maintained during the loading and insertion of the PIT tag.

In frogs and toads, PIT tags can be inserted subcutaneously after the area is cleaned as described earlier, or they can be inserted into the coelom with the use of the procedures described in the Surgically Invasive section of the chapter. For subcutaneous implantation, approximately 4 mm of skin on the ventral surface can be pinched and the tag inserted via syringe.[57] In Eastern Hellbenders *(Cryptobranchus alleganiensis alleganiensis)*, PIT tags were implanted in the dorsal side of the tail approximately 8 cm posterior to the hindleg.[58]

In reptiles, PIT tags are generally implanted subcutaneously, although implantation sites vary by taxa. For example, in crocodilians, PIT tags can be injected subcutaneously at the junction of the ninth and tenth ventral scale rows posterior to the cloaca.[49] In lizards, PIT tags can be inserted subcutaneously, through a small incision in the skin on the side of the animal[34] or anterior to the left rear leg in large lizards or tuatara.[59] In snakes of all sizes, PIT tags can be implanted subcutaneously between the second and third left dorsal scale rows, approximately two thirds of the way down the body.[50,60] They can also be inserted into the body cavity during transmitter placement. PIT tagging may not be appropriate for all species because tags may be expelled through the walls of the digestive tract of some species (e.g., Brown Water Snakes, *[Nerodia taxispilota]*[61]), and tags placed in the body cavity can migrate.[49] The frequency with which PIT tags are expelled or migrate within the body has not been quantified for any species.

PIT tags in adult freshwater turtles, terrapins, and tortoises can be injected into the loose skin at the shoulder or hind leg on either side of the body. Buhlmann and Tuberville[62] describe a method for implanting PIT tags in small aquatic turtle species such as *Sternotherus* and *Kinosternon* spp. They recommend holding the animal vertically and carefully inserting the syringe above a hind leg, to implant the tag adjacent and parallel to the bridge of the shell. Researchers have surgically implanted sterile PIT tags in hatchling and small turtles and tortoises by making a small incision into the inguinal skin just in front of the back leg, creating a small pocket under the skin with hemostats, and then inserting the PIT tag with the hemostats. Tissue glue is used to close the incision. Local anesthesia with lidocaine or bupivacaine can be used depending on the size of the patient. Care should be taken to avoid toxicity in small turtles. Dexmedetomidine alone or in combination with ketamine and/or an opioid agent is a good reversible sedative that can be used for this procedure. Dosage depends on the species. PIT tags appear to have high retention rates but may migrate from the implantation site; thus scanning the entire body for tags is recommended.

PIT tags are also commonly used to mark sea turtles. The minimum straight carapace length for PIT tag application is 30 cm. Tags are placed in the left front flipper either in the triceps superficialis muscle (shoulder area) or in the flexor carpi ulnaris (posterior aspect of the flipper, anterior and immediately distal to the second large scale). Tags should not be inserted through fibropapillomas or any abnormal skin. Infection rates are low provided that appropriate sterilization and site cleaning techniques are employed.[63] PIT tags are generally used as a secondary marking method in sea turtles because flipper tags are often lost.[64,65] Redundancy in marking methods is critical in sea turtles because of possible migration of PIT tags and the difficulty in effectively scanning such large animals. In addition, differences in PIT tag manufacturers used in different projects around the world may preclude detection.

As with other taxa, PIT tags would seem to have advantages over other marking methods because the tags are small, passive, and may last indefinitely. However, a study found higher levels of corticosteroids in lizards implanted with PIT tags than in those marked by toe clipping.[66] It is possible that such stress responses occur in other taxa, but this effect of marking has not been quantified sufficiently because most of the studies that have been conducted only measure survivorship of the individual and tag retention.

Shell Drilling and Notching. Adult turtles and tortoises can be permanently marked by notching the marginal scales of the carapace; appropriate clean techniques should be used (i.e., the area to be notched or drilled should be cleaned with betadine and alcohol at least once before drilling, and the drill bits should be soaked in an appropriate disinfectant between turtles).[67] Turtles and tortoises have 11 to 12 scales on each side of their carapace; scales at the anterior and posterior portion of the shell generally have a thin margin that can easily be notched with a triangular file (Figure 29-27) or Dremel tool or drilled with the use of a small drill bit (Figure 29-28).[68] Scales on the bridge connecting the carapace and plastron (scales 4 to 7) should not be filed because they are generally not flared and there is a risk of penetrating the body cavity. In addition, drilling holes directly through bone may cause lesions in the bone or bone marrow.

Several different numbering or alphabetical schemes can be derived when scute notches are made on turtles, but in general, scales in each of the four quadrants of the turtle (i.e., front right, front left, rear right, rear left) are assigned a series of numbers (e.g., 1s, 10s, 100s, and 1000s) or letters such that thousands of individuals can be uniquely marked[68] (Figure 29-29). Shell notching has been used successfully to

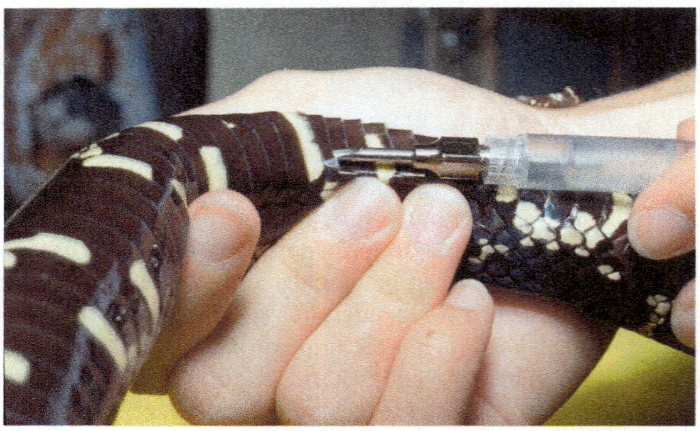

FIGURE 29-26 Subcutaneous injection of a passive integrated transponder (PIT) tag into an Eastern Kingsnake *(Lampropeltis getula)* with the use of a 12-gauge needle. *(Photo courtesy of D.E. Scott.)*

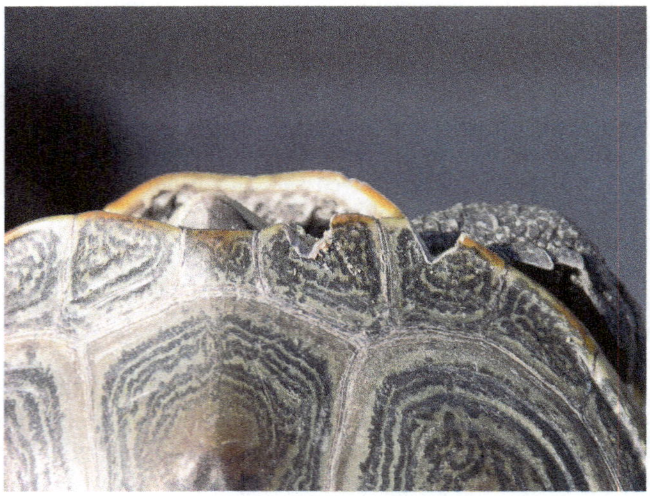

FIGURE 29-27 Shell marginal notched with a triangular file. *(Photo courtesy Dr. Terry M. Norton, Georgia Sea Turtle Center, Jekyll Island, Ga.)*

identify individual turtles over more than 25-year capture intervals (Gibbons W, Greene J: Unpublished data, 2001). Soft shell turtles lack bony marginal scales but can be marked by notching the margin of the shell[69,70] or by clipping claws.[67] Hatchling turtles can be marked with the same numeric and alphabetical system with the use of fingernail clippers to create a notch in the marginal scutes. Most chelonians tolerate notching of the shell without analgesia or sedation, but if a drill is used to create a hole in the shell, adequate sedation and analgesia is indicated. Dexmedetomidine alone or in combination with ketamine and/or morphine derivatives are good choices because they are effective and reversible.

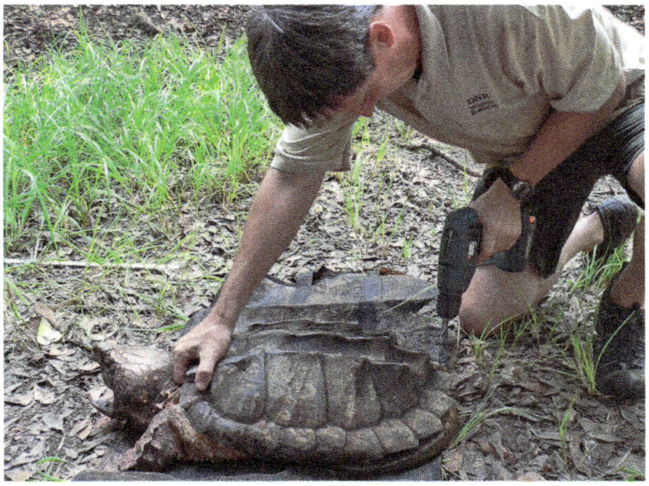

FIGURE 29-28 Use of a handheld drill to mark marginals on larger freshwater turtles. *(Photo courtesy Dr. Terry M. Norton, Georgia Sea Turtle Center, Jekyll Island, Ga.)*

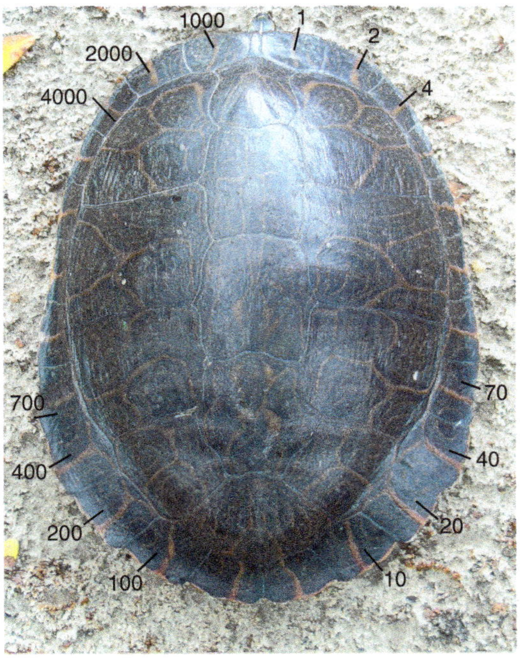

FIGURE 29-29 Example of a turtle shell marking scheme. Marginal scales should be notched such that the turtle can be individually identified. Combinations of scales (e.g., numbers 1 and 2 on the upper right quadrant of the carapace) can be notched to mark the turtle as number 3.

Shell notching does not work as well on sea turtles as on freshwater turtles because of their thick shells, extensive growth, and the frequency of marginal shell injury that can obscure marks. However, a cordless drill can be used to drill holes through the keratinous overlay in the supracaudals (Figure 29-30). As the turtle grows, holes in the keratin migrate toward the edge of the marginals. If a turtle is recaptured, the same drill pattern can simply be reapplied at the highest part of the keratin. On nesting female sea turtles, a flashlight can be shined beneath the shell to determine where the keratin layer extends beyond the bone. Shell notching is not possible on all species, such as Olive Ridley Sea Turtles *(Lepidochelys olivacea)* (Andrews K: Pers. observation, 2011). In other species, such as Loggerhead Sea Turtles *(Caretta caretta)*, drilling can be problematic because of high loads of epibiota that can prevent drilling or that can grow over holes and prevent positive identification (Andrews K: Pers. observation, 2011). However, this technique has proven effective and essential in a long-term saturation tagging project of Hawksbill Sea Turtles.[45] Many of the techniques used here are performed by biologists in the field studying large populations of reptiles and amphibians. As this field evolves veterinarians are becoming more involved and can assist biologists in making decisions about practical but appropriate analgesia for painful procedures and where clean and sterile techniques need to be utilized. These techniques are rarely indicated in clinical practice where individual pet reptiles are involved; however, it is helpful for veterinarians dealing with amphibians and reptiles to be familiar with the current identification practices that are performed.

Toe Clipping. Historically, frogs, salamanders, lizards, and juvenile crocodilians were often marked by removal of toes or *toe clipping*.[32,71] There is some controversy about the level of pain produced by this procedure and whether analgesia or sedation should be used when toe clipping is performed.[30] When large numbers of animals are processed, it may be impractical to provide such intensive care. Researchers using this technique should keep this in mind and consider seeking alternative identification methods when available. The advantage of toe clipping is the low cost and large numbers of unique marks available if individual digits and limbs are assigned

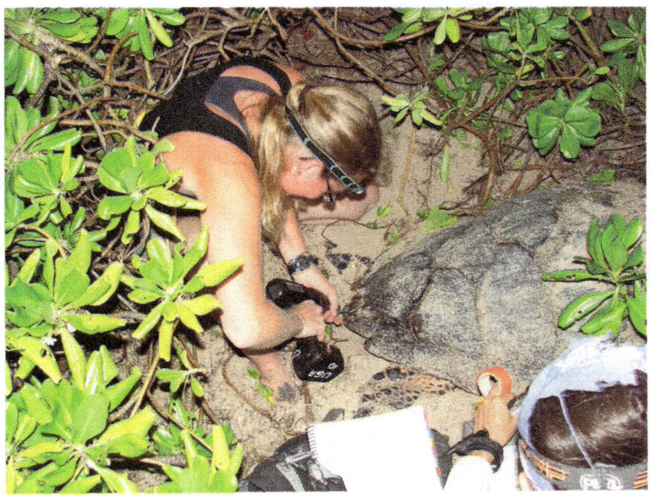

FIGURE 29-30 Use of a handheld drill to mark keratinous growth on subcaudals on marine turtles.

a different series of numbers. To facilitate recognition of a toe-clip mark versus a natural injury, researchers can remove multiple toes on different feet. Removal of adjacent toes should be avoided. The thumbs of adult male frogs, which are used in amplexus, should never be removed, nor should more than two digits on any one limb be removed. Scissors should be disinfected with an appropriate product (e.g., chlorhexidine) before use and between animals. A drop of tissue glue can be used to stop the bleeding. Excised toes can be preserved in ethanol for genetic analysis or skeletochronology.[72,73]

In addition to pain from the procedure, there is concern that toe clipping may affect survival of individuals. Studies have shown that the number of toes clipped may negatively affect frog survival,[74] particularly in arboreal species (e.g., tree frogs, *Hyla* spp.). However, a laboratory study on Squirrel Tree Frogs *(Hyla squirella)* found no difference in growth and survival after toe clipping.[75] Many salamanders and some frogs can regenerate toes quickly; thus the reliability of the method is further limited. Both toe clips and injectable fluorescent polymers (mentioned previously) have been used to mark individual amphibians[76]; the advantage of using both methods is increased reliability in identifying individuals over time, although the effects of such invasive marking methods on behavior and long-term survival are not known.[77]

Toe clipping is more effective in lizards and juvenile crocodilians than in amphibians because their toes do not regenerate. However, the technique may have negative effects on behavior of arboreal lizards, which have subdigital toe pads for clinging to vegetation.[78] In contrast, a number of studies have demonstrated that toe clipping does not affect sprint speed, which is a measure of fitness in terrestrial lizards.[79-81] The frequency of natural toe loss in lizards has been used as further evidence that toe clipping in lizards is unlikely to influence survival,[82] yet natural toe loss can preclude recognition of toe clips.[83] Although the technique is commonly used with juvenile alligators, natural toe loss from conspecific interactions is frequent and can reduce accuracy and detectability in recaptures.

Scale Clipping. Scale clipping is an inexpensive technique that is frequently used to mark snakes. Removal of the scale, with small sharp, sterile scissors, leaves a scar that persists after shedding and the marks can be accurately read for many years. The method was originally described for subcaudal scales,[84] but Brown and Parker[85] presented a marking system using ventral scales, which are larger and easier to remove than subcaudals.[86] Depending on the numbering system, the entire scale can be removed, or the left or right half of the ventral scale can be removed.[85] Application of tissue glue can prevent excessive bleeding. This technique can be used on snakes of all sizes, but fewer scales should be removed and smaller scissors may be required for neonates or small snake species. Local anesthesia with lidocaine or bupivacaine provides adequate analgesia for this procedure. A nonsteroidal antiinflammatory drug such as meloxicam provides postprocedure analgesia.

Scute Clipping. Tail scute clipping is one of the more common, affordable, and persistent methods of marking crocodilians. Detectability of clipped tail scutes is reduced with juveniles because of their accelerated growth rates, but overall, this technique is the most efficient in terms of ease of application and the ability to identify large numbers of individuals.[83] Enumeration systems vary and can consist of numeric or alphabetical ordering. Both left and right sides of dorsal scutes can be incorporated to increase the number of potential marks. A sterilized utility knife (X-Acto, Elmer's Products, Inc., Columbus, Ohio) or box cutter can be useful for making a clean cut in the least amount of time. Dull blades will result in multiple cuts to mark the animal, thereby increasing handling time and stress. The tail scute must be removed down into the muscle; the cut should be made just below where the scales merge with the adjoining scales (Figure 29-31). If the scute clipping is performed properly, a small amount of bleeding will occur and indicates that the mark will truly be permanent. Appropriate aseptic technique, as described earlier, should be used. Local anesthesia with lidocaine or bupivacaine will provide appropriate analgesia.

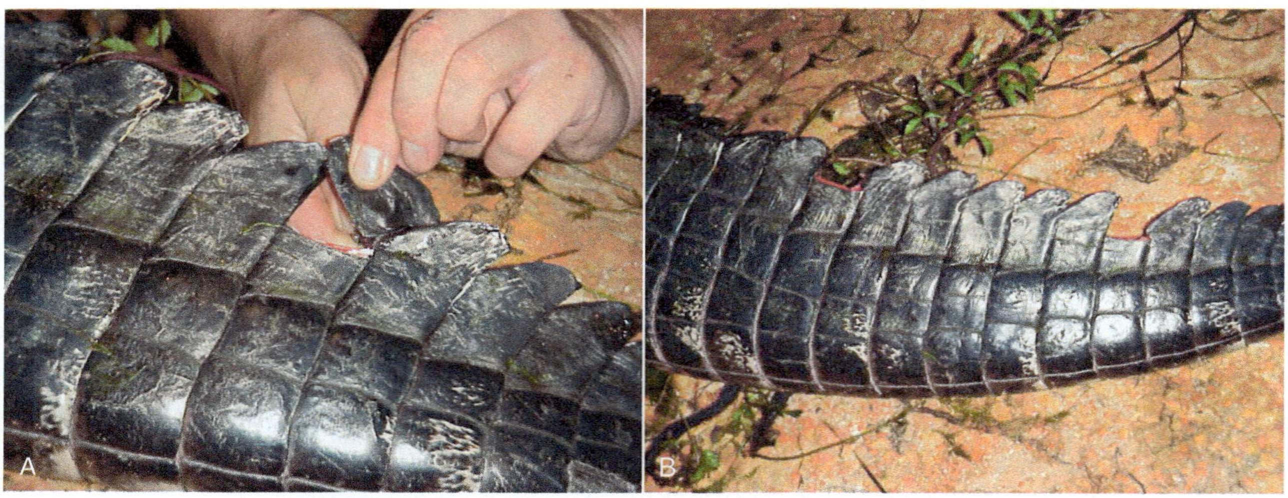

FIGURE 29-31 **A,** Removal of a scute on the tail of an American Alligator *(Alligator mississippiensis).* **B,** Completed pattern of a double clip on an American Alligator tail. *(Photo courtesy of C. Hagen.)*

Heat Branding. Heat branding is a fast, affordable, and straightforward method for marking snakes. Although the method was originally described as a method to mark amphibians and reptiles,[87] it is most appropriate for use with snakes.[88] It could be appropriate for some lizards with thick skin, but it was not effective in a pilot test with *Calotes* spp. (Whitaker N, Andrews K: Unpublished data, 2008). Pilot tests have been conducted on heat-branding in juvenile American Alligators, but the mark was insufficient for long-term identification (Tuberville T, Andrews K: Unpublished data, 2012). Disposable medical cautery units can be used to brand individual scales in patterns similar to those recommended for scale clipping[89]; however, the brands should also be applied to four to five lateral scales that correspond to the marked ventral scales to differentiate between marks and scars from natural injuries (Figure 29-32). High and low temperature settings are available on some cautery units; the low temperature units setting should be used with neonates or small snake species. This technique has been used successfully on a broad array of snake species and both neonates and adults.[89] If applied correctly, brands can persist for many years; however, long-term durability of the mark for longer lived species (e.g., *Crotalus* spp.) is not known. Cautery tips will last longer if overhanging scale material is trimmed off on keeled-scale snakes before branding.

Freeze Branding. Freeze branding, which alters the pigmentation of the scales, can also be used to mark lizards, snakes, and crocodilians.[90] Coolants include dry ice and ethyl alcohol or liquid halocarbon (Freon). Coolants can be applied to the skin with copper wire with a rounded tip or a synthetic sponge-tipped dowel for 20 to 30 seconds. Freeze branding has several shortcomings over heat branding. The marks are variable depending on the original color pattern of the animal and can be difficult to read.

Magnetized Wire Tags. Magnetized wire tags have been used to mark large numbers of sea turtles. They are less expensive than PIT tags, have high retention rates (95% to 100%),[91] and they appear to be effective for the lifetime of the animal.[92] Magnetized tags cannot be used to differentiate individuals unless used in conjunction with another marking

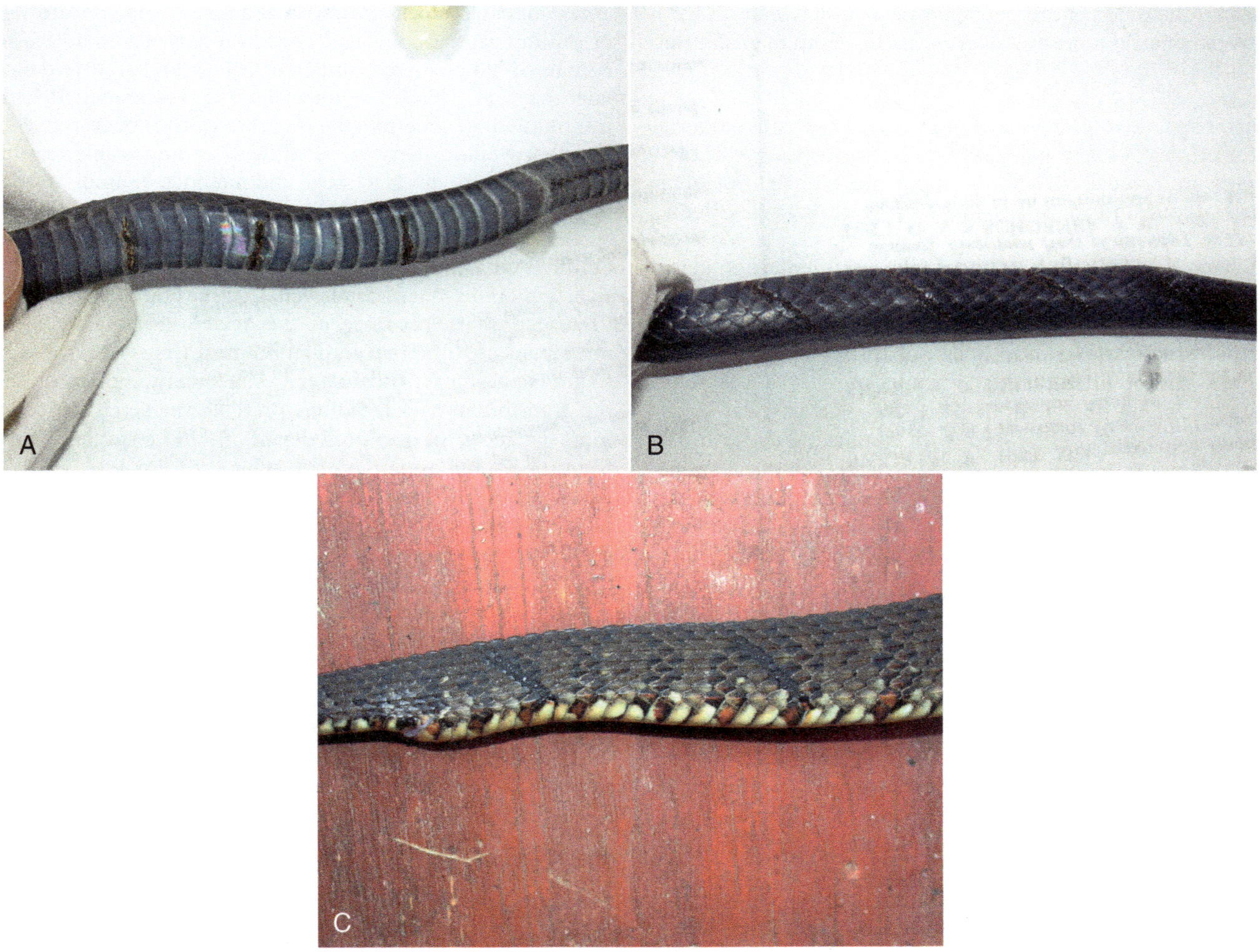

FIGURE 29-32 A, Ventral scale pattern after heat branding on a Black Racer *(Coluber constrictor).* This image displays code 146 (anal plate is skipped). **B,** Lateral scale pattern after heat branding for the same individual code as in **A. C,** Image of healed lateral marks from heat branding on a Banded Water Snake *(Nerodia fasciata). (Photos courtesy of J.D. Willson.)*

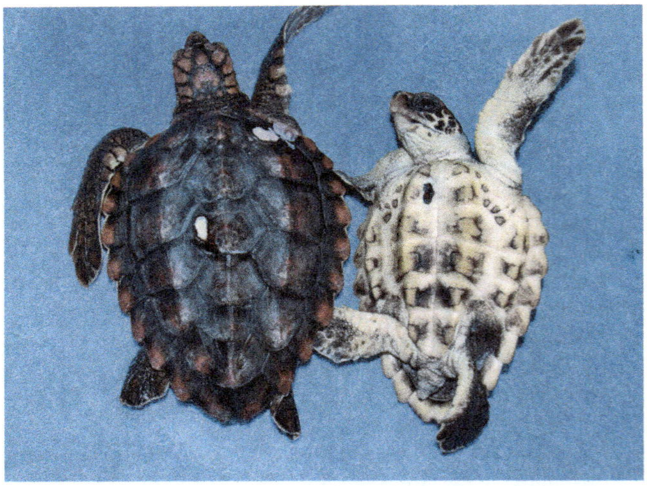

FIGURE 29-33 Carapacial and plastral placement of living tags. *(Photo courtesy Dr. Jynette Wyneken, Florida Atlantic University, Boca Raton, Fla.)*

technique.[93] Wire tags are typically placed in foreflippers[94] and require a magnetometer for field identification. Tags can also be detected on x-ray films. The disadvantage of this technique is that magnetometers can be expensive and may detect false-positive animals if there are other magnetic components in the area of the animal.[94]

Living Tags. Living tags have been used to identify cohorts or year-classes of hatchling and juvenile sea turtles.[36,95,96] Living tags are created by autografting a piece of light-colored plastron tissue into a darker scute on the carapace (Figure 29-33).[94] Tags grow with the turtle and appear as spots or streaks in older individuals. It does take a trained eye to identify a mark, particularly on adults that received the tags as hatchlings. However, living tags provided confirmation of the return of head-start Kemp's Ridley Sea Turtles to Padre Island National Seashore in Texas 11 years after release.[96]

Grafts can be obtained with the use of a surgical biopsy punch and can be secured with surgical glue.[95] Initial experimentation of the technique tested the use of melanin-destroying substances to emphasize the contrast of the plastral material from the carapace.[97] Generally, living tags are applied to different scutes to represent different year classes.[93,98]

RADIO TELEMETRY, SATELLITE TELEMETRY, BIOTELEMETRY, AND ARCHIVAL DATA RECORDERS

The purpose of this section is to introduce some basic principles of telemetry and describe techniques that have worked well for the authors and other researchers and likely have a broad application; an exhaustive review of the literature will not be provided. Amphibians and reptiles are difficult animals to study because they are often cryptic and wary. They also live in habitats that are often inaccessible and can spend considerable periods of time submerged in water or below ground. The ongoing advancement and miniaturization of electronic tagging technology has provided the means to effectively study these animals in the wild with minimal disturbance.[99] In addition, data on physiologic function (e.g., heart rate, body temperature, and feeding habits) may be assessed. Telemetry refers to an active transmission of data coming from an animal, with the objective of remotely collecting data on an animal's location, behavior and physiology, and characteristics of the environment.[88] Acoustic, electric, magnetic, and electromagnetic (e.g., visible light, radio wave, and microwave) forms of energy can be used to transmit data.[88]

The most commonly used spatial technology in herpetofauna is radio telemetry, which utilizes high-frequency radio waves. The equipment to conduct radio telemetry studies includes a transmitter, a power source (e.g., battery), and a transmitting antenna, all of which must be attached to the animal. Transmitter packages can be externally attached through a variety of methods or surgically implanted internally. Radio signals are detected by receiving antennae, which can be handheld, positioned on land at specific locations, or carried on land via vehicles, ships, planes, or satellites.[88] Satellite telemetry, including global positioning systems (GPS), enables information to be relayed from the transmitter to a receiver via satellites. Biotelemetry refers to the transmission of biological information from sensors on the animal, without direct contact between the transmitter and receiver. Internal physiologic data such as heart rate, body temperature, or electrocardiographic results, behavioral data such as diving time and depth, and environmental information such as ambient temperature, light, or salinity can all be relayed. Archival data recorders are self-contained biotelemetric units that collect and archive data for later recovery. This technology allows for researchers to gather information on wide-ranging (e.g., sea turtles) or secretive species that would otherwise be difficult or impossible to study. A wide range of designs, sizes, and methods of application are now available and allow for study of a variety of species.

Disadvantages and limitations of this technology include (1) high cost and complexity of use, (2) battery capacity and size limitations on transmission longevity and strength, and (3) the physical presence of the device may affect the animal's behavior. Internal implantation of transmitter packages requires anesthesia and surgery. Attachment and retention of the transmitter package often presents many challenges. In most instances, transmitting devices should eventually detach from the animal or be removed, which may require recapture. Recovery of archival recorders is required to retrieve data, which may also necessitate recapture and even another surgery. The researcher should select a transmitter package and attachment method appropriate to the animal. The general rule of thumb is that a transmitter package (i.e., battery, transmitter, and antenna) should not exceed 5% of the animal's body mass[86] and the attachment and placement should not impede the animal's movements, physiology, reproductive success, and survival. Tradeoffs between transmitter attachment methods and transmitter weight, transmitter longevity, and transmission range should be determined to optimize performance so that the particular study's objectives can be met.

Radio Telemetry: Nonsurgical Placement

Amphibians. Telemetry placement in amphibians is complicated by their generally small body size and sensitive skin. Most manufacturers can configure a transmitter based on the body size and life history of the focal species. However, projected battery life of the transmitter is limited by battery size, so small transmitters may need to be refurbished with a fresh

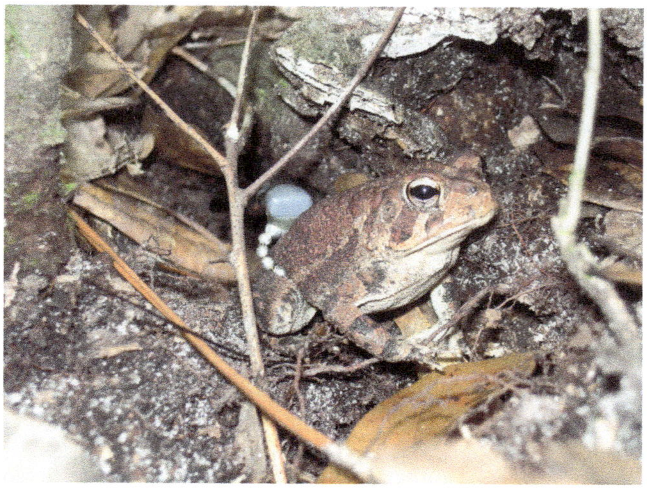

FIGURE 29-34 Southern Toad *(Anaxyrus terrestris)* with belt attachment of a radio transmitter package. *(Photo courtesy of S. Sterrett.)*

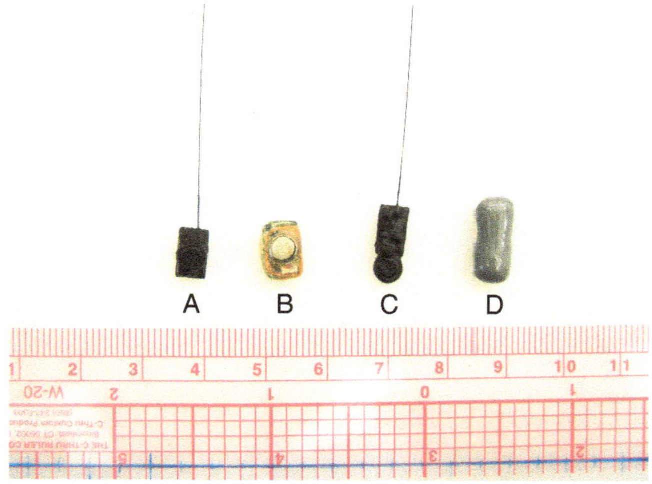

FIGURE 29-35 Different configurations for small radio transmitters used in amphibians. **A,** The transmitter has the battery mounted on top with a free hanging antenna. **B,** The transmitter has the antenna coiled around the battery, and the entire package is encapsulated in acrylic for implantation into the body cavity. **C,** The transmitter has the battery mounted at the end of the transmitter, creating a longer but thinner package, also with a free hanging antenna. **D,** A fully encapsulated transmitter with the same configuration as in *C.*

battery or replaced frequently (every 1 to 2 weeks to up to 3 months, depending on the size of the transmitter package). Transmitters may be attached externally to frogs with the use of belts or harnesses lined with small beads to prevent abrasion of the skin (Figure 29-34). The belt must have enough slack to prevent wear on the skin but must be tight enough to prevent the animal from jumping out of the harness or becoming entangled. For external transmitter placement, the antenna is loose and will trail behind the animal (Figure 29-35). Because of the body shape and fossorial habit of many salamanders, external attachment of transmitters is generally not used (see section on surgical placement of radio transmitters further on).

Reptiles

CROCODILIANS. In a recent publication, methods for acquisition and monitoring of behavioral and physiologic variables from free-ranging crocodilians through the use of data loggers and via satellite, radio, and acoustic telemetry were described.[100-104] Radio telemetry has been most widely used to track the movement patterns of crocodilians in addition to body temperatures and heart rates. The nuchal shield has been most commonly used as the site for transmitter attachment; however, measuring body temperature via radio telemetry requires that the transmitter be located internally either via ingestion[105] or by surgical implantation into the coelomic cavity.[106,107]

Archival tags (data loggers) have been used to record diving behaviors, fine-scale movement patterns, and heart rates of crocodilians.[108] Large volumes of data can be stored within these tags and downloaded at a later time. The greatest challenge with this technology is retrieving the tags. To maximize chances of retrieving them, researchers use other technologies simultaneously (e.g., radio telemetry or satellite telemetry) to locate the tag or animal. The tags are designed to release and float.[103] describe a technique using a tag and transmitter encased in a neoprene sleeve that incorporated a polystyrene float. The nuchal shield was used as the external attachment site so that the tag could surface each time the animal was on the surface. Manual restraint and a local anesthetic were used to place the tag. Holes were drilled through the center of four of the scutes to align with wires from the data package. The wires were threaded through the holes in a manner that minimized any loops of wire being exposed so that the telemetry package would not become snagged. Plastic-coated wire was secured with crimp sleeves.

A time-release mechanism was designed to deploy an archival tag in an effort to study Saltwater Crocodile *(Crocodylus porosus)* diving behaviors and fine-scaled movement patterns.[103] These animals inhabit waters with varying salinities from freshwater to saltwater, and it was very unlikely that they could be recaptured. The data-logging units were positioned on the nuchal shield with a similar attachment protocol as already described. Radio and acoustic telemetry were used to retrieve the archival tags. A novel self-release mechanism was designed and used a fluid-filled, spring-loaded syringe and hypodermic needle that could be set to release the tag for deployment periods of days to weeks. The spring-loaded syringe slowly advanced the plunger, and once the plunger moved past an islet on the flotation casing, the unit detached from the aluminum base plate, which eventually corroded off as the crimps dissolved. The time of release was controlled by the amount of fluid in the syringe, the viscosity of fluid, the gauge of needle, and the strength of the spring (Figure 29-36).

LIZARDS. Radio telemetry has been used to study aspects of behavior and spatial ecology in a variety of lizard species including Beaded Lizards *(Heloderma horridum),* Gila Monsters ([*Heloderma suspectum*]; Goode M: Unpublished data, 2011), Yarrow's Spiny Lizard *(Sceloporus jarrovi),* Lace Monitor *(Varanus varius),* Southern Alligator Lizard *(Eligaria multicarinata),* Land Mullet Skink *(Egernia major),* Eastern Bearded Dragon *(Pogona barbata),*[109] and Water Dragons *(Physignathus lesueurii).*[110] Goodman[109] reviewed a variety of telemetry techniques that have been used in West Indian iguanas *(Cyclura* spp.), including ingested transmitters, transmitters externally

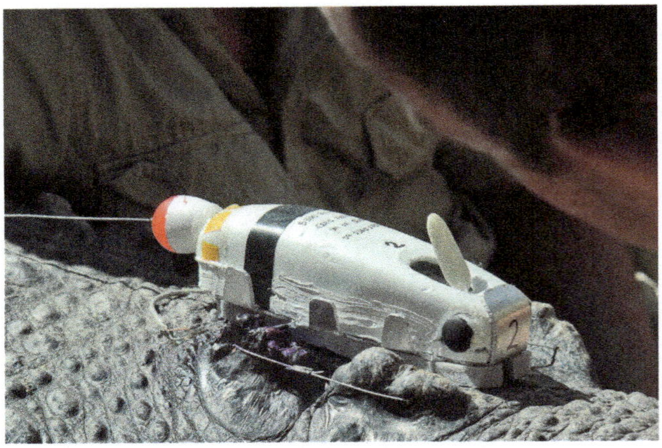

FIGURE 29-36 Data logger (archival tag) with self-release device attached to the nuchal scutes of an Estuarine crocodile (*Crocodylus porosus*). The data logger recorded water depth, acceleration in three dimensions, compass bearing, speed, and body temperature. *(Photo courtesy of C.E. Franklin.)*

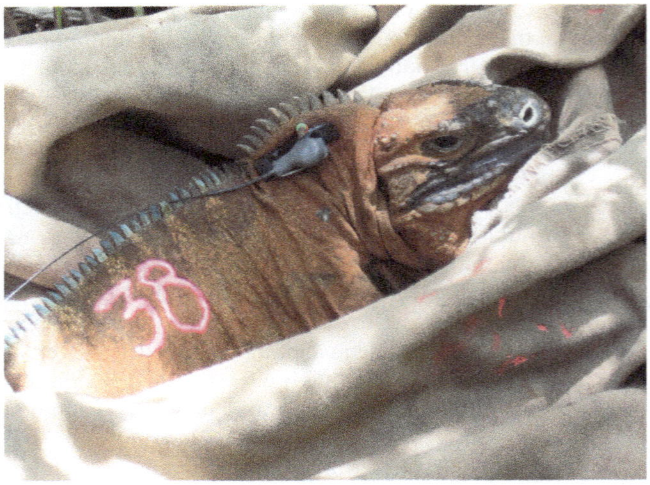

FIGURE 29-37 Caribbean iguana with radio transmitter sutured to the dorsal crest. *(Photo courtesy of Tandora Grant.)*

applied with duct tape, suture of transmitters to the dorsal crest (Figure 29-37), transmitter collars, belts, and harnesses (Figure 29-38), and use of various adhesives to attach transmitters. The signal range did not differ dramatically between most methods but did differ across habitats and among transmitter models, especially in relation to free antenna length. An additional consideration is the tradeoff between signal strength and battery life. Different researchers using the same model of transmitter may select reduced signal strength to increase battery life if the focal species is not wide-ranging; thus there was substantial variation in signal range and battery life among research projects.[109] Knapp and Owens[111] conducted radio telemetry on hatchling Andros Iguanas *(Cyclura cychlura cychlura)* by placing transmitters on the dorsal side of the pelvic girdle with test monofilament line wrapped around the lizard's body to secure it. This method may also be useful for hatchlings and small lizards of other species.

A harness to attach radio transmitters to Water Dragons was made by cutting a sheet of nylon mesh or fly screen in the shape of a square with two extending straps.[110] Cutting the square and straps to fit the individual lizard is critical: if they are too large, it may get caught on vegetation, and if too small, it may cause discomfort or abrasions to the skin. The radio transmitter was glued to the harness with adhesive (Super Glue; Super Glue Corp., Rancho Cucamonga, Calif) before attaching the harness to the animal. The square part of the harness was placed firmly on the lizard's back, above the forearms, while the straps were then pulled over the shoulders, crossed on the chest, and pulled up under the lizard's forearms. After pulling the straps snug, they were adhered to the square with Super Glue and to one another where they crossed on the chest. The mesh was held together at glue points with forceps. The harness was easily removed by cutting the straps with scissors. Water Dragons were monitored for up to 2 months without any harness losses or any noticeable problems for the lizards.

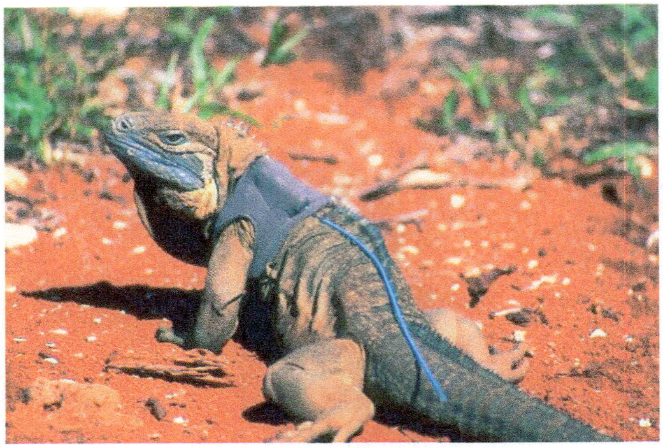

FIGURE 29-38 Caribbean iguana fitted with a harness transmitter. *(Photo courtesy of Rick Hudson.)*

SNAKES. Radio transmitters can be attached externally to snakes to collect short-term movement data.[112] The method is ideal for use with juvenile snakes or small-bodied species.[113] Transmitters should be attached dorsolaterally, approximately two thirds of the snout-to-vent length behind the head with adhesive (Super Glue) gel (Figure 29-39). Transmitters are typically shed during ecdysis and can be retrieved for use on another animal.

Freshwater Turtles, Terrapins, and Tortoises. The predominant way transmitters have been attached to turtles is by mounting the tag onto the carapace. Different techniques have varying levels of success depending on the life history traits, age, and size of the study animals (Figure 29-40). Boarman and collegues[114] reviewed 113 scientific papers, reports, and semitechnical articles on radio tracking projects with turtles and concluded that little information was available in the literature to evaluate the effects of transmitters on the study of animals. In this review, transmitters were attached to the carapace by a variety of methods including epoxy, silicone sealant, dental acrylic, and other types of adhesives. Additionally, there were descriptions of the transmitters being strapped on with harnesses or attached via bolts, wire, cable, or nylon ties or with monofilament line, which was passed through the holes drilled into the posterior carapace or marginal scutes. In these cases, the transmitter was either attached to

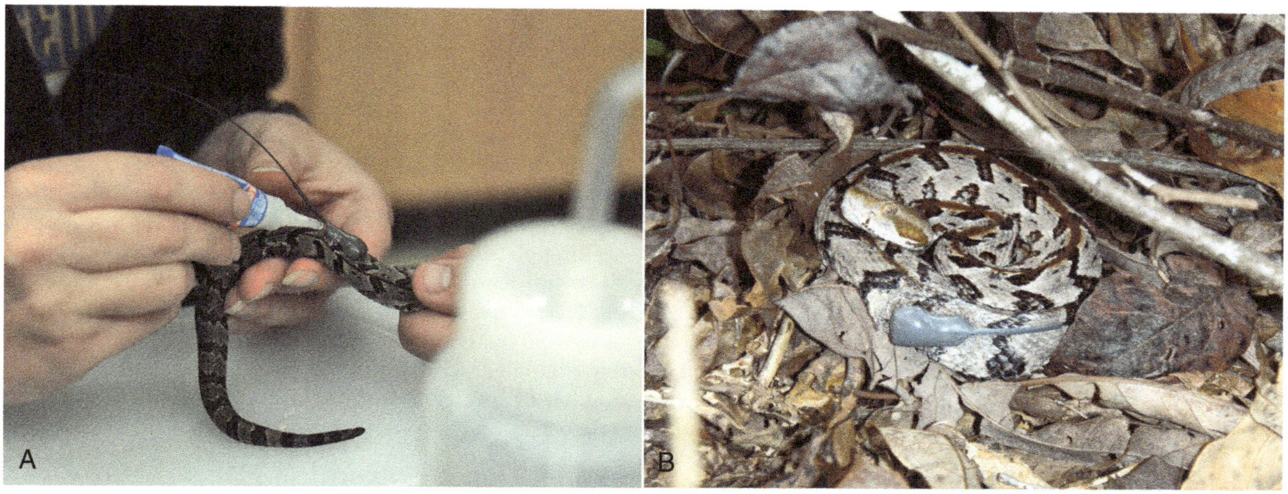

FIGURE 29-39 **A** and **B,** External attachment of a radio transmitter to a neonate Timber Rattlesnake *(Crotalus horridus). (Photos courtesy of E.M. Schlimm.)*

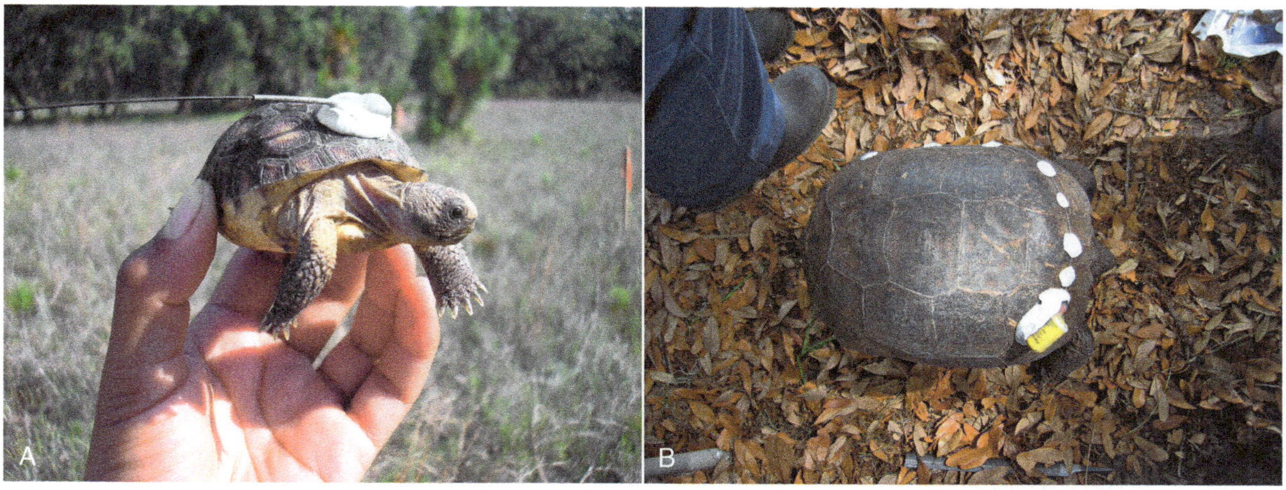

FIGURE 29-40 **A.** Juvenile Gopher Tortoise (*Gopherus polyphemus*) with radio transmitter on carapace. *(Photo courtesy Tracey D. Tuberville, Savannah River Ecology Laboratory, The University of Georgia, Athens, Ga).* **B.** Adult Gopher Tortoise with radio transmitter on carapace. *(Photo courtesy Dr. Terry M. Norton, Georgia Sea Turtle Center, Jekyll Island, Ga).*

the carapace or allowed to trail behind the turtles. There were many possible behavioral (e.g., mating disruptions) and physical problems that were potentially caused by transmitters. Shell deformities occurred on hatchling Gopher Tortoises because the epoxy holding transmitters encroached on growth areas.[115] This should be avoided when transmitters are placed on the carapace, especially in young, growing animals. Transmitters may become entangled in vegetation, usually between gaps between the shell and the transmitter or the antenna. Transmitters may attract the attention of predators and humans and therefore should be camouflaged in some way (Figure 29-41). Boarman and collegues[114] recommended a process for transmitter placement in Desert Tortoises that is applicable to other nonmarine chelonids:

1. Test the transmitter to confirm that it is functional.
2. Clean dirt off the carapace.
3. Preposition the transmitter to first left or right coastal scute and fit as flush to the carapace as possible.
4. To position the antenna, cut short sections of flexible 3-mm plastic tubing and attach each section to the first

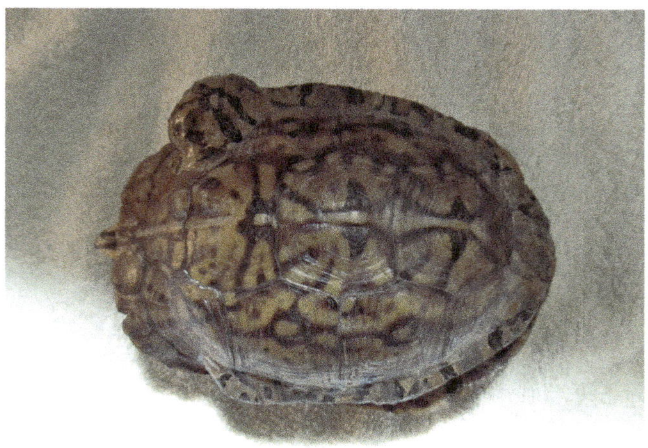

FIGURE 29-41 Radio transmitter and wrapped antenna that has been painted to camouflage the equipment on an Eastern Box Turtle *(Terrapene carolina).(Photo courtesy of J.E. Colbert.)*

four vertebral scutes using epoxy. Each section should be cut slightly shorter than its associated scute. Super Glue can be used to hold each section of tubing in place while quick drying, pliable putty epoxy is spread over each section of tubing in a continuous layer from the scute on the side of the tube to the scute surface on the opposite side of the tube. Avoid getting any epoxy on the scute sutures or neighboring scutes to allow for shell growth.

5. Place the antenna through the tube sections leaving approximately 50 to 120 mm hanging loose beyond the posterior of the animal.
6. Attach the transmitter with putty epoxy, using care not to bridge the scute margins and leaving no spaces between the transmitter and the carapace to get caught in vegetation.
7. Paint the transmitter and putty to reduce reflectivity and contrast.

In addition to these points, the transmitter placement site should be disinfected, as described earlier in the chapter. The transmitter should not be applied to an abnormal part of the shell (e.g., deformation or site of infection). The carapace can be roughened slightly with sandpaper or a Dremel tool before the epoxy is applied. The authors have had success with using a marine epoxy putty (WaterWeld; J-B Weld Company, Sulphur Springs, Tex) for the initial attachment of the transmitter and then coating it with a liquid epoxy (Power-Fast+, Fast Set Formula; Powers Fasteners, Inc. Brewster, NY). The epoxy putty alone may be successful for securing transmitters to terrestrial species, but it is recommended that liquid epoxy be used in aquatic species. A digital, distant-laser thermal monitoring device (Raynger ST; Raytek Corporation, Santa Cruz, Calif) is used to make sure the epoxy does not rise above 37.8°C (100°F) during the curing process. If necessary, the area is sprayed with cool water. In immature growing turtles, it is important not to cross scute suture lines to avoid interfering with the growth of the shell. Hatchling and juvenile tortoises can be radio tracked using small, lightweight radio transmitters attached to the costal scutes with silicon aquarium sealant (Dap; see Figure 29-40, *A*). This sealant is readily removed without damaging the shell of the tortoise.

Bolts and other fasteners can be used to attach radio transmitters to the carapace of aquatic turtles.[110] A surgical preparation and sterile technique should be used in this procedure because it requires drilling through the bone of the shell. Transmitter packages with aluminum plates with holes at either end for attachment and whip antennae are available through several manufacturers (e.g., Holohil Systems, LTD; Carp, Ontario, Canada; and Sirtrack, North Liberty, Iowa). The preferred site of attachment is on top of the posterior marginal scutes and underlying the peripheral bones of the carapace, typically in a region above one of the hindlimbs.[111] Attachment at this site is less likely to create drag or impede movement through substrate or vegetation. The most posterior scute should not be used because it will likely interfere with mating behavior. It is important to pre-place the transmitter on the shell to mark the spots to be drilled and to assess how the transmitter fits in relation to the curvature of the shell. If necessary, a small amount of epoxy can be used to create a flat surface for attachment. Holes drilled too close to the outside edge may break down from wear, allowing the fastener to slip, and holes drilled too close to the scute seams often result in excessive bleeding. For Pig-nosed Turtles *(Carettochelys insculpta)*, the epoxy was replaced with neoprene strips cut to the size of the transmitter, which softened the pressure of the transmitter against the shell. Additionally, Pig-nosed Turtles have no scutes, so it was critical to ensure that the holes were drilled on or near the seams between the marginal bones, which are clearly visible beneath the skin in this species. Tags were attached with stainless steel bolts and locking nuts threaded with nylon to prevent loosening and corrosion-resistant metal backing plates. The nut should be on top (transmitter side) to allow full leg movement and prevent abrasion of the skin on the legs. Gaps between the tag and the shell were filled with putty epoxy to prevent debris and vegetation from becoming entangled. This technique has been successful in a large number of species. Turtles have been tracked up to 3 years in some cases.

Radio Telemetry: Surgical Placement

Only healthy animals should be selected for surgical radio telemetry placement. The signal strength and frequency of the transmitter provided by the manufacturer should be verified with a receiver before placement in the animal to avoid implanting a nonfunctioning transmitter. Surgical procedures should be conducted during the appropriate time of year so that surgical sites can heal adequately. Anesthesia and surgeries should be conducted by a veterinarian with extensive experience with amphibians and reptiles using sterile technique. Although not ideal, individuals without a veterinary degree will likely continue to conduct surgeries but still must have IACUC approval. At a minimum, these individuals should receive specialized training in anesthesia, surgery, and sterile technique and have close consultation with an experienced veterinarian.

All telemetry devices and data loggers should be sterilized with either ethylene oxide gas or hydrogen peroxide plasma sterilization before implantation, as previously described for PIT tags. Arrangements can be made with local human hospitals, veterinary schools, or other specialty facilities if this is not available to the researcher. The benefits far outweigh the costs. Cold sterilization is not recommended.

General Guidelines for Amphibian Surgery. In general, because of their size, many amphibians are not well-suited for internal placement of telemetry packages. Internal placement of radio telemetry had been described for large frogs[116,117] and salamanders (e.g., Tiger Salamanders and Spotted Salamanders *[Ambystoma maculatum]*,[118] and the Eastern Hellbender[58]). Presurgical preparation of the patient includes ensuring good hydration and electrolyte balance by soaking the animal in a shallow water bath for 60 minutes before surgery. The amphibian can be weighed preoperatively and postoperatively to monitor hydration. The amphibian should be fasted before surgery for a minimum of 4 hours.[119] Appropriate analgesia and anesthesia should be used for internal transmitter placement and other invasive and potentially painful procedures. Although other anesthetic options are available, buffered tricaine methanesulfonate (MS-222; Argent Chemical Laboratories, Inc., Redmond, Wash) has been used widely by veterinarians and researchers for anesthesia in amphibians and appears to have a wide margin of safety.[119] After being anesthetized, the amphibian is removed from the anesthetic bath to avoid overdosing or prolonged anesthesia. Well-oxygenated clean water should be provided during anesthesia, and additional anesthetic can be added, if needed. Although amphibian skin secretions are known to have antimicrobial properties, sterile techniques should be followed. Because of the potential for toxicity from the various available antiseptics, it is recommended that the patient be rinsed with sterile water before placement of sterile drapes around the patient. Surgical instruments should be heat or gas sterilized. Anesthetized amphibians should not be released until they regain their ability to right themselves. A small incision is made into the skin, thin muscle layer, and coelomic lining to enter the coelomic cavity. The authors have used transmitters in which the antenna is tightly coiled around the battery and the entire package is encapsulated in acrylic (see Figure 29-35, *D*). The transmitter is placed into the coelom, and the incision is closed. The least reactive suture material should be used: polydioxanone (PDS) is recommended for internal sutures and nylon is recommended for skin sutures.[120] Internal transmitters will need to be removed or replaced, which is a consideration that researchers should be aware of when working with rare species, those that are difficult to capture, or species that are particularly susceptible to stress from invasive procedures.

PIT tags can also be implanted into the body cavity of frogs and salamanders, either by syringe or through a small (2-mm to 3-mm) incision in the skin with the use of surgical methods previously described (Figure 29-42). In salamanders, the tags can be inserted along the side of the body, approximately 5 mm anterior to the hindleg[121]; tags should be inserted anteriorly, parallel to the long axis of the body. Incisions can be closed with a small amount of tissue glue.

General Guidelines for Reptile Surgery. A presurgical health screening is recommended. Appropriate analgesia and anesthesia should be used and needs to be tailored to the particular reptile species undergoing surgery. In most cases, injectable sedatives and anesthetics will be followed by intubation and gas anesthesia. Appropriate cardiac and respiratory monitoring equipment should be available. Recommended suture material includes polydioxanone (PDS II; Ethicon, Inc., Somerville, NJ),

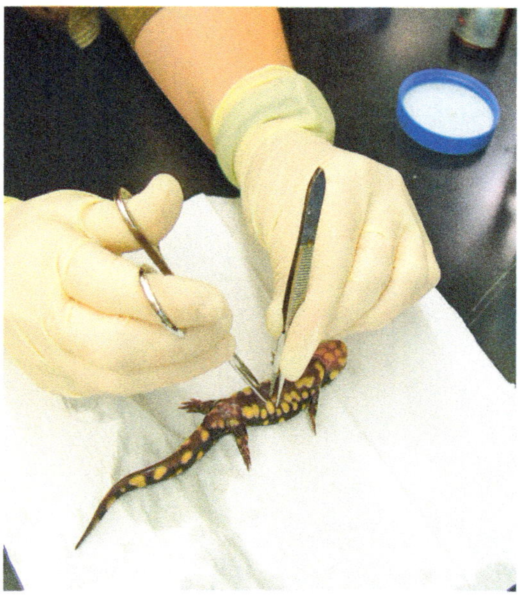

FIGURE 29-42 Surgical implantation of a passive integrated transponder (PIT) tag in an Eastern Tiger Salamander *(Ambystoma tigrinum)*.

an absorbable suture that is used internally and is made of a nonabsorbable nylon (Ethicon; Ethicon, Inc., Somerville, NJ) for the skin. A study conducted by Govett and collegues[122] found that PDS was the preferred suture material for sea turtles.

Radio transmitters used in all of the procedures described further on were manufactured by Holohil Systems, Ltd (Ontario, Canada), unless indicated otherwise. These transmitters are available in a variety of sizes, and the larger transmitters have longer battery life.

CROCODILIANS. Intracoelomic radio transmitter implantation in crocodilians has been conducted under injectable anesthesia with subsequent intubation and manual ventilation with a bag valve mask (Ambu bag).[100-104] A small skin incision was made between scales in the flank of the abdominal region, just posterior to the right hindlimb. Muscle layers beneath the skin were carefully separated to reveal the coelomic lining. Hemostats were used to secure the coelomic lining, and an incision was made to expose the coelom, where the transmitter was inserted. To avoid disturbance when the animals were tracked, the researchers used an automatic and continuous recording station positioned at least 100 m from the waterhole to simultaneously monitor up to 10 individuals. Radio signals from the temperature-sensitive transmitters were received by a four-piece Yagi aerial antenna, mounted 25 m directly above the waterhole that the crocodiles inhabited.[103]

Alternatively, using a similar surgical approach, researchers implanted a multichannel radio telemetry system to measure blood flow and pressure, electrocardiographic data, and body temperature in several captive American Alligators.[123] The technique has been reported to be promising for free-ranging crocodilians.[103]

The authors (TMN, KMA) have developed a technique for surgical implantation of radio transmitters in the muscle of the proximal tail of American Alligators. The technique has been used on six alligators to date. Anesthesia used included dexmedetomidine (Dexdomitor, 0.5 mg/mL; Phizer Animal Health, New York, N.Y.) at 0.010 to 0.15 mg/kg, ketamine (Ketaject, 100 mg/mL; Phoenix Inc, St. Joseph, Mo) at 5 mg/kg, and butorphanol (Butorphic, 10 mg/mL; Lloyd Laboratories, Inc, Shenandoah, Iowa) at 0.2 mg/kg given in combination intramuscularly. After 15 minutes, if deeper anesthesia was needed, propofol (PropoFlo, 20 mg/mL, Abbott Laboratories, North Chicago, Ill) was administered as a slow bolus intravenously to effect at 3 mg/kg. Lidocaine (2%; Butler Animal Health Supply, Dublin, Ohio) was infiltrated into the incision area. Intubation and ventilation with a bag valve mask were performed in all cases. Gas anesthesia can be used to further control anesthesia but has not been necessary with the injectable drug combination used. Atipamezole (Antisedan, 5 mg/mL; Pfizer Animal Health, New York, N.Y.) was used for reversal at the same volume as the dexmedetomidine, given half intramuscularly and half intravenously.

The skin was surgically prepared. A 3-cm to 5-cm skin incision was made between scales about a third of the way down from the dorsal aspect of the tail. Blunt dissection was used to create a pocket between muscle planes, where the transmitter was inserted (Figure 29-43). Holohil Systems Ltd. (Ontario, Canada) transmitters (Model SI-2, 50 mm × 11 mm, 36-month battery projected life) developed for snakes have been used. The antenna was threaded subcutaneously caudally with the use of rigid copper tubing as described in the Snakes section further on. Similarly, a small skin incision at the distal end of the tubing was made with the same technique. It is a bit more difficult to thread the tubing because of the stiffness of the scales; thus more than one incision was usually needed. The surgical site was closed using 2.0 PDS in a simple interrupted suture pattern for the muscle and skin.

To date, reliable signal transmission has been maintained for 12 to 24 months. Although full battery life has not been sustained for these tracked individuals, researchers (Andrews K: Unpublished data, 2010) also received faulty transmitters, so it is unclear whether the reduced battery life can be attributed to malfunctioning equipment or internal crimping of the antenna, which would thereby reduce signal transmission. Further, signal transmission is reduced in brackish water habitats, which could have reduced relocation of the animals. Regardless, the technique was proven effective, so data collection will continue with future individuals to further articulate the technique. Internal implantation of devices in American Alligators is the technique of choice in the field, where it is preferable that tracked individuals need not be visually identified.

A technique recently described subcutaneous implantation of temperature- or pressure-sensitive acoustic telemetry devices in Saltwater Crocodiles.[103] The animals ranged from 2 to 5 m in length. The crocodiles were manually restrained, and a local anesthetic was infiltrated into the surgical site. A 2-cm skin incision was made, and a small pocket was formed under the skin, along a skinfold, with the use of blunt-ended scissors

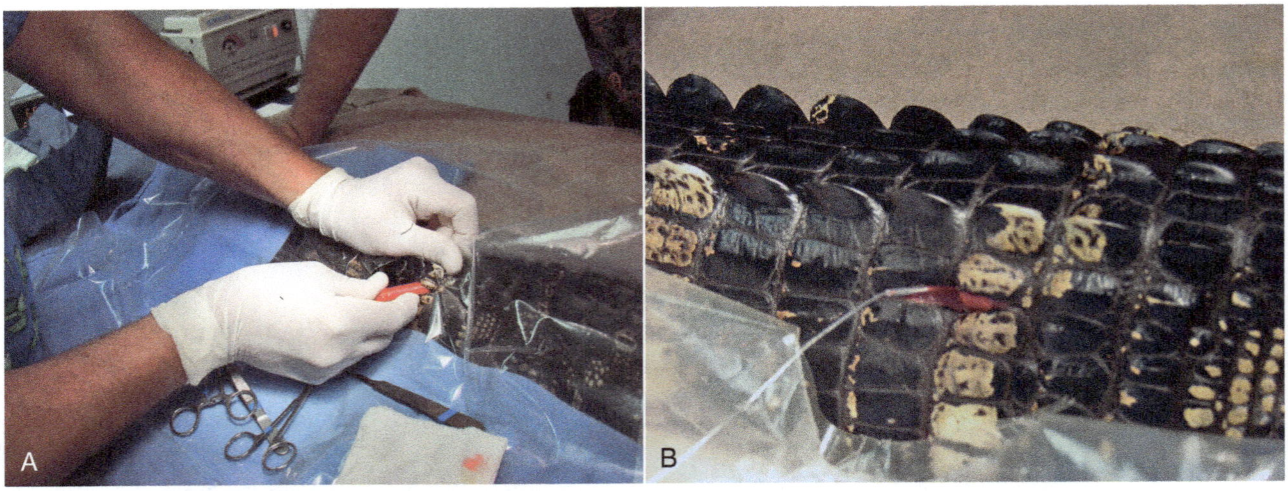

FIGURE 29-43 **A** and **B,** Surgical placement of a radio transmitter in an American Alligator *(Alligator mississippiensis)* tail. *(Photos courtesy Kimberly M. Andrews, Jekyll Island Authority, Georgia Sea Turtle Center and The University of Georgia, Savannah River Ecology Laboratory.)*

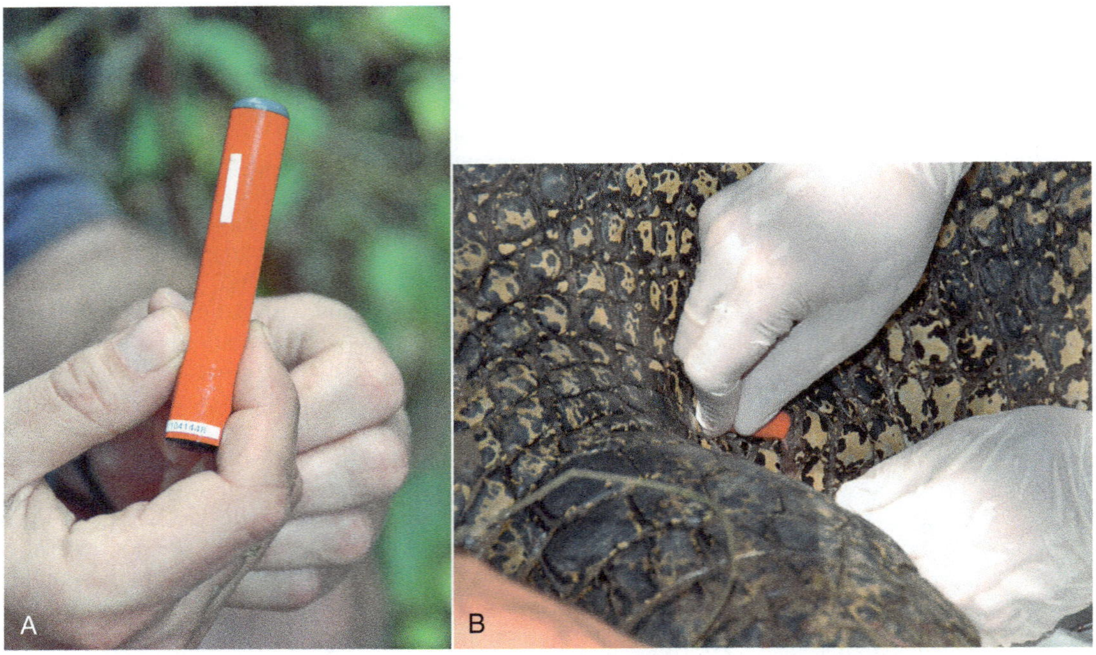

FIGURE 29-44 **A,** Vemco acoustic tag. **B,** Surgically implanting a temperature-sensitive or pressure-sensitive acoustic transmitter subcutaneously in a Saltwater Crocodile *(Crocodylus porosus)*. *(Photos courtesy of C.E. Franklin.)*

(Figure 29-44). The transmitter was then inserted (V16, Vemco-cylindrical, 72 mm long and 15 mm in diameter with rounded ends). The transmitter was positioned so that when the animal surfaced it remained well below the water. The researchers used fixed receiver stations. The technology has potential to be extremely useful in crocodiles because the signal transmission occurs through water and transmission operates irrespective of salinity. Furthermore, the transmitters can be programmed to have a life span of more than 10 years. A variety of sensors are available to measure temperature and pressure (water depth). The signals can be picked up by automatic stationary receivers or actively tracked. The authors reported excellent transmission; animals were detected more than 500 m away with the use of a directional hydrophone and active tracking receiver. At the time of the publication, the transmitters had been functioning well for more than 9 months. Further study is needed to evaluate transmitter retention time.

LIZARDS. An effective technique for surgically implanting transmitters in the coelom of Anegada Ground Iguanas (*Cyclura pinguis*) has been reported and has potential for use in other lizard species.[124] With this technique, two-point fixation of the transmitter to the internal body wall was achieved. Antenna placement in the coelom was a critical part of the procedure. Of 23 iguanas, 20 transmitted good signals for at least 10 months after surgery (Figure 29-45).

Another method was described by Doody and collegues[110] for surgical implantation of radiotransmitters in a semiaquatic monitor lizard (*Varanus mertensi*). Gas anesthesia was used. The site was aseptically prepared for implantation. A 2-cm to 3-cm skin incision was made longitudinally on the lateral side of the abdomen, approximately 2 to 3 cm anterior from the hindlimbs. Muscle was incised to gain access to the coelomic lining, which was then incised. Transmitters (Holohil Systems, Ontario, Canada, Model 2I-T, 3 g, 2.5 cm × 0.6 cm) with a 10-cm external whip antenna were inserted into the coelom. The transmitter was positioned longitudinally within the coelom. A thin-walled brass tube was threaded subcutaneously from the anterior point of incision along the lateral fold of the animal to just behind the head. The external antenna was positioned inside the tube, and the tube was removed through a small incision made just behind the head, leaving the antenna in place under the skin. Only minimal long-term effects were noted, according to the authors, over a 2-year study period. Fifty individuals were implanted, and 37 transmitted more than 16 days; 4 were tracked successfully for 2 years.

SNAKES. Radio telemetry devices have been surgically placed in the coelomic cavity of a variety of snake species by one of the authors (TMN). Complete healing takes approximately 4 to 8 weeks in reptiles maintained in ideal thermoregulatory conditions. The methodology that follows is a modification of that described previously.[125]

Snout-to-vent and snout-to-tail measurements are taken. The snout-to-vent measurement is divided by three; this distance is measured from the cloaca (vent) anteriorly and used for the incision site for transmitter placement. A permanent marker can be used to mark the skin incision site. The snake is prepared for sterile surgery in a routine fashion. A 3- to 5-cm lateral skin incision is made between the second and third scale rows and then reflected ventrally past the ribs so that an incision can be made in the coelomic lining, which allows access to the coelomic cavity. Care should be taken not to incise the air sac during this process so that the transmitter is not inserted into the respiratory system.

An appropriately sized transmitter should be selected. Temperature-sensitive transmitters are available from select manufacturers, or microtemperature data loggers (iButtons; Maxim Integrated Devices, Sunnyvale, Calif) that have been coated in multipurpose rubber coating (PlastiDip; Plasti Dip International, Blaine, Minn) can also be implanted intracoelomically caudal to the transmitter to record body temperatures. Sterilized copper tubing, a rigid dog urinary catheter, or a similar rigid sterile instrument is threaded subcutaneously anteriorly. The antenna is threaded into the lumen of the tubing. A small skin incision is made in the area of the

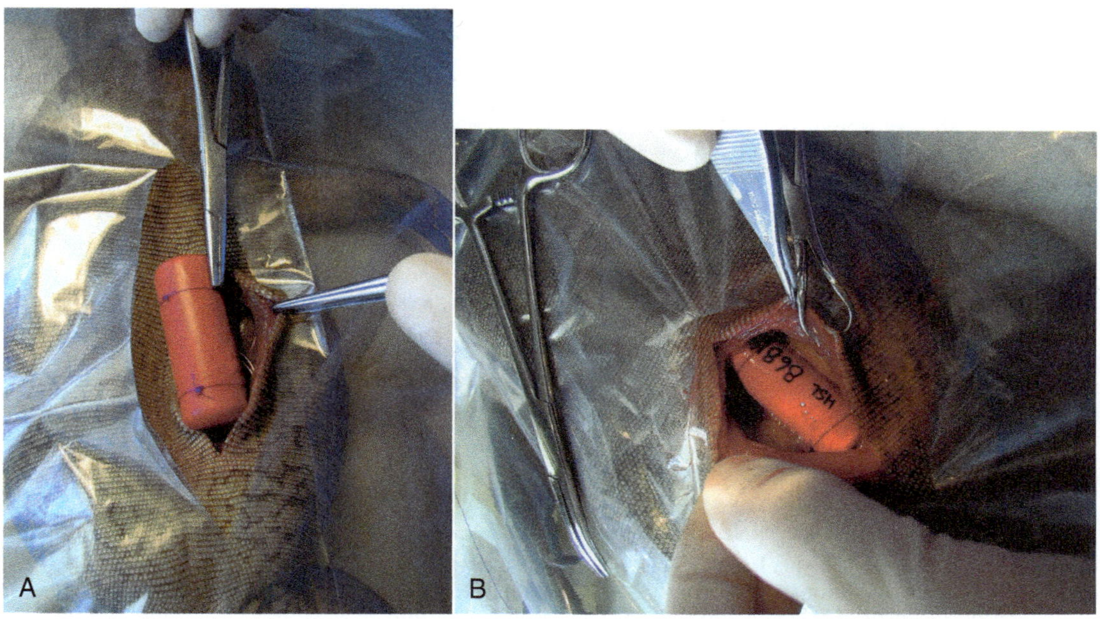

FIGURE 29-45 **A** and **B,** Surgical placement of radio transmitters in Caribbean iguanas. *(Photos courtesy of Fort Worth Zoo Animal Health.)*

anterior end of the tubing. The tubing is removed, leaving the antennae in place (see further on). The antenna can be anchored to musculature by one suture (placed approximately 0.5 cm anterior to the transmitter), which reduces the chances of the antennae protruding from the incision site. Care is taken to ensure that the antenna is not crimped where it enters the transmitter (Figure 29-46). An appropriate suture material and suture pattern should be used to close the surgical site as previously described in this chapter for other reptiles.

Some species of snakes, such as the Eastern Indigo Snake, are prone to developing bacterial infections at the transmitter site. Recent studies on the Eastern Massasauga Rattlesnake (*Sisturus catenatus catenatus*) indicate bacterial infections still occur with some frequency, despite proper incorporation of sterile techniques.[126]

Satellite Telemetry

Satellite telemetry has been used most extensively to study long-term large spatial movements and activities of sea turtles and estuarine crocodiles. This technique is especially important in the marine environment, where very high frequency (VHF) signals are greatly attenuated and distances to be covered are usually large.[127] The primary disadvantage of this technology is the cost of the transmitters and satellite time.

Most sea turtle tracking research that has been published has focused on postnesting females because of their accessibility. For example, a study was conducted on the Georgia coast to evaluate internesting intervals and postnesting migratory behavior in female Loggerhead Sea Turtles.[128] In this study, a variety of methodologies including acoustic, radio, and satellite telemetry were used to evaluate short- and long-term movement patterns, nest site fidelity, and interactions with shrimp trawl fishery (Figure 29-47). Comparisons between the distributions were used to produce potential management scenarios (closures and fleet reductions) designed to reduce the likelihood of interactions. Through application of predictive modeling, spatial closures were identified to have only limited merits as management options, whereas fleet reductions were most likely to produce actual decreases in interactions between turtles and shrimp trawlers during nesting seasons. Until recently, very limited information was available on the spatial ecology of male Loggerhead Sea Turtles during the breeding season. Arendt and colleagues evaluated the movement and diving patterns

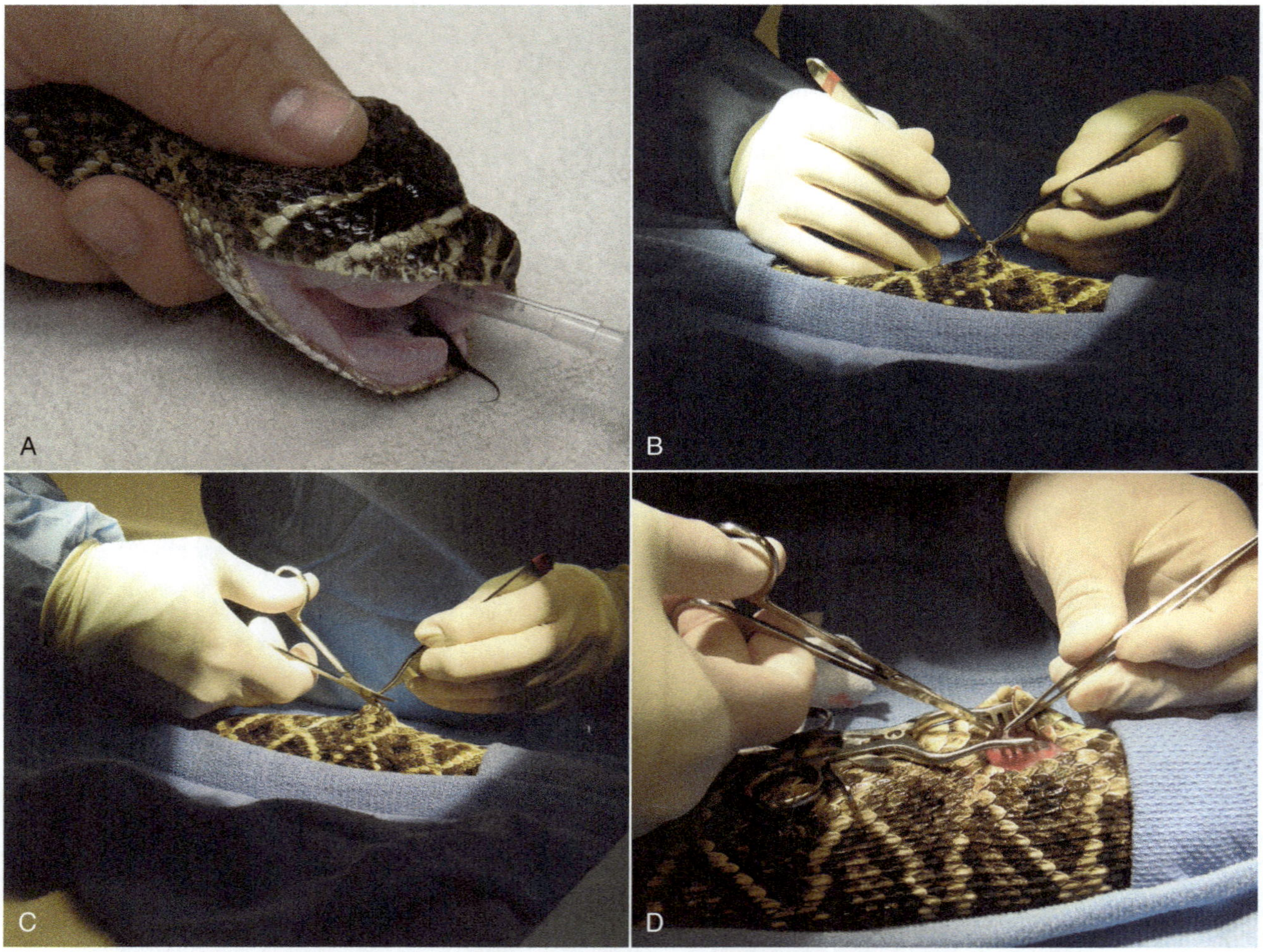

FIGURE 29-46 Surgical placement of a radio transmitter into the coelom of an Eastern Diamondback Rattlesnake *(Crotalus adamanteus)*. **A,** Isoflurane anesthesia is administered through an endotracheal tube. **B,** Initial stab incision into the skin with a scalpel blade. **C,** Skin incision is completed with scissors. **D,** Incision of coelomic lining with scissors. Retractors improve exposure.

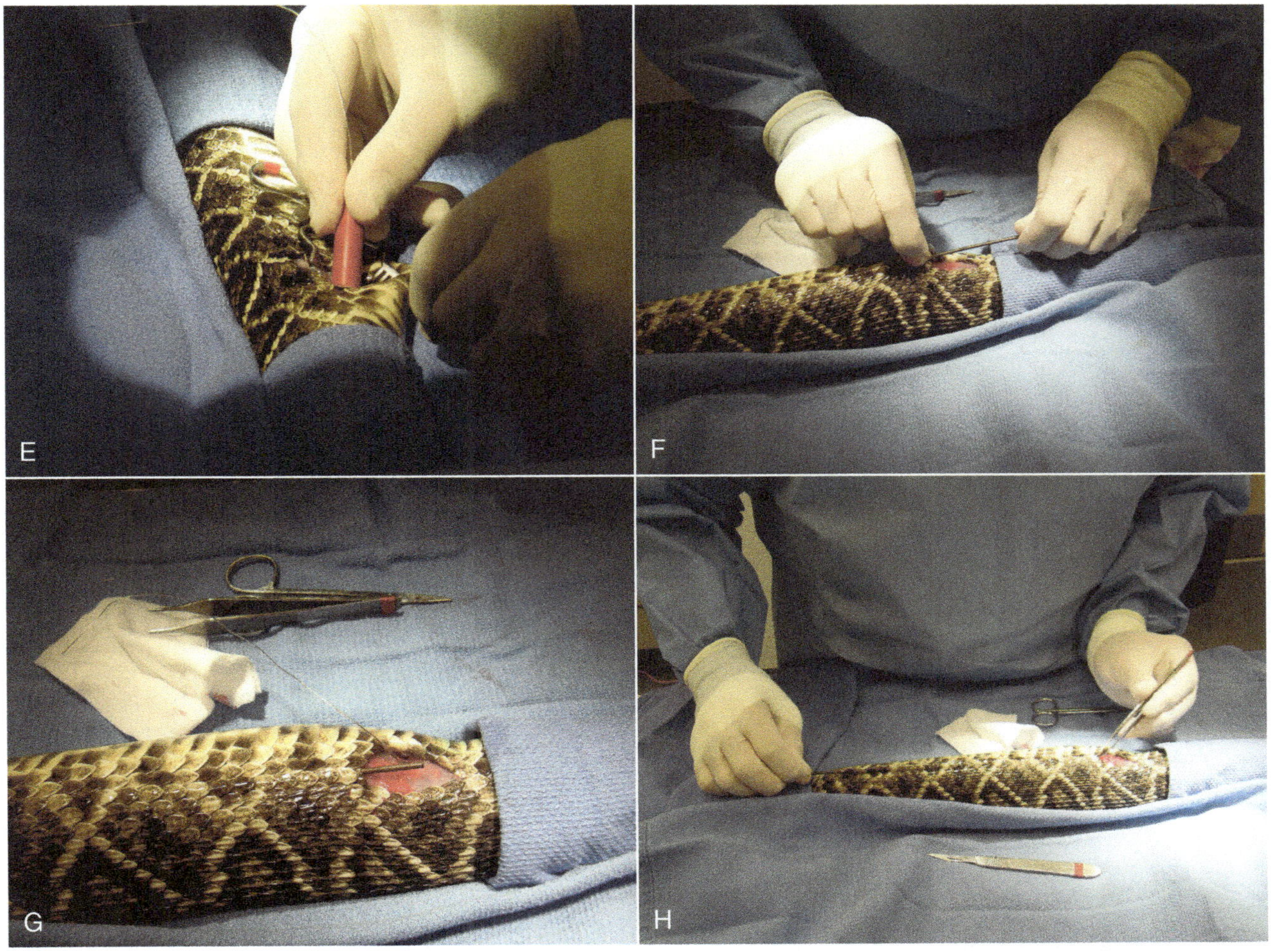

FIGURE 29-46, cont'd **E,** Radio transmitter is being placed into the coelom. **F,** Threading copper tubing subcutaneously. **G,** Copper tubing in place for threading antenna. **H,** Small incision is made to pull out the copper tubing while leaving the antenna in place.

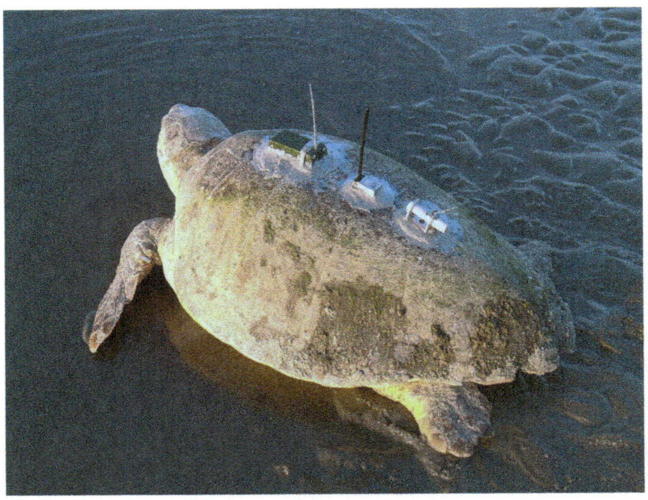

FIGURE 29-47 Loggerhead Sea Turtle *(Caretta caretta)* with satellite, sonic, and radio transmitters on carapace. *(Photo courtesy of Mark Dodd.)*

of resident and migrant adult male Loggerhead Sea Turtles during the breeding season in Cape Canaveral, Florida[129] and after dispersal postbreeding.[130] Satellite telemetry in this study provided critical information for assisting in future conservation management of this species that did not previously exist.

A variety of satellite attachment techniques have been used in sea turtles, including tethering of buoyant transmitter housing to the posterior end of the shell, attachment of "backpack" style transmitters to the anterior vertebral scute with fiberglass cloth and polyester resin, fiberglass filler, two-part epoxies, or putties, and combinations of these techniques.[131] Retention time of satellite tags has been and continues to be problematic. Integration of antifouling paints[132] and an alternative adhesive, Sonic-Weld steel-reinforced epoxy putty,[133] has increased retention time.

The Georgia Sea Turtle Center (GSTC) has utilized this technology to track rehabilitated Loggerhead Sea Turtles after release (Figure 29-48). Satellite placement techniques have been similar to those previously described,[134] except that the transmitter is partially covered with epoxy with only the saltwater switches exposed, as depicted in (Figure 29-49). A laser temperature gun is used to monitor the temperature of the epoxy; when it reaches above 37.8°C (100°F), water is used to reduce the temperature. Although these transmitters could

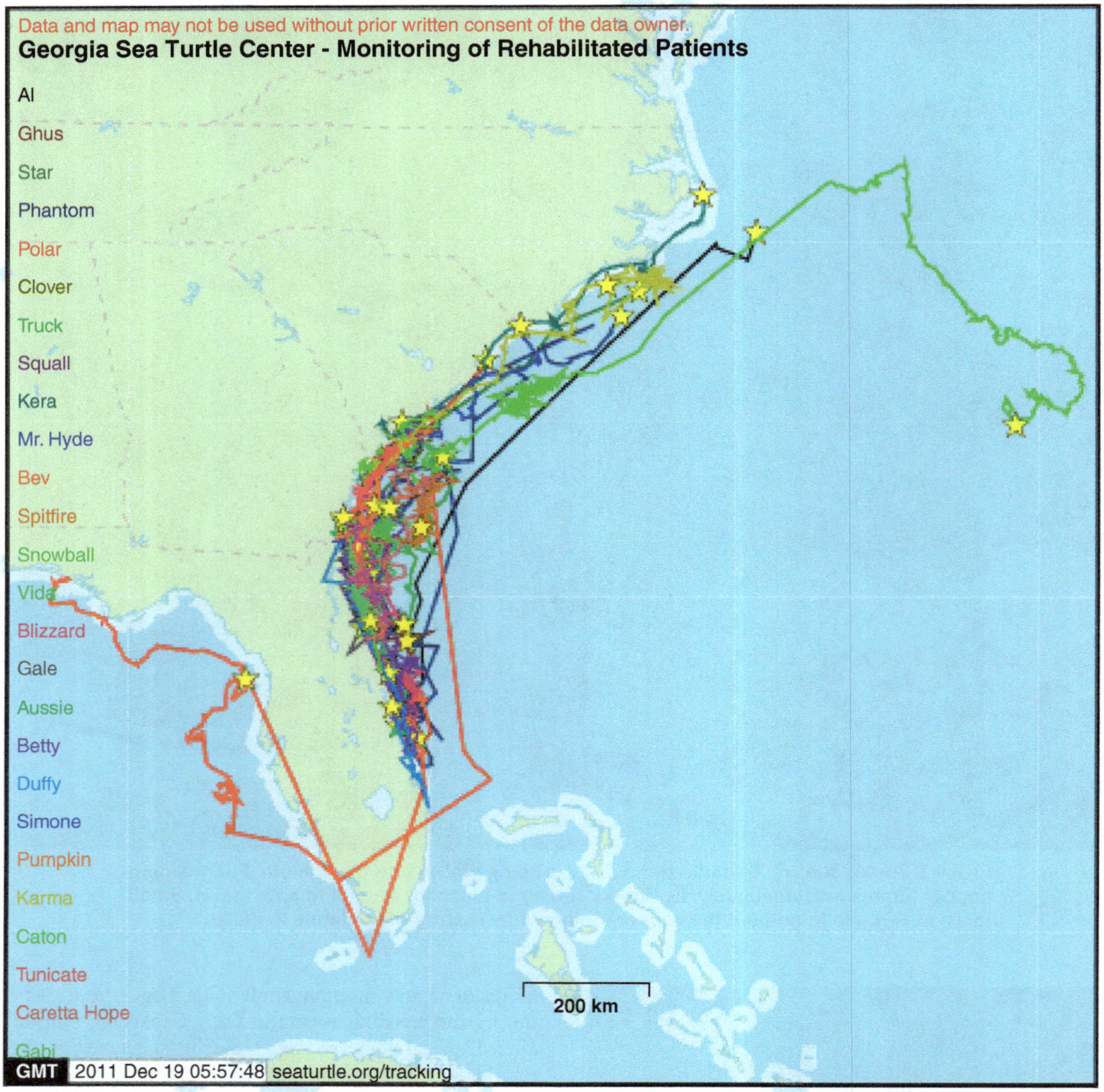

FIGURE 29-48 Satellite tracks of rehabilitated sea turtles released by the Georgia Sea Turtle Center.

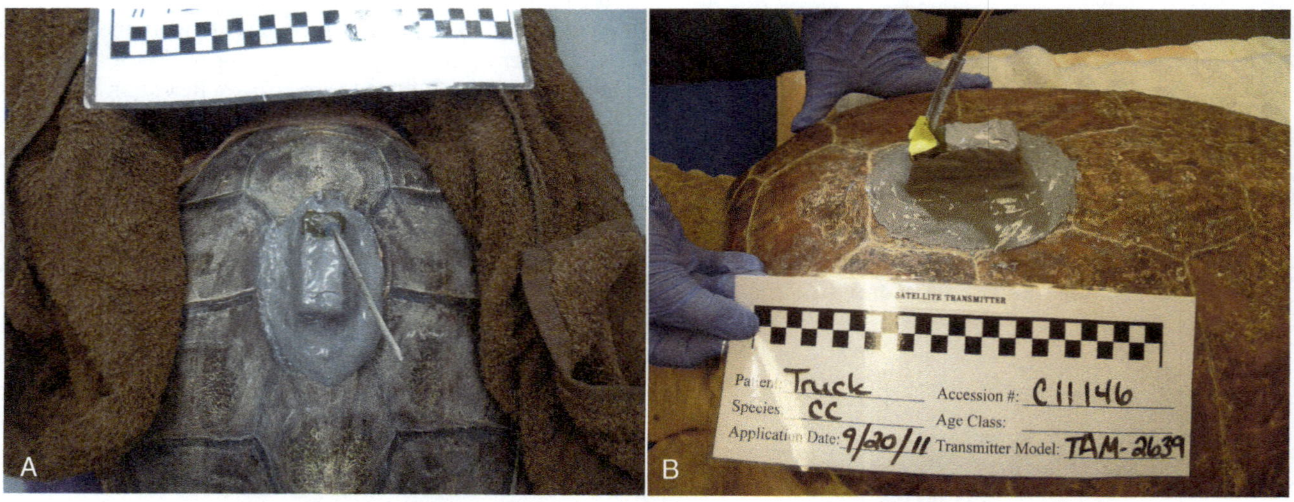

FIGURE 29-49 **A** and **B,** Satellite transmitter placed on a Loggerhead Sea Turtle *(Caretta caretta)* carapace.

theoretically last for 3 years, data collection for more than 1 year has been rare, most likely because of physical damage to the antennae or transmitters and/or biological fouling of the saltwater switch sensor. On October 13, 2011, a rehabilitated juvenile female Loggerhead Sea Turtle that had been released with a satellite transmitter from Jekyll Island, Georgia, United States, on July 13, 2009 was recovered by a research vessel near Cumberland Island, Georgia. The turtle was healthy and in good body condition, and the transmitter was still in place. The transmitter itself was covered with epibiota and was missing the antenna (Figure 29-50).

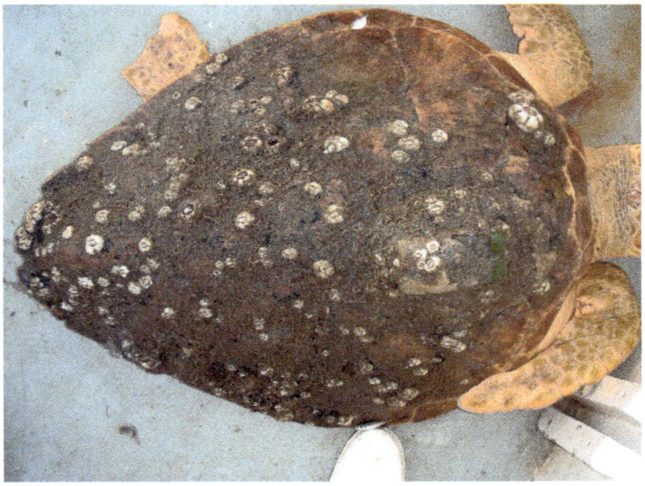

FIGURE 29-50 Rehabilitated Loggerhead Sea Turtle *(Caretta caretta)* released with a satellite transmitter was recaptured more than 2 years later.

Satellite telemetry has also been used successfully to study long range movements of estuarine crocodiles.[102] Before attachment of the device, the area around the nuchal shield was surgically prepared after a local anesthetic was administered. Two holes were drilled into each of four scutes in the nuchal shield, and wires were fed through the holes. A Kiwi-Sat 101 transmitter was attached to the scutes with the use of plastic coated stainless steel wire threaded through four steel loops on the sides of the transmitter and fastened with lead crimps (Figure 29-51). Fifty percent of the animals sent signals for more than 10 months, and four sent signals for more than 15 months.[102]

CONCLUSIONS

Capture techniques, marking of individuals for identification purposes, and telemetry placement techniques are used extensively in amphibian and reptile research and conservation activities. It is critical that veterinarians and biologists continue to work together to develop sound protocols that provide the vital information that this research sets out to obtain while causing minimal negative effects to the individual animals and populations that are being studied and preserved.

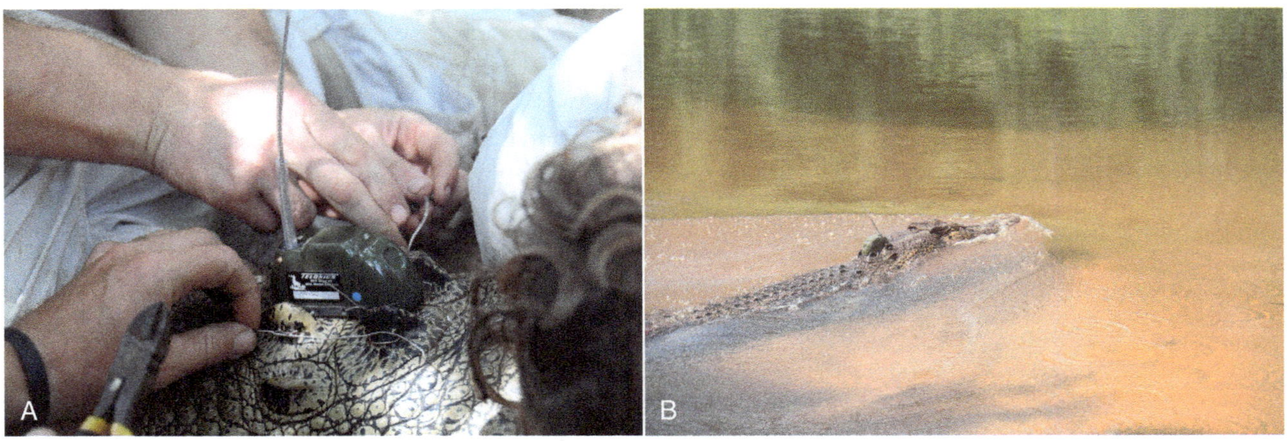

FIGURE 29-51 **A,** Satellite/GPS tag being attached to the nuchal scutes of an Estuarine crocodile *(Crocodylus porosus).* **B,** Satellite/GPS tag attached to the nuchal scutes of a 2.8 m female Saltwater Crocodile *(Crocodylus porosus). (Photos courtesy of C.E. Franklin.)*

REFERENCES

1. Fellers GM, Drost CA. Sampling with artificial cover. In: Heyer WR, Donnelly MA, McDiarmid RW, et al, eds. *Measuring and monitoring biological diversity: standard methods for amphibians*. Washington DC: Smithsonian Institution Press, 1994;146-150.
2. Muenz TK, Golladay SW, Vellidis G, et al. Stream macroinvertebrates and amphibians as indicators of ecosystem stress: a case study from the coastal plains. *J Environ Qual* 2006;35:1924-1968.
3. Kjoss VA, Livaitis JA. Comparison of two methods to sample snake communities in early successional habitats. *Wildl Soc Bull* 2001;29:153-157.
4. Pauley TK, Little M. A new technique to monitor larval and juvenile salamanders in stream habitats. *Banisteria* 1998;12:32-36.
5. Waldron JL, Dodd CK, Corser JD. Leaf litterbags: factors affecting capture of stream-dwelling salamanders. *Appl Herpetol* 2003;1:23-36.
6. Moulton CA, Fleming WJ, Nerney BR. The use of PVC pipes to capture hylid frogs. *Herpetol Rev* 1996;27:186-187.
7. Boughton RG, Staiger J, Franz R. Use of PVC pipe refugia as a sampling technique for hylid treefrogs. *Am Midl Nat* 2000;144:168-177.
8. Fogarty JH, Vilella FJ. Use of native forest and eucalyptus plantations by *Eleutherodactylus* frogs. *J Wildl Manage* 2003;67:186-195.
9. Bartareau TM. PVC pipe diameter influences the species and sizes of treefrogs captured in a Florida coastal scrub community. *Herpetol Rev* 2004;35:150-152.
10. Zacharow M, Barichivich JW, Dodd CK, Jr. Using ground-placed PVC pipes to monitor hylid treefrogs: capture biases. *Southeast Nat* 2003;2:575-590.
11. Borg CK, Hoss SK, Smith LL. A method for preventing flying squirrel mortality in PVC pipe treefrog refugia. *Wildl Soc Bull* 2004;32:1313-1315.
12. Shaffer HB, Alford RA, Woodward BD, et al. Quantitative sampling of amphibian larvae. In: Heyer WR, Donnelly MA, McDiarmid RW, et al, eds. *Measuring and monitoring biological diversity: standard methods for amphibians*. Washington DC: Smithsonian Institution Press, 1994;130-141.
13. Tucker AD, Fitzsimmons NN, Gibbons JW. Resource partitioning by the estuarine turtle *Malaclemys terrapin*: trophic, spatial, and temporal foraging constraints. *Herpetologica* 1995;51:167-181.
14. Vogt RC. New methods for trapping aquatic turtles. *Copeia* 1980;368-371.
15. Moll D, Moll EO. *The ecology, exploitation, and conservation of river turtles*. New York: Oxford University Press, 2004.
16. Dreslik MJ, Kuhns AR, Phillips CA. Structure and composition of a Southern Illinois freshwater turtle assemblage. *Northeast Nat* 2005;12:173-186.
17. Ream C, Ream R. The influence of sampling methods on the estimation of population structure in painted turtles. *Am Midl Nat* 1966;75:325-338.
18. Gamble T. The relative efficiency of basking and hoop traps for painted turtles *(Chrysemys picta)*. *Herpetol Rev* 2006;37:308-312.
19. Gibbons JW, Bennett, DH. Determination of anuran terrestrial activity patterns by a drift fence method. *Copeia* 1974;236-242.
20. Gibbons JW, Semlitsch RD. Terrestrial drift fences with pitfall traps: an effective technique for quantitative sampling of animal populations. *Brimleyana* 1981;7:1-16.
21. Burgdorf SJ, Rudolph DC, Conner RN, et al. A successful trap design for capturing large terrestrial snakes. *Herpetol Rev* 2005;36:421-424.
22. Steen DA, Smith LL, Bailey MA. Suggested modifications to Burgdorf et al's (2005) classic terrestrial snake trap design. *Herpetol Rev* 2010;41:320-321.
23. Johnson SA, Barichivich WJ. A simple technique for trapping *Siren lacertina, Amphiuma means*, and other aquatic vertebrates. *J Freshwater Ecol* 2004;19:263-269.
24. Luhring TM, Jennison CM. A new stratified aquatic sampling technique for aquatic vertebrates. *J Freshwater Ecol* 2008;23:445-450.
25. Chabreck RH. Methods of capturing, marking and sexing alligators, in *Proceedings*. Annu Southeast Assoc Game Fish Comm 1963;47-50.
26. Elsey RM, Trosclair PL III. A new live trap for capturing alligators. *Herpetol Rev* 2004;35:253-255.
27. Taylor RW. Human predation on the gopher tortoise *(Gopherus polyphemus)* in north-central Florida. *Bull Fla State Museum Biol Sci* 1982;28:79-102.
28. Burke RL, Cox J. Evaluation and review of field techniques used to study and manage gopher tortoises. In: Szaro RC, Severson KE, Patton DR, eds. *Management of amphibians, reptiles, and small mammals in North America*. Flagstaff, Ariz: US Department of Agriculture Forest Service, 1988;205-215.
29. Maier PP, Segars AL, Arendt MD, et al. Development of an index of sea turtle abundance based upon in-water sampling with trawl gear. Final project report to The National Marine Fisheries Service. National Oceanic and Atmospheric Administration, *Silver Springs, Md* March 31, 2004. Grant NA07FL0499.
30. Wright KM. Overview of amphibian medicine. In: Mader D, ed. *Reptile medicine and surgery*. 2nd ed. Philadelphia: WB Sanders Co, 2006;941-971.
31. McDonald DL, Dutton PH. Use of PIT tags and photoidentification to revise remigration estimates of leatherback turtles *(Dermochelys coriacea)* nesting in St. Croix, US Virgin Islands, 1979-1995. *Chelon Conserv Biol* 1996;2:148-152.
32. Ferner JW. A review of marking techniques for amphibians and reptiles. *Herpetol Circ No. 9*, 1979;1-41.
33. Jones SM, Ferguson GW. The effect of paint marking on mortality in a Texas population of *Sceloporus undulatus*. *Copeia* 1980;850-854.
34. Rodda GH, Bock BC, Burghardt GM, et al. Techniques for identifying individual lizards at a distance reveal influences of handling. *Copeia* 1988;905-913.
35. Gannon PJ, Secoy DM. Paint-marking the rattle of rattlesnakes. *Herpetol Rev* 1984;15:75-76.
36. Balazs GH. Factors to consider in the tagging of sea turtles. In: Eckert KL, Bjorndal KA, Abreu-Grobois FA, et al, eds. *Research and management techniques for the conservation of sea turtles*. Washington, DC: IUCN/SSC Marine Turtle Specialist Group, 1999;101-109.
37. Van Dam RP, Diez C. Home range of immature hawksbill turtles *(Eretmochelys imbricata* (Linnaeus)) at two Caribbean Islands. *J Exp Mar Bio Ecol* 1998;220:15-24.
38. Schultz JP. Sea turtles nesting in Surinam. *Zool Verhandelingen* 1975;143:61-62.
39. MacNeil JE, Dharmarajan G, Williams RN. SalaMarker: a code generator and standardized marking system for use with Visible Implant Elastomers. *Herpetol Conserv Biol* 2011;6:260-265.
40. Cecil SG, Just JJ. Use of acrylic polymers for marking of tadpoles (Amphibia, Anura). *J Herpetol* 1978;12:95-96.
41. Heard GW, Scroggie MP, Malone B. Visible implant alphanumeric tags as an alternative to toe-clipping for marking amphibians—a case study. *Wildl Res* 2008;35:747-759.
42. Bailey LL. Evaluating elastomer marking and photo identification methods for terrestrial salamanders: marking effects and observer bias. *Herpetol Rev* 2004;35:38-41.
43. Temsiripong Y. Growth and survival rates of wild and repatriated hatchling American alligators *(Alligator mississippiensis)* in central Florida lakes. MS Thesis, University of Florida, Tampa, 1999.
44. Balazs GH. Factors affecting the retention of metal tags on sea turtles. *Mar Turtle Newslett* 1982;20:11-14.
45. Richardson JI, Bell R, Richardson TH. Population ecology and demographic implications drawn from an 11-year study of nesting hawksbill turtles, *Eretmochelys imbricata*, at Jumby Bay, Long Island, Antigua, West Indies. *Chelon Conserv Biol* 1999;3:244-250.
46. Limpus CJ. Estimation of tag loss in marine turtle research. *Wildl Res* 1992;19:457-469.
47. Parmenter CJ. A preliminary evaluation of the performance of passive integrated transponders and metal tags in a population study of the flatback sea turtle *(Natator depressus)*. *Wildl Res* 1993;20:375-381.

48. Bjorndal KA, Bolten AB, Lagueux CJ, et al. Probability of tag loss in green turtles nesting at Tortuguero, Costa Rica. *J Herpetol* 1996;30:567-571.
49. Camper JD, Dixon JR. *Evaluation of a microchip marking system for amphibians and reptiles*. Austin, Texas: Parks and Wildlife Department, 1988.
50. Gibbons JW, Andrews KM. PIT tagging: simple technology at its best. *Bioscience* 2004;54:447-454.
51. Roark AW, Dorcas ME. Regional body temperature variation in corn snakes measured using temperature-sensitive passive integrated transponders. *J Herpetol* 2000;34:481-485.
52. Bittner TD, King RB, Kerfin JM. Effects of body size and melanism on the thermal biology of garter snakes *(Thamnophis sirtalis)*. *Copeia* 2002;477-482.
53. Charney ND, Letcher BH, Haro A, et al. Terrestrial passive integrated transponder antennae for tracking small animal movements. *J Wildl Manage* 2008;73:1245-1250.
54. Cucherousset J, Marty P, Pelozuelo L, et al. Portable PIT detector as a new tool for non-disruptively locating individually tagged amphibians in the field: a case study with Pyrenean brook salamanders *(Calotriton asper)*. *Wildl Res* 2008;35:780-787.
55. Hamed MK, Ledford DP, Laughlin TF. Monitoring non-breeding habitat activity by subterranean detection of ambystomatid salamanders with passive integrated transponder (PIT) tags and a radio frequency identification (RFID) antenna system. *Herpetol Rev* 2008;39:303-306.
56. Boarman WI, Beigel ML, Goodlett GC, et al. A passive integrated transponder system for tracking animal movements. *Wildl Soc Bull* 1998;26:886-891.
57. Ireland D, Osbourne N, Berrill M. Marking medium- to large-sized anurans with passive integrated transponders (PIT) tags. *Herpetol Rev* 2003;34:218-220.
58. Burgmeier NG, Sutton TM, Williams RN. Spatial ecology of the eastern hellbender *(Cryptobranchus alleganiensis alleganiensis)* in Indiana. *Herpetologica* 2011;67:135-145.
59. Moore JA, Daugherty CH, Godfrey SS, et al. Seasonal monogamy and multiple paternity in a wild population of a territorial reptile (tuatara). *Biol J Linnean Soc* 2009;98:161-170.
60. Keck MB. Test for detrimental effects of PIT tags in neonatal snakes. *Copeia* 1994;226-228.
61. Mills M, Hudson CJ, Berna HJ. Spatial ecology and movements of the brown water snake *(Nerodia taxispilota)*. *Herpetologica* 1995;51:412-423.
62. Buhlmann KA, Tuberville TD. Use of passive integrated transponder (PIT) tags for marking small freshwater turtles. *Chelon Conserv Biol* 1998;3:102-104.
63. Dutton P, McDonald D. Use of Pit tags to identify adult leatherbacks. *Mar Turtle Newslett* 1994;67:13-14.
64. Rivalan P, Godfrey MH, Prévot-Julliard A-C, et al. Maximum likelihood estimates of tag loss in leatherback sea turtles. *J Wildl Manage* 2005;69:540-548.
65. Balazs GH, Chaloupka M. Spatial and temporal variability in somatic growth of green sea turtles *(Chelonia mydas)* resident in the Hawaiian Archipelago. *Mar Biol* 2004;145:1043-1049.
66. Langkilde T, Shine R. How much stress do researchers inflict on their study animals? A case study using a scincid lizard, *Eulamprus heatwolei*. *J Exp Biol* 2006;209:1035-1043.
67. Cagle FR. A system of marking turtles for future identification. *Copeia* 1939;170-173.
68. Gibbons JW. Why do turtles live so long? *Bioscience* 1987;37:262-269.
69. Plummer MV. Collecting and marking. In: Harless M, Morlock H, eds. *Turtles: perspectives and research*. Toronto: John Wiley & Sons, Inc, 1979;45-60.
70. Plummer MV. A notching system for marking softshell turtles. *Herpetol Rev* 2008;39:64-65.
71. Donnelly MA, Guyer C, Juterbock JE, et al. Techniques for marking amphibians. In: Heyer WR, Donnelly MA, McDiarmid RW, et al, eds. *Measuring and monitoring biological diversity. standard methods for amphibians*, Washington DC: Smithsonian Institution Press, 1994;277-284.
72. Buhlmann KA, Mitchell JC. Age of adult eastern tiger salamanders *(Ambystoma tigrinum tigrinum)* in a Virginia sinkhole pond complex: implications for conservation. *J Elisha Mitchell Sci Soc* 2000;116:239-244.
73. Gonser RA, Collura RV. Waste not, want not: toe-clips as a source of DNA. *J Herpetol* 1996;30:445-447.
74. McCarthy MA, Parris KM. Clarifying the effect of toe clipping on frogs with Bayesian statistics. *J Appl Ecol* 2004;41:780-786.
75. Liner AE, Smith LL, Castleberry SB. Effects of toe-clipping on the survival and growth of *Hyla squirella*. *Herpetol Rev* 2007;38:143-145.
76. Hoffmann K, McGarrity ME, Johnson, SA. Technology meets tradition: a combined VIE-C technique for individually marking anurans. *Appl Herpetol* 2008;5:265-280.
77. Campbell TS, Irvin P, Campbell KR, et al. Evaluation of a new technique for marking anurans. *Appl Herpetol* 2009;6:247-254.
78. Bloch N, Irschick DJ. Toe-clipping dramatically reduces clinging performance in a pad-bearing lizard *(Anolis carolinensis)*. *J Herpetol* 2004;37:293-298.
79. Huey RB, Dunham AE, Overall KL, et al. Variation in locomotor performance in demographically known populations of the lizard *Sceloporus merriami*. *Physiol Zool* 1990;63:845-872.
80. Dodd CK Jr. The effects of toeclipping on sprint performance of the lizard *Cnemidophorus sexlineatus*. *J Herpetol* 1993;27:209-213.
81. Borges-Landáez PA, Shine R. Influence of toe-clipping on running speed in *Eulamprus quoyii*, an Australian scincid lizard. *J Herpetol* 2003;37:592-595.
82. Hudson S. Natural toe loss in southeastern Australian skinks: implications for marking lizards by toe-clipping. *J Herpetol* 1986;30:106-110.
83. Jennings ML, David DN, Porter KM. Effect of marking techniques on growth and survivorship of hatchling alligators. *Wildl Soc Bull* 1991;19:204-207.
84. Blanchard FN, Finster EB. A method of marking live snakes for future recognition, with a discussion of some problems and results. *Ecology* 1933;14:334-347.
85. Brown WS, Parker WS. A ventral scale clipping system for permanently marking snakes (Reptilia: Serpentes). *J Herpetol* 1976;10:247-249.
86. Silvy NJ, Lopez RR, Peterson MJ. Wildlife marking techniques. In: Braun CE ed. *Techniques for wildlife investigations and management*. 6th ed. Bethesda, Md: The Wildlife Society, 2005;339-376.
87. Clark DR Jr. Branding as a marking technique for amphibians and reptiles. *Copeia* 1971;148-151.
88. Mellor DJ, Beausoleil NJ, Stafford KJ. *Marking amphibians, reptiles and marine mammals: animal welfare, practicalities and public perceptions in New Zealand*. New Zealand Department of Conservation Te Papa Atawhai, 2004.
89. Winne CT, Willson JD, Andrews KM, et al. Efficacy of marking snakes with disposable medical cautery units. *Herpetol Rev* 2006;37:52-54.
90. Lewke RE, Stroud RK. Freeze branding as a method for marking snakes. *Copeia* 1974;997-1000.
91. Higgins BM, Robertson BA, Williams TD. Manual for mass wire tagging of hatchling sea turtles and the detection of internal wire tags. NOAA Technical Memorandum NMFS-SEFC-402. 1997.
92. Eckert SA, Crouse D, Crowder LB, et al. *Review of the Kemp's ridley sea turtle headstart experiment, 22-23 September 1992, Galveston, Texas*. Report submitted to the U. S. Department of Commerce, National Oceanic and Atmospheric Administration, National Marine Fisheries Service, Southeast Fisheries Science Center, Miami, Florida, 1992.
93. Fontaine C, Shaver D. Head-starting the Kemp's ridley sea turtle, *Lepidochelys kempii*, at the NMFS Galveston Laboratory, 1978-1992: a review. *Chelon Conserv Biol* 2005;4:838-845.
94. Fontaine CT, Revera DB, Williams TD, et al. Detection, verification and decoding of tags and marks in head-started Kemp's ridley sea turtles, *Lepidochelys kempii*. NOAA Technical Memorandum NMFS-SEFC-334. 1993.

95. Wood F, Wood J. Release and recapture of captive reared green sea turtles *(Chelonia mydas)* in the waters surrounding Grand Cayman. *Herpetol J* 1993;3:84-89.
96. Shaver DJ. Head-started Kemp's ridley turtles nest in Texas. *Mar Turtle Newslett* 1996;74:5-7.
97. Hendrickson LP, Hendrickson JR. A new method for marking sea turtles. *Mar Turtle Newslett* 1981;19:6-7.
98. Caillouet CW Jr, Fontaine CT, Williams TD, et al. The Kemp's ridley sea turtle headstart project: an annual report for fiscal year 1985. NOAA Technical Memorandum, NMFS-SEFC-174, 1986.
99. Wilson RP, Shepard ELC, Liebsch N. Prying into the intimate details of animal lives: use of a daily diary on animals. *Endang Species Res* 2007;3:123-137.
100. Campbell HA, Sullivan S, Read MA, et al. Ecological and physiological determinants of dive duration in freshwater crocodile. *Functional Ecology* 2010;24:103-111.
101. Campbell HA, Dwyer RG, Gordos M, et al. Diving through the thermal window: implications for a warming world. *Proceedings of the Royal Society Biological Sciences* published online 7 July 2010. doi: 10.1098/rspb.2010.0902.
102. Campbell HA, Watts ME, Sullivan S, et al. Estuarine crocodiles ride surface currents to facilitate long-distance travel. *J Anim Ecol* 2010;79:955-964.
103. Franklin CE, Read MA, Kraft PG, et al. Remote monitoring of crocodilians: implantation, attachment and release methods for transmitters and data-loggers. *Mar Freshwater Res* 2009;60:284-292.
104. Gordos MA, Hamann M, Schauble CS, et al. Diving behaviour of *Elseya albagula* from a naturally flowing and hydrologically altered habitat. *J of Zoology* 2007;272:458-469..
105. Grigg GC, Seebacher F, Beard LA, et al. Thermal relations of large crocodiles, *Crocodylus porosus*, free-ranging in a naturalistic situation. *R Soc London Biol Sci* 1998;265:1793-1799.
106. Seebacher F, Grigg GC. Pattern of body temperature in wild freshwater crocodiles, *Crocodylus johnstoni*: thermoregulation versus thermoconformity, seasonal acclimatization, and the effect of social interactions. *Copeia* 1997;549-557.
107. Seebacher F. Behavioural postures and the rate of body temperature change in wild freshwater crocodiles, *Crocodylus johnstoni*. *Physiol Biochem Zool* 1999;72:57-63.
108. Seebacher F, Franklin CE, and Read MA. Diving behaviour of a reptile *(Crocodylus johnstoni)* in the wild: interactions with heart rate and body temperature. *Physiol Biochem Zool* 2005;78:1-8.
109. Goodman RM, Knapp CR, Bradley KA, et al. Review of radio transmitter attachment methods for West Indian rock iguanas (genus *Cyclura*). *Appl Herpetol* 2009;6:151-170.
110. Doody JS, Roe JA, Mayes P, et al. Telemetry tagging methods for some freshwater reptiles. *Mar Freshwater Res* 2009;60:293-298.
111. Knapp CR, Owens AK. An effective new radio transmitter attachment technique for lizards. *Herpetol Rev* 2005;36:264-266.
112. Cobb VA, Green JJ, Worrall T, et al. Initial den location behavior in a litter of neonate *Crotalus horridus* (Timber Rattlesnakes). *Southeast Nat* 2005;4:723-730.
113. Linehan JM, Stohlgren KM, Schlimm EM et al. Dispersal patterns of neonate timber rattlesnakes *(Crotalus horridus)* in Southwestern Georgia. *Copeia* 2012;3:460-464.
114. Boarman WI, Goodlett T, Goodlett G, et al. Review of radio transmitter attachment techniques for turtle research and recommendations for improvement. *Herpetol Rev* 1998;29:26-33.
115. Butler JA, Bowman RD, Hull TW, et al. Movements and home range of hatchling and yearling gopher tortoises, *Gopherus polyphemus*. *Chelon Conserv Biol* 1995;1:173-180.
116. Werner JK. A radiotelemetry implant technique for use with *Bufo americanus*. *Herpetol Rev* 1991;22:94-95.
117. Seebacher F, Alford RA. Movement and microhabitat use of a terrestrial amphibian *(Bufo marinus)* on a tropical island: seasonal variation and environmental correlates. *J Herpetol* 1999;33:208-214.
118. Madison DM. The emigration of radio-implanted spotted salamanders, *Ambystoma maculatum*. *J Herpetol* 1997;31:542-551.
119. Wright KM, Whitaker BR. *Amphibian medicine and captive husbandry*. Malabar, Fla: Krieger Publishing Company, 2001.
120. Tuttle AD, Law JM, Harms CA, et al. Evaluation of gross and histologic reactions to five commonly used suture materials in the skin of the African clawed frog *(Xenopus laevis)*. *J Am Assoc Lab Anim Sci* 2006;45:22-26.
121. Ott JA, Scott DE. Effects of toe-clipping and PIT-tagging on growth and survival in metamorphic *Ambystoma opacum*. *J Herpetol* 1999;33:344-348.
122. Govett PD, Harms CA, Linder KE. Effect of four different suture materials on the surgical wound healing of loggerhead sea turtles, *Caretta caretta*. *J Herpetol Med Surg* 2004;14:4-10.
123. Axelsson M, Dang Q, Pitsillides K. A novel, fully implantable, multichannel biotelemetry system for measurement of blood flow, pressure, ECG and temperature. *J Appl Physiol* 2007;102:1220-1228.
124. Ferrell ST, Marlar AB, Alberts AC, et al. Surgical technique for permanent intracoelomic radiotransmitter placement in Anegada iguanas *(Cyclura pinguis)*. *J Zoo Wildl Med* 2005;36:712-715.
125. Reinert HK, Cundall D. An improved surgical implantation method for radio-tracking snakes. *Copeia* 1982;702-705.
126. Lentini AM, Crawshaw GJ, Licht LE. Pathologic and hematologic responses to surgically implanted transmitters in eastern massasauga rattlesnakes *(Sistrurus catenatus catenatus)*. *J Wildl Dis* 2011;47:107-125.
127. Read MA, Grigg GC, Irwin SR, et al. Satellite tracking reveals long distance coastal travel and homing by translocated estuarine crocodiles, *Crocodylus porosus*. *PLoS One* 2007;9:949-953.
128. Scott JA. Use of satellite telemetry to determine ecology and management of the loggerhead turtle *(Caretta caretta)* during the nesting season in Georgia. Unpublished MS Thesis. University of Georgia, Athens, 2006.
129. Arendt MD, Segars AL, Byrd JI, et al. Distributional patterns of adult male loggerhead sea turtles *(Caretta caretta)* in the vicinity of Cape Canaveral, Florida, USA during and after a major annual breeding aggregation. *Mar Biol* 2011;159:101-112.
130. Arendt MD, Segars AL, Byrd JI, et al. Migration, distribution, and diving behavior of adult male loggerhead sea turtles *(Caretta caretta)* following dispersal from a major breeding aggregation in the Western North Atlantic. *Mar Biol* 2011;159:113-125.
131. Seney EE, Higgins BM, Landry AM. Satellite transmitter attachment techniques for small juvenile sea turtles. *J Exp Mar Bio Ecol* 2010;384:61-67.
132. Seney EE. Population dynamics and movements of the Kemp's ridley sea turtle, *Lepidochelys kempii*, in the northwestern Gulf of Mexico. Unpublished PhD Dissertation. Texas A&M University, College Station, 2008.
133. Mansfield KL. Sources of mortality, movements and behavior of sea turtles in Virginia. Unpublished PhD Dissertation. College of William and Mary, Gloucester Point, Virginia, 2006.
134. Mitchell SV. Use of epoxy in telemeter attachment. In: Abreu-Grobois FA, Briseño-Dueñas R, Márquez R, et al, compilers, in *Proceedings*. 18th Int Sea Turtle Symp. U.S. Department of Commerce, NOAA Technical Memorandum, NMFS-SEFSC-436, 2000.

CHAPTER 30

Forensics in Reptile Investigation

Melinda D. Merck and
Douglas R. Mader

Veterinarians are becoming more involved with legal issues in herpetoculture. Whether it is evaluating abuse or assessing evidence for illegal trafficking, professional medical expertise is often needed.

Recognizing neglect and cruelty can be difficult. In some cases, cruelty (Figure 30-1) or neglect (Figure 30-2) may be obvious, but in others, what appears to be neglect can simply be a matter of timing. For example, an inspection of a pet store reveals a Monitor Lizard lying in a feces ridden water bowl. Is this the norm or did the animal happen to defecate moments before the observer noticed the situation (Figure 30-3)? Finally, what may appear to be cruelty may actually be ignorance/stupidity on the part of the owner (Figure 30-4,).

Although several publications have addressed forensics in herpetoculture and medicolegal aspects of herpetology in recent years,[1-11] there has yet to be a document that specifically defines "herp cruelty", in the United States. The United States Department of Agriculture (USDA) does not regulate reptiles and amphibians, and as such, there are no guidelines on caging, nutrition, husbandry requirements, or shipping (Figures 30-5 and 30-6) like there are for other mammals such as dogs and cats. Without written standards, at most, U.S. veterinarians evaluating neglect/cruelty cases can only offer an "opinion." In the United Kingdom herpetology protection falls under the 1911 Protection of Animals Act that was updated in 2007. The legally important term found within the act is "unnecessary suffering", for which many people have been prosecuted.

Often these opinions are based on the experience of the veterinarian making the observations. Two different veterinarians observing the same situation may yield two completely different opinions. It is imperative that standards are established; otherwise, the legal standard will be that of the person giving testimony.

Until such herp-specific guidelines are developed, veterinarians can use the "Five Freedoms" as a template for assessing the health and welfare of herps. The Five Freedoms evolved from the Report of the Technical Committee to inquire into the welfare of animals kept under intensive livestock husbandry systems (the Brambell Report, December 1965, HMSO London) (Box 30-1). These principles were and are relevant and suggest appropriate measures for any animal species kept by humans—specifically, that all animals must be protected from unnecessary suffering.

RECOGNITION AND REPORTING OF NEGLECT AND CRUELTY

Not all municipalities or governments require that veterinarians report animal abuse. In the United States, only about a dozen states require that animal neglect or cruelty is reported (see animallaw.info for a current list of U.S. states requiring mandatory reporting). In addition, the definition of *animal* varies from location to location. The state of Florida defines an *animal* as "any dumb creature." In this case, *animal* covers reptiles, amphibians, and fish, among others. Nonetheless, even in states where cruelty reporting is mandatory, reptiles and amphibians may not be covered if they are not considered under the definition of *animal*.

Veterinarians take an oath to prevent animal suffering when they graduate. Regardless of whether they are required by law to do so, veterinarians have an ethical responsibility to act when they see suspected neglect or cruelty cases.

As stated by Yoffe-Sharp,[12] veterinarians play many vital roles in cases brought to the attention of authorities, including the following:

- Recognizing and reporting suspected cases of animal abuse
- Acting as medical experts
- Assisting at crime scene investigations
- Collecting and documenting evidence

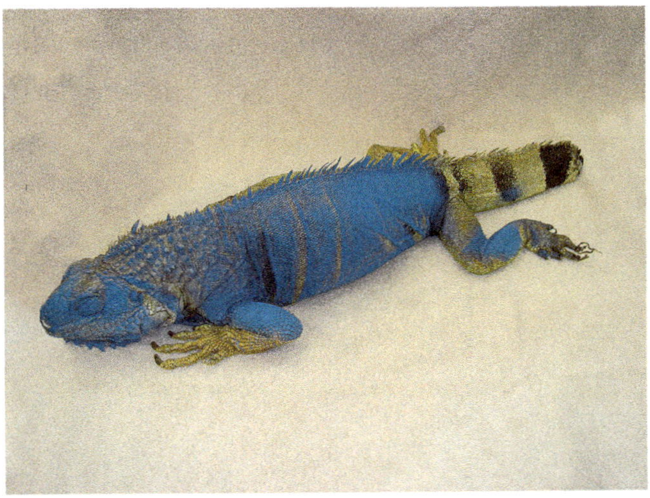

FIGURE 30-1 This iguana, a victim of animal cruelty, was painted blue and had its rear feet and tail cut off. *(Photo courtesy Dr. Douglas R. Mader, Marathon Veterinary Hospital, Marathon, Fla.)*

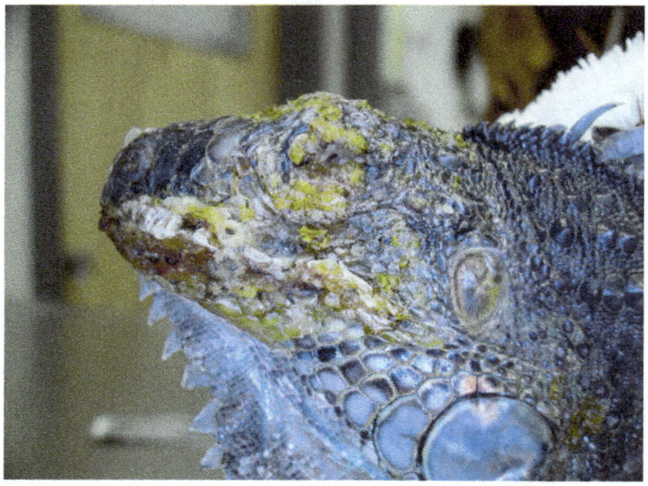

FIGURE 30-2 Neglect, such as seen in this iguana that was suffering from a severe mite infestation, can easily be confused with cruelty or abuse. *(Photo courtesy Dr. Douglas R. Mader, Marathon Veterinary Hospital, Marathon, Fla).*

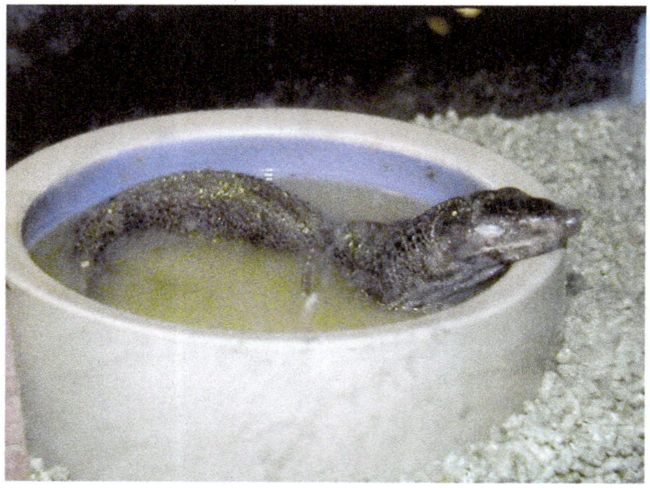

FIGURE 30-3 This photograph showing a monitor soaking in a feces-filled water bowl could be interpreted as evidence of neglect or cruelty. However, it could also illustrate the issue of timing, if the animal had defecated just moments before the photo was acquired. *(Photo courtesy Dr. Douglas R. Mader, Marathon Veterinary Hospital, Marathon, Fla.)*

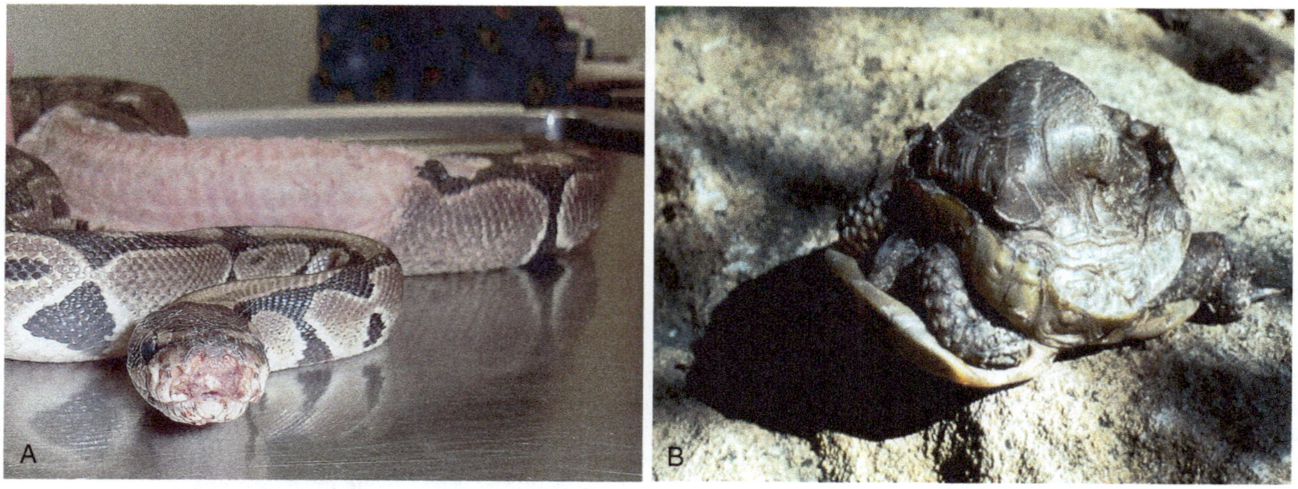

FIGURE 30-4 **A,** The owner placed a large, live rat unattended in the cage with this python that was not in a hunger state. As a result, the prey became the predator. **B,** This grossly deformed box turtle has been malnourished its entire life. Although, ostensibly, these cases look like abuse, in actuality, both of these cases are examples of ignorance on the part of the owner. *(Photos courtesy Dr. Douglas R. Mader, Marathon Veterinary Hospital, Marathon, Fla.)*

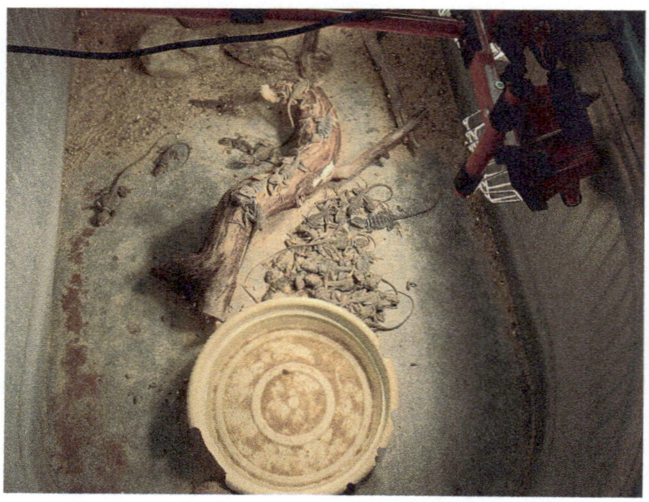

FIGURE 30-5 Evaluation of housing conditions may be a part of a herp-trained veterinarian's responsibility. *(Photo courtesy Dr. T. Tristin.)*

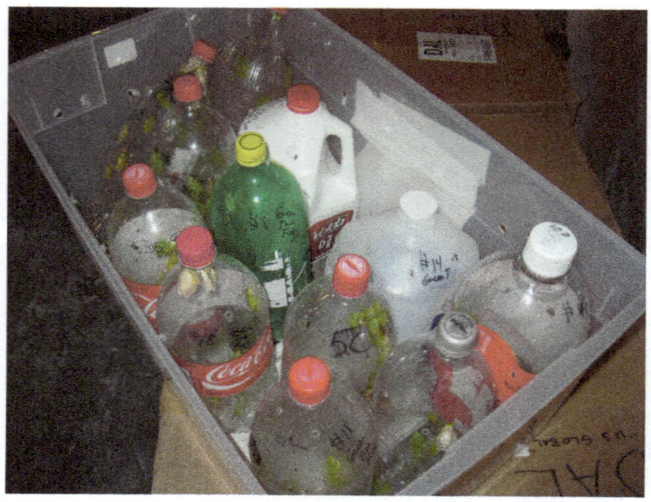

FIGURE 30-6 Improper shipping conditions for a collection of amphibians. *(Photo courtesy Dr. T. Tristin.)*

BOX 30-1 THE FIVE FREEDOMS

1. Freedom from Hunger and Thirst: by ready access to fresh water and a diet to maintain full health and vigor
2. Freedom from Discomfort: by providing an appropriate environment including shelter and a comfortable resting area
3. Freedom from Pain, Injury, or Disease: by prevention or rapid diagnosis and treatment
4. Freedom to Express Normal Behavior: by providing sufficient space, proper facilities, and company of the animal's own kind
5. Freedom from Fear and Distress: by ensuring conditions and treatment that avoid mental suffering

- Testifying as expert witnesses in court
- Recognizing suspected abuse and neglect of family members and reporting to appropriate authorities

In addition, specifically regarding herp cases, veterinarians' roles may include the following:

- Identifying species
- Distinguishing captive versus wild caught
- Identifying parasites of specimens (to determine origin)
- Assessing the health status of confiscated animals

Although reporting cruelty is not required in all U.S. states, the American Veterinary Medical Association (AVMA) advocates the responsibility of the veterinarian to report suspected cases of animal abuse, cruelty, and neglect to the appropriate authorities.[13] An excerpt from the AVMA Principles of Veterinary Medical Ethics[13] reads as follows: "Veterinarians and their associates should protect the personal privacy of patients and clients. Veterinarians should not reveal confidences unless required to by law or it becomes necessary to protect the health and welfare of other individuals or animals."

The AVMA Position Statement on Animal Abuse and Animal Neglect[13]:

The AVMA recognizes that veterinarians may observe cases of animal abuse or neglect as defined by federal or state laws or local ordinances. When these situations cannot be resolved by education, the AVMA considers it the responsibility of the veterinarian to report such cases to appropriate authorities. Disclosure may be necessary to protect the health and welfare of animals and people. Veterinarians should be aware that accurate record keeping and documentation of these cases are invaluable.

Similarly, the American Animal Hospital Association offers the following Position Statement on Animal Abuse[14]:

In order to encourage veterinarians and practice team members to be responsible leaders in their communities and to assist in the detection and reporting of animal abuse, the profession should educate its members to recognize, document, and report animal abuse, develop forensic models, promote legislation concerning reporting by veterinarians and collaborate with other animal and humane welfare groups and professionals within communities to eliminate the incidence of animal abuse.

RESPONSIBILITY OF THE VETERINARIAN

Yoffe-Sharp[12] recommends that veterinarians should

- Acquire a working knowledge of applicable laws pertaining to animal cruelty in their state, county, and community
- Know which agency in their jurisdiction is responsible for enforcement of animal cruelty laws and develop a working relationship with that agency
- Establish policies and procedures for recognizing and reporting abuse and provide training for all employees

DOCUMENTATION

The forensic examination is a process conducted for legal purposes that requires appropriate documentation. Everything associated with the case is subject to legal scrutiny that includes all notes, correspondence, photographs, radiographs, examination findings, reports, and the handling of evidence. These are all considered evidence and will be reviewed by the investigator, prosecutor, defense attorney, and judge. The use of forms is extremely useful in forensic cases to ensure procedures are followed completely and to meet the legal standard for evidence. These forms include chain of custody/evidence log, photo log, and live and necropsy examination.

Chain of Custody

Any evidence related to a crime must follow a chain of custody. This refers to a process of documentation in which the evidence is accounted for at all times, and there is a record of any alteration (e.g., testing; Figure 30-7). Evidence is anything collected or recorded from the animal and includes samples, photographs, radiographs, and the animal itself. It should be the investigating agency or their designee that transports the live or deceased animal to the veterinarian. When that is not possible, a courier service with tracking procedures may be used, and the chain of custody is still maintained.

All evidence must be properly collected, packaged, and labeled, and each item must be recorded in the evidence log (see Figure 30-7). All evidence should be kept in a locked cabinet with restricted access. If the evidence must be kept in a refrigerator or freezer without a lock, it should be located in an area with limited personnel access. A restricted access box may be placed inside the refrigerator or freezer, such as a metal lockbox, that will allow the evidence to be maintained under acceptable conditions. If the evidence is transferred to another person, location, or laboratory, it must be noted in the evidence log with the time, date, and a signature from the sender and/or recipient. This also applies to the body of the animal.

Whenever evidence needs to be transferred, including laboratory samples, chain of custody procedures should be followed. An evidence receipt form should be sent along with the evidence with instructions for the receiving agency/person to fill out the chain of custody section and fax it back (see Figure 30-7). It should be noted on any test request form that the samples are "Evidence," "Forensic Samples," or involve a "Criminal Investigation." This may assist the receiving laboratory to institute certain handling protocols and assign the appropriate person to perform the analysis.

If evidence is removed from storage it should be documented in the evidence log, including the purpose, if opened, and any testing or alteration. If necessary, a sealed evidence package should be opened in a different place from the original opening; the original seal needs to be preserved. This will later provide proof that the original seal was not broken. After the examination is complete, the item is placed back in the original package, sealed with evidence tape, signed, and dated. Evidence must be held until the legal case is over. Because additional legal avenues may be pursued after a case is closed, the prosecuting authority should be consulted before disposing of any evidence.

Photography and Videography

Photographic as well as possibly video documentation of all live and deceased animal examinations should be performed. The type of camera used is important; Polaroid and film cameras should no longer be used now that inexpensive digital cameras are prevalent. Digital cameras are ideal because the quality of the photograph is immediately evident, the photographs are digitally preserved, and they may be enhanced for further evaluation, if necessary. Digital SLR cameras with interchangeable lenses allow flexibility between long range and macro photography. With digital cameras, the pictures may be copied to a computer and preserved on a CD for authentication, and the digital card may be cleared and re-used. A minimum of three CDs should be made: one for the veterinarian, one for the lead investigator, and one for the prosecutor. Each disc should be labeled with the case number, date, and the photographer's name. A reference number should be assigned and multiples noted (e.g., the first CD of six designated "1 of 6," and the copy number (e.g., "copy 1"). The number of CDs and copies should be recorded in the evidence log. A copy of the photo log should be included with any CD copies.

There are some general guidelines regarding photography for legal cases. The photographs may need to be enlarged for court, so the resolution of the photographs should be high enough to prevent loss of detail. After a photograph is taken

Evidence Log/COC Record

Agency:________________
Case number:________________
Evidence holding location:________________

Item ID	Evidence description	Date	Initials	Purpose for removal/tests performed

Item ID____ Removal date______ Receipt date______
By__________ By__________
Release sign__________ Receipt sign__________

Item ID____ Removal date______ Receipt date______
By__________ By__________
Release sign__________ Receipt sign__________

Item ID____ Removal date______ Receipt date______
By__________ By__________
Release sign__________ Receipt sign__________

Item ID____ Removal date______ Receipt date______
By__________ By__________
Release sign__________ Receipt sign__________

Item ID____ Removal date______ Receipt date______
By__________ By__________
Release sign__________ Receipt sign__________

FIGURE 30-7 An evidence log.

with a digital camera, the image should be checked for quality and adjustments made as necessary. No photograph should ever be deleted; this is to prevent the appearance that exculpatory evidence was deleted. A photo may be altered only after the original is preserved. Any enhancements or alterations should be documented and saved separately from the original. Several photography software programs automatically record the alteration steps. Photographs should only be of items related to the case; no personal photos should be on the digital card. The photos should be professional: remember, they may end up in court. Care should be taken to avoid including personnel in the photographs, if possible. Hands in the photograph holding or pointing at the area of interest should be avoided; instruments should be used instead. All photographs should be taken at a 90-degree angle to the area of interest. The lighting should be evaluated for each photograph, and reflection off the object or tissue should be avoided. All photographs should be recorded in a photo log (Figure 30-8). The photos may be logged as they are being taken or after all photography is completed.

The photographs should begin with the case information, including the case number, date, and animal ID written on a card or dry-erase board. This first picture with the case and animal information may be taken with or without the animal in the photo. All photographs after this initial picture should only be of the examination of that animal. When cases involve multiple animals, this protocol will ensure consistency of the photographs and reduce the chance of errors. If additional photographs are needed of an animal that has already been photographed, the sequence starts again with the case and animal ID information card. General photos should be taken showing the entire body of the animal, that is, right and left side, front (facial), hind (rear), and dorsal and ventral (if possible) views.

Photo Log Sheet Page __ of __

Agency: ______________________

Case number: ______________________

Date of incident/exam: ______________________

Photographer: ______________________ Assisted by: ______________________

Digital CD copies: _____ Provided to: ______________________

Photo #(s)	Notes

FIGURE 30-8 A photo log.

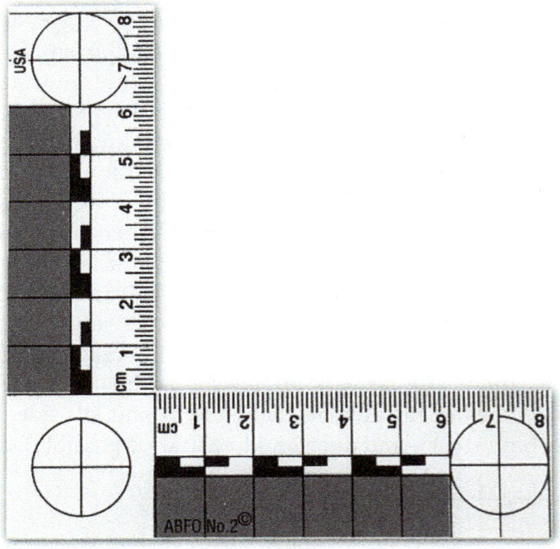

FIGURE 30-9 American Board of Forensic Odontology (ABFO) no. 2 photography scale. *(Photo courtesy Dr. Douglas R. Mader, Marathon Veterinary Hospital, Marathon, Fla.)*

Photographs, with and without scale, should be taken of any obvious lesions, abnormal physical findings, and any evidence found on the body.

For all photos, it is important to capture the context and location, starting with overall views, then medium views, and finally close-ups. Taking only a close-up view is not useful in court without the reference or context photos. This process of narrowing down the focus and showing perspective may take several photographs to achieve. When physical evidence on the body is photographed, an evidence marker should be in the photo, including the close-up views. Special markers, scales, and pointers for small evidence are available, or a piece of paper with a letter or number system can be created. The markers, with the ID number written on a piece of paper, may be reduced in size to accommodate close-ups. Close-up photographs should be taken with and without a photo scale to show that no evidence was obscured by the scale. The purpose of a photo scale is to show the size of the item. There are special photography scales, such as American Board of Forensic Odontology (ABFO) no. 2 scales (Figure 30-9), that also have symbols and a gray scale to allow correction for size distortion (elongation) and color discrepancies. If a photo scale is not available, other items with known sizes may be used, such as a coin or dollar bill. A macro lens may be used for clear close-ups of small lesions. Because of the sensitivity to movement of fine detail lenses, it is recommended that a mini-tripod be used for stability when photos are taken.

Video may be taken of the live animal examination. The video should begin with a shot of the case and animal ID number. It is preferable to have the time and date showing on the recording. Videography is most valuable when an animal shows obvious difficulty performing certain functions, such as those affected by neurologic or ambulatory problems. It is also helpful to show certain behaviors, such as vocalizing because of pain or severe brain injury. In starvation cases, it is useful to video the animal's response when first given water and food. It is best to videotape anything that can better be appreciated through live recording rather than still photos. The video may be copied to a DVD, and the same evidence procedures as for photography should be used.

Examination Documentation

When an animal is examined in a forensic case, the veterinarian is working on behalf of the court, and there must be full documentation of all the findings, including the positive and negative. From a legal standpoint, if it is not documented, it was not done. The examination should include written and photographic documentation. Radiographs are recommended for animal abuse cases for documentation of findings and determination of hidden injuries or disease. Digital radiographs are preferred, and CD copies should be made following the aforementioned photography protocol. Diagrams may be used to document injuries such as bruising and wounds. Videography may be helpful for documenting live animal examinations, especially where behavior of the animal is a factor in the case. It may also be helpful to have a recording device during examination of the animal for dictating findings. Some general considerations should be taken into account for all written documentation. Leaving blank areas on forms should be avoided; *N/A* or a strike through the item should, instead, be used if no entry is required. Editorial remarks on the record should also be avoided. Any errors should be corrected by drawing a single line through the entry, marking it "error," and dating and initialing it.

The top of the examination form should have the investigating agency or authority information including their case number and the lead investigator's name (Figure 30-10). The name of the examining veterinarian and any other parties present for the examination should be noted. The date and time of the examination should be recorded, including the time when the examination is concluded. No examination should be conducted without all the information from the investigators and/or owner, including crime scene findings and photographs, the investigator's reports, and any witness statements. This information provides the proper context in which the veterinarian can more accurately interpret the examination findings. Anything provided by the investigator should be documented on the form. A description of the animal, including species, sex, coloring, distinguishing marks, and estimated or known age, should be recorded. The basis for age determination should be defined on the document. Details of how the animal arrived should be noted for live and deceased examinations. This includes the person's name that transported the animal, the method of transport, and packaging details. For deceased animals, the external and internal packaging is recorded and photographs are taken as each layer of packaging is removed. Any tears or leakage of the packaging material should be noted, as well as the degree of decomposition. Any courier information on the package should be photographed and, if possible, removed and placed in the case file.

Because of the legal nature of the case and because the animal is considered evidence, several factors need to be taken into account regarding euthanasia of the victim and release or disposal of the body. If it is part of an active investigation, permission for euthanasia usually must be obtained from the investigating authority, who often defers to the veterinarian's recommendation. An exception to the permission requirement may include a situation in which the animal is in critical condition and euthanasia is urgently required for humane reasons.

Live Exam

Agency: ______________________

Officer: ______________________

Case #: ______________________

Examining veterinarian: ______________________

Date of exam: __________ Time: Start ______ Finish ______

Subject of exam: ______________________

Method of arrival: ______________________

Materials provided/reviewed: ______________________

____

Crime scene/forensic findings: ______________________

____

Examination findings: ______________________

Weight: ________ T: ________ MM/CRT: ________ Hydration: ________

Coat condition: __________ Parasites: ______________________

BCS: (1)Emaciated (2)Very thin (3)Thin (4)Lean (5)Ideal

(6)Mildly ovrwt (7)Ovrwt (8)Obese (9)Morbidly obese

EENM (eyes, ears, nose, mouth): ______________________

____

____

Ausc/Abd palp: ______________________

____

____

Perineal: ______________________

Musculoskeletal: ______________________

____

Additional findings: ______________________

____

____

Evidence of medical/surgical intervention: ______________________

____

Radiographic interpretation: ______________________

____

Evidence/samples collected and testing: ______________________

FIGURE 30-10 A live examination form.

For all euthanasia, the reason should be documented along with the doctor's name, date, and time of death. The handling of bodies after examination is also subject to evidence procedures. In human legal cases, the body is only released after the examination is completed, with photo documentation of the examination, and all procedures and testing are also completed. This includes the standard practice in which all tissues and samples submitted for testing are kept by the laboratories (e.g., fixed tissue and slides) for opposing counsel to conduct independent examination or testing. This is the legal right of the defendant, and failure to be able to exercise that right can result in the inadmissibility of the test results. The release and disposal of animal bodies may be handled the same way, provided the same requirements are met.

EVIDENCE COLLECTION AND PACKAGING

Appropriate equipment is needed for evidence collection and packaging. There is an Animal Cruelty Forensics Kit for veterinarians available from Tri-Tech Forensics (tritechforensics.com). Proper protocol for preventing contamination should be followed when collecting and packaging evidence. Gloves should be changed between handling of different evidence items to prevent cross-contamination. If the gloves were stored in such a manner that they could have been contaminated, the gloves may be rolled with a fresh lint roller tape to remove any trace evidence before continuing. Touching one's face, hair, or body before handling the evidence should be avoided. A mask may be worn to prevent contamination of DNA through coughing or sneezing. The item should be picked up or touched at areas where the suspect would not normally grab the item to protect fingerprint evidence. Sterile swabs should be used for evidence collection. Disposable or thoroughly cleaned tools should be used with evidence, and the tools should be cleaned before handling each new piece of evidence. Tools may be cleaned by rinsing with clean water and then drying with a clean tissue; the process should be repeated twice before sampling. Bleach should not be used when DNA evidence is collected.

Different types of evidence require different types of packaging and storage. The type of packaging chosen should be appropriate in size and material for the particular item and should be clean or new to avoid contamination. The goal is to preserve the integrity of the evidence. Clean paper evidence bags and envelopes are preferred over plastic, which may allow moisture to build up over time, thus damaging the evidence. However, plastic storage has been shown not to degrade DNA for up to 3 months.[15] Each item of evidence should be packaged separately. Evidence that is wet or moist needs to properly dry. The wet item may be wrapped in clean brown or butcher paper and then placed in a paper bag. Sharp objects should be packaged so that contamination or injury by puncturing is prevented when the objects are handled. Special evidence boxes and tubes are available from criminal investigation supply companies. Fragile items should be packaged carefully to prevent damage in handling and transport. Gunshot projectiles should be collected with the use of plastic instruments or gloved fingers to prevent damage to any ballistic evidence. They should then be packaged in a cardboard box so that damage or marks to the surface are prevented. Small items such as hair or fibers should be placed in coin envelopes or pharmaceutical folds and then placed in a larger envelope. A pharmaceutical fold can be created with a piece of clean paper that is trifolded from top to bottom, then trifolded again from side to side. The paper is unfolded and the collected item is placed in the center; the paper is then refolded, which secures the evidence. Samples of biological stains may be collected with the use of sterile swabs. For dry stains, a wet–dry technique may be used: moisten a sterile swab with distilled or sterile water, roll the swab on the area of interest to rehydrate the cells, then swab the moistened area with a dry sterile swab. Dry swabs may be placed in a paper envelope. If the swab is wet it should be allowed to air-dry or be placed inside a swab box, which allows the swab to breathe and dry safely. The entire swab box is then placed inside a paper envelope or bag to protect it from contamination while drying. Arson evidence requires special packaging to prevent vapors from escaping or being absorbed, such as when plastic containers are used. Instead, clean unused metal paint cans or special arson packaging containers from evidence collection supply companies should hold the evidence.

Forensic entomology has the greatest ability to give an accurate time of death through the arrival and succession of insects postmortem. It may also provide information on time of injury when maggots are found on live animals (myasis). The documentation, collection, and packaging of insect evidence is different than other types of evidence. The blow fly is the first insect to colonize on the body after death. It is important for the veterinarian to understand the life cycle of the blow fly to recognize various life cycle stages and collect appropriate samples. The developmental rate of the blow fly species present on the body is used to determine time of colonization, which is used to determine the minimum postmortem interval.

The blow fly first deposits eggs on the body, which hatch and develop to first-, second-, and third-instar larvae (maggots). They then go through a migratory phase, moving away from the body, then pupate into adult flies through a process called metamorphosis, leaving behind the empty pupa casing. The puparia are small and brown-colored with circular ridges on the surface. They are often mistaken for rat droppings, which have smooth surfaces. This developmental sequence is influenced by species, temperature, weather conditions, and season. As the number of maggots increases, they form a large mass, which raises the temperature of the body and within the mass itself. The temperature reading inside the maggot mass is important to obtain for the entomologist. The weather data from the closest weather station for the period in question should be submitted to the entomologist along with the samples for analysis.

Collection of entomologic samples from the body during examination should include all the different types of insect evidence, including adult insects. The oldest life cycles should be collected because they probably represent the earliest time of insect arrival and colonization. For all packaging, two labels should be created with the date and time, case number, location of the sample collected, and the sample number. These should be filled out in pencil to avoid any destruction of the writing. A double labeling system should always be used in which one label is placed inside the plastic container and the other is affixed to the outside of the container.

Blow fly egg masses should first be photographed and their location documented. Forceps should be used to break off a small piece of egg mass approximately the size of a dime; it should be collected from the center because the eggs at the edge may be desiccated and no longer viable. Each egg mass collected from each location on the body should be kept separate. The mass collected should be broken in half, and one half should be placed in 70% to 85% ethyl alcohol. The other half should be placed in a larval-rearing pouch. These pouches are made by taking a piece of aluminum foil and folding it to create a three-dimensional rectangular pouch, with the corners crimped together. A small piece of beef or pork liver should be placed inside as a feeding substrate should the larvae hatch. The top should also be crimped together, sealing the sample. This pouch should then be placed inside a plastic container for shipment; approximately 1 inch of soil or vermiculite should be placed in the bottom, and small air holes should be punched into the plastic top. This substrate absorbs any fluids that leak from the pouch and, for late stage larval samples, provides a burrowing substrate.

For maggot analysis, the oldest (largest) larvae should be collected because they are the ones that first hatched and, in turn, were the first eggs laid. A sample of the largest maggots and some of the next size down should be placed into hot or boiling water for 5 minutes to kill and blanch them, and the time of blanching should be documented. This process prevents the decomposition of the maggot. They should then be transferred to a vial of 70% to 85% isopropyl alcohol. They may also be placed in 70% to 85% isopropyl alcohol if hot water is not available for blanching. The vial should be double-labeled as described for egg masses: one label in the liquid and another affixed to the outside.

Another live sample of the maggots should be preserved in the larval-rearing pouches for examination. Too many maggots should not be placed in the pouch because they may die from lack of air. The migratory larvae may be found moving away from the body during the examination. Puparia, the metamorphosis stage, or pupa casings may or may not be found on the animal's body. Both migratory larvae and puparium samples are postfeeding and do not require a food substrate. They should be placed in a plastic container with vermiculite or sand on the bottom and a damp paper towel to prevent desiccation. Pupa casings are fragile and should be collected, placed in a dry vial with tissue paper for protection, and submitted for species identification. The presence of pupa casings indicates that at least a full life cycle of the fly has been completed.

DNA testing is commonly performed in forensic cases for species determination or when individualization is needed for a match to a questioned sample. The identification of species is especially important in the illegal trade of animals. Databases of exotic and rare species DNA have been developed to facilitate the investigations of these crimes. Mitochondrial DNA (mtDNA) is often used when the sample of nuclear DNA is too small or degraded. The mtDNA is unique in that it is maternally inherited and shared by all along the maternal line. Each source of DNA requires special collection and submission procedures. Sources of DNA include fresh collected blood, dried blood stains, wet blood stains, buccal (cheek) swabs, bones, teeth, hair, feathers, feces, muscle, organs, hide, saliva, semen, and urine. The DNA laboratory should be contacted before shipment of any samples to determine what tests will be needed and the priority of testing and to ensure that collection and submission procedures are followed. It is helpful to create a manual for DNA collection and packing based on the information provided by the laboratory and keep it readily available.

Clean latex or nitrile gloves should be worn during collection of DNA samples to avoid contamination. Procedures for biological sample collection and packing procedures should be followed. Care should be taken to avoid dirt or leaf material contamination, which can inhibit DNA analysis. Fresh blood collected by venipuncture should be placed into an EDTA or ACD tube, refrigerated, and shipped overnight to the laboratory. For buccal swabs, the swab is placed inside the cheek and swirled 10 times; two swabs should be collected from each animal. Fresh semen or urine should be placed in a leak-proof container and frozen. Dried saliva, semen, and urine evidence may be swabbed. Feces can also be used for DNA testing. Dried feces should be placed in a paper container, and wet feces should be collected in a leak-proof container and immediately frozen. Muscle, organ, and skin samples may be used for DNA, unless it has been more than 72 hours postmortem and/or the body has significantly decomposed.

Spleen, muscle (especially tongue), and liver are good sources for DNA. The fresh tissue should be frozen in an airtight container and shipped overnight with a cold pack. Paraffin-embedded tissue can be used for DNA. A 1-inch square piece of tissue should be submitted in a sealed container. Formalin-fixed tissues can possibly be used if the tissues have fixed for up to 10 days. When the soft tissue is too degraded, teeth are useful sources of DNA because the pulp of the teeth is well protected from decomposition. It is preferable to submit at least two teeth in good condition without any cracks or chips. If no teeth are available, then a 3-inch to 4-inch piece of long bone may be submitted. Do not clean or bleach the teeth or bone.

All evidence needs to be properly sealed, not only to protect it but also to visually show that the integrity of the evidence has been maintained. Evidence tape is made to easily tear and is not meant to hold bags closed or boxes together. Packing tape may be used to seal containers, and evidence tape may then be placed over it. The person who packaged the evidence then signs or places his or her initials and the date across the tape. In lieu of evidence tape, other tape such as duct tape or waterproof medical tape may be used as long as it can be written on. A sealed evidence package should always be opened in a different area than where it was initially sealed; the package should then be resealed with the use of standard packaging protocol.

The package should be properly labeled with the evidence number, case number, date, collection location, description of the item, time collected, collector's name, and signature. If the evidence contains biological fluids or tissue and/or poses a potential hazard to humans, it should be marked with a biohazard label. Each item of evidence is assigned an evidence identification number, and all evidence is recorded in the evidence log (see Figure 30-7). Certain evidence such as blood tubes, which need refrigeration, will change or degrade if not handled properly. Chain of custody procedures should be followed, and any transfer, storage, or transport of the evidence should be documented.

NONACCIDENTAL INJURIES

Nonaccidental injury (NAI) is the forensic term used to identify "the intentional harm of an animal." This includes but is not limited to willful neglect, infliction of injury, pain, or distress, and malicious killing of an animal.[16]

There are many different types of nonaccidental injuries. They include penetrating injuries, nonpenetrating injuries (e.g., blunt force trauma), burns, gunshot wounds, asphyxia, drowning, poisoning, ritualistic crime, and animal fighting injuries. Several factors need to be considered before the determination of accidental versus nonaccidental injury is made. Veterinarians must draw on their own experience with known accidental injuries and compare those findings to the evaluation.

The environment and husbandry for the animal directly affect the health of the animal and must be analyzed along with physical examination findings. Animal cruelty should be suspected in every case in which the history, crime scene findings, and environmental conditions do not support the examination findings. Aberrant findings should not be disregarded because they are often the key piece of evidence showing that the injuries sustained are nonaccidental.

Certain injuries, such as burns, can be difficult to determine. For instance, in some species of reptiles, burns do not always manifest immediately and, in fact, may not be apparent for more than a week, which may make proving causation difficult. Likewise, the usually thickened skin and surface scales of reptiles may mask bruising, which makes the association with blunt force trauma nearly impossible without necropsy or radiographic support.

All injuries or suspected abnormalities should be documented with written reports, as well as photographs, radiographs, and laboratory testing. If weapons or projectiles are involved, physical evidence should be collected and documented (Figure 30-11).

THE FORENSIC REPORT

The reports generated for any investigation are important. When a report is written, it is for the whole community: law enforcement, prosecutor, defense attorney, defendant, judge, and jury. These reports are legal documents and are examined throughout the legal process of the case. For criminal cases, they are submitted to the investigating and prosecuting agency. As the case progresses, the report is examined by the defense counsel, the defendant, their expert witness, and the judge. It is from these reports that decisions are made by both sides, including whether to prosecute and how to charge the defendant. The forensic report is used to map out defense and prosecution strategies and may be used to determine plea bargains or sentencing. On the basis of the contents and how the report is written, it can reveal how the veterinarian will testify. Of note, approximately 95% of criminal cases are resolved without a trial.

The purpose of the forensic report is to provide a clear understanding of the veterinary evidence. It should include information provided by investigating authorities and/or anyone else connected to the investigation, examination findings, procedures, samples/evidence collected, test submissions and results (medical and forensic), medical diagnoses, treatments and outcomes, and conclusions. The forensic report collates all the findings and their interpretation and provides a well-balanced professional opinion. The forensic report should be clear, methodical, and formatted in a logical manner.

Just as with the terminology used in giving testimony, the terminology used in the forensic report is also important. Unless there is medical or scientific proof that something occurred, the veterinarian may not be able to make certain statements. The best test to apply to any statement is, "how do you know?" Even with eyewitness statements, the information is still not necessarily considered fact. Statements made by the veterinarian should be based on a reasonable degree of scientific or medical certainty. Statements may also be made with an explanation for the basis and context. Absolute statements should be made with caution and only with certainty of the analysis. Peer discussion of findings may be helpful in consideration of all theories before reaching a conclusion.

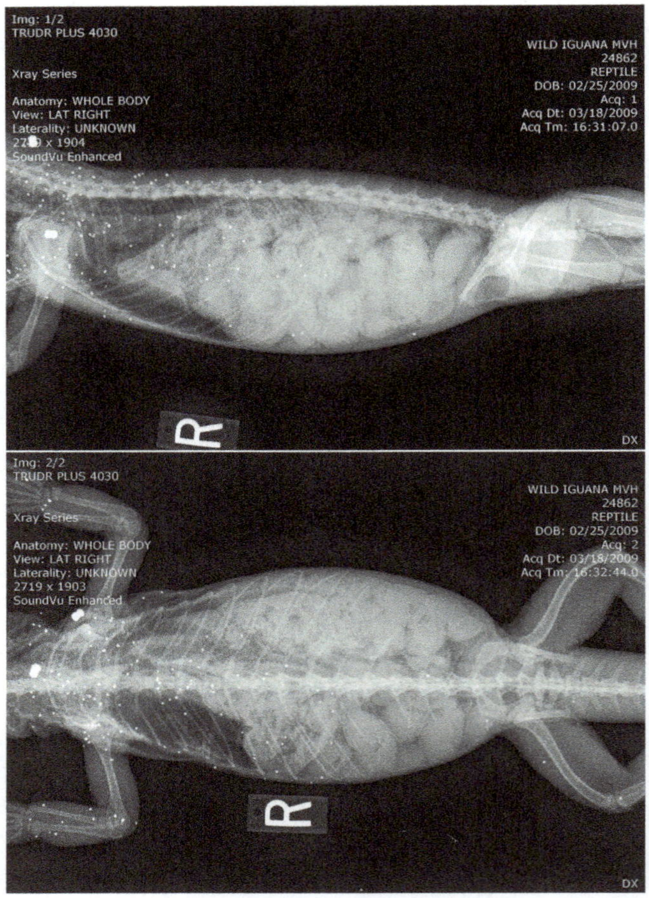

FIGURE 30-11 Material evidence should be saved and catalogued in cases of animals injured by physical objects, such as the pellets and BBs seen in these radiographs. *(Photo courtesy Dr. Douglas R. Mader, Marathon Veterinary Hospital, Marathon, Fla.)*

For multiple animal cases, each animal's findings may be listed in one report (see further on) or in separate reports. When separate reports are written, each report will be analyzed and compared, so it is important to have continuity of descriptions and terminology. Sometimes a report is needed before the receipt and analysis of all test results and the final determination of conclusions. In these cases, a verbal report may be given to the investigating officer, or a preliminary report may be issued. If a written preliminary report is required, it should be written with great caution and should not contain anything other than known facts, confirmed findings, and pending tests. Conclusions, if any, should be carefully drafted in preliminary reports and based only on confirmed information. If these conclusions change in the final report, the basis for the changes must be explained. Both the preliminary and final reports should be kept as separate files. They are both considered evidence and part of discovery material to be turned over to the opposing counsel. All electronic communications and documentation made at the scene or during the examination, laboratory results, forensic testing, expert consultations, photographs, radiographs, and any treatment or medical records must be preserved as evidence for the case.

The reports for animal cruelty cases should be titled Examination Report or Necropsy Report for a live or deceased

Examination Report

Agency: ____________________

Officer: ____________________

Case #: ____________________

Examining veterinarian: ____________________

Date of exam: ____________________

Subject of exam: ____________________

Reason for exam: ____________________

Method of arrival: ____________________

Crime scene/forensic findings: ____________________

Medical history: ____________________

Abbreviations: mm = mucous membranes; HLA = heart, lung auscultation; A = abdomen palpation; UR = unremarkable; BCS = body condition score

Definitions: ____________________

Body condition score : 1-3 = Too thin; 4-5 = Ideal; 6-9 = Overweight

Examination findings: ____________________

Evidence of injury: ____________________

Procedures and results: ____________________

Entomology findings: ____________________

Summary of findings: ____________________

Time of injury: __________

Mechanism of injury: ____________________

Cause of injury: ____________________

Contributory cause: ____________________

Manner of injury: ____________________

Conclusions: ____________________

[Name] ____________________ Date: __________

[Signature] ____________________

FIGURE 30-12 An examination report.

victim, respectively. For consultations, the report may be titled Expert Opinion Report. Microsoft Word document templates of report forms may be useful for creating templates for examination reports and necropsy reports (Figures 30-12 and 30-13).

Report Format

The following is a general description of recommended headings and subheadings to be used in forensic reports. It is appropriate to use medical terminology in the first sections of the report, but lay terminology should be used starting at the Summary of Findings section.

Heading

The top of the report should have information about the investigating agency, lead investigating officer, and case number. This should be followed by the examining veterinarian information, including the name, address, phone number, fax number, and date of the examination.

Subject of Examination

This section should contain a full description of the animal, including the species, breed, sex, known or estimated age, coloring, any distinguishing marks, and animal ID. The basis for the age determination, such as dentition, medical records,

Necropsy Report

Agency: ______________________

Investigator: ______________________

Case #: ______________________

Examining veterinarian: ______________________

Date of exam: __________

Subject of exam: ______________________

Reason for exam: ______________________

Method of arrival: ______________________

Description of packaging: ______________________

Materials provided/reviewed: ______________________

Crime scene/forensic findings: ______________________

Medical history: ______________________

ABBREVIATIO NS: mm = mucous membranes; HLA = heart, lung auscultation; A = abdomen palpation; UR = unremarkable; BCS = body condition score

Definitions: ______________________

Canine body condition score: 1-3 = Too thin; 4-5 = Ideal; 6-9 = Overweight

Examination findings: ______________________

External exam: ______________________

Rigor: ______________________

Decomposition: ______________________

Entomological evidence: ______________________

Body condition score: __________

Weight: __________

Coat condition: ______________________

Ectoparasites: ______________________

Head: ______________________

Chest: ______________________

Abdomen: ______________________

Perineum: ______________________

Legs: ______________________

Feet: ______________________

Tail: ______________________

FIGURE 30-13 A necropsy report.

Evidence of medical/surgical intervention: ____________________

____

Radiographic interpretation: ____________________

____

Internal exam: ____________________

Skin reflection: ____________________

Head: ____________________

Thoracic cavity: ____________________

Abdominal cavity: ____________________

Neck: ____________________

Respiratory tract: ____________________

Cardiovascular system: ____________________

Gastrointestinal tract: ____________________

Biliary tract: ____________________

Pancreas: ____________________

Spleen: ____________________

Adrenals: ____________________

Urinary tract: ____________________

Reproductive tract: ____________________

Musculoskeletal system: ____________________

Evidence of injury: ____________________

Procedures and results: ____________________

Entomology findings: ____________________

Summary of findings: ____________________

Survival period: ____________________

Time of death: ____________________

Mechanism of death: ____________________

Cause of death: ____________________

Contributory cause: ____________________

Manner of death: ____________________

Conclusions: ____________________

[Name] ____________________ Date: __________

[Signature] ____________________

FIGURE 30-13, cont'd

lack of ocular changes, or age-related color change, should be included. For the multiple animal examination report, the animal IDs are placed under the Examination Findings section.

Reason for Examination

This section should contain a sentence describing the reason for the examination or report. Some reasons include animal cruelty investigation or expert opinion analysis.

Material Provided/Reviewed

This section should contain a list of all material provided, including the source, that is associated with the animal or case. This may be materials provided by the investigating agency, attorney, or the owner.

Crime Scene/Forensic Findings

This section is the context for the analysis of the examination findings and should contain any crime scene or forensic findings. These may be from personal observations during on-scene investigation work by the veterinarian or information provided by the investigator. When the information is provided verbally by the investigator, it should be clearly noted. For example, "According to Officer (name) on (the date)," then the information that was conveyed verbally should follow. A summary of the information contained in the materials provided for review should be noted in this section. This includes photographs, videos, reports, and witness statements. Any conclusions from this information may be documented here or under the Conclusions section of the report. All weather data recorded at the scene or from a weather station should be documented here, including the time of the readings.

Medical History

Any known medical history should be documented in this section. This includes medical records and any treatments at another facility before the examination. It may include a verbal medical history provided by the owner or investigator, but it should be noted as such, as well as noting who provided that information. All medical history related to the victim's injuries should be described in this section, including initial examination findings, response or lack of response to treatment, all medications given, radiographic findings, and whether the animal died or was euthanized.

Abbreviations

It is appropriate to use medical abbreviations in the report provided that a key is included for clarity. This key may be modified on the basis of the abbreviations used by the veterinarian in the report.

Definitions

A section for definitions of the medical terms used in the report should be included for the benefit of the nonveterinarian reader. Some medical terms may be common enough for lay understanding and do not need to be defined. Any terminology unique to animals versus humans should be defined in this section or within the body of the report. The body condition scoring system that is used should also be included. A definition of each of the scores may be attached to the report.

Examination Findings

This section may have several subsections depending on the type of report, type of examination (live or deceased), nature of the injuries, and medical procedures performed.

External Examination

This section should include all the documented findings from the live animal examination form and the External Examination Findings section on the necropsy examination form (Figure 30-14). For the live animal, this subheading of External Examination may be eliminated under Examination Findings. An attempt at describing the body condition score (BCS) should be made. General reference to a defined BCS, such as the scale published by Purina for dogs and cats, should be provided here (see Figure 30-12). This can be extrapolated to herp specimens. For multiple animal reports, the findings for each animal can be listed in alphanumeric order by the animal ID. For each animal subject, examination information (e.g., age and sex), examination findings, and test results are documented with the use of abbreviations. The following line begins with Summary, and a list of the summary of findings in lay terms are noted (see Summary of Findings section further on). For large-scale cases, the list may be further broken down based on the crime scene location from where the animal was removed (Box 30-2).

Evidence of Injury

This section is optional and is most useful with complicated injuries such as multiple stab or gunshot wounds, animal bites, or other external injuries or obvious fractures. It is not necessary to repeat the descriptions in the external or internal examination sections. For gunshot cases, the trajectory description may be placed in this section or as a separate heading.

Photographs and Diagrams

Photographs and/or diagrams in the forensic report are extremely useful for illustrating examination findings. The photo selection should be the most representative of the injury, disease state, or abnormal finding. Diagrams may be inserted into the photo using Microsoft Word document tools to highlight or explain the areas of interest (Figure 30-15).

Medical Treatment and Results

For live animal examinations, any treatment or procedures performed should be recorded. Hospitalizations, medications, and treatment response, including a timeline, should be documented. The reasons for the animal's progress, recovery, or failure to respond to treatment should be addressed in this section.

Procedures and Results

All evidence collected from the animal, including samples, and tests conducted should be listed in this section. Any samples collected and held for possible future testing should be noted.

Entomology Findings

All entomologic evidence collected should be described in this section. The location of the collected insect evidence on the body should be noted. The weather data submitted with the insect samples should be kept as evidence in the case file. The results reported by the forensic entomologist should be listed in this section.

Necropsy Exam

Agency: ______________________

Officer: ______________________

Case #: ______________________

Examining veterinarian: ______________________

Date of exam: __________ Time: Start ______ Finish ______

Subject of exam: ______________________

Route of delivery: ______________________

Description of packaging: ______________________

Materials provided/reviewed: ______________________

____

Crime scene/forensic findings: ______________________

____

Examination findings: ______________________

External exam: ______________________

Decomposition score: ______________________

Rigor: ______________________

Lividity: ______________________

Rectal temp: ______________________

Entomological evidence: ______________________

BCS: (1)Emaciated (2)Very thin (3)Thin (4)Lean (5)Ideal

(6)Mildly ovrwt (7)Ovrwt (8)Obese (9)Morbidly obese

Weight: ________

Coat condition: ______________________

Ectoparasites: ______________________

Head: ______________________

____

Chest: ______________________

____

Abdomen: ______________________

____

Perineum: ______________________

____

Legs: ______________________

____

Feet: ______________________

FIGURE 30-14 An example of a necropsy examination form.

Continued

Tail: ______

Evidence of medical/surgical intervention: ______

Radiographic interpretation: ______

Internal exam: ______

Skin reflection findings: ______

Head: ______

Thoracic cavity: ______

Abdominal cavity: ______

Neck: ______

Respiratory tract: ______

Cardiovascular system: ______

Gastrointestinal tract: ______

Biliary tract: ______

Pancreas: ______

Spleen: ______

Adrenals: ______

Urinary tract: ______

Reproductive tract: ______

Musculoskeletal system: ______

Samples collected: ______

Additional comments: ______

FIGURE 30-14, cont'd

Summary of Findings

Beginning in this section of the report, every effort should be made to use lay terms instead of medical terms. All the pertinent findings should be listed numerically in this section. This should include examination findings (normal and abnormal), test results, and a summary of the injuries. Descriptive qualifiers such as *mild* or *severe* should be used to describe each finding. In neglect cases, for example, a summary list may include: "Emaciated (BCS 2/9), anemia, and retained skin". This section is also where the examination findings, materials reviewed, and the crime scene/forensic findings can be brought together. For example, in blunt force trauma cases, "Blunt force trauma to the snake's head, a minimum of 3 blows." If the investigator provides information about a particular weapon suspected of being used on the animal, a statement may be made regarding if the injuries are consistent with that weapon.

BOX 30-2 EXAMPLE OF A FORENSIC REPORT

Location A

ID A2D5-001: Python, adult, female, tan/black/gold, 6 kg, BCS 2/9, mm-grey, crt 2s, dz; Labwk: leukocytosis with azurophilia, anemia, hookworms

Summary

Emaciated, anemia, hookworms

Evidence of Medical and/or Surgical Intervention

This section should contain any findings of medical and/or surgical intervention on the animal such as intravenous catheters or chest tubes.

Radiographic Interpretation

Any radiographic procedures should be noted, and the views and the interpretation should be described.

Internal Examination

For the necropsy report, all the findings under this section on the necropsy examination form should be placed here.

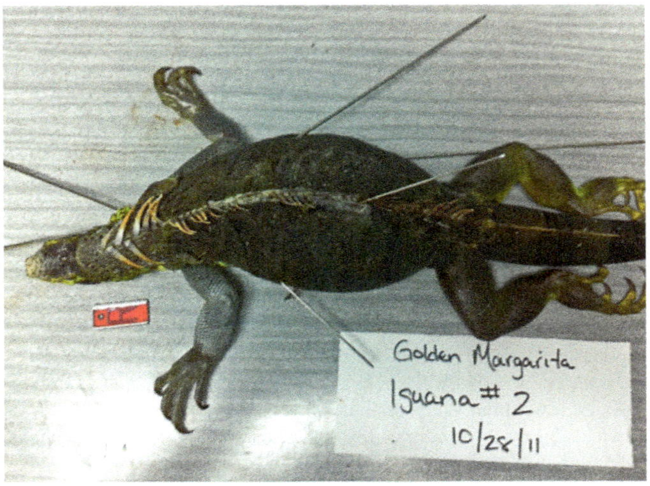

FIGURE 30-15 Photographs can be used to help demonstrate physical injuries such as the projectile tracts seen in this gunshot victim. *(Photo courtesy Eileen Slomka-McFarland LVT, Marathon Veterinary Hospital, Marathon, Fla.)*

For example, "Blunt force trauma to the snake's head, a minimum of 3 blows, consistent with a hammer." Unless there has been forensic evidence proving that particular weapon was used, the veterinarian does not know for a fact that it caused the injuries. At most, *consistent with* can be stated.

For a multiple animal report, the list should include the number of animals associated with the listed findings. For example, "Anemia (12 snakes)" should be written, with the total number of animals examined listed in parentheses next to the section title. For large-scale cases in which animals are listed under different crime scene locations, a location Summary of Findings should be listed followed by a total Summary of Findings for all the animals.

Survival Period

If any findings, including witness statements, indicate that the animal survived for a period of time before death, then the estimated time should be noted in this section. This may also be used on live animal examinations when an estimate may be made for the time of injury or disease. In this case, the estimate refers to the period the animal has survived after affliction of disease or trauma. The survival period estimate is often based on the examination findings and the veterinarian's experience and knowledge. The basis for the estimate, for example, medical findings or witness statement, should be documented.

Time of Death

The known or estimated time of death should be noted in this section. This may be based on the investigation findings, witness statements, and/or postmortem examination findings.[6] The basis for this determination should be documented. The term *unknown* is appropriate if determination of the time of death is not possible. The next section is known as the Death/Injury Statement. The final determinations regarding the death or injury are made in this section. For each category, the word *death* may be replaced with *injury* for the live examination report.

Mechanism of Death

This refers to the biochemical or physiologic abnormality or derangement that resulted in death (e.g., shock, septicemia, meningitis, pneumonia, etc.).

Cause of Death

This refers to the injury or disease that began a sequence of events that ultimately led to the death of the animal (e.g., gunshot wounds, stab wounds, blunt force trauma). The cause of death may be proximate or immediate. If the animal was euthanized, the cause of death is listed as euthanasia, and the cause of injury or disease that was the proximate reason for euthanasia is also listed.

Contributory Cause

This refers to any condition the animal had that could have contributed to death. For example, in a case in which the cause of death was multiple stab wounds, the mechanism of death was exsanguination and hypovolemic shock, and the contributory cause may be a clotting disorder that contributed to the hemorrhage. In the case of a starved, emaciated animal dying of hypothermia, the contributory cause would be starvation.

Manner of Death

This refers to the circumstances surrounding the death. Traditionally, the classifications in humans are homicide, suicide, accident, natural, or undetermined. In animals, the classifications are nonaccidental, accidental, natural, or undetermined.

Conclusions

This section is where the veterinarian ties all the examination and crime scene/forensic findings together. It should include everything listed in the Summary of Findings and the conclusions. This section should be a clear explanation of how the conclusions were reached and the basis for each. This section should contain factual findings, as well as the veterinary opinion of all the information documented in the report. It is important to know the language of the applicable laws so that, if applicable, appropriate statements can be made using the language found in that law. This is also the area that the veterinarian can educate the reader on the importance of certain findings, clarify any interpretations, and explain certain processes such as starvation. The pain and suffering of the animal should be thoroughly discussed. The use of terminology is important, such as *consistent with*. The terms *unique* and *indicative of* should be used cautiously and only with a strong basis. It is not appropriate to comment on whether the actions of the person who allegedly committed the acts in question were right or wrong. It is also not appropriate or within the veterinarian's purview to speculate in the report on a potential weapon without being asked to consider if a certain weapon could have been used. The veterinarian can only consider the information provided by the investigating agency or the persons for whom the report is being written. It is the strength of this final section that may reveal how the veterinarian will testify.

Finalization

The report should be finalized with the veterinarian's name, signature, and the date of the report.

SUMMARY

Forensic medicine has become more sophisticated in recent years. Sadly, more situations have also come to light in recent years in which this expertise has been needed. Illegal smuggling, hoarding, improper housing, and more require the professional assessment of trained veterinarians. With increasing prices seen in the reptile and amphibian trade, theft—and hence proof of ownership and lineage—has also been more of an issue. Veterinarians with proper training in herpetologic forensics will be in high demand.

REFERENCES

1. Baker BW. A brief overview of forensic herpetology. *Appl Herpetol* 2008;5:387–402.
2. Bauer AM. Geckos in traditional medicine: forensic implications. *Appl Herpetol* 2009;6:81–89.
3. Cooper ME. Forensics in herpetology—legal aspects. *Appl Herpetol* 2008;5:307-318.
4. Cooper JE. Methods in herpetological forensic work—post-mortem techniques. *Appl Herpetol* 2008;5:351-370.
5. Cooper JE. The estimation of *post-mortem* interval (PMI) in reptiles and amphibians: current knowledge and needs. *Herpetol J* 2012;22:91-96.
6. Frye FL. Establishing time of death in reptiles and amphibians, in *Proceedings*. Assoc Rept Amphib Vet 1999;23-25.
7. Frye FL. Methods in herpetological forensic work—sampling and standard laboratory techniques. *Appl Herpetol* 2008;5:339-350.
8. Hart M, Budgen P. Forensic record-keeping and documentation of samples. *Appl Herpetol* 2008;5:387-402.
9. McDowall IL. DNA technology and its applications in herpetological research and forensic investigations involving reptiles and amphibians. *Appl Herpetol* 2008;5:371-385.
10. Mitchell MA, Hernandez-Divers SJ. Methods in herpetological forensic work—clinical techniques. *Appl Herpetol* 2009;6:3-28.
11. Rothschild B. Scientifically rigorous reptile and amphibian osseous pathology: lessons for forensic herpetology from comparative and paleo-pathology. *Appl Herpetol* 2009;6:47-49.
12. Yoffe-Sharp BL, Loar LM. The veterinarian's responsibility to recognize and report animal abuse. *J Am Vet Med Assoc* 2009;234:732-737.
13. American Veterinary Medical Association Web site. Available at: www.avma.org.
14. American Animal Hospital Association Web site. Available at: www.aahanet.org.
15. Wilson A, Adams E. Studying the effects of plastic storage systems on DNA degradation of blood evidence, in *Proceedings*. 62nd Annu Sci Meet Am Acad Forens Sci, 22-27 February, 2010, Seattle, Washington.
16. McGuinness K, Allen M, Jones B. Non-accidental injury in companion animals in the Republic of Ireland. *Ir Vet J* 2005;58(7):392-396.

SUGGESTED READING

Cooper JE, Cooper ME. *Introduction to veterinary and comparative forensic medicine*. Oxford, England: Blackwell Publishers, 2007.

Cooper JE, Cooper ME. *Wildlife forensic investigation: principles and practice*. Boca Raton, Fla: CRC Press, 2013.

Merck M, ed. *Veterinary forensics: animal cruelty investigations*. 2nd ed. Ames, Iowa: John Wiley & Sons, 2013.

Warwick C, Frye FL, Murphy JB. *Health and welfare of captive reptiles*. London: Chapman and Hall, 1995.

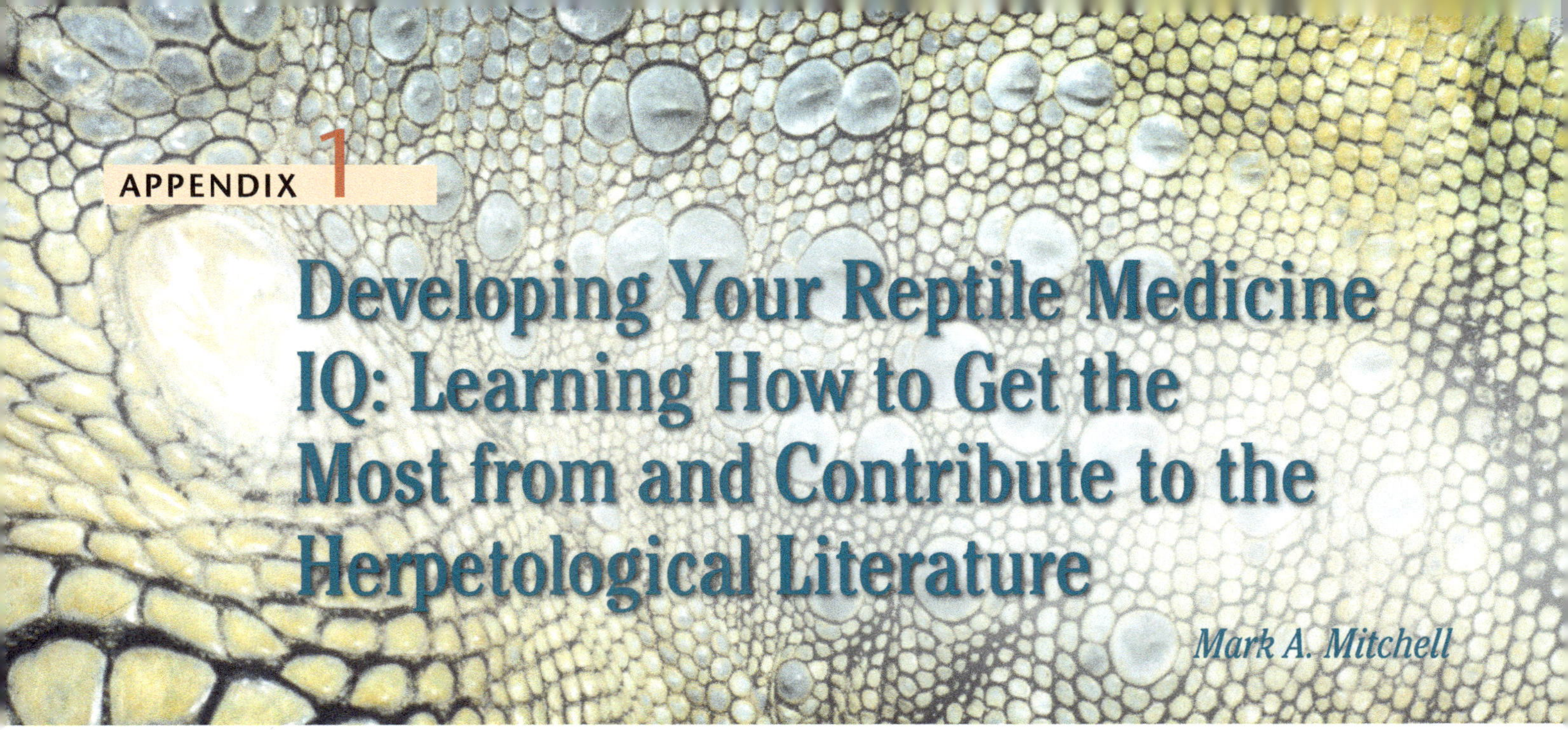

APPENDIX 1

Developing Your Reptile Medicine IQ: Learning How to Get the Most from and Contribute to the Herpetological Literature

Mark A. Mitchell

Veterinarians source knowledge in a number of different ways. As students, the majority of our knowledge is provided in the classroom. In Western civilization, students have become so reliant on this source of knowledge that they are less likely to pursue other resources (e.g., books or peer-reviewed literature). Certainly, the specialists (faculty) providing this knowledge have expertise in their fields, but the information being delivered is a subjective review of their own experiences. This type of knowledge sourcing is important, but it is only suitable earlier in our training as veterinary professionals. As we develop and begin careers in veterinary medicine, our ability to source knowledge changes. For many veterinary clinicians, their sources of knowledge come through continuing education presentations and books. Continuing education seminars, much like classroom teaching in veterinary school, are subjective. They represent a potentially good method of acquiring current, up-to-date knowledge regarding a field, but they remain a collection of the opinions and interpretations of the speaker. Books are also a relevant and quick source of knowledge, such as this text. However, they too are ultimately a collection of the authors' experiences and interpretations of the literature. Again, they represent an opportunity to obtain knowledge, but they have the potential for introducing the biases of the author. Additionally, by the time many books are published, the information provided is typically at least 1 to 2 years old. Ultimately, as we grow and develop as veterinarians, we need to rely on objective sources of knowledge. Although many of the previous examples rely on these types of information, the best opportunity we have for acquiring this type of information is to delve into the scientific literature itself. Peer-reviewed literature provides us our best opportunity to obtain objective data with minimal potential for misclassification bias. It is important to retain the caveat of *minimal* in such a description because even the peer-reviewed literature is not perfect. The primary limitations associated with this source of knowledge are related to the limitations of the reviewers and editorial staff. Not all of the individuals reviewing manuscripts are comfortable with the concepts of study design and statistical methods. If these things are not fully vetted at the review process, there is the potential for misclassification. This becomes important when we consider how we develop our knowledge. It can be likened to a foundation on a house. We hope to develop a solid foundation of knowledge based on objective, defendable information; however, it is possible that, through no fault of our own, we build a foundation with some weak supports. A number of reviewers for journals, as well as members of the editorial staff, may be uncomfortable with evaluating the statistical analysis used in a study. Unless a statistician is consulted, it is possible that flawed methods are being used to draw flawed conclusions. To minimize the likelihood for building a "weakened" knowledge base from which we rely on to manage our patients and clients, we need to become more self-reliant in our ability to objectively review the literature serving as our foundation of knowledge.

A typical peer-reviewed article is divided into four sections: Introduction, Materials and Methods, Results, and Discussion. There is certainly some degree of variability within this construct (e.g., separate Statistical Methods or Conclusion sections), but, for the most part, journals adhere to a format following this pattern. In the author's experience (subjective assessment), the majority of the peer reviewers of the journals for which he serves as editor (*Journal of Herpetological Medicine and Surgery* and *Journal of Exotic Pet Medicine*) and clinicians he trains are comfortable with reading and understanding the Introduction and Discussion sections of an article but are less confident in their ability to comprehend the statistical methods and thus the results. Likewise, many authors of peer-reviewed manuscripts are also not comfortable with these sections of their own works for the same reason. It is these types of limitations that can potentially introduce misclassification bias into the scientific literature and our own knowledge base. To minimize the potential for such a shortcoming, we need to develop some level of skill with interpreting these sections, along with the other components of the article. While it is beyond the scope of this article to provide a detailed review of statistics, it is possible to develop flow charts to show common patterns for interpreting whether data was handled correctly. It is important for veterinary clinicians to realize that becoming comfortable with statistics or study design comes with practice and experience; however, this should come

BOX A-1 TWELVE QUESTIONS USED TO DETERMINE THE VALUE OF A PEER-REVIEWED ARTICLE

What was the purpose of this study?
What were the objectives and hypotheses? Are they clearly defined?
Did the introduction satisfactorily present the research problem?
What type of study was used?
What type of data was collected?
Was the sample size sufficient?
Were the methods appropriate?
Was the statistical analysis correct?
Were the tables and graphs useful?
Were citations and references appropriate?
Were the conclusions correct?
What would you have changed about the study?

as no surprise to the readers of this text because many veterinarians working with reptiles and amphibians developed their skills using a basis of knowledge and practical experience acquired from nonherpetologic species (e.g., dogs, cats, and horses).

The purpose of this chapter is to provide the reader with a step-by-step approach for constructively analyzing a peer-reviewed article. The series of questions outlined in Box A-1 serve as the basis for this analysis. In addition to using these questions/methods for training veterinary professionals, the author also utilizes these methods for reviewing manuscripts for peer-reviewed journals. A secondary purpose of this chapter is to provide an outline for prospective veterinary clinicians to follow when conducting research. For the field of herpetologic medicine to develop, it will require clinicians to share the findings of their work. Historically, clinicians have contributed to the literature by publishing case reports; however, because there is a general lack of financial resources to study herpetologic medicine, it will require a grassroots effort from those in the field (or clinic) to generate scientific information to improve the way we practice medicine and surgery on these species. The information provided in this chapter can also be used by clinicians as a basis for formulating projects using data they collect at their own hospital.

QUESTION 1: WHAT WAS THE PURPOSE OF THE STUDY?

The purpose of a study should be clearly defined in the Introduction, providing the reader with an opportunity to determine a clear direction of the study. There are times when the Introduction does not appear to define a clear direction for the article; in these cases, it is important for the reader to understand that if the authors did not have a clear vision, the research itself might also be flawed. Being able to answer questions 2 and 3 will assist the reader in determining whether the author(s) have defined the direction of the research.

QUESTION 2: WHAT WERE THE OBJECTIVES AND HYPOTHESES? ARE THEY CLEARLY DEFINED?

Advancement in science occurs because researchers set objectives and hypotheses to answer specific questions of interest. Although it is generally expected that this approach is used in veterinary medicine, it is often difficult to discern the specific hypotheses being pursued by some authors because these directives are not clearly defined. Many articles do include objectives, but objectives are typically written as being less specific and more general in their direction. This generality can sometimes be seen in the limitations of the results, in that some authors only provide descriptive statistics or limited comparisons when more robust statistical methods could have been used. Additionally, in many examples, it appears that the hypotheses are generated after the research is completed and the data collected. In these cases, it is often difficult to answer certain hypotheses post-hoc. Whether graduate students are being taught or colleagues are consulting on a research study, the first question to ask regarding the research is, what are the hypotheses to be answered? By starting with specific hypotheses, it is possible to determine the type of study required to test the hypotheses, the sample size required for the study, and the statistical methods that will be required to complete the study. It is rare (<5%) for the specific hypotheses of research studies to be included in peer-reviewed articles in the exotic and zoologic medicine journals (Mitchell M: unpublished data Oct, 2012).

One of the more common reasons veterinary researchers misuse statistics is that they do not appear to have a solid grasp on their intended hypothesis(es). By specifically stating the hypothesis in the article,[1-6] it can be used as a guide for the reader to determine the direction of the study and evaluate the "correctness" of the methods. Remember, just because something is published does not mean it is correct. Studies have found a significant number of errors in published articles.[7] Although it is the intent of the peer-review process to catch and prevent the publication of incorrect information, it is ultimately a subjective review process. So what does this mean to the clinician trying to interpret the findings or place a value on the information provided in the article? It reinforces the importance of being able to understand the "methods" used for a study. If we can appreciate that a design is flawed, than we may be more cautious in how we use and apply the results from a particular study. If we do not, we are susceptible to building a foundation of knowledge with structural flaws.

For those developing research projects, it is best to define hypotheses based on some biologically relevant question. By starting with what is biologically (or clinically) relevant, it is easier to determine what type of data need to be collected and how they may be useful to the reader (or clinician). The hypothesis should define the outcome to be tested (dependent variable(s)) and any risk factors (independent variables). The number of hypotheses required will depend on how many different scientific questions the author hopes to answer. The primary limitation associated with the number of hypotheses that can be answered is associated with the size of the study population (sample size). When the sample size is small, the likelihood is increased for a Type II error (accepting a null hypothesis when it is false). To limit the likelihood for introducing error, researchers should focus on testing the most important question(s) with the sample size that is available (see Question 6: Was the sample size sufficient?).

QUESTION 3: DID THE INTRODUCTION SATISFACTORILY PRESENT THE RESEARCH PROBLEM?

The Introduction to an article should provide the reader with an overall review of the reason the research was done. Most Introductions comprise three paragraphs, although some are shorter (one to two paragraphs) and some are longer (more than three paragraphs).[8-13] Typically, the first paragraph (or section) of an Introduction will provide insight into the species or problem to be studied, the second paragraph (section) will indicate why there is need for the study, and the third paragraph (section) will outline the specific purpose or objectives of the study. This is also the point that the specific hypotheses to be tested should be introduced. Sufficient references to describe the material presented in the Introduction should be provided. It is important for the reader to evaluate the types of references used. In the herpetologic literature, many of the references are based on proceeding abstracts and book chapters. As stated earlier, while these references can certainly be invaluable, they are not rigorously peer reviewed. The date of the references should also be noted. It is important that citations include the original reference to a specific topic. It is not uncommon in the veterinary literature for a reference to cite the most recent report of a topic, rather than the original citation. When this occurs, there is the possibility for a loss of detail through the translation. The quality of an article can often be determined by the degree and/or extent that references are used.

QUESTION 4: WHAT TYPE OF STUDY WAS USED?

A number of different study types can be used to conduct research, from nonexperimental to experimental studies. It is important to recognize the different methods used to conduct these studies because the success of the research in each case is dependent on meeting the assumptions of the studies' inherent designs. For the individual reading the scientific literature, it is important to understand the various intricacies of each study type to ensure that the information being published is not biased by a flaw in the study design.

The most common types of studies used in clinical research are experimental or interventional studies. These types of studies typically are set up as true experimental studies and use preselected study subjects or are set up as clinical trials, in which patients presented to a practice are used as the study subjects. The former type of study is typically done in academia, and the latter is typically done at the clinic level. Clinical trials represent an excellent opportunity for practitioners to contribute to the scientific literature.

Experimental trials require the researcher/clinician to assign the exposure to the various study subjects. The *exposure* is typically defined as the independent risk factor being tested. Typically, one group is given a specific treatment or exposure, while another group serves as a control.[4,8,10,12,13] Although it is possible to evaluate multiple exposures in a study, it is best to limit them to minimize the potential for introducing error (e.g., Type II error). The primary limiting factor with this type of study, especially when multiple exposures are evaluated is sample size, which will be addressed later (see Question 6). An advantage of experimental studies is that the researcher/clinician also has control over selecting the study populations. Variability can be reduced by selecting animals on the basis of important biological characteristics such as species, sex, and age. Not controlling for these factors, especially with small sample sizes, can lead to erroneous conclusions. Individuals reading the literature should train themselves to look for these subtleties to ensure that they are not overinterpreting or underinterpreting the value of the published material. A primary disadvantage of clinical trials is related to the ethics of withholding treatment. It would be hard to explain to a client that their pet is not responding to a treatment because it was given a placebo. A common practice that can be done to eliminate this risk is to allow each animal to serve as its own control. Not only will this limit the possibility of causing an ethical dilemma in the design of the study but it will also reduce the sample size needed for a study because each animal serves as its own control (see Question 6). Another common shortcoming of these types of studies, especially in clinical trials, is the potential bias associated with the researchers interpretation of the results. Individuals designing studies—and those reading the literature—should be sure that some form of blinding is done in the trial. Although in veterinary medicine we are typically less concerned about placebo effects being introduced by our patients, the potential for them to be introduced by the client or researcher are possible. It is for this reason that studies should have some degree of blinding introduced (single or double blinding), in which the clinician evaluating the patient or the pathologist reading histopathologic slides is not familiar with the classification of the subjects. Another concern to be aware of is how a particular outcome is measured. It is best to limit the amount of subjective data being recorded. Subjective data (e.g., noncontrolled body condition scores, color of mucous membranes, or radiologist interpretations) allows each investigator an opportunity to provide their own interpretation of a particular measurement. It can be difficult to draw conclusions from such variable measures, especially when the sample size for the study is small. However, objective measures are also subject to variability, especially when different equipment is used. Unless studies are focused on validating results between equipment,[3] it is important for the study to use the same equipment across all study subjects to minimize the potential for introducing measurement bias. Finally, when clinical trials are performed, it is important to consider the potential influence of migration bias. When subjects are lost to follow-up, it can be difficult to determine what influence that loss can have on the end results. The literature may not describe or list this type of loss as "lost to follow-up." Again, it is often up to the individual reading the literature to tease out where these types of limitation may exist. Individuals planning studies and those reading the literature should consider the potential influence these types of potential biases can have on the end results of a study.

Nonexperimental studies are also commonly found in the herpetologic literature. Of these study types, cross-sectional and case-control studies are most common, whereas cohort studies are practically nonexistent because of the expense and time required for this type of study. Nonexperimental studies offer advantages over experimental studies because they can reduce the potential for ethical dilemmas (e.g., giving a placebo over a treatment) and study expense (e.g., cross-sectional and case-control studies can be done with the use of historical data). A primary disadvantage of these types of studies is that the researcher has less control over many of the variable being evaluated. For example, historical or retrospective case-control studies are limited to what may have been recorded in a patient's file. Cross-sectional studies represent those studies that take a snapshot in time of a population. Also termed *prevalence studies,* these are an excellent first attempt at evaluating certain risk factors (independent variables) against a specific outcome. Hematologic studies commonly use this type of study design to establish reference ranges for a particular species by sex, age, or some other independent factor.[1] Many clinicians with busy practices have the opportunity to characterize the prevalence of a disease in their patient population that could be used to explain a disease at a higher level (e.g., for all captive reptiles of that species within a country or elsewhere).[14] Similarly, these types of studies are also well-suited for characterizing disease status in wild populations of reptiles.[15-16] A disadvantage of cross-sectional studies is related to the fact that exposure and disease status are ascertained at the same time, which makes it impossible to determine when an exposure/disease occurred. Because of this, it is possible to overrepresent cases with a long duration of disease (e.g., serologic test results for diseases with a low mortality rate) and underreport cases with a short-term duration of illness (e.g., ranavirus infections: short duration, high mortality).[16-17] The limitations imposed by this study design can be overcome in the interpretation of the results. It is important for the reader and researcher not to overinterpret the results and assign a timeline when it is not possible. The case-control study is another nonexperimental study that can be quite useful in obtaining insight into associations between a dependent variable and variable risk factors. Most case-control studies are done from a historical or retrospective approach; therefore they are ideally suited for clinical practice. Whereas cohort studies are based on comparing different study populations by an exposure and waiting for an outcome to occur, case-control studies are based on knowing the outcomes associated with study populations and looking into which risk factors were different between the groups. An example of a study that could fit both study designs would be one that evaluated the likelihood of the development of secondary nutritional hyperparathyroidism (SNHP)(outcome variable) in a species of reptile based on the presence of vitamin D (independent variable/risk factor) in the diet/ultraviolet B light (UVB). A case-control study could be done by matching patients of that particular species with SNHP to those of the same species without SNHP. A comparison between the groups based on a number of descriptors could be done, with the presence or absence of vitamin D being the primary risk factor being assessed. It could be difficult to separate the presence or absence of vitamin D in some patients based on the level of detail obtained in the history, client knowledge regarding diets, longevity of the patient, loss to follow-up, or any other factors that can be lost through poor record keeping. If data were available, this type of study would require little expense short of time to review the records and analyze the data. A cohort study could also be done in a longitudinal fashion (over time) in which animals that are presented to a practice and that have a different risk toward vitamin D (presence/absence of UVB light and/or dietary forms) could be matched and followed up. A timeline would be established to determine the length of time the animals would be followed up to evaluate whether SNHP developed. Although this study type gives a researcher more control, it is more costly and timely; this is why these types of studies are rarely done in veterinary medicine and more commonly done in human medicine. All three of these examples of nonexperimental studies have advantages and disadvantages regarding their ability to provide reliable and accurate results related to a specific hypothesis(es), and the clinical researcher performing such a study or clinicians attempting to build their knowledge base from such material need to be aware of the potential pitfalls to avoid overinterpreting or underinterpreting the value of the research or publication.

QUESTION 5: WHAT TYPE OF DATA WAS COLLECTED?

There are three basic types of data a clinician can encounter: categorical, ordinal, and continuous. Categorical data are also commonly referred to as nominal data. This type of data is typically characterized as data that fit into "categories." Common examples of categorical data include data on seroprevalence (seropositive, seronegative), sex (male, female), and age by group and not year (juvenile, adult). Categorical data are straightforward and often the simplest type of data to collect. A limitation of this type of data is that it cannot be manipulated mathematically. Instead, this type of data is most often categorized as prevalence data and evaluated as proportions. An example of this can be found in a study that characterized the prevalence of *Salmonella* in Red-eared Slider (*Trachemys scripta elegans*) eggs and hatchlings before and after treating the eggs.[12] The outcome data in the study were reported as a prevalence per group and compared with the use of appropriate nonparametric statistics.

Ordinal data are ranked data that do not have uniform scales. These data are often misrepresented by mathematical manipulation. When something is characterized with the use of rank data, it is only possible for the data to fall into one of the designated categories. An example of this can be found in an article evaluating the clinical and cardiopulmonary effects of clove oil and propofol on Tiger Salamanders (*Ambystoma tigrinum*).[18] In the article, the various reflexes were coded with the use of an ordinal scale: 0, present; 1, slowed; 2, absent. With this type of data, each measurement could only be assigned a 0, 1, or 2. Some authors will determine means using ordinal data, but it is not appropriate. In the previously mentioned sample, a 1.2 or a 2.4 would have no meaning. While limitations remain with this type of data, it is possible to evaluate frequencies with ordinal measurements and nonparametric statistics.

The final type of data is interval or continuous data. This type of data has a known interval size and is measureable. The majority of the objective data we collect as clinicians falls into this category, including body weight, temperature, hematologic data (e.g., packed cell volume or white blood cell numbers), and biochemistry profiles, among others. Examples of this type of data are found in Mayer and colleagues[1] in reference to hematologic data from Crested Geckos (*Rhacodactylus ciliatus*). Continuous data are the one type of data that can be manipulated mathematically. This type of data is commonly reported with a measure of central tendency (e.g., mean and median) and a measure of variability (e.g., standard deviation [SD] and percentiles). Continuous data also allow for the most robust statistical comparisons, parametric statistics.

There are advantages and disadvantages to using each of these data types. As mentioned, categorical data are typically the easiest data type to collect but are limited regarding their potential for mathematical manipulation and statistical testing. Ordinal data, likewise, are limited as to what types of information they can provide but, in addition, are more limited by sample size than categorical data. Continuous data, being the most robust data type, are highly restricted by sample size. Continuous data with a high degree of variability (e.g., SD) from small study population can be very difficult to interpret and are often prone to Type II errors. Because of these limitations, both the researchers producing the science and clinicians reviewing the literature need to become comfortable with the inherent strengths and weaknesses associated with each type of data. Being aware of the limitations associated with the data will help minimize the risk that both the researchers and individuals reading the peer-reviewed literature will overinterpret the results, especially if they are misrepresented.

QUESTION 6: WAS THE SAMPLE SIZE SUFFICIENT?

Sample size is one of the primary reasons studies fail to accomplish their goal. Historically, sample sizes for studies would follow "apparently" acceptable numbers: n = 6, n = 12, n = ? Many Institutional Animal Care and Use Committees would allow researchers to use these types of numbers because they were used in previously published reports. Fortunately, this narrowed outlook is being replaced with an expectation that researchers can justify the number of study subjects they need to answer a specific hypothesis(es). The reason that sample size is important is related to the types of error that can occur if the study population in too small. There are two basic types of error that one should be concerned with regarding statistical comparisons: Type I errors and Type II errors. A Type I error is the probability of concluding that there is a significant difference between some comparison (reject the null hypothesis) when, indeed, there is no difference. Type I errors are typically not a major concern in most studies because the general probability (*P*) used for determining significance is <0.05 (i.e., there is a 5% chance or 1 in 20 chance of such an outcome occurring by chance alone). At some level this is a subjective approach, and most people use it because they are not comfortable moving away from it. As far as odds go, 0.05 is generally considered acceptable; however, there are times when the odds could be lower ($P < 0.01$) or higher ($P < 0.10$) and still be appropriate. The most likely situation for a Type I error exists when multiple comparisons are made with the use of the same data. An example might be if researchers analyzed herpesvirus status in a population of tortoises by comparing sex by herpes status, age by herpes status, and location (e.g., collection) of tortoises by herpes status. The animals in all three groups are represented in all three comparisons. If age really was an important determinant, but the study population from one location was much older than another, location may also appear significant. The likelihood of a Type I error can be minimized if a correction (e.g., Bonferroni) is applied. The Bonferroni correction reduces the *P* value. In the previous example with three independent groups (e.g., sex, age, and location), the new *P* value would be 0.016, so for anything to be significant the *P* value for the comparison would need to be less than 0.016.

The other type of error, Type II error, is the more important of the two errors. Type II error is the probability of concluding that no significant difference was found between some comparison (accept the null hypothesis) when, indeed, there is a difference. A Type II error is likely anytime $P > 0.05$ (if $P < 0.05$ is characterized as being the standard for significance). The reason that this is the more important of the two errors, in the author's opinion, is because it is more directly tied to sample size and the researcher has less direct control over it (e.g., Type I error can be controlled by altering *P* value, whereas Type II error requires larger sample sizes, which may be difficult to obtain for financial or logistic reasons). Because researchers may not be comfortable interpreting statistics and sample sizes in studies may be limited because of financial constraints and subject availability, there are times when Type II errors are unknowingly committed. The best way to determine whether a Type II error is possible is to evaluate the power associated with the comparison. *Power* is the probability of concluding that there is a difference between some comparison (reject null hypothesis) when there is one (e.g., opposite of Type II error). Power = 1 − β, where β is the false-negative rate (i.e., Type II error). The scale for power ranges from 0 to 100, where 100 is the highest power. A power value more than 0.80 is considered appropriate. Therefore, if a power analysis is performed, and it is more than 0.80 and $P > 0.05$, then it is just not likely that any difference between a comparison was likely to be significant. If power is less than 0.80 and $P > 0.05$, then the potential for a Type II error should be considered. To determine the risk for a Type II error, researchers should perform a power analysis. The author performs a post-hoc (after the statistical comparison is done) power analysis for any $P > 0.05$ and ≤ 0.10. This range is used because the *P* values approach 0.05, and the likelihood for Type II errors increase in these cases when sample sizes are small. Knowing and reporting that the power is low in these cases and explaining that a Type II error is possible provides some explanation as to why a difference did not exist when it possibly did exist but could not be determined because of a limited study sample size. The author believes that many authors erroneously conclude differences between comparisons do not exist when they do because of their discomfort moving away from $P < 0.05$. Veterinarians reading the peer-reviewed literature need to also become comfortable with what a *P* value represents. When *P* values are more than 0.05 but approach the value and the authors conclude "no significant difference" and nothing more, it is important to recognize that a difference may have existed and sample size may have played a role. Being aware of these types of issues will improve what clinicians gain from the literature and ensure a more solid foundation to their knowledge base.

A final note regarding a misconception about power relates to times when small sample sizes are used in a study but a significant difference exists (null hypothesis rejected). In Acierno and colleagues,[13] the total sample size of two groups of Red-eared Sliders was n = 12 (six in each group). The difference noted between 25-hydroxyvitamin D levels between the groups (one exposed to UVB light, the other not exposed to UVB light) was significant. A reviewer of the article asked whether the power and sample size were sufficient for the study. The simple answer was yes. In cases in which the null hypothesis is rejected ($P \leq 0.05$), the risk for a Type II error is nonexistent (Type I errors are a concern when the null hypothesis is rejected). Small sample sizes do not have to be a limiting factor; the difference between the groups being compared just needs to be large enough to be detectable. When data are highly variable, this can be difficult with small sample sizes. In the case of the aforementioned turtle study, the UVB-exposed turtles' 25-hydroxyvitamin D levels were all much higher than their conspecifics without UVB light.

The best way for a researcher to avoid the pitfalls associated with low sample size is to conduct an a priori estimate of a required sample size using baseline power (0.80) and alpha ($P = 0.05$) values for a comparison. With the advent of commercial statistical software, this can be done in minutes. A number of different software programs are capable of determining this estimate; however, the author has experience using MedCalc (Ostend, Belgium) and S-Plus (Palo Alto, Calif). When a sample size needed for a particular study is estimated, it is important to have some idea, a priori, of how large a difference is expected between two groups. In some cases, examples in the literature may help derive this information, whereas in others, it may only be possible to ask experts for opinions or derive a minimum expected difference. Regardless, this has the benefit of serving as a guide to estimating a sample size. Ultimately, the more precise and confident the researcher hopes to be with the end result, the larger the sample size needed to detect a desired difference. In cases in which sample size limitations exist because of financial or logistic reasons, a one-tailed approach versus a two-tailed approach can also be helpful when the null hypothesis is being characterized. A two-tailed directional hypothesis suggests that the outcome being compared between two groups could be higher or lower than the other, with no particular direction. A one-tailed directional hypothesis suggests that the researchers believe that one group will be directionally higher or lower (but not both) than the other group. The Red-eared Slider study is an excellent example of this. When the hypothesis was established, it was determined that a one-tailed directional hypothesis would be used: turtles in the UVB light group would have higher 25-hydroxyvitamin D values then non–UVB-exposed turtles. This was selected because the researchers wanted to confirm an expected hypothesis (that UVB light was important to this species) using a pilot study with a limited sample size. Because a one-tailed directional hypothesis was used, it was easier to confirm a difference if one indeed existed. The peer-reviewed literature would benefit greatly from all authors performing a priori sample size estimation. In addition to determining the feasibility of the research (e.g., whether an expected difference could be detected based on the number of study subjects and finances available), it would also prove useful in post-hoc analysis in ruling out Type II errors and thus the potential likelihood of misrepresenting a study's conclusions. In the case of studies comparing two populations (e.g., an experimental study comparing different egg washing treatments against *Salmonella* in turtle eggs and hatchlings), the a priori information needed would be the baseline power (0.80), alpha ($P = 0.05$), and the expected prevalences between the treatment groups. If, for example, an egg wash was expected to reduce the prevalence of *Salmonella* in eggs from a finding in untreated eggs (40% *Salmonella* positive) to less than 10%, the sample size required for the study would be 29 eggs treated in each group. Likewise, if a study was being done with continuous data, the sample size could be determined with the same power and alpha values and the expected difference between the two comparison groups and their expected SD. In the turtle UVB example, an expected difference of 25-hydroxyvitamin D levels could be 30 nmol/L and an expected SD for each group could be 17.5 nmol/L. The sample size required for such a comparison was 12 (six animals in each group). The author is careful to read whether a priori information regarding sample size is provided in the peer-reviewed literature. Seeing this type of forethought suggests that the researchers considered their hypotheses carefully. When this information is not provided, it is important to look closely at the Results and Discussion to determine whether any shortcomings in the conclusions are the direct result of a mistake in study design or whether the finding(s) was/were appropriate.

QUESTION 7: WERE THE METHODS APPROPRIATE?

Regardless of the study type, selection of the study subjects should be done with the use of some random selection criteria. Many studies report simply that the study subjects were "randomly" assigned, but no specifics are given as to how it was done. Not randomly allocating the subjects before starting a study can lead to misclassification bias, which will weaken the overall value of the results. A variety of methods can be used for randomly allocating study subjects. The simplest methods involve a coin flip or pulling numbers from a hat. More advanced methods include computer-generated numbers or random numbers tables. Because methods for randomizing subject distribution are readily available on the Internet (e.g., http://stattrek.com/Tables/Random.aspx), there is no reason they cannot commonly be used in herpetologic research. There are cases where randomly assigning subjects requires several important considerations (e.g., treatment group, age, sex). In these cases, a stratified randomization technique can be used. This method focuses on allocating subjects by the criteria of primary interest (e.g., exposure to a treatment or not) and then allocating based on other factors (e.g., age or sex). Veterinarians that are reading the literature and trying to interpret the results should consider whether the authors of a particular article identify the methods for subject allocation. Not randomly assigning the subjects can lead to assembly bias that may or may not be apparent in the published document. In these cases, this author is careful not to overinterpret the conclusions.

The type of test performed is another aspect of the methods section that should be examined. It is not uncommon for the methods section to be superficially reviewed because of an individual's inexperience with a specific testing method or field. Examples of this include molecular work and pathology. It is important for clinicians to become familiar with the scientific methods used to derive the results in an article, lest they accept what is written as truth and miss it being incorrect. This is especially important when the methods do not provide specific details. In some cases, references to a commercial laboratory or previously published article will be used to defend a set of methods. Each assay that is performed has a sensitivity and specificity associated with it. These test characteristics can vary in the same assay based on the laboratory performing them, which can have a significant impact on the end results. Additionally, differences in how a certain assay is performed can also cause dramatically different results. In Allender and colleagues,[19] serum samples from 26 Massasaugas (*Sistrurus catenatus*) were submitted to three different laboratories that used hemagglutination inhibition (HI) assays to screen for paramyxovirus. The test results among the three laboratories were very different: one laboratory reported 0% prevalence, another 100% prevalence, and yet another 56% prevalence. The assays did use different viral isolates; however, most clinicians submit their tests to laboratories without considering the influence of such a finding. Additionally, because sensitivity and specificity testing had not been done on the tests, it was not possible to interpret the "correctness" of each test. The discrepancy among the laboratories implies that the outcome for a case could be dramatically different depending on where the HI assay was run. In the herpetologic medicine peer-reviewed literature, very few articles evaluate agreement between different diagnostic tests and few articles describe the sensitivity and specificity of different assays; therefore clinicians using the peer-reviewed literature need to be sure they understand the methods being reported. If they are unfamiliar with them, it would behoove them to peruse the literature (specifically on the type of methods used) to determine their validity. If not, it is possible that clinical decisions to cull animals or allow them through quarantine could be incorrect.

QUESTION 8: WAS THE STATISTICAL ANALYSIS CORRECT?

Statistics. The mere mention of this word can make the most confident clinician cower. This should not be the case, but it is human nature to fear what we do not understand. As reptile and amphibian veterinarians, we should actually be well-suited to face this fear. We routinely help those in our community face their fears as they relate to species with which we work. Likewise, performing chi-square tests or odds ratios does not require much more than a basic understanding of arithmetic. We fear the unknown. If we learn how important statistics are to understanding the science we use to practice medicine, they become less of an unknown.

Clinicians can become comfortable with statistics once they put them in perspective. Statistics are to research what a diagnostic test (e.g., white blood cell count) is to a clinical case. Biostatisticians use statistics to rule in/rule out a hypothesis in the same fashion veterinarians use a diagnostic test to rule in/rule out a disease. As clinicians, we learn to apply certain diagnostic tests under certain conditions, and the same is done for statistics in research.

Because entire texts are dedicated to statistics, it is beyond the scope of this chapter to go into too much detail. However, the intent of this chapter is not to make the reader a competent biostatistician but more competent when reading the peer-reviewed literature. Knowing how to look for trends in the presentation of data, similar to looking for trends in the diagnostic approach in a case report, will provide a clinician with the skills to determine whether the statistical methods are being used in an appropriate manner.

Question 5 asked the question, "What type of data was collected?" This is the first step in directing the reader to the types of statistics that should be used to analyze data. Although the analysis of data can be complex, most of the statistics required for clinical research follows straightforward trends. Additionally, although several statistical tests can often be applied to make the same comparison, single, common examples can be used for simplification of the process. The two common types of statistics used are parametric and nonparametric. The primary difference between these two methods relates to the distribution of the data. Parametric statistics require that the data meet the assumption of normality (follow a Gaussian distribution). Nonparametric tests do not have the same assumption. When the three data types—continuous, ordinal, and categorical—are examined, only continuous data can meet the assumption of normality. Therefore (1) data that are categorical or ordinal should be analyzed with nonparametric statistics. For continuous data to be analyzed with parametric methods, it must meet the assumption of normality. (2) The authors should clarify whether the distribution of the data was analyzed for normality. The most common ways to assess normality include specific tests of normality (e.g., Shapiro-Wilk test or Kolmogorov-Smirnov test) or examination of the distribution of the data with other methods such as skewness, kurtosis, and normality plots.[1,6,8-10] Continuous data that do not meet the assumption of normality should be analyzed with nonparametric tests or should be transformed (e.g., log transformed) to meet the assumption of normality. If the authors do not clarify these types of information, it could mean that there are flaws in the results. Reporting of the results should also be considered in these cases. The measure of central tendency gives the reader an idea of where the data cluster around the central value. The three primary measures of central tendency are the mean (weighted average), median (middle value), and mode (most frequent value). When data are normally distributed, all three are similar. When data are not normally distributed, the median is the best representative of the central tendency. It is not uncommon for the mean to be reported regardless of distribution, and this is not, in this author's opinion, the best approach. Clinicians attempting to characterize a central tendency using skewed (not normal) data may find it difficult when relating the results to their own patients. Likewise, variability in data is often misrepresented. The SD describes dispersion around the mean. Data that are not normally distributed can have large SDs, and these large SDs can make it very difficult to relate to real-world cases. In cases in which data are not normally distributed, a better representation of central tendency is median and percentiles (e.g., 10% to 90% or 25% to 75%; these explain where 80% or 50% of the data lie, respectively). To truly maximize the value of the literature, clinicians should become comfortable in identifying the most appropriate methods for characterizing these types of descriptive statistics. Not only will it provide better relevance outside of the study population but it will also provide insight into the understanding of the methods and techniques used by the authors to either reaffirm or give pause to their results and conclusions.

The next step in assessing the statistics relates to the number of dependent variables and independent variables being tested.

For simplicity, this discussion is divided into two groups: one dependent variable or two or more dependent variables. Tables A-1 and A-2 give examples of common statistical tests used to analyze data with one dependent variable and two or more dependent variables by the different data types, respectively. Using these tables as a flow chart to determine whether statistics were evaluated correctly is an excellent first step. Another component of statistics not covered in the tables includes those cases in which multiple independent variables are evaluated simultaneously against a dependent variable. When two independent variables are present and the dependent variable is continuous and normally distributed, a two-way analysis of variance can be used. When two or more variables are present, regression analysis can be used. The type of regression analysis is based on the data type of the dependent variable: categorical, logistic regression; ordinal, ordinal regression; continuous, linear regression. Although the previous statistical methods focus on comparisons looking at association, there are also statistics used for correlation and agreement. Examples of statistics looking at correlation include Pearson's correlation coefficient (parametric data) and Spearman's rank correlation coefficient (nonparametric data), whereas kappa (categorical data), weighted kappa (ordinal data), and Bland-Altman plots (continuous data) are routinely used for agreement analysis. Clinicians who can associate these statistical tests with the data types will be better prepared to interpret the "correctness" of the statistical methods used to conduct a study.

QUESTION 9: WERE THE TABLES AND GRAPHS USEFUL?

Tables and graphs are routinely used to provide a visual aid in displaying data. For individuals preparing manuscripts, tables and graphs can be an excellent way to provide a synopsis of data without using a great deal of print. The author prefers tables over graphs in most cases because looking at the absolute numbers (data) provides a better gauge of the results; others may prefer graphs because they remove the numbers and are more "visually appealing." Regardless of preference, graphs can also be useful in showing visual trends.

QUESTION 10: WERE CITATIONS AND REFERENCES APPROPRIATE?

This is a highly relevant question relating to the herpetologic medicine literature. Although it is preferred that references for an article are derived from peer-reviewed literature, a majority of the references found in the herpetologic medicine peer-reviewed literature are from proceedings and book chapters. This tends to reduce the overall impact and strength associated with the field. Using non–peer-reviewed sources potentially introduces a greater degree of subjectivity into the outcome. Clinicians should become familiar with the literature so that they are aware of whether references used to defend a study are current and are the best standard for drawing the conclusions that are made. In a number of cases, peer-reviewed literature may not be available to reference for a particular subject, which leaves the authors to draw their conclusions using non–peer-reviewed materials.

QUESTION 11: WERE THE CONCLUSIONS CORRECT?

By answering questions 1 to 10, one should be able to determine whether the conclusions reported in a peer-reviewed article are valid. If questions cannot be answered (e.g., no obvious hypotheses; data distribution not evaluated; statistical comparisons not made, only descriptive statistics given), it is important to consider how these limitations might affect the conclusions drawn by the authors. As mentioned earlier in this chapter, veterinarians rely on the peer-reviewed literature to develop and build their knowledge. If our knowledge is restricted to only what we read and we do not recognize what is incorrect or incomplete, it can affect our clinical skills and, ultimately, the success we have with our patients.

TABLE A-1

Different Types of Statistical Tests Used for a Single Dependent Variable

No. of Independent Variables	Data Type: Categorical	Data Type: Ordinal	Data Type: Continuous
0	Binomial test	Wilcoxon signed rank test	One-sample *t* test
1	Fisher exact test/Chi-square test	Mann-Whitney test	Independent samples *t* test
≥2	R × C Chi-square test	Kruskal-Wallis analysis of variance	Analysis of variance

TABLE A-2

Different Types of Statistical Tests for Two or More Dependent Variables

No. of Dependent Variables	Data Type: Categorical	Data Type: Ordinal	Data Type: Continuous
2	McNemar test	Wilcoxon paired rank test	Paired sample *t* test
>2	Cochran *Q* test	Friedman test for repeated measures	Repeated measures analysis of variance

QUESTION 12: WHAT WOULD YOU HAVE CHANGED ABOUT THE STUDY?

This is a question every individual reading a peer-reviewed article should consider. For those who also conduct research or publish clinical reports, it gives insight into how they may better prepare their own work in the future. Considering this question also helps to open the reader's mind to many of the potential pitfalls discussed throughout this chapter. We are much more apt to note shortcomings in a study as we train ourselves to see how things could be different.

CONCLUSION

As veterinarians progress through their careers from their veterinary education through practice, their reliance on different sources of knowledge changes. Veterinary clinicians need to recognize the importance of using the peer-reviewed literature as a primary source of information. Although wading through the literature can seem daunting, it is hoped that the questions and information outlined in this chapter can serve as a guide for assisting the clinician in identifying what is important and how to avoid potential pitfalls when reading the literature.

REFERENCES

1. Mayer J, Knoll J, Wrubel K, et al. Characterizing the hematologic and plasma chemistry profiles of captive crested geckos (*Rhacodactylus ciliatus*). *J Herpetol Med Surg* 2012;21:68-75.
2. Labelle AL, Whittington JK, Breaux CB, et al. Clinical utility of a complete diagnostic protocol for the ocular evaluation of free-living raptors. *Vet Ophthalmol* 2012;15:5-17.
3. Burdick SB, Mitchell MA, Neil J, et al. Evaluation of two-point of care meters and a portable chemistry analyzer for measurement of blood glucose concentrations in juvenile white-tailed deer (*Odocoileus virginianus*). *J Am Vet Med Assoc* 2012;240:596-599.
4. Walden M, Mitchell MA. Evaluation of three treatment modalities against *Isospora amphiboluri* in inland bearded dragons (*Pogona vitticeps*). *J Exot Pet Med* 2012;21:213-218.
5. Redavid LA, Sharp CR, Mitchell MA, et al. Plasma lactate measurements in healthy cats. *J Vet Pharmacol Ther* 2012;22:580-587.
6. Stewart K, Mitchell MA, Norton T, et al. Measuring the level of agreement in hematologic and biochemical values between blood sampling sites in leatherback sea turtles (*Dermochelys coriacea*). *J Zoo Wildl Med* 2012;43:719-725.
7. Seigel D. Clinical trials, epidemiology, and public confidence. *Stat Med* 2003;22:3419-3425.
8. McFadden M, Bennett A, Mitchell MA. Evaluation of the histologic reactions to commonly used suture materials in the skin and musculature of ball pythons (*Python regius*). *Am J Vet Res* 2011;72:1397-1406.
9. Wojick KB, Langan JN, Mitchell MA. Evaluation of MS-222 (tricaine methanesulfonate) and propofol as anesthetic agents in Sonoran desert toads (*Bufo alvarius*). *J Herpetol Med Surg* 2011;20:79-83.
10. Acierno M, Mitchell MA, Roundtree M, et al. Effects of ultraviolet radiation on plasma 25-hydroxyvitamin D concentrations in corn snakes (*Elaphe guttata guttata*). *Am J Vet Res* 2008;69:294-297.
11. Vitousek M, Mitchell MA, Woakes AJ, et al. High costs of female choice in a lekking lizard. *PLoS One* 2007;57:140-146.
12. Mitchell MA, Adamson T, Singleton B, et al. Evaluation of a combination of sodium hypochlorite and polyhexamethylene biguanide as an egg wash for red-eared slider turtles (*Trachemys scripta elegans*) to suppress or eliminate *Salmonella* organisms on egg surfaces and in hatchlings. *Am J Vet Res* 2007;68:158-164.
13. Acierno M, Mitchell MA, Roundtree M, et al. Evaluating the effect of ultraviolet B radiation on 1,25 hydroxyvitamin D levels in red-eared sliders (*Trachemys scripta elegans*). *Am J Vet Res* 2006;67:2046-2049.
14. Kim DY, Mitchell MA, Bauer R. An outbreak of adenoviral infection in inland bearded dragons (*Pogona vitticeps*) coinfected with dependovirus and coccidial protozoa (*Isospora* sp.) *J Vet Diagn Invest* 2002;14:332-334.
15. Allender M, Mitchell MA, Phillips C, et al. Hematologic and biochemical ranges and selected viral titers in wild-caught Eastern Massasauga Rattlesnakes (*Sistrurus catenatus catenatus*). *J Wild Dis* 2006;42:107-114.
16. Wolf T, Mitchell MA, Roy A, et al. Seroprevalence of alphaviruses in chelonians from southeastern Louisiana. *J Herpetol Med Surg* 2009;18:5-8.
17. Allender MC, Mitchell MA, Torres T, et al.. Pathogenicity of frog virus 3-like virus in red-eared slider turtles (*Trachemys scripta elegans*) at two environmental temperatures. *J Comp Pathol* 2013;doi: 10.1016/j.jcpa.2013.01.007 [Epub ahead of print].
18. Mitchell MA, Riggs S, Singleton CB, et al. Evaluating the clinical and cardiopulmonary effects of clove oil and propofol on tiger salamanders (*Ambystoma tigrinum*). *J Exot Pet Med* 2009;18:50-56.
19. Allender MC, Mitchell MA, Dreslik MJ, et al. Measuring agreement and discord among hemagglutination inhibition assays against different ophidian paramyxovirus strains in Eastern massasauga (*Sistrurus catenatus catenatus*). *J Zoo Wildl Med* 2008;29:358-361.

APPENDIX 2

Reptile Viruses

Rachel E. Marschang and
Stephen J. Divers

POXVIRUSES

General characteristics:

DNA virus; large brick-shaped, enveloped virions up to 400 nm
Replicates in cytoplasm; hence ICIB
Very stable outside host; can remain infectious for years in organic debris
Horizontal transmission from environment or direct contact; many require damage to epithelium to invade host
Incubation in reptiles unknown; persistent infections postulated in crocodilians
In general, uninfected papules heal without scarring unless secondary infection
Treatment and control: debridement and wound cleansing, topical and, if warranted, systemic antimicrobials, supportive care (fluids, nutritional support, temperature), strict isolation, good hygiene, reduce stress (e.g., overcrowding), improve husbandry and nutrition
Autogenous vaccination in crocodiles
Resistant to many disinfectants; KOH, steam, NaOH, phenols likely to be effective
Standard quarantine procedures

Virus	Species	Clinical Signs	Pathology	Specific Diagnosis	Comments
Caiman poxvirus	Spectacled Caiman	1-3 mm gray-white papular skin lesions over entire body but especially on head; may coalesce to form patches	Edematous dermatitis, mononuclear cellular infiltrates and large eosinophilic ICIB in hypertrophied epithelial cells	Histopathology, EM	
Crocodile poxvirus	Nile Crocodiles, Saltwater Crocodiles, Freshwater Crocodiles	Especially in juveniles; 2-8 mm yellow-brown proliferative, diffuse skin lesions, especially around eyes (can cause blindness), nostrils, mouth, ventral neck and body, limbs and tail base; 2-5 mm brown blotches on gums and tongue	Multifocal hyperkeratosis, parakeratosis, large eosin ICIB	Histopathology, EM, PCR	Stress and poor water quality considered predisposing factors in outbreaks
Tegu poxvirus	Golden Tegu	Brown papular dermatitis	Eosin ICIB of epithelial cells	Histopathology, EM	Spontaneously resolved in 3-4 mo
Chameleon poxvirus	Flap-necked Chameleons	None	ICIB within monocytes and macrophages in spleen and liver	Histopathology, EM	Chlamydophila inclusions also identified
Tortoise poxvirus	Hermann's Tortoise	Papular skin lesions around the eyes		Histopathology, EM	

IRIDOVIRUSES

General characteristics:

DNA virus, 120-300 nm, icosahedra, may be enveloped
Replicates in cytoplasm , hence mostly ICIB
Viruses very likely can cross taxonomic divides
Very stable outside host; can remain infectious for months in water or organic debris
Treatment and control: supportive care (antimicrobials, fluids, nutritional support, temperature), strict isolation, good hygiene, reduce stress (e.g., overcrowding), improve husbandry and nutrition. Do not mix species! Infected animals may be a danger for other reptiles, amphibians, and fish.
Standard quarantine procedures

Virus	Species	Clinical Signs	Pathology	Specific Diagnosis	Comments
Ranavirus	Many different species; chelonians most commonly affected, including Hermann's Tortoises, Spur-thighed Tortoises, Gopher Tortoises, Box Turtles, Soft-shelled Turtles, Burmese Star Tortoises, Russian Tortoises, Red-eared Sliders, Egyptian Tortoises, Marginated Tortoises; Squamates also affected, including Green Pythons, Leaf-tailed Gecko, and Mountain Lizard	Either no signs before death or stomatitis, upper respiratory tract disease, rhinitis, conjunctivitis, tracheitis, respiratory distress, anorexia, lethargy, moribund, "red-neck disease," nasal discharge	Hepatitis, tracheitis, pneumonia, vasculitis, basophilic ICIBs sometimes described, granulomatous lesions frequently described	Virus isolation, PCR	Infections caused by various ranaviruses, some closely related to frog virus 3; ranaviruses appear to be very species-unspecific and may be able to switch hosts between animal classes, including reptiles, amphibians, and fish
Erythrocytic necrosis viruses	Many different squamate species, including free-ranging snakes and lizards	Ranging from no clinical signs to anemia and death	ICIBs in peripheral RBCs	EM	Undetermined clinical importance; a transmission study showed that infection in lacertid lizards kept at suboptimal temperatures could become systemic and lead to death
Invertebrate iridoviruses (IIV)	Usually infect many different species of insects, including some commonly fed to reptiles (e.g., crickets); have also been detected in various lizard species, including chameleons, Bearded Dragons, Frilled Lizard, and Green Iguana	Ranging from no clinical signs to skin lesions, cachexia, and death	None described	Virus isolation, PCR	Clinical significance of IIV infection in reptiles unknown; postulated infection from infected prey insects

HERPESVIRUSES

General characteristics:

Enveloped and pleomorphic, 100-200 nm
Nuclear replication; hence INIB
Cause latent infections
Horizontal transmission by direct contact: oculonasal and respiratory secretions, saliva, and feces
Commonly affect the gastrointestinal tract, respiratory tract, eye, and integument; secondary bacterial or mycotic infections common
Treatment and control: supportive care (broad spectrum antimicrobials, fluids, nutritional support, temperature, lesion debridement, nebulization), acyclovir, strict isolation, improve hygiene (sensitive to common disinfectants, such as sodium hypochlorite), reduce stress (e.g., overcrowding), improve husbandry and nutrition
Quarantine: 3-6 mo, VN/ELISA, PCR at beginning and end of quarantine
Any reptile infected with herpesvirus should be considered latently infected

Virus	Species	Clinical Signs	Pathology	Specific Diagnosis	Comments
Herpesviruses of Chelonians					
Herpesvirus of freshwater turtles	Pacific Pond Turtle, Painted Turtle, Map Turtle	Lethargy, anorexia, muscular weakness, edema	Ecchymotic hemorrhages on limbs, neck, plastron; limb and pulmonary edema; hepatomegaly and hepatic necrosis; splenic hypertrophy	INIB in liver, spleen, lung, kidney, and pancreas; EM	Antimicrobials to control secondary infections, acyclovir
Herpesvirus of tortoises	At least four different herpesviruses (TeHV1-4) found in different species of Testudinidae	Oculonasal discharge, regurgitation, anorexia, lethargy, rhinitis, stomatitis, dyspnea, conjunctivitis, pharyngitis, glossitis, pneumonia, ataxia, and lymphoproliferative diseases	Ulcerative, necrotizing, hyperplastic lesions of the oropharynx, GI and respiratory tracts, serous atrophy of fat, hepatic fatty degeneration, CNS involvement if severe	Large eosinophilic INIB in liver, spleen, lung, kidney, brain, GI tract; EM; ELISA; VN; PCR; virus isolation	Mortality up to 100%; antimicrobials to control secondary infections; acyclovir therapy; immunomodulators (e.g., Zylexis)
Gray-patch disease	Captive-bred/reared Green Sea Turtles, 56 days to 1 year old	Epizootics of small circular papular skin lesions, coalesce into patches, then ulcerate	Ulcerative/necrotizing lesions	Basophilic INIB in epidermal cells; EM; PCR	Predisposed by overcrowding and elevated temperatures; mortality 5% to 10% in severely affected individuals; acyclovir may be useful; outbreaks concentrate in January through August; disease experimentally reproduced
Lung, eye, trachea disease (LETD)	Green Sea Turtles older than 1 yr	Harsh respiratory sounds; ulcerations/caseous debris over globe, oropharynx, and trachea; buoyancy problems; develop over 2-3 wks	Keratitis, conjunctivitis, periglottal necrosis with mixed inflammatory infiltrate, necrotizing/caseous tracheitis, severe bronchopneumonia, multifocal white nodules on liver	Amorphous INIB in epithelial cells of trachea and lung; EM; PCR; virus isolation	High mortality over weeks or months; disease experimentally reproduced; virus survives for up to 120 h in seawater
Fibropapillomatosis	Free-ranging Green Sea Turtles; Pacific Ridley, Olive Ridley, Hawksbill, and Loggerhead rarely	Papillomatous tumors, gray to black, 2-20 cm, focal/multifocal, head, limbs, tail, plastron, carapace, cornea.; internal papillomas affecting kidney, liver, GI tract, lung; cachexia of free-ranging turtles	Fibropapillomas: marked hyperplasia of epidermis, vacuolation of cytoplasm, and ballooning degeneration of epidermal cells, proliferating fibroblasts in dermis	Eosinophilic INIB in fibropapilloma lesions; EM; PCR	Wide surgical removal of external lesions (internal lesions have poor prognosis); theorized causes are infection (herpesvirus) and environmental factors; disease experimentally reproduced; possible transmission by *Ozobranchus* leech (mechanical vector)

Loggerhead genital-respiratory HV (LGRV)	Free-ranging Loggerhead Sea Turtles	Ulcers in the trachea, around the cloaca, and on the base of the phallus	Epithelial hyperplasia, ballooning degeneration, INIB in epithelial cells, especially at the margins of ulcers	PCR	
Loggerhead orocutaneous HV (LOCV)	Free-ranging Loggerhead Sea Turtles	Ulcers and cutaneous plaques in the oral cavity	Epithelial hyperplasia, ballooning degeneration, INIB in epithelial cells, especially at the margins of ulcers	PCR	
Herpesviruses of Squamates					
Herpesvirus of boa constrictors	Two neonate Boa Constrictors	Clutch of 16, 9 stillborn, 6 died before 1 yr, 1 survived	Fatty degeneration of liver, multifocal hepatic and splenic necrosis, exudative glomerulonephritis	Amphophilic INIB in liver; EM	
Venom gland herpesvirus infection of elapids and viperids	Indian Cobra, Banded Krait, Siamese Cobra, Mojave Rattlesnake	Thick tenacious venom, swollen venom glands	Multifocal necrosis of columnar glandular epithelium, mixed inflammatory infiltration	INIB in venom and venom gland	
Iguana herpesvirus 1	Green Iguana	Subclinical anorexia, lethargy, brilliant green coloration, lymphocytosis, spontaneous hemorrhage	Lymphocytosis, splenomegaly; histiocytic infiltrates of liver, spleen, myocardium, and bone marrow	INIB; EM	Clinical signs of disease experimentally reproduced
Iguana herpesvirus 2	San Esteban Chuckwallas	Fibrotic gingival hyperplasia, death	Hemorrhagic and congested lungs, pale necrotic liver, necrotic spleen, empty GI tract	INIB in liver; PCR	
Herpesvirus of agamas	Agamas	None; died within 6 mo of capture	Hepatic and splenic necrosis, exudative pneumonia	INIB in liver and lung	
European green lizard herpesvirus	European Green Lizards	Cutaneous papillomas associated with bites from mating	Characteristic papillomatous lesions	INIB in papillomas	Also in conjunction with "papovavirus" and reovirus
Gerrhosaurid herpesviruses 1-3	Sudan Plated Lizards; Black-lined Plated Lizards	Stomatitis, dyspnea	Labial and periglottal stomatitis	INIB in oral epithelium; PCR	
Varanid HV 1	Green Tree Monitors	Proliferative stomatitis	Chronic proliferative gingivitis	PCR	
Herpesviruses of Crocodilians					
Herpesvirus of saltwater crocodiles	Saltwater Crocodiles	Crust on the abdominal skin	Degeneration of superficial keratinocytes, INIB in epithelial cells under and around the crust	EM	Poxvirus infection, biting and crowding also present in the group; evidence of herpesvirus infection found in only one animal of a group
Herpesvirus of alligators	American Alligators	Red nodules and petechial hemorrhages on cloacal mucosa	Lymphoid follicular aggregates (no INIB observed)	PCR	Etiology unclear because of lack of typical histologic changes in affected tissues

ADENOVIRUSES

General characteristics:

Nonenveloped, 70-90 nm
Nuclear replication; hence basophilic INIB
Usually host-adapted, causing few pathologic signs but causing disease in young; in adults, infections can become clinical with concomitant disease/stress
Commonly affect the GI and respiratory tract, liver, kidney, CNS; often asymptomatic
Disease rare in animals with functional immune system; concurrent bacterial, fungal, viral, or parasitic infections common
Horizontal and vertical transmission, generally by fecal–oral route
Treatment and control: supportive care (broad-spectrum antimicrobials, fluids, nutritional support, temperature), strict isolation, improve hygiene (removal of feces, persists in environment), treat underlying disease, reduce stress (e.g., overcrowding), improve husbandry and nutrition
Formalin, aldehyde, and iodophor disinfectants are effective
Quarantine: 6 months, strict hygiene (remove feces), PCR detection

Virus	Species	Clinical Signs	Pathology	Specific Diagnosis	Comments
Nile crocodile adenovirus	Nile Crocodiles	Underweight, no signs before death	Necrotizing enteritis, hepatic necrosis, congestion of lung, intestine, and kidney	Basophilic INIB in hepatocytes and crypt epithelial cells; EM	Diseases occurred in two animals in Zimbabwe
Agamid AdV	Bearded Dragons, Rankin Dragons	Ranging from none to failure to thrive, anorexia, paresis, coelomic distension, depression, lethargy	Subcutaneous, coelomic, intestinal, and perirenal petechial to ecchymotic hemorrhages; enlarged yellow mottled liver with necrosis and vacuolar hepatic lipidosis; interstitial, peritubular nephritis and tubular lipidosis; pancreatitis, and lung congestion	Basophilic INIB in liver, kidney, intestine, pancreas, bile ducts; EM; PCR	Concurrent coccidia and microsporidia; coinfection with other viruses, including dependovirus, IIV, reovirus, and ferlavirus
Varanid AdV	Water Monitors, Savannah Monitors	No signs, death	Hepatitis, proliferation of mucosal epithelial cells	Basophilic INIB in liver; EM; PCR	
Chameleonid AdV	Mountain Chameleon, Jackson's Chameleon, Veiled Chameleon	None to anorexia, tracheitis, esophagitis, opisthotonus, death in less than 3 days	Enteritis, tracheitis, esophagitis, mononuclear infiltrate	Basophilic INIB in epithelial cells of trachea, esophagus, enterocytes; EM; PCR	Mountain Chameleon was wild caught and strictly quarantined, so natural infections can occur
Helodermatid AdV 1 and 2	Mexican Beaded Lizards and Gila Monsters (also other lizard species)	Death of several animals	Not done	PCR, virus isolation (IgH-2)	
Eublepharid AdV	Fat-tailed Geckos, Leopard Geckos	Wasting, death	Enteritis, pancreatitis, INIB in intestine and pancreas	PCR	
Gekkonid AdV	Tokay Gecko	Weight loss, regurgitation	Not done	PCR	
Scincid AdV	Blue tongued Skink	Asymptomatic neonate	Not done	PCR	
Siadenovirus of chelonians	Sulawesi Tortoises, Impressed Tortoises, Burmese Star Tortoises	Anorexia, lethargy, mucosal ulcerations, nasal and ocular discharge, diarrhea, death	Enterocolitis, INIB in enterocytes	EM, PCR	Coinfection with amoeba, bacteria; high mortality rate

Leopard tortoise AdV	Leopard Tortoise	Biliverdinuria, wasting, episodes of hemorrhage	Not done	EM	Coinfection with a herpesvirus
Box turtle AdV	Box Turtle	Death	Degeneration of liver cells, INIB in hepatocytes	PCR	Coinfection with mycoplasma
Snake adenovirus 1	Cornsnakes, Boa Constrictors, probably many other species	Lethargy, dehydration, anorexia, dermatitis, regurgitation, head tilt, death	Edematous small intestine containing excessive mucus, hepatomegaly with mottling and necrosis, lung congestion	Large basophilic INIB in hepatocytes only; EM; viral isolation (VH-2); PCR	Concurrent infections with parasites, bacteria, retroviruses, reoviruses, ferlaviruses, parvoviruses, herpesviruses common
Snake AdV-2	Colubrid snakes, viperid snakes	Inappetence, death	Enteritis, INIB in epithelial cells of stomach and intestine	EM, PCR	
Snake AdV-3	Colubrid snakes	Inappetence, cachexia, head tilt, dehydration, death	Enteritis, INIB in epithelial cells of stomach and intestine	EM, PCR	

PAPILLOMAVIRUSES

General characteristics:
- DNA virus, 45-50 nm, nonenveloped, icosahedral
- Replicate in nucleus, producing INIB
- Papilloma viruses are generally highly host-specific and cause benign skin tumors (papillomas)
- Difficult to replicate in cell culture; identification with molecular techniques (sequencing, cloning, hybridization) with use of nucleic acid from lesions
- Horizontal transmission; suggested routes by epidermal trauma (e.g., biting during mating)
- Persist in the environment; inactivated by sodium hypochlorite, iodophors, and formaldehyde
- Treatment and control: surgical removal but often recur, prolonged treatment using salicylic acid, supportive care (e.g., topical antimicrobials), strict isolation, good hygiene, reduce stress (e.g., overcrowding), improve husbandry (i.e., reduce skin trauma from abrasive substrates; reduce aggression), and nutrition
- Potential for autogenous vaccines
- Standard quarantine procedures: 6 months

Virus	Species	Clinical Signs	Pathology	Specific Diagnosis	Comments
Bolivian side neck turtle papillomavirus	Bolivian Sideneck Turtles	Pale, flat to oval skin lesions, especially on head; focal to coalescing patches; plastron lesions typically ulcerate and secondarily infected	Thickened stratum corneum, hyperplastic, acanthotic epidermis, vacuolated nuclei	INIBs in epidermal cells; EM	
European green lizard papillomavirus	European Green Lizards	Firm, grey to black, 2-20-mm proliferative masses, especially on neck and tail base, not on ventrum	Hyperkeratotic, hyperplastic epidermal cells	INIBs in epidermal cells; EM	Herpesvirus and reovirus also demonstrated in lesions; surgical removal effective in mild cases
Russian tortoise papillomavirus	Russian Tortoise	Stomatitis		EM in lung wash	No virus detected in oral scrapings from the same animal
Caretta caretta papillomavirus 1	Loggerhead Sea Turtle	Small white papules on skin, resolved after several months		EM, PCR	
Chelonia mydas papillomavirus 1	Green Sea Turtle	Small white papules on skin, resolved after several months		EM, PCR	

PARVOVIRUSES

General characteristics:

- DNA virus, 18-26 nm, nonenveloped, icosahedral
- Replicate in nucleus, producing large, basophilic INIB
- Often in association with a helper virus, adenovirus or herpesvirus; all reptile parvoviruses have been found in association with other viruses
- Replicate in rapidly growing cells; hence predilection for intestinal tract; cause severe diarrhea
- Horizontal transmission by fecal–oral route; very stable outside host
- Inactivated by formalin or sodium hypochlorite; parvoviruses destroyed by 0.5% formaldehyde for 15 min
- Treatment and control: supportive care (antimicrobials, fluids, nutritional support, temperature), strict isolation, good hygiene, reduce stress (e.g., overcrowding), improve husbandry and nutrition
- Standard quarantine procedures

Virus	Species	Clinical Signs	Pathology	Specific Diagnosis	Comments
Kingsnake parvovirus	Juvenile Californian Mountain Kingsnake	Regurgitation, dehydration, death in less than 72 h	Gastroenteritis; pylorus and small intestine dilated and filled with pasty yellow ingesta; multifocal petechial hemorrhages of GI tract, serosa; intestinal mucosal edema and necrosis; crypt distension with sloughed enterocytes, hyperplasia, and villus blunting	Basophilic Cowdry type A INIB in enterocytes peripheral to necrosis; EM: parvovirus (15-18 nm) and adenovirus (65-70 nm)	Other snakes including adults of same species were unaffected; these juveniles were fed wild-caught fence lizards that were proposed as a possible source of infection
Bearded dragon dependovirus	Neonate Bearded Dragons	Nonspecific signs, death	Enteritis	Basophilic INIBs in liver and small intestine; EM: adenovirus in liver and intestine, dependovirus in liver	
Serpentine adeno-associated virus (SAAV), dependovirus	Boa Constrictor, Royal Python, Indonesian Pit Viper			Virus isolation in virus-host cells	Unknown clinical importance

CIRCOVIRUSES

General characteristics:

- Nonenveloped DNA viruses, approximately 12-21 nm
- Usually specific for one or few host species; mostly described in avian species
- Usually horizontal transmission by fecal–oral routes
- Extremely stable in the environment
- Treatment and control: none described

Virus	Species	Clinical Signs	Pathology	Specific Diagnosis	Comments
Turtle circovirus	Painted Turtle		Multifocal areas of necrosis in spleen and liver	EM	Single report in macrophages of affected turtle

"TORNOVIRUS"

General characteristics: Nonenveloped small DNA viruses
May represent a new genus of the family *Circoviridae* or a new viral family
Transmission routes unknown
Probably extremely stable in the environment
Treatment and control: none described

Virus	Species	Clinical Signs	Pathology	Specific Diagnosis	Comments
Sea turtle tornovirus (STTV1)	Green Sea Turtles	Sea turtles had severe fibropapillomatosis (also infected with a herpesvirus)	Extensive external and internal fibropapillomas	Metagenomics	STTV1 not believed to be the cause of fibropapillomatosis (see herpesviruses); may affect the immune system of infected sea turtles or may be an opportunistic pathogen

RETROVIRUSES

General characteristics: Nonenveloped, 95-110 nm
Variable effects from subclinical to acute neurologic disease and neoplasia; endogenous retroviruses have been demonstrated in many different reptilian species; some of these have been shown to be replication competent

Virus	Species	Clinical Signs	Pathology	Specific Diagnosis	Comments
Inclusion body disease-associated retrovirus	Boa Constrictors and Burmese Pythons	IBD: Pythons: acute; head tremors, opisthotonus, loss of righting reflex Boas: chronic; regurgitation, loose feces, stomatitis, dermatitis, dysecdysis, cutaneous neoplasia, leukemia, pneumonia, poor striking ability, dull mentation, anorexia, star-gazing, blindness, head tilt, disorientation	IBD: Acute: nonsuppurative meningoencephalitis (python > boa), hepatitis, hepatic lipidosis, ulcerative dermatitis, pneumonia Chronic: splenic/pancreatic fibrosis, pancreatic atrophy, fat/muscle atrophy; proliferative pneumonia, urate nephrosis, small intestine gas distension	EM, Virus isolation	The etiology of IBD is unknown, but believed to be viral. Retroviruses and, more recently, arenaviruses (see Arenaviruses) have been discussed as possible etiological agents.
Python endogenous retrovirus	*Python molurus, Python curtus*	IBD diagnosed in some cases but not all		Virus isolation; PCR	Highly expressed and species-specific endogenous retrovirus; not causally linked to any disease (including IBD)
Other retroviruses identified from snakes (with or without obvious pathology)	Jararacussu Viper, Russell's Viper, Cornsnake, California Kingsnake, Boa Constrictor, Brazilian Lancehead, Four-lined Chicken Snake, Burmese Python	Palpable mass in one snake, otherwise none	Normal venom and spleen, pericardial myxofibroma, embryonal rhabdomyosarcoma, leukemia, erythroleukosis, fibrosarcoma, lymphosarcoma, transitional cell carcinoma, adenocarcinoma, renal and mesenchymal tumors	Retroviruses detected by EM	Often type C retroviruses
Green sea turtle retrovirus	Green Sea Turtle	None to fibropapillomas	None to fibropapillomas	EM retrovirus in healthy and fibropapillomatosis cases; heart, lung	Reverse transcriptase activity higher in fibropapillomatosis cases; retrovirus may be precipitating factor for fibropapillomatosis

Tuatara retrovirus	Tuatara	None	None	PCR	Endogenous retrovirus
Crocodilian endogenous retroviruses	Crocodilians	None	None	PCR	Endogenous retroviruses

REOVIRUSES

General characteristics:
- Nonenveloped, RNA viruses, 70-85 nm, nearly spherical icosahedral particles
- Many are nonpathogenic; a few cause high morbidity and mortality, depending on host age, strain virulence, route of exposure, and concurrent disease
- Horizontal transmission by direct contact or excrement; incubation in reptiles unknown
- Diagnosis: EM, virus isolation, or PCR from tissues or swabs (but may be present in healthy animals)
- Treatment and control: supportive care (broad-spectrum antimicrobials, fluids, nutritional support, temperature), strict isolation, good hygiene, reduce stress (e.g., overcrowding), improve husbandry and nutrition
- Stable outside the host, especially in organic debris, resistant to many disinfectants; infectivity reduced by prolonged contact with high concentrations of iodine, ethanol, or formalin
- Standard quarantine procedures

Virus	Species	Clinical Signs	Pathology	Specific Diagnosis	Comments
Chinese viper reovirus	Chinese Vipers	Recently imported, no signs of disease before death	Hepatic necrosis, vacuolar degeneration of hepatocytes and enteritis; concurrent intestinal nematodiasis	EM of intestinal cells; virus isolation	
Rattlesnake reovirus	Western Rattlesnake	Incoordination, proprioceptive deficits, convulsions	No gross or histologic lesions	EM in brain, virus isolation	
Royal python reovirus	Royal Python	Moribund		EM, virus isolation	
Rough green snake reovirus	Rough Green Snake	Wasting, death	Necrotizing hepatitis	EM, PCR	
Ratsnake reovirus	Ratsnakes	Death	Pneumonia	Virus isolation	Experimental transmission led to pneumonia in infected juvenile Ratsnake
Reptilian reoviruses	Multiple snake and lizard species	Most commonly associated with lung and neurologic disease		Virus isolation, PCR	
Spur-thighed tortoise reovirus	Spur-thighed Tortoise	Stomatitis, death		Virus isolation	

RHABDOVIRUSES

General characteristics:
- Enveloped, bullet-shaped, 100-430 nm long and 45-100 nm in diameter, RNA viruses
- Some species multiply only in mammals, birds, fish, or arthropods; many have both arthropod and vertebrate hosts (arboviruses); some vertebrate viruses have a very broad host range
- Rhabdoviruses detected in reptiles have been arboviruses also capable of infecting mammals
- Not very stable in the environment; inactivated by standard disinfectants
- NOTE: may be zoonotic

Virus	Species	Clinical Signs	Pathology	Specific Diagnosis	Comments
Charlesville virus	Australian House Gecko	None	None	Virus isolation	
Marco, Timbo, and Chaco viruses	Teiid lizards	None	None	Virus isolation	

PARAMYXOVIRUSES

General characteristics:

- Enveloped, RNA viruses, pleomorphic, 150-300 nm
- Multiple strains may infect different reptile species; generally low host specificity
- Commonly affect the respiratory tract but also the brain and pancreas
- Horizontal transmission by direct contact, respiratory secretions, fomites
- Seroconversion takes at least 8 weeks
- Development of HI antibody does not correlate with cessation of virus shedding
- Treatment and control: supportive care (broad-spectrum antimicrobials, diazepam for seizures, fluids, nutritional support, temperature), strict isolation, improve hygiene to reduce fomite spread, reduce stress (e.g., overcrowding), improve husbandry and nutrition, and do not mix different species
- Sodium hypochlorite, lysol, phenol, formalin disinfectants are effective; if organic contamination, must use detergent first
- Quarantine: 4 months, strict hygiene, test for HI antibody at start and end; serial PCR on oral and cloacal swabs and transtracheal washes; eliminate ectoparasites (especially mites)

Virus	Species	Clinical Signs	Pathology	Specific Diagnosis	Comments
Ferlaviruses	Mainly viperidae (e.g., Fer-de-Lance, *Crotalus, Vipera, Bothrops, Trimeresurus, Bitis, Ophiophagus, Agkistrodon, Hydrodynastes*) but also reported in Elapidae, Colubridae, Boidae, Pythonidae; also in various lizard species (Caiman Lizards, Monitor Lizards, and a Knob-scaled Lizard); also detected in chelonians (occasionally Leopard Tortoise and Hermann's Tortoise)	Peracute: death Acute (1-3 days): severe respiratory disease, dyspnea, brown to hemorrhagic discharge from nostrils and trachea, opisthotonus, head tremors, loss of righting reflex, convulsions, star-gazing Chronic (weeks to > 1 yr): mild respiratory disease leading to chronic pneumonia, often secondary bacterial infections, progressive neurologic disease, hypophagia, anorexia, regurgitation, emaciation	Lung edema, hemorrhage, and hypertrophy; proliferation of type II alveolar cells; secondary bacterial infections and caseous pneumonia; hepatic necrosis, enlarged pancreas, multifocal gliosis, and perivascular cuffing in brain	Virus isolation (VH-2), PCR	Predisposed by poor husbandry, especially suboptimal temperature, old age; secondary bacterial pneumonias are common; concomitant adenovirus and reovirus infections; different species appear to differ in their susceptibility to infection with ferlaviruses as well as to their susceptibility to ferlaviral disease; viperids most affected; many lizard species and boas and pythons appear to be somewhat resistant
Sunshine Virus	Australian Pythons (Black-headed Pythons *[Aspidites melanocephalus]* and Jungle Carpet Pythons *[Morelia spilota cheynei]*)	Neurorespiratory disease	Not described	Virus isolation (VH-2), PCR	This virus has so far only been described in Australia; its prevalence there and in other parts of the world are not yet known; it differs distinctly from all previously described paramyxoviruses

ARENAVIRUSES

General characteristics:

Enveloped pleomorphic, 50-300 nm RNA viruses
Most arenaviruses infect mammals, with rodents as natural hosts. Some arenaviruse of rodents are zoonotic. Highly divergent arenaviruses have recently been detected in snakes with IBD
Not very stable in the environment; easily inactivated by standard disinfectants

Virus	Species	Clinical Signs	Pathology	Specific Diagnosis	Comments
California Academy of Sciences Virus (CASV), Golden Gate Virus (GGV), Collierville virus (CVV), Boa Av NL B3 Virus	Annulated Tree Boas (*Corallus annulatus*), Boa constrictor, Emerald Tree Boa (*Corallus caninus*)	IBD: Pythons: acute; head tremors, opisthotonus, loss of righting reflex Boas: chronic; regurgitation, loose feces, stomatitis, dermatitis, dysecdysis, cutaneous neoplasia, leukemia, pneumonia, poor striking ability, dull mentation, anorexia, star-gazing, blindness, head tilt, disorientation	IBD diagnosed in all snakes	Next generation sequencing, PCR	Arenaviruses have recently been detected by next generation sequencing in IBD positive boas and pythons in the United States and Europe appear to be the most likely cause of IBD in snakes. See section on retroviruses for earlier, alternate theories on the etiology of IBD

BUNYAVIRUSES

General characteristics:

Enveloped pleomorphic, 80-120 nm RNA viruses
Viruses in several genera, including the orthobunyaviruses, are capable of alternately replicating in vertebrates and arthropods
Different viruses are transmitted by mosquitoes, ticks, phlebotomine flies, and other arthropod vectors
Not very stable in the environment; easily inactivated by standard disinfectants
NOTE: may be zoonotic

Virus	Species	Clinical Signs	Pathology	Specific Diagnosis	Comments
Tortoise orthobunyvirus	Texas Soft-shelled Turtle *(Trionyx spinifera emoryi)*	None	None	Isolation in suckling mice	
Kowanyama virus	Australian skink	None	None	Virus isolation	

PICORNAVIRUSES

General characteristics:

Nonenveloped RNA viruses, 22-30 nm
Replication in cytoplasm
Usually specific for one or few host species
Horizontal transmission by fecal–oral, fomite, or airborne routes
Relatively stable in the environment; inactivated by virucidal disinfectants
Treatment and control: supportive care (broad-spectrum antimicrobials, fluids, nutritional support, temperature), strict isolation, improve hygiene (sensitive to common disinfectants [e.g., sodium hypochlorite]), reduce stress (e.g., overcrowding), improve husbandry and nutrition
Quarantine: at least 3-6 months; carrier status appears possible

Virus	Species	Clinical Signs	Pathology	Specific Diagnosis	Comments
Picornavirus of tortoises	Most commonly found in Spur-thighed Tortoises but also described in other species, including Marginated Tortoises, Hermann's Tortoises, Leopard Tortoises, and Egyptian Tortoises	Softening of the carapace in young animals, upper respiratory tract disease, stomatitis, ascites, death; also found in clinically healthy tortoises		Virus isolation	Often found together with other infectious agents (e.g., herpesviruses, mycoplasma)

Picornavirus of snakes	Aesculapian Snake, Boa Constrictor	Gastrointestinal disease	Enteritis	EM	Adenovirus also found in intestine of the Boa Constrictor, parvovirus-, adenovirus-, and herpesvirus-like viruses also found in the intestine of the Aesculapian Snake

CALICIVIRUSES

General characteristics:

- RNA virus, 35-40 nm, nonenveloped, icosahedral
- Replicate in cytoplasm; may find INIB and ICIB
- Transmission unknown
- Inactivated by sodium hypochlorite
- Diagnosis: histologic demonstration of inclusions, EM, PCR, virus isolation
- Treatment and control: supportive care (antimicrobials, strict isolation), good hygiene, reduce stress (e.g., overcrowding), improve husbandry and nutrition
- Standard quarantine procedures

Virus	Species	Clinical Signs	Pathology	Specific Diagnosis	Comments
Reptilian calicivirus Crotalus type 1	Aruba Rattlesnake, Rock Rattlesnake, Eyelash Viper	Diarrhea, lethargy, death	Enteritis, hepatitis	EM, virus isolation in vero cells from cloacal swabs	Isolated viruses not definitively associated with particular disease; virus recovered from cloacal swabs of healthy animals and in small intestine, liver, and kidney of diseased animals at necropsy; experimental infection in Western Rattlesnake did not produce pathognomonic disease

TOGAVIRUSES AND FLAVIVIRUSES

General characteristics:	RNA viruses, icosahedral enveloped particles, 40-70 nm Transmitted by arthropod vectors, especially mosquitoes and ticks Reptiles implicated in maintenance and transmission of WEE, EEE, VEE, JE, and West Nile viruses Serologic evidence of togaviruses in 25 species snakes, 14 species lizards, 12 species chelonia, 1 crocodilian Many reptiles serve as subclinical natural reservoirs: high viremia for improved vector infection and transmission; horizontal and vertical transmission Serologic activity documented in free-ranging reptiles; viremia ceases after solid immune response, often subclinical Unstable outside the host; inactivated by common disinfectants Diagnosis: serology, virus isolation, EM, PCR, immunoperoxidase staining with monoclonal antibodies Treatment and control: prevent contact with vectors (i.e., control arthropods or move outdoor reptiles inside during high vector prevalence), supportive care (antimicrobials, fluids, nutritional support, temperature), good hygiene, reduce stress (e.g., overcrowding), improve husbandry and nutrition Standard quarantine procedures; remove arthropods and control mosquitoes Attention: many of these viruses are zoonotic!

Virus	Species	Clinical Signs	Pathology	Specific Diagnosis	Comments
Western equine encephalitis (WEE) virus	Garter Snakes, Gopher Snakes, Blue Racers, Texas Tortoises	None	None	Virus isolation from blood, EM; serology: HI, VN	Cyclic viremia associated with temperature changes
Eastern equine encephalitis (EEE) virus	Garter Snakes, Spotted Turtles, Cuban Iguanas	None	None	Virus isolation, EM	Viremia lasted 36 days to > 6 mo
Japanese encephalitis (JE) virus	Soft-shelled Turtle, Skinks, Chinese Ratsnakes, various species have been shown to be susceptible to infection	None	None	Virus isolation, EM	Unknown clinical importance
West Nile virus	American Alligators, other crocodilians	Depression, lethargy, neurologic disease	Heterophilic lymphoplasmocytic meningoencephalomyelitis; coelomic effusion; fibronecrotic oral mucosal exudate, glossitis, necrotic stomatitis; enlarged pale liver with red mottling, hepatic lipidosis, necrotic hepatitis, splenitis; myocardial degeneration and necrosis, mild interstitial pneumonia, adrenalitis	Virus isolation, EM, PCR	High viremia, potential amplification hosts; 3.3% mortality
	Green Iguanas, Florida Gartersnakes, Red-ear Sliders	None	None	Virus isolation, EM	Low but detectable viral loads in blood, oral or cloacal swabs, and/or organs

AdV, Adenovirus; *CASV,* California Academy of Sciences Virus; *CNS,* central nervous system; *CVV,* Collierville virus; *DNA,* deoxyribonucleic acid; *EEE,* Eastern equine encephalitis; *EM,* electron microscopy; *GGV,* Golden Gate virus; *GI,* gastrointestinal; *HI,* hemagglutination inhibition; *IBD,* inclusion body disease; *ICIB,* intracytoplasmic inclusion bodies; *IIV,* invertebrate iridovirus; *INIB,* intranuclear inclusion bodies; *JE,* Japanese encephalitis; *KOH,* potassium hydroxide; *LETD,* lung, eye, trachea disease; *LGRV,* loggerhead genital-respiratory herpesvirus; *LOCV,* loggerhead orocutaneous herpesvirus; *NaOH,* sodium hydroxide; *PCR,* polymerase chain reaction; *RBCs,* red blood cells; *SAAV,* serpentine adeno-associated virus; *STTV,* sea turtle tornovirus; *VEE,* Venezuelan equine encephalitis; *VN/ELISA,* virus neutralization or enzyme-linked immunosorbent assay; *WBC,* white blood cells; *WEE,* Western equine encephalitis.

Adapted from Jacobson ER. Viruses and viral diseases of reptiles. In: Jacobson ER, ed. *Infectious diseases and pathology of reptiles.* Boca Raton: CRC Press, Taylor and Francis Group, 2007;395-460, Marschang RE. Viruses infecting reptiles. *Viruses* 2011;3:2087-2126, and Chapter 5, Clinical Virology, in this book.

APPENDIX 3

Reptile Formulary and Laboratory Normals*

James W. Carpenter, Eric Klaphake, and Paul M. Gibbons

TABLE 1

Antimicrobial, Antiviral, and Antifungal Agents[a]

Drug dosages are first listed by "most species," followed by dosages in snakes, lizards, chelonians, and crocodilians; feed and water dosages are generally listed last.

Agent	Dosage	Species/Comments
Acyclovir	≥80 mg/kg PO q24h[1]	Tortoises/PD; herpesvirus; poor oral absorption
	80 mg/kg PO q8h or 240 mg/kg/day PO[2]	Tortoises/herpesvirus; uncertain efficacy
Amikacin	—	Potentially nephrotoxic. Often used in combination with penicillins, cephalosporins or metronidazole
	3.48 mg/kg IM once[3]	Pythons/PD
	5 mg/kg IM then 2.5 mg/kg q72h[4]	Gopher snakes/PD; house at high end of optimum temperature range during treatment
	5 mg/kg IM then 2.5 mg/kg q72h[5,6]	Lizards
	2.5-3 mg/kg IM q72h × 5 treatments[7]	Sea turtles
	5 mg/kg IM q48h[8]	Gopher tortoises/PD; 30°C (86°F)
	2.25 mg/kg IM q72h[9]	Alligators/PD
Amoxicillin	22 mg/kg PO q12-24h[10,11]	Most species
Amphotericin B	0.5 mg/kg IV q48-72h[12]	Most species/nephrotoxic; can use in combination with ketoconazole; administer slowly
	0.5-1 mg/kg IV, ICe q24-72h × 14-28 days[10]	Most species/aspergillosis
	1 mg/kg IT q24h × 14-28 days[13]	Most species/respiratory infection; dilute with water or saline
	0.1 mg/kg intrapulmonary q24h × 28 days[14]	Greek tortoises/pneumonia
	1 mg/kg q24h ICe × 2-4 wk[15]	Crocodilians
	5 mg/150 mL saline × 1 h nebulization q12h × 7 days[16]	Most species/pneumonia
Ampicillin	3-6 mg/kg PO, SC, IM q12-24h[11,17]	Most species
	10-20 mg/kg SC, IM q12h[18]	Most species
	20 mg/kg IM q24h[19]	Chelonians
	50 mg/kg IM q12h[20,21]	Tortoises
Azithromycin	10 mg/kg PO q2-7d[22]	Ball pythons/PD; single-dose study; may cause nonregenerative anemia; *Mycoplasma, Cryptosporidium,* Giardia; location dictates dosage frequency: skin q3d; respiratory tract q5d; liver/kidneys, q7d
Carbenicillin	200 mg/kg IM q24h[23]	Carpet pythons/PD
	400 mg/kg IM q24h[24]	Snakes/PD; 30°C (86°F)
	400 mg/kg SC, IM q24h[5]	Lizards
	200-400 mg/kg IM q48h[19]	Chelonians: may cause skin sloughing in desert tortoises
	400 mg/kg IM q48h[25]	Chelonians/PD
Cefoperazone	100 mg/kg IM q96h[20]	Snakes/PD (24°C [75°F])
	125 mg/kg IM q24h[20]	Lizards/PD (24°C [75°F])

*All reptile formulary information has been modified from J. Carpenter. Exotic animal formulary. 4th ed. St Louis: Saunders, 2013, by permission.

TABLE 1—cont'd

Antimicrobial, Antiviral, and Antifungal Agents[a]

Agent	Dosage	Species/Comments
Cefotaxime	20-40 mg/kg IM q24h[17,19]	Most species
Ceftazidime	20-40 mg/kg SC, IM, q48-72h[6,20,26] 20 mg/kg SC, IM, IV q72h[5,27] 22 mg/kg IM, IV q72h[28]	Most species/in chameleons use q24h Snakes/PD; 30°C (86°F) Sea turtles
Ceftiofur sodium	2.2 mg/kg IM q48h[10] 5 mg/kg SC, IM q24h[29] 2.2 mg/kg IM q24h[10] 4 mg/kg IM q24h[10,17]	Snakes Lizards/PD Turtles Tortoises
Cefuroxime	100 mg/kg IM q24h[10,17]	Most species, snakes/30°C (86°F)
Cephalexin	20-40 mg/kg PO q12h[20]	Most species/unknown absorption
Cephalothin	20-40 mg/kg IM q12h[17,20,30]	Most species
Chloramphenicol	— 40 mg/kg PO, SC, IM q24h, or 20 mg/kg PO, SC, IM q12h[19,20,31] 40 mg/kg SC q24h[32] 50 mg/kg SC q12-72h[20,33]	Most species/public health concern Most species/20 mg/kg may be given q24h in larger crocodilians Snakes/PD (29°C [84°F]) Snakes/PD; q12h in indigo, rat, king snakes; q24h in boids, moccasin snakes; q48h in rattlesnakes; q72h in red-bellied water snakes
Chlortetracycline	200 mg/kg PO q24h[20,30]	Most species
Ciprofloxacin	10 mg/kg PO q48h[10] 11 mg/kg PO q48-72h[34]	Most species Pythons/PD
Clarithromycin	15 mg/kg PO q48-72h[35,36]	Tortoises/PD (mycoplasmosis)
Clindamycin	5 mg/kg PO q12h[30]	Most species
Danofloxacin	6 mg/kg SC, IM[37] 6 mg/kg SC q48h × 30d[38]	Loggerhead sea turtles Tortoises/mycoplasmosis
Doxycycline	5-10 mg/kg PO q24h × 10-45 days[30,31] 50 mg/kg IM, then 25 mg/kg q72h[21,39]	Most species/mycoplasmosis Tortoises 27°C (81°F)
Enrofloxacin	5-10 mg/kg q24h PO, SC, IM, ICe[30] 6.6 mg/kg IM q24h, or 11 mg/kg IM q48h[34] 10 mg/kg IM q48h[40] 5 mg/kg PO, IM q24h[41] 10 mg/kg IM q5d[42] 5 mg/kg IM q24-48h[43] 5 mg/kg IM q12-24h[45] 5 mg/kg IM q48h[7] 10 mg/kg IM q24h[21] 5 mg/kg IV q36-72h[46,47] Nasal flush 50 mg/250 mL sterile water; 1-3 mL/naris q24-48h[31]	Most species/IM is painful and may result in tissue necrosis/sterile abscesses; SC may cause skin discoloration/tissue necrosis Pythons/PD Snakes/PD Lizards/PD; marked pharmacokinetic variability with PO route Monitors/PD Chelonians, most species/PD; neurologic signs and diarrhea reported in a Galapagos tortoise[44] Chelonians/PD; q12h for *Pseudomonas* and *Citrobacter*, q24h for other bacteria Sea turtles Chelonians/PD Crocodilians/PD; mycoplasmosis Tortoises/URT syndrome; use until no more discharge (5-10 days); may use concurrently with parenteral antibiotics
Fluconazole	5 mg/kg PO q24h[48] 21 mg/kg SC once, then 10 mg/kg SC 5 days later[49,50]	Lizards/dermatophytosis Loggerhead sea turtles/PD
Gentamicin	— 2.5 mg/kg IM q72h[32,52] 2.5-3 mg/kg IM, then 1.5 mg/kg q96h[53] 3 mg/kg IM q>96h[54] 6 mg/kg IM q72-96h[55] 1.75-2.25 mg/kg IM q72-96h[9]	Nephrotoxic,[51] especially in snakes Snakes/PD Snakes/PD Turtles/PD (29°C [84°F]); lower dose may be more appropriate Turtles/PD (24°C,[75°F]) Crocodilians/PD; respiratory infection
Griseofulvin	20-40 mg/kg PO q72h × five treatments[56] 15 mg/kg PO q72h[57-59]	Most species/dermatitis; limited success Most species

Continued

TABLE 1—cont'd

Antimicrobial, Antiviral, and Antifungal Agents[a]

Agent	Dosage	Species/Comments
Itraconazole	5 mg/kg PO q24h[60]	Most species/some hepatotoxicity noted when used for *Chrysosporium* anamorph of *Nannizziopsis vriesii*
	10 mg/kg PO q24h[61]	Snakes
	5 mg/kg PO q24h[62]	Panther chameleons
	10 mg/kg PO q48h × 60 days[63]	Chameleons (Parson's)/osteomyelitis
	23.5 mg/kg PO q24h[64]	Lizards/PD; after 3-day treatment, therapeutic plasma concentration persists for 6 days beyond peak concentration; treatment interval not determined
	5 mg/kg PO q24h or 15 mg/kg PO q72h[65]	Kemp's Ridley sea turtles
Kanamycin	10-15 mg/kg IM, IV q24h (or divided doses)[10,11]	Most species/24°C (75°F); nephrotoxic
Ketoconazole	—	May use antibiotics concomitantly to prevent bacterial overgrowth; may use concurrently with thiabendazole
	15-30 mg/kg PO q24h × 14-28 days[17]	Most species
	25 mg/kg PO q24h × 21 days[66]	Snakes, turtles
	15 mg/kg q72h PO[57-59]	Most species
	15-30 mg/kg PO q24h × 14-28 days[67,68]	Chelonians/PD; systemic infection
	50 mg/kg PO q24h × 14-28 days[30]	Crocodilians
Lincomycin	5 mg/kg IM q12-24h[10]	Most species; nephrotoxic
	10 mg/kg PO q24h[10]	Most species
Marbofloxacin	10 mg/kg PO q48h[69]	Ball pythons/PD
Metronidazole	20 mg/kg PO q48h × ≥7 days[70]	Most species
	50 mg/kg PO q24h × 7-14 days[34]	Most species; potential side effects at this dose; lower dose may be prudent
	20 mg/kg PO q48h[71,72]	Snakes/PD
	20 mg/kg PO q24-48h[73]	Iguanas/PD
Oxytetracycline	6-10 mg/kg PO, IM, IV q24h[10,11]	Most species/may produce inflammation at injection site
	5-10 mg/kg IM q24h[35]	Tortoises/mycoplasmosis
	10 mg/kg IM, IV q5d[74]	Crocodilians/PD (27°C [81°F]); mycoplasmosis
Penicillin, benzathine	10,000-20,000 U/kg IM q48-96h[20]	Most species
Penicillin G	10,000-20,000 U/kg SC, IM, IV, ICe q8-12h[11]	Most species/infrequently used
Piperacillin	50-100 mg/kg IM q24h[10,11]	Most species/nephrotoxic
	50 mg/kg IM, then 25 mg/kg q24h[10,30]	Snakes
	100 mg/kg IM q48h[75]	Snakes/PD
	100-200 mg/kg SC, IM q24-48h[18]	Chameleons
	100 mg/10 mL saline × 30 min nebulization q12h[76]	Most species/pneumonia
Streptomycin	10 mg/kg IM q12-24h[11]	Most species/nephrotoxic; avoid with hepatic dysfunction
Sulfadiazine	25 mg/kg PO q24h[30]	Most species/nephrotoxic
Sulfadimethoxine	90 mg/kg IM, then 45 mg/kg q24h[11]	Most species/nephrotoxic
Thiabendazole	50 mg/kg PO q24h × 14 days[77]	Chelonians/pneumonia; dermatitis
Ticarcillin	50-100 mg/kg IM q24h[11]	Most species/nephrotoxic
	50-100 mg/kg IM, IV q24-48h[78]	Loggerhead sea turtles/PD
Tobramycin	—	Nephrotoxic
	2.5 mg/kg IM q24-72h[10,17]	Most species
	10 mg/kg IM q24-48h[10]	Chelonians/can be given q48h in tortoises
Trimethoprim/sulfadiazine	—	Avoid in renal dysfunction; compound parenteral form
	15-25 mg/kg PO q24h[30]	Most species
	20-30 mg/kg IM q24-48h[34]	Most species
	30 mg/kg IM q24h × 2 days, then q48h[10,11,20]	Most species/can administer PO, SC
Trimethoprim/sulfamethoxazole	10-30 mg/kg PO q24h[11]	Most species/ Avoid in renal dysfunction
Tylosin	5 mg/kg IM q24h × 10-60 days[10,17]	Most species/mycoplasmosis
Voriconazole	10 mg/kg PO[79]	Bearded dragons/no hepatotoxicity noted when used for *Chrysosporium* anamorph of *Nannizziopsis vriesii*
	5 mg/kg SC[80]	Red-eared sliders/exceeded MIC only until 4 h after injection; 26°C (78°F)

ICe, Intracoelomic; *IM,* intramuscular; *IT,* intrathecal; *IV,* intravenous; *MIC,* minimum inhibitory concentration; *PD,* pharmacodynamic; *PO,* by mouth; *SC,* subcutaneous; *URT,* upper respiratory tract.

[a]Because reptiles are ectothermic, pharmacokinetics of drugs are influenced by ambient temperature. Antimicrobial therapy should be conducted at the upper end of the patient's preferred (selected) optimum temperature zone.

TABLE 2

Antiparasitic Agents

Agent	Dosage	Species/Comments
Albendazole	50 mg/kg PO[30]	Most species/ascarids
Carbaryl powder (5%)	Lightly dust animal and environment; rinse after 1 h; repeat in 7 days[20,81]	Lizards; snakes/mites
Chloroquine	125 mg/kg PO q48h × 3 treatments[30]	Tortoises/hemoprotozoa
Emodepside (1.98%) + praziquantel (7.94%)	1.12 mL/kg[82,83]	Many species/PD; nematodes; cestodes; aquatic turtles must be kept dry 48 h after application; appears safe, but need more safety and efficacy data
Fenbendazole	—	May have antiprotozoan effect; may cause leukopenia, avoid with septicemia[84]
	25-100 mg/kg PO q14d × 1-4 treatments[16,39,85]	All species/nematodes
	50 mg/kg PO q24h × 3-5 days[20,86,87]	All species/nematodes (× 3 days); flagellates and giardia in chameleons (× 5 days)
	100 mg/kg once[88]	Tortoises/nematodes; ova still sheds for 30 days
Fipronil	Spray or wipe on then wash off in 5 min q7-10d prn[20,81]	Most species/mites, ticks; beware of reactions to alcohol carrier; needs safety evaluation[89]
Imidacloprid and moxidectin	0.2 mg/kg topical q14d × 3 treatments[90]	Lizards/eliminated hookworms and pinworms; needs safety and pharmacokinetic evaluation
Ivermectin	—	Do not use in chelonians,[91] crocodilians, indigo snakes, or skinks[30,39,87]
	0.2 mg/kg PO, SC, IM repeat in 14 days[5,92 93]	Snakes (except indigos), lizards (except skinks)[39]/nematodes,[94] mites; dilute with propylene glycol for oral use; colored animals may have skin discoloration at injection site; rare adverse effects reported in chameleons[5]; do not use within 10 days of diazepam or tiletamine/zolazepam; rare death and occasional nervous system signs, lethargy, or inappetence;[87] pentastomids in monitors (with dexamethasone)[92]
	5-10 mg/L water topical spray q3-5d up to 28 days[87]	Snakes (except indigos), lizards (except skinks)/mites; less effective than fipronil; spray on skin and in newly cleaned cage, then allow to dry before replacing water dish
Metronidazole	—	Protozoan (i.e., flagellates, amoebae) overgrowth; may stimulate appetite; may cause severe neurologic signs at doses >200 mg/kg[95]; death occurred in indigo and mountain king snakes at 100 mg/kg[16]; for small patients, injectable form can be administered PO; oral liquid not available in the United States but can be compounded
	40-100 mg/kg PO, repeat in 10-14 days[11]	Most species/flagellate overgrowth
	20 mg/kg PO q48h[71]	Corn snakes/PD; 28°C (82°F); protozoa
	40 mg/kg PO, repeat in 14 days[16,20]	Uracoan rattler, milk, tricolor king, and indigo snakes/flagellates
	40-60 mg/kg PO q7d × 2-3 doses[96]	Chameleons/flagellates; amoebae
	40-200 mg/kg PO, repeat in 14 days[97]	Geckos/ocular lesions (40 mg/kg) and SC lesions (200 mg/kg) caused by *Trichomonas*
	50 mg/kg PO q24h × 2-5 days[86]	Chameleons/when accompanied by increased gastrointestinal symptoms
	20 mg/kg ICe q48h[98]	Red-eared sliders/PD; ICe administration not recommended; needs further safety evaluation
	25 mg/kg PO q24h × 5 days or 50 mg/kg PO q14 days prn[99]	Chelonians (tortoises)/amoebae; use 25 mg/kg dosage for clinically ill cases
Paromomycin	35-100 mg/kg PO q24h × ≤28 days[11,16,93]	Most species/amoebae
	100 mg/kg PO q24h × 7 days, then 2 ×/wk × 3 mo[100]	Snakes/cryptosporidia; reduced clinical signs and oocyte shedding; does not eliminate the organism
	300-360 mg/kg PO q48h × 14 days[101]	Lizards (gila monsters)/cryptosporidia
	300-800 mg/kg PO q24h prn[102]	Geckos/cryptosporidia; reduced clinical signs; does not eliminate the organism
Permethrin	Environmental treatment, 1 s of spray/ft^2; wait until dry before returning animal to enclosure[81]	Lizards, snakes/mites; ticks; FDA approved; safe and effective; wash immediately if accidentally applied to skin
	Topical[81]	Tortoises/ticks

Continued

TABLE 2—cont'd

Antiparasitic Agents

Agent	Dosage	Species/Comments
Ponazuril	30 mg/kg PO q48h × 2 treatments[103,104]	Bearded dragons/coccidiosis
Praziquantel (also see Emodepside)	8 mg/kg PO, SC, IM, repeat in 14 days[5,18,30]	Most species/cestodes, trematodes; higher dosages have been administered[20]
	5-10 mg/kg PO q14d[86]	Chameleons/flukes may best be left untreated if not causing a problem
	25-50 mg/kg PO q3h × 3 treatments[105,106]	Sea turtles (green, loggerhead)/PD; spirorchidiasis
Pyrantel pamoate	5 mg/kg PO, repeat in 14 days[87]	Most species/nematodes
	25 mg/kg PO q24h × 3 days; repeat in 3 wk[20,107]	Most species/ascarids, hookworms, pinworms
Pyrethrin spray (0.09%)	Topical q7d × 2-3 treatments[81]	Most species/use water-based labeled for kittens and puppies; apply with cloth; can also spray cage, wash out after 30 min; use sparingly and with caution; pyrethroids are safer
Quinacrine	19-100 mg/kg PO q48h × 14-21 days[108]	Most species/some hematozoa
Quinine sulfate	75 mg/kg PO q48h × 14-28 days[108]	Most species/some hematozoa; toxic at >100 mg/kg q24h; ineffective against exoerythrocytic forms
Resmethrin spray/shampoo	Topical, repeat q≥10d prn[81]	Most species/mites; pyrethroid; safer than pyrethrins; use with care; spray (0.35%) or shampoo entire animal, rinse off immediately in running, tepid water; protect eyes (other than snakes) with 1 drop of mineral oil; lightly spray environment, wipe off in 5-10 min
Spiramycin	160 mg/kg PO q24h × 10 days, then 2×/wk for 3 mo[100]	Snakes/cryptosporidia; may reduce clinical signs and oocyte shedding; does not eliminate
Sulfadiazine, sulfamerazine	—	Most species/coccidia; watch renal dysfunction[95]
	75 mg/kg PO, then 45 mg/kg q24h × 5 days[11,86,108]	Most species/coccidia
	25 mg/kg PO q24h × 21 days[5,77,108]	Snakes, lizards/coccidian
Sulfadimethoxine	50 mg/kg PO q24h × 3-5 days, then q48h prn[87]	Most species/coccidia; watch renal dysfunction
	90 mg/kg PO, IM, IV, then 45 mg/kg q24h × 5-7 days[11,16,108]	Most species/coccidia
Sulfamethazine	50 mg/kg PO q24h × 3 days, off 3 days, on 3 days[108]	Most species/coccidia
	25 mg/kg PO, IM q24h × 21 days[109]	Most species/coccidia
	75 mg/kg PO, IM, IV, then 40 mg/kg q24h × 5-7 days[16,17]	Most species/coccidia; ensure adequate hydration and renal function
Toltrazuril 5%	5-15 mg/kg q24h × 3 days[110]	Bearded dragons/coccidia
	15 mg/kg q48h × 10 days; discontinue for 2 wk; repeat q48h × 10 days prn[111]	Tortoises/intranuclear coccidiosis; needs safety, efficacy, and pharmacokinetic study
Trimethoprim/sulfa	—	Most species/coccidia; avoid potentiated sulfa drugs in cases of dehydration or renal dysfunction[95]
	30 mg/kg PO q24h × 2 days, then q48h × 21 days[5,108]	Most species/coccidia
	30 mg/kg IM q24h × 2 days, then 15 mg/kg IM q48h × 10-28 days[108]	Most species/coccidia

FDA, U.S. Food and Drug Administration; *ICe,* intracoelomic; *IM,* intramuscular; *IV,* intravenous; *PD,* pharmacodynamic; *PO,* by mouth; *prn,* as required; *SC,* subcutaneous.

TABLE 3

Chemical Restraint/Anesthetic and Analgesic Agents

Agent	Dosage	Species/Comments
Acepromazine	0.05-0.25 mg/kg IM[31]	Most species/preanesthetic with ketamine
	0.1-0.5 mg/kg IM[112,113]	Most species/preanesthetic; reduce by 50% if used with barbiturates
Alphaxalone	—	Not available in the United States
	6-9 mg/kg IV, or 9-15 mg/kg IM[114]	Most species/good muscle relaxation; variable results; needs more evaluation; possible violent recovery;[115] avoid within 10 days of DMSO
	6-15 mg/kg IM, IV[116]	Most species
	9 mg/kg IV[117]	Snakes, lizards/induction; not effective for blotched blue-tongued skinks
	15 mg/kg IM[112]	Lizards, chelonians/induction,35-40 min; duration 15-35 min; good muscle relaxation
	24 mg/kg ICe[118]	Chelonians (red-eared sliders)/surgical anesthesia with good relaxation
Atipamezole	Same volume SC, IV, IP as medetomidine or dexmedetomidine[a,119,120]	Most species/medetomidine and dexmedetomidine reversal; severe hypotension in gopher tortoises IV[121]
Atropine	0.01-0.04 mg/kg SC, IM,[122] IV,[12] ICe[123]	Most species/preanesthetic; rarely indicated; for profound bradycardia[123]; may help prevent intracardiac shunting[57]; ineffective dose in green iguanas[124]
	0.5 mg/kg IM, IV, IT, IO[95]	Most species/bradycardia, decrease secretions, CPR
Bupivacaine	1-2 mg/kg local q4-12h prn[116]	Most species; 4 mg/kg max dose
Buprenorphine	0.005-0.02 mg/kg IM q24-48h[125]	Most species/analgesia
	0.1-1 mg/kg IM[126]	Most species/analgesia
Butorphanol	—	Combinations (see ketamine) follow; recent studies call into question use in providing analgesia in reptiles, including red-eared sliders, ball pythons, bearded dragons, and green iguanas; respiratory depression at high doses[127-129]
	0.4-1 mg/kg SC, IM[123]	Most species/analgesia; sedation; preanesthetic
	0.5-2 mg/kg IM or 0.2-0.5 mg/kg IV, IO[126]	Most species/preanesthetic
	1-1.5 mg/kg SC, IM[123]	Lizards/administer 30 min before isoflurane for smooth, shorter induction
	0.2 mg/kg IM[125,130]	Chelonians/tranquilizer
	20 mg/kg IM[131]	Cornsnakes/potential analgesia
Butorphanol (B)/midazolam (M)	(B) 0.4 mg/kg + (M) 2 mg/kg IM[132]	Most species/preanesthetic; administer 20 min before induction
Carprofen	1-4 mg/kg PO, SC, IM, IV q24h,[133] follow with half the dose q24-72h[134]	Most species/analgesia; nonsteroidal antiinflammatory
Dexmedetomidine[a]	—	α_2 agonist that has replaced medetomidine[a]
Diazepam	—	Combinations follow; muscle relaxation; give 20 min before anesthesia; potentially reversible with flumazenil; interaction with ivermectin
	0.5 mg/kg IM, IV[95]	All species/seizures
	0.2-0.8 mg/kg IM[123]	Snakes/use with ketamine for anesthesia with muscle relaxation
	0.2-2 mg/kg IM, IV[116]	Snakes, lizards
	2.5 mg/kg PO[123]	Iguanas/reduce anxiety that often leads to aggression
	0.2-1 mg/kg IM[116,123]	Chelonians/use with ketamine for anesthesia with muscle relaxation
Doxapram	5 mg/kg IM, IV[132] q10min prn	Most species/respiratory stimulant; reduces recovery time; reported to partially "reverse" effects of dissociatives[133]
	4-12 mg/kg IM, IV[123]	Most species/respiratory stimulant
	20 mg/kg IM, IV, IO[95]	Most species/respiratory stimulant
Epinephrine (1:1000)	0.5-1 mg/kg IV, IO, IT[95]	Most species/CPR, cardiac arrest
Fentanyl	2.5 μg/h patch to caudodorsal lumbar skin[135]	Prehensile-tailed skinks/no side effects reported after 24 h when skink blood levels reached human therapeutic levels; environmental temperature can significantly affect absorption

Continued

TABLE 3—cont'd

Chemical Restraint/Anesthetic and Analgesic Agents

Agent	Dosage	Species/Comments
Flunixin meglumine	0.1-0.5 mg/kg IM q12-24h[133]	Most species/analgesia; use max of 3 days
	1-2 mg/kg IM q24h × 2 treatments[136,137]	Lizards/nonsteroidal antiinflammatory; postsurgical analgesia
	0.5-2 mg/kg IM q12-24h[116]	Most species/nonsteroidal antiinflammatory; analgesia
Glycopyrrolate	0.01 mg/kg SC,[122] IM, IV[132]	Most species/preanesthetic; excess mucus; use with prolonged bradycardia; dose does not work in green iguanas[124]
Haloperidol	0.5-10 mg/kg IM q7-14d[138]	Boids/aggression management
Isoflurane	3%-5% induction[13]	Most species/inhalation anesthetic of choice in reptiles
	1%-3% maintenance[39]	
Ketamine	—	Muscle relaxation and analgesia may be marginal; prolonged recovery with higher doses; larger reptiles require lower dose; painful at injection site; safety questionable in debilitated patients; avoid with renal dysfunction; snakes may be permanently aggressive after ketamine anesthesia[115]; recommend only as preanesthetic before isoflurane for surgical anesthesia
	20-60 mg/kg IM, or 5-15 mg/kg IV[31]	Most species/muscle relaxation improved with midazolam or diazepam
	22-44 mg/kg SC, IM[115,139]	Most species/sedation
	55-88 mg/kg SC, IM[139]	Most species/surgical anesthesia; induction, 10-30 min; recovery, 24-96 h
	20-60 mg/kg SC, IM[122,140]	Snakes/sedation; induction, 30 min; recovery, 2-48 h
	60-80 mg/kg IM[39]	Snakes/light anesthesia; IPPV may be needed at higher doses
	30-50 mg/kg SC, IM[122,140]	Lizards/sedation; variable results
	20-60 mg/kg IM[113,140,141]	Chelonians/sedation; induction, 30 min; recovery, ≥24 h; potentially dangerous in dehydrated and debilitated tortoises
	25 mg/kg IM, IV[7]	Sea turtles/sedation
	38-71 mg/kg ICe[142]	Green sea turtles/anesthesia; induction, 2-10 min; duration, 2-10 min; recovery, <30 min
	60-90 mg/kg IM[112,140]	Chelonians/light anesthesia; induction, <30 min; recovery, hours to days; require higher doses than most other reptiles
	20-40 mg/kg SC, IM, ICe (sedation), to 40-80 mg/kg (anesthesia)[143]	Crocodilians/induction, <30-60 min; recovery, hours to days; in larger animals, 12-15 mg/kg may permit tracheal intubation[123]; not recommended alone in Nile crocodiles[144]
Ketamine (K)/butorphanol (B)	See (K) dosages + (B) ≤1.5 mg/kg IM[123]	Snakes/anesthesia with improved muscle relaxation
	(K) 10-30 mg/kg + (B) 0.5-1.5 mg/kg IM[123]	Chelonians/minor surgical procedures (i.e., shell repair)
Ketamine (K)/diazepam (D)	See (K) dosages + (D) 0.2-0.8 mg/kg IM[123]	Snakes/anesthesia with improved muscle relaxation
	(K) 60-80 mg/kg[112]+ (D) 0.2-1 mg/kg IM[123]	Chelonians/anesthesia; muscle relaxation
Ketamine (K)/medetomidine (M)[a]	—	Medetomidine no longer commercially available, can be compounded[a]; reverse with atipamezole
	(K) 10 mg/kg + (M) 0.1-0.3 mg/kg IM[145]	Most species
	(K) 3-8 mg/kg + (M) 0.025-0.08 mg/kg IV[146]	Giant tortoises (Aldabra)
	(K) 4 mg/kg + (M) 0.04 mg/kg IM[147]	Green sea turtles
	(K) 4-10 mg/kg + (M) 0.04-0.14 mg/kg IM[148]	Chelonians/sedation and muscle relaxation for shell repair
	(K) 5 mg/kg + (M) 0.05 mg/kg IV[149]	Loggerhead sea turtles/induction of anesthesia for intubation
	(K) 5-10 mg/kg IM + (M) 0.1-0.15 mg/kg IM, IV[150]	Tortoises (small-medium)
	(K) 10-20 mg/kg IM + (M) 0.15-0.3 mg/kg IM, IV[150]	Turtles (fresh water)
	(K) 5-10 mg/kg + (M) 0.1-0.15 mg/kg IM[151]	Alligators/adults
	(K) 10-15 mg/kg + (M) 0.15-0.25 mg/kg IM[151]	Alligators/juveniles

TABLE 3—cont'd

Chemical Restraint/Anesthetic and Analgesic Agents

Agent	Dosage	Species/Comments
Ketamine (K)/midazolam (M)	(K) 20-40 mg/kg + (M) ≤2 mg/kg IM[152]	Chelonians/sedation; muscle relaxation
	(K) 60-80 mg/kg[112] + (M) ≤2 mg/kg IM[123]	Chelonians/anesthesia; muscle relaxation
Ketoprofen	2 mg/kg SC, IM q24h[133]	Most species/analgesia; in green iguanas, IM, IV q24h; administration at this dose may be too frequent based on PK study[153]
Lidocaine (0.5%-2%)	2-5 mg/kg; local or topical[116,123]	Most species/local analgesia; infiltrate to effect, often used in conjunction with chemical; 10 mg/kg maximum dosage immobilization
Medetomidine[a]	—	Medetomidine is no longer commercially available but can be compounded[a]; poor immobilization alone, see combinations
Meloxicam	0.1-0.5 mg/kg PO, SC q24-48h[57-59]	Most species
	0.5 mg/kg PO, IM or 0.22 mg/kg IV[154]	Red-eared sliders/PK; found better absorption IM vs. PO;[154] after IV administration, plasma levels decreased rapidly
	0.2 mg/kg PO, IV q24h[155]	Green iguanas/PD
	0.1-0.2 mg/kg PO, IM q24h × 4-10 days[148]	Chelonians
Meperidine/Pethidine	5-10 mg/kg IM q12-24h[125]	Most species/analgesia; no noticeable effect in snakes, even at 200 mg/kg
	20 mg/kg IM q12-24h[133]	Most species/analgesia
	2-4 mg/kg ICe q6-8h[57]	Lizards
	2-4 mg/kg ICe[156]	Nile crocodiles/analgesia
Methohexital	5-20 mg/kg SC,[139] IV[12]	Most species/induction, 5-30 min; recovery, 1-5 h; use at 0.125%-0.5% concentration; much species variability; decrease dose 20%-30% for young\animals; avoid use in debilitated animals
	9-10 mg/kg SC,[157] ICe	Colubrids/induction, ≥22 min; recovery, 2-5 h; does not produce soft tissue irritation seen with other barbiturates; may need to adjust dosage in obese snakes
Metomidate	10 mg/kg IM[145,158]	Snakes/profound sedation; not available in the United States
Midazolam	—	See butorphanol, ketamine for combinations; can be reversed by flumazenil
	2 mg/kg IM[115,139]	Most species/preanesthetic; increases efficacy of ketamine; effective in snapping turtles; not in painted turtles[139]
	0.5-2 mg/kg[159]	Lizards
	1.5 mg/kg IM[160]	Turtles (red-eared sliders)/sedation; onset, 5.5 min; duration, 82 min; recovery, 40 min; much individual variability
Morphine	—	No effective analgesic dose in cornsnakes[129]
	1.5-6.5 mg/kg IM[128,129,131,148]	Red-eared sliders (long-lasting respiratory depression), freshwater crocodiles, *Anolis* lizards/may be effective thermal analgesia in bearded dragons
	10 mg/kg IM[129]	Crocodilians/analgesia
Oxymorphone	0.025-0.1 mg/kg IV[12]	Some species/analgesia; avoid in cases with hepatic or renal dysfunction; no noticeable effect in snakes, even at 1.5 mg/kg[115]
	0.05-0.2 mg/kg SC, IM q12-48h[125]	See previous dosage comments within Oxymorphone
Pentazocine	2-5 mg/kg IM q6-24h[125]	Analgesia

Continued

TABLE 3—cont'd

Chemical Restraint/Anesthetic and Analgesic Agents

Agent	Dosage	Species/Comments
Propofol	—	If administered in supravertebral sinus, be aware of potential submeningeal delivery[161]; anesthesia; rapid, smooth induction; 15-25 min anesthesia and restraint in most species; rapid, excitement-free recovery; administered IV/IO slowly; reduce dosages by as much as 50% in premedicated animals; apnea and bradycardia; intubation and IPPV generally required
	0.3-0.5 mg/kg/min IV, IO constant rate infusion or 0.5-1 mg/kg IV, IO periodic bolus[116]	Most species/maintenance anesthesia; must provide respiratory and thermal support
	5-10 mg/kg IV, IC[158,162]	Snakes
	3-5 mg/kg IV, IO[150,163]	Lizards/intubation and minor diagnostic procedures; may need additional dose in 3-5 min; less cardiopulmonary depression
	5-10 mg/kg IV, IO[164]	Iguanas/higher dose is recommended for induction for short duration procedures or intubation
	2 mg/kg IV[132]	Giant tortoises
	3-5 mg/kg IV[148]	Chelonians/sedation (i.e., shell repair)
	10 mg/kg IV[165]	Red-eared sliders/40-85 min anesthesia
	20 mg/kg IV[165]	Red-eared sliders/60-120 min anesthesia
	10-15 mg/kg IV[143]	Crocodilians/duration, 0.5-1.5 h; maintain with gas anesthetics; experimental IM with hyaluronidase
Sevoflurane	To effect[5,166]	Most species/anesthesia; rapid induction and recovery when intubated
Tiletamine/zolazepam	—	Sedation, anesthesia; severe respiratory depression possible—IPPV;[39] variable results; prolonged recovery; lower dose in heavier species; good for muscle relaxation before intubation[130,167]
	4-5 mg/kg SC, IM[139]	Most species/sedation; induction, 9-15 min; recovery, 1-12 h; adequate for most noninvasive procedures
	5-10 mg/kg IM[132]	Most species
	3 mg/kg IM[150]	Snakes/facilitates handling and intubation of large snakes; induction, 30-45 min; prolongs recovery
	10-30 mg/kg IM[112] to 20-40 mg/kg IM[13,168]	Snakes, lizards/induction, 8-20 min; recovery, 2-10 h; variable results; longer sedation and recovery times at 22°C (72°F) than at 30°C (86°F);[169] good sedation in boa constrictors at 25 mg/kg IM[169]; generally need to supplement with inhalational agents for surgical anesthesia; some snakes died at 55 mg/kg
	5-10 mg/kg IM, IV[123]	Large tortoises/facilitates intubation; if light, mask with isoflurane rather than redosing
	1-2 mg/kg IM[15]	Crocodilians/recovery takes several hours
	2-10 mg/kg IM[123]	Large crocodilians/may permit intubation
	10-40 mg/kg SC, IM, ICe[143]	Crocodilians, anesthesia
	15 mg/kg IM[170]	Alligators/induction, >20 min; minor procedures
Tramadol	11 mg/kg PO[171]	Bearded dragons
	5-10 mg/kg PO[172]	Red-eared sliders/thermal analgesia, higher doses may affect ventilation
Xylazine	—	Infrequently used; variable effects; potentially reversible with yohimbine
	0.1-1.25 mg/kg IM, IV[12]	Most species
	0.1-1 mg/kg IM[15]	Crocodilians/atipamezole better reversal
	1-2 mg/kg IM[113,143]	Nile crocodiles

CPR, Cardiopulmonary resuscitation; *IC,* intracardiac; *ICe,* intracoelomic; *IM,* intramuscular; *IO,* intraosseous; *IP,* intraperitoneal; *IPPV,* intermittent positive pressure ventilation; *IT,* intrathecal; *IV,* intravenous; *PD,* pharmacodynamic; *PK,* pharmacokinetic; *PO,* by mouth; *prn,* as required; *SC,* subcutaneous.

[a]Medetomidine is no longer commercially available, although it can be obtained from select compounding services. Dosages listed here are a guide for possible use with dexmedetomidine, an α_2 agonist that is the active optical enantiomer of the racemic compound medetomidine. It is used at half the dose of medetomidine but the same volume because of higher concentration. Although the same effects would be expected as with medetomidine, there are limited data on the efficacy and safety of dexmedetomidine in reptiles, and, to date, it appears to have been seldom used clinically in reptiles. The effects of the volume-to-volume use of the two drugs may not be equivalent, so the dose of dexmedetomidine may need to be adjusted based on clinical response.

TABLE 4

Hormones and Steroids

Agent	Dosage	Species/Comments
Arginine vasotocin	0.01-1 μg/kg IV, ICe[173] q12-24h × 2-3 treatments	Most species/dystocias; give 30-60 min after parenteral Ca; available for research; higher doses reported; 0.5 μg/kg commonly recommended
Calcitonin	1.5 U/kg SC q8h × 14-21 days prn[12]	Most species (e.g., iguanas)/severe NSHP; administer after Ca; avoid if hypocalcemic
	50 U/kg IM repeat in 14 days[30,174] 50 U/kg q7d × 2-3 doses[175,176]	Green iguanas/salmon calcitonin; do not give if hypocalcemic
Dexamethasone	0.6-1.25 mg/kg IM, IV[12]	Most species/shock (septic/traumatic)
	2-4 mg/kg IM, IV q24h × 3 days[177]	Most species/inflammatory, noninfectious respiratory disease
	0.3-1.5 mg/kg IM, IV, IO[59]	Chelonians/hyperthermia
Dexamethasone sodium phosphate	0.1-0.25 mg/kg SC, IM, IV[17]	Most species/shock (septic/traumatic)
Insulin	1-5 U/kg IM, ICe q24-72h[178]	Snakes, chelonians/doses adjusted based on response to therapy and serial blood glucose; ICe may take 24-48 h before response
	5-10 U/kg IM, ICe q24-72h[178]	Lizards, crocodilians/see previous dosage comments within Insulin
Leuprolide acetate	0.4 mg/kg IM[179]	Iguanas/did not suppress testosterone levels in males
Levothyroxine	0.02 mg/kg PO q48h[180]	Tortoises/hypothyroidism; stimulates feeding in debilitated tortoises
	0.025 mg/kg q24h in morning[181]	Tortoises/monitor T_4 levels
Methylprednisolone	1 mg/kg IV q24h[59]	Chelonians/ivermectin toxicity
Nandrolone	0.5-5 mg/kg IM q7-28d[182]	Most species/hepatic lipidosis
	1 mg/kg IM q7-28d[183]	Lizards/anabolic steroid; reduces protein catabolism; may stimulate erythropoiesis
Oxytocin	—	Dystocias; results variable; works well in chelonians, less in snakes and lizards; give 1 h after Ca administration
	1-10 U/kg IM[31,184]	Most species/higher dose is commonly used; may be repeated up to three treatments at 90 min intervals, increasing dosage
	2 U/kg IM q4-6h × 1-3 treatments[185]	Most species
	1-5 U/kg IM,[186] repeat in 1 h	Lizards/alternatively, 5 U/kg by slow IV or IO over 4-8 h[186]
	1-2,[187] 2-20,[17,67] or 10-20[188] U/kg IM	Chelonians
Prednisolone	2-5 mg/kg PO, IM[133]	Most species/analgesia (chronic pain)
	0.5 mg/kg q24h × 14 days, then q48h until PCV stable[57]	Lizards/autoimmune hemolytic anemia
Prednisolone sodium succinate	5-10 mg/kg IM, IV,[119] IO[183]	Most species/shock; hyperthermia; may help reduce nephrocalcinosis
Prednisone	0.5-1 mg/kg PO, SC, IM, IV[189]	Most species/lymphoma, leukemia, myeloproliferative disease
	0.8 mg/kg q48h[190]	Most species/chronic T-lymphocytic leukemia; combine with chlorambucil, but monitor uric acid levels
Stanozolol	5 mg/kg IM q7d prn[17]	Most species/anabolic steroid; management of catabolic disease states

Ca, Calcium; *ICe*, intracoelomic; *IM*, intramuscular; *IO*, intraosseous; *IV*, intravenous; *NSHPT*, nutritional secondary hyperparathyroidism; *PCV*, packed cell volume; *PO*, by mouth; *prn*, as required; *SC*, subcutaneous; T_4, thyroxine.

TABLE 5

Nutritional/Mineral/Fluid Support*

Agent	Dosage	Species/Comments
Calcium glubionate	10 mg/kg PO q12-24h prn[70]	All species/NSHPT
	360 mg/kg (1 mL/kg) PO q12-24h prn[39,174]	Most species/NSHPT; hypocalcemia; dystocia; ensure adequate UVB exposure and proper nutrition
Calcium gluconate	100 mg/kg SC, IM, ICe[191,192] q6-24h[39,174]	Most species/hypocalcemia (low ionized Ca); when patient is stable switch to oral Ca
Calcium gluconate/borogluconate	10-50 mg/kg SC, IM[70]	Most species/hypocalcemia; hypocalcemic dystocia
Calcium glycerophosphate/Calcium lactate	1-5 mg/kg SC, IM[70]	Most species/hypocalcemia; hypocalcemic dystocia
	10-25 mg/kg SC, IM[17]	Most species/hypocalcemia; dystocia
	10 mg/kg SC, IM, ICe q24h × 1-7 days[5,174]	Lizards (iguanas)/hypocalcemia
Electrolyte solutions	Voluntary drinking (whole body soak)[193]	All species/oral fluid therapy; early treatment of anorexia; dilute 1:1 with water; caution against drowning
	10-20 mL/kg via gavage or esophagostomy tube q24h[193]	All species/rehydration; when stable; first stage in supplemental nutrition
Hydroxyethyl starch	3-5 mL/kg slow IV or IO bolus prn[193,194]	All species/hypoalbuminemia; hypovolemic perfusion deficits; increased capillary permeability; use with crystalloids; reduce crystalloid volume 40%-60%; max volume 20 mL/kg[195]
Iodine	2-4 mg/kg PO q24h × 14-21 days, then q7d[17]	Herbivorous species/iodine deficiency (goiter); suggested daily dietary iodine 0.03 mg/kg BW[196]
Iron dextran	12 mg/kg IM 1-2 ×/wk × 45 days[197]	Crocodilians/iron deficiency; in other species for anemia[99]
Lactated Ringer's solution (LRS)	15-40 mL/kg SC, IV, IO prn[194]	Land turtles/fluid replacement; use extracoelomically after warming the patient; avoid lactate if hepatic insufficiency
Metronidazole	12.5-50 mg/kg PO[11]	Most species/appetite stimulant
	50-100 mg/kg PO[18]	Chameleons/appetite stimulant
Polymerized bovine hemoglobin	3-5 mL/kg slow IV or IO bolus prn[193,194]	All species/hemoglobin polymer; hypoalbuminemia; hemorrhage; severe anemia; hypovolemic perfusion deficits; increased capillary permeability; use with crystalloids; reduce crystalloid volume 40%-60%; max volume 20 mL/kg[195]
Replacement crystalloid solutions	10-30 mL/kg q24h or divided into 2-3 boluses several hours apart[198]	All species/ongoing regurgitation or severe diarrhea
	15-25 mL/kg/day PO, SC, IV, IO, ICe, EpiCe prn[136]	All species/replacement fluid therapy; warm to 29°C (84°F)[194]
Ringer's solution for reptiles:	10-20 mL/kg q24h[199]	All species/hypertonic dehydration or to prevent aminoglycoside nephrotoxicity
1 part Normosol-R + 2 parts 2.5% dextrose in 0.45% saline[197] or	15 (large reptiles) to 25 (small reptiles) mL/kg q24h or divided into 2 doses per day[136]	All species/hypertonic dehydration; warm fluids to 28°C (82°F)
1 part Normosol-R + 1 part 5% dextrose + 1 part 0.9% saline	20 mL/kg q12h[39]	Chelonians/severe dehydration
Selenium	0.028 mg/kg IM[5]	Lizards/deficiency; myopathy
Vitamin A	—	Overdose causes epidermal sloughing; greater risk with aqueous parenteral formulation[196,200,201]; may help infectious stomatitis
	1000-5000 U/kg IM q7-10d × 4 treatments[17]	Most species/hypovitaminosis A
	2000 U/30 g BW PO once, repeat in 7 days[201,202]	Chameleons/eye swelling, respiratory disease, hemipenile plugs, dysecdysis
	200-300 U/kg[196] SC, IM	Turtles/hypovitaminosis A; give in conjunction with PO vitamin A (2-8 U/g feed DM)

TABLE 5—cont'd

Nutritional/Mineral/Fluid Support*

Agent	Dosage	Species/Comments
Vitamins A, D_3, E	0.15 mL/kg IM, repeat in 21 days[31]	Most species/hypovitaminosis A, D_3, or E; contains alcohol and may sting when given; alcohol-free product can be compounded commercially
	0.3 mL/kg PO, then 0.06 mL/kg q7d × 3-4 treatments[188]	Box turtles/hypovitaminosis A; parenteral use may result in hypervitaminosis A and D; given PO may enhance Ca uptake
Vitamin B complex	0.3 mL/kg SC, IM q24h[99]	Most species/anorexia; hypovitaminosis B
	25 mg thiamine/kg PO q24h × 3-7 days[185]	Most species/appetite stimulant; hypovitaminosis B
Vitamin B_1 (thiamine)	50-100 mg/kg PO, SC, IM q24h[203]	Piscivores/thiamine deficiency from thawed fish
	30 g/kg feed fish PO[17]	Crocodilians/treat or prevent deficiency
Vitamin B_{12} (cyanocobalamin)	0.05 mg/kg SC, IM[17]	Snakes, lizards/appetite stimulant
Vitamin C	10-20 mg/kg SC, IM q24h[204,205]	All species/hypovitaminosis C; stomatitis; skin slough in snakes; supportive therapy for bacterial infections
Vitamin D_3	—	NSHPT; hypocalcemia; deficiency and excess may lead to soft tissue calcification
	1000 U/kg IM, repeat in 1 wk[39]	Most species/deficiency; use with oral calcium glubionate and carbonate, general dietary management, and UVB irradiation
	200 U/kg PO, IM q7d[5,174]	Lizards/PO safer than IM
	400 U/kg IM q7d × 3 treatments[175]	Green iguanas/NSHPT; use with calcitonin after normocalcemic; also give PO calcium
Vitamin E/selenium	1 U vitamin E/kg[196] IM	Piscivores/hypovitaminosis E; myopathy, anorexia, swollen subcutaneous nodules
	50 U vit E/kg + 0.025 mg selenium/kg IM[206]	Lizards/hypovitaminosis E (vitamin E/selenium)
Vitamin K_1	0.25-0.5 mg/kg IM[31]	Most species/hypovitaminosis K_1; coagulopathies

BW, Body weight; *Ca*, calcium; *DM*, dry matter; *ICe*, intracoelomic; *IM*, intramuscular; *IO*, intraosseous; *IV*, intravenous; *NSHPT*, nutritional secondary hyperparathyroidism; *PO*, by mouth; *prn*, as required; *SC*, subcutaneous; *UVB*, ultraviolet B.
*See also Table 10.

TABLE 6

Miscellaneous Agents

Agent	Dosage	Species/Comments
Allopurinol	10-20 mg/kg PO q24h[67,183,207]	Most species/gout; decreases production of uric acid;[208] long-term therapy; tortoises may respond best
	25 mg/kg PO q24h[209]	Green iguanas
	50 mg/kg PO q24h × 30 days, then q72h[210]	Chelonians/hyperuricemia
Aluminum hydroxide	100 mg/kg PO q12-24h[208]	Most species/hyperphosphatemia; decreases intestinal absorption of phosphorus; use cautiously in patients with gastric outlet obstruction
Amidotrizoate	7.5 mL/kg PO[211]	Tortoises/gastrointestinal contrast agent; give via gavage; mean transit times: 2.6 h at 30.6°C (87°F); 6.6 h at 21.5°C (71°F)
Aminophylline	2-4 mg/kg IM[12]	Most species/bronchodilator
Atropine	0.01-0.04 mg/kg IM, IV q8-24h[212]	Most species/dries up excess mucous secretions with infectious stomatitis
	0.1-0.2 mg/kg IM prn[31]	Most species/organophosphate toxicity prn
	0.2 mg/kg SC, IM[213]	Most species/respiratory distress associated with excessive secretions
Barium sulfate	5-20 mL/kg PO[214]	Most species/gastrointestinal contrast studies

Continued

TABLE 6—cont'd

Miscellaneous Agents

Agent	Dosage	Species/Comments
Calcium EDTA	10-40 mg/kg IM q12h[191]	Most species/heavy metal chelation; ensure hydration
Carboplatin	2.5-5 mg/kg IV, IC[189]	Most species/chemotherapy
Chlorambucil	0.1-0.2 mg/kg PO[189]	Most species/chemotherapy
Cimetidine	4 mg/kg PO, IM q8-12h[17]	Most species/gastric and duodenal ulceration; esophagitis; gastroesophageal reflux; may use in renal failure to increase phosphate loss
Cisapride	0.5-2 mg/kg PO q24h[30]	Most species/motility modifier; GI stasis; may be compounded in the United States; ineffective in desert tortoises at 1 mg/kg[215]
Cisplatin	0.5-1 mg/kg IV (prehydrate), IC, intralesional (in oil)[189]	Most species/chemotherapy
Cyclophosphamide	10 mg/kg SC, IM, IV, IC[189]	Most species/chemotherapy
Dioctyl sodium sulfosuccinate	1-5 mg/kg PO[216]	Most species/constipation; use 1:20 dilution
Doxorubicin	1 mg/kg IV q7d × 2 treatments, then q14d × 2 treatments, then q21d × 2 treatments[217]	Snakes/chemotherapy
Furosemide	2-5 mg/kg PO, IM, IV q12-24h[17,31,57-59]	Most species/diuretic for edema and pulmonary congestion, while lacking loop of Henle, may effect via other mechanisms
Hydrochlorothiazide	1 mg/kg q24-72h[183]	Lizards/promotes diuresis; monitor hydration status
Iodine compound	500 mg/kg IV, IO[183]	Lizards/IV urography; take radiographs 0, 5, 15, 30, and 60 min postinjection
Iohexol	5-20 mL/kg PO[89]	Most species/gastrointestinal contrast studies, nonionic, organic iodine solution; good alternative to barium;[214] faster transit time than barium; can be diluted 1:1 with water
Lactulose	0.5 mL/kg PO q24h[57,59,218]	Lizards, chelonians/hepatic lipidosis
L-Asparaginase	400 U/kg SC, IM, IC[187]	Most species/chemotherapy
Melphalan	0.05-0.1 mg/kg PO[187]	Most species/chemotherapy
Methimazole	2 mg/kg q24h × 30 days[200]	Snakes/excessive shedding from hyperthyroidism; limited effectiveness
Methotrexate	0.25 mg/kg IV, SC, PO[187]	Most species/chemotherapy
Metoclopramide	0.06 mg/kg PO q24h × 7 day[30,219]	Most species/stimulates gastric motility
	1-10 mg/kg PO q24h[220]	Tortoises/stimulates gastric motility; ineffective in desert tortoises at 1 mg/kg[215]
Milk thistle (*Silybum marianum*)	4-15 mg/kg PO q8-12h[57,59]	Lizards, chelonians/ hepatoprotectant
Pentobarbital	60-100 mg/kg IV, ICe[221,222]	Euthanasia
Pimobendan	0.2 mg/kg PO q24h[57]	Lizards
Potassium chloride	2 mEq/kg IV, ICe[174]	Most species/euthanasia; cardioplegic; administer after a euthanasia solution
Probenecid	250 mg/kg PO q12h[223]	Most species/gout; increases uric acid excretion; can be increased prn
S-Adenosylmethionine	30 mg/kg PO q24h[224]	Savannah monitors/liver disease
Sodium bicarbonate	0.5-1 mg/kg IV[30]	Most species/hypoxic acidosis postanesthesia
Sucralfate	500-1000 mg/kg PO q6-8h[12]	Most species/oral, esophageal, gastric, and duodenal ulcers
Tamoxifen 60-day time-release pellets	Pellets containing 5 mg tamoxifen implants, ICe[225]	Leopard geckos/inhibition of follicular development for 60 days if implanted before vitellogenesis
Vincristine	0.025 mg/kg IV[189]	Most species/chemotherapy

GI, Gastrointestinal; *IC*, intracavitary; *ICe*, intracoelomic; *IM*, intramuscular; *IV*, intravenous; *PO*, by mouth; *prn*, as required; *SC*, subcutaneous.

TABLE 7

Hematologic and Serum Biochemical Values[a]

Measurement	Boa constrictor (Boa constrictor)[226-228]	Emerald tree boa (Corallus caninus)[228]	Rainbow boa (Epicrates cenchria)[228]	Blood python (Python curtus)[228]	South Asian pythons (Python molurus ssp)[228]	Ball python (Python regius)[228,229]	Green tree python (Chondropython viridis)[228]	Jungle carpet python (Morelia spilota cheynei)[228,230]	Reticulated python (Python reticulatus)[228]
HEMATOLOGY									
PCV (%)	29 (10-45)	22.6 (6-57)	28 (11-40)	25 (15-49)	28 (18-36)	22 (10-30)	17 (8-27)	25 (10-46)	24 (18-30)
RBC ($10^6/\mu L$)	0.73 (0.16-2.1)	2.16 (0.54-5.05)	0.92 (0.34-1.74)	0.65	1.44 (0.65-6.9)	0.82 (0.12-1.31)	0.85 (0.4-1.3)	0.92 (0.54-1.3)	0.72 (0.41-1.25)
Hgb (g/dL)	9 (2.6-15.3)	8.2 (6.1-11.4)	10.6 (8-13.1)	—	9.4 (7-11)	8.0 (5.5-9.6)	5.9 (4-7)	9.3 (4-15.5)	10.7 (5.2-30)
MCV (fL)	393 (159-625)	237 (37-360)	292 (175-534)	340	275 (52-384)	381 (211-917)	229 (208-250)	282 (178-414)	343 (176-429)
MCH (pg)	132 (84-208)	120 (113-128)	160	—	93 (16-127)	82-139	100	114 (67-159)	138 (60-186)
MCHC (g/dL)	32 (22-42)	34 (30-36)	36 (33-40)	—	32 (29-35)	31 (25-40)	36 (33-40)	40 (24-53)	37 (29-45)
WBC ($10^3/\mu L$)	8.54 (0.88-22.6)	4.35 (0.48-10.6)	7.99 (1-35.2)	11.7 (1.13-42.5)	9.94 (2-19.8)	9.74 (1-26)	11.3 (3.5-22.1)	11.93 (1.72-34.1)	7.6 (1.8-17.7)
Heterophils ($10^3/\mu L$)	2.46 (0.21-12.3)	1.61 (0.18-5.36)	2.85 (0.03-10)	1.82 (0.31-3.99)	2.36 (0.42-6.84)	2.86 (0.37-10.80)	3.89 (0.86-6.63)	2.78 (0.29-11.3)	2.03 (0.5-4.02)
Lymphocytes ($10^3/\mu L$)	4.01 (0.16-18.5)	2.48 (0.14-8.27)	3.91 (0.1-32.4)	6.71 (0.34-33.6)	5.78 (0.34-18.6)	4.18 (0.13-14.10)	3.44 (0.21-11.2)	6.11 (0.6-19.7)	3.77 (0.42-11.9)
Monocytes ($10^3/\mu L$)	0.68 (0.02-6.55)	0.45 (0.06-2.12)	0.9 (0.03-3.06)	0.62 (0.13-2.12)	1.016 (0.06-5.01)	1.00 (0.01-3.20)	0.74 (0.04-2.35)	2.21 (0.06-8.79)	1.72 (0.11-6.76)
Azurophils ($10^3/\mu L$)	1.75 (0-5.76)	0.71 (0.1-1.84)	1.08 (0.11-4.44)	2.82 (0.27-6.8)	1.81 (0.26-4.8)	3.4 (0.3-13.26)	5.42 (0.97-13.9)	3.46 (0.09-18.04)	3.73 (1.07-6.88)
Eosinophils ($10^3/\mu L$)	0.26 (0.03-1.22)	0.07 (0.06-0.08)	0.11 (0.04-0.22)	0.08	0.45 (0.1-1.4)	0.25 (0.12-0.37)	0.16 (0.1-0.22)	0.19 (0.08-0.34)	0.68 (0.04-1.95)
Basophils ($10^3/\mu L$)	0.46 (0.03-2.77)	0.07 (0.03-0.14)	0.1 (0.02-0.27)	0.93 (0.32-1.83)	0.25 (0.08-1.08)	0.38 (0.05-1.12)	0.55 (0.07-1.8)	0.26 (0.05-1.76)	0.06 (0.06-0.7)
CHEMISTRIES									
ALP (U/L)	287 (43-1342)	128 (61-323)	27 (14-37)	44 (8-56)	105 (7-728)	61 (13-153)	209 (112-349)	40 (13-60)	64 (4-144)
ALT (U/L)	14 (0-37)	5 (1-10)	4 (1-6)	10 (3-17)	19 (0-40)	14 (5-26)	43 (8-132)	17 (6-38)	8 (0-29)
Amylase (U/L)	22 (5-67)	293 (160-470)	—	—	3255	2490 (1611-3368)	902 (564-1240)	—	1690 (416-2963)
AST (U/L)	35 (3-331)	30 (5-92)	43 (9-136)	56 (6-209)	22 (1-205)	55 (2-118)	27 (11-75)	16 (5-46)	34 (7-105)
Bilirubin, total (mg/dL)	0.2 (0-0.6)	0.2 (0.2-0.3)	0.4 (0-0.8)	0.3 (0.2-0.5)	0.6 (0-2)	0.4 (0-2.1)	0.2	0.5	0.3
BUN (mg/dL)	5 (0-34)	2 (0-4)	2 (1-3)	1 (0-2)	4 (1-14)	1 (0-3)	2 (0-2)	3 (2-3)	4 (0-12)
Calcium (mg/dL)	15.9 (9-27)	12.7 (10.3-17.4)	13.4 (11.3-18.9)	14.7 (13.5-16.2)	19 (9.9-34)	15.3 (10.8-22.2)	23.4 (10.3-80.1)	14.4 (12.8-16.5)	23.5 (8.6-78)
Chloride (mEq/L)	125 (108-139)	130 (119-138)	115 (94-128)	131 (123-138)	118 (101-135)	120 (109-130)	125 (119-130)	115 (109-123)	118 (104-129)
Cholesterol (mg/dL)	131 (34-314)	206 (116-343)	206 (140-314)	214 (76-445)	289 (146-445)	182 (23-302)	204 (116-360)	315 (264-386)	309 (257-356)
Creatine kinase (U/L)	526 (53-1728)	592 (157-985)	154 (31-745)	668 (327-1009)	494 (42-3093)	1318 (93-3108)	614	398 (27-1350)	1818 (356-8342)
Creatinine (mg/dL)	0.4 (0.1-1.6)	0.6 (0.4-0.9)	0.4 (0.1-0.7)	0.9 (0.5-1.3)	1.4 (0.1-16.9)	0.2 (0-0.5)	0.2 (0.2-0.5)	1.3 (0.3-3.7)	0.2 (0.1-0.4)
GGT (U/L)	4 (0-10)	2 (1-2)	5	8 (0-16)	9 (0-26)	5	78 (5-223)	31 (16-71)	38 (14-64)
Glucose (mg/dL)	37 (9-85)	27 (5-56)	17 (2-46)	30 (13-74)	24 (1-83)	23 (2-43)	—	32 (9-55)	22
Iron (µg/dL)	113 (103-122)	—	—	207 (49-364)	456 (20-5525)	371 (77-782)	206	306 ± 160	313 (43-1048)
LDH (U/L)	235 (16-877)	632 (76-1680)	401 (141-661)	4.9	—	—	—	330 (48-547)	—
Lipase (U/L)	2730	—	—	3.7 (3.1-4.5)	4.7 (2.9-9.1)	3.8 (0.9-7.2)	11.8 (4-26.3)	3.4 (2.1-6.1)	7.2 (2.5-14.58)
Magnesium (mEq/L)	2.95 (2.9-3)	—	—	6.3 (3.3-11.2)	4.8 (3.8-6.3)	7.1 (4.3-10.5)	5.3 (5.2-5.3)	6.1 (4.9-9)	6.6 (4.4-10.2)
Osmolarity (mOsm/L)	306	—	—	6.2 (3.6-8.1)	7.3 (4.2-10.5)	6.7 (3.2-10.5)	5.4 (3.9-6.9)	7.6 (5.9-10.9)	7.5 (6.1-9.8)
Phosphorus (mg/dL)	4.7 (2.6-11.7)	4.1 (1.8-8)	5.4 (3.8-7.7)	2.3 (1.6-2.8)	2.7 (1.7-3.9)	2.5 (1-8.4)	2 (1.3-2.7)	3.1 (2.8-3.3)	3.9 (1.9-7.2)
Potassium (mEq/L)	5.4 (3-10)	5 (3-8.7)	3.2 (1.2-5)	4.1 (3.1-4.9)	4.9 (2.4-6.7)	4.6 (2.1-9)	4.4 (3.4-5)	4.9 (4.2-5.5)	5.4 (3.7-8)
Protein, total (g/dL)	7 (4.3-10.8)	4.5 (2.6-7.2)	6.2 (3.7-8)	160 (155-164)	158 (151-165)	159 (146-173)	158 (157-159)	153 (150-158)	157 (142-169)
Albumin (g/dL)[b]	3.1 (1.9-5.3)	2.6 (2-3.6)	2.6 (1.8-3.6)	16 (13-22)	114 (16-532)	31	—	30	45
Globulin (g/dL)[b]	4 (2.2-6.9)	2.8 (1.8-3.6)	4.1 (2.8-5.8)	4.3 (2.1-7.1)	4.3 (1.3-18)	7.6 (1.1-23)	7.7 (1.6-20.4)	6.5 (1.9-23.7)	7.8 (3.5-17.4)
Sodium (mEq/L)	158 (130-171)	157 (148-167)	155 (137-163)						
Triglyceride (mg/dL)	103 (3-457)	24 (10-49)	72 (64-90)						
Uric acid (mg/dL)	4.7 (0-11.9)	4.7 (1.4-19.2)	7.2 (2.1-27.5)						

Continued

TABLE 7—cont'd

Hematologic and Serum Biochemical Values[a]

Measurement	Gopher snake (Pituophis catenifer)[228,231]	Cornsnake (Elaphe guttata)[228]	Yellow rat snake (Elaphe obsoleta quadrivitatta)[228,232]	Common kingsnake (Lampropeltis getula)[228]	Milk snake (Lampropeltis triangulum)[228]	Indigo snake (Drymarchon corais)[228,233]	Panther chameleon (Furcifer pardalis)[228]	Spiny-tailed lizard (Uromastyx spp)[228,234]	Blue-tongued skink (Tiliqua scincoides)[228]
HEMATOLOGY									
PCV (%)	25 (15-38)	32 (21-52)	24 (9-46)	29 (12-45)	26 (8-38)	24 (15-34)	27 (16-35)	29 (4.9-44.5)	31 (22-46)
RBC (10^6/μL)	0.67 (0.14-1.4)	1.21 (0.62-1.85)	0.77 (0.21-1.34)	3.11 (0.35-14)	0.89 (0.49-2)	0.62 (0.43-0.76)	0.83 (0.42-1.6)	0.78 (0.33-4.1)	1.1 (0.73-1.36)
Hgb (g/dL)	9.7 (4.3-12.3)	11.5 (9.7-13.5)	8.3 (2.8-15.2)	—	10.4 (6.9-11.9)	9.2 (7.3-11.1)	—	9.9 (3.3-17.4)	10.4 (6-13)
MCV (fL)	578 (246-1571)	315 (171-404)	361 (198-765)	304 (27.9-500)	377 (135-615)	369 (221-558)	330 (200-418)	415 (119-614)	299 (266-354)
MCH (pg)	111 (81-132)	127 (110-143)	121 (90-175)	—	119 (89-164)	258	—	133 (1.2-203)	98 (44-173)
MCHC (g/dL)	33 (27.5-36)	35 (32-40)	32 (26-54)	—	34 (29-45)	40 (33-46)	—	33 (22-41)	33 (16-57)
WBC (10^3/μL)	6.36 (1.56-11.5)	11.3 (1.02-31.4)	9.32 (0.37-25)	12.7 (1.46-42.2)	9.17 (1.25-24.7)	10.8 (2-26.9)	—	958 (290-2290)	—
Heterophils (10^3/μL)	1.62 (0.18-9.43)	2.7 (0.21-8.35)	1.93 (0.06-10.5)	1.63 (0.19-4.8)	1.14 (0.05-4.46)	1.96 (0.35-8.1)	6.18 (0.47-18.6)	3.1 (1-8.1)	7.3 (2.2-19.6)
Lymphocytes (10^3/μL)	3.39 (0.24-8.03)	5.61 (0.41-22.9)	4.05 (0.14-14.4)	7.5 (0.13-33.3)	5.92 (0.47-19.2)	6.26 (0.28-16.7)	1.57 (0.09-4.17)	2 (0.59-5.36)	2.45 (0.54-6.24)
Monocytes (10^3/μL)	0.88 (0.05-3.07)	0.93 (0.04-1.75)	1.5 (0.01-9.72)	0.8 (0.05-5.83)	1.15 (0.07-3.6)	1.5 (0.04-4.84)	2.96 (0.21-9.67)	0.99 (0.27-4.05)	2.75 (0.32-10.9)
Azurophils (10^3/μL)	0.94 (0.45-1.67)	2 (0.15-5.34)	3.05 (0.06-8.33)	3.26 (0.21-8.87)	1.58 (0.03-5.93)	1.58 (0.5-4.69)	—	0.04 (0-0.5)	0.84 (0.35-1.49)
Eosinophils (10^3/μL)	0.08 (0.05-0.12)	0.1 (0.08-0.12)	0.1 (0.01-0.22)	0.11 (0.02-0.22)	0.1 (0.01-0.25)	0.23 (0.13-0.43)	1.25 (0.08-3.74)	—	0.34 (0-1.08)
Basophils (10^3/vL)	0.15 (0.02-0.51)	0.55 (0.07-1.44)	0.26 (0.05-0.66)	0.42 (0.1-1.3)	0.33 (0.04-1.82)	0.4 (0.08-0.74)	—	0.04 (0-0.2)	1.5 (0.03-2.96)
							0.1 (0.07-0.13)	0.03 (0-0.33)	0.98 (0.11-2.24)
CHEMISTRIES									
ALP (U/L)	58 (9-170)	54 (23-75)	142 (37-858)	88 (23-152)	108 (70-168)	123 (80-161)	—	31 (5.9-139)	71 (39-101)
ALT (U/L)	22 (11-65)	34 (4-62)	13 (2-72)	18 (8-25)	8 (3-17)	10 (3-16)	—	11 (2.4-35)	20 (5-34)
Amylase (U/L)	344 (214-473)	458 (366-574)	1337 (630-2626)	848	665	—	—	134	—
AST (U/L)	53 (16-127)	43 (10-224)	29 (2-142)	54 (5-249)	46 (0-178)	46 (6-163)	10 (0-31)	73 (29-172)	50 (7-106)
Bilirubin, total (mg/dL)	0.4 (0.3-0.6)	0.7 (0.1-1)	0.2 (0.1-0.8)	0.4 (0.1-0.7)	0.4 (0.1-0.9)	2.1 (0.6-3.5)	—	0.3 (0.1-0.7)	—
BUN (mg/dL)	2.2 (1-5)	2 (0-6)	5 (0-20)	2 (0-4)	5 (2-14)	7 (0-22)	—	0.56 (0-3)	1 (0-2)
Calcium (mg/dL)	14.5 (11.1-17.6)	16.1 (13.5-19.6)	15.9 (11.3-73.2)	26.4 (12.3-60)	14.6 (12.4-17.6)	33 (12-59)[c,297]	10.3 (8.9-11.7)	9.9 (7.2-13.2)	14.2 (10.4-20.6)
Chloride (mEq/L)	134 (109-148)	124 (109-137)	118 (68-140)	115 (88-136)	127 (111-134)	119 (100-129)	—	126 (111-135)	113 (111-115)
Cholesterol (mg/dL)	265 (152-493)	433 (314-572)	377 (101-745)	409 (117-1083)	357 (154-563)	278 (116-397)	—	161 (64-295)	183 (72-429)
Creatine kinase (U/L)	669 (175-1763)	699 (91-2460)	221 (73-646)	500 (108-1112)	202 (92-332)	644 (68-1923)	—	1780 (141-10k)	2517 (73-5832)
Creatinine (mg/dL)	0.3 (0.1-0.6)	0.6 (0.2-2)	0.5 (0.2-1.3)	0.6 (0-1.6)	0.5 (0.3-1.1)	0.3 (0.2-0.3)	—	0.4 (0.1-3)	0.3 (0.1-0.6)
GGT (U/L)	10 (0-34)	5 (0-13)	9 (1-35)	9	8 (3-13)	15	—	8	8
Glucose (mg/dL)	88 (24-129)	56 (32-88)	66 (26-117)	46 (8-82)	54 (15-76)	46 (28-89)	294 (219-341)	200 (68-356)	127 (63-160)
Iron (μg/dL)	98	—	—	190 (30-488)	816 (18-2807)	313 (13-1055)	—	209 (22-899)	735 (364-1106)
LDH (U/L)	76 (20-191)	182 (48-444)	419 (4-5665)	6.2 (0.7-15.2)	8.6 (2.9-25)	7.4 (5.3-9)[c,297]	—	3.48 (2.1-10.2)	364
Lipase (U/L)	8 (5-17)	—	4 (3-4)	5.3 (2.8-9.2)	5.5 (3.3-9.7)	6.5 (3.8-14.3)	8.2 (5.5-9.8)	4.5 (1.3-10)	5.7 (2.8-7.7)
Magnesium (mg/dL)	3.2	—	2.5	7.5 (3.6-12)	6.8 (3.8-11.6)	8.6 (4.6-12.3)	—	3.7 (3-4.6)	5.7 (4.3-8.6)
Phosphorus (mg/dL)	4.1 (2.5-5.7)	4.5 (2.8-5.7)	3.7 (1.7-14.7)	2.9 (1.6-6.8)	2.3 (1.8-3)	2.5 (1.7-4.6)	5.8 (4.7-7.8)	4 (2.6-7.4)	6.2 (5.3-7.6)
Potassium (mEq/L)	4.7 (3.3-6.5)	6.7 (3.3-16.6)	4.7 (1.6-8.5)	4 (1.8-5.8)	5.3 (3.3-9)	3.8 (3.3-4.4)	2.5 (1.8-3.2)	2 (1.2-3.1)	2.2 (1.3-2.9)
Protein, total (g/dL)	5.3 (3.2-7.4)	6.8 (4.6-10.8)	6.4 (3.3-8.9)	163 (132-184)	167 (157-178)	157 (143-170)	3.5 (2.9-4.6)	2.9 (2.2-4.6)	4 (3.3-5.2)
Albumin (g/dL)[b]	2.4 (1.6-3.2)	3.6 (2.5-7.6)	2.3 (1.6-3.8)	149 (66-278)	428 (68-1620)	92 (76-118)	—	173 ± 4	149 (142-158)
Globulin (g/dL)[b]	3.1 (1.9-3.2)	3.9 (3.2-4.8)	4.1 (2.6-6.4)	5.7 (2.4-14.7)	6.3 (2.1-35.6)	8.6 (2.2-17.1)	—	175 (111-238)	—
Sodium (mEq/L)	171 (155-187)	165 (154-174)	164 (151-177)				9.4 (4-16.1)	2.94 (0.3-7.3)	3.8 (0.7-8.5)
Triglyceride (mg/dL)	27 (16-37)	331 (47-1118)	195 (21-1017)						
Uric acid (mg/dL)	6.7 (2-17.6)	7.2 (2.8-19.9)	7.6 (1.6-47)						

Measurement	Bearded dragon (Pogona vitticeps)[228,235]	Chinese (Asian) water dragon (Physignathus cocincinus)[236]	Green iguana (Iguana iguana)[228,237-242]	Green iguana (Iguana iguana) male[e,243,244]	Green iguana (Iguana iguana) female[e,243,244]	Green iguana (Iguana iguana) juvenile[e,243]	Prehensile-tailed skink (Corucia zebrata)[228,245]	Tegu lizard (Tupinambis spp)[f,228,246]	Green basilisk (Basiliscus plumifrons)[228]
HEMATOLOGY									
PCV (%)	30 (19-40)	35 (32-40)	25-38	34 (29-39)	38 (33-44)	38 (30-47)	35 (24-60)	25 ± 2.6	36 (29-41)
RBC ($10^6/\mu L$)	0.97 (0.68-1.21)	—	1-1.9	1.3 (1-1.7)	1.4 (1.2-1.8)	1.4 (1.3-1.6)	1.5 (0.66-3.28)	0.96 ± 0.14	—
Hgb (g/dL)	9.5 (6.7-12)	—	8-12	8.6 (6.7-10.2)	10.6 (9.1-12.2)	9.6 (9.2-10.1)	9.6 (7.4-11.6)	11.4 ± 1.6	8.9 (8.6-9.1)
MCV (fL)	311 (236-397)	—	165-305	266 (228-303)	270 (235-331)	—	263 (152-600)	261 ± 23	—
MCH (pg)	108 (81-140)	—	65-105	25 (23-28)	28 (25-31)	—	69 (42-111)	119 ± 12.5	—
MCHC (g/dL)	34 (24-45)	—	20-38	15 (11-25)	15 (8-25)	16 (8-22)	28 (17-56)	45.6 ± 3.4	26 (22-29)
WBC ($10^3/\mu L$)	8.14 (1.99-23)	13.5 (11.7-18.2)	3-10	3.6 (1-5.4)	3.2 (0.6-6.4)	2.2 (1-3.8)	12.4 (3.9-22.4)	16.8 ± 2.5	16.8 (6.1-31)
Heterophils ($10^3/\mu L$)	2.17 (0.35-4.99)	5.1 (3.9-6.9)	0.35-5.2	9.7 (5-16.5)	9.9 (5.2-14.4)	12.9 (6.2-17.2)	4.4 (1.02-6.4)	2.2 ± 0.45	8.9 (2.8-17.7)
Lymphocytes ($10^3/\mu L$)	4.68 (0.57-17)	7.2 (5.6-9.5)	0.5-5.5	1.3 (0.2-2.7)	1.2 (0.4-2.3)	0.4 (0.3-0.6)	2.7 (0.3-4.7)	7.5 ± 0.58	6.4 (1.8-10.7)
Monocytes ($10^3/\mu L$)	0.7 (0.03-2.72)	1.1 (0.4-1.9)	0-0.1	0.1- (0-0.3)	0.1 (0-0.2)	0.3 (0-0.4)	0.1 (0.0-1)	1 ± 0.41	1.5 (0.12-4)
Azurophils ($10^3/\mu L$)	0.53 (0.04-1.84)	0 (0-0.6)	0-1.7	0.4 (0.1-1)	0.5 (0.2-1.2)	0.5 (0.1-0.7)	2.8 (0.4-4.8)	1.8 ± 0.56	—
Eosinophils ($10^3/\mu L$)	0.15 (0.06-0.27)	0.2 (0.1-0.3)	0-1	100 (100-200)	100 (100-300)	100 (100-300)	0.6 (0-3)	4.1 ± 0.11	—
Basophils ($10^3/\mu L$)	0.39 (0.05-1.01)	0.5 (0.2-0.8)	0-0.5				1.9 (0.1-4.3)	0.4 ± 0.01	1.5
Fibrinogen (mg/dL)	180 (0-300)	—	0-300				—	133 (0-200)	—
CHEMISTRIES									
ALP (U/L)	151 (15-447)	—	40 (4-170)	39 (14-65)	59 (22-90)	—	154 (44-334)	160 ± 85	137 (77-230)
ALT (U/L)	12 (5-20)	—	21 (0-97)	32 (4-76)	45 (5-96)	—	9 (2-23)	33 ± 24	13 (5-21)
Amylase (U/L)	497	—	1815 (996-2988)	22 (12-30)	29 (19-41)	—	19 (0-76)	18 ± 14	60 (14-136)
AST (U/L)	27 (0-77)	16.5 (8-52)	52 (2-100)	33 (19-65)	40 (7-102)	41 (13-72)	0.2 (0-0.9)	0.3 ± 0.2	0.6 (0.5-0.8)
Bile acids (rest; μmol/L)	—	—	7.5 (2.6-30.3)	0.8 (0.1-1.4)	1.5 (0.3-3.1)	—	1 (0-2)	1 ± 1	5 (1-20)
Bile acids (7.5h; μmol/L)	—	—	32.5 (15.2-44.1)	11.3 (8.6-14.1)	12.5 (10.8-14)	14.3 (12.1-23.2)	13 (11-21)	12.2 ± 0.8	10.5 (9.8-11.2)
Bilirubin, total (mg/dL)	0.5 (0-3.7)	—	0.3 (0-4.9)	119 (115-124)	121 (113-129)	—	124 (123-129)	121 ± 7	127 (125-129)
BUN (mg/dL)	3 (1-7)	—	2 (0-10)	161 (82-214)	255 (204-347)	—	144 (11-252)	206 ± 67	957 (550-1393)
Calcium (mg/dL)	11.8 (8.6-27)	12.4 (11.6-13.3)	12 (6-18)[d]	19.9 (15.2-24.7)	19 (16-23)	—	210 (27-940)	641 ± 568	5355 (2691-9436)
Ionized Ca^{++} (mmol/L)	—	—	1.01-1.62	79 (36-162)	270 (81-512)	—	0.2 (0-0.7)	0.3 ± 0.1	0.4 (0.2-0.8)
Chloride (mEq/L)	130 (104-160)	—	117 (102-130)	166 (70-244)	170 (105-258)	273 (131-335)	0 (0-1)	7	—
Cholesterol (mg/dL)	513 (230-900)	—	104-333[d]	5.3 (3.2-7.6)	6.3 (2.8-9.3)	7.7 (4.3-9)	100 (70-122)	128 ± 30	174 (60-280)
Creatine kinase (U/L)	1211 (59-7000)	1747 (19-6630)	1876(174-8768)[d]	4 (2.8-6.1)	3.6 (2-5.8)	—	236 (42-1139)	540 ± 537	—
Creatinine (mg/dL)	0.3 (0.0-0.6)	—	0.5 (0.2-1.3)	5.4 (4.4-6.5)	6.1 (4.9-7.6)	5 (4.2-6.1)	361 (335-373)	—	—
GGT (U/L)	2 (1-2)	—	3 (0-10)	2 (1.3-3)	2.4 (1.5-3)	2.3 (2-2.8)	—	—	—
Glucose (mg/dL)	210 (139-291)	157 (112-243)	169-288	3.5 (2.5-4.4)	3.8 (2.8-5.2)	2.7 (2.2-3)	3.7 (2.8-6.7)	5.6 ± 2.1	9.5 (6.2-11.6)
Iron (μg/dL)	—	—	88-133	0.6 (0.4-0.9)	0.7 (0.3-1)	0.8 (0.7-0.9)	3.6 (1.4-5)	2.4 ± 1.4	2.9 (2.4-3.5)
LDH (U/L)	304 (35-628)	—	617 (36-7424)[d]	157 (152-162)	163 (156-172)	—	5.9 (3.8-9)	6.6 ± 1.3	5.7 (4-8.3)
Lipase (U/L)	—	—	21 (17-24)	10.2 (2.2-15.7)	0.26 (0.07-0.35)	—	2.4 (1.3-3.6)	3.6 ± 0.7	3.1 (2.6-3.5)
Magnesium (mEq/L)	—	—	2.4-4	2.7 (1.5-5.8)	3.6 (0.9-6.7)	3.3 (0.7-5.7)	4.8 (3.5-8)	—	—
Phosphorus (mg/dL)	5.7 (2.7-15.1)	5.7 (3.4-8.2)	5 (2.5-21)[d]				3.1 (1.9-5.4)	2.9 ± 1.2	2.9 (2.1-4.9)
Potassium (mEq/L)	3.6 (1-6.5)	4.2 (3.8-4.5)	1.3-3				158 (145-167)	159 ± 4	163 (145-172)
Protein, total (g/dL)	5 (3.6-6.4)	7 (6.6-7.5)	5.4 (4.1-7.4)[d]				93 (28-319)	31	285 (9-712)
Albumin (g/dL)[b]	2.6 (1.3-4.6)	2.2 (2.1-2.3)	2.1-2.8				1.6 (<0.3-3.1)	3.2 ± 2	10.9 (1-96.6)
Albumin (PEP; g/dL)[b]	—	—	1.8 (1.4-3.1)						
Globulin (g/dL)[b]	2.3 (1-4.4)	4.7 (4.5-5.3)	2.5-4.3[d]						
α (PEP; g/dL)[b]	—	—	0.9 (0.4-1.2)						
β (PEP; g/dL)[b]	—	—	2.2 (1.6-3.8)[d]						
γ (PEP; g/dL)[b]	—	—	0.3 (0.1-0.4)						
A/G Ratio	—	—	0.5 (0.41-0.78)						
Sodium (mEq/L)	153 (137-190)	150 (147-153)	158-183						
Triglyceride (mg/dL)	261 (93-437)	—	383 (7-1323)[d]						
Uric acid (mg/dL)	5.2 (1.6-11.4)	2.3 (1.9-2.7)	2.6 (0-8.2)[d]						
Vit D_3 (25-OH; nmol/L)	—	—	51-393[d]						

Continued

TABLE 7—cont'd

Hematologic and Serum Biochemical Values[a]

Measurement	Savannah monitor (Varanus exanthematicus)[228]	Water monitor (Varanus salvator)[228]	American alligator (Alligator mississippiensis)[228]	Dwarf caiman (Paleosuchus palpebrosus)[228]	Eastern box turtle (Terrapene carolina)[228,247,248]	Ornate box turtle (Terrapene ornata)[228]	Radiated tortoise (Astrochelys radiata)[228,249,250]	Red-footed tortoise (Chelonoidis carbonaria)[228]	Indian star tortoise (Geochelone elegans)[228]
HEMATOLOGY									
PCV (%)	31.2 (21-51)	33.2 (20-44)	24.7 (12-38)	22 (16-28)	26 (21-32)	26 (18-37)	10-51	29 (18-47)	21 (12-31)
RBC (10^6/μL)	1.23 (0.63-1.58)	0.98 (0.42-1.42)	0.57 (0.38-1.2)	0.66 (0.43-0.89)	0.49 (0.09-0.89)	0.62 (0.46-0.8)	0.3-1.1	2.1 (0.47-6.3)	0.37 (0.24-0.55)
Hgb (g/dL)	10.5 (6.2-13.2)	10.5 (9.8-11.5)	7.7 (5.7-11.3)	7.7 (6.2-8.8)	5.1	7.2 (6-9)	5.6 (4-8)	7.5 (7-7.9)	7.9 (6.9-8.5)
MCV (fL)	284 (229-382)	335 (227-595)	453 (230-762)	362 (180-535)	420 (229-1000)	408 (350-463)	454 (319-571)	347 (71-468)	—
MCH (pg)	94 (89-99)	140 (104-177)	146 (105-202)	98	102	122 (108-136)	108 (82-133)	136 (123-149)	—
MCHC (g/dL)	32 (26-38)	33 (30-40)	32 (23-44)	33 (23-38)	28 (26-29)	33 (31-33)	28 (26-33)	31 (29-32)	27 (26-28)
WBC (10^3/μL)	5.07 (1.2-11.3)	11.1 (2.9-26)	8.33 (1.75-20.8)	6 (2.7-13.5)	10.8 (8-13)	5.8 (2-11.1)	2.5-14	7.1 (2.2-13.4)	11.02 (0.75-31)
Heterophils (10^3/μL)	1.95 (0.38-4.06)	5.58 (2.09-11.1)	3.85 (0.65-16.7)	3 (1.4-6.2)	4.8 (1.7-9)[f]	1.8 (0.1-4.5)	0.7-8	1.8 (0.09-6.4)	4.09 (0.17-14.9)
Lymphocytes (10^3/μL)	2.12 (0.43-5.25)	3.43 (0.3-10.1)	3.18 (0.36-12.1)	2.57 (0.18-10.1)	4.9 (2.6-8.2)[f]	2.9 (1.5-5.6)	0.4-5.8	3.3 (0.23-6.1)	5.14 (0.16-17.6)
Monocytes (10^3/μL)	1.64 (0.06-6.67)	0.81 (0.06-3.38)	0.37 (0.04-0.84)	0.13 (0.03-0.23)	0.11 (0-0.4)[f]	0.06 (0.04-0.07)	0.02-0.5	0.18 (0.04-0.67)	0.38 (0.02-1.35)
Azurophils (10^3/μL)	0.11	2.26 (0.42-5.98)	0.64 (0.04-3.54)	0.52 (0-1.3)	—	0.25 (0.06-0.67)	0-0.82	0.98 (0.29-2.5)	0.72 (0.08-1.73)
Eosinophils (10^3/μL)	—	0.1	0.29 (0.04-1.02)	0.1 (0.05-0.18)	0.02 (0-0.1)[f]	0.96 (0.07-4.4)	0.03-0.82	0.5 (0.02-2.3)	0.96 (0.08-2.24)
Basophils (10^3/μL)	0.15 (0.07-0.28)	0.11 (0.06-0.14)	0.71 (0.04-3.23)	0.16 (0.05-0.48)	0.21 (0-0.4)[f]	0.42 (0.07-0.94)	0.1-2.5	1.4 (0.05-5.5)	0.76 (0.04-3)
Fibrinogen (mg/dL)	156 (100-300)	500 (200-700)	267 ± 115	100 (0-200)	—	—	117 (100-200)	—	—
CHEMISTRIES									
ALP (U/L)	89 (5-675)	187 (35-410)	46 ± 29	11 (6-16)	62 (29-102)	26 (15-37)	72-392	84 (39-173)	174 (38-379)
ALT (U/L)	70 (7-374)	36 (4-138)	49 ± 42	45 (24-71)	7 (2-14)	30 (25-33)	0-17	18 (4-63)	5 (0-15) 1235
Amylase (U/L)	—	1021 (265-1868)	471 ± 335	533	160	—	—	—	87 (12-296)
AST (U/L)	22 (1-78)	38 (5-239)	314 ± 158	78 (17-139)	124 (2-620)	62 (33-201)	25-348	238 (97-616)	—
Bilirubin, total (mg/dL)	0.1 (0-0.3)	0.1 (0-0.3)	0.2 ± 0.2	0.2 (0-0.6)	0.5 (0.1-1)	0.3 (0.1-0.4)	0.3-31.3	—	0.2 (0-0.4)
BUN (mg/dL)	1 (0-5)	3 (0-6)	3 ± 3	1 (0-2)	49 (20-102)	47 (4-65)	0-0.5	0.5 (0.1-1.1)	4 (0-11)
Calcium (mg/dL)	14.6 (11.9-17.5)	14.4 (8.5-22)	11.2 ± 2.2	10.7 (9.7-11.4)	13.6 (6.5-26.4)	11.1 (8-13.6)	2-34	17 (4-53)	12 (9.3-17.6)
Chloride (mEq/L)	116 (105-124)	110 (100-128)	109 ± 21	113 (99-126)	106 (101-112)	108 (96-115)	8.6-18	12.7 (9.5-15.8)	104 (90-112)
Cholesterol (mg/dL)	116 (49-231)	94 (22-291)	128 ± 73	147 (68-344)	240 (65-496)	155 (125-185)	91-112	100 (89-119)	128 (77-252)
Creatine kinase (U/L)	764 (150-3048)	772 (176-1818)	2663 ± 2493	1984 (37-9890)	463 (37-898)	918 (88-3100)	56-154	146 (47-284)	1496 (144-8518)
Creatinine (mg/dL)	8.7 (0-67)	0.5 (0-1)	0.4 ± 0.2	0.3 (0-0.4)	0.4	1 (0.2-2.4)	33-5666	360 (43-996)	0.3 (0.2-0.5)
GGT (U/L)	7 (1-11)	24 (7-48)	6 ± 7	84 (29-187)	84 (33-153)	71 (8-113)	0.1-0.5	0.4 (0.2-1.3)	4 (0-5)
Glucose (mg/dL)	118 (90-159)	115 (42-215)	92 ± 42	221 (80-485)	206 (111-313)	362 (300-424)	5 (0-11)	28 (7-130)	109 (39-199)
Iron (μg/dL)	—	242 (111-429)	—	—	3.5	—	21-93	94 (17-171)	—
LDH (U/L)	427 (29-3699)	693 (34-3588)	522 ± 541	303 (301-304)	—	—	60	107	438 (12-863)
Lipase (U/L)	—	—	12	3.8 (3.2-5.1)	4 (1.6-8.2)	3.6 (2.7-4.8)	213-6444	401 (242-534)	5
Magnesium (mEq/L)	3.1	2.5 (2.2-2.7)	—	4.1 (3.7-4.5)	5.6 (3-9.7)	7.2 (6-8.8)	5-50	—	4.1 (2.7-5.7)
Osmolarity (mOsmol/L)	332 (319-345)	—	—	5.1 (3.6-6.9)	5.6 (2.7-7.5)	4.9 (2.8-7.6)	2.5-7	3.8 (1.8-5.8)	5.2 (3.9-5.9)
Phosphorus (mg/dL)	4.6 (3.1-7.5)	5.8 (3-10)	4.3 ± 1.6	1.4 (1.1-1.7)	2.2 (1.2-3.2)	2.3 (1.6-3.4)	3.1-5.8	5.4 (3.7-6.8)	4.7 (3.9-5.9)
Potassium (mEq/L)	4.2 (3.2-5.7)	4.6 (3.5-6.5)	4.1 ± 0.9	2.2 (1.8-2.5)	—	—	3-6.6	5.2 (3.3-7.4)	2.1 (1.5-3.1)
Protein, total (g/dL)	6.7 (4.2-8.6)	7.6 (5.2-11.9)	5.4 ± 1.2	4.1 (3.5-5.2)	3.4 (2.5-4.7)	2.7 (1.2-4.2)	0.6-2.4	1.9 (1.3-3.4)	—
Albumin (g/dL)[b]	2.1 (1.5-3.5)	2.4 (1.2-3.4)	1.7 ± 0.3	147 (140-153)	144 (138-149)	140 (132-160)	0.9-2.4	—	2.7 (2.3-3.1)
Albumin (PEP; g/dL)[b]	3.2 (3.1-3.3)	3.1 (3-3.2)	—	92 (9-174)	—	—	1.4-3.2	3.1 (2-5.3)	—
Globulin (g/dL)[b]	4.9 (3.4-6.6)	4.9 (3.2-7.3)	3.7 ± 0.9	2.4 (0.7-4.5)	1.6 (0.5-3.1)	2.2 (0.6-5.6)	0.1-0.5	—	—
α-1 (PEP; g/dL)[b]	—	0.1	—				0.6-1.9	—	—
α-2 (PEP; g/dL)[b]	—	0.9 (0.8-1)	—				0.6-1.5	—	—
β (PEP; g/dL)[b]	—	0.9	—				0.4-0.9	—	128 (122-133)
γ (PEP; g/dL)[b]	—	4.7 (2.6-6.8)	—				121-146	131 (116-155)	60 (27-110)
Sodium (mEq/L)	156 (149-165)	156 (142-176)	144 ± 26				26-303	246 (28-480)	3.3 (1-8.1)
Triglyceride (mg/dL)	135 (17-476)	35 (6-78)	241 ± 360				0.3 (0-0.6)	0.8 (0.3-1.3)	
Uric acid (mg/dL)	6.7 (1.2-18)	5.8 (1-16.6)	1.7 ± 1.1						

Measurement	Desert tortoise (Gopherus agassizii)[228, 251-254]	Gopher tortoise (Gopherus polyphemus)[255]	Russian tortoise (Testudo horsfieldii)[256,257]	African spurred tortoise (Centrochelys sulcata)[228]	Leopard tortoise (Stigmochelys pardalis)[228]	Galapagos tortoise (Chelonoidis nigra)[228]	Sliders (Trachemys scripta ssp)[228, 258-260]	Painted turtle (Chrysemys picta)[228,259,260]	Green sea turtle (Chelonia mydas)[228,261]
HEMATOLOGY									
PCV (%)	15-39	23 (15-30)	23 (22-34)	28 (9-48)	22 (7-60)	19 (11-27)	29 (25-33)	28 (24-30)	37 (27-49)
RBC (10⁶/μL)	0.28-1.34	0.54 (0.24-0.91)	—	0.9 (0.43-1.28)	0.82 (0.58-1.06)	0.39 (0.28-0.6)	0.84 (0.33-2.21)	0.57 (0.41-0.68)	1.94
Hgb (g/dL)	3.6-10.3	6.4 (4.2-8.6)	—	10.2 (6.4-15.7)	16.1 (8.8-28)	6 (4.1-9.9)	11.1 (10-12.2)	11.2 (10.7-11.7)	10.7
MCV (fL)	197-688	—	—	386 (201-575)	279 (179-379)	528 (280-667)	409 (179-697)	271 (183-365)	155
MCH (pg)	39-189	—	—	133 (91-165)	83	169 (111-222)	108	—	55
MCHC (g/dL)	19-35	—	—	35 (24-62)	44 (42-46)	31 (25-37)	30	—	36
WBC (10³/μL)	0.97-10.9	15.7 (10-22)	8.5 (5-12.5)	7.97 (1.2-25.6)	10.23 (1.3-23)	7.72 (0.3-33.1)	13.7 (1.2-25.5)	6.7 (1.2-12.9)	11.7 (2.9-18)
Heterophils (10³/μL)	0.49-7.3	4.7 (1-12.5)[g]	3.7 (1.3-4.6)	3.44 (0.32-9.62)	4.25 (0.21-12.8)	2.82 (0.27-20.4)	5 (0.95-14)	2.2 (0.17-4.26)	3.5 (0.9-6.6)
Lymphocytes (10³/μL)	0-3.8	8.9 (3.2-17.4)[g]	4.7 (3.6-7.6)	3.68 (0.19-13.7)	2.7 (0.72-6.6)	4.24 (0.09-25.5)	3.3 (0.25-7.88)	1.6 (0.23-3.46)	6.7 (1.2-10.1)
Monocytes (10³/μL)	0-0.57	1.1 (0.3-2.9)[g]	0.01 (0-0.02)	0.64 (0.06-2.25)	0.38	0.16 (0.01-0.58)	0.24 (0.14-0.38)	0.26	0.62 (0.11-1.3)
Azurophils (10³/μL)	0-0.9	—	0.05 (0.03-0.12)	0.25 (0.02-0.54)	—	0.36 (0.03-1.97)	0.58 (0.23-1.33)	0.51 (0.25-0.77)	1.2 (0.17-2.7)
Eosinophils (10³/μL)	0-0.95	—	0.05 (0.02-0.06)	0.35 (0.03-1.41)	0.1 (0.09-0.12)	0.42 (0.02-5.18)	1.53 (0.17-5.9)	0.55 (0.09-1.03)	0.42 (0.08-1.08)
Basophils (10³/μL)	0-4.3	0.94 (0.2-2.4)[g]	0.05 (0.02-0.08)	0.3 (0.02-0.54)	0.21 (0.18-0.24)	0.54 (0.01-2.72)	3.8 (0.31-8)	2.17 (0.04-4.86)	0.18 (0.08-0.34)
CHEMISTRIES									
ALP (U/L)	43-176	39 (11-71)	498 (181-1188)	36 (12-59)	121 (54-173)	96 (30-302)	395 (201-677)	208	6-67
ALT (U/L)	21 (0-66)	15 (2-57)	1 (0-2)	13 (1-71)	8	7 (0-28)	14 (1-66)	—	31 (5-82)
AST (U/L)	41-106	136 (57-392)	20 (12-32)	—	—	167 (20-523)	493 (411-535)	152	534
Bile acids (μmol/L)	0-5.4	—	—	108 (34-401)	110 (41-344)	56 (19-187)	183 (108-350)	0.1	74-245
Bilirubin, total (mg/dL)	0-0.9	0.02 (0-0.1)	0.015 (0-0.09)	0.4 (0-2.6)	0.1	0.3 (0-1)	0.2 (0.1-0.5)	37	0.03-0.2
BUN (mg/dL)	0-4	30 (1-130)	12 (4-17)	3 (0-6)	41 (6-72)	14 (2-42)	25 (4-54)	10 (8.8-11.4)	93 (54-154)
Calcium (total; mg/dL)	9.3-14.7	12 (10-14)	13.2 (9.9-19.5)	12.1 (6.6-20)	12.2 (9.1-20.4)	12.6 (4.8-41)	13.4 (10-18)	85	8-8.8
Ionized calcium (mmol/L)	—	—	1.28 (1-1.6)	106 (93-123)	—	96 (83-119)	102 (81-107)	—	101-121
Chloride (mEq/L)	94-112	102 (35-128)	—	160 (69-394)	189 (164-237)	225 (78-506)	162 (106-227)	—	221 (142-354)
Cholesterol (mg/dL)	56-233	76 (19-150)	109 (25-210)	1518 (291-6205)	359 (223-704)	1262 (216-8090)	3095 (392-4856)	—	326-2729
Creatine kinase (U/L)	2262 (944-3880)	160 (32-628)	123 (6-344)	0.3 (0.1-0.4)	0.6	0.2 (0.1-0.5)	0.3 (0.2-0.5)	76 (76-84)	0.1 (0-0.4)
Creatinine (mg/dL)	0.11-0.37	0.3 (0.1-0.4)	—	14 (3-19)	—	6 (0-10)	7 (0-21)	—	6 (0-21)
GLDH (U/L)	—	—	1 (0.6-1.5)	142 (54-277)	91 (48-132)	144 (38-445)	84 (52-138)	412	67-178
Glucose (mg/dL)	92-165	75 (55-128)	59 (40-86)	81 (80-82)	—	73 (8-593)	—	—	362 (117-600)
LDH (U/L)	25-250	273 (18-909)	—	1315 (258-1980)	446 (346-546)	719 (197-1884)	1713 (371-5763)	4.8	75-477
Magnesium (mEq/L)	2.1 (1.8-2.4)	4.1 (3.3-4.8)	—	3.9 (1.5-7.8)	4 (2.5-6.6)	4.6 (2-10.3)	6 (1-15)	3.1 (2.8-3.1)	—
Phosphorus (mg/dL)	1-6.3	2.1 (1-3.1)	2.6 (1.3-3.9)	5 (3.6-8.5)	6.7 (5.4-7.4)	5.3 (3.2-8.1)	2.2	2.9 (2.6-3.2)	4.8-12.2
Potassium (mEq/L)	3.5-4.7	5 (2.9-7.)	5.3 (1.9-7.2)	3.9 (1.6-7)	3.2 (1.6-5.9)	4.8 (2.4-8.3)	5.2 (3.7-7.5)	2.4 (2.4-4.4)	4.9-11.1
Protein, total (g/dL)	3-4.6	3.1 (1.3-4.6)	3 (2.5-4.6)	1.5 (0.6-2)	1.1 (0.5-1.5)	1.8 (0.8-3.1)	4.1 (3.5-4.7)	1.2	3-7.1
Albumin (g/dL)[b]	1.2-2.2	1.5 (0.5-2.6)	1.6 (1.2-2.3)	2 (1.0-2.9)	1.5 (1.1-1.8)	3.2 (1.2-5.7)	4.6 (2.8-6.1)	1.2	2.1-6.2
Albumin (PEP; g/dL)[b]	—	—	—	138 (121-155)	141 (135-149)	128 (114-141)	2 (1.6-2.5)	143	0.7-1.8

Continued

TABLE 7—cont'd

Hematologic and Serum Biochemical Values[a]

Measurement	Desert tortoise (Gopherus agassizii)[228, 251-254]	Gopher tortoise (Gopherus polyphemus)[255]	Russian tortoise (Testudo horsfieldii)[256,257]	African spurred tortoise (Centrochelys sulcata)[228]	Leopard tortoise (Stigmochelys pardalis)[228]	Galapagos tortoise (Chelonoidis nigra)[228]	Sliders (Trachemys scripta ssp)[228, 258-260]	Painted turtle (Chrysemys picta)[228,259,260]	Green sea turtle (Chelonia mydas)[228,261]
CHEMISTRIES—cont'd									
Globulin (g/dL)[b]	1.2-2.6	—	1.4 (1.3-2.3)	—	—	2 (1-2)	2.6 (1.2-3.7)	—	1.5-4.7
α-1 Glob (PEP; g/dL)[b]	1	—	—	163 (53-388)	—	271 (29-1345)	137 (124-144)	2 (1.2-2)	139-158
α-2 Glob (PEP; g/dL)[b]	1	—	—	—	—	29	304 (30-664)		492 (124-932)
β Glob (PEP; g/dL)[b]	0.6	—	—	5.2 (2.1-10.5)	3.2 (0.5-15.3)	2.3 (0.5-7.4)	1.2 (0.6-3.2)		1 (0.2-1.5)
γ Glob (PEP; g/dL)[b]	—	—	—						
Sodium (mEq/L)	122-139	138 (127-148)	138 (131-149)						
Triglyceride (mg/dL)	0-425	—	—						
Uric acid (mg/dL)	2.7-7.2	3.5 (0.9-8.5)	1.2 (0.8-3.9)						
Vitamin A (μg/mL)	0.2-0.6	—	—						
Zinc (ppm)	0.4-3.7	—	—						

A/G ratio, Albumin/globulin ratio; *ALP,* alkaline phosphatase; *ALT,* alanine aminotransferase; *AST,* aspartate aminotransferase; *BUN,* blood urea nitrogen; *GGT,* gamma-glutamyl transpeptidase; *Hgb,* hemoglobin; *LDH,* lactate dehydrogenase; *MCH,* mean corpuscular hemoglobin; *MCHC,* mean corpuscular hemoglobin concentration; *MCV,* mean corpuscular volume; *PCV,* packed cell volume; *PEP,* protein electrophoresis; *RBC,* red blood cell; *WBC,* white blood cell.

[a]Listed values are mean (min-max), unless a single value indicates n = 1 or a range that is not enclosed in parentheses indicates a reported reference range.

[b]Albumin is measured by colorimetry (e.g., bromocresol green), and globulin value is calculated unless otherwise indicated.

[c]Remarkably high reference ranges for Ca (mean, 159 mg/dL; range, 30-337 mg/dL) and P (mean, 35 mg/dL; range, 8-69) have also been reported.[233]

[d]Can be elevated in gravid females; vitamin D_3 is higher in female green iguanas.[242]

[e]These data were obtained from iguanas housed outdoors with unfiltered sunlight.

[f]Adults.

[g]Calculated from data.

TABLE 8

Environmental, Dietary, and Reproductive Characteristics of Reptiles[137,199,262-267]

Species	Environmental Preference: Temperature[a-c]	Environmental Preference: RH (%)	Diet[d]	Method of Reproduction[e]	Gestation/ Incubation Period (Days)[f]
SNAKES					
Ball (Royal) python *(Python regius)*	25-30°C (77-86°F)	70-80 (use humidity box)[g]	C	Ov	90
Boa constrictor *(Boa constrictor)*	28-34°C (82-93°F)	50-70 (use humidity box)[g]	C	V	120-240
Garter snake *(Thamnophis sirtalis)*	22-30°C (72-86°F)	60-80 (use humidity box)[g]	C	V	90-110
King snake *(Lampropeltis getula)*	23-30°C (73-86°F)	50-70 (use humidity box)[g]	Op/c	Ov	50-60
Sand boa (*Eryx* sp)	25-30°C (77-86°F)	20-30	C	V	120-180
LIZARDS					
Bearded dragon *(Pogona vitticeps)*	27-30°C (80-85°F)	— (use humidity box)[g]	I: young; H: adult	Ov	65-90
Green anole *(Anolis carolinensis)*	23-29°C (73-84°F)	70-80	I/c	Ov	60-90
Green iguana *(Iguana iguana)*	29-38°C (84-100°F)	60-80	H	Ov	73
Jackson's chameleon *(Chamaeleo jacksonii)*	21-27°C (70-81°F)	50-70	I	V	90-180
Leopard ground gecko *(Eublepharis macularius)*	25-30°C (77-86°F)	20-30 (use humidity box)[g]	I	Ov	55-60
Australian Water dragon *(Physignathus lesueurii)*	25-34°C (77-93°F)	80-90; Need water with filter[h]	I/om	Ov	90
CHELONIANS					
Common box turtle *(Terrapene carolina)*	24-29°C (75-84°F)	60-80 (use humidity box)[g]	C/f	Ov	50-90
Desert tortoise *(Gopherus agassizii)*	25-30°C (77-86°F)	— (use humidity box)[g]	H	Ov	84-120
Greek tortoise *(Testudo graeca)*	20-27°C (68-81°F)	30-50 (use humidity box)[g]	H/om	Ov	60
Painted turtle *(Chrysemys picta)*	23-28°C (73-82°F)	80-90; Need water with filter[h]	H/I/o	Ov	47-99
Red-eared slider *(Trachemys scripta elegans)*	22-30°C (72-86°F)	80-90; Need water with filter[h]	C	Ov	59-93
Russian tortoise *(Testudo horsfieldii)*	21-32°C (70-90°F)	— (use humidity box)[g]	H	Ov	56-84
CROCODILIAN					
American alligator *(Alligator mississippiensis)*	30-35°C (86-95°F)	80-90; Need water with filter[h]	C/p	Ov	62-65

C, Carnivorous; *F*, frugivorous; *H*, herbivorous; *I*, insectivorous; *O*, molluscavorous; *Om*, omnivorous; *Op*, ophiophagus; *Ov*, oviparous; *P*, piscivorous; *RH*, relative humidity; *V*, viviparous.

[a]Temperatures shown are ideal ambient daytime temperature gradients. These should be allowed to fall by approximately 5°C (9°F) during the night. "Hot-spot" temperatures should generally be 5°C (9°F) greater than the highest temperature shown.

[b]Preferred daytime temperature range for other commonly housed captive snakes are rosy boa *(Lichanura trivirgata)*, 27-29.5°C (81-85°F); green tree python *(Morelia viridis)*, 24-28°C (75-82°F); carpet python *(Morelia spilota)*, 27-29.5°C (81-85°F); cornsnake *(Elaphe guttata)*, 25-30°C (77-86°F); black rat snake *(Elaphe obsoleta)*, 25-29°C (77-84°F); gopher/bullsnake *(Pituophis melanoleucus)*, 25-29°C (77-84°F).

[c]Preferred daytime temperature range for other commonly housed captive lizards are day gecko (*Phelsuma* sp), 29.5°C (85°F); chameleons (montane) (*Chamaeleo* spp), 21-27°C (70-81°F); chameleons (lowland) (*Chamaeleo* spp), 27-29°C (81-84°F); blue-tongued skink (*Tiliqua* sp), 27-29.5°C (81-85°F); monitor lizards (*Varanus* spp), 29-31°C (84-88°F); tegus (*Tupinambis* spp), 27-30°C (81-86°F).

[d]Uppercase letters denote principal dietary requirements. Lowercase denotes secondary preference.

[e]Temperature-dependent.

[f]Can have long hatch times dependent on incubation parameters.

[g]This simulates humid underground burrow. Use dark colored plastic container with cut entrance, moistened paper towels, or sphagnum moss.

[h]Need to set up water component like fish tank with proper filter (use one for koi or turtles), pump, water quality testing, dechlorinator.

TABLE 9

Urinalysis Values of Chelonians[267-270]

Measurement	Normal Values	Abnormal Values
Specific gravity	1.003-1.014 (mean, 1.008)	Up to 1.034
pH	Herbivores: alkaline Omnivores: 5-8	Acidic[a]
Color	Colorless to pale yellow with white urates	Dark yellow, yellow-brown, yellow-green
Turbidity	Clear	Cloudy
Protein	Trace proteinuria	Increased proteinuria
Glucose	Glucosuria up to 30 mg/dL	Glucosuria can be higher than 50 mg/dL with anorexia
Renal casts	None	Various types present
Calcium, phosphorus, ammonia, urea, creatinine	Detectable in urine	Significantly increased in urine of *Testudo* spp. with renal disease
AST, CK, LDH	Detectable in urine	Significantly increased in urine of *Testudo* spp. with renal disease
Crystals	Amorphous urates/ammonium biurates	Many other crystals found in renal failure; uric acid crystals in gout; bilirubin and tyrosine crystals in liver disease

AST, Aspartate aminotransferase; *CK,* creatine kinase; *LDH,* lactate dehydrogenase.
[a]May be associated with hibernation, anorexia, and improper diet.

TABLE 10

Selected Products and Guidelines Used in Force-Feeding Anorectic or Debilitated Reptiles[a,b]

Agent	Guidelines	Species/Comments
Alfalfa pellets (e.g., iguana or rabbit pellets) or powder (Alfalfa Powder, NOW Foods)	Blend (1:4) with electrolyte solution or water; 20 mL/kg PO q48h (lizards) to q84h (chelonians)[29,271]	Herbivorous reptiles/administer via gavage; may clog feeding tube; for iguanas, may gavage equal volume of water on alternate days until patient is stable and eating[271]; soaked pellets can also be hand-fed (especially by owner)
Baby foods	Vegetable; blend in with other food sources	Herbivorous reptiles/administer via gavage; for some species, some fruit baby food can be added
	Meat (small amount); blend in with other food sources	Omnivorous species/administer via gavage
Dog/cat food, canned (a/d, Hill's; Maximum-Calorie Iams; Nutritional Recovery Formula, Eukanuba)	30 mL/kg PO q7-14d[38,159]	Carnivorous species/administer via gavage; although low protein (8.5%), some concern over high purine and vitamin A levels (probably OK unless concurrent renal disease); in dehydrated animals, dilute 1:1 with physiologic solution, oral human electrolyte solutions (pediatric: Pedialyte, Ross; Gatorade); once stabilized, small whole animals (lubricated with egg white) can be force-fed
Electrolyte solutions (Pedialyte, Ross; Gatorade)	15-25 mL/kg PO q24h	Most species
High protein powders (Carnivore Care, Oxbow Pet Products; Emeraid Carnivore, Lafeber)	Mix as labeled, generally to pancake batter consistency; feed small amount to start (see bag suggestion) once daily	Insectivorous and carnivorous species/once reconstituted, can be mixed 1:1 with an alfalfa or timothy product for true omnivorous reptiles; administer via gavage
Timothy hay-based powder (Herbivore Critical Care Fine Grind, Oxbow Pet Products; Emeraid Herbivore, Lafeber)	Mix as labeled, generally to pancake batter consistency; feed small amount to start (see bag suggestion) once daily	Herbivorous species/once reconstituted, can be mixed 1:1 with an alfalfa or timothy product for true omnivorous reptiles; administer via gavage

[a]General guidelines for force-feeding: generally provide nutrition after rehydration of patient; needs may vary with specific disease (e.g., low protein with renal disease); force-feeding volumes are frequently started at a low/modest level and gradually brought up to the desired level (for patients with severe disease/cachexia, transition should be very gradual); concurrent to force-feeding and hydrating a patient, highly palatable food items should be provided for voluntary food intake.
[b]Dietary fiber supplements (alfalfa pellets or powder; barley powder; purified cellulose) should be an integral part of enteral therapy for herbivorous reptiles.

TABLE 11

Selected Sources of Diets and Other Commercial Products for Reptiles[a,b]

FOODS AND SUPPLEMENTS			
Fluker Farms	800-735-8537	www.flukerfarms.com	
Drs Foster & Smith	800-381-7179	www.drsfostersmith.com	
Kaytee	800-529-8331	www.kaytee.com	
Mazuri	800-227-8941	www.mazuri.com	
Oxbow Animal Health	800-249-0366	www.oxbowanimalhealth.com	
Pretty Pets	800-356-5020	www.prettybird.com	
Reliable Protein Products	480-361-3940	www.zoofood.com	
Repashy Superfoods	855-737-2749	www.store.repashy.com	
Rep-Cal	800-406-6446	www.repcal.com	
San Francisco Bay Brand	510-792-7200	http://sfbb.com	
Sticky Tongue Farms	951-244-3434	www.stickytonguefarms.com	
Tetra Fauna	800-423-6458	www.tetra-fish.com	
T-Rex Products	800-991-8739	www.t-rexproducts.com	
Zoo Med Laboratories	888-496-6633	www.zoomed.com	
ZuPreem	800-345-4767	www.zupreem.com	
LIVE/FROZEN FOODS FOR CARNIVORES			
American Rodent Supply	317-899-1599	www.americanrodent.com	Frozen mice, rats
Big Cheese Rodents	800-887-0921	www.bigcheeserodents.com	Frozen mice, rats
Carolina Mouse Farm	864-944-6192	—	Frozen mice, rats
The Gourmet Rodent	352-472-9189	www.gourmetrodent.com	Frozen mice, rats, rabbits, chicks
Hoosier Mouse Supply	317-831-1219	www.hoosiermousesupply.com	Live (local) and frozen mice, rats
Komodo Reptiles	914-788-8722	www.komodoreptiles.com	Live (local) and frozen mice, rats
Mouse Factory	800-720-0076	—	Live and frozen mice, rats
Perfect Pets Inc	800-366-8794	www.perfectpet.net	Frozen mice, rats, hamsters, gerbils, guinea pigs, rabbits, chicks
Rodent Pro	812-867-7598	www.rodentpro.com	Frozen mice, rats, rabbits, guinea pigs, chicks, quail
LIVE FOODS FOR INSECTIVORES			
Arbico Organics	800-827-2847	www.arbico-organics.com	Crickets, fly pupae, mealworms, waxworms, superworms
Bassett's Cricket Ranch	800-634-2445	www.bcrcricket.com	Crickets, mealworms
The Drosophila Co	954-227-3966	http://www.jtresser.com/flypaper.html	Fruit flies
Fluker Farms	800-735-8537	www.flukerfarms.com	Crickets, mealworms, fruit flies, hissing cockroaches
Ghann's Cricket Farm	800-476-2248	www.ghann.com	Crickets, soldier fly larvae
Grubco	800-222-3563	www.grubco.com	Crickets, superworms, mealworms, fly larvae
Knutson's	800-248-9318	www.knutsonlivebait.com	Night crawlers, crickets, mealworms
Komodo Reptiles	914-788-8722	www.komodoreptiles.com	Crickets, superworms, goliath worms, fruit flies, mealworms, nightcrawlers
Millbrook Cricket Farm	800-654-3506	www.millbrookcrickets.com	Crickets, mealworms, superworms
Mulberry Farms	760-731-6088	www.mulberryfarms.com	Silkworm larvae
The Phoenix Worm Store	—	www.phoenixworm.com	Soldier fly larvae
Rainbow Mealworms	800-777-9676	www.rainbowmealworms.net	Crickets, mealworms, cockroaches
Russell's Cricket Farm	234-738-3663	www.livecrickets.com	Crickets, mealworms, superworms
Sunshine Mealworms	800-322-1100	—	Mealworms, crickets, superworms
Top Hat Cricket Farm	800-638-2555	www.tophatcrickets.com	Crickets, mealworms, superworms, hornworms, waxworms
Topline Whlse Dist Co.	888-922-0464	—	Nightcrawlers, redworms, hissing cockroaches
LIGHTS			
Duro-Test Lighting	800-289-3876	—	Vita-Lite fluorescent
Fluker Farms	800-735-8537	www.flukerfarms.com	Incandescent, heat
General Electric	800-435-4448	www.gelighting.com	Incandescent, heat
Hikari Sales USA	800-621-5619	www.hikariusa.com	UVB fluorescent
Mac Industries, Inc	252-241-4584	www.reptileuv.com	Mega-ray UVB
Philips	800-555-0050	www.lighting.philips.com	Incandescent, heat
Sylvania	978-777-1900	www.sylvania.com	350BL blacklights
T-Rex Products	800-991-8739	www.t-rexproducts.com	Mercury vapor UVB, incandescent, heat

Continued

TABLE 11—cont'd

Selected Sources of Diets and Other Commercial Products for Reptiles[a,b]

Zilla	888-255-4527	www.zilla-rules.com	Incandescent, heat, UVB fluorescent
Zoo Med Laboratories	888-496-6633	www.zoomed.com	Incandescent, heat, mercury vapor UVB, fluorescent UVB
HEATING DEVICES			
Avitec	800-646-2473	www.avitec.com	Conical ceramic heat emitters, thermostats
The Bean Farm	877-708-5882	www.beanfarm.com	Heat tape, heat pads
Big Apple Pet Supply	800-922-7753	www.bigappleherp.com	Thermostats
Fluker Farms	800-735-8537	www.flukerfarms.com	Under-cage heat pads
Helix Controls	760-726-4464	www.helixcontrols.com	Thermostats, heat tape, heat panels
LLL Reptile	888-547-3784	http://lllreptile.com	Pearlco conical ceramic heat emitters
Zilla	888-255-4527	www.zilla-rules.com	Conical ceramic heat emitters, thermostats
Zoo Med Laboratories	888-496-6633	www.zoomed.com	Thermostats, rheostats, heat pads, tape, cables
HUMIDITY DEVICES			
Exo Terra (Hagen)	800-724-2436	www.exo-terra.com	Ultrasonic fogger, Monsoon rainfall
Humidifirst	561-752-1936	www.humidifirst.com	Mist Pac ultrasonic humidifiers
Zoo Med Laboratories	888-496-6633	www.zoomed.com	Ultrasonic fogger, Repti fogger, Habba mist, Hygro-Therm humidity controller
ENVIRONMENTAL SENSING AND MONITORING DEVICES			
Exo Terra (Hagen)	800-724-2436	www.exo-terra.com	Remote digital thermometers, hygrometers
FLIR	866-477-3687	www.flir.com	Infrared thermography
Onset Computer Corp.	800-564-4377	www.onsetcomp.com	HOBO data loggers
Raytek	800-227-8074	www.raytek.com	Digital infrared thermometer
Solartech	800-798-3311	www.solarmeter.com	Solarmeter 6.2 UVB meter
Zilla	888-255-4527	www.zilla-rules.com	Digital infrared thermometer
Zoo Med Laboratories	888-496-6633	www.zoomed.com	Hygro-Therm humidity/heat monitor and controller

[a]Many pet stores sell live and frozen food for reptiles, as well as many of the products listed.
[b]Numerous sources of information were used to compile this table, particularly Internet sources.

REFERENCES

1. Gaio C, Rossi T, Villa R, et al. Pharmacokinetics of acyclovir after a single oral administration in marginated tortoises, *Testudo marginata*. *J Herpetol Med Surg* 2007;17:8-11.
2. McArthur S. Problem solving approach to common diseases of terrestrial and semi-aquatic chelonians. In: McArthur S, Wilkinson R, Meyer J, eds. *Medicine and surgery of tortoises and turtles*. Oxford, UK: Blackwell Publishing Ltd, 2004;309-377.
3. Johnson JH, Jensen JM, Brumbaugh GW, et al. Amikacin pharmacokinetics and the effects of ambient temperature on the dosage regimen in ball pythons *(Python regius)*. *J Zoo Wildl Med* 1997;28:80-88.
4. Mader DR, Conzelman GM, Baggot JD. Effects of ambient temperature on half life and dosage regimen of amikacin in the gopher snake. *J Am Vet Med Assoc* 1985;187:1134-1136.
5. Barten SL. The medical care of iguanas and other common pet lizards. *Vet Clin North Am Small Anim Pract* 1993;23:1213-1249.
6. Stahl SJ. Pet lizard conditions and syndromes. *Semin Avian Exot Pet Med* 2003;12:162-182.
7. Whitaker BR, Krum H. Medical management of sea turtles in aquaria. In: Fowler ME, Miller ME, eds. *Zoo & wild animal medicine: current therapy*. 4th ed. Philadelphia: WB Saunders Co, 1999;217-231.
8. Caligiuri R, Kollias GV, Jacobson E, et al. The effects of ambient temperature on amikacin pharmacokinetics in gopher tortoises. *J Vet Pharm Therapeut* 1990;13:287-291.
9. Jacobson ER, Brown MP, Chung M, et al. Serum concentration and disposition kinetics of gentamicin and amikacin in juvenile American alligators. *J Zoo Anim Med* 1988;19:188-194.
10. Diver SJ. Empirical doses of antimicrobial drugs commonly used in reptiles. *Exot DVM* 1998;1:23.
11. Frye FL. *Reptile care: an atlas of diseases and treatments*. Neptune City, NJ: TFH Publications, Inc, 1991;1-637.
12. Frye FL. *Reptile clinician's handbook*. Malabar, Fla: Krieger Publishing, 1994.
13. Jenkins JR. A formulary for reptile and amphibian medicine, in *Proceedings*. 4th Annu Avian/Exot Anim Med Symp, University of California, Davis, 1991;24-27.
14. Hernandez-Divers SJ. Pulmonary candidiasis caused by *Candida albicans* in a Greek tortoise *(Testudo graeca)* and treatment with intrapulmonary amphotericin B. *J Zoo Wildl Med* 2001;32:352-359.
15. Lloyd M. Crocodilia. In: Fowler ME, Miller RE, eds. *Zoo and wild animal medicine*. 5th ed. Philadelphia: Elsevier Saunders; 2003;59-70.
16. Jacobson ER. Use of chemotherapeutics in reptile medicine. In: Jacobson ER, Kollias GV Jr, eds. *Exotic animals*. New York: Churchill Livingstone, 1988;35-48.
17. Gauvin J. Drug therapy in reptiles. *Semin Avian Exot Pet Med* 1993;2:48-59.
18. Jenkins JR. Husbandry and diseases of Old World chameleons. *J Small Exot Anim Med* 1992;1:166-171.

19. Page CD, Mautino M. Clinical management of tortoises. *Compend Cont Educ Pract Vet* 1990;12:79-85.
20. Funk RS. A formulary for lizards, snakes, and crocodilians. *Vet Clin North Am Exot Anim Pract* 2000;3:333-358.
21. Spörle H, Gobel T, Schildger B. Blood levels of some anti-infectives in the spur-thighed tortoise (*Testudo hermanni*), in *Proceedings*. 4th Intl Colloq Path Med Rept Amphib 1991;120-128.
22. Coke RL, Hunter RP, Isaza R, et al. Pharmacokinetics and tissue concentrations of azithromycin in ball pythons (*Python regius*). *Am J Vet Res* 2003;64:225-228.
23. Holz PH, Burger JP, Baker R, et al. Effect of injection site on carbenicillin pharmacokinetics in the carpet python, *Morelia spilota*. *J Herpetol Med Surg* 2002;12:12-16.
24. Lawrence K, Needham JR, Palmer GH, et al. A preliminary study on the use of carbenicillin in snakes. *J Vet Pharmacol Therapeut* 1984;7:119-124.
25. Lawrence K, Palmer GH, Needham JR. Use of carbenicillin in 2 species of tortoise (*Testudo graeca* and *Testudo hermanni*). *Res Vet Sci* 1986;40:413-415.
26. White SD, Bourdeau P, Bruet V, et al. Reptiles with dermatological lesions: a retrospective study of 301 cases at two university veterinary teaching hospitals (1992-2008). *Vet Dermatol* 2010;22:150-161.
27. Lawrence K, Muggleton PW, Needham JR. Preliminary study on the use of ceftazidime, a broad spectrum cephalosporin antibiotic, in snakes. *Res Vet Sci* 1984;36:16-20.
28. Stamper MA, Papich MG, Lewbart GA, et al. Pharmacokinetics of ceftazidime in loggerhead sea turtles (*Caretta caretta*) after single intravenous and intramuscular injections. *J Zoo Wildl Med* 1999;30:32-35.
29. Benson KG, Tell LA, Young LA, et al. Pharmacokinetics of ceftiofur sodium after intramuscular or subcutaneous administration in green iguanas (*Iguana iguana*). *Am J Vet Res* 2003;64:1278-1282.
30. Stein G. Reptile and amphibian formulary. In: Mader DR, ed. *Reptile medicine and surgery*. Philadelphia: WB Saunders Co, 1996;465-472.
31. Jenkins JR. Medical management of reptile patients. *Compend Cont Educ Pract Vet* 1991;13:980-988.
32. Bush M, Smeller JM, Charache PN, et al. Preliminary study of antibiotics in snakes, in *Proceedings*. Annu Conf Am Assoc Zoo Vet 1976;50-54.
33. Clark CH, Rogers ED, Milton JL. Plasma concentrations of chloramphenicol in snakes. *Am J Vet Res* 1985;46:2654-2657.
34. Klingenberg RJ. Therapeutics. In: Mader DR, ed. *Reptile medicine and surgery*. Philadelphia: WB Saunders Co, 1996;299-321.
35. Johnson JD, Mangone B, Jarchow JL. A review of mycoplasmosis infections in tortoises and options for treatment, in *Proceedings*. Annu Conf Assoc Rept Amphib Vet 1998;89-92.
36. Wimsatt J, Johnson J, Mangone BA, et al. Clarithromycin pharmacokinetics in the desert tortoise (*Gopherus agassizii*). *J Zoo Wildl Med* 1999;30:36-43.
37. Marin P, Bayon A, Fernandez-Varon E, et al. Pharmacokinetics of danofloxacin after single dose intravenous, intramuscular, and subcutaneous administration to loggerhead turtles *Caretta caretta*. *Dis Aquat Organ* 2008;82:231-236.
38. Mader DR: Pers. com., 2011.
39. Boyer TH. *Essentials of reptiles: a guide for practitioners*. Lakewood, Colo: AAHA Press, 1998;1-253.
40. Young LA, Schumacher J, Papich MG, et al. Disposition of enrofloxacin and its metabolite ciprofloxacin after intravascular injection in juvenile Burmese pythons (*Python molurus bivittatus*). *J Zoo Wildl Med* 1997;28:71-79.
41. Maxwell LK, Jacobson ER. Preliminary single-dose pharmacokinetics of enrofloxacin after oral and intramuscular administration in green iguanas (*Iguana iguana*), in *Proceedings*. Annu Conf Am Assoc Zoo Vet 1997;25.
42. Hungerford C, Spelman L, Papich M. Pharmacokinetics of enrofloxacin after oral and intramuscular administration in savannah monitors (*Varanus exanthematicus*), in *Proceedings*. Annu Conf Am Assoc Zoo Vet 1997;89-92.
43. Prezant RM, Isaza R, Jacobson ER. Plasma concentrations and disposition kinetics of enrofloxacin in gopher tortoises (*Gopherus polyphemus*). *J Zoo Wildl Med* 1994;25:82-87.
44. Casares M, Enders F. Enrofloxacin side effects in a Galapagos tortoise (*Geochelone elephantopus nigra*), in *Proceedings*. Annu Conf Am Assoc Zoo Vet 1996;446-448.
45. Raphael BL, Papich M, Cook RA. Pharmacokinetics of enrofloxacin after a single intramuscular injection in Indian star tortoises (*Geochelone elegans*). *J Zoo Wildl Med* 1994;25:88-94.
46. Helmick KE, Papich MG, Vliet KA, et al. Pharmacokinetics of enrofloxacin after single-dose oral and intravenous administration in the American alligator (*Alligator mississippiensis*). *J Zoo Wildl Med* 2004;35:333-340.
47. Martelli P, Lai OR, Krishnasamy K, et al. Pharmacokinetic behavior of enrofloxacin in estuarine crocodile (*Crocodylus porosus*) after single intravenous, intramuscular, and oral doses. *J Zoo Wildl Med* 2009;40:696-704.
48. Wissman MA, Parsons B. Dermatophytosis of green iguanas (*Iguana iguana*). *J Small Exot Anim Med* 1993;2:133-136
49. Harms CA, Lewbart GA, Beasley J. Medical management of mixed nocardial and unidentified fungal osteomyelitis in a Kemp's Ridley sea turtle, *Lepidochelys kempii*. *J Herpetol Med Surg* 2002;12:21-26.
50. Mallo KM, Harms CA, Lewbart GA, et al. Pharmacokinetics of fluconazole in loggerhead sea turtles (*Caretta caretta*) after single intravenous and subcutaneous injections, and multiple subcutaneous injections. *J Zoo Wildl Med* 2002;33:29-35.
51. Montali RJ, Bush M, Smeller JM. Pathology of nephrotoxicity of gentamicin in snakes: model for reptilian gout. *Vet Pathol* 1979;16:108-115.
52. Bush M, Smeller JM, Charache P, et al. Biological half-life of gentamicin in gopher snakes. *Am J Vet Res* 1978;39:171-173.
53. Hilf M, Swanson D, Wagner R, et al. A new dosing schedule for gentamicin in blood pythons (*Python curtus*): a pharmacokinetic study. *Res Vet Sci* 1991;50:127-130.
54. Beck K, Loomis M, Lewbart G, et al. Preliminary comparison of plasma concentrations of gentamicin injected into the cranial and caudal limb musculature of the eastern box turtle (*Terrapene carolina carolina*). *J Zoo Wildl Med* 1995;26:265-268.
55. Raphael B, Clark CH, Hudson R Jr. Plasma concentration of gentamicin in turtles. *J Zoo Anim Med* 1985;16:136-139.
56. Rossi J. Practical reptile dermatology, in *Proceedings*. North Am Vet Conf 1995;648-649.
57. Jepson L. Lizards. In: *Exotic animal medicine: a quick reference guide*. Philadelphia: Saunders/Elsevier, 2009;268-314.
58. Jepson L. Snakes. In: *Exotic animal medicine: a quick reference guide*. Philadelphia: Saunders/Elsevier, 2009;315-357.
59. Jepson L. Turtles and tortoises. In: *Exotic animal medicine: a quick reference guide*. Philadelphia: Saunders/Elsevier, 2009;358-411.
60. Martel A, Hellebuyck T, Van Waeyenberghe L. Treatment of infections with *Nannizziopsis vriesii*, an emergent reptilian dermatophytea, in *Proceedings*. Annu Conf Assoc Rept Amphib Vet 2009;69-70.
61. Mitchell M. Ophidia. In: Fowler ME, Miller RE, eds. *Zoo and wild animal medicine*. 5th ed. Philadelphia: Saunders/Elsevier, 2003;82-91.
62. Heatley J, Mitchell M, Williams J, et al. Fungal periodontal osteomyelitis in a chameleon, *Furcifer pardalis*. *J Herpetol Med Surg* 2001;11:7-12.
63. Bicknese E, Pessier A, Boedeker N. Successful treatment of fungal osteomyelitis in a Parson's chameleon (*Calumma parsonii*) using surgical and anti-fungal treatments, in *Proceedings*. Annu Conf Assoc Rept Amphib Vet 2008;86.
64. Gamble KC, Alvarado TP, Bennett CL. Itraconazole plasma and tissue concentrations in the spiny lizard (*Sceloporus* sp.) following once-daily dosing. *J Zoo Wildl Med* 1997;28:89-93.
65. Manire CA, Rhinehart HL, Pennick GJ, et al. Steady-state plasma concentrations of itraconazole after oral administration in Kemp's ridley sea turtles, *Lepidochelys kempi*. *J Zoo Wildl Med* 2003;34:171-178.

66. Jacobson ER. Antimicrobial drug use in reptiles. In: Prescott JF, Baggot JD, eds. *Antimicrobial therapy in veterinary medicine.* Ames: Iowa State University Press, 1993;543-552.
67. Mautino M, Page CD. Biology and medicine of turtles and tortoises. *Vet Clin North Am Small Anim Pract* 1993;23:1251-1270.
68. Page CD, Mautino M, Derendorf H, et al. Multiple dose pharmacokinetics of ketoconazole administered orally to gopher tortoises (*Gopherus polyphemus*). *J Zoo Wildl Med* 1991;22:191-198.
69. Coke RL, Isaza R, Koch DE, et al. Preliminary single-dose pharmacokinetics of marbofloxacin in ball pythons (*Python regius*). *J Zoo Wildl Med* 2006;37:6-10.
70. Funk RS, Diethelm G. Reptile formulary. In: Mader DR, ed. *Reptile medicine and surgery.* 2nd ed. St. Louis: Saunders/Elsevier, 2006;1119-1139.
71. Bodri MS, Rambo TM, Wagner RA, et al. Pharmacokinetics of metronidazole administered as a single oral bolus to red rat snakes, *Elaphe guttata. J Herpetol Med Surg* 2006;16:15-19.
72. Kolmstetter CM, Cox S, Ramsay EC. Pharmacokinetics of metronidazole in the yellow rat snake, *Elaphe obsoleta quadrivitatta. J Herpetol Med Surg* 2001;11:4-8.
73. Kolmstetter CM, Frazier D, Cox S, et al. Pharmacokinetics of metronidazole in the green iguana, *Iguana iguana. Bull Assoc Rept Amphib Vet* 1998;8:4-7.
74. Helmick KE, Papich MG, Vliet KA, et al. Pharmacokinetic disposition of a long-acting oxytetracycline formulation after single-dose intravenous and intramuscular administrations in the American alligator (*Alligator mississippiensis*). *J Zoo Wildl Med* 2004;35:341-346.
75. Hilf M, Swanson D, Wagner R, et al. Pharmacokinetics of piperacillin in blood pythons (*Python curtus*) and in vitro evaluation of efficacy against aerobic gram-negative bacteria. *J Zoo Wildl Med* 1991;22:199-203.
76. Murray MJ. Pneumonia and lower respiratory tract disease. In: Mader DR, ed. *Reptile medicine and surgery.* 2nd ed. St Louis: Saunders/Elsevier, 2006;865-877.
77. Jacobson E, Kollias GV Jr, Peters LJ. Dosages for antibiotics and parasiticides used in exotic animals. *Compend Cont Educ Pract Vet* 1983;5:315-324.
78. Manire CA, Hunter RP, Koch DE, et al. Pharmacokinetics of ticarcillin in the loggerhead sea turtle (*Caretta caretta*) after single intravenous and intramuscular injections. *J Zoo Wildl Med* 2005;36:44-53.
79. Van Waeyenberghe L, Baert K, Pasmans F, et al. Voriconazole, a safe alternative for treating infections caused by the *Chrysosporium* anamorph of *Nannizziopsis vriesii* in bearded dragons (*Pogona vitticeps*). *Med Mycol* 2010;48:880-885.
80. Innis C, Young D, Wetzlich S, et al. Plasma voriconazole concentrations in four red-eared slider turtles (*Trachemys scripta elegans*) after a single subcutaneous injection, in *Proceedings.* Annu Conf Assoc Rept Amphib Vet 2008;72.
81. Fitzgerald KT, Vera R. Acariasis. In: Mader DR, ed. *Reptile medicine and surgery.* 2nd ed. St. Louis: Saunders/Elsevier, 2006;720-738.
82. Mehlhorn H, Schmahl G, Frese M, et al. Effects of a combination of emodepside and praziquantel on parasites of reptiles and rodents. *Parasitol Res* 2005;97(Suppl 1):S65-S69.
83. Schilliger L, Betremieux O, Rochet J, et al. Absorption and efficacy of a spot-on combination containing emodepside plus praziquantel in reptiles. *Rev Med Vet (Toulouse)* 2009;160:557-561.
84. Neiffer DL, Lydick D, Burks K, et al. Hematologic and plasma biochemical changes associated with fenbendazole administration in Hermann's tortoises (*Testudo hermanni*). *J Zoo Wildl Med* 2005;36:661-672.
85. Klingenberg RJ. A comparison of fenbendazole and ivermectin for the treatment of nematode parasites in ball pythons, *Python regius. Bull Assoc Rept Amphib Vet* 1992;2:5-6.
86. Klingenberg RJ. Diagnosing parasites of Old World chameleons. *Exot DVM* 2000;1(6):17-21.
87. Klingenberg RJ. *Understanding reptile parasites.* Irvine, Calif: Advanced Vivarium Systems, 2007;1-200.
88. Giannetto S, Brianti E, Poglayen G, et al. Efficacy of oxfendazole and fenbendazole against tortoise (*Testudo hermanni*) oxyurids. *Parasitol Res* 2007;100:1069-1073.
89. Carpenter JW: Pers. observation, 2011.
90. Groza A, Mederle N, Darabus G. Advocate-therapeutical solution in parasitical infestation in frillneck lizard (*Chlamydosaurus kingii*) and bearded dragon (*Pogona vitticeps*). *Lucrari Stiintifice—Universitatea Stiinte Agricole Banatului Timisoara, Med Vet* 2009;42:105-108.
91. Teare JA, Bush M. Toxicity and efficacy of ivermectin in chelonians. *J Am Vet Med Assoc* 1983;183:1195-1197.
92. Flach EJ, Riley J, Mutlow AG, et al. Pentastomiasis in Bosc's monitor lizards (*Varanus exanthematicus*) caused by an undescribed *Sambonia* species. *J Zoo Wildl Med* 2000;31:91-95.
93. Wilson SC, Carpenter JW. Endoparasitic diseases of reptiles. *Semin Avian Exot Pet Med* 1996;5:64-74.
94. Luppi M, Costa M, Malta M, et al. Treatment of *Rhabdias labiata* with levamisole and ivermectin in boa constrictor (*Boa constrictor amarali*). *Veterinaria Noticias* 2007;13:61-65.
95. Mitchell MA. Therapeutics. In: Mader DR, ed. *Reptile medicine and surgery.* 2nd ed. St Louis: Saunders/Elsevier, 2006;631-664.
96. Stahl SJ. Clinician's approach to the chameleon patient, in *Proceedings.* North Am Vet Conf 2006;1667-1670.
97. Miller HA, Brandt PJ, Frye FL, et al. *Trichomonas* associated with ocular and subcutaneous lesions in geckos, in *Proceedings.* Annu Conf Assoc Rept Amphib Vet 1994;102-107.
98. Innis C, Papich M, Young D. Pharmacokinetics of metronidazole in the red-eared slider turtle (*Trachemys scripta elegans*) after single intracoelomic injection. *J Vet Pharm Therapeut* 2007;30:168-171.
99. Gibbons PM: Pers. observation, 2011.
100. Cranfield MR, Graczyk TK. Cryptosporidiosis. In: Mader DR, ed. *Reptile medicine and surgery.* 2nd ed. St. Louis: Saunders/Elsevier, 2006;756-762.
101. Paré JA, Crawshaw GJ, Barta JR. Treatment of cryptosporidiosis in Gila monsters (*Heloderma suspectum*) with paromomycin, in *Proceedings.* Annu Conf Assoc Rept Amphib Vet 1997;23.
102. Coke RL, Tristan TE. *Cryptosporidium* infection in a colony of leopard geckos, *Eublepharis macularius,* in *Proceedings.* Annu Conf Assoc Rept Amphib Vet 1998;157-163.
103. Bogoslavsky B. The use of ponazuril to treat coccidiosis in eight inland bearded dragons (*Pogona vitticeps*), in *Proceedings.* Annu Conf Assoc Rept Amphib Vet 2007;8-9.
104. Mitchell MA. Ponazuril. *J Exot Pet Med* 2008;17:228-229.
105. Adnyana W, Ladds PW, Blair D. Efficacy of praziquantel in the treatment of green sea turtles with spontaneous infection of cardiovascular flukes. *Aust Vet J* 1997;75:405-407.
106. Jacobson E, Harman G, Laille E, et al. Plasma concentrations of praziquantel in loggerhead sea turtles (*Caretta caretta*) following oral administration of single and multiple doses, in *Proceedings.* Annu Conf Assoc Rept Amphib Vet 2002;37-39.
107. McFarlen J. Commonly occurring reptilian internal parasites, in *Proceedings.* Annu Conf Am Assoc Zoo Vet 1991;120-127.
108. Willette-Frahm M, Wright KM, Thode BC. Select protozoal diseases in amphibians and reptiles. *Bull Assoc Rept Amphib Vet* 1995;5:19-29.
109. Girling SJ, Raiti P. *BSAVA manual of reptiles.* 2nd ed. Quedgeley, Gloucester, UK: British Small Animal Veterinary Association, 2004.
110. Doneley B. Caring for the bearded dragon, in *Proceedings.* North Am Vet Conf 2006;1607-1611.
111. Praschag P, Gibbons P, Boyer T, et al. An outbreak of intranuclear coccidiosis in Pyxis spp. Tortoises. *Proc 8th Annu Symp Conserv Biol Tortoises Freshwater Turtles* 2010;42-43.
112. Millichamp NJ. Surgical techniques in reptiles. In: Jacobson ER, Kollias GV Jr, eds. *Exotic animals.* New York: Churchill Livingstone, 1988;49-74.
113. Page CD. Current reptilian anesthesia procedures. In: Fowler ME, ed. *Zoo & wild animal medicine: current therapy.* 3rd ed. Philadelphia: WB Saunders Co, 1993;140-143.

114. Lawton MPC. Anaesthesia. In: Benyon PH, Lawton MPC, Cooper JE, eds. *Manual of reptiles*. Ames, Iowa: Iowa State University Press, 1992;170-183.
115. Bennett RA. A review of anesthesia and chemical restraint in reptiles. *J Zoo Wildl Med* 1991;22:282-303.
116. Schumacher J, Yelen T. Anesthesia and analgesia. In: Mader DR, ed. *Reptile medicine and surgery*. 2nd ed. St Louis: Saunders/Elsevier, 2006;442-452.
117. Scheelings TF, Holz P, Haynes L, et al. A preliminary study of the chemical restraint of selected squamate reptiles with alfaxalone, in *Proceedings*. Annu Conf Assoc Rept Amphib Vet 2010;114-115.
118. Hackenbroich C, Failing K, Axt-Findt U, et al. Alphaxalone-alphadolone anesthesia in *Trachemys scripta elegans* and its influence on respiration, circulation and metabolism, in *Proceedings*. 2nd Conf Euro Assoc Zoo Wildl Vet 1998;431-436.
119. Fleming GJ. Capture and chemical immobilization of the Nile crocodile *(Crocodylus niloticus)* in South Africa, in *Proceedings*. Annu Conf Assoc Rept Amphib Vet 1996;63-66.
120. Smith JA, McGuire NC, Mitchell MA. Cardiopulmonary physiology and anesthesia in crocodilians, in *Proceedings*. Annu Conf Assoc Rept Amphib Vet 1998;17-21.
121. Dennis PM, Heard DJ. Cardiopulmonary effects of a medetomidine-ketamine combination administered intravenously in gopher tortoises. *J Am Vet Med Assoc* 2002;220:1516-1519.
122. Boyer TH. Clinical anesthesia of reptiles. *Bull Assoc Rept Amphib Vet* 1992;2:10-13.
123. Schumacher J. Reptiles and amphibians. In: Thurman JC, Tranquilli WJ, Benson GJ, eds. *Lumb and Jones' veterinary anesthesia*. 3rd ed. Baltimore, Md: Williams & Wilkins, 1996;670-685.
124. Pace L, Mader DR. Atropine and glycopyrrolate, route of administration and response in the green iguana *(Iguana iguana)*, in *Proceedings*. Annu Conf Assoc Rept Amphib Vet 2002;79.
125. Heard DJ. Principles and techniques of anesthesia and analgesia for exotic practice. *Vet Clin North Am Small Anim Pract* 1993;23:1301-1327.
126. Bennett RA, Divers SJ, Schumacher J, et al. Roundtable: anesthesia. *Bull Assoc Rept Amphib Vet* 1999;9:20-27.
127. Schnellbacher R. Butorphanol. *J Exot Pet Med* 2010;19:192-195.
128. Sladky KK, Kinney ME, Johnson SM. Effects of opioid receptor activation on thermal antinociception in red-eared slider turtles *(Trachemys scripta)*. *Am J Vet Res* 2009;70:1072-1078.
129. Sladky KK, Miletic V, Paul-Murphy J, et al. Analgesic efficacy and respiratory effects of butorphanol and morphine in turtles. *J Am Vet Med Assoc* 2007;230:1356-1362.
130. Raphael BL. Chelonians. In: Fowler ME, Miller RE, eds. *Zoo and wild animal medicine*. 5th ed. Philadelphia: Saunders/Elsevier, 2003;48-58.
131. Sladky KK, Kinney ME, Johnson SM. Analgesic efficacy of butorphanol and morphine in bearded dragons and corn snakes. *J Am Vet Med Assoc* 2008;233:267-273.
132. Bennett RA. Reptile anesthesia. *Semin Avian Exot Pet Med* 1998;7:30-40.
133. Lawton MPC. Pain management after surgery, in *Proceedings*. North Am Vet Conf 1999;782.
134. McArthur SDJ, Wilkinson RJ, Barrows MG. Tortoises and turtles. In: Meredith A, Redrobe S, eds. *BSAVA manual of exotic pets*. 4th ed. Gloucestershire, GB: British Small Animal Veterinary Association, 2002;208-222.
135. Gamble KC. Plasma fentanyl concentrations achieved after transdermal fentanyl patch application in prehensile-tailed skinks, *Corucia zebrata*. *J Herpetol Med Surg* 2008;18:81-85.
136. Boyer TH. Emergency care of reptiles. *Vet Clin North Am Exot Anim Pract* 1998;1:191-206.
137. Stahl SJ. Reproductive disorders of the green iguana, in *Proceedings*. North Am Vet Conf 1998;810-813.
138. Stegman N, Heatley JJ. The use of haloperidol in mitigation of human-directed aggression in boid snakes, in *Proceedings*. Annu Conf Assoc Rept Amphib Vet 2010;113.
139. Bennett RA. Anesthesia. In: Mader DR, ed. *Reptile medicine and surgery*. Philadelphia: WB Saunders Co, 1996;241-247.
140. Johnson JH. Anesthesia, analgesia, and euthanasia of reptiles and amphibians, in *Proceedings*. Annu Conf Am Assoc Zoo Vet 1991;132-138.
141. Holz P, Holz RM. Evaluation of ketamine, ketamine/xylazine, and ketamine midazolam anesthesia in red-eared sliders (*Trachemys scripta elegans*). *J Zoo Wildl Med* 1994;25:531-537.
142. Wood FE, Critchley KH, Wood JR. Anesthesia in green the sea turtle, *Chelonia mydas*. *Am J Vet Res* 1982;43:1882.
143. Lloyd ML. Crocodilian anesthesia. In: Fowler ME, Miller RE, eds. *Zoo & wild animal medicine: current therapy*. 4th ed. Philadelphia: WB Saunders Co, 1999;205-216.
144. Lane T. Crocodilians. In: Mader DR, ed. *Reptile medicine and surgery*. 2nd ed. St. Louis: Saunders Elsevier, 2006;100-117.
145. Divers SJ. Anesthetics in reptiles. *Exot DVM* 1999;1(3):7-8.
146. Lock BA, Heard DJ, Dennis P. Preliminary evaluation of medetomidine/ketamine combinations for immobilization and reversal with atipamezole in three tortoise species. *Bull Assoc Rept Amphib Vet* 1998;8:6-9.
147. Helmick KE, Bennett RA, Ginn P, et al. Intestinal volvulus and stricture associated with a leiomyoma in a green turtle *(Chelonia mydas)*. *J Zoo Wildl Med* 2000;31:221-227.
148. Fleming G. Clinical technique: chelonian shell repair. *J Exot Pet Med* 2008;17:246-258.
149. Chittick EJ, Stamper MA, Beasley JF, et al. Medetomidine, ketamine, and sevoflurane for anesthesia of injured loggerhead sea turtles: 13 cases (1996-2000). *J Am Vet Med Assoc* 2002;221:1019-1025.
150. Heard DJ. Advances in reptile anesthesia, in *Proceedings*. North Am Vet Conf 1999;770.
151. Heaton-Jones TG, Ko J, Heaton-Jones DL. Evaluation of medetomidine-ketamine anesthesia with atipamezole reversal in American alligators *(Alligator mississippiensis)*. *J Zoo Wildl Med* 2002;33:36-44.
152. Bienzle D, Boyd CJ. Sedative effects of ketamine and midazolam in snapping turtles. *J Zoo Wildl Med* 1992;23:201-204.
153. Tuttle AD, Papich M, Lewbart GA, et al. Pharmacokinetics of ketoprofen in the green iguana *(Iguana iguana)* following single intravenous and intramuscular injections. *J Zoo Wildl Med* 2006;37:567-570.
154. Rojo-Solís C, Ros-Rodriguez JM, Valls M. Pharmacokinetics of meloxicam (Metacam) after intravenous, intramuscular, and oral administration in red-eared slider turtles *(Trachemys scripta elegans)*, in *Proceedings*. Joint Conf Am Assoc Zoo Vet/Am Assoc Wildl Vet 2009;228.
155. Divers SJ, Papich MG, McBride M, et al. Pharmacokinetics of meloxicam following intravenous and oral administration in green iguanas *(Iguana iguana)*. *Am J Vet Res* 2010;71:1277-1283.
156. Allen DG, Pringle JK, Smith D. *Handbook of Veterinary Drugs*. Philadelphia: JB Lippincott Co, 1993;534-567.
157. Nichols DK, Lamirande EW. Use of methohexital sodium as an anesthetic in two species of colubrid snakes, in *Proceedings*. Joint Conf Am Assoc Zoo Vet/Assoc Rept Amphib Vet 1994;161-162.
158. Schaeffer DO. Anesthesia and analgesia in nontraditional laboratory animal species. In: Kohn DF, Wixson SK, White WJ, et al, eds. *Anesthesia and analgesia in laboratory animals*. New York: Academic Press,1997;338-378.
159. Schumacher J. Lacertilia. In: Fowler ME, Miller RE, eds. *Zoo and wild animal medicine*. 5th ed. Philadelphia: Saunders/Elsevier, 2003;73-81.
160. Oppenheim YC, Moon PF. Sedative effects of midazolam in red-eared sliders *(Trachemys scripta elegans)*. *J Zoo Wildl Med* 1995;26:409-413.
161. Quesada RJ, Aitken-Palmer C, Conley K, et al. Accidental submeningeal injection of propofol in gopher tortoises *(Gopherus polyphemus)*. *Vet Rec* 2010;167:494-495.
162. Anderson NL, Wack RF, Calloway L. Cardiopulmonary effects and efficacy of propofol as an anesthetic agent in brown tree snakes, *Boiga irregularis*. *Bull Assoc Rept Amphib Vet* 1999;9:9-15.

163. Heard DJ. Advances in reptile anesthesia and medicine, in *Proceedings*. Annu Conf Assoc Avian Vet/Avian Specialty Advanced Prog/Small Mam Rept Prog 1998;113-119.
164. Bennett RA, Schumacher J, Hedjazi-Haring K, et al. Cardiopulmonary and anesthetic effects of propofol administered intraosseously to green iguanas. *J Am Vet Med Assoc* 1998;212:93-98.
165. Ziolo M, Bertelsen M. Effects of propofol administered via the supravertebral sinus in red-eared sliders. *J Am Vet Med Assoc* 2009;234:390-393.
166. Rooney MB, Levine G, Gaynor J, et al. Sevoflurane anesthesia in desert tortoises *(Gopherus agassizii)*. *J Zoo Wildl Med* 1999;30:64-69.
167. Fleming GJ. Crocodilian anesthesia. *Vet Clin North Am Exot Anim Pract* 2001;4:119-145.
168. Schobert E. Telazol use in wild and exotic animals. *Vet Med* 1987;82:1080-1088.
169. Stirl R, Krug P, Bonath KH. Tiletamine/zolazepam sedation in boa constrictors and its influence on respiration, circulation, and metabolism, in *Proceedings*. Conf Euro Assoc Zoo Wildl Vet 1996;115-119.
170. Clyde VL, Cardeilhac PT, Jacobson ER. Chemical restraint of American alligators *(Alligator mississippiensis)* with atracurium or tiletamine-zolazepam. *J Zoo Wildl Med* 1994;25:525-530.
171. Greenacre CB, Massi K, Schumacher JP, et al. Comparative antinociception of various opioids and non-steroidal anti-inflammatory medications versus saline in the bearded dragon *(Pogona vitticeps)* using electrostimulation, in *Proceedings*. Annu Conf Rept Amphib Vet 2008;87.
172. Baker BB, Sladky KK, Johnson SM. Evaluation of the analgesic effects of oral and subcutaneous tramadol administration in red-eared slider turtles. *J Am Vet Med Assoc* 2011;238:220-227.
173. Lloyd ML. Reptilian dystocias review—causes, prevention, management, and comments on the synthetic hormone vasotocin, in *Proceedings*. Annu Conf Am Assoc Zoo Vet 1990;290-296.
174. Bennett RA. Management of common reptile emergencies, in *Proceedings*. Annu Conf Assoc Rept Amphib Vet 1998;67-72.
175. Mader DR. Metabolic bone diseases. In: Mader DR, ed. *Reptile medicine and surgery*. 2nd ed. St Louis: Saunders/Elsevier, 2006; 841-851.
176. Mader DR. IME—Use of calcitonin in green iguanas, *Iguana iguana*, with metabolic bone disease. *Bull Assoc Rept Amph Vet* 1993;3:5.
177. Schumacher J. Respiratory diseases of reptiles. *Semin Avian Exot Pet Med* 1997;6:209-215.
178. Stahl SJ. Diseases of the reptile pancreas. *Vet Clin North Am Exot Anim Pract* 2003;6:191-212.
179. Kirchgessner M, Mitchell M, Domenzain L, et al. Evaluating the effect of leuprolide acetate on testosterone levels in captive male green iguanas *(Iguana iguana)*. *J Herpetol Med Surg* 2009;19:128-131.
180. Norton TM, Jacobson ER, Caligiuri R, et al. Medical management of a Galapagos tortoise *(Geochelone elephantopus)* with hypothyroidism. *J Zoo Wildl Med* 1989;20:212-216.
181. Franco KH, Hoover JP. Levothyroxine as a treatment for presumed hypothyroidism in an adult male African spurred tortoise *(Centrochelys* [formerly *Geochelone*] *sulcata)*. *J Herpetol Med Surg* 2009;19:42-44.
182. Hernandez-Divers SJ, Cooper JE. Hepatic lipidosis. In: Mader DR, ed. *Reptile medicine and surgery*. 2nd ed. St. Louis: Saunders/Elsevier, 2006;806-813.
183. Divers SJ. Clinician's approach to renal disease in lizards, in *Proceedings*. Annu Conf Assoc Rept Amphib Vet 1997;5-11.
184. Faulkner JE, Archambault A. Anesthesia and surgery in the green iguana. *Semin Avian Exot Pet Med* 1993;2:103-108.
185. Antinoff N, Bauck L, Boyer TH, et al. *Exotic animal formulary*. 2nd ed. Lakewood, Colo: AAHA Press, 1999.
186. Divers SJ. Medical and surgical treatment of pre-ovulatory ova stasis and post-ovulatory egg stasis in oviparous lizards, in *Proceedings*. Annu Conf Assoc Rept Amphib Vet 1996;119-123.
187. Boyer TH. Emergency care of reptiles. *Semin Avian Exot Pet Med* 1994;3:210-216.
188. Boyer TH. Common problems of box turtles (*Terrapene* spp) in captivity. *Bull Assoc Rept Amphib Vet* 1992;2:9-14.
189. Mauldin GN, Done LB. Oncology. In: Mader DR, ed. *Reptile medicine and surgery*. 2nd ed. St Louis: Saunders/Elsevier, 2006;299-322.
190. Georoff TA, Stacy NI, Newton AN, et al. Diagnosis and treatment of chronic T-lymphocytic leukemia in a green tree monitor *(Varanus prasinus)*. *J Herpetol Med Surg* 2009;19:106-114.
191. Norton TM. Chelonian emergency and critical care. *Semin Avian Exot Pet Med* 2005;14:106-130.
192. Rivera S. Health assessment of the reptilian reproductive tract. *J Exot Pet Med* 2008;17:259-266.
193. Gibbons PM. Critical care nutrition and fluid therapy in reptiles, in *Proceedings*. 15th Annu Intl Vet Emerg Crit Care Symp 2009;91-94.
194. Mader DR, Rudloff E. Emergency and critical care. In: Mader DR, ed. *Reptile medicine and surgery*. 2nd ed. St Louis: Saunders/Elsevier, 2006;533-548.
195. Wellehan JFX, Gunkel CI. Emergent diseases in reptiles. *Semin Avian Exot Pet Med* 2004;13:160-174.
196. Donoghue S. Nutrition. In: Mader DR, ed. *Reptile medicine and surgery*. 2nd ed. St. Louis: Saunders/Elsevier, 2006;251-298.
197. Suedmeyer WK. Iron deficiency in a group of American alligators: diagnosis and treatment. *J Small Exot Anim Med* 1991;1:69-72.
198. Kirchgessner M, Mitchell MA. Chelonians. In: Mitchell MA, Tully TN Jr, eds. *Manual of exotic pet practice*. St. Louis: Saunders/Elsevier, 2009;207-249.
199. Jarchow JL. Hospital care of the reptile patient. In: Jacobson ER, Kollias GV Jr, eds. *Exotic animals*. New York: Churchill Livingstone, 1988;19-34.
200. Millichamp NJ. Ophthalmology. In: Girling SJ, Raiti P, eds. *BSAVA manual of reptiles*. 2nd ed. Quedgeley, Gloucester: British Small Animal Veterinary Association, 2004;199-209.
201. Stahl SJ. Captive management, breeding, and common medical problems of the veiled chameleon *(Chamaeleo calyptratus)*, in *Proceedings*. Annu Conf Assoc Rept Amphib Vet 1997;29-40.
202. Harkewicz KA. Dermatologic problems of reptiles. *Semin Avian Exot Pet Med* 2002;11:151-161.
203. Calvert I. Nutritional problems. In: Girling SJ, Raiti P, eds. *BSAVA manual of reptiles*. 2nd ed. Quedgeley, Gloucester: British Small Animal Veterinary Association, 2004;289-308.
204. Fraser MA, Girling SJ. Dermatology. In: Girling SJ, Raiti P, eds. *BSAVA manual of reptiles*. 2nd ed. Quedgeley, Gloucester: British Small Animal Veterinary Association, 2004;184-198.
205. Mehler SJ, Bennett RA. Upper alimentary tract disease. In: Mader DR, ed. *Reptile medicine and surgery*. 2nd ed. St Louis: Saunders/Elsevier, 2006;924-930.
206. Farnsworth RJ, Brannian RE, Fletcher KC, et al. A vitamin E-selenium responsive condition in a green iguana. *J Zoo Anim Med* 1986;17:42-43.
207. Raiti P. Veterinary care of the common kingsnake, *Lampropeltis getula*. *Bull Assoc Rept Amphib Vet* 1995;5:11-18.
208. Mader DR. Gout. In: Mader DR, ed. *Reptile medicine and surgery*. Philadelphia: WB Saunders Co, 1996;374-379.
209. Hernandez-Divers SJ, Martinez-Jimenez D, Bush S, et al. Effects of allopurinol on plasma uric acid levels in normouricaemic and hyperuricaemic green iguanas *(Iguana iguana)*. *Vet Rec* 2008;162:112-115.
210. Koelle P. Efficacy of allopurinol in European tortoises with hyperuricemia, in *Proceedings*. Annu Conf Assoc Rept Amphib Vet 2001;185-186.
211. Meyer J. Gastrographin as a gastrointestinal contrast agent in the Greek tortoise *(Testudo hermanni)*. *J Zoo Wildl Med* 1998;29:183-189.
212. Messonnier S. Formulary for exotic pets. *Vet Forum* 1996;Aug:46-49.
213. Rossi JV. Emergency medicine of reptiles, in *Proceedings*. North Am Vet Conf 1998;799-801.
214. Carpenter JW. Radiographic imaging of reptiles, in *Proceedings*. North Am Vet Conf 1998;873-875.
215. Tothill A, Johnson J, Branvold H, et al. Effect of cisapride, erythromycin, and metoclopramide on gastrointestinal transit time in the desert tortoise, *Gopherus agassizii*. *J Herpetol Med Surg* 2000;10:16-20.

216. Gillespie D. Reptiles. In: Birchard SJ, Sherding RG, eds. *Saunders manual of small animal practice.* Philadelphia: WB Saunders Co, 1994;1390-1411.
217. Rosenthal K. Chemotherapeutic treatment of a sarcoma in a corn snake, in *Proceedings.* Joint Conf Am Assoc Zoo Vet/Assoc Rept Amphib Vet 1994;46.
218. Stahl SJ. Medical management of bearded dragons, in *Proceedings.* North Am Vet Conf 1999;789-792.
219. Divers SJ. Constipation in snakes with particular reference to surgical correction in a Burmese python *(Python molurus bivittatus),* in *Proceedings.* Annu Conf Assoc Rept Amphib Vet 1996;67-69.
220. Wright KM. Common medical problems of tortoises, in *Proceedings.* North Am Vet Conf 1997;769-771.
221. American Veterinary Medical Association Web site. AVMA guidelines on euthanasia. Available at: www.avma.org/issues/animal_welfare/euthanasia.pdf. Accessed May 6, 2011.
222. Burns RB, McMahan W. Euthanasia methods for ectothermic vertebrates. In: Bonagura JD, ed. *Kirk's current veterinary therapy XII: small animal practice.* Philadelphia: WB Saunders Co, 1995;1379-1381.
223. Plumb DC. Probenecid. In: Plumb DC, ed. *Plumb's veterinary drug handbook.* 6th ed. Ames, Iowa: Blackwell Publishing, 2008;1028-1030.
224. Naples LM, Langan JN, Mylniczenko ND, et al. Islet cell tumor in a Savannah monitor *(Varanus exanthematicus). J Herpetol Med Surg* 2009;19:97-105.
225. DeNardo DF, Helminski G. Birth control in lizards? Therapeutic inhibition of reproduction, in *Proceedings.* Annu Conf Assoc Rept Amphib Vet 2000;65-66.
226. Chiodini RJ, Sundberg JP. Blood chemical values of the common boa constrictor *(Constrictor constrictor). Am J Vet Res* 1982;43:1701-1702.
227. Machado CC, Silva LFN, Ramos PRR, et al. Seasonal influence on hematologic values and hemoglobin electrophoresis in Brazilian *Boa constrictor amarali. J Zoo Wildl Med* 2006;37:487-491.
228. Teare JA. Physiological data reference values project. International Species Information System (ISIS), Apple Valley, Minn, 2010.
229. Johnson JH, Benson PA. Laboratory reference values for a group of captive ball pythons *(Python regius). Am J Vet Res* 1996;57:1304-1307.
230. Centini R, Klaphake E. Hematologic values and cytology in a population of captive jungle carpet pythons, *Morelia spilota cheynei,* in *Proceedings.* Annu Conf Assoc Rept Amphib Vet 2002;107-111.
231. Mader DR, Horvath CC, Paul-Murphy J. The hematocrit and serum profile of the gopher snake *(Pituophis melanoleucas catenifer). J Zoo Anim Med* 1985;16:139-140.
232. Ramsay EC, Dotson TK. Tissue and serum enzyme activities in the yellow rat snake *(Elaphe obsoleta quadrivitatta). Am J Vet Res* 1995;56:423-428.
233. Drew ML. Hypercalcemia and hyperphosphatemia in indigo snakes *(Drymarchon corais)* and serum biochemical reference values. *J Zoo Wildl Med* 1994;25:48-52.
234. Naldo JL, Libanan NL, Samour JH. Health assessment of a spiny-tailed lizard (*Uromastyx* spp.) population in Abu Dhabi, United Arab Emirates. *J Zoo Wildl Med* 2009;40:445-452.
235. Ellman MM. Hematology and plasma chemistry of the inland bearded dragon, *Pogona vitticeps. Bull Assoc Rept Amphib Vet* 1997;7:10-12.
236. Mayer J. Characterizing the hematologic and plasma chemistry profiles of captive Chinese water dragons, *Physignathus cocincinus. J Herpetol Med Surg* 2005;15:45-52.
237. Dennis PM, Bennett RA, Harr KE, et al. Plasma concentration of ionized calcium in healthy iguanas. *J Am Vet Med Assoc* 2001;219:326-328.
238. Divers SJ, Redmayne G, Aves EK. Haematological and biochemical values of 10 green iguanas *(Iguana iguana). Vet Rec* 1996;138:203-205.
239. Gimenez M, Saco Y, Pato R, et al. Plasma protein electrophoresis of *Trachemys scripta* and *Iguana iguana. Vet Clin Pathol* 2010;39:227-235.
240. Hernandez-Divers SJ, Knott CD, MacDonald J. Diagnosis and surgical treatment of thyroid adenoma-induced hyperthyroidism in a green iguana *(Iguana iguana). J Zoo Wildl Med* 2001;32:465-475.
241. McBride M, Hernandez-Divers SJ, Koch T, et al. Preliminary evaluation of pre- and post-prandial 3[alpha]-hydroxy bile acids in the green iguana, *Iguana iguana. J Herpetol Med Surg* 2006;16:129-134.
242. Nevarez JG, Mitchell MA, Le Blanc C, et al. Determination of plasma biochemistries, ionized calcium, vitamin D_3, and hematocrit values in captive green iguanas *(Iguana iguana)* from El Salvador, in *Proceedings.* Annu Conf Assoc Rept Amphib Vet 2002;87-91.
243. Harr KE, Alleman AR, Dennis PM, et al. Morphologic and cytochemical characteristics of blood cells and hematologic and plasma biochemical reference ranges in green iguanas *J Am Vet Med Assoc* 2001;218:915-921.
244. Judd HL, Laughlin GA, Bacon JP, et al. Circulating androgen and estrogen concentrations in lizards *(Iguana iguana). Gen Comp Endocrinol* 1976;30:391-395.
245. Wright KM, Skeba S. Hematology and plasma chemistries of captive prehensile-tailed skinks *(Corucia zebrata). J Zoo Wildl Med* 1992;23:429-432.
246. Troiano J, Gould E, Gould I. Hematological reference intervals in Argentine lizard *Tupinambis merianae. Comp Clin Pathol* 2008;17:169-174.
247. Diethelm G, Stein G. Hematologic and blood chemistry values in reptiles. In: Mader DR, ed. *Reptile medicine and surgery.* 2nd ed. St. Louis: Saunders/Elsevier, 2006;1103-1118.
248. Fudge AM. Laboratory reference ranges for selected avian, mammalian, and reptilian species. In: Fudge AM, ed. *Laboratory medicine: avian and exotic pets.* Philadelphia: WB Saunders Co, 2000;375-400.
249. Marks SK, Citino SB. Hematology and serum chemistry of the radiated tortoise *(Testudo radiata). J Zoo Wildl Med* 1990;21:342-344.
250. Zaias J, Norton T, Fickel A, et al. Biochemical and hematologic values for 18 clinically healthy radiated tortoises *(Geochelone radiata)* on St Catherines Island, Georgia. *Vet Clin Pathol* 2006;35:321-325.
251. Alleman AR, Jacobson ER, Raskin RE. Morphologic and cytochemical characteristics of blood cells from the desert tortoise *(Gopherus agassizii),* in *Proceedings.* Annu Conf Assoc Rept Amphib Vet 1996;51-55.
252. Christopher MM, Berry KH, Wallis IR, et al. Reference intervals and physiologic alterations in hematologic and biochemical values of free-ranging desert tortoises in the Mojave Desert. *J Wildl Dis* 1999;35:212-238.
253. Dickinson VM, Jarchow JL, Trueblood MH. Hematology and plasma biochemistry reference range values for free-ranging desert tortoises in Arizona. *J Wildl Dis* 2002;38:143-153.
254. Gottdenker NL, Jacobson ER. Effect of venipuncture sites on hematologic and clinical biochemical values in desert tortoises *(Gopherus agassizii). Am J Vet Res* 1995;56:19-21.
255. Taylor RW Jr, Jacobson ER. Hematology and serum chemistry of the gopher tortoise, *Gopherus polyphemus. Comp Biochem Physiol A* 1982;72:425-428.
256. Knotkova Z, Doubek J, Knotek Z, et al. Blood cell morphology and plasma biochemistry in Russian tortoises *(Agrionemys horsfieldi). Acta Vet Brno* 2002;71:191-198.
257. Mathes KA, Holz A, Fehr M. Blood reference values of terrestrial tortoises (*Testudo* spp.) kept in Germany. *Tierarztl Prax Ausg K Klientiere Heimtiere* 2006;34:268-274.
258. Crawshaw GJ, Holz P. Comparison of plasma biochemical values in blood and blood-lymph mixtures from red-eared sliders, *Trachemys scripta elegans. Bull Assoc Rept Amphib Vet* 1996;6:7-9.
259. Gaumer A, Goodnight CJ. Some aspects of the hematology of turtles as related to their activity. *Am Midland Nat* 1957;58:332-340.
260. Jacobson ER. Evaluation of the reptile patient. In: Jacobson ER, Kollias GV Jr, eds. *Exotic Animals.* New York: Churchill Livingstone, 1988;1-18.
261. Flint M, Morton JM, Limpus CJ, et al. Development and application of biochemical and haematological reference intervals to identify unhealthy green sea turtles *(Chelonia mydas). Vet J* 2010;185:299-304.

262. Barrie MT. Chameleon medicine. In: Fowler ME, Miller RE, eds. *Zoo & wild animal medicine: current therapy*. 4th ed. Philadelphia: WB Saunders Co,1999;200-205.
263. Cunningham AA, Gill C. Management in captivity. In: Benyon PH, Lawton MPC, Cooper JE, eds. *Manual of reptiles*. Ames: Iowa State University Press, 1992;14-31.
264. Dundee HA, Rossman DA. *The amphibians and reptiles of Louisiana*. Baton Rouge: Louisiana State University Press, 1989;270-272.
265. Harless M, Morlock H. *Turtles—perspectives and research*. New York: John Wiley & Sons, 1979;356-366.
266. McKeown S. General husbandry and management. In: Mader DR, ed. *Reptile medicine and surgery*. Philadelphia: WB Saunders Co, 1996;9-19.
267. Gibbons PM, Horton SJ, Brandl SR. Urinalysis in box turtles, Terrapene spp, in *Proceedings*. Annu Conf Assoc Rept Amphib Vet 2000;161-168.
268. Innis CJ. Observations on urinalysis of clinically normal captive tortoises, in *Proceedings*. Annu Conf Assoc Rept Amphib Vet 1997;109-112.
269. Koelle P. Urinalysis in tortoises, in *Proceedings*. Annu Conf Assoc Rept Amphib Vet 2000;111-113.
270. Koelle P, Hoffmann R. Urinalysis in European tortoises—part II, in *Proceedings*. Annu Conf Assoc Rept Amphib Vet 2002;117.
271. Stahl SJ. Common Diseases of the Green Iguana. Proc North Am Vet Conf 1998;806-809.

APPENDIX 4

Abridged Formulary for Amphibians

†Kevin Wright, James W. Carpenter, and Ryan S. DeVoe

Note: All dosages should be considered ones that have been used by the author(s) and appear to be effective in one or more species; at worst, dosages may have no grossly observable unexpected deleterious effect. Because of the paucity of data in a limited number of amphibian species, caution is advised when a medication is used on an unfamiliar species.

Note: Water baths containing antibiotics or topical applications may not provide as consistent distribution as parenteral administration. Subcutaneous administration in anurans can be through the (dorsal) lymph sac.

Bold items are commonly used medication. ***Bold italicized*** entries indicate pharmacokinetic data or data originating from the cited articles published in peer-reviewed periodicals or major conference proceedings.

†Deceased.

TABLE 1

Antimicrobial Agents Used in Amphibians

Agent	Dosage	Species/Comments
Amikacin	***5 mg/kg IM q36h***[a]	Bullfrogs
	5-10 mg/kg SC, IM, ICe q24-48h	
Ceftazidime	20 mg/kg SC, IM q48-72h	
Chloramphenicol	50 mg/kg SC, IM, ICe q12-24h	Caution: even miniscule exposure carries risk of aplastic anemia in susceptible individuals; wear disposable gloves when handling
	20 mg/L bath changed daily	
Ciprofloxacin	10 mg/kg ICe, PO q24h	
	500-750 mg/75 L as 6-8 hour bath q24h	May be used for large numbers of animals
Doxycycline (Psittavet, Vetafarm)	50 mg/kg IM q7d	Broad-spectrum antibiotic, part of quadrant therapy; may have antiinflammatory effect; chlamydophilosis
Doxycycline (Vibramycin, Pfizer)	10-50 mg/kg PO q24h	African clawed frogs/chlamydophilosis
Doxycycline 1% topical gel, compounded	Apply topically q8-12h, not to exceed 10 mg/kg per day	Useful for localized lesions; may have anti-inflammatory effect
Enrofloxacin (Baytril, Bayer)	***5-10 mg/kg PO, SC, IM q24h***[a]	Bullfrogs
		ICe and topical routes also used but without PD
Enrofloxacin and silver sulfadiazine solution (Baytril Otic, Bayer)	Apply topically to lesions q12h	May have some antifungal effect but does not appear effective on chytrid
Gentamicin	***2.5 mg/kg IM q72h***[b]	Coldwater mudpuppies *(Necturus)*; more frequent dosing may be needed if temperature >4°C (39.2°F)
	3 mg/kg IM q24h at 22.2°C (72°F)[c]	Leopard frogs/PD; at higher temperatures, serum concentrations will be lower
	Intracameral injection once, not to exceed 4 mg/kg	Panophthalmitis
Metronidazole and metronidazole benzoate	10 mg/kg PO q24h × 5 to 10 days	For chronic diarrhea
	20 mg/kg PO q48h × 20 days	Anaerobic infections
	50 mg/kg PO q24h × 3 days	Flagellates and amoebas

Continued

TABLE 1—cont'd

Antimicrobial Agents Used in Amphibians

Agent	Dosage	Species/Comments
Ofloxacin 0.3% ophthalmic solution	1 ggt q2-4h × 10 days	Keratitis; may also be applied topically to wounds
Oxytetracycline	***50-100 mg/kg IM q48***[a]	Bullfrogs/especially useful in cases of chlamydiosis (use up to 30 days)
	50 mg/kg PO q24h	
	100 mg/L × 1-hour bath	
Silver sulfadiazine (Silvadene Cream 1%, Marion)	Topical q24h	Antibiotic cream
Trimethoprim/sulfate	15-20 mg/kg IM q48h	Chronic diarrhea

gtt, Drop; *IM,* intramuscular; *ICe,* intracoelomic; *PD,* pharmacodynamics; *PO,* per os (by mouth); *SC,* subcutaneous.
Adapted from [a]Letcher J, Papich M. Pharmacokinetics of intramuscular administration of three antibiotics in bullfrogs *(Rana catesbeiana)*, in *Proceedings.* Annu Conf Assoc Rept Amphib Vet/Am Assoc Zoo Vet 1994;79-93; [b]Stoskopf MK, Arnold J, Mason M. Aminoglycoside antibiotic levels in the aquatic salamander *(Necturus necturus)*. *J Zoo Anim Med* 1987;18:81-85; and [c]Teare JA, Wallace RS, Bush M. Pharmacology of gentamicin in the leopard frog *(Rana pipiens)*, in *Proceedings.* Annu Conf Am Assoc Zoo Vet 1991;128-131.

TABLE 2

Antifungal Agents Used in Amphibians

Agent	Dosage	Species/Comments
Amphotericin B	1 mg/kg ICe q24h	Internal mycoses
Benzalkonium chloride	2 mg/L × 1-hour bath q24h	Saprolegniasis
Chloramphenicol (straight chemical)	***20 ppm as continuous bath replaced fresh daily for up to 30 days***[a]	Chytridiomycosis; safe for larvae, recent metamorphs, and adults; confirm negative result by real-time PCR; caution: even miniscule exposure carries risk of aplastic anemia in susceptible individuals; wear disposable gloves when handling
	30 ppm as continuous bath replaced fresh daily for up to 30 days[b]	
Florfenicol (straight chemical)	30 ppm as continuous bath replaced fresh daily for up to 30 days	Chytridiomycosis; safe for larvae, recent metamorphs, and adults; confirm negative result by real-time PCR
Fluconazole	60 mg/kg PO q24h	
Itraconazole	***0.01% in 0.6% salt solution as 5 min bath q24h×11 days***[c]	Topical route best choice to treat chytridiomycosis; do not use with larvae
	10 mg/kg PO q24h	
Nystatin 1% cream	Topical	Cutaneous mycoses
Temperature elevation	***37°C (98.6°F) for 16h***[d]	Chytridiomycosis; lower temperatures (down to 30°C [86°F]) may be effective with longer duration

ICe, Intracoelomic; *PCR,* polymerase chain reaction; *PO,* per os (by mouth).
Adapted from [a]Bishop PJ, Spear R, Poulet R, et al. Elimination of the amphibian chytrid fungus *Batrachochytrium dendrobatidis* by Archey's frog *Leiopelma archeyi. Dis Aquat Organ* 2009;84:9-15; [b]Pessier AP, Mendelson JR, eds. *A manual for control of infectious diseases in amphibian survival assurance colonies and reintroduction programs.* Apple Valley, Minn: IUCN/SSC Conservation Breeding Specialist Group. Available at: http://czaw.org/manual-control-infectious-diseases-amphibian-survival-assurance-colonies-and-reintroduction-programs. Accessed Dec 31, 2010; [c]Nichols DK, Lamirander EW, Pessier AP, et al. Experimental transmission and treatment of cutaneous chytridiomycosis in poison dart frogs *(Dendrobates auratus* and *Dendrobates tinctorius)*, in *Proceedings.* Annu Conf Am Assoc Zoo Vet/Internatl Assoc Aquat Anim Med 2000;42-44; and Woodhams DC, Alford RA, Marantelli G. Emerging disease of amphibians cured by elevated body temperature. *Dis Aquat Organ* 2003;55:65-67.

TABLE 3

Antiparasitic Agents Used in Amphibians

Agent	Dosage	Species/Comments
Benzalkonium chloride	2 mg/L × 1-hour bath q24h to effect	Protozoa
Distilled water	3-hour bath	Protozoa
Febantel (in combination with pyrantel pamoate and praziquantel; Drontal Plus, Bayer)	0.01 mL/1 g (10 mL/kg) PO q2-3 weeks	Nematodes, cestodes, possibly trematodes
Fenbendazole	50 mg/kg PO q24h × 3 to 5 days, repeat in 14 to 21 days	Nematode
	50-100 mg/kg PO, repeat in 2 to 3 weeks prn	
Ivermectin		Caution: may cause flaccid paralysis with overdosage; caffeine or physostigmine may ameliorate effects[53]
	0.2-0.4 mg/kg PO, SC, repeat q14d prn	Nematodes, including lungworms; mites
	2 mg/kg topically, repeat in 2 to 3 weeks	Especially useful for small specimens[54] and *Rana* spp[20]
	10 mg/L as 60-min bath, repeat q14d prn	Best route for treating mites
Levamisole		May cause paralysis in some species at suggested dosages; caffeine or physostigmine may ameliorate effects
	100 mg/L × ≥72-hour bath	Nematodes, including subcutaneous nematodes in aquatic amphibians; water soluble form is available through aquaculture supply companies
	100-300 mg/L × 24-hour bath, repeat in 1 to 2 weeks	
Metronidazole	50 mg/kg PO q24h × 3 to 5 days	Confirmed cases of amoebiasis and flagellate overload
	100-150 mg/kg PO, repeat in 2-3 weeks or prn	Protozoa (e.g., *Entamoeba, Hexamita, Opalina*)
Paromomycin (Humatin, Parke Davis)	50-75 mg/kg PO q24h	Gastrointestinal protozoa
Ponazuril	30 mg/kg PO q12h × 3 days, repeat in 3 weeks; often more effective at 30 mg/kg PO q24h × 30 days; may work with less frequent treatments	Coccidia but not *Cryptosporidium*; may have some effect on unidentified protozoan cysts
Praziquantel	8-24 mg/kg PO, SC, ICe, topically, repeat q14d	Trematodes, cestodes
	10 mg/L × 3-hour bath, repeat q7-21d	Trematodes, cestodes
Pyrantel pamoate	5 mg/kg PO q14d	Nematodes
Ronidazole	10 mg/kg PO q24h × 10 days	Flagellated protozoa, amoebas
Salt (sodium chloride)a	4 to 6 g/L continuous bath	Ectoparasitic protozoa
	6 g/L × 5-10 min bath q24h × 3 to 5 days	Ectoparasitic protozoa
	25 g/L × ≤10 min bath	Ectoparasitic protozoa
Selamectin (Revolution, Pfizer)	***6 mg/kg topically***[b]	Bullfrogs

ICe, Intracoelomic; *PO,* per os (by mouth); *prn,* as needed; *SC,* subcutaneous.
Adapted from [a]Marcec R, Mitchell MA, Kirshenbaum BS, et al. Clinical and physiologic effects of sodium chloride baths in axolotls, *Ambystoma mexicanum,* in *Proceedings.* ARAV, Seattle, Wash 2011;1; [b]D'Agostino JJ, West G, Boothe DM, et al. Plasma pharmacokinetics of selamectin after a single topical administration in the American bullfrog *(Rana catesbeiana). J Zoo Wildl Med* 2007;38:51-54.

TABLE 4

Chemical Restraint/Anesthetic/Analgesic Agents Used in Amphibians

Agent	Dosage	Species/Comments
Buprenorphine (Buprenex, Reckitt and Colman)	***38 mg/kg SC***[a]	Analgesia >4 hours; ED_{50} in leopard frogs
Clove oil (eugenol)	***0.3 mL/L (≈310-318 mg/L)***[b]	Anesthesia; deep anesthesia after 15-min bath; caused reversible gastric prolapse in 50% of leopard frogs
	0.45 mL/L (≈473 mg/L)[c]	Anesthesia; deep anesthesia induced in 80% of tiger salamanders
	0.35 mL/L (350 mg/L)[d]	Anesthesia for short surgical procedures in African clawed frogs
Fentanyl	***0.5 mg/kg SC***[a]	Analgesia >4 hours; ED_{50} in leopard frogs
Isoflurane		Anesthesia; induction chamber; inhalant of choice
	3% to 5% induction, 1% to 2% maintenance	Terrestrial species
	Topical mixture of isoflurane (3 mL), KY jelly (3.5 mL), and water (1.5 mL)[e]	*Bufo* spp (0.035 mL/g BW), African clawed frogs (0.025 mL/g BW)/ induce in closed container; once induced, remove excess from animal
	0.28 mL/100 mL bath[e]	Induce in closed container
	Bubbled into water to effect[e]	Aquatic species
Ketamine		May have long induction and recovery times; does not provide good analgesia so may not be suited for major surgical procedures; other agents preferred; see lidocaine
	50-150 mg/kg SC, IM	Most species
Lidocaine 1% to 2%	Local infiltration	All/local anesthesia; with or without epinephrine; 2% lidocaine in combination with ketamine has been used for minor surgeries; use with caution
Meloxicam	0.4 to 1.0 mg/kg PO, SC, ICe q24h	Analgesia
Morphine	***38-42 mg/kg SC***[a]	Analgesia >4 hours
Nalorphine	***122 mg/kg SC***[a]	Analgesia >4 hours
Naloxone	***10 mg/kg SC titrate to effect***[a]	Antagonist for buprenorphine, butorphanol, codeine, fentanyl, morphine
Naltrexone	***1 mg/kg SC titrate to effect***[a]	Antagonist for buprenorphine, butorphanol, codeine, fentanyl, morphine
Pentobarbital sodium	60 mg/kg IV, ICe	Euthanasia; ICe is preferred route; can also be administered in lymph sacs in anurans
Propofol	***88 mg/L***[f]	Light anesthesia in African clawed frogs but did not eliminate pain response; narrow margin of safety with death at 175 mg/L
	35 mg/kg ICe[c]	Deep anesthesia in 83% of tiger salamanders
	60-100 mg/kg ICe[g]	Euthanasia
Sevoflurane	Topical application	Rapid recovery unless constant reapplication
	Topical mixture of sevoflurane (5 mL) + water soluble jelly (5 mL)	

TABLE 4—cont'd

Chemical Restraint/Anesthetic/Analgesic Agents Used in Amphibians

Agent	Dosage	Species/Comments
Tricaine methanesulfonate (MS-222) (Finquel, Argent)		Anesthesia; buffer the acidity by adding sodium bicarbonate to the solution to a pH of 7.0-7.1; aerate water to prevent hypoxemia; remove from bath on induction or overdosing can readily occur; following bath, place terrestrial amphibians on moist towel or in very shallow water to recover; some species can be induced at much lower concentrations than listed here; in some cases, anesthesia can be maintained by dripping a dilute solution of this drug (100-200 mg/L) over the skin or by covering animal with a paper towel moistened with the anesthetic
		Most species/may be irritating administered SC, IM (neutral solution is preferred)
	50-200 mg/kg SC, IM, ICe[h]	Leopard frogs
	100-200 mg/kg ICe	Bullfrogs
	100-400 mg/kg ICe	Larvae/induction
	100-200 mg/L bath to effect	Tadpoles, newts/induction in 15-30 min
	200-500 mg/L bath to effect[h]	Frogs, salamanders/induction in 15-30 min
	0.5-2 g/L bath to effect	Most gill-less adult species (unless very large)/ induction
	1 g/L bath to effect	Toads/induction in 15-30 min
	2-3 g/L bath to effect	Euthanasia; can be administered ICe or in lymph sacs
	10 g/L bath	

BW, Body weight; ED_{50}, effective dose for 50% of the population; *ICe,* intracoelomic; *IM,* intramuscular; *IV,* intravenous; *SC,* subcutaneous.
Adapted from [a]Machin KL. Amphibian pain and analgesia. *J Zoo Wildl Med* 1999;30:2-10; [b]Lafortune M, Mitchell MA, Smith JA. Evaluation of clinical and cardiopulmonary effects of clove oil (eugenol) on leopard frogs, *Rana pipiens. J Herpetol Med Surg* 12(4):13-18, 2001; [c]Mitchell MA, Riggs SM, Singleton CB, et al. Evaluating the clinical and cardiopulmonary effects of clove oil and propofol in tiger salamanders *(Ambystoma tigrinum). J Exot Pet Med* 2009;18:50-56; [d]Guénette SA, Hélie P, Beaudry F, et al. Eugenol for anesthesia of African clawed frogs *(Xenopus laevis). Vet Anaesth Analg* 2007;34:164-170; [e]Stetter MD, Raphael B, Indiviglio F, et al. Isoflurane anesthesia in amphibians: comparison of five application methods, in *Proceedings.* Annu Conf Am Assoc Zoo Vet 1996;255-257; [f]Guénette SA, Beaudry F, Vachon P. Anesthetic properties of propofol in African clawed frogs *(Xenopus laevis). J Am Assoc Lab Anim Sci* 2008;47(5):35-38; [g]von Esse FV, Wright KM. Effect of intracoelomic propofol in White's tree frogs, *Pelodryas caerulea. Bull Assoc Rept Amphib Vet* 1999;9:7-8; [h]Downes H. Tricaine anesthesia in amphibia: a review. *Bull Assoc Rept Amphib Vet* 1995;5:11-16.

TABLE 5

Miscellaneous Agents Used in Amphibians

Agent	Dosage	Species/Comments
Amphibian Ringer's solution (ARS)	6.6 g NaCl, 0.15 g KCl, 0.15 g $CaCl_2$, and 0.2 g $NaHCO_3$ in 1 L water	For treating hydrocoelom and subcutaneous edema; place animal in shallow ARS bath until stabilized (≈24 hours or more); replace with fresh solution daily; may need to wean animal off ARS by placing it in gradually more dilute solutions; hypertonic solution created by using 800-950 mL water instead of 1 L and may be more effective for some cases of hydrocoelom; up to 10 g of glucose may be added per liter, but then solution must be made fresh daily
Atropine	0.1 mg SC, IM prn	Organophosphate toxicosis
Caffeine	Use caffeinated tea bag; steep (soak) until solution is "weak tea"; place amphibian in shallow bath, replace q6h	Stimulant; may help reverse ivermectin or levamisole toxicosis, or excessively deep anesthesia
Calcium glubionate	1 mL/kg PO q24h	Nutritional secondary hyperparathyroidism
Calcium gluconate	100-200 mg/kg SC	Hypocalcemic tetany
	2.3% continuous bath (with 2-3 IU/mL vitamin D_3)	Nutritional secondary hyperparathyroidism

Continued

TABLE 5—cont'd

Miscellaneous Agents Used in Amphibians

Agent	Dosage	Species/Comments
Critical care diets		
Carnivore Critical Care (Oxbow)	3% bodyweight PO q24-72h	Dosage is approximate; may be more appropriate to offer larger volume less frequently for easily stressed animals
Emeraid for Carnivores (Lafeber)	3% BW PO q24-48	Dosage is approximate; may be more appropriate to offer larger volume less frequently for easily stressed animals
Dexamethasone	1.5 mg/kg SC, IM	Vascularizing keratitis
	1.5 mg/kg IM, IV	Shock
Dextrose 5% solution	Bath	For treating hydrocoelom and subcutaneous edema; place animal in shallow bath until stabilized (≈24 hours or more); replace with fresh solution daily; may need to wean animal off dextrose by placing it in gradually more dilute solutions; 7.5% to 10% solutions may be more effective for some cases of hydrocoelom
Doxycycline	1.25-2.5 mg/kg PO, SC, ICe q24h	Antiinflammatory
	1% gel topically q12h	Antiinflammatory
Hetastarch (6% in 0.9% saline)	Bath not to exceed 1 hour without reassessment	May help with initial treatment of some hydrocoelom
Meloxicam	0.4 to 1.0 mg/kg PO, SC, ICe q24h	Antiinflammatory; presumptive analgesia; adjunct therapy for septicemia
	0.5% gel topically q24h; do not exceed 0.4 mg/kg	Antiinflammatory for localized wounds
Methylene blue	2 mg/mL bath to effect	Nitrite and nitrate toxicoses
Oxygen	100% for up to 24 hours	Adjunct treatment for septicemia, toxicoses
Physostigmine (ophthalmic drops)	1 drop/50 g topically q1-2h to effect	May ameliorate flaccid paralysis from ivermectin or levamisole toxicosis
Prednisolone sodium succinate	5-10 mg/kg IM, IV	Shock
Sodium thiosulfate	1% solution as continuous bath to effect	Halogen toxicosis
Vitamin A (Aquasol A, 50,000 U/mL, Mayne Pharma)	Dilute 1:9 with sterile water; make fresh weekly; apply 1 drop from a tuberculin syringe with 27-g needle to amphibians under 5 g; 1 drop from tuberculin syringe without needle is about 200 U and useful for 15-30 g BW; for larger animals, try 1 drop per 10 g BW; topically q24h × 14 days, then q4-7d	Hypovitaminosis A; given the plethora of organ systems that hypovitaminosis A may affect, it is reasonable to institute vitamin A supplementation of any clinical ill amphibian, particularly ones with signs similar to "short tongue syndrome", swollen eyelids, evidence of infectious dermatitis, hydrocoelom, or simply, failure to thrive
	1 U/g PO daily × 14 days	
Vitamin A gel caps (10,000 U/cap)	Dilute 1:9 with corn oil to yield 1000 U/mL, give 1 U/g PO q24h × 14 days, then q7d	Hypovitaminosis A; given the plethora of organ systems that hypovitaminosis A may affect, it is reasonable to institute vitamin A supplementation of any clinical ill amphibian, particularly ones with signs similar to "short tongue syndrome", swollen eyelids, evidence of infectious dermatitis, hydrocoelom, or simply, failure to thrive
Vitamin B_1	25 mg/kg feed fish	Deficiency resulting from thiaminase-containing fish
Vitamin D_3	2 to 3 U/mL continuous bath (with 2.3% calcium gluconate)	Nutritional secondary hyperparathyroidism
	100-400 U/kg PO q24h	
Vitamin E (alpha-tocopherol)	1 mg/kg PO, IM q7d	Steatitis

BW, Body weight; *ICe*, intracoelomic; *IM*, intramuscular; *IV*, intravenous; *PO*, by mouth; *prn*, as needed; *SC*, subcutaneous.

APPENDIX 5

Weights and Measures Conversions

WEIGHTS AND MEASURES CONVERSIONS

Weights

1 milligram (mg) = 1000 micrograms (mcg or µg)
1 grain (gr) = 64.8 mg (≈65 mg)
1 gram (g) = 15.43 grains (≈15 grains) = 1000 mg
1 kilogram (kg) = 1000 g
1 ounce (oz) = 28.35 g (≈30 g)
1 pound (lb) = 454 g = 16 oz = 0.45 kg
2.2 lbs = 1 kg

Liquid Measures

1 drop = 0.05 (1/20) milliliter (mL)
1 cubic centimeter (cc) = 1 mL
1 liter (L) = 1000 mL
1 teaspoon (tsp) = 5 mL
1 tablespoon (Tbsp) = 15 mL
1 fluid ounce (fl oz) = 29.57 mL (≈30 mL)
1 quart = 2 pints = 32 fl oz (≈0.95 L)
1 gallon = 4 quarts = 3.785 L
1 cup = 8 fl oz = 237 mL = 16 Tbsp

Imperial Pint

1 imperial pint = ⅛ imperial gallon
= ½ imperial quart
= 4 imperial gills
= 20 imperial fluid ounces
= 568.26125 millilitres
≈ 568 mL
≈ 34.677429099 cubic inches
≈ 1.2009499255 U.S. liquid pints

Linear Measures

1 millimeter (mm) = 0.039 inches (in)
1 centimeter (cm) = 0.39 in
1 meter (m) = 39.37 in
1 in = 2.54 cm
1 foot (ft) = 30.48 cm
1 yard (yd) = 91.44 cm

APPENDIX 6

Celsius Versus Fahrenheit Conversions

Celsius Versus Fahrenheit Conversions

°C	°F	°C	°F
0	32.0	26	78.8
1	33.8	27	80.6
2	35.6	28	82.4
3	37.4	29	84.2
4	39.2	30	86.0
5	41.0	31	87.8
6	42.8	32	89.6
7	44.6	33	91.4
8	46.4	34	93.2
9	48.2	35	95.0
10	50.0	36	96.8
11	51.8	37	98.6
12	53.6	38	100.4
13	55.4	39	102.2
14	57.2	40	104.0
15	59.0	41	105.8
16	60.8	42	107.6
17	62.6	43	109.4
18	64.4	44	111.2
19	66.2	45	113.0
20	68.0	46	114.8
21	69.8	47	116.6
22	71.6	48	118.4
23	73.4	49	120.2
24	75.2	50	122.0
25	77.0		

Note: Equivalents of Celsius (Centigrade) and Fahrenheit temperature scales. Temperature formulas: °C = 5/9 (°F – 32) and °F = (°C x 9/5) + 32.

APPENDIX 7

U.S./IU (Blood Values) Conversion

U.S./IU (Blood Values) Conversion

	Conventional (U.S.) Unit	Conversion Factor	SI Unit
HEMATOLOGY			
Red blood cell count	$10^6/\mu L$	1	$10^{12}/L$
Hemoglobin	g/dL	0.1	g/L
MCH	pg/cell	1	pg/cell
MCHC	g/dL	0.1	g/L
MCV	μm^3	1	fl
Platelet count	$10^3/\mu L$	1	$10^9/L$
White blood cell count	$10^3/\mu L$	1	$10^9/L$
PLASMA CHEMISTRY			
Alkaline phosphatase	μ/L	1	IU/L
ALT (SGPT)	μ/L	1	IU/L
Albumin	g/dL	10	g/L
Ammonia (NH_4)	μg/dL	0.5871	μmol/L
Amylase	μ/L	1	IU/L
AST (SGOT)	μ/L	1	IU/L
Bilirubin	mg/dL	17.1	μmol/L
Calcium	mg/dL	0.2495	mmol/L
Carbon dioxide	mEq/L	1	mmol/L
Chloride	mEq/L	1	mmol/L
Cholesterol	mg/dL	0.02586	mmol/L
Cortisol	μg/dL	27.59	nmol/L
Creatine kinase	μ/L	1	IU/L
Creatinine	mg/dL	88.4	μmol/L
Fibrinogen	mg/dL	0.01	g/L
Glucose	mg/dL	0.05551	mmol/L
Iron	μg/dL	0.1791	μmol/L
Lipase			
Sigma Tietz	μ/dL	280	IU/L
Cherry Crandall	μ/L	1	IU/L
Lipid, total	mg/dL	0.01	g/L
Osmolality	mOsm/kg	1	mmol/kg
Phosphate (as inorganic P)	mg/dL	0.3229	mmol/L
Potassium	mEq/L	1	mmol/L
Protein, total	g/dL	10	g/L
Sodium	mEq/L	1	mmol/L
Thyroxine (T_4)	μg/dL	12.87	nmol/L
Urea nitrogen	mg/dL	0.357	mmol/L*
Uric acid	mg/dL	59.48	μmol/L

ALT, Alanine aminotransferase; *AST,* aspartate aminotransferase; *MCH,* mean corpuscular hemoglobin; *MCHC,* mean corpuscular hemoglobin count; *MCV,* mean cell volume; *SGOT,* serum glutamate oxaloacetate transaminase; *SGPT,* serum glutamate pyruvate transaminase; *SI,* International System of Units; *U.S.,* United States.

*Urea.

Modified from *The Merck veterinary manual.* 8th ed. Whitehouse Station, NJ: Merck and Co. 1998, as adapted from *The SI manual in health care.* Canada: Metric Commission, 1981.

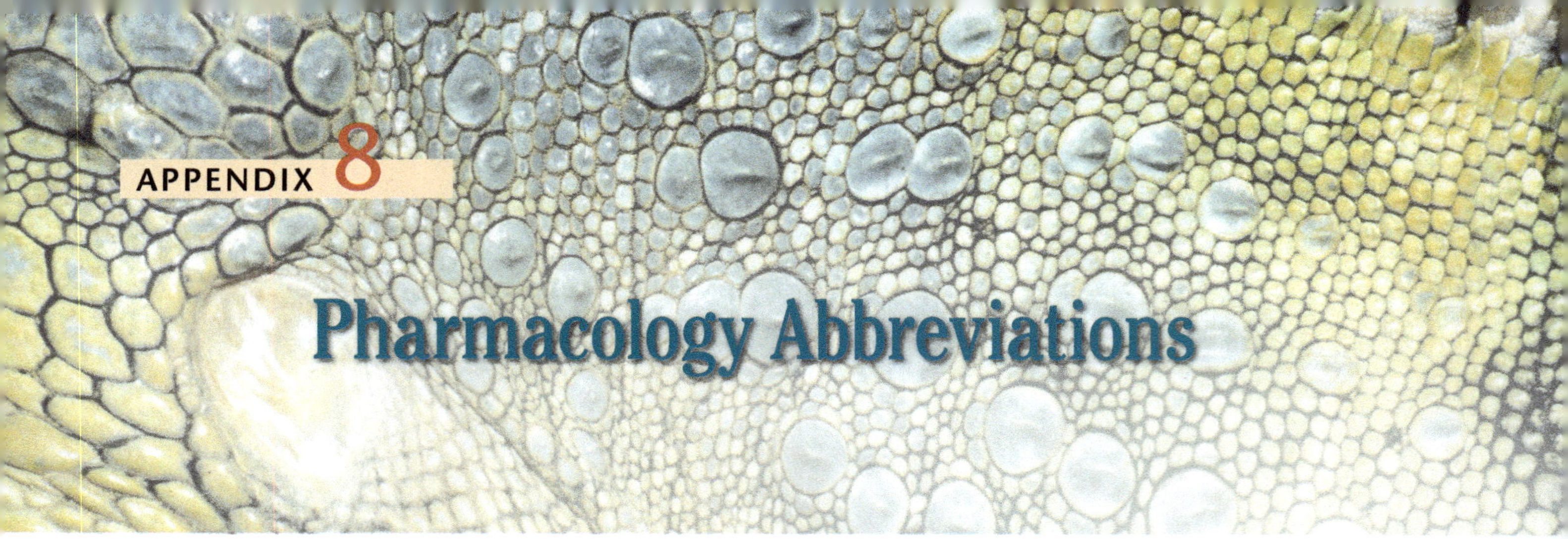

APPENDIX 8

Pharmacology Abbreviations

Pharmacology Abbreviations

Abbreviation	Definition
ac	before meals
ad	right ear
ad lib	at pleasure
adm	administer
aq	water
as	left ear
au	both ears
bid	twice a day
c	with
cap(s)	capsule(s)
cc	cubic centimeter
disp	dispense
fl oz	fluid ounce
g (gm)	gram
gr	grain
gtt(s)	drop(s)
h (hr)	hour
hs	at bedtime
IC	intracardiac
ICe	intracoelomic
IM	intramuscularly
inj	inject
IV	intravenously
kg	kilogram
lb	pound
mg	milligram
mL	milliliter
od	right eye
os	left eye
ou	both eyes
oz	ounce
pc	after meals
PO	by mouth
prn	as needed
q	every
qd	every day
q4h	every 4 hours, etc
q24h	once a day
qid	four times a day
qod	every other day
qs	a sufficient quantity
®	registered trademarked name
SC (SQ)	subcutaneously
sig:	instructions to patient
sol'n	solution
stat	immediately
susp	suspension
tab(s)	tablet(s)
Tbs (Tbsp)	tablespoon
tid	three times a day
tsp	teaspoon
ut dict	as directed

APPENDIX 9

Reptile and Amphibian History Form

PATIENT DETAILS

REPTILE AND AMPHIBIAN HISTORY FORM

A detailed history is essential to provide the most appropriate veterinary care for your animal. Please complete this form as accurately as possible. If there is anything you are unsure about you can discuss it in more depth with the veterinary staff during your appointment.

PATIENT DETAILS

Patient's name or identification:______________________________

Common and/or scientific species name:______________________________

Date of birth: _________ or est. age: ____________ Sex: M ☐ F ☐ neutered/spayed ☐ unknown ☐

Origin: captive bred ☐ wild caught import ☐ unknown ☐

How long have you had this animal?______________________________

From where did you obtain this animal?______________________________

Does your herp have any history of breeding or laying eggs? N ☐ Y ☐ Please give details ______________________________

____

When did your herp last shed? ____________________ How often has your herp been shedding? ______________

Do you have any other herps or pets? N ☐ Y ☐ Please give details ______________________________

Have you or your herp had any contact with other herps in the last 30 days? N ☐ Y ☐ Please give details__________

____

When was the last herp added to your collection? ______________________________

REASON FOR PRESENTATION TODAY

What is the primary complaint or what signs you have noticed? How long have these problems been present?

____

What health problems has your herp had previously?______________________________

____

When and why did you last see a veterinarian? ______________________________

Has your herp received any treatment in the last 30 days? N ☐ Y ☐ Please give details (what was used, dosage, how often, duration? ______________________________

Have you noticed any change in your herp's behavior? N ☐ Y ☐ Please give details ______________________________

____

Have any other animals or persons in the household had any illness in the last 30 days? ______________________________

____

CAGE ENVIRONMENT

What type of cage is used? arboreal (tall, climbing) ☐ terrestrial ☐ aquatic ☐ Cage size: ____________________

What is the cage made of? plastic/fiberglass ☐ wooden ☐ metal ☐ glass ☐ other:____________________

What is the floor substrate? paper ☐ corncob ☐ sand ☐ AstroTurf ☐ bark ☐ other:____________________

What decor and furnishings are present? ____________________

Is there additional ventilation (grills or mesh)? N ☐ Y ☐ Please give size/details____________________

Are bathing facilities provided? N ☐ Y ☐ Please give details____________________

How often is the cage cleaned?____________________

What cleaning/disinfectant agents are used?____________________

What heating equipment is used?

Ceramic/infrared ☐ power_____W thermostat control: N ☐ Y ☐

Spot light/bulb ☐ power_____W thermostat control: N ☐ Y ☐

Heat mat ☐ size:________________ under cage ☐ or inside cage ☐ thermostat control: N ☐ Y ☐

Aquarium water heater ☐ power_____W thermostat control: N ☐ Y ☐

Other heaters; please give details____________________

Are the heat sources screened from the animals? N ☐ Y ☐ Please give details ____________________

Can the animal(s) touch or access the heat source? N ☐ Y ☐ Please give details ____________________

Is additional lighting provided inside the cage? N ☐ Y ☐

If yes, what type of light is used? light bulb ☐ fluorescent strip light ☐

What is the model and manufacturer? ____________________

When was the light last replaced? ____________________

Are the lights screened from the animals? N ☐ Y ☐ Please give details ____________________

Can the animal(s) touch or access the lights? N ☐ Y ☐ Please give details ____________________

How many hours of light are provided each day? ____________________

Is there ever access to direct sunlight (not through glass or plastic)? N ☐ Y ☐

If yes, how many hours per day or per week? ____________________

Do you measure the humidity in the cage? N ☐ Y ☐ If yes, what is the humidity level? ____________________

What are the daytime temperatures? Hottest area, basking area = ____________ Coolest area = ____________

What are the nighttime temperatures? Hottest area, basking area = ____________ Coolest area = ____________

Are these temperatures measured using a thermometer? N ☐ Y ☐

Does anyone in the household smoke? N ☐ Y ☐ Do you use any aerosolized products? N ☐ Y ☐

Have there been changes in the herp's environment in the last 3 months? N ☐ Y ☐ Please give details ____________

____

DIET

How often do you feed your herp? ____________________

Indicate which foods are eaten and in what amounts (by number, weight, or approx. volume):

Plant material: vegetables ☐ type and amount per feed ____________________

frozen/thawed ☐ fresh ☐ other ☐

flowers ☐ type and amount per feed ____________________

frozen/thawed ☐ fresh ☐ other ☐

fruits ☐ type and amount per feed ____________________

frozen/thawed ☐ fresh ☐ other ☐

Insects: crickets ☐ ________ locusts ☐ ________ mealworms ☐ ________ waxworms ☐________

earthworms ☐ ________ others ____________________

Rodents: mice ☐ type and number per feed ____________________ freshly killed ☐

rats ☐ type and number per feed ____________________ frozen/thawed ☐

Birds or fish: Please give details ____________________ live prey ☐

Do you feed any wild animals to your herp? N ☐ Y ☐ Please give details ____________________

Any other food items fed? Please give details ____________________

Do you use any nutritional supplements? N ☐ Y ☐ If yes, what, how much, and how often ____________________

____

What water supply do you provide? tap water ☐ bottled water ☐ rain/river water ☐ other water source ☐ ________

How is water provided? bowl ☐ dripper system ☐ spray ☐ How often ____________________

How often is the water changed?____________________

Do you use any water supplements? N ☐ Y ☐ Please give details ____________________

Have you noticed any changes in feeding or drinking behavior? Please give details ____________________

____

Have you noticed any changes in droppings (fecal material, urine and urates)? Please give details ____________________

____

Any other comments or information ____________________

____

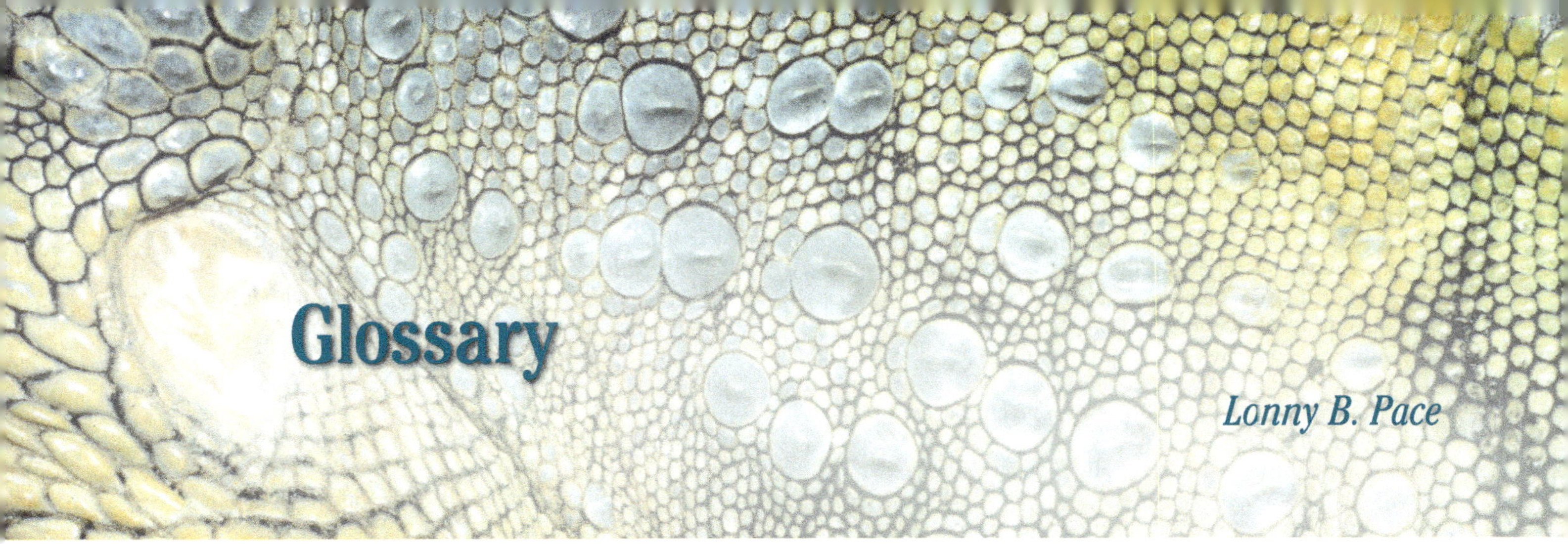

Glossary

Lonny B. Pace

aberrant Deviating from the normal form, structure, or course
abiotic All nonliving components of the environment (e.g., weather and geology)
acrodont With teeth fused to the summit of the jawbones
Ad libitum As one wishes or pleases
adipose Fat
aerobic Living or active only in the presence of oxygen
albumen The white protein part of an egg
allantochorion An embryonic membrane
allantois A sac in the developing egg that primarily functions as a vessel for waste products
ambient External or outside
ambient temperature The surrounding temperature
amelia Congenital pathology in which the affected individual has no limbs
amniote A tetrapod that arises developmentally from an amniotic egg (e.g., reptiles, birds, and mammals)
amphophilic Staining with both basic and acidic dyes
amplexus Amplex (v.), amplectant (adj.), amplectic (adj.). The copulatory behavior of frogs in which the male sits on the female's back and grasps her with his forelimbs; amplexus can be inguinal (forefeet grasping body immediately in front of hindlimbs), axillary (immediately behind forelimbs), cephalic (on head or neck), straddled (male sits on shoulders of female while frogs are vertical and sperm flows down the female's back), or glued (male is attached to females back by adhesive substance). In amplexus, the cloacae of the male and female are adpressed, and sperm and eggs are extruded simultaneously. Amplexus is absent in some frogs.
anamniote A tetrapod that lacks an amniotic egg in its development (e.g., amphibians)
anemia Below-normal levels of erythrocytes, hemoglobin, or hematocrit
anomaly Anomalies (pl.). Abnormality or birth defect
anorexia Loss of appetite
anterior The front or head end of an animal
anthelmintic A medicine that kills or ejects worms, usually of the intestines
anthropogenic Adjective describing human influence, usually pertaining to the natural environment
anthropomorphic Attributing human qualities or emotions to animals
antibody Any of a large number of proteins of high molecular weight that are produced normally by specialized white blood cells (B lymphocyte cells) after stimulation by an antigen and act specifically against the antigen in an immune response
anticoagulant Any substance that prevents or retards the clotting of blood
antigen Any substance, usually protein or carbohydrate (as a toxin or enzyme), capable of stimulating an immune response
antiseptic Preventing infection; any substance that prevents the growth of microorganisms
antivenene Serum produced to combat the effects of (snake) venom
anurans Order of frogs and toads
arcade Parts of the skull roof that separate the orbits and the temporal openings
archosaurs The clade of reptiles whose surviving members are crocodiles and birds
aspirate The act of sucking up, sucking in, or withdrawing fluids or gases from a body cavity (e.g., lungs, thorax, peritoneum, urinary bladder)
atrophy The physiologic or pathologic reduction in size of a cell, tissue, organ, or region in the body
auditory meatus The ear canal, either external or internal
autoinfection Infection by an organism within the body
autolysis The destruction of cells by enzymes within them that occurs after death or by some diseases
autotomy The voluntary shedding of parts of the body in animals, usually in defense. Autotomy of the tail is common in many lizard species.
axilla Axillary (adj.). At the forelimb insertion
bacteriophage A virus that infects bacteria
bacteriostasis Bacteriostatic (adj.). Inhibition of the growth of bacteria without destruction
basal Pertaining to the most fundamental, basic, lowest, least, or deepest level
Bidder's organ An organ found cranial to the kidney in the true toad *(Bufo)* family. The function of the organ is incompletely understood.
bifurcate Forked; divided into, or the site of, two parts or branches
bilateral Pertaining to two sides
biological clock An internal biological rhythm that is responsible for periodic changes in an animal's behavior
biopsy The removal and examination of tissue, cells, or fluids from the living body
biota Biotic (adj.). All living components of the environment
bipedal Moving on two limbs
brackish Slightly salty (e.g., water in marshes near seas)

brill The transparent immovable spectacle that covers the eye in snakes and some lizards
brumation Brumate (v.). A period of prolonged cool temperature without actual hibernation. This is the new term that is being used in reptiles. It replaces the old term, *hibernation,* which should only be used in mammals.
buccal The mouth cavity
calcareous Of, like, or containing calcium
calculi Any abnormal stony deposit formed in the body (e.g., bladder, kidney)
canker An ulcer like sore, especially in the mouth.
cannibalism Eating one's own kind
carapace The upper shell of a turtle (and other animals with horny protective coverings)
carbohydrate An organic compound that comprises the starches, sugars, celluloses, and dextrins
cardiovascular Pertaining to the heart and the blood vessels as a unified body system
carnivore Carnivorous (adj.). A flesh-eating organism
carotenoid Group of plant-based fat soluble nutrients, some of which are precursors to Vitamin A
carrion Decaying flesh of a dead body that may serve as food for scavenging animals
caseous Cheesy; of or like cheese
cataract Opacity of the crystalline lens or capsule of the eye
cathartic Purgative; in medicine, a substance used to stimulate the evacuation of the bowels
catheter A rigid or flexible tube used to pass fluids into or out of a body cavity, passage, or vessel
caudally Toward the tail
caudate Adjective to describe an animal with a tail or a tail-like appendage. Scientific name for a salamander
cecum The cavity in which the large intestine begins and into which the ileum opens
cellulitis Inflammation of connective tissue
cervical Of the neck
chaetae Chitinous bristle or seta found in some species of annelid worms for the purpose of locomotion
chemotherapy The treatment or prevention of disease with the use of drugs
chimaera Literally, monster
chitin Chitinous (adj.). The structural material of some animals, mainly those in the phylum Arthropoda
chlamydophilosis Disease caused by *Chlamydophila psittaci* (formerly *Chlamydia psittaci*). Commonly regarded as psittacosis or chlamydiosis in avian patients
chytridiomycosis Disease of amphibians caused by the water fungi *Batrachochytrium dendrobatidis*
chytrids Fungi of the division Chytridiomycota to which *Batrachochytrium dendrobatidis* belongs
cilia Cilium (sing.). Hairlike cytoplasmic processes of cells, comprised of microtubules, that serve in locomotion or in the movement of substances.
clade A phylogenic term referring to a single phylum or branch with a single ancestor
classification Node name or node-based name. This classification category name labels a clade that stems from the immediate common ancestor of two or more designated descendants.
cloaca A common chamber for the passage of feces, urine, and reproductive material
cnidarians Of the phylum Cnidaria
coelomic cavity The cavity of most higher multicellular animals in which the visceral organs are suspended
coevolution Evolution of two separate but interdependent species as they adapt to each other
coliforms Gram-negative non–spore-forming rods found within the intestinal tract of many vertebrates
conduction The transmission of heat (and electricity) by the passage of energy from particle to particle
congenital Existing before or at birth
consensus PCR PCR with flanking primers to amplify repeat regions from a number of species
conspecifics Conspecific (adj.). Individuals or populations of the same species
constriction A method used by some snakes to overpower prey that uses the application of pressure from the coils to cause asphyxia
convection A transference of heat caused by the differences in density of air as a result of temperature; the upward movement of warm light air
coprophageous Eating feces
copulation Copulate (v.). The act of sexual intercourse; coitus
core temperature Temperature within the body
cortex The outer portion of an organ situated just beneath the capsule
cranial Of, toward, or pertaining to the skull
crepuscular Active at dawn or dusk
cross feeding Transferring an uneaten food animal from one snake's cage to another
crotalid Any member of the rattlesnake family Crotalidae
crustacean An aquatic arthropod that includes the shrimp, crab, barnacle, and lobster
cryptic Hidden
culture The growth of microorganisms on artificial media
curettage The process of cleaning or scraping tissues from body surfaces
cutaneous Of, belonging to, or involving the skin
cyst A structural form in the life cycle of certain parasites in which they form a protective wall; a saclike structure in the body that, when abnormal, is filled with fluid or diseased matter
cytology The study of cell structure
debride The cutting away of tissue: the cutting away of dead or contaminated tissue from a wound to prevent infection; chemical agents may be used to achieve similar results
decapitation Removal of the head
decongestant A medication used to relieve congestion, as in nasal passages
definitive host A host in which sexual maturation of a parasite occurs
dehydrate To remove water, as in the body
digenetic Relating to the subclass Digenea (trematode worms); phenotypic effect of two nonallelic genes
disarticulation Separation at a joint
disinfectant Any substance used to destroy pathogens
display A ritualized pattern of behavior directed at other animals for sexual, territorial, or protective motives
distal Toward the tip of an extremity (i.e., closest to the body)
diuretic Any substance that increases the flow of urine
diurnal Active in daytime
dorsal Pertaining to the back part of the body
dorsal ventral Extending in a direction from the dorsal surface to the ventral surface

double clutching Producing two clutches in less than 1 year; used for pythons and boas, although clutch refers to eggs
duct A small enclosed tube conducting fluid
durophagous Eating hard-bodied prey; often used in herpetology for snakes and lizards that prey on skinks or related lizards armored with osetoderms beneath scales
dysecdysis Unable to slough off outer epidermis
dyspnea Labored breathing
dystocia Slow or difficult labor
ecdysis Sloughing off outer epidermis
ectoparasite An organism that lives on another organism (host)
ectotherm An animal that regulates its body temperature by using energy derived from external sources. This term accurately describes the thermogenic behavior of most reptiles.
ectromelia Congenital pathology in which the affected individual has no limbs or imperfect limbs
edema Excessive accumulation of fluid in cells, tissues, or cavities of the body that results in swelling
edentate Lacking teeth
encephalomyelitis Inflammation of the brain and spinal cord
encyst To form a cyst
endemic Restricted to or constantly present in a particular locality
endogenous Originating from within; internally
endothelium The epithelium lining of internal cavities of the body
endotherm An animal whose thermal energy is a byproduct of its own metabolism. This includes mammals, birds, and some reptiles. For example, female pythons regulate their body temperature during egg brooding cycles with shivering thermogenesis.
enteric Intestinal
enzootic Affecting animals in a certain area, climate, or season
erythrocyte Red blood cell
estivate The act of becoming dormant to survive hot, dry conditions
ethologic Relating to behavior
etiology Etiological (adj.). The scientific study of the causes of disease.
euthanize Euthanasia (n.). To kill painlessly; painless death
excreta Waste matter eliminated (excreted) from the body, especially feces and urine
exogenous Coming from outside the animal
exoskeleton Any hard external supporting structure of a body
exostosis The condition of a bone having a rugose surface, commonly arising from the fusion of bone and dermis or osteoderms
exsanguinate To remove the circulating blood
extant The state of a population or species of being alive now; not extinct
exudate Any substance discharged through pores, incisions, etc
fang A large specialized tooth adapted for the injection of poison into prey
femoral pores A number of hollow scales arranged on the underside of the thighs in many lizards. Usually better developed in males, they can be used in some species as a means of gender identification. Their function is not understood.
fertilization The penetration of the ova's cell membrane by the sperm and the fusion of the sperm and ovum pronuclei to reestablish a diploid state
fertilization, external The condition in which the sperm and ovum come in contact outside the reproductive tract or cloaca of a female
fertilization, internal The condition in which the sperm and ovum come in contact within the reproductive tract or cloaca of a female
fibropapilloma Fibroadenoma; a benign tumor that contains both fibrous and glandular elements
fibrosis Abnormal increase in fibrous connective tissue
filarial Pertaining to parasitic nematodes in the superfamily Filarioidea. Adults live in the vertebrate host's circulatory or lymphatic systems, the connective tissues, or serous cavities; larval forms (microfilaria) are found in the bloodstream or lymph spaces.
firmicutes Taxonomic phylum within the kingdom Bacteria; primarily gram positive.
flagella Flagellum (sing.). A tail-like structure on microorganisms and sperm used for propelling the organism
flora The entire plant life of any geographic area
folivore Folivorous (adj.). A foliage-eating organism
follicle The structure in the ovary that contains the developing ovum
footcandle A unit of illumination equal to the amount of light produced one foot away from a single candle
fossorial Living underground; not all fossorial animals are burrowers, but instead they may use preexisting holes and cavities in the earth.
frugivore Frugivorous (adj.). A fruit-eating organism
fungus Fungi (pl.). A parasite that feeds on living organisms or dead organic material; includes mold, mildew, rust, smut, and the mushroom
fuzzies Newborn rodents that have just begun to grow hair
gait The pattern of limb movement
gastroenteritis Inflammation of the stomach and intestines
genital pore An external opening to the male or female reproductive structures
gingiva Gingival (adj.). The mucous membranes and underlying soft tissue that surround a tooth and the gums
gnathotheca The horny covering of the lower mandible of the beak
goiter Enlargement of the thyroid gland
gonad An ovary or testis
gout A disease characterized by an excess of uric acid in the blood and deposits of uric salts in various tissues, especially the viscera and joints
grade A group of organisms that possess a similar adaptive level of organization
gram negative Pertaining to microorganisms that appear pink microscopically after the Gram's stain process is completed
granulation Formation into granules, such as new capillaries on the surface of a wound
granuloma Granulomatous (adj.). A mass or nodule of chronically inflamed tissue with granulations that is usually associated with an infective process
gravid Pregnant
gular Of or pertaining to the throat
Harderian gland A gland situated at the inner junction of the eyelids (inner canthus) in vertebrates but especially in those with a well-developed nictitating membrane
hatchling An animal recently hatched from an egg. The duration of the hatchling state is variable, although its end in reptiles might be fixed by the disappearance of the yolk-sac scar.

heartwater A disease of ruminants caused by infection with *Ehrlichia [Cowdria] ruminantium*
heliophilic Sun-loving
heliothermic Deriving heat from the sun
helminth Refers to worms of the platyhelminthes, nematoda, or annelida
hemagglutination inhibition assay Variance of a hemagglutination assay that measures antibodies in serum
hematocrit The portion of blood cells to the volume of blood
hematologic Referring to the blood, its nature, functions, and disease
hemipenes The paired sex organ of the male, typical in lizards and snakes. The singular term is *hemipenis,* not *hemipene.*
hemipenis Hemipenes (pl.). Either one of the paired copulatory organs situated laterally in a cavity at the base of the tail of snakes and lizards
hemorrhagic Heavy bleeding or characterized by blood
hepatotoxic Any substance that is injurious or lethal to liver cells
herbivore Herbivorous (adj.). A plant-eating organism
herpetologist One who studies reptiles and amphibians
herpetology The study of amphibians and reptiles
herpitliary An outside enclosure used for keeping both amphibians and reptiles in near-natural conditions
herptile A name used to collectively describe an amphibian or reptile
heterodont Processing teeth of several types (e.g., tearing, cutting, crushing, grinding)
Hexacanth embryo Pertaining to the six-hooked Eucestoda larva (oncosphere) within an egg
hexon gene Gene encoding the hexon surface protein of the adenovirus
hibernaculum An artificial or natural place where certain animals spend the winter in a dormant condition
hibernation The act of spending the cold winter months in a state of torpor. This is a mammalian term and is no longer used for reptiles.
homeotherm An animal whose body temperature is relatively consistent (±2°C). Some reptiles can regulate their body temperature within a narrower range than this, especially during periods of activity.
homeothermic The ability of an organism to maintain itself at a constant temperature
homodont Processing teeth of a single type
homoxenous Living within only one host during a parasite's life cycle
hormone Any chemical substance produced by an organ or cells of an organ that is carried by bloodstream or other body fluids to cells for a specific regulatory effect
hybrid The usually sterile young produced as a result of a cross mating between two different species
hybridization Cross-breeding
hydration Fluid replacement
hydroscopic Having the capacity to absorb or take up fluids from bodily tissue
hyperplasia An abnormal increase in the number of cells that compose a tissue or organ
hyperthermia The elevation of the body temperature via exogenous sources (e.g., the treatment of disease with inducing fever)
hypertonic Excessive or above normal in tone or tension, especially muscles; having an osmotic pressure greater than that of physiologic salt solution or of any other solution taken as a standard
hypoglycemia An abnormally low concentration of sugar in the blood
hypotensive Abnormally low blood pressure
hypothermia Abnormally low body temperature
hypoxia Hypoxic (adj.). An abnormal condition that results from oxygen deficiency
illumina sequencing Method of DNA sequencing (developed by a company who was acquired by the company Illumina)
IM Intramuscular
immunohistochemistry The use of immunologic methods and histochemistry to analyze tissues
immunosuppressive The action of inactivating a specific antibody by various agents to permit the acceptance of a foreign substance by an organism
inanition A state of starvation
inbreeding Reproduction of the same or closely related genetic material
inclusion body A minute foreign particle within a cell (e.g., a virus)
indigenous Naturally of, or belonging to, a region or country; innate; inherent; inborn
inflammation The body's reaction to injury, characterized clinically by heat, swelling, redness, and pain
insectivore An insect-eating organism, although commonly used for an organism that eats any arthropod
intergrade An animal that may show the mixed characteristics of two different subspecies at the border of their respective ranges
intermediate host An organism that harbors the asexual or intermediate phases of a parasite
intracelluar Within the cell
intravenous Within or into the veins
intussusception Telescoping, slipping, prolapsing, or passage of one part of the intestine into another
IV Intravenous
Jacobson's organ A pair of organs situated in the anterior part of the palate that corresponds with and is closely allied to the internal nares. Used to smell the contents of the mouth and may be used in conjunction with the forked tongue.
karyomegaly Enlargement of the nucleus
keratitis Inflammation of the cornea
kilogram (kg) One thousand grams (1000 g) or 2.2 pounds
kinesis The ability of a lizard to raise the upper part of the skull through movement of the quadrate
Koch's postulates The four criteria required to associate microbes with disease, as postulated by Robert Koch and Friedrich Loeffler
labial Pertaining to the lips
larva Larvae (pl.). The free-living immature form of any animal that changes structurally when it becomes an adult
lateral Away from the midline of the body; on the side
lavage The irrigation or washing out of an organ
lethargy Pathologic drowsiness
leukocyte White blood cell
life cycle Stages through which an organism passes, generation after generation
lumen The cavity or channel within a tubular structure or organ
major histocompatibility complex A group of genes that code for proteins found on the surfaces of cells that help the immune system recognize foreign substances

malnutrition Poor nourishment that results from improper diet
manu Hand or forefoot
medial Toward the midline of the body
medulla The central portions of certain organs (e.g., adrenal glands)
melanism A condition in which an animal possesses an unusually abundant amount of dark pigment in the skin such as to make it appear black; fairly common in certain lizard and snake species
melena The discharge of feces colored black by altered or digested blood
meningoencephalitis Combined inflammation of the membranes that cover the brain (meninges) and the spinal cord
mesomycetozoal Of the clade Mesomycetozoa, typically parasites of frogs, salamanders, and fish
mesonephros The adult kidney of fishes and amphibians
metabolism Metabolic (adj.). The process of assimilating food into complex elements that are then dissimilated into simple ones to produce energy
metagenomics Field of study allowing the identification of genes from all organisms in a sampled environment through parallel DNA sequencing
metanephric Pertaining to the permanent kidney of reptiles, birds, and mammals that develops from an excretory organ lying behind the mesonephros in an embryo. In higher vertebrates, the mesonephros develops into the epididymis and vas deferens.
meter A unit of length in the metric system equal to 39. 37 inches
MHC genotypes The genotype of the major histocompatibility complex
microfilaria Microfilaria (pl.). First-stage juvenile of any filariid nematode that is viviparous and is usually found in the blood or tissue fluids of the definitive host
microflora Flora of a small area; in medicine, the microorganisms of the intestines
micron (μ) One-thousandth of a millimeter (1/1000 mm)
milligram (mg) One one-thousandth of a gram (1/1000 g)
milliliter (mL) One one-thousandth of a liter (1/1000 L); is equal to one cubic centimeter (1 cc)
minimum and maximum critical temperatures The upper and lower thermal tolerance limits, where the righting reflex is lost in 50% of animals
molluscivore Molluscivorous (adj.). A mollusk-eating organism
monogenetic Pertaining to animals without alternating asexual and sexual generations
monophyletic Relating to descent from a single ancestor or a single taxon
monotypic Having only one type (e.g., a genus consisting of only one species or the feeding of only one food type).
montane Mountain dwelling
morbidity A diseased state or condition
morph A particular body form or colored group of individuals. Morph is used regularly in discussion of polymorphism and variation of individuals within a population of species.
morphology The study of an organism's form or shape or the shape of one or more of an organism's parts
mucosa Mucosal (adj.). Mucous membrane; the membrane lining body cavities that come in contact with air
mycobacterial Pertaining to rod-shaped, aerobic, gram-positive bacteria of the family Mycobacteriaceae (e.g., an infection)
mycotic dermatitis Inflammation of the skin from a fungus infection
mycotoxin A toxin produced by a fungus
myiasis A condition that results from the invasion of tissues or organs of humans and other animals by dipterous larva
myoglobin The respiratory pigment of muscle fibers; differs from blood hemoglobin in that it has a higher affinity for oxygen and a lower affinity for carbon dioxide
myxozoal Members of the phylum Myxozoa, which are primarily intracellular parasites
nanometer (nm) A unit of length equal to one-billionth of a meter
nares Nasal passages; the nostrils
necropsy Examination of a dead animal; postmortem examination
necrosis The death of tissue
necrotizing dermatitis Inflammation of the skin that results in the death of the tissue
nectivore A nectar-eating organism
neonate Neonatal (adj.). A newly born infant
neoplasm A tumor or aberrant new growth of abnormal cells or tissues
neotropic Neotropical (adj.). Of the zoogeographic region that includes South America, the West Indies, Central America, and tropical Mexico
nephritis An acute or chronic disease of the kidneys characterized by inflammation, degeneration, and fibrosis
nephrotoxic A toxic substance that destroys the cells of the kidneys
neurotoxic A toxic substance that destroys the cells of nerve tissue
nictitating membrane Thin transparent conjunctival tissue in certain vertebrates (e.g., birds and reptiles), called the third eyelid, that serves to protect the eyeball without obscuring vision
nocturnal Active at night
nodule A small node
nonpathogenic Not causing disease
obligatory Required; necessary
occlude To prevent the passage of
occult Concealed from observation; not apparent without symptoms; hidden
ocular Of or pertaining to the eye
olfaction The sense of smell
oligochaetes Segmented worms from the order Oligochaeta
omnivore Omnivorous (adj.). Any animal that feeds on both plant and animal matter
ompA genes A chlamydial gene that encodes the major outer membrane protein
oocyst Cyst stage of apicomplexans containing sporozoites, resulting from sporogony
oogenesis The process of egg formation
opalinids Of the suborder Ophidia
operculum Opercular (adj.). A lid or covering
opisthotonic spasm Describes a condition in which the head (and lower limbs of animals other than snakes) is bent backward while the body is arched forward
opportunistic Referring to any organism that is incapable of inducing disease in a healthy host but is able to produce infections in a less resistant or injured host
oral disc The anterior area or the oral area of invertebrates; term describing the circumoral elements of a tadpole

organic Derived from or pertaining to living organisms
osteoderm A bony deposit in the form of a plate or scale found in the dermal layers of the skin
osteoid Bone-like; young hyaline bone matrix in which calcium salts are deposited
osteomalacia A bone disease characterized by a softening as a result of a deficiency of calcium
osteomyelitis Infection of the bone marrow or bone structure, usually caused by a bacterium (e.g., *Staphylococcus*)
oviparous Oviparously (adj.). Producing eggs that hatch after leaving the body of the female
oviposit To lay eggs
oviposition The act of laying or depositing eggs in specific sites
ovoviviparous Having nonshelled eggs that hatch internally
ovulation Release of mature eggs or ova
ovum An egg, in both pythons and boas, regardless of whether it is fertilized, the plural is ova
palate The roof of the mouth that separates the oral cavity from the nasal cavity
palentine The main bone plate in the palate
palpate To examine by touching
palpebra Palpebral (adj.). Pertaining to the eyelids
palpebral membrane A transparent "eye" lid that lies beneath the true eyelids and can extend horizontally from its resting position in the inner corner of the eye to the outer corner
panophthalmitis Inflammation of all the tissues of the eyeball
paramyxovirus Also known as OPMV, ophidian paramyxovirus infection has been isolated in a wide variety of reptilian and mammalian cell types; clinical signs of illness are variable, from going unnoticed altogether to loss of appetite, muscle tone, or equilibrium; in one epizootic, a snake underwent violent convulsions.
paraphyletic Relating to a taxonomic group that includes some but not all of the descendants from a common ancestor
parasite Any organism that lives in or on another organism (host) to obtain some advantage but contributes nothing useful in return
parasiticide A substance or agent used to destroy parasites
paratenic host A host in which a parasite survives without undergoing further development; a transport host
parenteral Brought into the body in a way other than the digestive tract (e.g., via injection)
parietal eye A vestigial "third eye" situated in the center of the skull between the parietals; a sensory structure capable of light reception that may serve as a temperature detector
parthenogenesis Parthenogenetic (adj.). Reproduction with the development of an unfertilized egg, seed, or spore
parthenogenetic Describing a method of reproduction in which the ova develop without fertilization by the male gamete, producing offspring genetically identical to the parent
parturition The act of giving birth
pathogen Pathogenic (adj.). An organism producing or capable of producing disease
perinatal Pertaining to the period shortly before and after birth
periocular Surrounding the eye
peristalsis Rhythmic muscular contractions often associated with the gastrointestinal tract or other tubular structures
pes Foot, specifically the hind foot
petecchial Referring to the minute rounded spot(s) of hemorrhage on body surfaces, such as skin, mucous and serous membranes, or on the cross-sectioned surface of an organ
phenotype The external appearance of a living organism
pheromone A chemical signal secreted by one animal that conveys specific information to another animal, usually a conspecific, and often elicits a specific behavioral or physiologic response
photoperiod The number of daylight hours best suited to an organism for proper growth and maturation
phylogeny The evolutionary history of species or taxonomic group
pinkies Newborn rodents without hair
plastron The under or ventral shell of a chelonian
plethodontidae Family of lungless salamanders
pleurodont With teeth set in a cavity on the inner side of the jawbone
poikilotherm An animal whose body temperature is variable. This is not the same as an ectotherm; indeed, many mammals, particularly those that undergo hibernation, could correctly be termed *poikilothermic*.
polar capsules Ovoid bodies found in some myxosporean parasites that contain a long spirally coiled thread that is suspected to aid in the attachment of the spore to the new host
polymelia Congenital pathology in which the affected individual has more than the normal number of limbs
polyphyodont With teeth that are replaced more than once
posterior Posteriorly (adj.). Situated behind or to the back of a part
postmetamorphic Period of life after changing form
postmortem After death
postpartum The period of time after parturition
POTZ Preferred optimum temperature zone. The range of temperatures within which a specific ectotherm functions optimally overall. It is the thermal environment within which a reptile engages in normal activities. Important to note is that all physiologic functions have a temperature at which they function optimally, but within a species, not all functions are optimized at the same temperature. The term *POTZ* is somewhat misleading because it implies a conscious choice. *Activity temperature range (ATR)* may be a better term because it is less anthropomorphic.
prehensile Adapted for holding or grasping
premaxilla The teeth-bearing bone at the front of the upper jaw
primary host First or main host
primer A short sequence of DNA or RNA, usually about 10 nucleotides long, that initiates DNA synthesis
primitive A character or condition that is the same as an ancestral character or condition
probe hybridization Technique used to detect certain nucleotide sequences by creating a complementary strand
proboscis An elongated structure located at the anterior end of the organism
progeny Children; descendants; offspring
proglottid Any of the segments of a tapeworm's body; each segment has both male and female reproductive organs
prolapse The falling down or sinking of a part or viscous procidentia from its usual position (e.g., forceful extrusion of the cloaca associated with straining)
prophylaxis Prevention or protection against disease
proteobacteria Major taxonomic phylum within the kingdom Bacteria, which are exclusively gram-negative bacteria
proteolytic The breaking down of proteins to form more simple substances

proteroglyphous Appertaining to snakes with canalized venom fangs at the front of the upper jaw that are usually fixed (e.g., in the Elapidae)
protozoa Unicellular eukaryotes in the Kingdom Protista
pseudomonads Of the genus *Pseudomonas*
pupa Pupae (pl.). An insect in the stage of development between the larval and adult forms
purgative A substance used to stimulate evacuation of the bowels (a cathartic)
purse-string suture A running stitch placed in a circle and pulled together to close an opening
purulent Consisting of, containing, or forming pus
pyrosequencing Method of DNA sequencing
qPCR Quantitative or real-time PCR, which combines detection and amplification in a single step
quadrate The part of the upper jaw that forms the point of articulation
quadrupedal Moving on four limbs
quarantine The act of isolating individuals, for purposes of examination, for the duration of the incubation period of most diseases from which they may have been exposed
radiograph Radiographically (adj.). To make a photograph on a sensitive film with projection of roentgen rays through a part of the body
raphe A seam or ridge
recrudescence The reappearance or regrowth
rectilinear locomotion A mode of limbless locomotion dependent on a wavelike pattern of rib movement
regurgitation The return of food from the stomach
renal–portal system Referring to the anatomic variation of reptiles whereby blood leaving the tail and pelvic limbs of these animals passes through the kidneys before returning to the heart
reservoir host An animal that provides a parasite with a suitable environment and, while doing so, serves as a source of infection for other animals
restriction fragment length polymorphism A method used to follow particular DNA sequences
reticulated Having a pattern of color that resembles a net
retinol Animal-derived form of Vitamin A
rhabditiform Larval form
rhamphotheca The horny covering or sheath of the beak
rhinotheca The horny covering or sheath of the upper mandible of the beak
rhizoid Rootlike filaments from the thallus of fungus
rolling circle amplification DNA amplification technique
rostral Pertaining to or resembling a beak or projection
rupicolous Living on walls or rocks
saline solution A salt solution. Physiologic saline solution contains 0.9 g sodium chloride to 100 mL water
salmonellosis Infection of an organism in the genus *Salmonella* (e.g., septicemia, gastroenteritis, food poisoning)
saltatory Moving by jumping, either bipedally or quadrupedally
saurian Reptile in the order Sauria; lizard
sauropsids A clade of amniotes that encompasses all reptiles and birds both current and extinct
SC or SQ Subcutaneous
scansorial Climbing in bushes, shrubs, and other relatively low growing vegetation; capable of climbing but not arboreal
scolex Head of a tapeworm
scute A horny, chitinous, or bony external plate or scale, as on the shell of a turtle or the underside of a snake; also called scutum
selected body temperature (Ts) The temperature selected by an individual when placed in an artificial thermal gradient. This varies over time because the temperature selected mirrors the optimal temperature for the physiologic function perceived as most important at that time. It is synonymous with preferred body temperature (Tp). This is sometimes expressed as a range of temperatures that reflects the middle 50% to 67% of the body temperatures measured during an animal's circadian temperature fluctuation.
self-limiting A disease that is limited by its own characteristics rather than outside influence
septicemia Septicemic (adj.). A disease spread throughout the body via the bloodstream by pathogenic microorganisms and their toxic products
sequelae A pathologic condition that results from a disease
serpentine A mode of limbless undulatory locomotion in which all portions of the body pass along the same path and use the same frictional surfaces for pushing the body forward
sexual dimorphism The condition in which the male and female of a species show obvious differences in color or structure
sidewinding A specialized mode of serpentine locomotion in which only two parts of the body touch the ground simultaneously
sister group The taxon sharing the most recent common ancestor with another taxon; a pair of taxa sharing the same common ancestor
SOLiD sequencing Method of DNA sequencing (developed by Life Technologies)
somatic Pertaining to the framework of the body but not to the viscera
spargana Sparganum (sing.) Cestode plerocercoids of unknown identity
species A taxonomic group of individuals similar in morphology and physiology
spermatophore A mucoid pedestal to support the sperm packets of some male salamanders; produced in the cloaca
sphenodontid The reptile clade whose last surviving members are the tuatara in New Zealand
spurious Not true or genuine; false
sputum Salvia, mucus, etc., that is spit out of the mouth
squamate The clade of the scaled reptiles consisting of the lizards (including snakes)
steatitis Inflammation of adipose tissue
stem name or stem-based name This classification category name labels a clade of all taxa that are more closely related to a specified set of descendants than to any other taxa
stomatitis Inflammation of the oral cavity
stress A condition in animals in which psychologic effects reduce resistance to disease; applies particularly to newly captured wild specimens
subcaudal Scales after the cloaca on the snake's ventral surface
subcutaneous SC, SQ; under the skin
subspectacular Referring to the area just beneath the fixed transparent watch glasslike covering (spectacle; eye cap) of the eye in snakes and some lizards
substrate In zoology, the ground or other solid material on which an animal moves or is fastened
SVL Snout-vent length; straight-line distance from the tip of the snout to the anterior edge of the vent
symbiont Symbiotic (adj.). Any organism involved in a parasitic, commensalistic, or mutualistic relationship with its "host"

symbiosis The interaction of organisms whereby one lives on, in, or with another
symmetrical Exhibiting corresponding characteristics on opposite sides of a plane
sympatric Occurring in the same geologic area
symphysis The joining of two bones with interlocking parts
syndrome A set of signs or a series of events that occur together and often point to a single disease or condition as the cause
Taqman PCR Real-time PCR utilizing Taq polymerase and a method that resembles the video game Pac-Man
taxa Taxon (sing.). A group or category, at any level, in a system for classifying plants or animals
taxonomy The study of the theory, rules, and procedure of classification
tectorial membrane A membrane in the inner ear that covers a patch of sensory hairs
tepid Moderately warm
teratogenic Tending to produce anomalies of formation or teratism; causing birth defects
terrestrial Mainly ground dwelling
thallus Undifferentiated fungal body; may also refer to plant, algae, or lichen
thecodont Having teeth inserted in sockets
therapeutic Serving to cure or to heal; a curative
thermoreceptor A heat-detecting organ (e.g., the “pit” in Pit Vipers)
thermoregulate To control temperature
thermoregulation The process used by ectotherms to maintain their preferred body temperature by moving in and out of areas of environmental warmth
thiaminase An enzyme present in raw fish (and in certain bacteria) that causes the cleavage of thiamine, rendering it unavailable to the body
thigmotherm An animal that derives its energy by thermal conduction from items in the environment. This applies to many crepuscular reptiles
TL Tail length or total length. For tail length, the distance from the posterior edge of the vent to the tip of the tail; for total length, the distance from the tip of the snout to the tip of the tail.
tomia Tomium (pl.). The cutting edge of a beak
torpid A state of being dormant or inactive
toxicofera Clade of reptiles based on the evolution of the venom gland
tractable Tame; able to be handled
transient Temporary
transport host Host in which a parasite survives without undergoing further development; also known as a paratenic host
tumor A swelling on some part of the body, especially a mass of new tissue growth independent of its surrounding structures, having no physiologic function
tympanum Tympana (pl.). Eardrum
ulcer Ulcerate (v.). An open sore on the skin or mucous membrane that often discharges pus
undulatory A group of limbless locomotion patterns in which the body moves through a series of curves
urate A salt of uric acid
uric acid A product of protein metabolism that is present in the blood and urine of animals living in arid areas
vent The external opening of the cloaca
venter Ventral (adj.). The underside or lower surface of an animal
ventral Pertaining to the belly
vermiculite Alteration of mica, producing hydrous silicate minerals that occur in tiny leafy scales that expand greatly when heated
vermin Verminous (adj.). Any animal regarded as objectionable by humans (e.g., flies, roaches, lice, rats)
vertebrate An animal that possesses a spinal column
vertical transmission The transmission of a trait, disease, etc., from parent to offspring across the placenta
vestigial Referring to a remnant of something formerly present or more fully developed
virus A vast group of minute infectious structures that rely totally on living cells for reproduction and metabolism
viscous Glutinous; sticky; semifluid; having high viscosity
vitellogenesis Development of the yolk part of an egg in the ovary
viviparous Those species that bear live offspring in an advanced state of development
Wolffian duct One of a pair of tubes or ducts that carry urine from the primitive or embryonic kidney to the exterior or to a primitive bladder. In some amphibian species the duct carries both urine and sperm, but most amphibians develop a separate tube to carry urine from the kidney.
xanthophylls Yellow carotenoid pigments in both plants and animals
xenomas A tumor that develops secondary to an infection of a fungus or protist of which microsporidia is the most commonly implicated
xeric Habitat with low moisture level or water availability; adapted to dry or arid conditions
yeast Single-celled ascomycete
yolk Aspherical mass of (usually) yellow nutritive fluid enclosed by the yolk sac and supportive of the developing embryo
zoonoses Diseases that may be transmitted to man from animals.
zoospores A motile flagellated asexual spore of alga or lower fungus

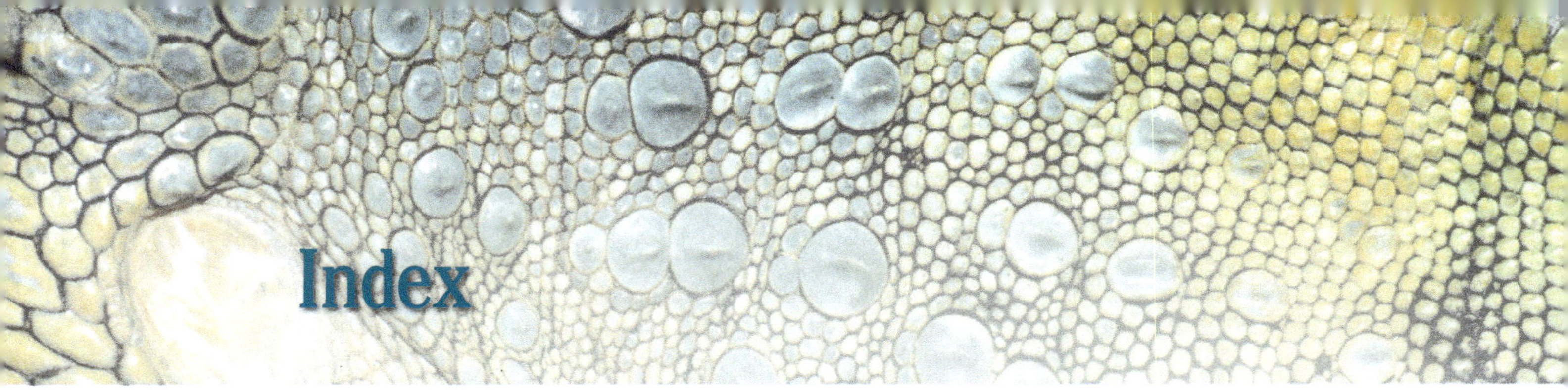

Index

Page numbers followed by *f* indicate figures; *t*, tables; and *b*, boxes.

C

D

E

F

G

M

U

V

W

X